a LANGE medical book

Greenberger's
CURRENT
Diagnosis & Treatment
Gastroenterology,
Hepatology, & Endoscopy

Fourth Edition

Editors

Sonia Friedman, MD
Associate Professor of Medicine, Harvard Medical School
Associate Physician, Division of Gastroenterology, Hepatology and Endoscopy
Brigham and Women's Hospital
Boston, Massachusetts

Richard S. Blumberg, MD
Professor of Medicine, Harvard Medical School
Vice-Chair for Research in Department of Medicine
Brigham and Women's Hospital
Boston, Massachusetts

John R. Saltzman, MD
Professor of Medicine, Part-time, Harvard Medical School
Physician, Division of Gastroenterology, Hepatology and Endoscopy
Brigham and Women's Hospital
Boston, Massachusetts

Mc
Graw
Hill

New York   Chicago   San Francisco   Athens   London   Madrid
Mexico City   Milan   New Delhi   Singapore   Sydney   Toronto

Greenberger's CURRENT Diagnosis & Treatment: Gastroenterology, Hepatology, & Endoscopy, Fourth Edition

3 4 5 6 7 8 9 LCR 27 26 25 24 23

ISBN 978-1-260-47343-8
MHID 1-260-47343-0
ISSN 1946-3030

Notice

Medicine is an ever-changing science. As new research and clinical experience broaden our knowledge, changes in treatment and drug therapy are required. The authors and the publisher of this work have checked with sources believed to be reliable in their efforts to provide information that is complete and generally in accord with the standards accepted at the time of publication. However, in view of the possibility of human error or changes in medical sciences, neither the authors nor the publisher nor any other party who has been involved in the preparation or publication of this work warrants that the information contained herein is in every respect accurate or complete, and they disclaim all responsibility for any errors or omissions or for the results obtained from use of the information contained in this work. Readers are encouraged to confirm the information contained herein with other sources. For example and in particular, readers are advised to check the product information sheet included in the package of each drug they plan to administer to be certain that the information contained in this work is accurate and that changes have not been made in the recommended dose or in the contraindications for administration. This recommendation is of particular importance in connection with new or infrequently used drugs.

This book was set in Minion Pro by KnowledgeWorks Global Ltd.
The editor was Jason Malley.
The production supervisor was Catherine Saggese.
Project management was provided by Tasneem Kauser, KnowledgeWorks Global Ltd.
Cover images: Top Inset Photo by flywish/Shutterstock; Bottom Inset Photo by Alpha Tauri 3D Graphics/Shutterstock.

This book is printed on acid-free paper.

Contents

Color insert appears between pages 400 and 401.

Authors

Francesco Alessandrino, MD
Assistant Professor in Clinical Radiology, Department of Radiology, University of Miami Leonard M. Miller School of Medicine, Miami, Florida
falessandrino@med.miami.edu
State-of-the-Art Imaging of the Gastrointestinal System

Jessica R. Allegretti, MD, MPH
Assistant Professor of Medicine, Harvard Medical School, Boston, Massachusetts; Associate Director, Crohn's and Colitis Center, Division of Gastroenterology, Hepatology and Endoscopy, Brigham and Women's Hospital, Boston, Massachusetts
jallegretti@bwh.harvard.edu
Acute Diarrheal Disorders

Gyorgy Baffy, MD, PhD
Associate Professor of Medicine, Harvard Medical School, Boston, Massachusetts; Chief, Section of Gastroenterology, VA Boston Healthcare System, Boston, Massachusetts
gbaffy@bwh.harvard.edu
Approach to Abnormal Liver Tests
Drug-Induced Liver Disease

Peter A. Banks, MD
Professor of Medicine, Harvard Medical School, Boston, Massachusetts; Director of the Center for Pancreatic Disease, Division of Gastroenterology, Brigham and Women's Hospital, Boston, Massachusetts
pabanks@bwh.harvard.edu
Acute Pancreatitis
Chronic Pancreatitis

Ronald Bleday, MD
Associate Professor of Surgery, Harvard Medical School, Boston, Massachusetts; Vice Chairman for Quality and Safety, Department of Surgery, Brigham and Women's Hospital, Boston, Massachusetts; Chief, Section of Colon and Rectal Surgery, Brigham and Women's Hospital & Dana-Farber Cancer Institute, Boston, Massachusetts
rbleday@bwh.harvard.edu
Inflammatory Bowel Disease: Surgical Considerations

Richard S. Blumberg, MD
Professor of Medicine, Harvard Medical School, Boston, Massachusetts; Vice-Chair for
Research in Department of Medicine, Brigham and Women's Hospital, Boston, Massachusetts
rblumberg@bwh.harvard.edu
Inflammatory Bowel Disease: Immunologic Considerations & Therapeutic Implications

Jennifer X. Cai, MD, MPH
Instructor in Medicine, Harvard Medical School, Boston, Massachusetts; Associate Physician, Division of Gastroenterology, Hepatology and Endoscopy, Brigham and Women's Hospital, Boston, Massachusetts
jxcai@bwh.harvard.edu
Disorders of Gastric & Small Bowel Motility

David L. Carr-Locke, MA, MD
Professor of Medicine, Weill Cornell Medicine, New York, New York; Clinical Director, Center for Advanced Digestive Care, New York Presbyterian Hospital, New York, New York
dac9184@med.cornell.edu
Endoscopic Retrograde Cholangiopancreatography (ERCP)

Mariana Castells, MD, PhD
Professor of Medicine, Harvard Medical School, Boston, Massachusetts; Director Mastocytosis Center, Brigham and Women's Hospital, Boston, Massachusetts
mcastells@bwh.harvard.edu
Mast Cell Disorders

Walter W. Chan, MD, MPH
Assistant Professor of Medicine, Harvard Medical School, Boston, Massachusetts; Director, Center for Gastrointestinal Motility, Division of Gastroenterology, Hepatology and Endoscopy, Brigham and Women's Hospital, Boston, Massachusetts
wwchan@bwh.harvard.edu
Gastroesophageal Reflux Disease
Disorders of Gastric & Small Bowel Motility
Chronic Constipation & Fecal Incontinence

Darwin L. Conwell, MD, MS
Professor of Medicine, The Ohio State University College of Medicine, Columbus, Ohio; Director, Gastroenterology, Hepatology and Nutrition; Co-Director, Digestive Disease Center, The Ohio State University Wexner Medical Center, Columbus, Ohio
darwin.conwell@osumc.edu
Acute Pancreatitis

Alan J. Cubre, MD
Instructor in Medicine, Harvard Medical School, Boston, Massachusetts; Associate Physician, Division of Abdominal Imaging and Intervention, Brigham and Women's Hospital, Boston, Massachusetts
acubre@bwh.harvard.edu
State-of-the-Art Imaging of the Gastrointestinal System

Rahul S. Dalal, MD, MPH
Research Fellow in Medicine, Harvard Medical School, Boston, Massachusetts; Clinical and Research Fellow, Division of Gastroenterology, Hepatology and Endoscopy, Brigham and Women's Hospital, Boston, Massachusetts
rsdalal@bwh.harvard.edu
Acute Diarrheal Disorders

Punyanganie S. de Silva, MBBS, MPH
Assistant Professor of Medicine, Harvard Medical School, Boston, Massachusetts; Associate Physician, Division of Gastroenterology, Hepatology and Endoscopy, Brigham and Women's Hospital, Boston, Massachusetts
pdesilva@bwh.harvard.edu
Gastrointestinal & Biliary Complications of Pregnancy

Russell D. Dolan, MD
Research Fellow in Medicine, Harvard Medical School, Boston, Massachusetts; Clinical and Research Fellow, Division of Gastroenterology, Hepatology and Endoscopy, Brigham and Women's Hospital, Boston, Massachusetts
rddolan@bwh.harvard.edu
Endoscopic Management of Acute Biliary & Pancreatic Conditions
Endoscopic Retrograde Cholangiopancreatography (ERCP)
Gastrointestinal Foreign Bodies
Endoscopic Ultrasound

Colston Edgerton, MD
Assistant Professor of Surgery, Division of Foregut and Metabolic Surgery, Medical University of South Carolina, Charleston, South Carolina
edgertoc@musc.edu
Endoscopic & Surgical Treatment of Obesity

Sonia Friedman, MD
Associate Professor of Medicine, Harvard Medical School, Boston, Massachusetts; Associate Physician, Brigham and Women's Hospital, Boston, Massachusetts
sfriedman1@bwh.harvard.edu
Inflammatory Bowel Disease: Medical Considerations
Irritable Bowel Syndrome

Shilpa Grover, MD, MPH
Assistant Professor of Medicine, Part-time, Harvard Medical School, Boston, Massachusetts; Director, Onco-Gastroenterology Program, Division of Gastroenterology, Hepatology and Endoscopy, Brigham and Women's Hospital, Boston, Massachusetts
sgrover@bwh.harvard.edu
Acute & Chronic Gastrointestinal Toxicities of Oncologic Therapy

Sanchit Gupta, MD, MS
Research Fellow in Medicine, Harvard Medical School, Boston, Massachusetts; Advanced IBD Fellow, Division of Gastroenterology, Hepatology and Endoscopy, Brigham and Women's Hospital, Boston, Massachusetts,
sgupta34@bwh.harvard.edu
Polypectomy

Matthew J. Hamilton, MD
Assistant Professor of Medicine, Harvard Medical School, Boston, Massachusetts; Associate Physician, Division of Gastroenterology, Hepatology and Endoscopy, Brigham and Women's Hospital, Boston, Massachusetts
mjhamilton@bwh.harvard.edu
Mast Cell Disorders
Eosinophilic Esophagitis

Nikroo Hashemi, MD, MPH
Assistant Professor of Medicine, Harvard Medical School, Boston, Massachusetts; Associate Physician, Division of Gastroenterology, Hepatology and Endoscopy, Brigham and Women's Hospital, Boston, Massachusetts
nhashemi@bwh.harvard.edu
Liver Neoplasms
Liver Transplantation

Jennifer L. Irani, MD
Assistant Professor of Surgery, Harvard Medical School, Boston, Massachusetts; Associate Surgeon, Division of General and Gastrointestinal Surgery, Brigham and Women's Hospital, Boston, Massachusetts
jirani@bwh.harvard.edu
Inflammatory Bowel Disease: Surgical Considerations

Kunal Jajoo, MD
Assistant Professor of Medicine, Harvard Medical School, Boston, Massachusetts; Clinical Director, Division of Gastroenterology, Hepatology and Endoscopy, Associate Physician, Brigham and Women's Hospital, Boston, Massachusetts
kjajoo@bwh.harvard.edu
Mesenteric Vascular Disease
Barrett Esophagus
Polypectomy

David X. Jin, MD, MPH
Instructor in Medicine, Harvard Medical School, Boston, Massachusetts; Associate Physician, Division of Gastroenterology, Hepatology and Endoscopy, Brigham and Women's Hospital, Boston, Massachusetts
djin@bwh.harvard.edu
Acute Pancreatitis
Autoimmune Pancreatitis

Pichamol Jirapinyo, MD, MPH
Instructor in Medicine, Harvard Medical School, Boston,
  Massachusetts; Director, Bariatric Endoscopy Fellowship
  and Associate Director, Bariatric Endoscopy, Division of
  Gastroenterology, Hepatology and Endoscopy, Brigham
  and Women's Hospital, Boston, Massachusetts
pjirapinyo@bwh.harvard.edu
Endoscopic & Surgical Treatment of Obesity

Walter M. Kim, MD, PhD
Lecturer in Medicine, Part-time, Harvard Medical School,
  Boston, Massachusetts; Division Chief, Gastroenterology,
  Lemuel Shattuck Hospital, Jamaica Plain, Massachusetts;
  Associate Physician, Division of Gastroenterology,
  Hepatology and Endoscopy, Brigham and Women's
  Hospital, Boston, Massachusetts
wkim@bwh.harvard.edu
Intestinal Malabsorption & Nutrition

Lawrence Kogan, MD
Resident, Division of General Internal Medicine,
  Warren Alpert Brown Medical School of Brown
  University, Providence, Rhode Island
lkogan@lifespan.org
*Acute & Chronic Gastrointestinal Toxicities of Oncologic
  Therapy*

Joshua R. Korzenik, MD
Assistant Professor of Medicine, Harvard Medical School,
  Boston, Massachusetts; Director, Crohn's and Colitis
  Center, Division of Gastroenterology, Hepatology and
  Endoscopy, Brigham and Women's Hospital, Boston,
  Massachusetts
jkorzenik@bwh.harvard.edu
Intestinal Malabsorption & Nutrition

Navin L. Kumar, MD
Assistant Professor of Medicine, Harvard Medical School,
  Boston, Massachusetts; Associate Physician, Division of
  Gastroenterology, Hepatology, and Endoscopy, Brigham
  and Women's Hospital, Boston, Massachusetts
nlkumar@bwh.harvard.edu
Mesenteric Vascular Disease
Diverticular Diseases of the Colon

Alice A. Lee, MD
Clinical Research Fellow, Division of Gastroenterology,
  Hepatology and Endoscopy, Brigham and Women's
  Hospital and Harvard Medical School, Boston,
  Massachusetts
Alee93@bwh.harvard.edu
Autoimmune Pancreatitis

Linda Lee, MD
Associate Professor of Medicine, Harvard Medical School,
  Boston, Massachusetts; Medical Director of
  Endoscopy, Division of Gastroenterology, Hepatology
  and Endoscopy, Brigham and Women's Hospital,
  Boston, Massachusetts
llee@bwh.harvard.edu
Endoscopic Ultrasound

Edward Lew, MD, MPH
Assistant Professor of Medicine, Harvard Medical School,
  Boston, Massachusetts; Staff Gastroenterologist, VA
  Boston Healthcare System, Boston, Massachusetts
edward.lew@med.va.gov
Peptic Ulcer Disease
Zollinger-Ellison Syndrome (Gastrinoma)

Michael Li, MD, MPH
Transplant Hepatology Fellow, Division of
  Gastroenterology and Hepatology, University of
  California, San Francisco, California
michael.li@ucsf.edu
Autoimmune Liver Disorders
Drug-Induced Liver Disease

Ramona Lim, MD
Instructor in Medicine, Harvard Medical School, Boston,
  Massachusetts; Associate Physician, Division of
  Gastroenterology and Fish Center for Women's Health,
  Brigham and Women's Hospital,
  Boston, Massachusetts; Associate Physician, Cancer
  Genetics and Prevention Program, Dana-Farber Cancer
  Institute, Boston, Massachusetts
rlim@bwh.harvard.edu
Colorectal Cancer Screening
Video Capsule Endoscopy & Deep Small Bowel Enteroscopy

Anne F. Liu, MD
Lecturer on Medicine, Part-time, Harvard Medical School,
  Boston, Massachusetts; Gastroenterologist, Division of
  Gastroenterology, Hepatology and Endoscopy, Brigham
  and Women's Harbor Medical Associates, Braintree,
  Massachusetts
afliu@bwh.harvard.edu
Irritable Bowel Syndrome
Viral Hepatitis
Nonalcoholic Fatty Liver Disease

Wai-Kit Lo, MD, MPH
Assistant Professor of Medicine, Harvard Medical School, Boston, Massachusetts; Associate Director, Center for Gastrointestinal Motility, Division of Gastroenterology, Hepatology and Endoscopy, Brigham and Women's Hospital, Boston, Massachusetts; Associate Director of Clinical Motility, VA Boston Healthcare System, Boston, Massachusetts
wlo@bwh.harvard.edu
Eosinophilic Esophagitis

Nayna A. Lodhia, MD
Instructor in Medicine, Harvard Medical School, Boston, Massachusetts; Associate Physician, Division of Gastroenterology, Hepatology and Endoscopy, Brigham and Women's Hospital, Boston, Massachusetts
nlodhia@bwh.harvard.edu
Chronic Constipation & Fecal Incontinence

Frederick L. Makrauer, MD
Assistant Professor of Medicine, Part-time, Harvard Medical School, Boston, Massachusetts; Associate Physician, Center for Crohn's and Colitis, Brigham and Women's Hospital, Boston, Massachusetts
fmakrauer@bwh.harvard.edu
Acute Abdominal Pain: Basic Principles & Current Challenges

Hiroshi Mashimo, MD, PhD
Associate Professor of Medicine, Harvard Medical School, Boston, Massachusetts; Director, GI Motility Service, VA Boston Healthcare System, Boston, Massachusetts
hiroshi_mashimo@hms.harvard.edu
Oropharyngeal & Esophageal Motility Disorders

Julia McNabb-Baltar, MD, MPH
Assistant Professor of Medicine, Harvard Medical School, Boston, Massachusetts; Associate Physician, Co-Director, Center for Pancreatic Disease, Division of Gastroenterology, Hepatology and Endoscopy, Brigham and Women's Hospital, Boston, Massachusetts
jmcnabb-baltar@bwh.harvard.edu
Chronic Pancreatitis
Tumors of the Pancreas

Vanessa Mitsialis, MD
Instructor in Medicine, Harvard Medical School, Boston, Massachusetts; Associate Physician, Brigham and Women's Hospital, Boston Massachusetts
vmitsialis@bwh.harvard.edu
Inflammatory Bowel Disease: Immunologic Considerations & Therapeutic Implications

Molly L. Perencevich, MD
Assistant Professor of Medicine, Harvard Medical School, Boston, Massachusetts; Associate Physician, Brigham and Women's Hospital, Boston Massachusetts
mperencevich@bwh.harvard.edu
Acute Abdominal Pain: Basic Principles & Current Challenges
Functional Dyspepsia

Rachel Placzek, PA-C
Physician Assistant, Division of Gastroenterology, Hepatology and Endoscopy, Brigham and Women's Hospital, Boston, Massachusetts
rplaczek@bwh.harvard.edu
Liver Diseases in Pregnancy

Malcolm K. Robinson, MD
Associate Professor of Surgery, Harvard Medical School, Boston, Massachusetts; Surgical Director, Perioperative Services, Vice Chair for Clinical Operations, Department of Surgery, Director, Nutrition Support Service, Brigham and Women's Hospital, Boston, Massachusetts
mkrobinson@bwh.harvard.edu
Endoscopic & Surgical Treatment of Obesity

Nicolette Rodriguez, MD, MPH
Research Fellow in Medicine, Harvard Medical School, Boston, Massachusetts; Clinical and Research Fellow, Division of Gastroenterology, Hepatology and Endoscopy, Brigham and Women's Hospital, Boston, Massachusetts
njrodriguez@bwh.harvard.edu
Colorectal Cancer Screening
Hereditary Gastrointestinal Cancer Syndromes

Anna Rutherford, MD, MPH
Assistant Professor of Medicine, Harvard Medical School, Boston, Massachusetts; Clinical Director of Hepatology, Associate Physician, Division of Gastroenterology, Hepatology and Endoscopy, Brigham and Women's Hospital, Boston, Massachusetts
arutherford@bwh.harvard.edu
Liver Diseases in Pregnancy
Acute Liver Failure

Marvin Ryou, MD
Assistant Professor of Medicine, Harvard Medical School, Boston, Massachusetts; Associate Physician, Division of Gastroenterology, Hepatology and Endoscopy, Brigham and Women's Hospital, Boston, Massachusetts
mryou@bwh.harvard.edu
Portal Hypertension & Esophageal Variceal Hemorrhage
Primary Sclerosing Cholangitis & Congenital Disorders of the Biliary System

Jordan Sack, MD, MPH
Instructor in Medicine, Harvard Medical School, Boston, Massachusetts; Associate Physician, Division of Gastroenterology, Hepatology and Endoscopy, Brigham and Women's Hospital, Boston, Massachusetts
jsack@bwh.harvard.edu
Approach to Abnormal Liver Tests
Complications of Cirrhosis: Ascites & Hepatic Encephalopathy
Liver Transplantation

John R. Saltzman, MD
Professor of Medicine, Part-time, Harvard Medical School, Boston, Massachusetts; Physician, Brigham and Women's Hospital, Boston, Massachusetts
jsaltzman@bwh.harvard.edu
Acute Upper Gastrointestinal Bleeding
Acute Lower Gastrointestinal Bleeding

Benjamin Smith, MD
Assistant Professor of Medicine, Harvard Medical School; Director of Endoscopy and Attending Physician, Faulkner Hospital, Boston, Massachusetts; Affiliate Staff, Brigham and Women's Hospital, Boston, Massachusetts
bnsmith@bwh.harvard.edu
Diverticular Diseases of the Colon
Metabolic Liver Diseases

Scott B. Snapper, MD, PhD
Professor of Medicine and Egan Family Professor of Pediatrics in the Field of Transitional Medicine, Harvard Medical School, Boston, Massachusetts; Chief, Division of Gastroenterology, Hepatology and Nutrition and Wolpow Family Chair and Director, IBD Center, Boston Children's Hospital, Boston, Massachusetts; Physician, Crohn's and Colitis Center, Brigham and Women's Hospital, Boston, Massachusetts
Scott.Snapper@childrens.harvard.edu.
Inflammatory Bowel Disease: Immunologic Considerations & Therapeutic Implications

Daniel J. Stein, MD, MPH
Instructor in Medicine, Harvard Medical School, Boston, Massachusetts; Associate Physician, Division of Gastroenterology, Hepatology and Endoscopy, Brigham and Women's Hospital, Boston, Massachusetts
djstein@bwh.harvard.edu
Video Capsule Endoscopy & Deep Small Bowel Enteroscopy

Elena M. Stoffel, MD, MPH
Associate Professor of Internal Medicine, University of Michigan Medical School, Ann Arbor, Michigan; Director, Cancer Genetics Clinic, Division of Gastroenterology, Department of Internal Medicine, University of Michigan, Ann Arbor, Michigan
estoffel@med.umich.edu
Hereditary Gastrointestinal Cancer Syndromes

Andrew C. Storm, MD
Assistant Professor of Medicine, Mayo Clinic School of Medicine, Rochester, Minnesota
Storm.Andrew@mayo.edu
Endoscopic Management of Acute Biliary & Pancreatic Conditions
Gastrointestinal Foreign Bodies

Sapna Syngal, MD, MPH
Professor of Medicine, Harvard Medical School, Boston, Massachusetts; Director, Gastroenterology, Dana-Farber/Brigham and Women's Cancer Center, Boston, Massachusetts; Director of Research, Genetics and Prevention Division, Dana-Farber Cancer Institute, Boston, Massachusetts
sapna_syngal@dfci.harvard.edu
Colorectal Cancer Screening
Hereditary Gastrointestinal Cancer Syndromes

Christopher C. Thompson, MD, MSc
Professor of Medicine, Harvard Medical School, Boston, Massachusetts; Director of Endoscopy, Division of Gastroenterology, Hepatology and Endoscopy, Co-Director, Center for Weight Management and Wellness, Brigham and Women's Hospital, Boston, Massachusetts
cthompson@hms.harvard.edu
Endoscopic Management of Acute Biliary & Pancreatic Conditions
Endoscopic Retrograde Cholangiopancreatography (ERCP)
Gastrointestinal Foreign Bodies

Jerry S. Trier,* MD
Professor of Medicine, Emeritus, Harvard Medical School, Boston, Massachusetts; Senior Physician, Honorary Staff, Division of Gastroenterology, Department of Medicine, Brigham and Women's Hospital, Boston, Massachusetts
Acute Diarrheal Disorders

*Deceased

Kathleen Viveiros, MD
Instructor in Medicine, Harvard Medical School, Boston,
  Massachusetts; Associate Physician, Division of
  Gastroenterology, Hepatology and Endoscopy, Brigham
  and Women's Hospital, Boston, Massachusetts
kviveiros@bwh.harvard.edu
Nonalcoholic Fatty Liver Disease
Complications of Cirrhosis: Ascites & Hepatic
  Encephalopathy
Portal Hypertension & Esophageal Variceal Hemorrhage

Alexander S. Vogel, MD
Research Fellow in Medicine, Harvard Medical School,
  Boston, Massachusetts; Clinical and Research
  Fellow, Division of Gastroenterology, Hepatology and
  Endoscopy, Brigham and Women's Hospital, Boston,
  Massachusetts
asvogel@bwh.harvard.edu
Metabolic Liver Diseases
Alcohol-Associated Liver Disease

Rachel W. Winter, MD, MPH
Instructor in Medicine, Harvard Medical School, Boston,
  Massachusetts; Associate Physician, Brigham and
  Women's Hospital, Boston, Massachusetts
rwinter@bwh.harvard.edu
Inflammatory Bowel Disease: Medical Considerations

Stephen D. Zucker, MD
Associate Professor of Medicine, Harvard Medical School,
  Boston, Massachusetts; Director of Hepatology,
  Division of Gastroenterology, Hepatology and
  Endoscopy, Brigham and Women's Hospital, Boston,
  Massachusetts
szucker@bwh.harvard.edu
Viral Hepatitis
Autoimmune Liver Disorders
Primary Sclerosing Cholangitis & Congenital Disorders of the
  Biliary System
Gallstone Disease

Preface

In 2002, after nearly 40 years as Chairman of Medicine at University of Kansas, Dr. Norton Greenberger (Nortie) joined the faculty of Harvard Medical School within the Division of Gastroenterology, Hepatology and Endoscopy at Brigham and Women's Hospital. Dr. Greenberger was one of the most distinguished gastroenterologists in the United States who had devoted his academic career to education and clinical care. He served as the President of the American Gastroenterological Association and was recipient of the Friedenwald Medal from the same organization. As an educator, reflecting his own personal discipline, it is estimated he trained 3000 young physicians at the University of Kansas Medical Center alone. Within two years at Brigham and Women's Hospital, he received the Jerry S. Trier, MD, Award in Education, the highest honor bestowed on a faculty member by the trainees. He was also a remarkable editor who has informed generations of gastroenterologists through his many affiliations. He succeeded Franz Ingelfinger as editor of the gastroenterology section of the *Yearbook in Medicine* in 1969 and continued this editorial responsibility for 28 years. In 1984, Nortie Greenberger and Frank Moody were the founding editors of the *Yearbook of Digestive Diseases*, which they continued until 1997. Together, they surveyed several thousand articles per year and identified the 250 key articles in Gastroenterology and Hepatology. The *Yearbook of Digestive Diseases* was widely read by gastroenterologists and surgeons and was regarded as an outstanding single-volume summary of important articles in the field. As co-editor of the yearbooks, Dr. Greenberger influenced young gastroenterologists nationally with his incisive comments about key papers. In 1970, he began his 50-year association with the well-known internal medicine textbook *Harrison's Principles of Internal Medicine*. He was principal author of chapters on malabsorption, acute and chronic pancreatic diseases, and gallbladder and biliary tract diseases, including in the most recent addition. It is not surprising therefore when he arrived at the Brigham and Women's Hospital in 2002, he had a vision for a new textbook on gastroenterology. Working with the publishers at McGraw Hill he established a new vehicle for educating gastroenterologists and students throughout the world which would be a singular volume of succinct chapters written by domain experts from our faculty at Brigham and Women's Hospital that was informative, up to date and not encyclopedic. From this emerged *CURRENT Diagnosis & Treatment Gastroenterology, Hepatology, & Endoscopy* which Dr. Norton Greenberger edited. This endeavor has been remarkably successful and is now in its fourth edition and has been translated into 9 different languages. Sadly, Dr. Greenberger passed away on March 21, 2020 leaving this legacy to others at Brigham and Women's Hospital to maintain in this new version that has been renamed *Greenberger's CURRENT Diagnosis & Treatment Gastroenterology, Hepatology, & Endoscopy*. Led by Dr. Sonia Friedman and Dr. John Saltzman, this fourth edition aims to carry on the goals of Dr. Greenberger's original purpose. It is divided into sections that cover all the critical elements associated with the current practice of gastroenterology, hepatology and endoscopy. In so doing, it is our aim to provide our colleagues and students with a concise compendium that is accessible and informative for anyone interested in this broad topic, whether it is medical students, residents, fellows, or even practicing gastroenterologists. We hope that you find this as enjoyable to read as it was for us and colleagues to write and edit.

Richard S. Blumberg, MD

Acute Abdominal Pain: Basic Principles & Current Challenges

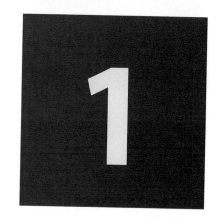

Molly L. Perencevich, MD
Frederick L. Makrauer, MD

ESSENTIAL CONCEPTS

▶ A careful and thorough history and physical exam remain essential to achieving and sustaining maximally safe, humane and cost-effective patient care.

▶ Advanced age, immunosuppression, and pregnancy may lead to atypical presentations of acute abdominal pain.

▶ In addition to surgical causes of abdominal pain, nonsurgical and functional causes should be considered.

▶ Socioeconomic factors and physical and sexual abuse should be considered in the assessment of patients with recurrent and unexplained acute abdominal pain.

▶ Race, ethnicity, gender, and other disparities and bias can impact the quality of patient care. Providers must be aware of these factors and seek to mitigate them.

▶ Narcotic pain medication will not obscure the recognition of key physical findings and may improve diagnostic accuracy by relaxing the patient. It should not be withheld from a patient with acute abdominal pain.

▶ The reduction of cumulative ionizing radiation, particularly in the imaging of inflammatory bowel disease (IBD), remains a high priority.

▶ Abdominal computed tomography (CT) is the most commonly performed imaging study for acute abdominal pain, although other studies may be recommended first depending on the clinical scenario.

▶ Magnetic resonance imaging (MRI) can be useful in evaluation of the biliary system and as a means of assessing bowel wall inflammation without ionizing radiation. However, exams can be challenging for critically ill patients and those with altered mental status, interpretation can be more difficult than CT, and it is more expensive than CT.

▶ Ultrasound is readily available, transportable, noninvasive and has no ionizing radiation. However, for the evaluation of the bowel and retroperitoneum, and in the presence of obesity, it is less sensitive than CT and MRI.

▶ Acute appendicitis is a common cause of acute abdominal pain with typical and atypical presentations.

General Considerations

Acute abdominal pain is generally defined as pain located in the abdomen that has occurred over a relatively short period of time, typically over several days. It is a common complaint in emergency departments (EDs), accounting for 5–10% of all ED visits. Appendicitis, cholecystitis, and choledocholithiasis, intestinal obstruction, pancreatitis, mesenteric ischemia, bowel perforation, and diverticulitis account for two-thirds of hospital admissions for acute abdominal pain and are associated with significant morbidity and mortality. Complications from interventional procedures as well as oncological therapy will also be encountered more frequently in major referral institutions. The cause of acute, nontraumatic abdominal pain remains unclear at the time of discharge in up to 30% of patients, particularly young women and the elderly.

There are racial and ethnic disparities in the evaluation and management of patients presenting with acute abdominal pain. Examples of inequity include Latinx and Black patients having longer wait times, less diagnostic imaging, reduced pain management, longer time from diagnosis to appendectomy, and use of less invasive surgical techniques. Efforts should be made to ensure all patients receive high quality care for acute abdominal pain. They include systematic changes, as well as a better understanding of implicit bias in health care professionals.

Our chapter focuses on the basic principles and challenges for the clinician in the evaluation and diagnosis of acute abdominal pain in adults. The patient with acute abdominal pain remains a clinical challenge for even the most-seasoned

Table 1–1. Common causes of acute abdominal pain.

Common Conditions	Key Diagnostic Test(s)
Acute appendicitis	Ultrasound, CT scan
Acute cholecystitis	Ultrasound
Choledocholithiasis, cholangitis	Ultrasound, MRCP, ERCP
Acute diverticulitis	CT scan
Acute pancreatitis	Serum amylase/lipase, CT scan
Bowel perforation	CT scan
Acute mesenteric ischemia	CT angiogram, MR angiogram
Ischemic colitis	CT scan, colonoscopy
Intestinal obstruction	Abdominal X-ray, CT scan
Sigmoid volvulus	CT scan, barium enema
Functional abdominal pain syndrome and Irritable bowel syndrome	History and physical exam, Rome criteria
Acute abdominal pain in women: • Pelvic inflammatory disease • Ectopic pregnancy • Adnexal pathology	HCG Pelvic examination Ultrasound
Biliary duct or pancreatic duct rupture	MRCP, ERCP (technetium-99 sulfur colloid scan)

CT, computed tomography; ERCP, endoscopic retrograde cholangiopancreatography; HCG, human chorionic gonadotropin; MRCP, magnetic resonance cholangiopancreatography; MR, magnetic resonance.

health care provider given the varied causes of abdominal pain (Tables 1–1 and 1–2). Successful management depends firstly on the clinician's clear understanding of the anatomy and physiology of gastrointestinal pain and a commitment to an independent and thorough medical history and physical examination of every patient. Laboratory and radiographic data are also important, but they cannot replace a well-performed excellent history and physical examination. Structured data collection, clinical scoring systems, and online decision-making tools may be helpful in measuring disease severity and guiding management. However, the clinician is encouraged to regularly seek the advice of trusted colleagues and current published guidelines, to "think outside of the box" and to always consider the *atypical* presentation of diseases, including common nongastrointestinal and extra-abdominal disorders. It must be remembered that all information is dated, and that new insights and experience should always be pursued.

▶ **Atypical Presentations**

Acute abdominal pain may present in atypical fashion in patients who are obtunded, septic, or immunosuppressed, elderly or very young, or in pregnancy. It may be very difficult to obtain an accurate history due to multiple sources of medical care, isolation from family members, and altered mental status. Physical and laboratory findings may be subtle in the presence of malnutrition, medications such as β-blockers, and hypothermia, diminished T-cell function or leukocyte response. In fact, altered mental status, oliguria, and hypotension may be the sole indicators of serious intra-abdominal disease. The elderly often have atypical presentations that represent a clinical challenge in the ED and must be evaluated with an abundance of caution. They require admission 50% of the time, and of those admitted, 33% eventually undergo surgery. At discharge, upwards of 40% still do not have a clear diagnosis.

▶ **Functional Disorders**

Functional disorders, such as irritable bowel syndrome (IBS) and functional abdominal pain syndrome (FAPS), are common and must always be considered. Constitutional symptoms are usually absent in functional gastrointestinal disorders. Symptoms are often chronic with episodes of acute worsening, but patients can present with severe abdominal pain. Obstacles to proper diagnosis include clinician and institutional inexperience, as well as psychosocial, anatomical, and pathophysiological factors. Patients with functional abdominal pain can undergo unnecessary repeated imaging and even surgery. However, patients with functional abdominal pain can also develop other causes of abdominal pain that may require imaging, so a careful history and exam should be performed with each encounter. Careful reflection and frequent re-examination of the abdomen in patients with a history of undiagnosed acute abdominal pain are strongly advised.

Opioid bowel dysfunction, including narcotic bowel syndrome (NBS), is increasingly common, particularly in the IBD and FAPS patient populations. NBS is thought to be mediated by central nervous system dysfunction in the setting of chronic opioid use. Patients with NBS may have paradoxical worsening of pain with the increase in narcotic dose.

Johnson TJ, Weaver MD, Borrero S, et al. Association of race and ethnicity with management of abdominal pain in the emergency department. *Pediatrics.* 2013;4:e851–e858. [PMID: 24062370]

Kurlander JE, Drossman DA. Diagnosis and treatment of narcotic bowl syndrome. *Nat Rev Gastroenterol Hepatol.* 2014;11: 410–418. [PMID: 24751914]

Macaluso CR, McNamara RM. Evaluation of acute abdominal pain in the emergency department. *Int J Gen Med.* 2012;5:789–797. [PMID: 23055768]

McDamara R, Dean AJ. Approach to acute abdominal pain. *Emerg Med Clin North Am.* 2011;29:159–173. [PMID: 21515174]

Natesan S, Lee J, Volkamer, et al. Evidence-based medicine approach to abdominal pain. *Emerg Med Clin North Am.* 2016; 34:165–190. [PMID: 27133239]

Scarborough JE, Bennett KM, Pappas TN. Racial disparities in outcomes after appendectomy for acute appendicitis. *Amer J Surg.* 2012;204:11–17. [PMID: 22154135]

Table 1–2. Less common causes of acute abdominal pain.

Category	Key Diagnostic Feature(s)
Metabolic/Endocrine	
Diabetic ketoacidosis	High serum glucose; ketoacidosis
Hyperthyroidism	High T_4, low TSH
Hypercalcemia	High serum calcium
Hypokalemia	Low serum potassium
Hypophosphatemia	Low serum phosphate
Addison disease	Low serum cortisol, elevated ACTH
Porphyria	High porphobilinogen and delta-ALA
Familial Mediterranean fever	Duration 1–3 days; pleuritis and peritonitis
Vascular/Cardiopulmonary	
Median arcuate ligament syndrome	MRA or CTA
Myocardial ischemia/infarction	Abnormal ECG, high troponin
Aortic dissection	Widened mediastinum and diagnostic CT angiogram
Pneumonia/pleurisy	Chest radiograph
Pulmonary embolus	Wells score, high D-dimer, CT angiography
Drug/Toxin	
Salicylate	Tinnitus, confusion, mixed respiratory alkalosis and metabolic acidosis
Anticholinergics	Confusion, dilated pupils, tachycardia, ileus, urinary retention
Tricyclic antidepressants (TCAs)	Delirium, anticholinergic symptoms, ECG changes, serum/urine TCA level
Cocaine	Tachycardia, hypertension, systemic end-organ ischemia, positive toxic screen
Heavy metals	Renal, neurologic toxicity, 24-hour urine assay
Vasculitis/Connective Tissue	
Systemic lupus erythematosus (SLE)	>4 of 11 SLE criteria
Systemic vasculitis	Multiorgan disease with positive P-ANCA and ANA, low complement

Category	Key Diagnostic Feature(s)
Scleroderma	Skin changes, Raynaud phenomenon, and visceral disease, Scl-70
Hematologic/Immunologic	
Sickle cell crisis	History, periarticular pain, effusions
IgA vasculitis (formerly called Henoch-Schönlein purpura)	Skin biopsy: leukocytoclastic vasculitis with IgA and C3 deposition
Hemolytic uremic syndrome	ARF with schistocytes on smear
Hereditary angioneurotic edema	Low C1 esterase inhibitor level
Systemic mast cell disease	High serum tryptase, urinary histamine, and prostaglandin D_2; increased tissue mast cells; abnormal bone marrow biopsy
Mast cell activation syndrome	Serologic markers as above
Food allergy	History, increased IgE level, challenge; mucosal eosinophilia
Thrombotic thrombocytopenic purpura	Fever, confusion, thrombocytopenia, schistocytes
Infectious	
Staphylotoxin	Fever, hypotension, rash (CDC case definition)
Bornholm disease	Fever, rash, spasmodic pain, enterovirus (coxsackie/echo)
Yersinia enterocolitica	Diarrhea, fever, positive stool culture, ileal inflammation
Tuberculous mesenteritis	Fever, fatigue, diarrhea, RLQ mass and ascites, positive biopsy
Dengue fever	Fever, hemolytic anemia, myalgias/arthralgias, low platelets, high LFTs, positive serology
Malaria	Fever, chill, diaphoresis, hemolytic anemia, myalgia, cough, multiorgan disease, RBC smear
Musculoskeletal	
"Slipping rib" (lower rib margin) syndrome	Production of pain with rib compression only on affected side (Hook sign)
Rectus sheath hematoma/neuroma	Carnett sign, CT
Chronic abdominal wall pain syndrome	Carnett sign

(Continued)

Table 1–2. Less common causes of acute abdominal pain (Continued)

Category	Key Diagnostic Feature(s)	Category	Key Diagnostic Feature(s)
Neuropsychiatric		Narcotic bowel syndrome	Recent acceleration or taper of chronic narcotic dose
Herpes zoster	Unilateral, painful vesicular rash in dermatomal distribution, positive DFA of lesion or PCR of fluid	**Renal**	
		Nephrolithiasis/ ureterolithiasis	Hematuria and positive CT
Abdominal migraine	Adolescents, cyclic occurrence		
Temporal lobe seizures	Adolescents, aura, abnormal EEG	Papillary necrosis	Hematuria, obstructive uropathy, diabetes, sickle cell disease
Radiculopathy	Mechanical pain in dermatomal distribution, positive MRI		

ACTH, adrenocorticotropic hormone; ANA, antinuclear antibody; ARF, acute renal failure; CDC, Centers for Disease Control and Prevention; CT, computed tomography; CTA, CT angiography; delta-ALA, delta-aminolevulinic acid (test); DFA, direct fluorescent antibody; ECG, electrocardiogram; EEG, electroencephalogram; IgA, immunoglobulin A; IgE, immunoglobulin E; LFTs, liver function tests; MRA, magnetic resonance angiography; MRI, magnetic resonance imaging; P-ANCA, perinuclear antineutrophilic cytoplasmic antibody; PCR, polymerase chain reaction (amplification); RBC, red blood cell; RLQ, right lower quadrant; RUQ, right upper quadrant; T4, thyroxine; TSH, thyroid-stimulating hormone.

Shah AA, Zogg CK, Zafar SN, et al. Analgesic access for acute abdominal pain in the emergency department among racial/ethnic minority patients: a nationwide examination. *Med Care.* 2015;53:1000–1009. [PMID: 26569642]

Shan A, Baumann G, Gholamrezanezhad. Patient race/ethnicity and diagnostic imaging utilization in the emergency department: a systematic review. *J Am Coll Radiol.* 2020;18:795–808. [PMID: 33385337]

Spangler R, Pham TV, Khoujah D, et al. Abdominal emergencies in the geriatric patient. *Int J Emerg Med.* 2014;7:43. [PMID: 25635203]

EVALUATION OF THE ACUTE ABDOMEN

The Medical History

"More errors in diagnosis are traceable to a lack of acumen in eliciting or interpreting symptoms than have ever been caused by failure to hear a murmur, feel a mass or take an electrocardiogram." — F. Dennette Adams, 1958

The clinician must always listen carefully to the patient, with minimal interruption, demonstrating patience, respect and empathy. Evaluation of acute abdominal pain must always begin with eliciting the patient's presenting circumstances, the perception of pain severity, location, quality (including radiation), timing (onset, frequency, duration, past experience), trigger(s), and modifiers. The pain history can be organized by the acronym "OPQRST" (Table 1–3). The Visual Analog Scale with facial diagrams can be used to objectify the patient's degree of pain.

Identification of the *region* of the abdomen in which the patient experiences distress narrows the choice of organ responsible for pain (Figure 1–1). Abdominal pain can be caused by inflammation or damage to nerve fibers (*neuropathic* pain) or non-nerve tissues (*nociceptive* pain). There are two types of nociceptive pain: *visceral* pain (due to an inflamed viscera) and *somatic* pain (due to localized peritoneal irritation). Visceral pain is described as the slow-onset of poorly localized, dull discomfort, while somatic pain is described as a sudden, sharp, well-localized, lateralizing pain. The clinician must also remember that visceral pain may also be experienced simultaneously in an additional location, distant from the affected organ (*referred*), and mimicking somatic pain. This phenomenon is explained by sensory autonomic fibers sharing a spinal cord segment with an unrelated spinothalamic pathway. Genetic factors that impact cellular pathways may account for variability in abdominal pain perception. *Visceral hyperalgesia* and *impaired inhibitory nociception* also moderate pain perception.

Multiple studies in functional gastrointestinal disorders suggest the clinical presentation of pain results from complex interactions between biologic, psychological, and social factors. Factors that may impact a patient's pain perception and interaction with the health care system include social stress, cultural experience, a history of trauma/abuse, and adverse prior medical experiences.

Table 1–3. OPQRST: A mnemonic for describing pain.

O	Onset
P	Precipitants and modifiers
Q	Quality
R	Radiation
S	Severity (with Visual Analog Scale facial expressions)
T	Timeline

Data from Macaluso CR, McNamara RM. Evaluation and management of acute abdominal pain in the emergency department, *Int J Gen Med.* 2012;5:789-797.

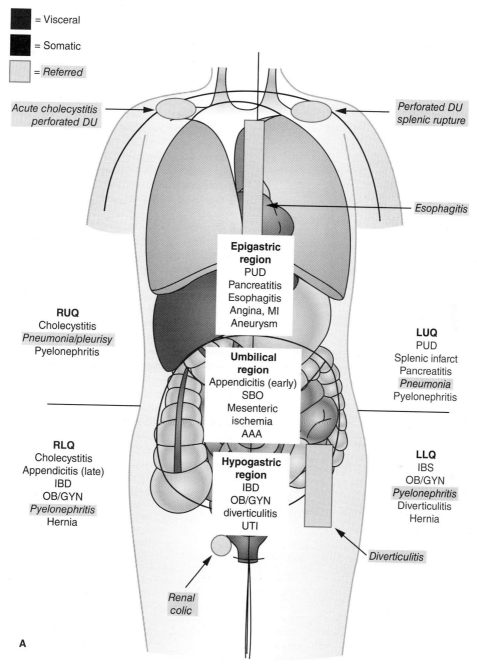

■ = Visceral

■ = Somatic

□ = *Referred*

Acute cholecystitis perforated DU

Perforated DU splenic rupture

Esophagitis

Epigastric region
PUD
Pancreatitis
Esophagitis
Angina, MI
Aneurysm

RUQ
Cholecystitis
Pneumonia/pleurisy
Pyelonephritis

LUQ
PUD
Splenic infarct
Pancreatitis
Pneumonia
Pyelonephritis

Umbilical region
Appendicitis (early)
SBO
Mesenteric ischemia
AAA

RLQ
Cholecystitis
Appendicitis (late)
IBD
OB/GYN
Pyelonephritis
Hernia

Hypogastric region
IBD
OB/GYN
diverticulitis
UTI

LLQ
IBS
OB/GYN
Pyelonephritis
Diverticulitis
Hernia

Diverticulitis

Renal colic

A

▲ **Figure 1–1.** Anatomy of abdominal pain: most frequent pain sites. **A.** Anterior view. **B.** Posterior view. AAA, abdominal aortic aneurysm; DU, duodenal ulcer; IBD, inflammatory bowel disease; IBS, irritable bowel syndrome; LLQ, left lower quadrant; LUQ, left upper quadrant; MI, myocardial infarction; OB/GYN, obstetric/gynecologic conditions; PUD, peptic ulcer disease; RLQ, right lower quadrant; RUQ, right upper quadrant; SBO, small bowel obstruction; UTI, urinary tract infection. (Reproduced with permission of Frederick L. Makrauer, MD.)

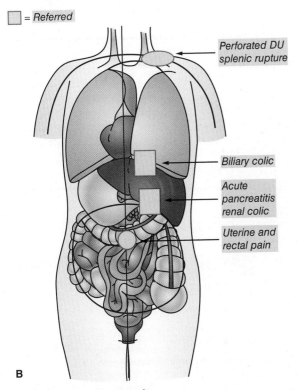

= *Referred*

Perforated DU splenic rupture

Biliary colic

Acute pancreatitis renal colic

Uterine and rectal pain

B

▲ **Figure 1–1.** *(Continued)*

Camilleri M. Genetics of human gastrointestinal sensation. *Neurogastroenterol Motil*. 2013;25:458–466. [PMID: 23594334]

Macaluso CR, McNamara RM. Evaluation of acute abdominal pain in the emergency department. *Intl J Gen Med*. 2012;5:789–797. [PMID: 23055768]

Van Outdenhove L, Levey RL, Crowell MD, et al. Biopsychosocial aspects of functional gastrointestinal disorders: how central and biopsychosocial aspects of functional gastrointestinal disorders contribute to the development and expression of functional gastrointestinal disorders. *Gastroenterology*. 2016;150:1355–1367. [PMID: 27144624]

▶ The Physical Examination

Physical examination of the patient with acute abdominal pain remains an important diagnostic tool; with a proper history, it will yield the correct initial diagnosis in at least 50% of patients. Narcotic pain medication may alter the physical findings but not to a degree that will affect diagnostic accuracy or management and it should not be withheld from the patient suffering from pain.

Vital signs are important to help determine whether a patient is critically ill. The abdominal exam includes inspection, auscultation, percussion, and palpation. Evidence of peritoneal irritation is suggestive of a surgical etiology of the pain. Pain out of proportion to physical findings should raise a concern for mesenteric ischemia. The value of the digital rectal examination in the evaluation of the acute abdominal pain is limited; its benefit is more obvious in the subacute office setting when neoplasm, IBD or sexually transmitted disease may be encountered. The abdominal exam may be different in the setting of pregnancy. Cardiac, pulmonary, vascular, gynecologic, and testicular exams should also be performed when relevant.

There are several bedside exam maneuvers (or "signs") that can be helpful in the evaluation of abdominal pain (Table 1–4). Having a patient cough or do a heel drop can be used to evaluate for peritoneal irritation. Murphy's sign, an inspiratory arrest during right upper quadrant palpation, is associated with acute cholecystitis. Abdominal wall pain, whether due to a rectus sheath hematoma, muscle tear, or postoperative neuroma, can be elicited by the Carnett sign. In eliciting the Carnett sign, the patient with pain and tenderness during palpation is re-examined after the abdominal wall is tensed using neck flexion (thus isolating the abdominal viscera and peritoneal cavity from the pressure of the examiner's hands). If the patient's discomfort *worsens*, it suggests a disorder of the abdominal wall. If it *lessens*, an intraabdominal process is more likely. Discomfort caused by a so-called slipping rib (or, lower rib margin syndrome) can be elicited by curling the fingers under the costal margin (usually left) while applying gentle pressure. Whenever safe and comfortable for the patient, abdominal wall hernias should always be pursued with the patient in the upright position.

The importance of the physical examination should continue to be emphasized as part of clinical care, despite reliance on abdominal imaging. Serial abdominal exams can identify important changes in the status of a patient, and they should be accurately recorded in the medical chart. If possible, diagramming the pain's location and radiation is also useful for subsequent observations by multiple clinicians.

Kessler D, Bauer SJ. Utility of the digital rectal examination in the emergency department: a review. *J Emerg Med*. 2012;43:1196–1204. [PMID: 22883714]

Ranji SR, Goldman LE, Simel DL, et al. Do opiates affect the clinical evaluation of patients with acute abdominal pain? *JAMA*. 2006;296:1764–1774. [PMID: 17032990]

Shian B, Larson ST. Abdominal wall pain: clinical evaluation, differential diagnosis, and treatment. *Am Fam Physician*. 2018;98:429–436. [PMID: 30252418]

▶ Laboratory Studies

A pregnancy test must always be performed in every woman of childbearing age. Complete blood count (CBC), liver enzymes, lipase, and urinalysis are commonly performed, but are most helpful when abnormal.

Misinterpretation of basic laboratory tests can lead to costly errors in diagnosis and patient management. Overinterpretation (eg, leukocytosis in a patient on corticosteroids)

Table 1–4. Abdominal examination: useful signs.

Abdominal Exam Sign	Disorder	Description
Carnett sign	Abdominal wall tenderness	In supine position: If discomfort is from abdominal wall (hernia, hematoma, tear), lifting head and shoulders (or raising legs in extension) will *increase* pain and tenderness. If discomfort is intra-abdominal in origin, the pain will *decrease, or not change.*
Closed eyes sign	Non-organic pain	During abdominal palpation, if pain/tenderness is organic, the eyes will be wide open. If the pain is (non-organic) functional, the eyes will more often remain closed.
Cough (Dunphy sign), or heel drop[a]	Peritoneal irritation	Cough (any position) or quick drop to heals (standing) triggers immediate, sharp, discomfort well-localized to the inflamed area.
Hook sign	Slipping rib syndrome	The clinician places the fingers under the lower costal margin and pulls the hand in an anterior direction. Pain or clicking indicates a positive test.
Murphy sign	Acute cholecystitis	Inability to deeply inspire (respiratory arrest) due to pleuritic pain with palpation of the right subcostal area (as the inflamed gallbladder comes in contact with the examiner's hand).
Obturator sign[a]	Deep pelvic inflammation	Pain on passive internal rotation of hip with the right knee in flexion.
Psoas sign[a]	Retroperitoneal inflammation	Pain on passive extension of the right hip with patient in the right lateral decubitus position.
Rovsing sign[a]	Right lower quadrant inflammation	Pain in the right lower quadrant when palpating the left lower quadrant.
Taxi test	Peritoneal inflammation	Similar to "Dunphy sign." Immediate, sharp discomfort well-localized to the inflamed area when traveling on uneven road surfaces.

[a] Particularly useful in diagnosing appendicitis.
Carnett JB. Intercostal neuralgia as a cause of abdominal pain and tenderness. *J Surg Gynecol Obstet.* 1926;42:625.
Gray DW, Dixon JM, Collin J. The closed eyes sign: an aid to diagnosing non-specific abdominal pain. *BMJ.* 1988;297:837.
Dunphy JE, Botsford TW. Examination of the abdomen: acute appendicitis. In: Physical Examination of the Surgical Patient. 1953:123.
Cyriax EF. On various conditions that may simulate the referred pains of visceral disease, and a consideration of these from the point of view of cause and effect. Practitioner. 1919;102:314.
Murphy JB. The diagnosis of gall-stones. The Medical News (London). 1903;82: 825.
Cope VZ. The thigh-rotation or obturator test: a new sign in some inflammatory conditions. *Br J Surg.* 1919;7:537.
Cope Z. Method of diagnosis: (II) The examination of the patient. Determination of illiopsoas rigidity. In: Silen W, ed. Cope's early diagnosis of the acute abdomen. 17th ed. Oxford: Oxford University Press; 1921. 42.
Rovsing T. Indirect elicitation of the typical pain at McBurney's point: a contribution to the diagnosis of appendicitis and typlitis. *Zentrablatt für Chirurgie.* 1907;34:1257.

or under-interpretation (eg, normal white blood cell count in a patient who is elderly, immunosuppressed or on chemotherapy) of results is not uncommon. White blood cell count and hematocrit may be normal in a patient with an incipient intra-abdominal catastrophe. Biomarkers of inflammation such as CRP are neither adequately sensitive nor specific. A normal serum lactic acid does *not* exclude active mesenteric ischemia, and a normal urinalysis does not exclude nephrolithiasis. It must always be remembered that elderly, immunosuppressed, or pregnant patients are often sicker than they appear and their laboratory studies suggest that.

Clinical Scores and Other Tools

A variety of scoring systems are available for the clinical assessment of patients with specific types of abdominal pain. An example is the use of the BISAP (bedside index of severity in acute pancreatitis) score in the management of acute pancreatitis. BISAP assigns points for five common indicators (blood urea nitrogen [BUN] >25 mg/dL, impaired mental status, SIRS, age >60, and pleural effusion) to provide a reliable means of determining pancreatitis severity and prognosis. In IBD, the Harvey Bradshaw Index (HBI, for Crohn) and Mayo Clinical Score (for ulcerative colitis), provide well-studied, reproducible noninvasive measures of disease activity for evaluation and treatment. The authors urge great caution in considering clinical scores as the sole measure for assessing high-risk patients who are significantly ill.

Computer-Aided Decision Support (CADS) has the potential to aid in diagnosis and standardize evaluation of patients with acute abdominal pain. However, all tools should be used only in the context of a full evaluation and as a supplement to clinical judgment.

Cooper JG, West RM, Clamp SE, Hassan TB. Does computer-aided clinical decision support improve the management of acute abdominal pain? *Emerg Med J.* 2011;28:553–557. [PMID: 21045220]

Kerner C, Carey K, Baillie C, et al. Clinical predictors of urgent findings on abdominopelvic CT in emergency department patients with Crohn's disease. *Inflamm Bowel Dis.* 2013;19:1179–1185. [PMID: 23552763]

Mounzer R, Langmead CJ, Wu BU, et al. Comparison of existing clinical scoring systems to predict persistent organ failure in patients with acute pancreatitis. *Gastroenterology.* 2012;142:1476–1482. [PMID: 22452289]

Imaging Studies

Imaging has an important role in the evaluation and management of patients with acute abdominal pain. The value of cross-sectional imaging continues to increase with improved sensitivity and specificity, reduced ionizing radiation and the development of intravenous and oral contrast agents which better assess acute or chronic mucosal inflammation. The clinician's choice of imaging study must always consider the patient's differential diagnosis, clinical condition, possibility of pregnancy, cumulative radiation dose in addition to the study's value, safety, ease of interpretation, availability, cost and local expertise.

Abdominal X-ray can provide rapid information but is most helpful when ureterolithiasis, bowel obstruction or perforation is suspected. Abdominal CT remains the "gold standard" in nonpregnant patients because of its high sensitivity and specificity in the global evaluation of acute abdominal pain. However, attention should be paid to the cumulative dose of ionizing radiation with repeated CT studies over time, particularly in patients with chronic abdominal pain and IBD. In IBD, the highest cumulative radiation exposure is encountered in patients with penetrating-type Crohn's disease.

Ultrasound (abdominal/pelvic) can be rapidly used and does not have radiation exposure. It should be the study of choice whenever possible in the young and pregnancy. Ultrasound is particularly helpful in the evaluation of abdominal aortic aneurysm, gallbladder disease, ureterolithiasis, ovarian pathology and ectopic pregnancy, and disturbance of portal venous flow. It may also be helpful in appendicitis.

MRI is also free of ionizing radiation and provides detailed cross-sectional information. It is particularly helpful in the evaluation of biliary and pancreatic pathology with MR cholangiopancreatography (MRCP). It can also effectively identify small bowel inflammation with MR enterography (MRE), and this should be considered in the evaluation of patients with IBD in the appropriate clinical setting. Nevertheless, MRI has certain disadvantages compared with CT. Gadolinium should be avoided in pregnancy. Also, MRI may be less available, requires more time than CT (challenging for critically ill patients and those with altered mental status), can be more difficult to interpret than CT, and is more expensive than CT.

Angiography (CT, MR, and interventional angiography) must be readily available in institutions that regularly evaluate the abdominal vasculature for possible mesenteric ischemia.

The proper choice of the most effective abdominal imaging method depends on the patient's clinical presentation and differential diagnosis. This process is further discussed in subsequent chapters.

Cartwright SL, Knudson MP. Diagnostic imaging of acute abdominal pain in adults. *Am Fam Physician.* 2015;91:452–459. [PMID 25884745]

Karla MK, Francis IR. Personalized dose reduction for computed tomography scanning: size matters, so does prior radiation exposure. *Clin Gastroenterol Hepatol.* 2010;8:231–232. [PMID: 20005984]

Khandelival A, Fasih N, Kielar A. Imaging of acute abdomen in pregnancy. *Radiol Clin North Am.* 2013;51:1005–1022. [PMID: 24210441]

Nguyen GC, Low D, Chong RY, et al. Utilization of diagnostic imaging and ionizing radiation exposure among an inflammatory bowel disease inception cohort. *Inflamm Bowel Dis.* 2020;26:898–906. [PMID: 31560042]

Additional Comments

The use of laparoscopy as a diagnostic tool, particularly in young and pregnant women, should be at the coordinated discretion of the patient's team of gynecologist/obstetrician, gastroenterologist and surgeon.

Table 1–5 includes several key considerations to keep in mind during the evaluation of patients with acute abdominal pain.

ACUTE APPENDICITIS

General Considerations

Acute appendicitis serves as an ideal illustrative example of how the application of the preceding general principles can strengthen proper diagnosis and care of the patient with the acute abdomen. The pathogenesis of acute appendicitis is infection secondary to luminal obstruction due to fecolith, lymphoid hyperplasia, infection, or tumor. Uncommonly, deformity of the appendiceal ostium during colonoscopy can present as "delayed," or "chronic," appendicitis.

Table 1–5. Key considerations in the evaluation of acute abdominal pain.

Approach every patient as an individual, with respect for their beliefs and experience.
Listen! Generate your own history, physical, and conclusions.
Always consider extra-abdominal, non-surgical, and functional diseases.
The elderly and the immunosuppressed are often sicker than they appear.
Pain, followed by vomiting, consider bowel obstruction.
Pain >> abdominal findings, consider ischemia.
Routine lab studies may be normal in the presence of an acute abdomen.
In women of childbearing age, always perform a pregnancy test.
Cross-sectional imaging should be considered as the "gold standard."
Lack of free air on imaging does not exclude obstruction.

In the United States, over 250,000 patients are admitted annually with the diagnosis of appendicitis, with a lifetime individual risk of 7–8%. It affects men slightly more than women, with the highest incidence found in the second and third decades of life. World-wide, appendectomy is the most commonly performed emergency operation but the reported incidence has dropped by more than 50% in the past three decades, for unclear reasons. With advancements in imaging leading to more timely diagnosis, the mortality rate is now less than 1%.

The perforation rate can reach 50–70% when diagnosis is delayed more than 24 hours. A complicated presentation and course is more likely with advanced age, pregnancy, obesity, smoking, and increased appendix length. Racial and ethnic disparities have been identified in appendiceal perforation rate, delayed diagnosis and imaging, use of analgesia, and time interval to appendectomy. Insurance and socioeconomic status may also influence perforation rate. Mortality is higher in the elderly than in the general population.

Goyal MK, Chamberlain JM, Webb, M, et al. Racial and ethnic disparities in the delayed diagnosis of appendicitis among children. *Acad Emerg Med.* 2020 Sept 29. Online ahead of print. [PMID: 32991770]

Goyal MK, Kuppermann N, Cleary SD, et al. Racial disparities in pain management in children with appendicitis in emergency departments. *JAMA Pediatr.* 2015;169:996–1002. [PMID: 26366984]

Ingraham AM, Cohen ME, Bilimoria KY, et al. Effect of delay to operation on outcomes in adults with acute appendicitis. *Arch Surg.* 2010;145:886–892. [PMID: 20855760]

Scarborough JE, Bennett KM, Pappas TN. Racial disparities in outcomes after appendectomy for acute appendicitis. *Am J Surg.* 2012;204:11–17. [PMID: 22154135]

▶ **Clinical Findings**

A. Symptoms and Signs

History and abdominal examination will vary depending on the location of the appendix. The "classic" presentation (acute periumbilical pain migrating to McBurney point, followed by nausea and vomiting) occurs in only 30–60% of patients. Other symptoms may also include gaseousness, altered bowel movements, and fatigue. Fever may be low grade or absent. The atypical location of the appendix in the third trimester of pregnancy represents a particular diagnostic challenge (see below).

The patient can appear relatively well or can be quite ill. Physical examination reveals variable tenderness at McBurney's point. Psoas and obturator signs can be used to evaluate for a retrocecal or pelvic appendicitis (see Table 1–4). The psoas sign is pain on passive extension of the right hip (with the patient in the right lateral decubitus position). The obturator sign is pain on passive external rotation of the hip with the right knee in flexion. Signs of peritoneal irritation can be found.

A palpable mass is uncommon, and more consistent with enteritis, gynecological disorders (uterine fibroid, tubal abscess or pregnancy, or ovarian cyst), Crohn's disease and benign or malignant tumor (adenocarcinoma of the cecum or appendix, carcinoid, lymphoma and, rarely, pseudomyxoma peritonei).

B. Laboratory Findings

A mild leukocytosis is common in acute appendicitis. Chemistry studies and urinalysis are usually normal. CRP can be elevated.

C. Clinical Scores

Clinical scores are not routinely used in the evaluation and management of acute appendicitis. The Alvarado score is a combination of clinical and laboratory parameters which has neither the sensitivity nor specificity adequate to determine the value of either CT or appendectomy. We do not recommend making a diagnosis of acute appendicitis based exclusively on clinical criteria unless appropriate imaging is not available.

D. Imaging Studies

1. Issues and controversies—The advantage of preoperative imaging, with CT or ultrasound, has been debated. Detractors cite delay in surgery, prolonged operating time, and increased length of stay and cost without the benefit of a reduction in negative appendectomy rate. However, in patients with a high clinical probability of appendicitis, almost one-third will be found to have another diagnosis or a normal scan. We recommend, therefore, that preoperative imaging (CT, MRI, or ultrasound) be performed in *all* patients with suspected acute appendicitis, even with high-probability clinical presentations.

2. Ultrasound—Ultrasound has a sensitivity of 85% and a specificity of 90% for acute appendicitis. Results are highly operator dependent. Findings that suggest acute appendicitis include diameter greater than 6 mm, thickened wall, noncompressibilty, and an appendicolith. There may also be a blind-ended lumen, not to be confused with an open-ended salpinx or gonadal vein. The patient may be tender on compression of the appendix with the ultrasound probe. Ultrasound should only be used as the sole imaging modality in patients with a high probability of appendicitis. False-positive results are common in patients with IBD, cecal diverticulitis, and pelvic inflammatory disease. The value of ultrasound is also limited in morbidly-obese patients, after perforation, or with retrocecal appendix location where it is inaccessible to luminal compression.

Ultrasound should be considered the study of choice in children and women of childbearing age, vulnerable to ionizing radiation. Ultrasound may also yield helpful information regarding adnexal anatomy.

3. CT Scan—Contrast-enhanced CT scan is commonly performed in the evaluation of acute appendicitis. The sensitivity is 96–98% and the specificity is 96%, particularly if an appendicolith is demonstrated. Positive findings include diameter greater than 6 mm, thickened wall with enhancement, periappendiceal fat stranding, and appendicolith. An air-filled appendix on CT essentially excludes acute appendicitis. Oral contrast is not recommended in the setting of possible ileus and may delay time to performing the scan.

Focal thickening of the terminal ileum or cecum may easily be confused with Crohn's disease, and an infected right fallopian tube may be mistaken for a dilated appendiceal lumen. Epiploic appendagitis will appear as an ovoid fat-attenuation focus with hyperattenuating rim near the colonic serosa. Infectious enteritis should be easily differentiated by the diffuseness of bowel wall thickening and contrast enhancement, in the presence of a normal-appearing appendix. Other less common mimics of appendicitis include mucocele of the appendix, ovarian disorders, and endometriosis. An advantage of CT over ultrasound is the ability to visualize the entire abdomen, demonstrating an alternative diagnosis in 15% of cases. An additional 15% of patients will have a normal abdominal CT.

4. MRI—MRI is generally recommended in patients for whom CT is not advised, such as pregnant women and older children in whom an ultrasound did not provide a diagnosis. The sensitivity is 95% and specificity is 92% for acute appendicitis. IV gadolinium contrast can be used, although it is contraindicated in pregnant patients.

Dahabreh IJ, Adam GP, Halladay CW, et al. Diagnosis of right lower quadrant pain and suspected acute appendicitis. *Rockville (MD): Agency for Healthcare Research and Quality (US)*; 2015 Dec. Report No.: 15(16)-EHC025-EF. [PMID: 27054223]

Kim K, Kim SY, Kim YH, et al. Low-dose abdominal CT for evaluating suspected appendicitis. *N Engl J Med.* 2012;366:1596–1605. [PMID: 22533576]

Ohle R, O'Reilly F, O'Brien KK, et al. The Alverado score for predicting acute appendicitis: a systematic review. *BMC Med.* 2011;9:139. [PMID: 22204638]

Raja AS, Wright C, Sodickson AD, et al. Negative appendectomy rate in the era of CT: an 18-year perspective. *Radiology.* 2010;256:460–465. [PMID: 20529988]

Differential Diagnosis

The differential diagnosis of acute appendicitis is broad, reflecting classical and atypical presentations of the disorder. It includes mesenteric lymphadenitis, bacterial enteritis, acute cecal diverticulitis, Crohn's disease, cholecystitis, epiploic appendagitis, Meckel diverticulitis, ureteral calculus, and gynecologic disorders including acute salpingitis, ruptured ovarian follicle (mittelschmerz), and ruptured ectopic pregnancy. Epiploic appendagitis will be discussed below. The remaining disorders are reviewed in ensuing chapters.

Treatment

A. Overview

Surgery has been recognized since 1886 as the definitive treatment for appendicitis. Active debate continues regarding the proper timing, use of antibiotics, and choice of operative technique (ie, open vs laparoscopic appendectomy) and which variables should influence these decisions. Recent data suggests that for selected patients, outpatient therapy with antibiotics is comparatively safe and effective.

The incidence of negative appendectomy has dropped to 3.5% with improved and more widely used preoperative imaging but it still may reach 20–30% in selected patient groups. For example, women aged 15–45 with preexisting IBS may have a 20% negative appendectomy rate due to the similarity of presentation with multiple other acute lower abdominal and pelvic pain disorders. The negative rate may reach more than 30% in pregnancy with restricted use of CT imaging and the atypical RUQ location of the appendix in the third trimester (see Figure 7–5).

B. Antibiotics

A third-generation intravenous cephalosporin may be initiated preoperatively in patients who are mildly ill. Sicker patients with signs of perforation and sepsis require broader coverage for anaerobes, including *Bacteroides*. Continuation of antibiotics postoperatively will depend on the surgical findings and the patient's clinical response. Antibiotic therapy as the sole treatment for uncomplicated acute appendicitis appears to be safe but is associated with a cumulative incidence of appendectomy of 27.3% at 1 year, and 43.4% after 5 years. Antibiotics alone should be used with caution in patients who are elderly, debilitated or suffering from any contraindication to surgery such as acute myocardial infarction.

Flum DR and CODA Collaborative. A randomized trial comparing antibiotics with appendectomy for appendicitis. *N Engl J Med.* 2020;383:1907–1919. [PMID: 33017106]

Salminen P, Tuominen R, Paajanen H, et al. Five-year follow-up of antibiotic therapy for uncomplicated acute appendicitis in the APPAC randomized clinical trial. *JAMA.* 2018;320:1259–1265. [PMID: 30264120]

Jaschinski T, Mosch CG, Eikermann M, et al. Laparoscopic versus open surgery for suspected appendicitis. *Cochrane Database Syst Rev.* 2018;11:CD001546. [PMID: 30484855]

Jones AE, Phillips AW, Jarvis JR, et al. The value of routine histo-pathological examination of appendectomy specimens. *BMC Surg.* 2007;7:17. [PMID: 17692116]

C. Interventional Radiology

Appendiceal rupture or abscess can be found in up to 25% of patients at presentation. When an abscess is present, CT-guided drainage and dedicated parenteral antibiotic therapy should be considered as the preferred alternative to immediate appendectomy. Interval appendectomy after resolution of the collection should then be performed at a later date. The timing must rest with the surgeon, after consultation with the gastroenterologist and radiologist.

D. Surgery

Appendectomy remains the treatment of choice for acute appendicitis, whether open or laparoscopic. Prevention of perforation is the major goal and the rate of perforation remains one of the major quality-of-care indicators in most institutions. A brief delay to obtain additional history, perform preoperative diagnostic studies and begin antibiotics does not increase the risk and may actually benefit the patient. Adjunctive antibiotic therapy should be administered at the discretion of the surgeon.

The role, timing, and choice of surgical approach remains the most debated aspect of management. Ultimately, the decision depends upon the condition of the patient and the surgeon's experience. The surgeon must first consider the degree of diagnostic certainty, imaging evidence for complicating disease, stage of appendicitis, and experience with the technique. Laparoscopic appendectomy, though more expensive than the open approach, remains the operation of choice for uncomplicated patients. Patients have fewer wound infections, less pain, and shorter hospital stays compared with those undergoing open laparotomy, but may have a greater chance of postoperative abscess. It is the safest approach in obese patients.

In women, particularly during pregnancy, there appears to be an advantage to laparoscopic appendectomy. It can identify unrelated gynecologic pathology and reduce the rate of negative appendectomy which is inversely proportional to fetal health and also a benchmark for quality of care (see Appendicitis in Pregnancy). In men, the benefit of laparoscopic appendectomy is less well-established.

Histology of the resected appendix can yield useful data in 2% of cases and should always be performed. Unexpected findings can include carcinoid, Crohn's disease, endometriosis, parasite, and other benign and malignant tumors.

UNIQUE PRESENTATIONS OF APPENDICITIS

1. Appendicitis in Pregnancy

Appendicitis is the most common nonobstetrical surgical disease during pregnancy, occurring in approximately 1 out of 800–1500 pregnancies. Initial diagnosis is inaccurate 25–50% of the time with treatment delayed by the normal effects of pregnancy including nausea, vomiting, discomfort and anatomical alteration created by the gravid uterus. The result is a higher perforation rate associated with excess morbidity, preterm delivery, and fetal loss. In contrast, physiological leukocytosis, without a left shift, may be misinterpreted. While maternal mortality remains near zero, the 12–55% risk of perforation can increase fetal loss from a baseline of 2–3% up to 20%. Hence, early surgical intervention is the recommended treatment strategy for appendicitis during pregnancy.

Ultrasound is the first imaging method of choice. If ultrasound is inconclusive (most commonly in the third trimester), CT or MRI without gadolinium is used. The risk of fetal harm from ionizing radiation is highest before week 25. Gadolinium contrast with MRI is contraindicated in pregnancy. The clinical judgment of the managing medical-surgical team, the standards in one's own institution, the patient's preference, and published guidelines must always factor into the clinician's choice of investigation.

The rate of negative appendectomy is higher in pregnant, than nonpregnant, women and carries an increased risk for fetal loss. The surgeon's goal of eliminating negative appendectomy during pregnancy with improved preoperative assessment must always be weighed against the potential for complications associated with preoperative imaging and any delay in surgical therapy. Laparoscopic appendectomy by an experienced surgeon appears safe and effective.

Abbasi N, Patenaude V, Abenhaim HA. Management and outcomes of acute appendicitis in pregnancy-population-based study of over 7000 cases. *BJOC.* 2014;121:1509–1514. [PMID: 24674238]

2. Atypical Appendicitis

Retrocecal (ileal) appendicitis presents with less pain and rigidity due to shielding from the abdominal wall and may present as an antalgic gait or a positive psoas sign (see Table 1–4). Classic localization of discomfort to the RLQ may be ill-defined due to the lack of appendix contact with the peritoneum. *Pelvic appendicitis* is characterized by severe, constant pain in the contralateral LLQ, with fecal and urinary urgency. Abdominal tenderness is variable, but severe tenderness on pelvic and rectal examination may be present. *Elderly appendicitis* is infrequent, and pain is vague, presenting in the RLQ in only 20% of patients. There may be no fever. The abdominal examination may yield only a nontender mass. The white blood cell count can be lower than expected. An incorrect diagnosis is made in up to 54% of elderly patients and, compared with younger patients, mortality is four to eight-fold greater.

Proper management of atypical appendicitis relies on a high index of suspicion, careful patient assessment, and the findings on cross-sectional imaging.

Spangler R, Pham TV, Khoujah D, et al. Abdominal emergencies in the geriatric patient. *Int J Emerg Med.* 2014;7:43. [PMID: 25635203]

3. Late ("Delayed") Appendicitis

Late (or Delayed) Appendicitis is defined as presentation following more than 72 hours of symptoms. It occurs most often in the elderly, 4% of children, and 6% of women of child-bearing age. Diagnosis in the latter group can be obscured by other, unrelated symptoms common in pregnancy including abdominal wall and pelvic soft tissue pain, nausea, chronic constipation, and other co-morbidities.

A phlegmon may be palpable in the RLQ or be seen on CT, usually with an abscess component. Accurate diagnosis is difficult due to the surrounding inflammatory response. Crohn's disease, infection, and neoplasm are part of the differential diagnosis. Malignancy (carcinoid, appendiceal and colonic adenocarcinoma, lymphoma, ovarian cancer, and, rarely, pseudomyxoma peritonei) may be present in 1% of cases. Studies of late appendicitis are all retrospective, having occurred largely before advanced CT imaging was widely available. Thirty percent of patients required a drainage procedure as their initial surgery, and appendectomy was usually postponed until abdominal sepsis could be controlled.

Patients should be kept fasting with intravenous fluids and antibiotics. A nontoxic patient (without tachycardia, abdominal rigidity, or oliguria) should avoid immediate surgical intervention, if possible, to await reduced local inflammation and improve diagnostic accuracy. The decision to employ percutaneous drainage of an abscess depends on fluid bacteriology, collection size and consistency, accessibility as well as the patient's ability to cooperate without general anesthesia. Percutaneous drainage as the sole treatment for delayed appendicitis is not recommended because the recurrence rate for abscess without appendectomy is 5–20%. Colonoscopy has a role in the preoperative and postoperative management of patients who are stable and have clinical and radiographic features of ileocolonic Crohn's disease or neoplasm. The appendix can often be involved in ileocolonic Crohn's disease and appendicitis may precede the diagnosis.

No clinical criteria have been developed to predict the clinical outcome of delayed appendectomy or the ideal timing of appendectomy. Curative surgery, ideally laparoscopy, is usually performed within 2–3 months.

4. Chronic ("Recurrent" or "Subacute") Appendicitis

Five to ten percent of patients with acute appendicitis may relate a history of a previous attack, and 1.5% will have had symptoms for more than 3 weeks. Such observations have led to the description of a subset of patients with so-called chronic appendicitis. The literature is entirely retrospective, and no clinical distinction has been drawn between patients having a normal appendix at appendectomy and those with an inflamed appendix. Fibrosis with luminal obliteration has been described but not fistula or abscess. The role of appendectomy for such patients is controversial because they appear to represent a distinct clinical group without the poor prognosis found in "late" or "delayed" appendicitis.

5. Epiploic Appendagitis

Epiploic appendagitis is a very uncommon, severely painful condition that may mimic classic appendicitis with the acute onset of RLQ or LLQ pain often after eating or exercise. It arises usually in previously healthy men in the fourth to fifth decades. Fever and obstructive symptoms are uncommon. Less common manifestations are incarceration (20%) and obstruction (10%). Risk factors are obesity, hernia, and physical inactivity. It can mimic acute appendicitis, diverticulitis, mesenteritis, or omental infarction. Pain is due to torsion and ischemia of one or more of the approximately 100 epiploic (or omental) appendages that arise from the serosal surface of the colon. These appendages are composed of adipose tissue with a vascular stalk, 0.5–5 cm in length and oriented in two rows.

The white blood cell count is normal. Preoperative diagnosis is uncommon even with the availability of Ultrasound and cross-sectional imaging. CT findings consist of 2–4 cm, oval, fat-density lesions with surrounding inflammation and central attenuation. Unlike diverticulitis, colon wall thickness and diameter are normal. It is important to make the diagnosis so as to avoid unnecessary surgery. The prognosis is considered excellent but there has been one report of a 40% recurrence rate. Surgery, performed electively for recurrent symptoms, involves resection of only the inflamed appendages.

Majajan P, Basu T, Pai CW, et al. Factors associated with potentially missed diagnosis of appendicitis in the emergency department. *JAMA Netw Open.* 2020;3:e200612. [PMID: 32150270]

Schnedl WJ, Krause R, Tafeit E, et al. Insights into epiploic appendagitis. *Nat Rev Gastroenterol Hepatol.* 2011;8:45–49. [PMID: 21102533]

Inflammatory Bowel Disease: Immunologic Considerations & Therapeutic Implications

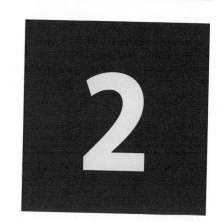

Vanessa Mitsialis, MD

Scott B. Snapper, MD, PhD

Richard S. Blumberg, MD

ESSENTIAL CONCEPTS

▶ Gut-associated lymphoid tissues (GALT) are characterized by a unique structure, physiologic inflammation, a tendency to suppress immune responses (oral tolerance), and production of secretory immunoglobulins.

▶ The immune response as orchestrated by GALT has two major arms: innate (rapid, hard-wired) and adaptive (delayed in onset with memory). The immune response is complemented by intrinsic barrier features of the intestinal mucosa as well as checked by numerous regulatory pathways to promote tolerance.

▶ Inflammatory bowel disease (IBD) is a chronic inflammatory condition of the intestines thought to arise from a dysregulated response to commensal microbes within the intestine. This condition is affected by a complex interplay of host genetic risk, aberrant immune responses, and environmental factors.

▶ The mucosal immune system is altered in IBD and is characterized by an abundance of proinflammatory mediators from cells associated with adaptive immunity (eg, T helper cells) and innate immunity (eg, macrophages, dendritic cells) which are expanded in IBD mucosa. There is evidence that nonimmune cells, such as epithelial and stromal cells, are also reprogrammed in IBD and play a significant role in the propagation of dysregulated immune responses.

▶ Historic paradigms regarding differential T helper cell responses in Crohn's disease versus ulcerative colitis have evolved with the use of large-scale and multidimensional immunophenotyping of human tissue. Both diseases seem to share many common immunological features.

▶ Therapies targeting specific cytokines, such as Tumor necrosis factor (TNF) and IL12/23, have revolutionized IBD treatment. However, the failure of many other cytokine-targeting therapies demonstrates the nuanced and pleiotropic effects of these mediators in IBD.

▶ Therapy targeting immune cell trafficking to intestinal tissue has proven successful in IBD and shows continued promise. However, the cumulative repertoire of therapies at this time for IBD is limited and many patients suffer with refractory disease.

▶ Increased understanding of IBD immunopathogenesis is essential to the ongoing development of therapeutic agents increasingly being administered in a logical, mechanism-based manner.

▶ General Considerations

Clinically, IBD is a chronic inflammatory condition of the intestines characterized by remission and relapses and distills clinically into one of two major subtypes of disease: ulcerative colitis (UC) and Crohn's disease (CD). Both diseases have a general commonality in their pathogenesis and are derived from a dysregulated mucosal immune response to antigenic components of the normal commensal microbiota that reside within the intestine.

At its core, IBD represents a disturbed relationship between the commensal microbiota, the intestinal epithelium, and the host immune system associated with dysregulation of inflammatory pathways. This interplay is increasingly recognized to be influenced by poorly understood environmental factors and genetic elements that affect the lifetime risk of developing this disorder. *Although genetic factors have been clearly established to be related to disease pathogenesis, identified through the study of rare monogenic forms of IBD in addition to genome-wide association studies in the broader IBD population, environmental factors known to affect disease course, such as tobacco smoke and appendectomy, are not well understood. These factors are unlikely in and of themselves to cause the disease but instead likely modify the genetically defined or undefined aspects of the most critical components that underlie the immunopathogenesis of this disease: intestinal bacteria, epithelial barrier, and mucosal immune response.* Of the latter three factors, the best understood influence—which has, to date, generated the most information resulting in novel and exciting new forms of therapy—involves the mucosal immune response associated with these disorders. *For this reason, a discussion of the immunopathogenesis of IBD not only is important for understanding the pathophysiology of these diseases but also provides a basis for understanding both the mechanisms and the rationale for using the wide variety of therapeutic approaches that have recently been developed or are soon to be developed for the treatment of these diseases.*

GENERAL PRINCIPLES OF GUT-ASSOCIATED LYMPHOID TISSUES AND THE MUCOSAL IMMUNE RESPONSE

The mucosa of the gastrointestinal tract, with a large surface area compounded by hierarchical folds, is the human body's largest interface between host and external environment. In addition to exposure to dietary antigens and pathogenic microbes, the human intestine is home to thousands of unique commensal bacterial species, most of which are congregated within the colon and distal small intestine where IBD most commonly occurs. The normal intestinal mucosal immune response to these antigens is highly specialized, balancing tolerance of benign microbiota with detection and eradication of pathogenic stimuli. The complex orchestration of antigen surveillance and associated immune cell response occurs in compartments organized throughout the intestine known as GALT. Given the extent of GALT—indeed, the body's most massive lymphoid "organ" —the human intestinal mucosal surface has been thought to exist in a state of controlled, or physiologic, inflammation, poised to react to pathogens but restrained just enough to enable oral tolerance (Table 2–1).

▷ Characteristics of GALT

GALT is spatially distributed such that the *induction* of immune responses occurs in discrete, organized lymphoid structures while the immune *effector action* occurs diffusely in the intestinal lamina propria and epithelium. Excluding the appendix, organized GALT is comprised of lymphoid follicles, which in aggregated form include Peyer's patches (located primarily in the terminal ileum), and in smaller form include isolated lymphoid follicles (ILF) scattered

Table 2–1. Unique characteristics of gut-associated lymphoid tissue.

1. Physiologic inflammation
2. Special types of organized lymphoepithelial structures (eg, Peyer patches)
3. Oral tolerance
4. Immunoglobulin A production and secretion

throughout the small intestine and colon. Crytopatches are even smaller clusters of immune cells nestled in between epithelial crypts. Diffuse GALT is comprised of the immune cells diffusely distributed within the intestinal lamina propria as well as the intraepithelial lymphocytes that reside within the epithelial layer. These specialized immune compartments are complemented by nonimmune and mechanical host defenses comprising the intestinal epithelial barrier system.

▷ Organized GALT

Organized GALT tissues, unlike lymph nodes, lack afferent lymphatics and are dedicated constitutively to the germinal center response. Instead of encountering antigen via afferent lymphatics, Peyer's patches and ILF are spatially located directly beneath a highly specialized follicle-associated epithelium (FAE), characterized by lack of microvilli and the presence of the so-called microfold cell (M cell). M cells take up luminal antigens and present them to dendritic cells (DCs) via their basolateral membrane through transcytosis. Antigen-presenting DCs then interact with naïve T cells in the "T cell zone" (the outermost portion of the follicle) where primed T cells express CXCR5, become follicular helper cells (Tfh cells), and migrate to the germinal center of the follicle. In the germinal center, Tfh cells as well as follicular DCs will prime B cells to undergo somatic hypermutation and affinity maturation into antibody-producing plasma cells. Primarily IgA-producing plasma cells, along with other lymphocytes, will then home to the lamina propria via expression of trafficking receptors including CCR9 and α4β7 (the latter being the target of anti-integrin therapy efficacious for both UC and CD). *Organized GALT tissues are therefore mainly inductive sites where antigens, especially bacterial antigens, are taken up, processed, and presented by DCs for the education of the GALT-associated lymphocytes.*

▷ Diffuse GALT

Diffuse GALT is comprised of the immune cells that infiltrate the lamina propria and the epithelial layer (intraepithelial lymphocytes, or IELs) distributed diffusely throughout the small and large intestine. Numerous immune cell subsets exist in the lamina propria including from the innate (eg, macrophages, DCs, natural killer cells, innate lymphoid cells, neutrophils, basophils, eosinophils, mast cells) and adaptive (eg, T cells, B cells, plasma cells) arms of the immune system. *The mainstay of the mucosal humoral response occurs in this compartment, whereby IgA-producing plasma cells, having matured in nearby germinal centers and having migrated into the lamina propria, secrete IgA into the intestinal lumen through epithelial transcytosis, neutralizing cognate antigen.* Circulating lymphocytes and leukocytes are able to access the lamina propria, as well as organized GALT structures, through high endothelial venules (HEV), which are specialized endothelial cells that express ligands for gut homing receptors, such as MAdCAM-1, enabling adhesion and dia-pedesis of immune cells through the endothelium into the surrounding tissue. *Diffuse GALT tissue is the main effector site of the mucosal immune response, where activated immune cells derived from nearby follicles or from the circulation orchestrate their response to antigenic stimuli originating from the gut lumen* (Figure 2–1).

Innate & Adaptive Immune Responses

The lymphocytes and leukocytes infiltrating the lamina propria and the epithelial layer are the main effectors of the immune response to luminal antigen. The complex interplay

between them spans both major arms of the immune sys-tem. These are the innate and adaptive (or specific) immune systems. *Innate immune cells are hard-wired to respond to a variety of nonhost antigens (typically microbial structures), whereas adaptive immune cells such as T and B cells typically undergo a maturation process to be highly selective and have immune memory for specific antigens.*

The innate immune system contains a pattern recogni-tion system that provides a hard-wired and rapid response to pathogen-associated or damage-associated molecular patterns (PAMPs or DAMPs). PAMPs typically represent microbial structures, such as the microbial outer mem-brane component lipopolysaccharide (LPS), while DAMPs

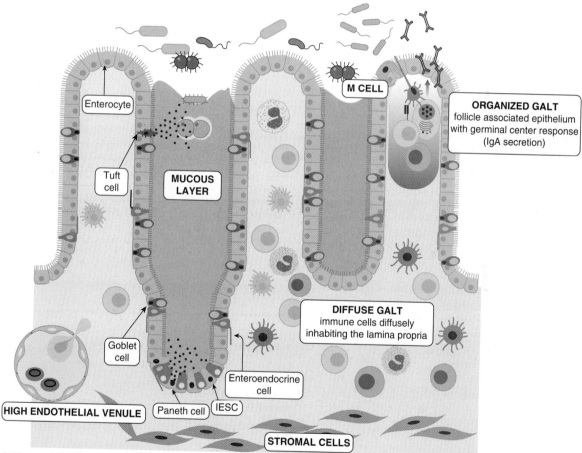

▲ **Figure 2–1. Fundamentals of GALT.** Featured is a schematic of the intestinal epithelium including the one-cell-thick epithelial layer composed of enterocytes and several highly specialized cells including goblet cells (secrete mucous), Paneth cells (secrete anti-microbial peptides), Tuft cells (secrete anti-helminthic chemicals), enteroendocrine cells, and intestinal epithelial stem cells (IESCs). In follicle-associated epithelium there are highly specialized M cells involved in antigen presentation and subsequent germinal center response, culminating in IgA production and secretion by plasma cells into the intestinal lumen. These discrete patches of lamina propria dedicated to the germinal center response make up organized GALT, whereas the immune cells diffusely inhabiting the lamina propria make up diffuse GALT. Depicted are high endothelial venules (HEVs) out of which leukocytes can traffic into the lamina propria, as well as stromal cells which provide essential components of the extracellular matrix.

represent structures related to nearby host cell death or distress, such as extracellular adenosine triphosphate (ATP). A classic group of pattern recognition receptors found on a wide variety of innate immune cells are toll-like receptors (TLRs), which bind to microbial structures as diverse as LPS or microbial DNA. Another major class of pattern recognition receptors includes the nucleotide oligomerization domain (NOD)-like receptors (NLRs), which recognize microbial structures such as muramyl dipeptide from the peptidoglycans of gram-negative and gram-positive bacteria. As will be discussed, NOD2 gene variants have been highly associated with CD, underscoring the importance of this hard-wired sensing system in mucosal immune homeostasis. Pattern-recognition receptors are distributed on virtually all cell types but are especially congregated on professional (eg, DCs, macrophages, and B cells) and non-professional (eg, intestinal epithelial cells) antigen-presenting cells (APCs).

Unlikely innate immunity, adaptive immunity has a delayed response and is characterized by immune memory. Adaptive immune cells, including T and B cells, require specific interactions with APCs in order to receive the signal to mature and proliferate. In their naïve state, T and B cells circulate with a uniquely arranged T (TCR) and B (BCR) cell receptor specific to a particular antigen. If the TCR or BCR binds to its cognate antigen presented on an APC (and if the lymphocyte-APC interaction supplies key activation signals), the T or B cell will undergo clonal expansion and activation to propagate an immune response. After the initial response, there will remain long-lived T and B cells that retain memory for that specific antigen, able to trigger a faster and robust response for future encounters. The innate and adaptive arms of the immune system act in concert to both promote and regulate each other in the generation of a balanced and effective immune response (Table 2–2).

▶ Role of Nonimmune Cells in the Immune Response

Nonimmune cells also play a key role in the orchestration of the immune response in the intestinal mucosa. In addition to lymphocytes and leukocytes, the lamina propria includes a rich network of supporting stromal cells with diverse functions including fibroblasts, smooth muscle cells, endothelial cells, pericytes, and glial cells. Fibroblasts, although primarily responsible for the creation and maintenance of the collagen-rich extracellular matrix, have been found to express HLA-DR/MHC II molecules (antigen presenting receptors classically found on professional APCs) as well as TLRs, suggesting they actively engage with antigens as well as with DAMPs/PAMPs. They are also able to secrete cytokines when activated, likely exerting modulating effects on nearby immune cells.

Similarly, the single-cell thick intestinal epithelial layer, comprised of enterocytes, goblet cells, Paneth cells, tuft cells, and enteroendocrine cells, plays its own specialized role in the immune response beyond the actions of its IELs. While goblet cells secrete mucin and other glycans to create a protective luminal mucous layer, Paneth cells secrete anti-microbial peptides and tuft cells secrete chemical substances thought to have anti-helminth effects. Pluripotent IESCs reside at the base of epithelial crypts and by differentiation into these various epithelial cell subsets, provide a reservoir for ongoing epithelial renewal. The mechanical integrity of the epithelial

Table 2–2. Innate and adaptive immunity.

Type of Immunity	Receptor	Ligand	Cell Type
Innate immunity (rapid, hard wired)	TLR2	Peptidoglycan	Macrophages
	TLR4	LPS	Macrophages/IEC
	TLR5	Flagellin	Macrophages/IEC
	TLR9	Bacterial DNA	Dendritic cells
	CRP	Bacterial carbohydrate	Serum
	NOD2	Muramyl dipeptide	Dendritic cells/IEC
Adaptive or specific immunity (delayed with memory)	TCR	HLA plus peptide	T cell
	BCR	Immunoglobulin	B cell
	CD28 (co-stimulatory)	CD80, CD86	T cell
	CTLA4 (inhibitory)	CD80, CD86	T cell

BCR, B-cell receptor; CRP, C-reactive protein; CTLA4, cytotoxic T lymphocyte–associated protein 4 (CD152); HLA, human leukocyte antigen; IEC, intestinal epithelial cell; IL-23R, interleukin-23 receptor; LPS, lipopolysaccharide; NOD2, nucleotide oligomerization domain–containing protein 2; TCR, T-cell receptor; TLR, toll-like receptor.

lining is further mediated by tight junctions which serve to both enable absorption of nutrients and keep out pathogenic invaders. As previously mentioned with respect to highly specialized M cells, epithelial cells also likely participate in antigen presentation and are known to express HLA-DR/MHC II as well as pattern-recognition receptors. Although more remains to be elucidated regarding the role of stromal cells and the epithelium in the immune response, these cells clearly participate in a dynamic way with professional immune cells in mediating mucosal immune homeostasis.

Checks and Balances

The intestinal mucosal immune response requires tight regulation in order to react appropriately to pathogens while at the same time being able to tolerate commensal and nonpathogenic dietary microbes. The innate and adaptive immune arms come equipped with an array of checks and balances to dampen inappropriate inflammatory responses. A main player is the regulatory T cell (Treg) which exerts suppressive effects on nearby effector T cells and APCs through a variety of mechanisms including anti-inflammatory cytokine secretion (eg, IL10, TGFβ, IL35) and inhibitory receptor signaling. In conventional T cells (ie, non-Tregs), a brake mechanism during T cell-APC interaction occurs via engagement of T cell inhibitory receptors, such as CTLA4 and PD-1, with cognate receptors on DCs. Regulatory or anti-inflammatory programs across essentially all immune cells are thought to exist, giving rise to B-regulatory cells, anti-inflammatory macrophage subsets and beyond. From an epithelial perspective, there is evidence that in response to commensal microorganisms, epithelial cells engage in TLR signaling that leads to cytoprotective effects, highlighting not only immune-modulating functions of epithelial cells but also the importance of commensal bacteria in mucosal immune homeostasis and tolerance. Similarly, subsets of fibroblasts residing in lymphoid tissue can exert suppressive effects on T cells via engagement of the T cell inhibitory receptor PD-1, further emphasizing the regulatory role of nonimmune cells in the immune response.

Dillon A, Lo DD. M Cells: intelligent Engineering of Mucosal Immune Surveillance. *Front Immunol.* 2019;10:1499. Published 2019 Jul 2. [PMID: 31312204]

Fletcher AL, Acton SE, Knoblich K. Lymph node fibroblastic reticular cells in health and disease. *Nat Rev Immunol.* 2015;15(6):350–361. [PMID: 25998961]

Habtezion A, Nguyen LP, Hadeiba H, et al. Leukocyte trafficking to the small intestine and colon. *Gastroenterology.* 2016;150(2):340–354. [PMID: 26551552]

Medzhitov R. Recognition of microorganisms and activation of the immune response. *Nature.* 2007;449(7164):819–826. [PMID: 17943118]

Nowarski R, Jackson R, Flavell R. The stromal intervention: regulation of immunity and inflammation at the epithelial-mesenchymal barrier. *Cell.* 2017;168(3):362–375. [PMID: 28129537]

Peterson LW, Artis D. Intestinal epithelial cells: regulators of barrier function and immune homeostasis. *Nat Rev Immunol* 2014;14:141–153. [PMID: 24566914]

Rakoff-Nahoum S, Hao L, Medzhitov R. Role of toll-like receptors in spontaneous commensal-dependent colitis. *Immunity* 2006;25:319–329. [PMID: 16879997]

Senda T, Dogra P, Granot T, et al. Microanatomical dissection of human intestinal T-cell immunity reveals site-specific changes in gut-associated lymphoid tissues over life. *Mucosal Immunol.* 2019;12(2):378–389. [PMID: 30523311]

Suzuki K, Kawamoto S, Maruya M, et al. GALT: organization and dynamics leading to IgA synthesis. *Adv Immunol.* 2010;107:153–185. [PMID: 21034974]

PATHOGENESIS OF INFLAMMATORY BOWEL DISEASE

General Principles

The major operating paradigm of our current understanding of IBD is that this disease represents hyperreactivity or loss of (oral) tolerance of the mucosal immune system to one's own mucosal microbiota. This is consistent with the general localization of the disease, both UC and CD, to the regions of the intestine where microbes are mostly present. This concept is mainly derived from observations from numerous animal models of IBD, as well as a lesser number of human clinical studies. The link between intestinal microorganisms and the host immune response is clear, as manifested in mouse models of IBD where germ-free mice are protected from disease, as well as in human disease, where antibiotic therapy has not only been found to be associated with CD but also part of the treatment strategy. IBD likely represents a dysregulated mucosal immune response in a genetically susceptible host to commensal microbial antigens. Additional, poorly understood environmental factors including external (ie, diet, tobacco smoke, NSAIDs, enteropathogen, and antibiotic exposures) as well as internal (ie, host anatomy, eg, appendectomy) also play a role in the dysregulation of the mucosal immune response underlying IBD pathogenesis.

Genetics

It has been known for decades that IBD in humans has a strong genetic basis, with initial publications in 1963 reporting that both UC and CD often affected multiple members of the same families. Subsequent studies have estimated that the risk of a first degree relative of an IBD patient having IBD is at least 10-fold that of healthy subjects. Over the years, twin studies have consistently shown a higher concordance of CD in monozygotic twins than in dizygotic twins, further highlighting the genetic underpinnings of the disease. According to one meta-analysis, the risk that both monozygotic twins will develop CD is 20–50% (several hundred times greater than the risk of CD in the general population) whereas the risk in dizygotic twins ranged from 0 to 7%. Genetic risk appears to be an important, if not an essential, variable in driving the causation of IBD.

The genetic contribution to the development of IBD exists on a continuum. At one extreme are the forms of IBD that have a monogenic basis and typically develop during the early periods of life. This includes early onset (<10 years of age), very early onset (<6 years of age), and infantile (1–2 years of age) types of IBD that derive from environmental interactions with, in some cases, highly penetrant single gene defects. At this time only a handful of genes are known to be associated with an IBD-predominant syndrome when mutations are present or inherited in a Mendelian manner. This list includes genes related to suppressive signaling in T cells, such those encoding IL10 and the IL10 receptor (*IL10*, *IL10RA*, and *IL10RB*) as well as LRBA, involved in trafficking of the inhibitory T cell receptor CTLA4 to the cell surface. Others on this list include genes related to epithelial integrity, including *TTC7A* mutations, associated with enhanced apoptosis of epithelial cells and disruption of epithelial apicobasal polarity. IBD-like phenotypes can also occur as part of syndromes associated with inborn errors of immunity affecting multiple organ systems. One example includes mutations in *FOXP3* (the transcription factor associated with Treg development and function) which causes Immune dysregulation, Polyendocrinopathy, and Enteropathy (IPEX) syndrome.

The majority of IBD, however, occurs in the second and third decades of life and represents a complex genetic disorder in which approximately 10% of cases may have an inheritable genetic factor based on a positive family medical history. In these cases, the number of genes involved in the pathogenesis is unknown but likely to be a significant number. *Genome-wide association studies (GWAS) and candidate gene studies with DNA sequencing have identified more than 250 IBD susceptibility loci throughout the human genome highlighting the existence of critical pathways in the pathogenesis of these disorders.* These pathways span key components of innate (both hematopoietic and nonhematopoietic) and adaptive immunity including bacterial sensing (in GWAS, up to 30% of CD patients have variants in the pattern recognition receptor gene *NOD2*), autophagy and the unfolded protein response (eg, *ATG16L1* and *XBP1*), epithelial barrier function, and tolerance. The genes identified to-date seem to associate with specific functional pathways that may be shared by CD and UC, as well as other immune-mediated diseases such as multiple sclerosis, type 1 diabetes mellitus, asthma, and others (Figure 2–2).

Epigenetics

GWASs have highlighted IBD-associated variants in numerous protein-encoding genes, the study of which has further informed our understanding of IBD pathogenesis. However, the vast majority of IBD-associated variants map to noncoding regions of DNA, including those known as DNA regulatory elements (DREs). These are regions of DNA that regulate the expression of genes, and include enhancer/promoter regions, silencer/insulator regions, as well as genetic material encoding microRNAs or long noncoding RNAs which themselves serve as regulators of transcription. Although it is difficult to disentangle the effects of particular genetic variants when they occur in these regions of noncoding DNA, they likely have far ranging and important consequences. Beyond mutation or variation in genetic material, additional, epigenetic structural changes affecting chromatin also likely play a major role in the reprogramming of the immune response in IBD. Epigenetic modifications to chromatin, typically through histone modification affecting the accessibility of DNA for transcriptional activity on a cellular level, have been found to be altered in IBD intestinal mucosa, with one study identifying different transcriptional profiles in CD patients resulting from different chromatin accessibility states. Although epigenetic variation is so far poorly understood in the context of IBD pathogenesis, it likely is of critical importance in mucosal inflammatory programs, linking cell-external cues with transcriptional fine-tuning on a cellular level.

Environment

The environmental factors that contribute to IBD pathogenesis are also poorly understood, but conclusions have been drawn primarily through large scale association studies in humans and animal models of IBD. Even in infancy, there may be environmental factors such as vaginal delivery and breastfeeding that seem to offer protection from subsequent development of IBD although the data is not entirely conclusive. Tobacco smoking has long been recognized as a factor associated with worse CD outcomes but paradoxically seems to be protective for UC-related inflammation. Diet also seems to play a role in microbiome and immune system dysregulation. This has been inferred from studies of immigrants from low-incidence countries to high IBD-incidence countries, whose children gain the same risk of developing IBD as children of families living in the same country for multiple generations. It has also been shown in human studies that a diet high in fats (especially saturated fats) and sugars is associated with IBD as is a diet low in fiber (ie, low in fresh fruits and vegetables). Animal models have complemented these findings, demonstrating that mice fed a high fat diet have increased intestinal inflammation and disturbed epithelial barrier function.

A recent umbrella review of meta-analyses of environmental associations in human IBD further identified smoking (CD), urban living (CD and IBD), appendectomy (CD), tonsillectomy (CD), antibiotic exposure (IBD), oral contraceptive use (IBD), consumption of soft drinks (UC), vitamin D deficiency (IBD), and non-Helicobacter pylori Helicobacter species (IBD) as associated with increased risk, and physical activity (CD), breastfeeding (IBD), bed sharing (CD), tea consumption (UC), high levels of folate (IBD), high levels of vitamin D (CD) and H. pylori infection (CD, UC, and IBD) as protective. *It is likely that these environmental triggers manipulate the human intestinal microbiome and*

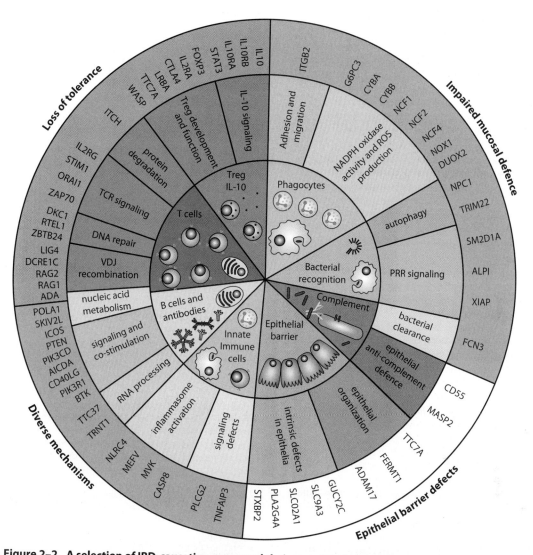

▲ **Figure 2–2. A selection of IBD-causative genes and their associated mucosal pathways.** Featured is a list of genes associated with monogenic forms of IBD (outer ring) along with the pathways thought to be disrupted by their mutations. PRR = pattern recognition receptor. Treg = T regulatory cell. (Reproduced with permission from Pazmandi J, Kalinichenko A, Ardy RC, et al: Early-onset inflammatory bowel disease as a model disease to identify key regulators of immune homeostasis mechanisms. *Immunol Rev.* 2019;287(1):162–185.)

metabolome, thereby propagating immunologic repercussions affecting mucosal integrity through a mix of genetic and epigenetic factors. One illustrative example relates to the aryl hydrocarbon receptor (AHR), a metabolite receptor expressed by immune cells in the intestinal mucosa with genetic variation associated with IBD in GWAS studies. Studies in mice have shown that alteration in tryptophan levels in the intestine via introduction of tryptophan-metabolizing bacteria affects AHR signaling with downstream effects on epithelial integrity, demonstrating a link between environmental (ie, dietary or bacterial) metabolites with immune signaling.

▶ Microbiome

Whether changes in the intestinal microbiome play a causative role in IBD pathogenesis or whether they reflect a consequence of disease remains unclear. Certainly, genetic predisposition seems to influence the human intestinal microbiome, as has been demonstrated through microbiome analyses of dizygotic and monozygotic twin cohorts as well as the fact that many IBD-associated genes relate to bacterial handling in the gut, including *NOD2, CARD9, ATG16L1, IRGM,* and *FUT2.* Genetic implication in microbiome composition is further underscored by the fact that healthy individuals who have a high burden of variants in bacterial-handling genes have stool microbiome profiles similar to those of IBD patients. The composition of the human microbiome has also been found to fluctuate quite rapidly based on diet, with one study demonstrating that several days of an animal-based diet was found to increase bile-tolerant bacterial organisms and decrease species which metabolize plant polysaccharides.

Most of what we know regarding the human intestinal microbiome relates to its bacterial composition, which has been phylogenetically profiled through the use of 16S rRNA sequencing or via shotgun metagenomic sequencing in health and in disease. The vast majority (>90%) of human intestinal commensal bacteria belong to one of two phyla—*Bacteriodetes* and *Firmicutes*—with additional less populous phyla including *Proteobacteria*, *Actinobacteria*, and *Verrucomicrobia*. Overall, studies of IBD patients have demonstrated a decrease in microbiome taxonomic diversity compared to healthy controls. Multiple studies have shown that IBD is associated with a decrease in obligate anaerobe species such as *Faecalibacterium prausnitzii* and *Roseburia* spp (both of which belong to the *Clostridia* family of *Firmicutes* and produce butyrate), and an increase in facultative anaerobes belonging to the *Enterobacteriaceae* family of *Proteobacteria*, such as *Escherichia coli*. Much less is known regarding the mycobiome (commensal fungi) or virome (commensal viruses) in IBD although IBD seems to be associated with reduced mycobiome diversity and alterations in the virome as well.

The content of the commensal microbiome—not only the various microbial species including bacteria, fungi, and viruses—but also the metabolic activity thereof, is likely to be significantly immunologically relevant. Gut bacteria produce small chain fatty acids (SCFAs) such as butyrate, acetate, and propionate upon breaking down dietary fiber, and it has been found that there is a decrease in butyrate and butyrate-producing bacteria in the IBD intestine. This may be quite relevant in disease modulation given that SCFAs have been shown to have effects on the mucosal immune response, including regulating Tregs and enhancing anti-bacterial activity of macrophages. Whereas SCFAs are decreased in the IBD intestine, other studies have shown an increase in other bacterial products including sphingolipids and bile acids. Sphingolipids have been found to exert pleiotropic effects on the intestinal mucosa including serving as a chemoattractant to lymphocytes, as will be discussed. Although still poorly understood, the human microbiome and dysbiosis thereof likely plays a significant role in modulation and perpetuation of IBD-related inflammation.

Agrawal M, Corn G, Shrestha S, et al. Inflammatory bowel diseases among first-generation and second-generation immigrants in Denmark: a population-based cohort study. *Gut.* 2020;70(6):1037–1043. [PMID: 32895335]

David LA, Maurice CF, Carmody RN, et al. Diet rapidly and reproducibly alters the human gut microbiome. *Nature.* 2014;505(7484):559–563. [PMID: 24336217]

Franzosa EA, Sirota-Madi A, Avila-Pacheco J, et al. Gut microbiome structure and metabolic activity in inflammatory bowel disease. *Nat Microbiol* 2019;4:293–305. [PMID: 30531976]

Gevers D, Kugathasan S, Denson LA, et al. The treatment-naive microbiome in new-onset Crohn's disease. *Cell Host Microbe* 2014;15:382–392. [PMID: 24629344]

Goodrich JK, Waters JL, Poole AC, et al. Human genetics shape the gut microbiome. *Cell.* 2014;159(4):789–799. [PMID: 25417156]

Halme L, Paavola-Sakki P, Turunen U, Lappalainen M, Farkkila M, Kontula K. Family and twin studies in inflammatory bowel disease. *World J Gastroenterol.* 2006;12(23):3668–3672. [PMID: 16773682]

Imhann F, Vich Vila A, Bonder MJ, et al. Interplay of host genetics and gut microbiota underlying the onset and clinical presentation of inflammatory bowel disease. *Gut* 2018;67:108–119. [PMID: 27802154]

Jostins L, Ripke S, Weersma RK, et al. Host-microbe interactions have shaped the genetic architecture of inflammatory bowel disease. *Nature.* 2012;491:119–124. [PMID: 23128233]

Kirsner JB, Spencer JA. Family occurrences of ulcerative colitis, regional enteritis, and ileocolitis. *Ann Intern Med.* 1963;59:133–144. [PMID: 14049341]

Kobayashi KS, Chamaillard M, Ogura Y, et al. Nod2-dependent regulation of innate and adaptive immunity in the intestinal tract. *Science.* 2005;307:371–374. [PMID: 15692051]

Lewis JD, Abreu MT. Diet as a trigger or therapy for inflammatory bowel diseases. *Gastroenterology* 2017;152:398–414 e6. [PMID: 27793606]

Meddens CA, van der List ACJ, Nieuwenhuis EES, et al. Non-coding DNA in IBD: from sequence variation in DNA regulatory elements to novel therapeutic potential. *Gut* 2019;68:928–941. [PMID: 30692146]

Orholm M, Munkholm P, Langholz E, Nielsen OH, Sørensen TI, Binder V. Familial occurrence of inflammatory bowel disease. *N Engl J Med.* 1991;324(2):84–88. [PMID: 1984188]

Pazmandi J, Kalinichenko A, Ardy RC, et al. Early-onset inflammatory bowel disease as a model disease to identify key regulators of immune homeostasis mechanisms. *Immunol Rev* 2019;287:162–185. [PMID: 30565237]

Piovani D, Danese S, Peyrin-Biroulet L, et al. Environmental risk factors for inflammatory bowel diseases: an umbrella review of meta-analyses. *Gastroenterology* 2019;157:647–659 e4. [PMID: 31014995]

Weiser M, Simon JM, Kochar B, et al. Molecular classification of Crohn's disease reveals two clinically relevant subtypes. *Gut* 2018;67:36–42. [PMID: 27742763]

MUCOSAL INFLAMMATORY SIGNATURES OF IBD

▶ General Principles

It remains incompletely understood how the previously noted genetically imposed risk factors, along with even less well-understood environmental factors, result in the development of IBD. However, through modulation of the intestinal epithelial cell barrier and immune cell function, the end result is a profound dysregulation of the homeostatic state of controlled intestinal inflammation and microbiome handling. This final outcome likely also alters the composition of the microbiome itself. Numerous studies have interrogated the nature of the inflammatory reprogramming in IBD intestinal mucosa, in humans as well as animal models, and have identified specific adaptive and innate immune cell responses characteristic of UC and CD inflammation.

UC is a diffuse superficial disease confined to the colonic mucosa, affecting the rectum and extending more proximally in a contiguous pattern of inflammation through part of, or through the entire, colon. This contrasts with the typical phenotypic pattern of CD, which is often characterized by penetrating inflammation that can be complicated by intestinal fibrosis or fistulization, and can affect any part of the intestine, large or small, in discontinuous fashion. Given that the nature of inflammation can be grossly different between UC (superficial, colonic, contiguous) and CD (penetrating, pan-intestinal, patchy) it is not entirely surprising that some distinct immunologic features have been identified specific to each disease on a mucosal level. *However, historical paradigms regarding differential immune responses in UC versus CD are slowly disassembling in the wake of more recent large-scale, multi-dimensional immunophenotyping studies in human IBD tissue. Overall, it appears that there is considerable overlap in the inflammatory hallmarks of these diseases with ongoing efforts to disentangle disease-specific pathways.*

Histopathologic Observations

Histopathologic analysis of active IBD intestinal tissue has for years been an essential component of diagnostic assessment and has revealed patterns of epithelial architectural disturbance and immune cell infiltration characteristic of both UC and CD. Both forms of IBD are typically characterized by the presence of *active inflammation*—defined by the presence of neutrophilic infiltration into crypts (cryptitis) or within crypt lumens (crypt abscesses) or within the epithelium with or without mucosal ulceration; and *chronic changes*, characterized by crypt architectural distortion (crypt length shortening or branching), infiltration of lymphocytes and plasma cells into the lamina propria, or Paneth cell metaplasia (presence of Paneth cells in the left colon where they are normally absent). Certain findings are thought to be more associated with UC than CD, including mucous layer depletion (indeed, a reduction in mucin-producing goblet cells has been associated with UC in many studies) and diffuse chronic inflammation and crypt distortion across multiple or all biopsied areas. Other findings are found to be more associated with CD, including presence of patchy, active inflammation sometimes without chronic changes and the presence of granulomas—organized collections of phagocytes including macrophages and DCs, as well as lymphocytes, forming multinucleated aggregates known as giant cells.

Local Immune Reprogramming

The changes in the mucosal landscape of the human IBD intestine have now been studied far beyond mere histopathologic assessment, with deep interrogation into the phenotypic and functional characteristics of the immune, epithelial, and stromal cell compartments that make up the intestinal mucosa. Historically, significant focus has been applied to the study of immune cell reprogramming in IBD, especially regarding T cell responses, outlined below. As scientific understanding progresses, more and more attention is being paid to the deep interconnectedness of hematopoietic and nonhematopoietic mucosal compartments, whose cross-talk is critical in propagating and mediating the interchange of inflammatory signaling originating at the epithelial interface.

One of the more explored paradigms in immune cell reprogramming in IBD relates to CD4-positive T helper (Th) cell polarization. T cells leave the thymus and migrate into peripheral tissues, such as the intestines, as naïve cells with a unique TCR specific for a particular and as-of-yet unencountered antigen. When T cells interact with a professional APCs (eg, DCs) which bear their cognate antigen (signal 1) and provide the appropriate co-stimulatory signal (signal 2), they are induced to deviate to one of several polarized fates under the control of cytokine stimuli in the microenvironment. Importantly, these T cell-programming cytokines are typically produced by the innate immune system, including by hematopoietic lineage cells such as APCs but also nonhematopoietic cells such as epithelial and stromal cells. Thus, cytokines associated with innate immune responses (eg, IL12, IL23) guide the adaptive immune response to one of the several outcomes (Figure 2–3).

Depending on the cytokine cocktail of their microenvironment, primed CD4+ T cells become polarized to adopt a specific inflammatory program including, but not limited to, so-called Th1, Th2, or Th17 responses, in addition to Treg phenotypes. These Th responses are themselves characterized by specific cytokine programs within Th cells, governed in part by specific transcription factors (eg, Tbet-mediated transcription in Th1 cells leading to Th1 production of IFNG and TNF). Recently, immunophenotyping studies of human IBD intestinal tissue using single-cell analytic techniques have expanded upon previous observations that Tregs in the IBD intestine seem to take on an inflammatory phenotype, including the production of pro-inflammatory cytokines such as TNF, IFNG, and IL17A, suggesting that the normal suppressive function of Treg signaling may be rewired in IBD. It is these inflammatory T cell responses—potentially affecting both Th cells and Tregs—that are thought to play a part in propagating IBD-related mucosal inflammation.

Less well-understood IBD-related immunologic reprogramming involves other adaptive (eg, B cells and plasma cells) and innate immune cells. For years it has been observed that there is an increase in local IgG in the inflamed gastrointestinal tract, and more recently it has been found that

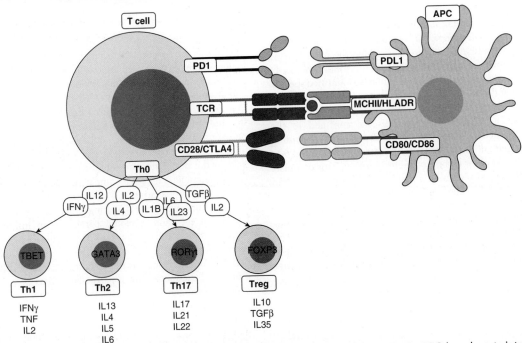

▲ **Figure 2–3. The APC: lymphocyte interaction and Th cell differentiation.** Pictured is the APC: lymphocyte interaction whereby antigen is presented by the APC via MCHII/HLADR and recognized by a cognate T cell receptor (TCR) (signal 1). A costimulatory signal (signal 2) is essential to propagate the response, and is supplied by the interaction of CD28 and CD80/86. Checkpoints are supplied by inhibitory receptors including CTLA4 and PD1/PDL1. If the naïve T helper cell is activated, it will undergo differentiation from Th0 to one of a number of cell fates, orchestrated by the cytokines in the environment. Key transcription factors for Th1, Th2, Th17, and Treg fates are features along with characteristic cytokines associated with each T cell type.

anti-commensal IgG is enriched in the stool of patients with colitis (as opposed to IgA-bound microbes), further implicating aberrant anti-microbial humoral responses in IBD pathogenesis. Innate immune cells responding to IgG-bound antigen in the intestine have been found to undergo a program of pro-inflammatory signaling including production of IL1B, a cytokine trigger for Th17 polarization. Recent single-cell transcriptional and proteomic studies in human IBD tissue have also identified activated phenotypes affecting innate immune cells (eg, inflammatory mononuclear phagocytes expressing TNF, IL1B, IL1A, and oncostatin-M), and stromal cells (including IL11-producing inflammatory fibroblasts and activated endothelial cells) (Figure 2–4).

Castro-Dopico T, Dennison TW, Ferdinand JR, et al. Anti-commensal IgG drives intestinal inflammation and Type 17 immunity in ulcerative colitis. *Immunity* 2019;50:1099–1114 e10. [PMID: 30876876]

DeRoche TC, Xiao SY, Liu X. Histological evaluation in ulcerative colitis. *Gastroenterol Rep (Oxf)*. 2014;2(3):178–192. [PMID: 24942757]

Feakins RM. Ulcerative colitis or Crohn's disease? Pitfalls and problems. *Histopathology*. 2014;64(3):317–335. [PMID: 24266813]

Kinchen J, Chen HH, Parikh K, et al. Structural remodeling of the human colonic mesenchyme in inflammatory bowel disease. *Cell*. 2018;175(2):372–386.e17. [PMID: 30270042]

Martin JC, Chang C, Boschetti G, et al. Single-cell analysis of Crohn's disease lesions identifies a pathogenic cellular module associated with resistance to anti-TNF therapy. *Cell* 2019;178:1493–1508 e20. [PMID: 31474370]

Mitsialis V, Wall S, Liu P, et al. Single-cell analyses of colon and blood reveal distinct immune cell signatures of ulcerative colitis and Crohn's disease. *Gastroenterology*. 2020;159(2):591–608. e10. [PMID: 32428507]

Parikh K, Antanaviciute A, Fawkner-Corbett D, et al. Colonic epithelial cell diversity in health and inflammatory bowel disease. *Nature*. 2019;567(7746):49–55. [PMID: 30814735]

Smillie CS, Biton M, Ordovas-Montanes J, et al. Intra- and intercellular rewiring of the human colon during ulcerative colitis. *Cell* 2019;178:714–730 e22. [PMID: 31348891]

Ungaro R, Mehandru S, Allen PB, et al. Ulcerative colitis. *Lancet*. 2017 29;389(10080):1756–1770.

Zhu J, Yamane H, Paul WE. Differentiation of effector CD4 T cell populations. *Annu Rev Immunol*. 2010;28:445–489. [PMID: 20192806]

CYTOKINES IN IBD AND THERAPEUTIC IMPLICATIONS

▶ Beyond Th1 and Th2

Historically, UC has been thought to be characterized by a Th2-driven inflammatory response, mediated by classic Th2-associated cytokines (eg, IL-4, IL-5, and IL-13) while CD has been thought to be characterized by a Th1 response mediated by IFNG, TNF, and IL2. This dichotomy was originally derived from early studies assessing select cytokine expression from IBD tissue, noting increased *IL5* transcripts in UC tissue and increased *IL2* and *IFNG* in CD tissue. However, with the advent of next generation sequencing technology, and high-resolution single cell analyses (ie, multi-parameter flow cytometry, mass cytometry [CyTOF], single cell RNA-sequencing [scRNA-seq]) applied to dissociated cells derived from human tissue, investigators have discovered significantly more nuanced and interconnected patterns of inflammation beyond this paradigm, building off pathways implicated in GWAS.

Much of the investigation has focused on cytokine signatures in human IBD tissue. Recent studies have consistently found expansion of IL17A+ lymphocytes, including Th17 cells but also IL17A+ CD8+ T cells, in active UC mucosa. Other studies have found a mixed Th1-17 response in IBD characterized by expansion of CD4+ T cells co-expressing IFNG and IL17A, reported in both UC and CD. Recently, a meta-analysis of multiple datasets of transcriptomes of IBD tissue samples reported a list of significantly regulated cytokines in UC, CD, and non-IBD; the vast majority of significantly regulated cytokines were found to be upregulated in both UC and CD compared to control tissue, and only a handful were either up- or down-regulated in UC or CD alone. Cytokines found to be upregulated in both UC and CD tissue include the classic Th1- and Th17-associated

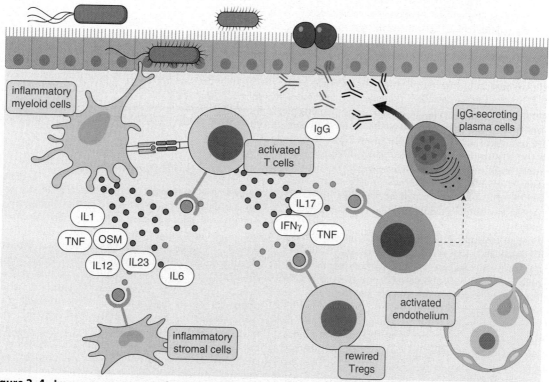

▲ **Figure 2–4. Immune reprogramming in the IBD intestine.** Featured are a series of cellular hallmarks associated with the IBD intestine, as have been identified from cumulative work assessing protein and transcriptional expression in translational studies. The IBD intestine appears to be characterized by inflammatory myeloid cells (including macrophages and dendritic cells) expressing pro-inflammatory mediators such as IL1, TNF, OSM, IL12/23, and IL6. These pro-inflammatory cytokines are likely sensed by the majority of cell types in the surrounding microenvironment, and likely reprogram the fate of Th cells, Tregs, B cells, stromal cells, and endothelial cells. T cells are activated in IBD tissue and express pro-inflammatory cytokines such as IL17, IFNG, and TNF (as have IBD-associated Tregs). Plasma cells in the IBD intestine have been found to secrete IgG in addition to IgA. (Data from Kinchen et al, 2018; Martin et al, 2019; Mitsialis et al, 2020; Smillie et al 2019.)

cytokines IL17A, IFNG, TNF, but also oncostatin-M (OSM), IL1B, IL1A, IL6, IL26, TNFSF13, TGFB1, TGFB2, TFB3, IL33, EBI3, LIF, and CSF1. Cytokines regulated in UC alone include TL1A, IL23A, IL16, IL34 (upregulated) and IL29, IL2, and IL37 (downregulated). Cytokines regulated in CD alone include CSF2, CSF3, IL27, IL11, IL22, IL12A, IL17F (upregulated) and IL32, IL21, and TSLP (downregulated). Further investigation into these differential patterns of cytokine expression is needed, including mechanistic experimentation, to clarify their role in disease pathogenesis.

TNF Blockade and Lessons Learned

TNF was the first cytokine to be specifically targeted with biologic therapy in IBD more than 20 years ago. Initial studies at that time demonstrated an increase in TNF in IBD mucosa, serum, and stool, and subsequent studies have shown TNF+ lymphocytes/leukocytes to be expanded in the IBD intestine and blood. However, the discrete effects of anti-TNF therapy on a mucosal level are not fully understood despite the efficacy of these medications (ie, infliximab, adalimumab, certolizumab, golimumab) in UC and/or CD. Our limited understanding is only further underscored by the fact that etanercept, an anti-TNF therapy used in rheumatoid arthritis among other rheumatologic conditions, has not been proven to be efficacious in IBD. Whereas other anti-TNF therapies are antibodies targeting soluble or membrane-bound TNF, etanercept is a decoy TNF receptor that may therefore modulate TNF signaling in a critically distinct way. Nevertheless, given the efficacy of antibodies targeting TNF for IBD, investigation into targeting related pathways is ongoing. Currently, early phase clinical trials are underway investigating the efficacy of anti-tumor necrosis like ligand 1A (TL1A) therapy, another cytokine found to be enriched in IBD mucosa.

Although targeting TNF on the basis of its enrichment in IBD tissue and stool revolutionized the arsenal of IBD therapy nearly 30 years ago, targeting other cytokines based on similar principles has not necessarily proved fruitful. This goes for IL17, to be discussed below, but also for IFNG, IL6, IL13, all of which have been found to be upregulated in IBD and targeted with biologic therapy without success (and, in some cases, resulting in worsening of IBD) or with serious adverse effects. Nevertheless, as will be discussed, therapy targeting the cytokines IL12/IL23 (ustekinumab) did join the ranks of anti-TNF blockade as one of a handful of biologic therapies efficacious for IBD (and the only other approved biologic therapy specifically targeting cytokines). Lessons learned from attempts to block key cytokine pathways in IBD suggest that most cytokines likely have pleiotropic effects on mucosal immune homeostasis and interfering with a fine-tuned signaling cascade may in some cases cause more harm than good.

The IL17: IL23 Axis

One cytokine network felt to be highly relevant to IBD and autoimmunity relates to Th17 and associated responses in the intestinal mucosa, mediated by the IL17-IL23 axis. The pro-inflammatory cytokine IL23, secreted by activated APCs such as macrophages and DCs, stimulates a range of so-called Type-17 lymphocytes including CD4+ Th17 cells but also other innate-like T cells expressing the RORgt transcription factor, such as gamma-delta T cells, natural killer T cells and innate lymphoid cells type 3 (ILC3). Type 17 cells respond to IL23 by secreting a Th17 program of cytokines including IL17 and IL22. Both IL17 and IL22 are thought to have pleiotropic effects on the surrounding microenvironment, including propagation of inflammation but also homeostatic effects—including promotion of epithelial integrity. Agents blocking IL17 signaling have not had efficacy in CD, and there are reports of anti-IL17 agents used for psoriasis exacerbating IBD, further underscoring the multimodality of this pathway in mucosal autoimmunity. On the other hand, agents targeting IL23 (specifically, the p40 subunit of the cytokine) have proven to be quite efficacious for both UC and CD (ie, ustekinumab). Multiple studies are currently investigating the use of monoclonal antibodies targeting the p19 subunit of IL23 or the IL23 receptor as treatments for IBD, emphasizing the enthusiasm for and promise of anti-IL23 therapeutics. The importance of this pathway is further highlighted by a number of IBD-associated genes including *IL17RA*, *IL23R*, *IL12B* (encoding the p40 subunit of IL23), *RORC* (the gene encoding RORgt), and *IL6ST* (IL6-STAT3 signaling mediates *RORC* expression), among others.

IL1 and the Inflammasome

Another highly relevant cytokine in IBD is IL1 and its associated family. IL1 is a classic pro-inflammatory cytokine that is released from cells (typically macrophages and DCs) upon inflammasome activation. The inflammasome is a higher-order assembly of proteins that comes together once a cell typically receives two danger signals—either a DAMP or a PAMP plus extracellular ATP—that then potentiates a series of events, including the cleavage of pro-IL1B to its mature form as well as the activation of IL18, another IL1 family member. IL1B exits the cell and mediates inflammatory events in the surrounding microenvironment, including activation of ILC3 signaling. One study analyzing a cohort of UC, CD, and non-IBD subject intestinal tissue using single-cell analyses identified expansion of IL1B+ macrophages in both UC and CD tissue but specific expansion of IL1B DC subsets in CD. Patients with loss of function mutations in *IL10RA* or *IL10RB* (encoding the IL10 receptor) who have infantile onset IBD have been found to have excessive IL1B production in macrophages and have been successfully treated with anti-IL1 therapy. These patients have extracolonic disease including perianal disease, suggesting a Crohn's-like phenotype. Exploration of anti-IL1 therapy (and/or targeting other components of the inflammasome) in IBD and especially in CD is likely a promising pathway in IBD therapeutics. Therapy targeting IL36, an IL1-family cytokine, is currently underway in clinical trials (in UC).

Oncostatin M and the Immune-Stromal Network

A series of investigations has identified the cytokine oncostatin-M (OSM) as associated with IBD inflammation and resistance to anti-TNF therapy. OSM is an IL6-family cytokine that is secreted by inflammatory myeloid cells and is sensed by fibroblasts via the OSM receptor (a heterodimeric receptor encoded by *OSMR* and *IL6ST*, both IBD-associated genes). This circuit is associated with inflammatory fibroblasts bearing a transcriptomic signature associated with resistance to anti-TNF therapy in UC, also characterized by *IL11*, *IL13RA2*, and *TNFRSF11B* expression. Pretreatment intestinal OSM transcript levels have been shown to be significantly higher in IBD patients who go on to be resistant to anti-TNF therapy compared to those who respond. Anti-oncostatin M therapy is currently being evaluated as part of a phase II clinical trial in CD.

JAK-STAT Signaling: A Common Pathway for Cytokines

Many cytokines, but also colony stimulating factors, certain hormones, and interferons, bind multi-subunit receptors on the cell surface that then exert their signaling effects through the phosphorylation of JAK and STAT proteins. Many of the cytokines that signal in this manner are integrally related to the T cell effector response as well as T cell differentiation, including IL2, IL4, IL5, IFNG, IL12, IL23, and IL10. Other cytokines that utilize JAK-STAT signaling are integral in the innate immune/stromal/epithelial response including IL6, IL11, OSM, and IL22. Different JAK proteins (ie, JAK1, JAK2, JAK3) are phosphorylated depending on the identity of the upstream cytokine receptor, which then in turn phosphorylate various STAT proteins (ie, STAT1–STAT6) which have DNA-binding ability and induce downstream transcriptional programs. The pan-JAK inhibitor tofacitinib is efficacious in UC, however given the breadth of pathway signaling disruption with JAK inhibition, pan-JAK inhibitors have been found to have an array of potential side effects affecting other nonmucosal programs, including cytopenias, thromboembolic events, and hyperlipidemia. Multiple studies are being conducted now using selective JAK inhibitors in IBD, including the selective JAK1 inhibitors filgotinib and upadacitinib in both UC and CD. Therapy targeting TYK2, a JAK-family member, is in early clinical trials in UC.

Promoting Anti-Inflammatory Pathways

Enhancing cytokine activity (as opposed to blockade) has been trialed for a series of purportedly beneficial/anti-inflammatory cytokines including administration of recombinant IL10, IL11, and IFNB, as well as enhancing TGFB through anti-SMAD7 therapy (Mongersen), all without success. Nevertheless, investigation via this avenue of cytokine manipulation continues. Relevant clinical trials include the use of a recombinant IL22:human IgG4 fusion protein, IL22Fc, to promote IL22 signaling in IBD in the hopes of improving epithelial integrity and healing. Other promising clinical trials involve the use of recombinant low-dose IL2 therapy in IBD as a means of promoting Treg activity. IL2 is a growth factor for both Treg and non-Treg T cells; by virtue of high affinity IL2-receptor expression on Tregs, IL2, when administered in low doses, seems to preferentially expand Treg populations and was successful in inducing and maintaining remission in moderate-to-severe UC in an early phase clinical trial (unpublished). Interestingly, daclizumab and basilixumab, agents which block the formation of the high affinity IL2 receptor on T cells, did not prove efficacious in IBD. Once again, this story highlights the rich complexity of cytokine signaling pathways in the maintenance of immune homeostasis and the need to more deeply understand the manifold pleiotropic effects of these mediators in the hopes of successfully harnessing therapeutic potential.

Danese S, Vermeire S, Hellstern P, et al. Randomised trial and open-label extension study of an anti-interleukin 6 antibody in Crohn's disease (ANDANTE I and II). *Gut.* 2019;68(1):40–48. [PMID: 29247068]

Feagan BG, Sandborn WJ, Gasink C, et al. Ustekinumab as induction and maintenance therapy for Crohn's disease. *N Engl J Med.* 2016;375(20):1946–1960. [PMID: 27959607]

Graham DB, Xavier RJ. Pathway paradigms revealed from the genetics of inflammatory bowel disease. *Nature.* 2020;578(7796): 527–539. [PMID: 32103191]

Herrlinger KR, Witthoeft T, Raedler A, et al. Randomized, double blind controlled trial of subcutaneous recombinant human interleukin-11 versus prednisolone in active Crohn's disease. *Am J Gastroenterol.* 2006;101(4):793–797. [PMID: 16635225]

Hueber W, Sands BE, Lewitzky S, et al. Secukinumab, a human anti-IL-17A monoclonal antibody, for moderate to severe Crohn's disease: unexpected results of a randomised, double-blind placebo-controlled trial. *Gut.* 2012;61(12):1693–1700. [PMID: 22595313]

Kim SC, Tonkonogy SL, Albright CA, et al. Variable phenotypes of enterocolitis interleukin 10-deficient mice monoassociated with two different commensal bacteria. *Gastroenterology.* 2005;129:891–906. [PMID: 15825073]

Leppkes M, Neurath MF. Cytokines in inflammatory bowel diseases - Update 2020. *Pharmacol Res.* 2020;158:104835. [PMID: 32416212]

Martin JC, Chang C, Boschetti G, et al. Single-cell analysis of Crohn's disease lesions identifies a pathogenic cellular module associated with resistance to anti-TNF therapy. *Cell.* 2019;178(6): 1493–1508.e20. [PMID: 31474370]

Mitsialis V, Wall S, Liu P, et al. Single-cell analyses of colon and blood reveal distinct immune cell signatures of ulcerative colitis and Crohn's disease. *Gastroenterology.* 2020;159(2):591–608.e10. [PMID: 32428507]

Mullin GE, Maycon ZR, Braun-Elwert L, et al. Inflammatory bowel disease mucosal biopsies have specialized lymphokine mRNA profiles. *Inflamm Bowel Dis.* 1996;2(1):16–26. [PMID: 23282452]

Pena-Rossi C, Schreiber S, Golubovic G, et al. Clinical trial: a multicentre, randomized, double-blind, placebo-controlled, dose-finding, phase II study of subcutaneous interferon-beta-1a in moderately active ulcerative colitis. *Aliment Pharmacol Ther.* 2008;28(6):758–767. [PMID: 19145731]

Reinisch W, de Villiers W, Bene L, et al. Fontolizumab in moderate to severe Crohn's disease: a phase 2, randomized, double-blind, placebo-controlled, multiple-dose study. *Inflamm Bowel Dis.* 2010;16(2):233–242. [PMID: 19637334]

Reinisch W, Panés J, Khurana S, et al. Anrukinzumab, an anti-interleukin 13 monoclonal antibody, in active UC: efficacy and safety from a phase IIa randomised multicentre study. *Gut.* 2015;64(6):894–900. [PMID: 25567115]

Rothenberg ME, Wang Y, Lekkerkerker A, et al. Randomized Phase I Healthy Volunteer Study of UTTR1147A (IL-22Fc): a potential therapy for epithelial injury. *Clin Pharmacol Ther.* 2019;105(1):177–189. [PMID: 29952004]

Salas A, Hernandez-Rocha C, Duijvestein M, et al. JAK-STAT pathway targeting for the treatment of inflammatory bowel disease. *Nat Rev Gastroenterol Hepatol.* 2020;17(6):323–337. [PMID: 32203403]

Sandborn WJ, Su C, Sands BE, et al. Tofacitinib as induction and maintenance therapy for ulcerative colitis. *N Engl J Med.* 2017;376(18):1723–1736. [PMID: 28467869]

Sands BE, Feagan BG, Sandborn WJ, et al. Mongersen (GED-0301) for active Crohn's disease: results of a phase 3 study. *Am J Gastroenterol.* 2020;115(5):738–745. [PMID: 31850931]

Shouval DS, Biswas A, Kang YH, et al. Interleukin 1β mediates intestinal inflammation in mice and patients with interleukin 10 receptor deficiency. *Gastroenterology.* 2016;151(6):1100–1104. [PMID: 27693323]

Smillie CS, Biton M, Ordovas-Montanes J, et al. Intra- and inter-cellular rewiring of the human colon during ulcerative colitis. *Cell* 2019;178:714–730 e22. [PMID: 31348891]

Targan SR, Hanauer SB, van Deventer SJ, et al. A short-term study of chimeric monoclonal antibody cA2 to tumor necrosis factor alpha for Crohn's disease. Crohn's disease cA2 study group. *N Engl J Med.* 1997;337:1029–1035. [PMID: 9321530]

Tilg H, van Montfrans C, van den Ende A, et al. Treatment of Crohn's disease with recombinant human interleukin 10 induces the proinflammatory cytokine interferon gamma. *Gut.* 2002;50(2):191–195. [PMID: 11788558]

West NR, Hegazy AN, Owens BMJ, et al. Oncostatin M drives intestinal inflammation and predicts response to tumor necrosis factor-neutralizing therapy in patients with inflammatory bowel disease [published correction appears in Nat Med. 2017 Jun 6;23 (6):788]. *Nat Med.* 2017;23(5):579–589. [PMID: 28586341]

ADDITIONAL THERAPEUTIC TARGETS IN IBD

As has been discussed in this chapter, the intestinal mucosal immune response is characterized by multiplexed interactions between numerous immune and nonimmune compartments, spanning hematopoietic, stromal and epithelial cell populations, in response to luminal antigens. Although the crux of the immune response is thought to originate with the APC: lymphocyte interaction, the propagation of the response critically affects the surrounding tissue microenvironment. Although in healthy intestinal tissue this response is appropriately modulated and plastic, in the IBD intestine, poorly understood immune, genetic, and environmental factors coalesce to perpetuate aberrant responses and lead to chronic, pathologic inflammation. The majority of investigation and therapeutic targeting in IBD has revolved around cytokine signaling in immune cells, as discussed above, which strategizes in part to abrogate the initial signaling cascades downstream of the APC: lymphocyte interaction. However, this focus represents only the tip of the iceberg of potential avenues of immune manipulation in the human intestine. Additional strategies include disrupting the trafficking of immune cells to sites of inflammation, discussed below, as well as innovative—but nevertheless inchoate—ways of modulating the immune response in the tissue microenvironment more broadly.

▶ Targeting the APC: Lymphocyte Interaction

The sentinel event of the mucosal immune response revolves around the APC: lymphocyte interaction, during which antigen—typically derived from bacterial products—is presented by an APC and recognized by a cognate TCR (or BCR). This interaction, as has been discussed, then triggers the proliferation of clonal populations of lymphocytes, all of which are primed to recognize and respond to said antigen. The T helper program of these population is deeply influenced by the cytokines in the microenvironment, many of them secreted by innate immune cells. In turn, differentiated and activated T helper cells secrete their own pro-inflammatory cytokines as a part of effecting the immune response, with critical implications for the tissue microenvironment and signaling events affecting both adaptive and innate immune compartments.

Targeting the APC: lymphocyte interaction has had disappointing results for the treatment of IBD although has proven quite successful in other diseases. A key brake system for the propagation of T cell activation and proliferation involves checkpoint inhibitors—receptors that when engaged serve to halt APC: lymphocyte signaling. One such receptor, CTLA4, has been targeted through the use of a decoy receptor, abatacept, which serves to engage cognate receptor and enhance this brake system. Abatacept, despite efficacy in rheumatoid and psoriatic arthritis, has been trialed without success in IBD. Interestingly, *blockade* of CTLA4 signaling (ipilimumab) and other checkpoint inhibitors (eg, PD1, PDL1) is commonly used in various cancers to enhance T cell-mediated tumor destruction but is associated with the induction of colitis which mimics IBD (a colitis which, in fact, can be treated with anti-TNF therapy). Therapy to specifically block T cells (visilizumab) and B cells (rituximab) has not proven successful in IBD. Nevertheless, nonbiologic approaches for depleting proliferating lymphocytes, such as the use of thiopurines and in part methotrexate, are successful and routinely used in the treatment of IBD.

Cellular Trafficking

In addition to anti-TNF therapy and anti-IL12/23 therapy, the other biologic therapy routinely used and found to be efficacious for CD and UC targets the α4β7 integrin (vedolizumab). α4β7 integrin is expressed by immune cells, and when in circulation is the ligand for MAdCAM1, expressed by HEVs enabling adhesion and, ultimately translocation from the circulation into the lamina propria. Vedolizumab is though to be highly "gut-specific" in terms of the reach of its effects, considering α4β7 is utilized primarily for gut-homing. As a result, it is thought to have less systemic side effects than other biologic therapies, including possibly less immunosuppression. Related therapies include natalizumab, targeting α4 integrin which is not gut-specific (also traffics immune cells to the central nervous system) and as a result has been associated with the development of progressive multifocal leukoencephalopathy due to JC virus infection. Despite the efficacy of α4β7 and α4 blockade, recently the anti-β7 antibody etrolizumab was not successful in clinical trials in IBD, for unclear reasons. Nevertheless, the enthusiasm for similar therapies continues and currently biologic therapy targeting MAdCAM1 is under investigation.

Recently, a nonbiologic, small molecule therapy agonizing the sphingosine-1-P signaling pathway, ozanimod, has been approved for the treatment of UC. Sphingosine-1-P (S1P) is a secreted lipid mediator that, among other pleiotropic effects, modulates lymphocyte egress from lymph nodes through a concentration gradient (S1P concentrations are relatively high in the blood and lymph but low in lymph node tissue). S1P binds to a family of G-protein coupled receptors on lymphocytes, a subset of which, when activated, orchestrate the egress of lymphocytes from lymph nodes into the circulation from where they can traffic to sites of tissue inflammation including the IBD intestine. S1P structural analogs, like ozanimod, overwhelm the natural S1P gradient and ultimately result in rapid S1P receptor internalization and destruction, sabotaging pathway signaling. Targeting this lymphocyte trafficking pathway via ozanimod and/or future therapeutics represents a significant expansion in our arsenal of therapies in IBD.

Other Therapies

A number of other avenues continued to be explored regarding broadly manipulating the intestinal microenvironment in IBD to achieve mucosal immune regulation. Significant interest in targeting microbial dysbiosis as a modality of restoring immune homeostasis, for example, has led to trials of fecal-microbial transplantation in IBD, with some preliminary successes in UC although investigation with large scale clinical trials is still lacking. Similarly, probiotic therapy, although potentially beneficial in UC and in pouchitis (inflammation of a surgically-created intestinal pouch following curative total proctocolectomy for UC) has not been shown to be of benefit in CD. Therapies meant to manipulate broad inflammatory programs ranging from mesenchymal-derived exosomes to micro-RNA therapy are also being actively investigated in IBD although a deep understanding of underlying mechanisms is still evolving (Table 2–3).

Conclusion

Critically understanding the mechanism of action of IBD therapies is helping to shape our understanding of IBD pathogenesis, and vice versa. Despite ongoing efforts and continually evolving technological lenses, our synthetic understanding of the grand orchestra of mucosal immune homeostasis remains piecemeal at best. Many of the therapies we have developed for IBD treatment have been borne out of key observations from human studies and animal models of disease—but the failure of many more therapies borne from the same practice serves as a cautionary tale, highlighting the delicate nature of the pleiotropic immune pathways that tether tolerance to pathologic inflammation. The more insight we gain from large-scale studies in humans, leading to targeted mechanistic modeling, the more equipped we will be to identify those molecular patterns that represent causal pathways rather than mere biomarkers of disease. With evolving data-driven approaches and technology, along with many promising new therapeutics in the pipeline, we will likely enter a new era of IBD treatment that not only will expand our arsenal of therapies but integrate patient-specific characteristics (eg, genetics, microbiome, active signaling pathways) to restore and maintain health.

Costello SP, Hughes PA, Waters O, et al. Effect of fecal microbiota transplantation on 8-week remission in patients with ulcerative colitis: a randomized clinical trial. *JAMA*. 2019;321(2):156–164. [PMID: 30644982]

Feagan BG, Greenberg GR, Wild G, et al. Treatment of ulcerative colitis with a humanized antibody to the α4β7 integrin. *N Engl J Med*. 2005;352:2499–2507. [PMID: 15958805]

Gionchetti P, Rizzello F, Helwig U, et al. Prophylaxis of pouchitis onset with probiotic therapy: a double-blind, placebo-controlled trial. *Gastroenterology*. 2003;124:1202–1209. [PMID: 12730861]

Leiper K, Martin K, Ellis A, et al. Randomised placebo-controlled trial of rituximab (anti-CD20) in active ulcerative colitis. *Gut*. 2011;60(11):1520–1526. [PMID: 21471566]

Sandborn WJ, Colombel JF, Enns R, et al. Natalizumab induction and maintenance therapy for Crohn's disease. *N Engl J Med*. 2005;353(18):1912–1925. [PMID: 16267322]

Sandborn WJ, Colombel JF, Frankel M, et al. Anti-CD3 antibody visilizumab is not effective in patients with intravenous corticosteroid-refractory ulcerative colitis. *Gut*. 2010;59(11):1485–1492. [PMID: 20947884]

Sandborn WJ, Colombel JF, Sands BE, et al. Abatacept for Crohn's disease and ulcerative colitis. *Gastroenterology*. 2012;143(1):62–69.e4. [PMID: 22504093]

Sandborn WJ, Feagan BG, Wolf DC, et al. Ozanimod induction and maintenance treatment for ulcerative colitis. *N Engl J Med*. 2016;374(18):1754–1762. [PMID: 27144850]

Table 2–3. Inflammatory bowel disease—therapeutic implications.

Target	Mechanism	Therapeutic Agent
Antigen	Eliminate pathogenic bacterial strain	Antibiotic/probiotic (in use)
Lymphocyte/APC interactions	Manipulate T-cell activation Lymphocyte depletion	Azathioprine/6-MP (in use) Anti-CD3 (visilizumab) (unsuccessful) CTLA4 decoy (abatacept) (unsuccessful) Anti-CD20 (rituximab) (unsuccessful)
Cytokines, membrane receptors and associated signaling	↓ Proinflammatory cytokines	Anti-TNF (infliximab, adalimumab, certolizumab pegol, golimumab) (in use) Anti-IL-12/IL-23p40 (ustekinumab) (in use) Anti-TNF (etanercept) (unsuccessful) Anti-IFNG (fontolizumab) (unsuccessful) Anti-IL-13 (anrukinzumab) (unsuccessful) Anti-IL-23p19 (mirikizumab) (in trial) Anti-TL1A (in trial) Anti-IL-17A (secukinumab) (unsuccessful) Anti-IL36 (spesolisumab) (in trial) Anti-OSM (in trial) Nonselective JAK inhibitor (tofacitinib) Selective JAK inhibitors (filgotinib, upadacitinib) (in trial) TYK2 inhibitor (in trial)
Cytokines and membrane receptors	↑ Anti-inflammatory cytokines	Low-dose IL2 (in trial) High affinity IL2 receptor blockade (daclizumab, basilixumab) (unsuccessful) TGFβ via anti-SMAD7 (mongersen) (unsuccessful) Recombinant IL10 (unsuccessful) Recombinant IL11 (unsuccessful) Recombinant IFNβ (unsuccessful)
Cellular recruitment	Block leukocyte trafficking	Anti-α4β7 (vedolizumab) (in use) Anti-α4 (natalizumab) (associated with PML, in use) Anti-β7 (etrolizumab) (unsuccessful) Anti-MAdCAM1 (ontalimumab) (in trial) S1P agonism (ozanimod)
Inflammatory mediators	Block inflammatory signaling	Mesalamines (in use) miRNA therapy (in trial) MSC therapy (in trial)
Barrier function and repair	↑ Epithelial barrier and restitution	IL22Fc (in trial)

APC, antigen-presenting cell; IFN, interferon; IL, interleukin; JAK1/3, Janus associated kinase; MAdCAM1, mucosal addressin cell adhesion molecule 1; MP, mercaptopurine; mRNA, micro RNA; MSC, mesenchymal stem cell; PML, progressive multifocal leukoencephalopathy; R, receptor; S1P, sphingosine-1-phosphate; SMAD7, SMAD family member 7; TL1A, tumor necrosis like ligand 1A; TNF, tumor necrosis factor.

Inflammatory Bowel Disease: Medical Considerations

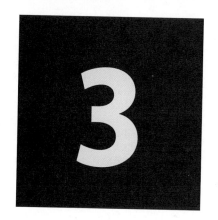

Rachel W. Winter, MD, MPH

Sonia Friedman, MD

ESSENTIALS OF DIAGNOSIS

- ▶ Crohn's disease and ulcerative colitis are chronic inflammatory diseases with well-described epidemiologic and clinical features.

- ▶ Genetic factors, immune dysregulation, and microbial gut flora all influence disease susceptibility.

- ▶ No single symptom, physical finding, or test result can diagnose inflammatory bowel disease (IBD); the diagnosis is based on consistent findings obtained from the history, physical examination, and laboratory, endoscopic, histologic, and radiologic studies.

- ▶ Multiple conditions can mimic IBD; infectious pathogens are a particular concern.

- ▶ Intestinal complications may occur in IBD, many of which may be more common depending on the disease type, location, severity, or duration; extraintestinal complications also occur, typically in association with active disease.

- ▶ Patients with long-standing colitis are at increased risk of developing colorectal cancer (CRC) and should be evaluated for dysplastic changes predictive of subsequent or synchronous malignancy.

- ▶ 5-Aminosalicylates, steroids, antibiotics, immunomodulators, and biologics are mainstays of therapy; the choice of appropriate medication is based on multiple variables, including disease type, location, and severity and patient characteristics.

General Considerations

IBD, including Crohn's disease (CD) and ulcerative colitis (UC), is a chronic inflammatory disease of the gastrointestinal (GI) tract. The immunologic basis of IBD is discussed in Chapter 2. This chapter addresses the diagnosis and medical treatment of IBD. Surgical considerations are discussed in detail in Chapter 4.

Epidemiology

Crohn's disease and ulcerative colitis affects millions of individuals worldwide. The highest reported prevalence is in Europe and North America (286 per 100,000 for UC and 319 per 100,000 for CD). While the incidence of IBD in North America and Europe has been stable or decreasing, the incidence has been increasing in countries that are recently industrialized such as Brazil and in other countries in Asia, Africa, and South America. Since the 1990's, it has been reported that immigration to Western countries is associated with new onset IBD. Increased risk of IBD among second-generation immigrants compared to first generation immigrants was reported in 1999. More recent studies have shown that immigrants who arrived in the United States after 1995 are diagnosed with IBD at younger ages and in a shorter time after immigration as compared to those who arrived from 1980 to 1994.

Crohn's disease and ulcerative colitis typically present at a relatively young age, often in adolescence, though individuals may be diagnosed at any age. The median age of diagnosis for Crohn's disease and ulcerative colitis is the third and fourth decades of life, respectively. Studies have suggested a second, smaller peak in incidence of IBD in the sixth and seventh decades, although this association is clearer for ulcerative colitis than for Crohn's disease. IBD is more prevalent in urban areas than rural areas, among Jewish people and Caucasians, though prevalence is increasing among other races and ethnicities, and is increased in higher socioeconomic classes.

Etiology

The cause of IBD is not entirely clear, though genetic, environmental, dietary, microbial, and immunologic factors clearly exist. While individuals with a family history of IBD are at increased risk, concordance rates among monozygotic twins for ulcerative colitis (6–18%) and Crohn's disease (50%) indicate that genetics are not the major factor in disease manifestation. One nationwide study showed that children born to mothers with UC have an increased risk of developing IBD (Hazard ratio [HR] 4.63, [3.49–6.160]). The HR of IBD among children born to mothers with Crohn's disease was 7.70, (5.66–10.47). Specific genetic markers that increase susceptibility to IBD are discussed in Chapter 2 along with a more complete discussion of the immunopathology of IBD.

Animal studies have demonstrated that the presence of commensal gut bacteria is necessary for IBD to occur. In theory, the subsequent enteritis or colitis results from a dysregulated or inappropriate immune response to flora tolerated by healthy individuals. Other environmental factors appear important as well. Cigarette smoking increases the risk for Crohn's disease but is protective for ulcerative colitis. Both oral contraceptive and nonsteroidal anti-inflammatory medications (NSAID's) have been implicated as risk factors for IBD, although the association remains controversial. Various diets are proposed as causes or remedies for IBD, but no rigorous scientific evidence demonstrates any specific diet causing IBD. A recent publication showed an association between consumption of diets with high inflammatory potential with an increased risk of Crohn's disease but not ulcerative colitis. Studies evaluating effects of dietary therapy on mucosal healing are challenging to design and control. Data have shown efficacy of exclusive enteral nutrition (EEN) and Crohn's disease exclusion diet with partial EEN in Crohn's disease. Additional diets commonly tried among patients with IBD include the specific carbohydrate diet and paleo diet, though evidence showing a positive effect in large controlled studies is lacking.

Carr I, Mayberry J. The effects of migration on ulcerative colitis: a three-year prospective study among Europeans and first- and second- generation South Asians in Leicester (1991–1994). *Am J Gastroenterol.* 1999;94:2918–2922. [PMID: 10520845]

Damas O, Avalos D, Palacio A, et al. IBD is presenting sooner after immigration. *Aliment Pharmacol Ther.* 2017;46(3):303–309.

Jølving LR, Nielsen J, Beck-Nielsen SS, et al. The association between maternal chronic inflammatory bowel disease and long-term health outcomes in children - A Nationwide Cohort Study. *Inflamm Bowel Dis.* 2017;23(8):1440–1446. [PMID: 28719543]

Levine A, Wine E, Assa A, et al. Crohn's disease exclusion diet plus partial enteral nutrition induces sustained remission in a randomized controlled trial. *Gastroenterology.* 2019;157:440–450. [PMID: 31170412]

Lo C-H, Lochhead P, Khalili H, et al. Dietary inflammatory potential and risk of Crohn's disease and ulcerative colitis. *Gastroenterology.* 2020;159(3):873–883. [PMID: 32389666]

Ng S, Shi H, Hamidi N, et al. Worldwide incidence and prevalence of inflammatory bowel disease in the 21st century: a systematic review of population-based studies. *Lancet.* 2018; 390(10114):2769–2778. [PMID: 29050646]

▶ Clinical Findings

Signs/Symptoms of Crohn's Disease

Crohn's disease most commonly affects the small bowel and/or colon, although the inflammation may affect any part of the GI tract from mouth to anus. Inflammation is transmural and can lead to complications including perforating disease and/or stricturing. Crohn's disease is characterized by one of three phenotypes: inflammatory, stricturing, or penetrating/fistulizing. The phenotype may change throughout the course of disease as an individual diagnosed initially with inflammatory Crohn's disease may subsequently develop strictures, fistulae, and/or abscesses. Among patients with small bowel involvement, over 90% have inflammation of the terminal ileum. The rectum is commonly spared from inflammation in individuals with Crohn's disease, which may facilitate distinguishing the diagnosis in newly symptomatic and untreated individuals. Crohn's disease is characterized by "skip areas" or patchy inflammation throughout the GI tract, in which areas of inflamed mucosa are adjacent to areas of normal mucosa. Isolated upper GI tract Crohn's disease, involving only the esophagus, stomach or duodenum is rare in the absence of more distal disease. Crohn's perianal disease, including abscesses and fistulae, may occur as isolated disease or in conjunction with ileal and/or colonic involvement.

Signs and symptoms of Crohn's disease often depend on the phenotype and disease location. Onset is typically insidious and clinical presentation can vary. For many patients, the clinical course is characterized by recurring episodes of symptomatic disease interspersed with periods of remission. Individuals with a stricture, or narrowing, of the intestine may have symptoms of abdominal pain after eating, abdominal distention, nausea/vomiting or may present with a bowel obstruction. Symptoms of fistulizing disease depend on the location of the fistula and whether an abscess develops. Abscesses may cause pain, fevers or other infectious symptoms. A fistula to the bladder may result in fecaluria or pneumaturia, whereas internal fistulae may drain to another area of the bowel or to the skin. Inflammation of the small bowel over time may result in nonbloody diarrhea due to malabsorption, weight loss, and/or vitamin and nutritional deficiencies. Iron deficiency and vitamin B12 deficiency are associated with fatigue. Inflammation involving the colon may present with symptoms similar to that of UC and may include hematochezia, tenesmus, crampy abdominal pain, and diarrhea.

Onset of ileal or ileocolonic Crohn's disease with involvement of the terminal ileum in the right lower quadrant may mimic acute appendicitis with right lower quadrant pain, fever, labs notable for leukocytosis, exam with tenderness and possible palpable mass and imaging consistent with ileal inflammation. In women with lower quadrant pain, an ovarian cyst or gynecologic etiology of symptoms should also be considered.

On exam of a patient with Crohn's disease, abdominal tenderness may be present, especially in the right lower quadrant if ileal inflammation is present. Patients with stricturing disease may have abdominal distention and those with a small bowel obstruction may also have tympany and high-pitched bowel sounds. Perianal fistulae can be visualized on careful perianal exam.

Signs/Symptoms of Ulcerative Colitis

Ulcerative colitis is characterized by inflammation of the mucosal layer of the colon and typically involves the rectum and extends proximally. Inflammation may be limited to the rectum or may extend to involve the entire colon, but usually occurs in a continuous pattern. Occasionally, patients may have distal colonic inflammation and a "cecal patch" of periappendiceal inflammation. This neither represents a true skip lesion suggestive of Crohn's disease, nor does it change the classification of disease extent to pancolitis. Ulcerative colitis is described by the extent of disease involvement: ulcerative proctitis, left-sided ulcerative colitis, or pan colitis. About 20% of patients have inflammation affecting their entire colon. Mild inflammation in the terminal ileum, often called backwash ileitis, may be seen among patients with right sided colonic and cecal involvement. Deep ileal ulcers, long segments of ileal inflammation or stricturing disease are more consistent with Crohn's disease and not ulcerative colitis. Disease extent of UC at diagnosis may change over time as inflammation may progress proximally with longer duration of disease and untreated inflammation. Of note, while continuous inflammation is typically seen at diagnosis, patients on medical therapy may have apparent skip lesions or rectal sparing due to partial healing of the colon and this should be recognized as a treatment effect and not a manifestation of/ change in diagnosis to Crohn's disease.

Individuals with ulcerative colitis often present with acute symptoms of rectal bleeding, tenesmus, urgency, mucous in the stool, and crampy abdominal pain. Patients may also report diarrhea and abdominal pain. They often report increased frequency of bowel movements and may awaken at night to defecate. Nausea and weight loss may occur in more severe disease. Individuals with hypoalbuminemia and severe inflammation involving the entire colon are at risk for developing toxic megacolon and have increased risk of perforation.

Lab Findings: Crohn's Disease and Ulcerative Colitis

No single laboratory test is diagnostic for Crohn's disease or ulcerative colitis. Patients with rectal bleeding or ileal inflammation may have anemia and/or iron deficiency. Malabsorption may also cause other vitamin and mineral deficiencies such as calcium, magnesium, vitamin B12, vitamin D, and folate. Leukocytosis and thrombocytosis are common and may reflect systemic inflammation. Serum albumin may also be low in the setting of malnutrition/malabsorption or protein-losing enteropathy. Inflammatory markers such as C-reactive protein (CRP) and erythrocyte sedimentation rate (ESR) are nonspecific markers of inflammation that are frequently elevated in Crohn's disease and ulcerative colitis.

Stool studies may aid in the diagnosis of IBD and also are commonly ordered to monitor disease and assess the etiology and severity of a flare among patients with an established diagnosis of IBD. Stool studies may reveal excess fat, indicative of malabsorption, or fecal leukocytes, indicative of gut inflammation. Stool studies for infectious pathogens, including standard stool culture, ova and parasites, and *Clostridium difficile*, should be negative. Fecal calprotectin, a marker of inflammation in the stool, is a more specific marker of inflammation in the GI tract but may not be as accurate if inflammation is only present in the proximal GI tract. Fecal lactoferrin, another marker of inflammation in the stool, is less commonly ordered but can also be used to assess inflammation. Lactoferrin is the major component of secondary granules in neutrophils and inhibits bacterial proliferation by iron binding. It is stable in the stool for 7 days. Calprotectin is present in neutrophils, monocytes, and macrophages. It comprises 60% of the cytosolic protein in neutrophils and also is stable in the stool for 7 days. In addition to their use in assessing for and monitoring inflammation, these stool markers can also help distinguish IBD from irritable bowel syndrome (IBS), potentially gauge disease activity, predict flare, and monitor and/or assess response to treatment. Since the stool tests are specific to the GI tract, they may be more reliable than CRP and ESR, which may be affected by other infectious and inflammatory conditions including, but not limited to, viral infections, rheumatologic diseases, and pregnancy.

▶ Radiographic Findings

Standard abdominal plain films can be useful for detecting obstructive disease and megacolon, but otherwise have a limited role in Crohn's disease and ulcerative colitis.

Magnetic resonance imaging (MRI) and computed tomography (CT) of the abdomen and pelvis are most commonly ordered as they allow for imaging of the bowel wall as well as extraluminal disease such as abscesses or inflammatory masses. MRI is preferred over CT for routine surveillance or monitoring of small bowel inflammation not only to minimize exposure to radiation, but also because mucosal enhancement identifies specific area of inflammation. MR enterography, which allows for detailed visualization of the bowel wall, is often recommended for patients with Crohn's disease and MR pelvis can provide detailed visualization of perianal fistulous tracts. CT scans may be more useful for detecting abscesses.

Additional small bowel imaging modalities may be useful among individuals with Crohn's disease but are less commonly utilized. Small bowel series can characterize small bowel mucosal disease, including strictures, ulcerations, and fistulae. Enteroclysis, although more sensitive, is limited by patient discomfort, increased radiation exposure, and is technically demanding. Barium enema remains an option for imaging colonic disease, especially to help delineate obstructive or fistulizing disease but is less commonly ordered than MRI and CT scans.

More commonly used in Europe, small bowel ultrasound (SBUS) is another useful modality for imaging small bowel CD. In experienced hands, SBUS is at least as sensitive as MRE and CTE for detecting small bowel CD. It is best suited for distal small bowel assessment, as the sensitivity of detecting lesions within the duodenum and proximal jejunum may be lower due to anatomical position. The limitations of SBUS include availability and operator experience.

Ripollés T, Poza J, Suarez Ferrer C et al. Evaluation of Crohn's disease activity: development of an ultrasound score in a multicenter study. *Inflamm Bowel Dis*. 2021;27(1):epub only. [PMID: 32507880]

Endoscopic Examination

Colonoscopy remains the mainstay in diagnosing and assessing Crohn's disease and ulcerative colitis as it allows direct visualization of colonic and ileal mucosa as well as mucosal biopsies. Strictures may form in patients with ulcerative colitis, but are less common than in patients with Crohn's disease and should always be thoroughly evaluated for malignancy. Patients with strictures that cannot be traversed endoscopically should be referred for surgery.

Endoscopic findings in ulcerative colitis often are first identified in the rectum and extend proximally and in a continuous pattern to include any length of colon from a short segment of the colon (sometimes limited only to the rectum) to the entire colon. Inflamed mucosa may be characterized by erythema, edema, granularity, and ulceration.

Hallmark endoscopic findings of Crohn's disease include ulcerations (erosions, aphthous ulcers and/or deeper ulcers), erythema, and granularity. Strictures may also be appreciated on colonoscopy. Abnormal/inflamed mucosa often occurs in a noncontinuous fashion, often described as "skip lesions," which can be helpful in distinguishing colonic Crohn's disease from ulcerative colitis. The rectum is often uninvolved and does not show inflammation at the time of diagnosis of Crohn's disease. Fistulae may be appreciated on colonoscopy in individuals with Crohn's disease, but they can be challenging to identify and are best seen on radiographic imaging. Histologic features of Crohn's disease include noncaseating granulomas and crypt abscesses, though these features are not required for a diagnosis.

Video capsule endoscopy (VCE) may be performed among patients with Crohn's disease in order to visualize small bowel mucosa. Common findings include ulcerations, ranging from small, shallow aphthous ulcers to deep ulcers. These may occur anywhere throughout the GI tract. One known complication of VCE is capsule retention, especially among patients with known stricturing small bowel disease. Prior to proceeding with VCE, it is recommended that patients have imaging to confirm absence of stricture and/or a patency capsule to document passage of the disintegrating capsule before the video capsule is swallowed.

Extraintestinal Manifestations

IBD may also cause extraintestinal complications. Common extraintestinal manifestations include dermatologic, rheumatologic, and ophthalmologic complications, and are prevalent among about one-third of patients with IBD. Extraintestinal manifestations may or may not parallel disease activity of the GI tract.

Dermatologic: Dermatologic manifestations include pyoderma gangrenosum and erythema nodosum. Pyoderma gangrenosum is characterized by painful purple ulcerations, often induced by trauma (Figure 3–1). This may or may not parallel IBD disease activity. Erythema nodosum, which typically parallels IBD disease activity, appears as painful, nonulcerated nodules that classically occur on the lower extremities (Figure 3–2). Other dermatologic conditions associated with IBD include Sweet's syndrome, vasculitis and aphthous stomatitis. Individuals with Crohn's disease may rarely develop cutaneous Crohn's disease.

Rheumatologic: Rheumatologic/musculoskeletal manifestations include arthritis and ankylosing spondylitis. Patients with IBD and especially those with a history of malabsorption or chronic steroid use may be at increased risk for osteoporosis and osteopenia and also osteonecrosis. Patients should have a baseline bone density scan.

Ophthalmologic: Uveitis, episcleritis, scleritis, iritis, and conjunctivitis are the more common ophthalmologic complications of IBD. Symptoms of uveitis include pain, redness, and photophobia. Scleritis most commonly presents with pain.

Hepatobiliary: Hepatobiliary diseases may occur concomitantly with IBD as a patient may have a diagnosis of both autoimmune liver disease and IBD, and patients with IBD, in particular those with UC, are at increased risk for development of primary sclerosing cholangitis (PSC), a disorder of the intra- and extrahepatic bile ducts characterized by fibrosis and inflammation of the ducts, which can lead to hepatic failure and cirrhosis. Individuals with PSC and IBD are at increased risk for colon cancer and should undergo annual surveillance. Regular monitoring of liver tests among all patients with IBD is recommended. Patients with PSC also carry a high risk for cholangiocarcinoma and should have yearly imaging to screen the biliary tree. PSC is further discussed in Chapter 49.

Colorectal: In addition to extraintestinal manifestations, individuals with ulcerative or Crohn's colitis are at increased risk for CRC. This risk increases 8–10 years after diagnosis. Chromoendoscopy may be performed for surveillance.

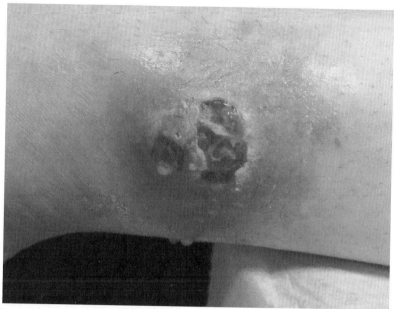

▲ **Figure 3-1.** Pyoderma gangrenosum of the lower extremity. Reproduced with permission from Avery Lachance, M.D.

Complications

Crohn's disease: Complications of inflammation and fibrosis in the GI tract include malabsorption, strictures, and fistulas. As discussed previously, chronic inflammation and fibrosis can result in narrowing of the lumen of the GI tract. Recurrent inflammation may lead to a fibrotic stricture, causing pain, distention and discomfort, and also increased risk for small bowel obstruction. Malabsorption/nutritional deficiencies may occur depending on the length of involved

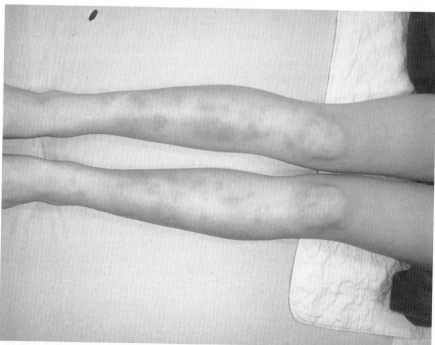

▲ **Figure 3-2.** Erythema nodosum of the lower extremities. Reproduced with permission from Avery Lachance, M.D.

bowel and the area of affected bowel. Patients with involvement of the terminal ileum are at increased risk for iron and vitamin B12 deficiencies.

Ulcerative colitis: Toxic megacolon, a severe complication of ulcerative colitis, is defined by a diameter >6 cm of the transverse or right colon and loss of haustration. Clinical symptoms may include abdominal pain, diarrhea, and fever. Urgent colectomy may be recommended if the colonic dilation does not resolve with conservative management as patients with significantly distended colons are at increased risk for perforation. Patients must be monitored closely, especially since clinical signs of perforation and peritonitis may be masked if a patient is being treated with steroids. Colonic strictures occur in 5–10% of patients. While strictures may be benign, they may also represent underlying malignancy and any patient with a stricture that cannot be traversed and fully evaluated endoscopically should be evaluated for surgical resection. Individuals with severe or refractory UC may undergo colectomy. Those who undergo ileal pouch anal anastomosis are at risk for pouchitis, or inflammation of the J pouch. This may be treated with probiotics, antibiotics, or biologics in refractory cases.

Individuals with a history of colonic inflammation for at least 8–10 years are at increased risk for CRC. This risk is greater among patients with untreated inflammation. All patients with a diagnosis established at least 8–10 years prior are recommended to undergo surveillance colonoscopy every 2 years. Patients with PSC are recommended to undergo annual surveillance.

▶ Differential diagnosis of IBD

As discussed, an individual suspected to have a new diagnosis of IBD should undergo endoscopic and radiologic evaluation in addition to laboratory and comprehensive history and physical. Equally important to obtaining studies that can aid in confirming a diagnosis of IBD is eliminating other possible etiologies of the patient's symptoms. Nonspecific symptoms of IBD, such as abdominal discomfort, diarrhea, tenesmus, and rectal bleeding, among others, may be due to other medical conditions and it is important to consider these in the differential diagnosis when evaluating a patient for possible IBD.

Infectious colitis and C. difficile: Infectious pathogens can mimic IBD and it is recommended that stool studies be sent for culture, ova and parasites and *C. difficile. Yersinia enterocolitica* can cause terminal ileitis and may mimic ileal Crohn's disease. Campylobacter may present with nausea, vomiting, and watery or bloody diarrhea, similar to onset or flare of ulcerative colitis. Similarly, shigellosis, which causes abdominal pain, fever and watery diarrhea, may present with symptoms suggestive of UC. *C. difficile,* which results in symptoms of watery diarrhea, abdominal discomfort, and tenesmus, may mimic IBD though may also occur concomitantly with a flare of IBD, and it is therefore important to test for *C. difficile*

in any patient with worsening of diarrhea suggestive of flare. Mycobacterial infection may present with distal ileal or cecal inflammation; diagnosis can be made with biopsy and culture. Cytomegalovirus (CMV) more commonly occurs in the esophagus or colon, though may also infect the small bowel. Symptoms of CMV include bloody diarrhea, abdominal pain, and may include fever and weight loss. Diagnosis can also be made by biopsy. Less common infections that may have presentations similar to IBD include herpes simplex virus, HIV/AIDS and ova and parasites including *Entamoeba histolytica, Necator americanus* (causes hookworm), *Trichuris trichiura* (whipworm), and *Strongyloides stercoralis.* Further discussion of infectious pathogens affecting the GI tract can be found in Chapter 5.

Diverticulitis: Diverticulitis may present with abdominal pain, fever, elevated inflammatory markers, leukocytosis, and recurrent diverticulitis may lead to fistula formation. Acute diverticulitis or fistula resulting from diverticular disease may be difficult to differentiate from Crohn's disease on imaging. However, individuals with diverticulitis rarely present with rectal bleeding and endoscopic and histologic findings should differ as colonic mucosa in areas without diverticula should be normal.

Irritable Bowel Syndrome: IBS is a chronic functional disorder of the GI tract. Symptoms include abdominal discomfort, increased gas and bloating and constipation, diarrhea or both. Patients with IBS do not have inflammation of the GI tract, and thus radiographic and endoscopic studies will be normal, as will inflammatory markers including fecal calprotectin.

Ischemic colitis: Ischemic colitis, which results from decreased blood flow to the colon, often presents with abdominal pain, urgency, and hematochezia. It occurs more commonly in elderly individuals and those with vascular disease. Endoscopic findings are often notable for a normal appearing rectum with clear delineation to an area of inflamed mucosa, often in the descending colon and affecting the splenic flexure.

Microscopic colitis: Microscopic colitis, which includes lymphocytic colitis and collagenous colitis, presents with chronic watery, nonbloody diarrhea, and abdominal cramps or bloating. Individuals may experience fecal incontinence. The endoscopic appearance of microscopic colitis is normal, though biopsies will show increased intraepithelial lymphocytes or increased deposition of subepithelial collagen. Risk factors for microscopic colitis include use of acid blockers (proton pump inhibitors and H2 blockers), NSAID's (ibuprofen) and selective serotonin reuptake inhibitors.

Celiac: Celiac disease, an immunologic reaction to gluten, may present with abdominal discomfort, bloating, change in bowel habits, and nutritional deficiencies similar to those seen in Crohn's disease. Obtaining serum tissue transglutaminase, serum IgA and biopsies of the duodenal bulb and second portion of the duodenum during upper endoscopy can help differentiate celiac disease from IBD. It is important to assess for celiac disease before a patient initiates a gluten free diet, as endoscopic/histologic findings and serologies may normalize with elimination of gluten from the diet. There are patients who have both celiac disease and IBD.

Malignancy: CRC may present with iron deficiency anemia, abdominal discomfort, rectal bleeding, change in bowel habits, among other symptoms. While colonoscopy is recommended to establish a diagnosis of IBD, it is important to remember that CRC may present like IBD and full colonoscopy, rather than flexible sigmoidoscopy, should be performed if a patient has not recently had a full colonoscopy.

Medication Use: NSAID's are known to increase risk for GI inflammation and bleeding. NSAID's can cause inflammation, erosions, and ulcerations and may mimic IBD or exacerbate IBD among those with an established diagnosis. A thorough history including use of over the counter medications is important to evaluate for NSAID use.

Immune checkpoint inhibitors: Immune checkpoint inhibitors (ICI) have become more commonly used in the therapy of many types of malignancy. ICI-colitis often presents with profuse watery diarrhea. Endoscopically, the mucosa often appears normal, though diagnosis can be made histologically. Further discussion of the complications of ICI can be found in Chapter 10.

▶ **Medical Therapy of Crohn's Disease and Ulcerative Colitis**

Maintenance Therapy

5-ASA: The 5-aminosalicylate medications are recommended for treatment of mild to moderate ulcerative colitis (Table 3–1). These medications can be administered orally or rectal (as suppositories or enemas). Side effects of sulfasalazine include rash, fever, agranulocytosis, hepatitis, and pancreatitis. Daily folic acid is recommended with administration of sulfasalazine. There are many brands of mesalamine, with differences in the area of the GI tract that is targeted and the frequency of dosing. *Pentasa* delivers mesalamine throughout the entire GI tract as capsule disintegration occurs in the stomach, allowing release of medication from the proximal small bowel through the colon. *Delzicol* and *Asacol* release in the distal small bowel. *Lialda* releases throughout the colon, and *Apriso* and *Balsalazide* release in the terminal ileum and colon. *Lialda* and *Apriso* are once-daily dosing, which may result in improved compliance. Side effects of mesalamine include headache and a paradoxical reaction of worsening diarrhea and abdominal discomfort. Renal impairment and pancreatitis are rare complications. Rectal formulations of mesalamine include *Rowasa* enemas and *Canasa* suppositories which may be effective in treating distal inflammation.

Thiopurines: Azathioprine and mercaptopurine are purine analogs that may be prescribed as monotherapy or in combination with another biologic medication. They may be used to achieve and/or maintain remission. Azathioprine is converted to mercaptopurine, which is metabolized to the active product thioinosinic acid. Improvement in inflammation may occur as early as 2–3 weeks, though may take up to 6 months. Dosing typically is 1–1.5 mg/kg per day for mercaptopurine and 2–2.5 mg/kg per day for azathioprine. Medication levels can be monitored by measuring levels of 6-thioguanine (goal therapeutic range 235–450 pg/m) and 6-methyl-mercaptopurine. Liver tests and blood counts must be monitored every few months as side effects can include

Table 3–1. Oral 5-ASA preparations.

Preparation	Formulation	Delivery	Dosing per day
Azo-bond			
Sulfasalazine (500 mg) (Azulfidine)	Sulfapyridine-5-ASA	Colon	3–6 g (acute)
Balsalazide (750 mg) (Colazal)	Aminobenzoyl-alanine–5-ASA	Colon	2–4 g (maintenance)
			6.75–9 g
Delayed-release			
Mesalamine (400, 800 mg) (Delzicol, Asacol HD)	Eudragit S (pH 7)	Distal ileum-colon	2.4–4.8 g (acute)
			1.6–4.8 g (maintenance)
Mesalamine (1.2 g) (Lialda)	MMX mesalamine (SPD476)	Ileum-colon	2.4–4.8 g
Controlled-release			
Mesalamine (250, 500, 1000 mg) (Pentasa)	Ethylcellulose microgranules	Stomach-colon	2–4 g (acute)
			1.5–4 g (maintenance)
Delayed- and extended-release			
Mesalamine (0.375 g) (Apriso)	Intellicor extended-release mechanism	Ileum-colon	1.5 g (maintenance)

hepatitis and leukopenia; additional side effects include pancreatitis and nausea. It is practice to test for a thiopurine methyltransferase (TPMT) mutation prior to starting a thiopurine as patients homozygous for this mutation should not be treated with thiopurines.

Tumor necrosis antagonists (infliximab, adalimumab, certolizumab pegol, golimumab): The introduction of infliximab, a chimeric immunoglobulin G monoclonal antibody directed against tumor necrosis factor (TNF), revolutionized the medical therapy of moderate to severe Crohn's disease and ulcerative colitis. The importance of TNF as a proinflammatory cytokine in IBD has long been appreciated (see Chapter 2). Administered intravenously (starting dose 5 mg/kg) at weeks 0, 2, and 6, infliximab is effective for achieving and maintaining remission in Crohn's disease and ulcerative colitis. Like the thiopurines, it is steroid sparing and effective in healing fistulae. Infliximab also can maintain remission in IBD, though even among patients who initially respond to therapy with anti-TNF medications, they may subsequently either lose response or develop antibodies to the medications, rendering the medications ineffective. For patients who are losing response to infliximab, the dose may be increased to 10 mg/kg with no change in the infusion interval and/or the interval to next infusion may be shortened to every 4 or 6 weeks. Infliximab trough levels and antibodies are now standard of care to check after the initial loading doses and prior to making any dose adjustment. There is ongoing debate about proactive versus reactive monitoring of drug levels. Antibody formation is thought to be mediated by reaction to the immune system's identification of infliximab as a foreign protein. Patients with no antibodies and subtherapeutic trough levels will benefit from decreasing the interval between infusions or increasing the dose whereas patients with high antibodies and low trough levels are thought to have lost response to the medication. A landmark trial comparing steroid-free remission in immunomodulator-naïve patients treated with combination of azathioprine and infliximab therapy showed statistically significant improvement in combination therapy over infliximab or azathioprine monotherapy up to 26 weeks.

In addition to infliximab, adalimumab and certolizumab pegol are approved for treatment of moderate to severe Crohn's disease, and adalimumab and golimumab are approved for treatment of moderate to severe ulcerative colitis. Both adalimumab (induction dose of 160 mg subcutaneously [SQ], followed by 80 mg SQ at week 2, then 40 mg SQ every 2 weeks) and certolizumab pegol (400 mg SQ at weeks 0, 2, and 4, followed by 400 mg SQ every 4 weeks) provide a similar response and remission rates as infliximab. Multicenter trials have demonstrated that both adalimumab and certolizumab pegol are effective in maintaining a clinical response in 50–60% of patients at 6 months or 1 year and remission in 25% of patients at 1 year. Additionally, among patients who have lost their response to infliximab, approximately 35% of patients will regain response with adalimumab or certolizumab therapy over 12 weeks. Similar to infliximab,

laboratory values for serum trough and drug antibodies are available commercially for adalimumab.

As foreign proteins, these agents can generate an immune response in terms of antibody formation against the drug itself, particularly if administered intermittently. For this reason, continuous therapy is the current standard of care. Loss of response to one medication does not necessarily mean a loss of response to the class.

Infection is the most serious complication with anti-TNF biologic agents. Patients are particularly vulnerable to tuberculosis and should be screened carefully for this prior to initial administration. Patients with latent hepatitis B are vulnerable to reactivation and patients who are not immune to Hepatitis B should receive at least the first dose of vaccine prior to initiating therapy with an anti-TNF medication. Reports have also been published of cases of histoplasmosis among patients receiving anti-TNF therapy in areas with histoplasmosis is endemic. Anti-TNF therapy should be held in the setting of pyogenic infections. Concern has been raised about possible increased risk of lymphoma, although this remains very uncommon. Less serious adverse effects include infusion or injection reactions, lupus-like reaction, psoriasis, drug-induced lupus, and serum sickness.

Vedolizumab: Vedolizumab is a humanized immunoglobulin GI monoclonal antibody to α4β7 integrin. α4β7 interrupts the inflammatory cascade by modulating lymphocyte trafficking. Unlike natalizumab, which is now very rarely prescribed for IBD, vedolizumab is selective for receptors in the GI tract and does not penetrate the blood-brain barrier minimizing the risk of progressive multifocal leukoencephalopathy (PML) or JC virus. Vedolizumab may be used as a first-line medication among patients with moderate to severe Crohn's disease or ulcerative colitis. While a clinical response to vedolizumab may be appreciated within a few weeks of initiating the medication, complete response may not occur until 3–6 months after starting treatment. A recent study comparing vedolizumab to adalimumab among patients with ulcerative colitis showed superiority of vedolizumab in achieving clinical and endoscopic remission. Arthralgias and headache appear to be the most common adverse reactions.

Ustekinumab: Ustekinumab is a fully human IgG1 monoclonal antibody that blocks interleukins 12 and 23 and is approved for treatment of moderate to severe Crohn's disease and ulcerative colitis. It is administered intravenously for the first dose; subsequent doses are subcutaneous. The UNITI trial showed rates of remission at 44 weeks of 53.1% among patients with Crohn's disease who received ustekinumab every 8 weeks compared to 35.9% among those who received placebo. The UNIFI trial which enrolled patients with ulcerative colitis showed 44-week maintenance rates of 43.8% among participants who received ustekinumab compared to 24% who received placebo.

Tofacitinib: Tofacitinib is a competitive JAK inhibitor approved to treat moderate to severe ulcerative colitis. Tofacitinib is effective as both induction and maintenance therapy and effects are usually seen within the first few weeks of therapy.

Initial studies showed remission rates of 34.3% with 5 mg and 40.6% with 10 mg at 52 weeks (OCTAVE Sustain). Dosing starts at 10 mg twice daily and may be decreased to 5 mg twice daily. Patients prescribed tofacitinib must be monitored closely. In addition to monitoring liver tests and blood counts, fasting lipid panels should be routinely checked. Patients are recommended to be vaccinated against herpes zoster.

Methotrexate: Methotrexate is a folic acid antagonist that has shown to be effective for achieving remission. It may be delivered subcutaneously or orally, though subcutaneous administration is often more effective. Common side effects include nausea, hepatitis, pancytopenia, and hepatic fibrosis. Patients with known liver disease should avoid this medication and labs must be monitored every 3 months. Patients taking methotrexate are recommended to also take a folic acid supplement. Methotrexate is an abortifacient and should be discontinued at least 3 months prior to a woman trying to conceive.

Antibiotics: Antibiotics may be used to treat Crohn's disease though are not recommended for long-term maintenance therapy. They are not recommended for treatment of ulcerative colitis, though may be prescribed to patients who have had a colectomy, as pouchitis often responds to antibiotic therapy. The most commonly prescribed antibiotics include ciprofloxacin, metronidazole, and rifaximin.

Dual Therapy: The practice of prescribing dual biologic agents for severe refractory IBD or to treat extraintestinal manifestations not controlled with one agent alone has recently been reported. While data are limited and reported as case reports or case series, dual targeted therapy may be an effective therapy for select patients. The most commonly used agents are vedolizumab with either ustekinumab or tofacitinib.

Nutritional/Dietary Therapies

It has long been hypothesized that diet contributes to the pathogenesis of IBD, but specifics regarding how diet may increase risk for IBD are unknown. Diet has also been shown to be effective in managing IBD, though controlled studies are difficult to conduct. Crohn's disease in particular, has been shown to be responsive to dietary interventions such as EEN. Crohn's disease also often improves with total parenteral nutrition (TPN) which effectively results in bowel rest. These therapies have been shown to be as effective as glucocorticoids in inducing remission. While EEN may be continued long-term, it is not optimal long-term therapy due to difficulty for patients to fully comply for extended periods of time. Partial EEN, as described in the Crohn's Disease Exclusion Diet, is well tolerated and thus may offer a long-term diet solution but additional data regarding efficacy are needed[6]. Studies evaluating the effect of diet in ulcerative colitis are fewer, and efficacy of diet in UC is largely based on anecdotal data. Diets that have been tried, with varying degrees of effectiveness, are the Mediterranean diet, Specific Carbohydrate Diet, Paleo diet, and IBD Anti-Inflammatory Diet (IBD-AID). Additional investigation into diet on achieving and maintain remission in IBD are warranted.

Colombel JJF, Sandborn WWJ, Reinisch W, et al. Infliximab, azathioprine, or combination therapy for Crohn's disease (SONIC study). *N Engl J Med.* 2010;362:1383–1395. [PMID: 20393175]

Dolinger MT, Spencer EA, Lai J, et al. Dual biologic and small molecule therapy for the treatment of refractory pediatric inflammatory bowel disease. *Inflamm Bowel Dis.* 2021;27(8):1210–1214. [PMID: 33125058]

Feagan BG, Sandborn WJ, Gasink C, et al. Ustekinumab as induction and maintenance therapy for Crohn's disease. *NEJM.* 2016;375:1946–1960. [PMID: 27959607]

Privitera, G, Onali S, Pugliese D, et al. Dual targeted therapy: a possible option for the managemnt of refractory inflammatory bowel disease. *JCC.* 2020;1–2. [PMID: 32674156]

Sands BE, Peyrin-Biroulet L, Loftus EVJ, Danese S, Colombel J-F. Vedolizumab versus adalimumab for moderate-to-severe ulcerative colitis. *NEJM.* 2019;381:1215–1226. [PMID: 31553834]

Sands BE, Sandborn WJ, Panaccione R, et al. Ustekinumab as induction and maintenance therapy for ulcerative colitis. *NEJM.* 2019;381:1201–1214. [PMID: 31553833]

▶ Treatment of Acute Inflammation

Glucocorticoids: Patients with acute inflammation due to Crohn's disease or ulcerative colitis often respond to oral or parenteral administration of glucocorticoids. Prednisone dosing often starts at 40 mg/daily before being tapered and may be prescribed at the time of diagnosis or an acute flare. Parenteral steroids are often dosed at 40–60 mg/day of methylprednisolone or 300 mg/day of hydrocortisone. Medications are usually administered q8–12 hours. Side effects of steroids are numerous and include, but are not limited to hyperglycemia, sleep disturbance, osteonecrosis, osteoporosis, fluid retention, irritability, and emotional disturbances and adrenal insufficiency. Budesonide is an oral steroid that has minimal systemic absorption and thus minimal glucocorticoid side effects. Two formulations exist: 3 mg tablets of Entocort are released in the terminal ileum to treat ileo-colonic disease; 9 mg tablets of Uceris is released in the colon to treat colitis. Entocort is usually prescribed at 9 mg/daily with a subsequent taper. While glucocorticoids may be very effective at inducing remission and treating acute inflammation, they are not recommended for maintenance therapy. Rectal steroid therapies in the form of enemas and suppositories are also available for treatment of distal colonic inflammation.

▶ Cyclosporine and Tacrolimus

Cyclosporine (CSA) and tacrolimus are calcineurin inhibitors and may be used to treat hospitalized patients with severe ulcerative colitis or Crohn's disease. They are best begun in a hospitalized patient who has failed intravenous corticosteroids within 7 days. Toxicities limit their long-term use. Nephrotoxicity and opportunistic infections are prime concerns. Seizures are also possible; for this reason, CSA should be avoided in patients with low cholesterol (<100 mg/dL) or hypomagnesemia. Given as a continuous infusion (2–4 mg/kg/day), CSA can induce a short-term response in patients. A comparison of CSA with infliximab as treatment for severe UC showed similar response rates between those treated with CSA compared to those treated with infliximab. Given similar response rates though significant possible toxicities and side effects of CSA, more health care providers elect to induce remission in UC with infliximab over CSA. Long-term follow up at median of 5.4 years showed that colectomy-free survival was independent of initial induction medication. A small study of 20 patients showed that combination therapy of either CSA or tacrolimus with vedolizumab was safe and effective at inducing clinical remission in patients with Crohn's disease and ulcerative colitis up to 52 weeks, though larger studies are needed.

Christensen B, Gibson P, Micic D, et al. Effective use of calcineurin inhibitors with vedolizumab in refractory inflammatory bowel disease. *Clin Gastroenterol Hepatol.* 2019;17(3):486–493.

Laharie D, Bourreille A, Branche J, et al. Ciclosporin versus infliximab in patients with severe ulcerative colitis refractory to intravenous steroids: a parallel, open-label randomised controlled trial. *Lancet.* 2012;380(9857):1909–1915. [PMID: 23063316]

Laharie D, Bourreille A, Branche J, et al. Long-term outcome of patients with steroid-refractory acute severe UC treated with ciclosporin or infliximab. *Gut.* 2018;67(2):237–243. [PMID: 28053054]

▶ Surgical Management of IBD

Surgery in Crohn's disease is frequently required to address complications of stricturing, penetrating, or fistulizing disease. Because recurrence at anastomotic sites is common, surgery is not recommended as a primary treatment strategy. Surgery for ulcerative colitis offers a therapeutic option as total proctocolectomy resects the diseased tissue and eliminates the necessity of medical therapy for colitis. Surgery is indicated in fulminant disease, severe medically refractory disease, and when colitis-associated dysplasia or malignancy is detected. Colectomy does not preclude other complications, such as PSC or pouchitis. An ileal pouch-anal anastomosis (IPAA) is the current surgery of choice in the elective setting. Total proctocolectomy with end ileostomy is also a reasonable choice and may be more appropriate given the clinical setting. Surgical considerations in the treatment of Crohn's disease and ulcerative colitis, surgical complications and pouchitis are discussed in detail in Chapter 4.

Disease Monitoring

Disease monitoring will likely depend on the prescribed medications as many of the immunosuppressing and biologic medications require more frequent monitoring of blood counts and liver tests. Fecal calprotectin can be used both to assess for disease inflammation/flare and also to monitor for remission in patients who do not have active symptoms. Patients with small bowel Crohn's disease may be followed by MRI if the involved area is not visible on endoscopy or colonoscopy. VCE may also be performed if the patient does not have a small bowel stricture and enables visualization of small bowel mucosa. Intestinal ultrasound has become increasingly used as an alternative imaging method as it provides a low-cost, noninvasive, and well-tolerated modality by which to monitor bowel inflammation. As mentioned previously, all patients with colonic inflammation for 8–10 years should undergo routine surveillance for CRC.

Health Maintenance

Health maintenance is also partially dependent on the medications with which a patient is treated, though recommendations regarding vaccinations and cancer surveillance have been recommended.

Vitamins/minerals: All patients should be evaluated for vitamin D deficiency at the time of diagnosis and annual screening is recommended. Patients with small bowel inflammation or those who have undergone ileal resection should be monitored for vitamin B12 and iron deficiency. Patients with more significant malabsorption may be at risk for additional nutritional deficiencies such as copper or zinc.

Vaccinations: All patients with IBD should receive the annual flu vaccine. Note that patients on immunosuppressing medications should not receive the live inhaled intranasal flu vaccine; the trivalent or quadrivalent inactivated flu vaccine is safe for patients regardless of type of medication. Pneumonia vaccines (Prevnar-13 and Pneumovax 23) are recommended for those on immunosuppressing medications. Vaccination for herpes zoster should be considered for all adults over age 50 and is also recommended for patients >65 years old or those who are prescribed tofacitinib. Adolescents should receive the vaccination for meningococcus as per routine vaccination guidelines. Hepatitis serologies should be checked prior to starting therapy with a biologic, and the first does of the Hepatitis B vaccine should be given prior to starting a biologic if a patient is not immune. In addition, history of exposure to tuberculosis must be evaluated prior to starting immnosuppressive medications (Table 3–2).

Dermatologic care: All patients with IBD should undergo screening for melanoma. In particular, those on immunosuppressing medications such as thiopurines and TNF antagonists are recommended to undergo annual screening for skin cancer.

Gynecologic care: Women on immunosuppressive therapy should to undergo annual screening for cervical cancer.

Mental Health: All patients should be screened for depression and anxiety.

Farraye FA, Melmed GY, Lichtenstein GR, Kane S V. ACG clinical guideline: preventive care in inflammatory bowel disease. *Am J Gastroenterol.* 2017;112:241–258. [PMID: 28071656]

Table 3-2. Vaccine Recommendations for Patients with Inflammatory Bowel Disease

Vaccine	Thiopurine therapy	Anti-TNF combination	Anti-TNF monotherapy	Ustekinumab Vedolizumab Tofacitinib
Standard dose quadrivalent influenza vaccine, inactivated	Age 18–64 years			Age 18–64 years
High dose trivalent influenza vaccine, inactivated	≥65 years	Age 18–64 years; Age >65 years	Age 18–64 years; Age >65 years	Age ≥65 years
Pneumococcal conjugate vaccine 13 valent (PCV 13)	All ages	All ages	All ages	All ages
Pneumococcal polysaccharide vaccine 23 valent (PPSV23)	All ages	All ages	All ages	All ages
Recombinant zoster vaccine (RZV)	≥50 years	≥50 years	≥50 years	≥50 years

Consider RZV for age 18–49 years on anti-TNF or tofacitinib therapy

Other recommended vaccines:	
Hepatitis B vaccine (Hep B)	All ages: 3-dose series on 0, 1, 6 month schedule or 2-dose series (hepB-CpG) at 0 and 1 month.
Either vaccine series	Check HBsAb 4–6 weeks after completing series.
Human papillomavirus vaccine (HPV)	Three doses 0, 1–2, and 6 month schedule for all ages <26 years. Age 27–45 years, 3 doses if likely to have new sexual partners.
Tetanus-diphtheria-acellular Pertussis (Td/Tdap)	If previously immunized, single dose of Tdap, then Td or Tdap every 10 years. A Tdap during each pregnancy during third trimester.
Meningococcal vaccines	Adults with risk factors should receive immunization.

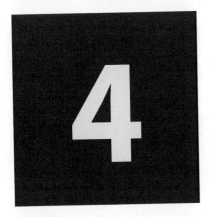

Inflammatory Bowel Disease: Surgical Considerations

Jennifer L. Irani, MD

Ronald Bleday, MD

ESSENTIAL CONCEPTS

Ulcerative Colitis

▶ Surgery is indicated when (1) chronic intractable disease is not controlled with medication, or drug side effects are too severe; (2) patients with severe colitis require an urgent procedure; or (3) dysplasia or cancer is present.

▶ Most patients needing surgery are candidates for an ileoanal pouch anastomosis (IPAA); the main considerations are age, gender, type of job, and lifestyle.

▶ In most patients undergoing IPAA, a temporary diverting loop ileostomy is constructed to decrease the likelihood of pelvic sepsis.

▶ The procedure of choice for acute fulminant colitis is total colectomy with end ileostomy.

Crohn's Disease

▶ In general, surgery is indicated for complications (ie, abscess, fistula, perforation, obstruction); considerations include symptom severity, medical treatment failure or side effects, and operative risk.

▶ Most patients found to have Crohn's disease at laparotomy for suspected appendicitis require early ileocolic resection.

▶ Surgery for symptomatic intestinal fistulas requires removal of the diseased segment, and the "innocent bystander" often does not require removal.

▶ Surgical procedures for treatment of fistula-in-ano include fistulotomy, long-term draining setons, endoanal flap closure, and ligation of intersphincteric fistula tract, if the rectal mucosa is normal.

▶ General Considerations

The term *inflammatory bowel disease* (IBD) encompasses a collection of gastrointestinal diseases that medical and surgical specialists treat in a collaborative fashion. Chapter 2 discusses genetic and immunologic factors influencing the development of IBD. Chapter 3 describes medical therapy for IBD. This chapter discusses the indications and types of surgery used for ulcerative colitis and Crohn's disease.

In general, these diseases are first treated with medications, and surgery is recommended after medical therapy has been exhausted. However, with certain presentations (eg, anal abscess, toxic colitis), surgery is the first line of therapy, with medication often given after a procedure. Our purpose in this chapter is to survey the surgical procedures used in the treatment of IBD and to discuss indications and timings relating to their use.

Armuzzi A, Ahmad T, Ling KL, et al. Genotype-phenotype analysis of the Crohn's disease susceptibility haplotype on chromosome 5q31. *Gut.* 2003;52:1133–1139. [PMID: 12864271]

Malik TA. Inflammatory bowel disease: historical perspective, epidemiology, and risk factors. *Surg Clin North Am.* 2015;95(6):1105–1122. [PMID:26596917]

ULCERATIVE COLITIS

Ulcerative colitis is usually successfully treated medically; however, it is estimated that between 15% and 30% of patients with ulcerative colitis will ultimately require surgery. Indications for surgery include medically refractory disease (including patients in whom the side effects of the medication are too severe to be endured), severe acute colitis (including hemorrhage and perforation), and cancer or dysplasia of the colorectal mucosa. Given that ulcerative colitis is a disease limited to the colon and rectum, one needs to remember that it is possible to "cure" this disease with surgical intervention.

Further, in most patients, success rates of surgical therapy are high, and sphincter-sparing options exist. Despite the use of new therapies such as biologics and small molecules, the incidence of surgery has not significantly changed in the past few years.

Before discussing the specific indications for surgery, several general issues relating to the patient with colitis need to be reviewed.

1. Ileal Pouch Anal Anastomosis (IPAA) or Ileostomy?—

When surgery is recommended for a patient with colitis, the surgeon needs to assess whether the patient is ultimately a candidate for a sphincter-sparing surgery that avoids a permanent ileostomy. Most patients are candidates for an ileo-anal procedure (see later discussion), but some are not. The main considerations in determining whether a patient should have an ileostomy or a sphincter-sparing procedure include age, gender, type of job, and lifestyle. For example, an older woman who has had several children may at presentation to the surgeon already have some fecal incontinence issues. As difficult as it may be for the patient's body image, recommending an ileoanal procedure in this patient would do her a disservice because it is highly likely that there would be significant fecal leakage and hygiene issues. Further, if a patient has a job or hobby that does not allow for access to a bathroom, an ileostomy may provide for a better quality of life than an ileoanal procedure.

2. Emotional support and education—

When surgery is recommended, the patient—and on occasion the medical team—may feel a sense of failure. In addition, the patient often has a significant fear of the procedure and the possible need for a permanent ostomy. The medical team, surgeon, and support staff need to be cognizant of this perception. Reassurance and education about the upcoming process is the best approach. Availability of support staff, such as an ostomy nurse, and discussions with previous patients who have undergone the procedure are extremely helpful in improving the patient's outlook on the surgery.

3. Immunosuppression—

The ill colitis patient is often referred to the surgeon after all immunosuppressive options have been exhausted. Surgical outcomes regarding infection and wound healing can be significantly affected by immunosuppressive medications. The gastroenterologist, surgeon, and patient should discuss whether any medications can be stopped before the procedure without risk of a significant disease flare. It often is not realistic to wean a patient off all immunosuppressive medications prior to surgery. In particular, many patients require and should remain on corticosteroids if these medications are necessary to avoid a significant exacerbation of a flare. Although patients undergoing surgery for IBD are at increased risk of developing surgical site infections (SSI), recent studies have shown that the addition of biologics to the treatment of ulcerative colitis has not increased the risks of postoperative complications.

4. Nutrition—

IBD and especially severe colitis can lead to weight loss, protein loss, and malnutrition. The value of intravenous nutrition preoperatively has not been reviewed in many years, and may not be beneficial compared to oral nutrition. Choice of operation is also affected by the nutritional status of the patient.

5. Medical comorbidities—

Although colitis usually affects younger patients, the medical comorbidities of the patient need to be reviewed because they may affect the type of procedure recommended. In particular, patients with colitis have an increased incidence of thrombotic complications in the postoperative period; therefore, a low threshold should be set for investigating any preoperative risk or postoperative symptoms for venous thrombosis either of the extremities or the intestinal venous system.

6. Bowel preparation—

Bowel preparation is recommended in any patient undergoing a colon resection. Recent studies have shown that mechanical preparation with oral antibiotics decreases the risk of SSI. We therefore recommend, when possible, that colitis patients undergo mechanical bowel preparation with oral antibiotics followed by administration of preoperative intravenous antibiotics to cover aerobic and anaerobic bacteria.

Oshima T, Takesue Y, Ikeuchi H, et al. Preoperative oral antibiotics and intravenous antimicrobial prophylaxis reduce the incidence of surgical site infections in patients with ulcerative colitis undergoing IPAA. *Dis Colon Rectum.* 2013;56:1149–1155. [PMID: 24022532]

Seo M, Okada M, Yao T, Furukawa H, Matake H. The role of total parenteral nutrition in the management of patients with acute attacks of inflammatory bowel disease. *J Clin Gastroenterol.* 1999;29(3):270–275. [PMID: 10509955]

▶ Indications for Surgery

A. Acute Colitis

Ideally operations for ulcerative colitis should be performed in a staged and deliberate manner. However, some patients develop severe acute colitis, requiring emergent surgical intervention.

Acute colitis is a term used to describe a series of signs and symptoms that include rapid onset of abdominal pain, bloody diarrhea, abdominal distention and tenderness, anorexia, fever, tachycardia, leukocytosis, and low urine output. It is important to remember that most of these patients use corticosteroids and other immunosuppressive agents that may mask the severity of many clinical symptoms. Severe colonic dilation or toxic megacolon is a feared complication of therapy that can lead to perforation, stool spillage, sepsis, and even death. Although acute colitis may occur in patients with known ulcerative colitis, it can also present as the heralding sign of colonic pathology in a patient not previously diagnosed with ulcerative colitis. Surgery is indicated for patients who exhibit signs of visceral perforation, generalized peritonitis, sepsis, or massive gastrointestinal bleeding. In addition, patients who do not improve despite maximized medical therapy after approximately 72 hours often require emergent operation. Other patients, who improve with medical treatment while NPO but who then deteriorate once an oral diet is resumed, often require surgery. The differential diagnosis of acute colitis includes *Clostridium difficile* infection, infectious diarrhea, and cytomegalovirus colitis. These conditions can coexist with and complicate ulcerative colitis. It is important to rule out these diseases, when possible, because their successful medical treatment can avoid an urgent or emergent surgical procedure. At times, however, the combination of baseline colitis and these secondary colitides necessitates an emergency procedure.

The choice of operation for an emergent procedure is discussed later in this chapter. In most cases, the goal of the surgeon is to "get in and get out." Typically, a total colectomy with ileostomy and Hartmann pouch (the oversewn rectum) is performed. This procedure can be completed quickly, removes about 90% of the large intestine, and avoids a complex pelvic dissection and anastomosis. The procedure also does not eliminate further treatment options for the patient; for instance, a sphincter-sparing ileoanal anastomosis can still be performed at a later date.

B. "Subacute" Colitis: Failure of Medical Therapy

Subacute colitis describes a disease pattern in which the patient is neither acutely ill with an unmistakable indication for resection, nor in remission and symptom free. Patients who experience symptoms of chronic intractable disease such as recurring acute colitis, steroid dependence, chronic fecal urgency, growth retardation, persistent active disease, or complications of medical therapy (eg, diabetes, hypertension, peptic ulcer disease, psychosis, myopathy, osteonecrosis, and cataracts) often benefit from surgical intervention. The long-term side effects of some of the new biologic medications have not yet been determined, and the patient, gastroenterologist, and surgeon need to balance the risks of long-term medical therapy against those of surgery. Again, it should be emphasized that one can "cure" ulcerative colitis with surgery, and most patients have an excellent quality of life without the need for medications. However, a small percentage of patients fail surgical therapy with a sphincter-sparing procedure and require an ileostomy, and some develop pouchitis, a postoperative condition that is rarely debilitating but can require chronic treatment.

C. Dysplasia or Cancer

In addition to the failure of medical management, dysplasia or cancer is an indication for surgery in patients with ulcerative colitis. Patients with IBD are at increased risk of colorectal cancer (CRC). The risk of CRC in ulcerative colitis depends on the duration of the disease, extent of disease and age at onset. A population-based study in the United States estimated that the risk of cancer was significantly increased in those with extensive disease or pancolitis (standardized incidence ratio [SIR] 2.4, 95% CI 0.6–6.0). In addition, patients with ulcerative colitis complicated by primary sclerosing cholangitis (PSC) may be at increased risk for CRC compared with those without PSC. A case-control study in which cases and controls were matched for the extent and duration of disease found that the risk of CRC was reduced with use of anti-inflammatory agents (including aspirin, nonsteroidal anti-inflammatory drugs, and 5-aminosalicylic acid [5-ASA] agents) and by surveillance colonoscopy, while it was increased in patients with a history of postinflammatory pseudopolyps.

Patients with disease extending to the hepatic flexure or more proximally have the greatest risk of CRC. Compared with an age-matched population, the risk begins to increase 8–10 years after the onset of symptoms. The approximate cumulative incidence of CRC is 5–10% after 20 years and 12–20% after 30 years of disease. Lower rates of CRC have also been found, and the risk may be decreasing over time with improved medical therapy and surveillance.

In one series, the absolute risk of CRC in patients with pancolitis was 30% after 35 years of disease. The risk was increased in those with the onset of symptoms prior to age 15. However, in other reports, the age of onset of colitis did not increase the risk of CRC after adjusting for the longer period of time that young patients were at risk and the extent of the disease.

Most studies have found that the risk of CRC increases after 15–20 years (~ one decade later than in pancolitis) in patients with colitis confined to the left colon (ie, distal to the splenic flexure). However, rates of CRC and dysplasia similar to those seen in patients with pancolitis have been described. Finally, patients with ulcerative proctitis and proctosigmoiditis are probably not at increased risk for CRC.

Although optimal surveillance strategies for colon cancer in patients with IBD vary by medical society, the following recommendations for patients with ulcerative colitis have been issued by American Society for Gastrointestinal Endoscopy (ASGE). All patients should undergo colonoscopy within 8 years of developing symptoms, and repeat every 1–3 years. However, the presence of active inflammation, anatomic abnormality (stricture, multiple pseudopolyps), history of dysplasia, family history of CRC in first-degree relative, or PSC merits annual surveillance. The American Gastroenterological Association (AGA) and American College of Gastroenterology (ACG) have slightly varied recommendations.

With new endoscopic technologies, the optimal surveillance strategy varies by organization, but often involves high-definition while light colonoscopy with random biopsies or chromoendoscopy with targeted biopsies.

Clarke WT and Feuerstein JD. Colorectal cancer surveillance in inflammatory bowel disease: practice guidelines and recent developments. *World J Gastroenterol.* 2019;25(30):4148–4157. [PMID:31435169]

Lutgens MW, van Oijen MG, van der Heijden GJ, Vleggaar FP, Siersema PD, Oldenburg B. Declining risk of colorectal cancer in inflammatory bowel disease: an updated meta-analysis of population-based cohort studies. *Inflamm Bowel Dis.* 2013; 19(4):789–799. [PMID: 23448792]

SCENIC international consensus statement on surveillance and management of dysplasia in inflammatory bowel disease. *Gastrointest Endosc* 2015;81:489–501.e26

Shergill AK, Lightdale JR, Bruining DH, et al. The role of endoscopy in inflammatory bowel disease. *Gastrointest Endosc.* 2015;81(5):1101–1121.e1113. [PMID: 25800660]

Velayos FS, Loftus EV Jr, Jess T, et al. Predictive and protective factors associated with colorectal cancer in ulcerative colitis: a case-control study. *Gastroenterology.* 2006;130:1941–1949. [PMID: 16762617]

▶ Surgical Options

The choice of operation(s) for a patient with ulcerative colitis is dependent on the presenting condition (emergent vs urgent vs elective), general issues previously discussed, and the experience of the surgeon. The choices include proctocolectomy and creation of an ileoanal anastomosis with a pouch (IPAA), proctocolectomy with end ileostomy, proctocolectomy and continent ileostomy (Koch pouch or variation), and in rare cases, total abdominal colectomy with ileorectal anastomosis.

Another surgical issue is how to stage these procedures. Can the procedure be completed in one operation, or does it require a two-stage or three-stage approach? Finally, in patients undergoing IPAA, should the anorectal mucosa that lines the sphincter complex and distal rectal wall just proximal to the dentate line be "stripped," or should 0–3 cm of this mucosa be left intact and the pouch stapled to this anorectal cuff?

Many factors are taken into account when the surgeon and patient choose an operation, including age, comorbidities, patient size, extent of disease, and patient preference. Ultimately, however, surgery results in complete removal of the colon and rectum, and near complete removal of the proximal anal mucosa, which effectively eliminates the disease.

A. Emergency Surgery

When an emergency operation is indicated, the best surgical option consists of total colectomy, end ileostomy, and the Hartmann pouch (stapling or sewing off the stump of the rectum). As mentioned, this procedure avoids a pelvic dissection, removes most of the large intestine, avoids an anastomosis, and does not eliminate any future options. The procedure also is used in patients in whom the diagnosis of ulcerative colitis is not clear. If the differential diagnosis includes Crohn's disease, indeterminate colitis, or *C difficile* or other infectious colitis, this procedure should be performed;

the eventual surgical choice can then be discussed after the pathologist has been able to examine the whole specimen. On extremely rare occasions, the surgeon's only option is a diverting ileostomy. The indication for this procedure is a patient who is hemodynamically unstable on the operating room table.

B. Ileoanal J Pouch Procedure

In the ileoanal J pouch procedure, the colon and rectum are removed in either one or two stages, and a reservoir is created using the distal ileum. This reservoir or pouch is then anastomosed to the anus in one of two ways: either with a hand-sewn anastomosis combined with stripping of the distal rectal mucosa down to the dentate line, or with a specialized stapling device that leaves 0–3 cm of distal rectum. The pouch procedure (IPAA) is a very attractive option because it not only removes the diseased areas, but it also allows the patient to remain continent and with normal anal defecation. It is usually performed as a two-stage operation: the first stage involves a complete proctocolectomy with ileoanal J pouch anastomosis and temporary diverting ileostomy, and the second (final) stage involves removal of the diverting ileostomy and restoration of intestinal continuity. The IPAA can also be performed after a patient has had emergency surgery (see later discussion). Once a patient has recovered sufficiently, both medically and psychologically, from an emergency total colectomy, the surgeon can proceed to removal of the remaining rectum and creation of the pouch. After creation of the IPAA a temporary diverting ileostomy is fashioned, and then later taken down. This series of procedures would be a 3-stage approach.

The purpose of the pouch in the IPAA is to provide a reservoir for stool as a means of decreasing the frequency of bowel movements. There are several different configurations for an ileoanal pouch. The most common shape is the J pouch, so named because it resembles the letter "J." The J pouch is created by folding the end of the oversewn ileum back on itself by 12–15 cm and then creating a common channel between the limbs via the apex of the J. The procedure can be performed with a surgical stapling device, which is quick and reliable. The pouch has an increased capacity, which then allows for a decreased frequency of bowel movements. The J pouch is anastomosed to the anus or very distal rectum through the opening at the apex that had been used to create the reservoir.

Several other pouch configurations (S, W, Q, etc) exist; however, one pouch shape rarely has an advantage over another. The S pouch is the only other configuration that is commonly used. To create an S pouch, the distal ileum is folded on itself three times for 8–10 cm, with the most distal limb having a short "spout." The spout is anastomosed to the anus. The key technical issue with the S pouch is to make sure the spout is not too long, since this can lead to difficulties in emptying of the pouch. Typically the spout is no longer than 2 cm.

In most patients, after creation of the pouch and the ileoanal anastomosis, a temporary diverting loop ileostomy is constructed.

The goal is to decrease the pelvic sepsis rate from a suture line leak either at the ileoanal anastomosis or along the suture or staple lines of the pouch. Pelvic sepsis rates and sequela may decrease when a temporary diverting ileostomy is used. Because pelvic sepsis can lead to poor pouch function and, in women, can lead to significant rates of infertility, the diversion is nearly always performed (ie, in >95% of all patients undergoing IPAA). In carefully selected patients, however, this temporary diversion can be eliminated. These patients tend to be thin and well nourished, tend to undergo a stapled anastomosis, and are not receiving immunosuppressive medications. The majority of pouches are performed as part of a 2-stage or 3-stage procedure, and are individualized based on patient factors such as nutrition status, comorbities, disease severity, indication for operation, use of corticosteroids, and also surgeon preference.

Pachler FR, Bisgaard T, Mark-Christensen A, Toft G, Laurberg S, et al. Impact on Fertility After Failure of Restorative Proctocolectomy in Men and Women With Ulcerative Colitis: A 17-Year Cohort Study. *Dis Colon Rectum.* 2020;63(6):816–822. [PMID:32149783]

C. Total Proctocolectomy and End Ileostomy

The IPAA is not suitable for all patients. For example, in patients who do not have sufficient anal sphincter function, an ileoanal J pouch may lead to involuntary soilage and leakage of stool. In these patients, the best surgical option is proctocolectomy with end ileostomy. This procedure removes all of the large bowel, including the colon, rectum, and anal glands, which are lined with columnar mucosa, thereby removing any subsequent risk of inflammation or carcinoma. It is usually performed as a one-stage procedure and, because there are no suture or staple lines, is often performed without major septic complications.

The disadvantage of the procedure is that it obligates the patient to a permanent ileostomy. Any stoma can have an effect on the patient's body image; however, this decrease in quality of life is counterbalanced by the overall increase in well-being that results from elimination of the disease. Additionally, for patients who have had problems with fecal incontinence, an ostomy can bring a significant improvement in quality of life.

Total proctocolectomy and end ileostomy are indicated in the following cases: poor anal sphincter control, those who need chemoradiation for cancer treatment, body habitus (ie, obese patients) that precludes an IPAA, prior small bowel resection, severe dysplasia or cancer in the distal rectal mucosa, and patient preference.

D. Continent Ileostomy

Another surgical option for patients with ulcerative colitis is total proctocolectomy and continent ileostomy. This procedure combines a total proctocolectomy with complex pouch and nipple configuration of the distal ileum. The nipple valve is sutured flush with the abdominal skin, and the pouch is then emptied using a catheter at regular intervals. Although ideal in theory, the continent ileostomy is associated with many complications, including fistulization, valve necrosis, prolapse of the valve, extrusion of the valve, dessusception, and incontinence. Additionally, the continent pouch uses significant amounts of distal ileum and if revised or removed, can result in significant loss of small bowel. This procedure is usually performed only at specialized centers, and its complexity and complication rate make it a rare choice for patients who need surgery for colitis.

E. Total Abdominal Colectomy with Ileorectal Anastomosis

In select patients with limited rectal involvement, compliant rectum, and no dysplasia or cancer, total abdominal colectomy with ileorectal anastomosis can be considered. This spares the patient a pelvic dissection and the associated potential complications such as sexual and urinary dysfunction, and decreased fertility in women, and usually allows for better postoperative function compared to IPAA. However, patients must be vigilant with surveillance endoscopy, and understand the potential need for medical therapy for proctitis. Completion proctectomy may become necessary in a significant number of patients for refractory disease or dysplasia/cancer.

F. Laparoscopic Approach

As with all colonic surgery, laparoscopic techniques can be applied to surgery for ulcerative colitis. The use of laparoscopic instruments does not, however, lead to a significant difference in hospitalization. Although the time to discharge may be decreased in patients undergoing a segmental colon resection, in those undergoing total colectomy or total proctocolectomy, the length of stay is often the same for both laparoscopic and open surgery. The laparoscopic procedure does have some advantage in cosmesis. The overall length of the small incisions is less than the incision length for open surgery, and sometimes the main laparoscopic incision can be placed low on the abdomen in a transverse manner so it can be hidden below a belt or panty line. The laparoscopic procedure is best reserved for thin patients who are undergoing an elective procedure. Larson and colleagues studied the functional outcome of laparoscopic-assisted versus open IPAA and found equivalent results for frequency and consistency of stool, medication usage, daytime and nocturnal incontinence, and quality of life in regard to social life, home life, family, travel, sports, recreation, and sex life.

Andersson P, Norblad R, Soderholm JD, Myrelid P. Ileorectal anastomosis in comparison with ileal pouch anal anastomosis in reconstructive surgery for ulcerative colitis–a single institution experience. *J Crohn's Colitis.* 2014;8(7):582–589. [PMID: 24315777]

Abdalla M, Norblad R, Olsson M, et al. Anorectal function after ileorectal anastomosis is better than pelvic pouch in selected ulcerative colitis patients. *Dig Dis Sci.* 2020;65(1):250–259. [PMID: 31372911]

Ishii H, Hata K, Kishikawa J, et al. Incidence of neoplasias and effectiveness of postoperative surveillance endoscopy for patients with ulcerative colitis: comparison of ileorectal anastomosis and ileal pouch-anal anastomosis. *World J Surg Oncol.* 2016;14:75. [PMID: 26960982]

Larson DW, Dozois EJ, Piotrowicz K, et al. Laparoscopic-assisted vs. open ileal pouch-anal anastomosis: functional outcome in a case-matched series. *Dis Colon Rectum.* 2005;48:1845–1857. [PMID: 16175324]

G. Fertility Considerations in Female Patients

Female patients requiring restorative proctocolectomy are usually in their reproductive years at the time of surgery. Cornish and colleagues reviewed the effect of restorative proctocolectomy on sexual function, urinary function, fertility, pregnancy, and delivery. They found that the incidence of dyspareunia increases after restorative proctocolectomy. There was a decrease in fertility, although pregnancy was not associated with an increase in complications. Vaginal delivery is safe after restorative proctocolectomy, and pouch function after delivery returns to pregestational function within 6 months.

Cornish JA, Tan E, Teare J, et al. The effect of restorative proctocolectomy on sexual function, urinary function, fertility, pregnancy and delivery: a systematic review. *Dis Colon Rectum.* 2007;50:1128–1138. [PMID: 17588223]

CROHN'S DISEASE

Crohn's disease can affect the entire gastrointestinal tract, from mouth to anus. It may be confined to the colon alone or involve only the anal canal. Segmental involvement, rectal sparing, fistulas, perianal disease, strictures, and abscess formation are all characteristics of granulomatous colitis. Characteristic "fat creeping" (subserosal extension of fat around the surface of the bowel) and prominent vascularity in the serosa are characteristics of the disease seen on gross inspection. The disease usually affects the bowel in a segmental fashion, leaving so-called skip lesions. Ulcerations and bowel wall thickening occur with areas of sparing in between pathologic areas. Fistulas often form in Crohn's disease and may involve small or large bowel, bladder, vagina, uterus, ureter, or skin, most commonly originating from the mesocolic (rather than antimesocolic) border of the bowel. Histologically, the three primary findings in Crohn's colitis are transmural inflammation and fibrosis, granulomas, and narrow, deeply penetrating ulcers or fissures.

The majority of patients with Crohn's disease require surgery during the course of their disease; surgical interventions are required in up to two thirds of CD patients during their lifetime. In general, surgery is indicated primarily for complications of the disease, including abscess, fistula, perforation, stricture, obstruction, perianal disease, dysplasia or cancer. The decision to operate involves consideration of symptom severity, medical treatment failure or side effects, and operative risks.

Crohn's disease involves the small bowel in 80% of patients. Ileocolitis is present in about 50% of patients, and 25% have ileitis alone. Twenty-five percent of patients have disease limited to the colon. One third of patients have perianal disease.

Gajendran M, Loganathan P, Catinella AP et al. A comprehensive review and update on Crohn's disease. *Dis Mon* 2018;64(2):20–57. [PMID: 28826742]

▶ Abscess

Intra-abdominal abscess may form as a result of perforation of the bowel, most commonly seen in the ileocecal area. Antibiotics and percutaneous drainage (abscess >3cm) are the mainstays of initial treatment. Surgical drainage is reserved for failure or inability to drain percutaneously. Successful percutaneous drainage may obviate the need for future surgical resection, but is often used as a bridge to surgical resection, often resulting in a decrease in complications.

Free perforation with uncontrolled sepsis and peritonitis with hemodynamic instability is an indication for immediate surgery.

▶ Fistula

Given the transmural nature of Crohn's disease, enteric fistulas may form from diseased bowel to other organs or skin. Initial management involves imaging, control of sepsis/abscess if present, resuscitation, antibiotics, and skin protection. Some asymptomatic internal fistulas (ie, between closely adjacent loops of bowel) may not necessarily require treatment. Symptomatic fistulas, however, require treatment, and this involves resection of the diseased bowel, and either repair of the uninvolved ("innocent bystander") organ, or simply allowing healing by secondary intention. Intestinal bypass should be avoided because it leaves behind persistent disease in the bypassed segment, and hence risk of abscess, perforation, bacterial overgrowth or malignancy. Enterocutaneous fistulas can cause significant morbidity and mortality, and require a multidisciplinary approach including surgeons, gastroenterologists, wound care nurses, and nutritionists. Initial management includes resolution of sepsis, resuscitation, nutrition optimization, medical therapy, and local skin care. Surgical intervention should be delayed until the patient's condition is optimized.

Hirten RP, Shah S, Sachar DB, et al. The management of intestinal penetrating Crohn's disease. *Inflamma Bowel Dis.* 2018;19;24(4):752–765. [PMID: 29528400]

Stricture

Patients with Crohn's disease can develop strictures from intestinal fibrosis, and although it can involve any intestinal segment, it most commonly involves the terminal ileum and ileocolonic region. Anastomotic strictures can also occur. Surgery is indicated when the structuring leads to obstruction, or when cancer is found or suspected. If endoscopic dilation is not possible or indicated, surgery in the form of stricturoplasty or resection is warranted. Endoscopic dilation may be considered for anastomotic strictures, or short (<5cm) strictures without fistula, abscess, or malignancy, especially when bowel preservation is needed. Repeat dilation is often needed.

Stricturoplasty may be indicated in patients with diffuse fibrotic stricture involvement of the small bowel, prior extensive small bowel resection, short bowel syndrome, and recurrent strictures within 12 months of previous operation. Contraindications to striicuroplasty include presence of phlegmon, abscess, fistula, preoperative malnutrition, suspected carcinoma, and multiple strictures in a short segment. The type of stricturoplasty performed depends on number and type of strictures present, as well as length of stricture. The Heineke-Mikulicz stricturoplasty is most commonly performed, and is ideal for short strictures less than 10 cm in length. Safety and efficacy of stricturoplasty compared to resection have been similar. The risk of Crohn's disease recurrence is similar for stricturoplasty and resection.

Stricturoplasty is not recommended for colonic strictures. Colonic strictures that cannot be endoscopically surveyed thoroughly require oncologic segmental resection given the risk of malignancy.

Ambe R, Campbell L, Cagir B. A comprehensive review of stricureplasty techniques in Crohn's disease: types, indications, comparisons, and safety. *J Gastrointest Surg* 2012;16(1):209–217 [PMID: 21909847]

Chan WPW, Mourad F, Leong RW. Crohn's disease associated strictures. *J Gastroenterol Hepatol.* 2018;33(5):998–1008. [PMID: 29427364]

Cancer and Dysplasia

There is an increased risk of colorectal carcinoma in patients with Crohn's compared to the general population, 0.5/1000 patient years duration in the United States, or about 2- to 3-fold increase. Possible risk factors include, younger onset IBD, longer disease duration, extent of disease, PSC, severity of inflammation, and family history of CRC. Colonoscopic surveillance should be tailored appropriately. Total proctocolectomy is generally recommended once cancer is found given the risk of multifocal dysplasia and metachronous cancers. Although there is ongoing debate regarding dysplasia, the presence of high grade dysplasia is often considered an indication for total proctocolectomy as well. Management of low grade dysplasia found on colonoscopy is controversial and must be tailored to the patient.

Carchman E. Crohn's Disease and the Risk of Cancer. *Clin Colon Rectal Surg.* 2019;32(4):305–313. [PMID: 31275078]

Kiran RP, Nisar PJ, Goldblum JR, et al. Dysplasia associated with Crohn's colitis: segmental colectomy or more extended resection? *Ann Surg* 2012;256(2):221–226. [PMID: 22791098]

Ileocolic Disease

Ileocecal Crohn's disease may masquerade as appendicitis. Traditionally, patients found to have terminal ileitis at laparotomy for presumed appendicitis, and who have a normal cecum, undergo appendectomy, leaving the diseased ileum in place. However, recent studies demonstrate that the majority of patients found to have Crohn's disease at laparotomy for appendicitis required early ileocolic resection; therefore, the traditional advice to leave the diseased bowel in place may be reconsidered.

The ileocecal region is the most common site of Crohn's disease. The diagnosis of ileocolic Crohn's disease may be delayed up to 1 year. The second surgery rate for ileocolic disease is 44% over 10 years, and the rates have not changed significantly with the introduction of biologics and other therapies given postoperatively as "maintenance" therapy.

Surgical Options for Colonic Crohn's

If emergency surgery is indicated, such as in the case of toxic megacolon or acute fulminant colitis, total colectomy with end ileostomy is the procedure of choice. Complex pelvic dissection should be avoided as well as anastomosis.

In patients with Crohn's colitis, depending on the focality of disease, either a segmental colectomy or total colectomy can be performed. In a meta-analysis comparing segmental colectomy with total colectomy for colonic Crohn's disease, there was earlier recurrence after segmental colectomy.

For patients with proctitis without colonic involvement, a proctectomy with intersphincteric dissection is performed.

In patients with refractory disease of both the colon and rectum, or who have malignant lesions in either the colon or rectum, a total proctocolectomy with end ileostomy is the procedure of choice. Ileal pouch anal anastomosis is generally not recommended in patients with Crohn's disease given the high rate of pouch failure.

Tekkis PP, Purkayastha S, Lanitis S et al. A comparison of segmental vs subtotal/total colectomy for colonic Crohn's disease: a meta-analysis. *Colorectal Dis.* 2006;8(2):82. [PMID: 16412066]

Yamamoto T, Watanabe T SO. Surgery for luminal Crohn's disease. *World J Gastroenterol.* 2014;20(1):78–90. [PMID: 24415860]

Perianal Crohn's Disease

The rectum and anal region can be involved in this chronic IBD, either together (as rectal and perianal Crohn's disease) or as separate entities, and the perianal disease often heralds the onset of intestinal symptoms of Crohn's disease. Perianal disease on its own has a better prognosis than disease associated with rectal involvement. However, it is important that definitive diagnosis be confirmed by histologic examination, as ulcerative colitis and Crohn's disease share similar features. Perianal involvement is present in 3.8–80% of patients, as seen in literature reviews (refer to Armuzzi and colleagues; McClane and Rombeau, listed later), and it recently has been cited as a distinct phenotype of Crohn's disease by identification of a susceptibility locus on chromosome 5.

There is a wide spectrum of presentation of perianal disease, with the perianal skin appearing bluish in active disease. Superficial ulcers may extend into the anal canal or be present on edematous fleshy tags protruding from the anal verge. These ulcers may be painless, whereas deep cavitating ones in the upper anal canal can be painful, causing abscesses and fistulas. The anus can be distorted with fistulizing disease and is sometimes described as a "watering can anus." Pain and swelling are common findings, and individuals with fistulas have persistent purulent discharge, pain, and possibly bleeding as well as fever and a preceding history of abscess development. The external opening on the skin is evident, and on digital rectal examination, anoscopy, or proctoscopy, an indurated area in the anal canal corresponding to the internal opening may be obvious. The involved rectal mucosa has a characteristic thickened, nodular feel and a congested and granular appearance.

Perianal Crohn's disease can manifest as edematous skin tags, fissures, abscesses, fistulas, and strictures. Long-standing perianal disease increases the risk for anal squamous cell cancer and adenocarcinoma.

An assessment of perianal Crohn's disease activity can be made by inquiring about discharge, pain, restriction of sexual activity, type of perianal disease, and degree of induration. A thorough assessment of intestinal pathology should be undertaken to determine the extent and severity of the disease, because terminal ileal disease sometimes manifests as a perianal fistula, and at other times, medical treatment of intestinal disease improves the outcome or healing of local surgery of perianal disease. Finally, pelvic MRI may be helpful in evaluation of complex perianal disease.

Armuzzi A, Ahmad T, Ling KL, et al. Genotype-phenotype analysis of the Crohn's disease susceptibility haplotype on chromosome 5q31. *Gut.* 2003;52:1133–1139. [PMID: 12865271]

Basu A, Wexner SD. Perianal Crohn's disease. *Curr Treat Options Gastroenterol.* 2002;5:197–206. [PMID: 12003714]

McClane SJ, Rombeau JL. Anorectal Crohn's disease. *Surg Clin North Am.* 2001;81:169–183. [PMID: 11218163]

Indications for Surgery

Traditionally, owing to poor or delayed healing, a conservative approach to the management of perianal Crohn's disease has been followed. Surgical procedures range from simple suppurative drainage to proctocolectomy and ileostomy, the latter reserved for intractable disease or complications associated with intestinal disease.

Indications for local surgery in perianal Crohn's disease include the drainage of pus in abscesses, bothersome fistulas-in-ano that are refractory to medical or nonsurgical management, rectovaginal fistulas, and, in severe proctitis, anal stenosis, or severe recurrent abscesses, proctectomy. It is important to note that medical therapy alone or surgical therapy alone does not have as high a success rate in the treatment of anal fistulae in Crohn's disease as does a combined approach. Surgery, antibiotics, and medical therapy, especially the use of anti-tumor necrosis factor agents used in sequence or combination have shown the best results.

Sciaudone G, Di Stazio C, Limongelli P, et al. Treatment of complex perianal fistulas in Crohn's disease: infliximab, surgery or combined approach. *Can J Surg.* 2010;53:299–304. [PMID: 20858373]

Surgical Options

Abscess

A common emergency presentation of perianal Crohn's disease is abscess formation requiring incision and drainage to allow maximum drainage of sepsis (Figure 4–1). Appropriate antimicrobial coverage is needed when significant cellulitis surrounds the abscess, or the patient is immunocompromised or has cardiac valvular pathology. A cruciate incision or an elliptical excision of skin overlying the area of maximum fluctuance is undertaken under general anesthesia if the abscess cavity is large. Any loculations are then gently broken up with a digit, and the wound is loosely packed (Figure 4–1A). This approach should suffice for superficial abscesses. For deep or high abscesses, placement of a mushroom or Malecot catheter allows adequate drainage and thus prevents premature closure of the surgical incision (Figure 4–1B).

At this time an examination to find any fistulas is undertaken under anesthesia. Usually a probe is inserted through the external opening to delineate the fistulous tract. If any resistance to the passage of the probe is encountered, care is taken to avoid creating false passages. If the internal opening is not evident, injection of dilute methylene blue dye or hydrogen peroxide into the external opening with an angiocatheter may facilitate visualization. The track, if found, is curetted, and a loose seton is inserted to allow drainage. The seton is a thread of foreign material that is passed through

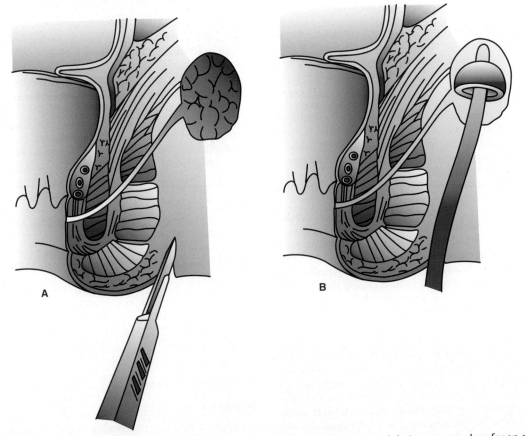

▲ **Figure 4–1.** Surgical approach to perianal abscess drainage. **A.** Simple incision and drainage procedure for an abscess. **B.** Incision and drainage followed by placement of a mushroom drainage catheter for an abscess. (Reproduced with permission from Schwartz DA, Pemberton JH, Sandborn WJ. Diagnosis and treatment of perianal fistulas in Crohn's disease. *Ann Intern Med.* 2001;135(10):906–918.)

a fistula tract and tied into a loop. (Silastic tubing or a vessel loop is preferred because they are soft and can remain in place for prolonged periods.) Drainage of sepsis decreases the risk of further abscess formation and avoids iatrogenic incontinence due to division of any sphincteric muscle, particularly in high anal fistula.

These simple procedures alleviate pain and improve the quality of life in most patients. They also permit magnetic resonance imaging or endoanal ultrasonographic imaging of the anus to delineate more complex fistula tracks or distorted anorectal anatomy. Later, as the sepsis resolves, a more definitive surgical procedure may be undertaken.

Some patients require long-term seton drainage because of the risk of complications that may occur with surgery (eg, delayed wound healing and incontinence). However, healing of the perianal pathology occurs with removal of the seton in some patients (Figure 4–2).

Surgical procedures for treating fistula-in-ano in patients with Crohn's disease vary, depending on the severity of symptomatology and the complexity of the fistulous track. The

following guidelines are suggested: (1) Asymptomatic fistulas need not be treated immediately. However, they often reclose at the level of the skin, and placement of a draining seton is often required to keep the tract open. (2) Simple, low fistulas may be treated by fistulotomy. (3) Complex fistulas may be well palliated with long-term draining setons. (4) Complex fistulas may be treated with advancement flap closure if the rectal mucosa is grossly normal (or with placement of a porcine plug, or with a LIFT [ligation of intersphincteric fistula tract] procedure.)

Simple low fistulas with a single external opening can be treated medically (antibiotics, anti-NF alpha), and often do not require surgical intervention.

Seton Placement

A loose draining seton is often the first step in perianal fistulizing Crohn's disease, combined with medical treatment. The seton promotes drainage and prevents recurrence of abscess. Medications include antibiotics, azathioprine/6-mercaptopurine, anti-TNF-α therapy (infliximab, adalimumab), or other biological

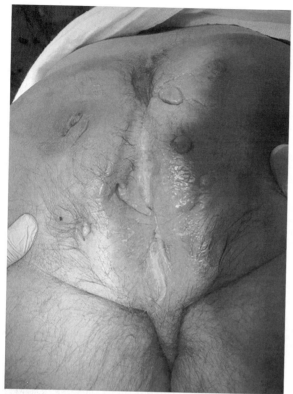

▲ **Figure 4–2.** Photo of perianal fistulas in a patient with perianal Crohn's disease. (Reproduced with permission from Vitaliy Poylin, MD.)

agents. This approach can achieve a complete or partial healing in the majority of cases. The seton is removed after several doses of biologic; exact timing is subjective. For more complex disease, setons may be left in much longer. Cutting setons should be avoided in Crohn's disease.

Fistulotomy

Fistulotomy involves laying open the fistula tract and merging it with the anal canal. This allows the tissues to heal from the inside out. Primary fistulotomy in Crohn's disease patients with low, simple fistulas demonstrates excellent healing rates, particularly in the absence of rectal disease. The procedure is contraindicated for complex and high fistulas where division of a large proportion of the anorectal sphincter would be necessary.

Person B, Wexner SD. Management of perianal Crohn's disease. *Curr Treat Options Gastroenterol.* 2005;8:197–209. [PMID: 15913509]

Rojanasakul A, Pattanaarun J, Sahakitrungruang C, et al. Total anal sphincter saving technique for fistula-in-ano; the ligation of intersphincteric fistula tract. *J Med Assoc Thai.* 2007;90:581–586. [PMID: 17427539]

Rutgeerts P. Review article: treatment of perianal fistulizing Crohn's disease. *Aliment Pharmacol Ther.* 2004;20(suppl 4):106–110. [PMID: 15352905]

Schwartz DA, Pemberton JH, Sandborn WJ. Diagnosis and treatment of perianal fistulas in Crohn's disease. *Ann Intern Med.* 2001;135:906–918. [PMID: 11712881]

Singh B, McMortenson NJ, Jewell DD, et al. Perianal Crohn's disease. *Br J Surg.* 2004;91:801–814. [PMID: 15227686]

Endoanal Advancement Flap

In patients with rectal-sparing disease and no inflammation, endoanal advancement flap may be an option. It is usually attempted after seton drainage so there is a mature tract.

An endoanal advancement flap consists of anal mucosa, submucosa, and usually part of the underlying circular muscle. The base of the flap should be twice the width of its apex to ensure adequate blood supply for healing. A curvilinear flap is most commonly used. It involves a semicircular incision starting at the dentate line and continuing proximally for 4–5 cm. The fistula tract is cored out, and the fistula is closed in layers, with mobilization of the flap. The diseased distal portion of the flap is trimmed before the flap is sutured to the mucosal edge of the anus. Success rates have been reported around 64% with incontinence rates around 9%.

Ali Soltani A, Kaiser AM. Endorectal advancement flap for cryptoglandular or Crohn's fistula-in-ano *Dis Colon Rectum* 2010;53(4):486–495 [PMID: 20305451]

An anocutaneous flap is another option for closing the internal opening. It has the theoretical advantage of not involving any sphincter and can be a more feasible option than an endoanal flap if the internal opening is located distally or if the anal canal is changed by stenosis or scarring after previous surgery or inflammation.

Ligation of Intersphincteric Fistula Tract (LIFT)

In this procedure, the surgeon divides the transphincteric fistula tract in the intersphincteric groove after a mature fistula tract has formed with use of a draining seton. Success rates in small studies with Crohn's patients are not as high as in non-Crohn's patients, and are <50%.

Emile SH, Kahn SM, Adejumo A et al. Ligation of intersphincteric fistula tract (LIFT) in treatment of anal fistula: An updated systematic review, meta-analysis, and meta-regression of the predictors of failure *Surgery.* 2020;167(2):484–492. [PMID: 31648932]

Fecal diversion—Diversion of the fecal stream by the creation of an ileostomy or a colostomy has been employed to manage anal fistulas in Crohn's disease, an approach first reported by Truelove. A loop defunctioning stoma, which should be easy to reverse, is constructed either laparoscopically or by open surgery. The decrease in fecal flow through the rectum and across the fistula tract allows the rectal mucosa to heal and the fistula to close. Creation of the stoma may improve the results of subsequent anal procedures, and also allows the patient to adjust to the prospect that life with a stoma is feasible. Symptomatic improvement after diversion is not predictable, and new manifestations of perianal Crohn's disease can develop. Approximately 50% of patients with symptomatic perianal Crohn's disease require permanent fecal diversion.

There are limited indications for fecal diversion in Crohn's disease. These include severe perianal sepsis, deep persistent anal ulceration, and complex anorectal or rectovaginal fistula, as well as complications refractory to medical and local surgical measures. In some patients, fecal diversion can be considered before commencement of combination medical therapy. Initially there is a high rate of perianal healing with reversal of the stoma in patient with rectal-sparing disease. However, in individuals with rectal or colonic Crohn's involvement, restoration of bowel continuity almost invariably leads to recurrence of perianal symptoms, eventually necessitating proctectomy.

Galandiuk S, Kimberling J, Al-Mishlab TG, et al. Perianal Crohn's disease: predictors of need for permanent diversion. *Ann Surg.* 2005;241:796–801. [PMID: 15849515]

Yamamoto T, Allan RN, Keighley MR. Effect of fecal diversion alone on perianal Crohn's disease. *World J Surg.* 2000;24:1258–1262. [PMID: 11071572]

Proctectomy

Patients with active anorectal disease who fail to respond to medical and previous surgical therapy may require proctectomy with end colostomy. Rates of 10–18% have been reported. Patients who also have colonic involvement require proctocolectomy with permanent end ileostomy. In ill or high-risk patients, this may be performed in two stages, with colectomy and end ileostomy comprising the first procedure, followed by completion proctectomy. In contrast to an abdominoperineal resection for rectal cancer, an intersphincteric dissection may be considered for the perineal component, as this leaves a smaller, more vascularized wound that heals with less morbidity. However, deep fistulating disease or sepsis may make this impossible. When a tension-free closure is not possible, the use of rectus abdominis, gluteal myocutaneous, and gracilis transposition flaps promote healing.

A recognized complication of proctectomy is a persistent perineal sinus. In such cases, it is important to rule out pelvic sepsis or an enteroperineal fistula, which would require resection of the affected bowel. Some patients experience phantom sensations after proctectomy that are analogous to those occurring after limb amputation. Explanation and reassurance is usually sufficient to allay patients' concerns.

Persistent perineal pain after proctectomy can be troublesome and may be caused by a neuroma.

Rius J, Nessim A, Noguerasa JJ, et al. Gracilis transposition in complicated perianal fistula and unhealed perineal wounds in Crohn's disease. *Eur J Surg.* 2000;166:218–222. [PMID: 10755336]

Plug and Glue

For longer, more complex fistulae with no evidence of anal sepsis, a porcine plug can be placed in the tract. The tract is usually curetted of all granulation tissue, and the plug is sutured to the anorectal wall with the rectal mucosa covering the plug. The conically shaped plug, made of porcine collagen, is pulled into the primary tract through the internal opening until it fills out the whole length of the tract. Both ends of the plug are secured with sutures, and at the internal opening, the end of the plug is covered with mucosa and also preferably with internal sphincter. The remaining external opening is left open for drainage. Champagne and colleagues reported a success rate of 83% with a median follow-up of 12 months for high cryptoglandular anal fistulas, and the method has also been used in a smaller group of patients with Crohn's fistulas reported by O'Connor and colleagues. However the exact place that these modalities have in the management of Crohn's fistula remains unclear, but their use does not preclude other surgical procedures should the treatment fail. Success rates are low, and the plug is often extruded.

Recent innovative therapy involves the use of adhesive products. Several studies have reported on fibrin glue treatment of anal fistula using both autologous fibrin tissue adhesives and commercially available fibrin glue. The adhesive is instilled in the fistula tract after curetting, and sometimes irrigation of the tract, to allow glue adhesion to the tissue. Insertion of the fibrin glue is continued until glue appears at the internal opening of the fistula. The sealant not only acts as a closing plug for the fistula, but also as the substrate for the in-growth of fibroblasts. The technique is not suitable for fistulas with extensions.

The reported success rates in patients have varied from 40% to 85%, with a mean of 67% for the various materials. Buchanan and colleagues reported long-term healing of only 14%, whereas Sentovich showed a healing rate of 60% when all patients had a draining seton preoperatively and the internal opening was closed with a suture at the time of glue instillation. In a later review by Swinscoe and colleagues of 12 studies, the overall healing rate was 53%. However, in patients with Crohn's disease, fistula results have been considerably lower. Recent data have shown no value in using fibrin glue over fistula surgery without glue. Currently, we do not recommend or use fibrin glue for the treatment of fistulae. All of these techniques for complex fistulae have a lower success rate with Crohn's disease. Success is improved when there is no evidence of anorectal sepsis and with quiescent rectal disease.

Lewis RT and Bleier JIS. Surgical Treatment of anorectal Crohn's disease. *Clin Colon Rectal Surg.* 2013;26(2):90–99. [PMID: 24436656]

Fissures

While idiopathic fissures occur in the posterior midline (90%) or anterior midline (10%), Crohn-associated fissures can occur anywhere in the anal canal, often off midline (Figure 4–3). Anal fissures in Crohn's disease may be asymptomatic, while ulcers are more likely to be painful. Medical management is the mainstay of treatment, including vasodilators and botulinum toxin. Lateral internal sphincterotomy is generally avoided given the risk of nonhealing wounds and incontinence.

Hemorrhoids and Skin Tags

Asymptomatic fissures, hemorrhoids, and skin tags in Crohn's patients should be left alone, and if surgery is requested, the patient should be informed of complications such as poor healing, stenosis, incontinence, and ulcer formation. Anal ulcers are likely to be worsened by surgery, and a trial with medical therapy should be instituted to promote healing. Symptomatic strictures should be cautiously dilated with Hegar dilators or an endoscopic balloon, as perforation is a risk. The stricture may be primary or occur as a complication of anorectal or ileal pouch surgery performed on the basis of an incorrect preoperative diagnosis of ulcerative colitis or indeterminate colitis. Severe strictures that do not respond to dilation may require an advancement flap (in low anal strictures) or ultimately fecal diversion or proctectomy (in anorectal stenosis).

Given the unpredictable disease process of perianal Crohn's fistulas and the variety of surgical options, management should be individually tailored, using combined medical and surgical approaches to offer the patient an improved quality of life.

Buchanan GN, Bartram CI, Phillips RK, et al. Efficacy of fibrin sealant in the management of complex anal fistula: a prospective trial. *Dis Colon Rectum.* 2003;46:1167–1174. [PMID: 12972959]

Champagne BJ, O'Connor LM, Ferguson M, et al. Efficacy of anal fistula plug in closure of cryptoglandular fistulas: long term follow-up. *Dis Colon Rectum.* 2006;49:1817–1821. [PMID: 17082891]

Cintron JR, Park JJ, Orsay CP, et al. Repair of fistulas-in-ano using fibrin adhesive: long-term follow-up. *Dis Colon Rectum.* 2000;43:944–949. [PMID: 10910240]

Johnson EK, Gaw JU, Armstrong DN. Efficacy of anal fistula plug vs. fibrin glue in closure of anorectal fistulas. *Dis Colon Rectum.* 2006;49:371–376. [PMID: 16421664]

Lindsey I, Smilgin-Humphreys MM, Cunningham C, et al. A randomized, controlled trial of fibrin glue vs. conventional treatment for anal fistula. *Dis Colon Rectum.* 2002;45:1608–1615. [PMID: 12473883]

Loungnarath R, Dietz DW, Mutch MG, et al. Fibrin glue treatment of complex anal fistulas has low success rate. *Dis Colon Rectum.* 2004;47:432–436. [PMID: 14978618]

O'Connor L, Champagne BJ, Ferguson MA, et al. Efficacy of anal fistula plug in closure of Crohn's anorectal fistulas. *Dis Colon Rectum.* 2006;49:1569–1573. [PMID: 16998638]

Pogacnik JS and Salgado G. Perianal Crohn's disease. *Clin Colon Rectal Surg.* 2019;32(5):377–385. [PMID: 31507348]

Sentovich SM. Fibrin glue for anal fistulas: long-term results. *Dis Colon Rectum.* 2003;46:498–502. [PMID: 12682544]

Swinscoe MT, Ventakasubramaniam AK, Jayne DG. Fibrin glue for fistula-in-ano: the evidence reviewed. *Tech Coloproctol.* 2005;9:89–94. [PMID: 16007368]

Cancer

Patients with long-standing Crohn's disease, like those with ulcerative colitis, are at increased risk of developing adenocarcinoma as well as squamous cell carcinomas. This increased risk has been attributed to an early onset and prolonged duration of disease. The incidence of carcinoma is much lower in patients with perineal Crohn's disease. Patients with adenocarcinoma require proctectomy. Those with squamous cell carcinoma may be considered for chemoradiotherapy; however, the functional outcome may be unsatisfactory. Therefore, proctectomy may be the preferred option. The diagnosis is usually made based on examination of biopsy specimens and brushings of the curetted fistulous tract.

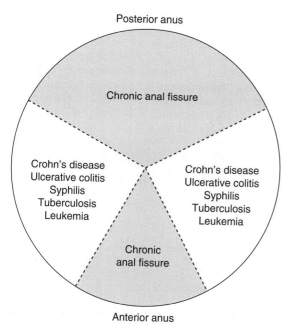

Posterior anus

Chronic anal fissure

Crohn's disease
Ulcerative colitis
Syphilis
Tuberculosis
Leukemia

Crohn's disease
Ulcerative colitis
Syphilis
Tuberculosis
Leukemia

Chronic anal fissure

Anterior anus

▲ **Figure 4–3.** Common locations of chronic anal fissures and other anal conditions.

Acute Diarrheal Disorders

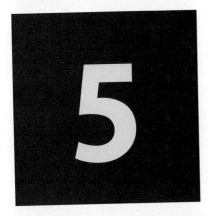

Rahul S. Dalal, MD, MPH

Jerry S. Trier, MD

Jessica R. Allegretti, MD, MPH

ESSENTIALS OF DIAGNOSIS

▶ High fever, frequent bloody stools, severe abdominal pain, dehydration, and no improvement after 3–4 days of initial supportive treatment are worrisome features.

▶ Sigmoidoscopy and biopsy are indicated in patients with bloody dysenteric stools and tenesmus lasting more than 3–4 days.

▶ Upper endoscopy and biopsy are indicated in patients with persistent diarrhea and evidence of malabsorption.

▶ Routine stool cultures aid in identifying *Salmonella*, *Shigella*, and *Campylobacter* but rarely provide useful information if diarrhea develops 2–3 days after hospitalization.

▶ Clinical features of shigellosis, salmonellosis, and *Campylobacter* colitis (diarrhea, tenesmus, fever, abdominal cramps) often overlap.

▶ Consider *Clostridioides difficile* infection after both recent and remote (within 3 months) use of antibiotics and if diarrhea develops during hospitalization.

▶ Severe *C difficile* infection is categorized by a white blood cell count >15,000/mm^3 and a serum creatinine >1.5mg/dL.

▶ Consider enterohemorrhagic *Escherichia coli* (*E coli* O157:H7) in patients with bloody diarrhea, abdominal pain, leukocytosis, and little or no fever, especially if uremia or microangiopathic anemia develops; if suspected, avoid antibiotics.

▶ Giardiasis and cryptosporidiosis are best diagnosed using stool immunoassays directed against *Giardia* and *Cryptosporidium* antigens which are more sensitive than microscopic stool examination.

ACUTE DIARRHEA

▶ General Considerations

Acute diarrheal diseases remain a major global public health problem, responsible for nearly 2 million deaths annually. Most deaths occur in low-income countries and many occur in infants and young children. The majority of acute diarrheal episodes reflect gastrointestinal infections, but medications, food intolerances, or the abrupt onset of chronic disease may be causative (Table 5–1). In the United States, acute diarrheal diseases are a major health and economic problem resulting in between 150 and 300 million total episodes, 900,000 hospitalizations, and approximately 6000–12,000 deaths per year.

Acute diarrheal diseases are second only to respiratory infections as a cause of time lost from work in the United States. As a symptom, diarrhea can be defined as an increase in frequency, volume, and often urgency of the passage of stool and as a decrease in stool consistency. More objectively as a sign, diarrhea is the passage of three or more unformed stools in 24 hours or an increase in stool mass to greater than 250 g in 24 hours. Acute diarrheal disease is generally defined as having begun within 14 days of presentation; diarrhea that persists for between 14 and 30 days is considered persistent and diarrhea that lasts more than 30 days is considered chronic.

DuPont HL. Acute infectious diarrhea in immunocompetent adults. *N Engl J Med*. 2014;370(16):1532–1540. [PMID: 24738670]

Thielman NM, Guerrant RL. Clinical practice. Acute infectious diarrhea. *N Engl J Med*. 2004;350:38–47. [PMID: 14702526]

GBD 2016 Diarrhoeal Disease Collaborators. Estimates of the global, regional, and national morbidity, mortality, and aetiologies of diarrhoea in 195 countries: a systematic analysis for the Global Burden of Disease Study 2016. *Lancet Infect Dis*. 2018;18(11):1211–1228. [PMID: 30243583]

Table 5–1. Major causes of acute diarrhea.

Viral infections
Bacterial infections
Parasitic infections
Medication related
 Laxatives
 Antibiotics
 Antacids
 Nonsteroidal anti-inflammatory agents
 Nutritional supplements
 Others (colchicine, gold, and many more)
Food related
 Allergies (shellfish)
 Additives (sulfites)
 Sorbitol
 Carbohydrate intolerances
Abrupt onset of chronic disease
 Inflammatory bowel disease
 Celiac disease
 Irritable bowel syndrome

▶ Pathogenesis

A. Normal Absorption and Secretion

Under normal circumstances, adults ingest approximately 2 L of fluid per day. An additional 7 L of endogenous secretions from salivary, gastric, pancreatic, biliary, and enteric sources enter the intestine for an approximate 24-hour load of 9 L. Ingested nutrients are dissolved or suspended in this 9-L fluid load. The healthy small intestine will absorb about 7.5 L, largely in the duodenum and jejunum. Of the 1.5 L that traverse the ileocecal valve, the colon absorbs approximately 1.3 L, resulting in a stool mass of no more than 200 g/24 hours. The maximum absorptive capacity of the small intestine is about 12 L and that of the colon, 4–6 L, for a total of 18 L; roughly double the normal daily fluid load.

B. Major Mechanisms of Diarrhea

An increased fluid load sufficient to overwhelm the intestinal and colonic absorptive capacity of about 12 L usually results in diarrhea. Excessive endogenous fluid secretion is the usual culprit, but excessive fluid intake may contribute. Examples of diseases that cause diarrhea by excessive secretion include cholera, toxigenic *E coli* infection, or, rarely, a vasoactive intestinal peptide-secreting tumor (Table 5–2).

Table 5–2. Major mechanisms of diarrhea.

Enhanced mucosal secretion
Impaired epithelial absorptive and digestive activity
Increased permeability of the epithelial barrier
Decreased absorptive surface
Altered motility
Increased intraluminal osmolarity

Epithelial cell absorptive and digestive function in the small and large intestine is impaired and permeability of the epithelial barrier is increased by the mucosal damage caused by a variety of gastrointestinal viral, bacterial, and protozoal infections. In addition, the available absorptive surface may be reduced as in, for example, rotavirus and norovirus enteritis and in giardiasis. Increased intraluminal osmolality is a cause of acute diarrhea. Ingestion of poorly absorbed or nonabsorbable laxatives such as magnesium citrate or magnesium hydroxide or polyethylene glycol 3350 are the classic examples, but impaired nutrient absorption in some intestinal infections contributes to diarrhea by increasing intraluminal osmolality. All of the mechanisms detailed above may be causative in acute diarrheal diseases in which there is substantial mucosal inflammation as occurs in most invasive and some toxigenic bacterial enterocolitides. If mucosal inflammation is mild or absent, as in cholera, enhanced fluid secretion, altered permeability, enhanced motility, or, in the case of laxative ingestion, increased intraluminal osmolality are the major mechanisms.

▶ Clinical Findings

A. Symptoms and Signs

A careful history and physical examination are crucial in the evaluation of patients presenting with acute diarrhea and should provide information as to the possible nature, underlying cause, and severity of the diarrhea. Historical points that should be explored include (1) any recent travels; (2) the nature of recent food ingestion, including type, preparation (fully cooked, rare, or raw), and location (home, restaurant, or street vendor); (3) occurrence of a similar illness among recent contacts; (4) medication history, especially new medications or past or current use of antibiotics; (5) sexual history; and (6) predisposing conditions, such as compromised immune status.

The character of the diarrhea also provides clues as to the site of involvement by the process causing the diarrhea. A large stool volume with little urgency, no tenesmus, and only a moderate increase in stool number suggests involvement primarily of the small intestine and more proximal colon, whereas frequent, low-volume dysenteric stools containing blood and mucus associated with urgency and tenesmus suggest disease involving the rectum and distal colon. Although a patient's subjective description of the nature of the diarrhea is helpful, examination of the stool by the clinician is most useful.

On physical examination, the presence or absence of fever should be determined. Hypotension, orthostasis, tachycardia, poor skin turgor, and dry mucous membranes indicate dehydration, a major cause of morbidity and mortality in acute diarrheal diseases, especially in the young and the elderly. A careful abdominal examination is essential to assess for evidence of localized abdominal infections (eg, appendicitis or diverticulitis) that may be associated with diarrhea. The abdomen should also be assessed for distention, which might suggest megacolon, and for the presence of peritoneal signs.

Switaj TL, Winter KJ, Christensen SR. Diagnosis and management of foodborne illness. *Am Fam Physician.* 2015;92(5):358–365. [PMID: 26371569]
DuPont HL. Approach to the patient with infectious colitis. *Curr Opin Gastroenterol.* 2012;28:39–46. [PMID: 22080825]

B. Laboratory Findings

The majority of patients with acute diarrhea in developed countries have relatively mild, self-limited illness, which resolves in a day or two and requires no specific diagnostic studies. A major goal of the initial assessment, including the history and physical examination, is to identify patients who have more serious disease meriting prompt and specific diagnostic studies and aggressive treatment (Figure 5–1). Worrisome features include high fever (>101.3°F), dehydration, frequent bloody stools with tenesmus (dysentery), severe abdominal pain, an immunosuppressed host, and no improvement in or progression of symptoms after 3–4 days of supportive treatment (see Figure 5–1). Useful tests for further evaluation include assessment of stool for fecal leukocytes or leukocyte markers such as lactoferrin or calprotectin, stool culture, blood culture, stool examination for ova and parasites, stool testing for *C difficile* toxin, endoscopy and mucosal biopsy, and in selected cases, abdominal imaging studies.

1. Fecal leukocytes, stool lactoferrin, and stool calprotectin—Examination of stool suspensions stained with methylene blue for the presence of fecal leukocytes is a time-honored test for evaluation of patients with acute diarrhea. Neutrophils are usually present in patients with dysenteric stools (containing blood and mucus) caused by infection with invasive bacteria (Table 5–3) and colitides unassociated with infection, as can occur in acute onset or during acute exacerbations of inflammatory bowel disease (IBD). In other words, the presence of neutrophils indicates the presence of an inflammatory colitis or enterocolitis but not its cause. Thus, the test lacks specificity for infectious colitis, and its reported sensitivities for invasive bacterial infections are only in the range of 60–70%, in part because the presence of neutrophils in stools is variable in patients with diarrhea caused by *Salmonella* or *Yersinia* infection. Fecal leukocytes are usually absent from the watery stools caused by viral infections and toxin-producing bacteria with exceptions being *C difficile*- and cytomegalovirus-induced enterocolitis, in which fecal neutrophils may be present (see Table 5–3). Fecal leukocytes are destroyed in the setting of amebiasis, therefore the presence of bloody diarrhea in the absence of fecal leukocytes can suggest this etiology.

Despite its limitations, fecal leukocyte testing remains worthwhile and, if positive, helps select patients who merit more extensive diagnostic evaluation and possibly empiric

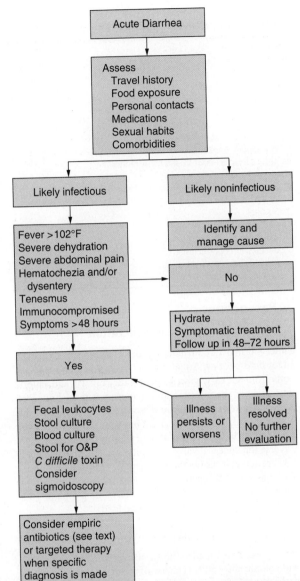

▲ **Figure 5–1.** Algorithm showing the approach to the patient with acute diarrhea. O&P, ova and parasites.

antibiotic therapy. Fecal lactoferrin and fecal calprotectin, surrogate markers for fecal neutrophils, can be measured using latex agglutination and enzyme-linked immunosorbent assay (ELISA). The tests have been used most widely in assessing patients with IBD. They appear to be more sensitive, less observer dependent, but more costly than the conventional fecal leukocyte assay. Falsely positive results for fecal lactoferrin may occur in breast-fed infants.

2. Stool culture—The indications for and cost-effectiveness of obtaining stool cultures from patients with acute diarrhea are still being debated. However, there is general consensus

Table 5–3. Fecal leukocytes in infectious diarrhea.[a]

Usually Present	Usually Absent	Variable
Shigellosis	Noroviruses	Salmonellosis
Campylobacter	Rotavirus	Noncholera vibrios
Invasive Escherichia coli	Vibrio cholerae	Clostridium difficile
	Enterotoxic E coli	Yersinia
	Enterohemorrhagic E coli	Cytomegalovirus
	Staphylococcus or Bacillus cereus food poisoning	
	Giardiasis	
	Amoebiasis	

[a]Fecal leukocytes are also present in noninfectious colitides such as active ulcerative colitis.

that too many are obtained. Most surveys report an incidence of positive stool cultures in only 1.5–3% of submitted stools with an estimated cost of more than $1000 per positive culture. As indicated earlier, most episodes of acute diarrhea are self-limited and resolve within 48–72 hours, often before the results of a stool culture are available. Stool cultures are rarely informative in nonimmunosuppressed patients who develop diarrhea 3 or more days after hospitalization.

Stool cultures should be obtained from patients with severe dehydration, fever exceeding 102°F (38.9°C), dysenteric stools, and stools that contain neutrophils, and from those in whom the culture may ultimately guide therapy. Stool cultures should also be obtained from all immunosuppressed patients who develop diarrhea or patients with other severe comorbidities, including acute IBD flares. Stool cultures should be obtained for epidemiologic purposes from food service workers or if an outbreak of diarrheal disease is suspected.

Once obtained, the stool specimen should be sent to the laboratory as soon as possible to minimize false-negative results. The clinician should also be cognizant of which organisms are identified by the particular laboratory performing the culture. In some laboratories, only *Salmonella*, *Shigella*, and *Campylobacter* are identified during routine processing. Hence, the clinician should specify other organisms if suspected, such as *Yersinia*, enterohemorrhagic *E coli* (EHEC), *Aeromonas*, or noncholera *Vibrio*, so that proper media and culture conditions are used.

3. Blood culture—Blood cultures should be obtained from patients with high fever, those with shaking chills, and those who are immunosuppressed.

4. Stool examination for ova and parasites—The yield of positive examinations for ova and parasites is low among patients with acute diarrhea as most parasitic infestations that cause diarrhea cause symptoms lasting several weeks or more. Indications for assessment include diarrhea that persists for more than 2 weeks, a history of travel to areas endemic for parasitic disease, exposure of children to day care centers or summer camps, a concomitant history of immunosuppression (HIV, chemotherapy, immunosuppressive

drugs), known IBD, men who have sex with men, and unexplained peripheral eosinophilia. As ova and parasites can be passed intermittently, optimal testing requires prompt examination of each of three specimens collected on separate days. If giardiasis or cryptosporidiosis is suspected, ELISAs or immunochromatographic assays that detect *Giardia* and/or *Cryptosporidium* antigens are superior to conventional microscopic examination of the stool, with sensitivity of 80–90% and >90% specificity.

5. *Clostridioides difficile* toxin—The recently reported rising incidence and increased morbidity and mortality of *C difficile* colitis (see later discussion) underscores the importance of *C difficile* toxin testing of the stool for timely diagnosis and implementation of therapy for this important disease. Groups at risk and, hence, indications for the test include patients who have received recent or even distant antibiotic therapy, patients who develop diarrhea in a hospital or other institutional setting, immunosuppressed patients, and patients with IBD with worsening diarrhea. Community-acquired cases even in the absence of known recent antibiotic use are being increasingly recognized.

The cytotoxicity assay using cultured fibroblasts has been the gold standard for testing for *C difficile* toxin, with sensitivity of approximately 70–90% and almost absolute specificity. However, the test is costly and requires 2–3 days for completion. More commonly used available testes are enzyme immunoassays (EIAs) for *C difficile* toxins A and B, EIA for clostridial glutamate dehydrogenase (GDH) which screen for clostridia but not its toxins, polymerase chain reaction (PCR) for toxin genes which have high sensitivity but have been associated with false positives and direct culture of *C difficile*, the latter of use for epidemiologic studies. A stepwise approach is now recommended, first screening with a highly sensitive test with either clostridial GDH or PCR for toxin genes, followed by a specific test, the EIA for toxin A and B.

Crobach MJ, Dekkers OM, Wilcox MH, Kuijper EJ. European Society of Clinical Microbiology and Infectious Diseases (ESCMID): data review and recommendations for diagnosing *Clostridium difficile*-infection (CDI). *Clin Microbiol Infect.* 2009;15(12):1053–1066. [PMID: 19929972]

DuPont HL. Diagnosis and management of *Clostridium difficile* infection. *Clin Gastroenterol Hepatol.* 2013;11:1216–1223. [PMID: 23542332]

Riddle MS, DuPont HL, Connor BA. ACG Clinical Guideline: diagnosis, treatment, and prevention of acute diarrheal infections in adults. *Am J Gastroenterol.* 2016;111(5):602–22. [PMID: 27068718]

C. Endoscopy and Biopsy

Sigmoidoscopy and biopsy can be very useful in selected patients with acute diarrhea. Sigmoidoscopy is indicated in patients with bloody, dysenteric stools and tenesmus lasting more than 3–4 days. The endoscopic appearance of the mucosa is often indistinguishable in patients with acute infectious diarrhea caused by invasive organisms compared with patients with IBD, but in such patients, it provides some information as to extent and severity of disease. Additionally, rectosigmoid biopsies may help distinguish acute infectious diarrhea from diarrhea caused by an acute flare of IBD (Plates 1 and 2). Sigmoidoscopy can also help exclude ischemic colitis, which may present with abdominal pain and bloody diarrhea. Sigmoidoscopy can provide a rapid, tentative diagnosis of *C difficile* colitis if the characteristic pseudomembranous lesions are present, although important to note these are not typically present in patients with IBD even when *C difficile* is the cause of the diarrhea. Additionally, sigmoidoscopy can provide rapid diagnosis of amoebiasis if secretions from the edge of ulcers are examined microscopically and the organism is seen. Mucosal biopsy from immunosuppressed patients may detect cytomegalovirus or herpetic proctocolitis. Upper endoscopy is indicated in patients with persistent diarrhea and malabsorption and, through examination of duodenal aspirates and mucosal biopsies, may detect parasitic infections including giardiasis, cryptosporidiosis, *Cystoisospora* infection, and occasionally strongyloidiasis.

Shen B, Kahn K, Ikenberry SO, et al. ASGE Guidelines. The role of endoscopy in management of patients with diarrhea. *Gastrointest Endosc.* 2010;71:887–892. [PMID: 20346452]

D. Imaging Studies

Imaging studies are usually not required in patients with uncomplicated acute diarrhea. An abdominal flat and upright film may be useful if there is worrisome abdominal distention in order to screen for toxic megacolon, which can occur in *C difficile* colitis and colonic amoebiasis. On occasion, computed tomography (CT) or ultrasound scan of the abdomen and pelvis may be indicated, if there is associated severe abdominal pain, tenderness, or evidence of peritoneal irritation as may occur in, for example, *Yersinia* enterocolitis, to exclude a focal intra-abdominal or pelvic process.

▶ Treatment

A. General Principles

Some general principles of treatment of acute diarrhea are summarized next. When specific therapy of a defined cause of acute diarrhea is indicated as, for example, for *C difficile* colitis, such treatment is described later, in the section titled "Acute Diarrheal Disease Caused by Specific Infections."

B. Treatment of Dehydration

Oral rehydration therapy will suffice in most patients who develop acute diarrhea. In milder cases, juices, broth, and water along with salted crackers usually suffice. If dehydration is more severe, oral rehydration fluids should be utilized. The World Health Organization (WHO) recommends the following formula per liter of water:

    2.6 g sodium chloride

    2.5 g sodium bicarbonate or 2.9 g trisodium citrate

    1.5 g potassium chloride

    13.5 g glucose or 27 g sucrose

Several oral rehydration solutions in addition to that recommended by the WHO are commercially available. Rehydrate closely mimics WHO oral rehydration solutions, whereas others (Pedialyte, Enfalyte) contain less sodium and may require intake of a larger volume. Maintaining a 1:1 molar ratio of sodium to carbohydrate facilitates sodium transport in diarrheal diseases in which the enteric sodium–glucose cotransport mechanism remains intact as, for example, in cholera or enterotoxigenic *E coli* (ETEC) infection. Some clinicians favor preparations formulated with complex carbohydrates such as rice-based solutions (CeraLyte). The WHO recommends zinc supplementation of oral rehydration solutions for children (10 mg/day for infants <6 months old; 20 mg/day for children >6 months old), but there are no recommendations for adults due to lack of data.

Intravenous hydration is often over-utilized in developed countries such as the United States. However, if diarrhea is massive and dehydration severe, especially in infants and young children, the elderly, and patients unable to rehydrate orally due to nausea, vomiting, or other comorbidities, intravenous rehydration is indicated. Serum electrolyte levels should be closely monitored, and imbalances corrected.

Aisenberg GM, Grimes RM. Computed tomography in patients with abdominal pain and diarrhoea: does the benefit outweigh the drawbacks? *Intern Med J.* 2013;43(10):1141–1144. [PMID: 24134171]

Atia A, Buchman AI. Oral rehydration solutions in non-cholera diarrhea: a review. *Am J Gastroenterol.* 2009;104:2596–2604. [PMID: 19550407]

Ofei SY, Fuchs GJ 3rd. Principles and practice of oral rehydration. *Curr Gastroenterol Rep.* 2019;21(12):67. [PMID: 31813065]

C. Antidiarrheal Drugs

The antimotility agent loperamide can be used with caution to provide symptomatic relief in patients without high fever, colonic distention, or dysenteric stools. The usual dose is 4 mg initially followed by 2 mg every 4–6 hours, as required for persistent diarrhea, not to exceed 16 mg/24 hours. Absorption may be increased by prolonging contact time of luminal contents with mucosa, although oral fluid intake should be continued. Fluid may pool in the gut lumen as antimotility agents do not decrease intestinal secretion. Diphenoxylate has also been used but is less desirable as it crosses the blood-brain barrier and has central opiate actions. Antimotility drugs should generally be avoided in patients with dysentery, and no antimotility drug should ever be used if the possibility of toxic megacolon is a concern. Moreover, there is some evidence that suggests that the use of antimotility agents, while reducing the number of stools, may prolong the course of some enteric infections, including those caused by *Shigella* and ETEC, perhaps by prolonging the time required for clearance of causative organisms and toxins from the gut. Bismuth subsalicylate reduces stool number, but there is no evidence that fecal fluid losses are decreased significantly.

D. Empiric Antibiotic Therapy

Although a controversial topic, antibiotics are overutilized in acute infectious diarrhea. Most episodes are self-limited and clear within 2–4 days or less without specific therapy; hence, most patients would derive little or no benefit and risk potential harm if antibiotics were indiscriminately prescribed. Their use predisposes to the development of resistant organisms. They provide no benefit in viral diarrhea caused by rotaviruses or noroviruses and may be harmful in EHEC infections, prolong fecal excretion of nontyphoidal *Salmonella*, and precipitate *C difficile* colitis. Their benefit in *Yersinia*, *Campylobacter*, and *Aeromonas* infections is controversial.

Generally accepted indications for the use of an empiric antibiotic include fever greater than 102°F (38.9°C) and chills, febrile dysentery, traveler's diarrhea that is severe or affects an individual in whom a shortened duration of illness is urgent, individuals with severe dehydration and prolonged, severe diarrhea (1 week or more), and the immunocompromised host. Quinolones are widely used for empiric treatment; macrolides such as azithromycin or erythromycin and, for travelers, rifaximin are alternatives.

Antibiotics should be avoided in patients with bloody stools, abdominal pain, but little or no fever until EHEC has been excluded from consideration.

E. Specific Antibiotic Therapy

Recommendations regarding antibiotic therapy for specific pathogens that cause acute infections are discussed in the next section.

Pawlowski SW, Warren CA, Guerrant R. Diagnosis and treatment of acute or persistent diarrhea. *Gastroenterology.* 2009;136: 1874–1886. [PMID: 19457416]

ACUTE DIARRHEAL DISEASE CAUSED BY SPECIFIC INFECTIONS

As indicated previously, most acute diarrheal disease is caused by transmissible infectious viruses, bacteria, or parasites. Infectious organisms cause disease by a number of mechanisms (Table 5–4). Some actually invade and proliferate in the intestinal epithelium, underlying mucosa, and lymphoid follicles. Others produce tissue-damaging cytotoxins while in the lumen and in contact with the epithelium. Still others elaborate enterotoxins that produce profound functional alterations but no detectable histologic lesion. Some adhere to the epithelial surface and induce epithelial damage and mucosal inflammation without invasion. Finally, still others produce toxins in vitro that, when ingested, induce symptomatic gastrointestinal illness.

The human host has defenses that resist enteric infections. Gastric acid secretion reduces bacterial colonization of the proximal small intestine, and there is evidence that individuals who have had acid-reducing gastric surgery are more susceptible to nontyphoidal salmonellosis and selected other enteric infections. Normal gastric motility is a defense factor; stasis predisposes to intestinal intraluminal bacterial proliferation, and there is evidence that the use of antimotility agents prolongs diarrhea caused by some enteric pathogens. The normal intestinal flora itself is protective. Its alteration by antibiotic therapy predisposes to *C difficile* colitis and reduces the number of organisms required to produce nontyphoidal salmonellosis. Antibodies secreted into the intestinal lumen by the intestine and via the biliary tract appear to play a protective role in reducing colonization of pathogens in the gut.

Table 5–4. Mechanisms of intestinal infections and infestations.

Mechanisms	Examples
Invasive	Rotavirus *Campylobacter* *Salmonella* *Shigella*
Cytotoxic	*Clostridium difficile* Enterohemorrhagic *Escherichia coli*
Enterotoxic	*Vibrio cholerae* Enterotoxigenic *E coli*
Enteroadherent	Enteropathogenic *E coli* Giardiasis
Toxin produced in vitro	*Bacillus cereus* *Staphylococcus aureus*

DuPont HL. Acute infectious diarrhea in immunocompetent adults. *N Engl J Med.* 2014;370(16):1532–1540. [PMID: 24738670]

Musher DM, Musher BL. Contagious acute gastrointestinal infections. *N Engl J Med.* 2004;351:2417–2427. [PMID: 15575058]

1. Viral Infections

A. Noroviruses

Noroviruses are caliciviruses—small, single-stranded RNA viruses that, despite extensive efforts, have not been cultured (Table 5–5). It is estimated that these viruses produce approximately 19–21 million episodes of illness, 56,000–71,000 hospitalizations, and 570–800 deaths annually in the United States. Noroviruses are the leading cause of foodborne disease in the United States. With advent of effective rotavirus vaccines, norovirus disease is now the most common cause of viral gastroenteritis in children as well as adults. Epidemic outbreaks in hospitals, nursing homes, in schools from catered food, in restaurants, and on cruise ships have been widely publicized, but endemic cases also occur. Transmission is via the fecal-oral route through contaminated food and water, from virus-contaminated environmental surfaces, and direct person-to-person contact. After ingestion, noroviruses bind to histo-blood group antigens on the enterocyte surface. The histo-blood group antigens are a major determinant of host susceptibility; nonsecretors are resistant to infection by a majority of strains of norovirus. Histologic studies of volunteers have shown that after ingestion, noroviruses induce a mild to moderate mucosal enteritis in susceptible individuals that peaks in severity approximately 48 hours after viral ingestion and resolves completely within 4–6 weeks or earlier. Lesions of the gastric mucosa were not detected after ingestion of Norwalk agent.

The incubation period is usually 12–48 hours, and clinical symptoms may include nausea, vomiting, watery diarrhea, and abdominal cramps. Fever, if present, is usually mild (<101.5°F [38.6°C]). The duration of clinical symptoms is short, usually ranging from a few hours to 3 days. The characteristic histologic lesion has been observed in asymptomatic volunteers after norovirus ingestion, providing evidence that some infections are subclinical. Routine laboratory studies remain normal unless severe dehydration develops, in which case elevations of blood urea nitrogen and creatinine and leukocytosis may be seen.

The diagnosis depends on the epidemiology and clinical features. A reverse transcription PCR assay and diagnostic immunoassays are available and are used largely to identify outbreaks but are not generally used to diagnose individual patients.

Treatment is supportive and consists of oral rehydration with carbohydrate–electrolyte solutions (see earlier discussion) and, in a small minority of patients with severe dehydration, by intravenous hydration. Symptomatic treatments such as bismuth subsalicylate and loperamide can be used but are usually not needed, and there is little evidence that they significantly influence fecal fluid losses. There is no effective antiviral agent. Attempts to develop an effective vaccine are ongoing and some early phase 2 studies are encouraging.

The prognosis is excellent for this generally self-limited disease, although deaths may occur in association with norovirus gastroenteritis, largely in debilitated, elderly patients with significant comorbidities or in very young children. Appropriate hand hygiene is essential to limit transmission. Similar to the prevention of *C difficile* transmission, soap and water are preferred over alcohol-based hand sanitizers because alcohol does not kill norovirus.

Table 5–5. Viral gastroenteritis.

Feature	Noroviruses	Rotavirus
Size	27 nm	70 nm
Nucleic acid	SS RNA	DS RNA
Age	>2 years	Infants, young children
Transmission	Fecal-oral: food, water	Fecal-oral
Pathologic findings	Mild enteritis	Mild to severe enteritis
Incubation	1–2 days	1–3 days
Duration	1–3 days	5–7 days
Diagnostics	RT-PCR and immunoassays are available; used largely to identify outbreaks	Commercial ELISA, latex agglutination, and RT-PCR assays useful for diagnosis
Treatment	Rehydration as needed	Vigorous rehydration
Vaccine	Several investigational vaccines are being tested	RotaTeq, Rotarix

ELISA, enzyme-linked immunosorbent assay; RT-PCR, reverse transcriptase polymerase chain reaction.

Glass RI, Parashar UD, Estes MK. Norovirus gastroenteritis. *N Engl J Med.* 2009;361:1776–1185. [PMID: 19864676]

Hall AJ, Lopman BA, Payne DC, et al. Norovirus disease in the United States. *Emerg Infect Dis.* 2013;19:1198–1205. [PMID: 23876403]

O'Brien SJ, Sanderson RA, Rushton SP. Control of norovirus infection. *Curr Opin Gastroenterol.* 2019;35(1):14–19. [PMID: 30346315]

Robilotti E, Deresinski S, Pinsky BA. Norovirus. *Clin Microbiol Rev.* 2015;28(1):134–164. [PMID: 25567225]; PMCID: PMC4284304.

B. Rotaviruses

Rotaviruses are a major cause of infectious diarrhea worldwide, accounting for more than 200,000 deaths each year. In the United States, prior to the widespread use of rotavirus vaccines, approximately 2.7 million children developed rotavirus gastroenteritis yearly, resulting in over 50,000 hospitalizations and an estimated 30 deaths. However, there is increasing evidence that with the introduction of effective vaccines in 2006, the incidence of rotavirus infection has decreased dramatically by over 80%.

Rotaviruses are double-stranded RNA viruses (see Table 5–5) whose classification is complex. There are several groups, which, in turn, may contain subgroups and multiple serotypes. Most but not all disease in humans is caused by group A. The virus invades, proliferates in, and destroys enterocytes, resulting in the passage of abundant virions in the stool of infected individuals for 7–10 days; however, virions can be shed for up to 3–4 weeks. Significant enteritis develops, with patchy shortening or even complete loss of villi, crypt hyperplasia, and inflammation of the lamina propria.

Symptomatic illness is more common in winter and occurs largely in infants and young children. Watery diarrhea, which can be profuse, and vomiting are the major symptoms, accompanied by fever in 50% or more of cases. Reinfections in older children and adults are usually asymptomatic or mild but can occasionally cause severe symptoms. Dehydration is a hazard—especially in infants, if diarrhea is accompanied by vomiting that precludes adequate oral fluid intake—and is the major cause of morbidity and death. The illness generally lasts from 4 to 7 days, but more protracted diarrhea has been reported. The diagnosis can be established by demonstrating rotavirus antigen in the stool by specific ELISA, latex agglutination, or PCR assays.

Hydration is the cornerstone of therapy and can often be achieved with oral rehydration regimens containing sugar, salt, and water or commercial oral rehydration formulations unless diarrhea is profuse and accompanied by vomiting, in which case intravenous rehydration may be lifesaving. The American Academy of Pediatrics does not recommend symptomatic therapy, including antimotility drugs, bismuth subsalicylate, and probiotics, for children younger than 5 years. The overall prognosis is excellent, with the vast majority of patients recovering completely within 7–10 days, except as noted earlier.

A pentavalent human-bovine reassortant rotavirus vaccine (RotaTeq) and a monovalent attenuated human rotavirus vaccine (Rotarix) are licensed in the United States. Vaccination is recommended for all infants who have no contraindications. There appears to be a very small increase in the risk of intussusception during the first week after administration of the first vaccine dose but experts agree that the benefits of vaccination greatly outweigh this risk.

Crawford SE, Ramani S, Tate JE, et al. Rotavirus infection. *Nat Rev Dis Primers.* 2017;3:17083 [PMID: 29119972]

Glass RI, Parashar UD. Rotavirus vaccines—balancing intussusception risks and health benefits. *N Engl J Med.* 2014;370: 568–570. [PMID: 24422677]

Kahn MA, Bass DM. Viral infections: new and emerging. *Curr Opin Gastroenterol.* 2010;26:26–30. [PMID: 19907323]

Payne DC, Boom JA, Staat MA. Effectiveness of pentavalent and monovalent rotavirus vaccines in concurrent use among US children <5 years of age, 2009-2011. *Clin Infect Dis.* 2013;57: 13–20. [PMID: 23487388]

C. Other Viruses

Enteric adenovirus causes a rotavirus-like endemic gastroenteritis primarily in children younger than 2 years. Its incubation period is longer than that of rotavirus, but it appears to be less contagious. Astrovirus also causes endemic gastroenteritis primarily in children but also among elderly and immunocompromised adults; occasional multicase outbreaks have been described. Clinically, gastroenteritis caused by adenovirus and astrovirus resembles that caused by rotavirus and norovirus, and the principles of therapy are the same. Diarrhea may also accompany enterovirus and coxsackievirus infections, although manifestations involving other systems often overshadow any accompanying diarrhea.

Whereas cytomegalovirus infections of the gastrointestinal tract notoriously affect immunocompromised patients, as discussed in Chapter 10, occasional cases of cytomegalovirus colitis have been described in apparently immunocompetent adults. In one study, 12 cases over a wide age range were described. Presenting features included hematochezia, diarrhea, and abdominal pain. Endoscopy generally revealed well-demarcated ulcers, and one patient died due to CMV pneumonia (8.3%). When diagnosed, antiviral therapy with agents such as ganciclovir or foscarnet is indicated.

Olortegui MP, Rouhani S, Yori PP, et al. Astrovirus infection and diarrhea in 8 countries. *Pediatrics.* 2018;141(1):e20171326. [PMID: 29259078]

Seo TH, Kim JH, Ko SY, et al. Cytomegalovirus colitis in immunocompetent patients: a clinical and endoscopic study. *Hepatogastroenterology.* 2012;59(119):2137–2141. [PMID: 23435132]

2. Bacterial Infections

Although specific bacterial infections are discussed on the following pages, the presentation of patients with *Shigella*, invasive *E coli*, *Campylobacter*, nontyphoidal *Salmonella*, and in some instances EHEC enterocolitis may be clinically indistinguishable. As a result, the decision about whether or not to begin empiric antibiotic treatment can be difficult. Although antibiotics may be of benefit in a few infections (shigellosis, invasive *E coli*), they have undesirable effects in others (EHEC, uncomplicated nontyphoidal *Salmonella* enterocolitis) and predispose to *C difficile* colitis. Hence, potential benefits versus risks must be weighed carefully.

A. Shigellosis

Shigella species are a major cause of dysenteric infectious colitis, with an estimated annual incidence of 450,000 in the United States. Four pathogenic species have been identified (*Shigella dysenteriae*, *Shigella flexneri*, *Shigella sonnei*, and *Shigella boydii*). Young children are often affected via outbreaks in day care and preschool environments. Disease is caused by direct person-to-person fecal-oral spread or by ingestion of contaminated food or water. The *Shigella* species are acid-resistant; hence, a very small inoculum (≤100 bacteria) can produce disease. The bacteria invade and spread through the epithelium, produce several enterotoxins, including Shiga toxin (*S dysenteriae*), and induce severe, acute inflammation of the mucosa (see Plate 1) probably by causing the release of proinflammatory cytokines. There is no available vaccine.

After an average 3-day incubation period, patients usually develop watery diarrhea, which often rapidly progresses to dysenteric stools with mucus and blood, tenesmus, and, usually, fever. Some patients also develop nausea and vomiting. The severity varies and ranges from watery stools without dysentery or significant fever to severe dysentery with more than 20 low-volume stools per day, abdominal cramps, tenesmus, and high fever. Sigmoidoscopy in patients with dysentery caused by shigellosis is usually grossly indistinguishable from that observed with other dysenteric infections (*Campylobacter*, nontyphoidal *Salmonella*) or a flare of idiopathic IBD. Biopsy can be useful in distinguishing infectious proctocolitis from a flare of idiopathic proctocolitis in that chronic changes such as crypt distortion and dropout are absent despite the presence of substantial inflammation, most prominently in the upper half of the mucosa (compare Plate 1 with Plate 2). Stools from the majority of patients contain neutrophils, and the diagnosis is established by stool culture.

In previously healthy individuals who are not immunosuppressed, shigellosis is usually self-limited and clears within about 1 week without treatment. Antibiotic therapy shortens the duration of symptoms and the fecal shedding of *Shigella* organisms by about 2–3 days and should be considered if fever is high and dysentery is severe or the stool cultures are positive, especially in infants and young children but also in adults. Antibiotic therapy is clearly indicated in patients with bacteremia (<10%), food handlers, elderly or malnourished patients with comorbidities, and the immunosuppressed. If possible, it should be guided by the antibiotic sensitivity of the *Shigella* species isolated from stool or blood culture. If antibiotic susceptibility is unknown, the current treatment of choice is a fluoroquinolone in adults, although reports of resistance to quinolones are appearing especially in Asia, and azithromycin in children younger than 18 years of age. There are reports of decreased susceptibility to azithromycin among men who have sex with men and the HIV population in the United States. Most species remain sensitive to ceftriaxone. In all patients, supportive measures such as hydration are important, but antimotility agents are not recommended as they may prolong symptoms and fecal shedding of *Shigella*.

Gastrointestinal complications are uncommon, but rectal prolapse, toxic megacolon, and even intestinal perforation have been reported. The most common gastrointestinal complication of this and other intestinal bacterial infections appears to be postinfectious irritable bowel syndrome, which occurs in as many as 10% of patients (see Chapter 24). Systemic complications include a sterile reactive arthritis occurring usually 1–2 weeks after the onset of gastrointestinal symptoms. In rare instances associated with *S dysenteriae* infection, the hemolytic uremic syndrome (HUS) with microangiopathic anemia, thrombocytopenia, and acute renal failure develops. In addition, seizures associated with high fever may occur, especially in infants and young children.

Kotloff KL, Riddle MS, Platts-Mills JA, Pavlinac P, Zaidi AKM. Shigellosis. *Lancet*. 2018;391(10122):801–812. [PMID: 29254859]

Kosek M, Yori PP, Olortegui MP. Shigellosis update: advancing antibiotic resistance, investment empowered vaccine development, and green bananas. *Curr Opin Infect Dis*. 2010;23:475–480. [PMID: 20689423]

Heiman KE, Karlsson M, Grass J, et al. Notes from the field: Shigella with decreased susceptibility to azithromycin among men who have sex with men - United States, 2002-2013. *MMWR Morb Mortal Wkly Rep*. 2014;63(6):132–133. [PMID: 24522098]; PMCID: PMC4584870

Shiferaw B, Soglghan S, Palmer A, et al. Antimicrobial susceptibility of Shigella isolates in Foodborne Diseases Active Surveillance Network (FodNet) sites, 2000-2010. *Clin Infect Dis*. 2012;54(suppl 5):S458–S463. [PMID: 22572670]

B. Nontyphoidal Salmonellosis

Salmonella organisms that cause disease in humans are a zoonosis widely distributed throughout the animal kingdom. Salmonellosis is one of the most common causes of foodborne enterocolitis in the United States. Most of the estimated 1.35 million annual cases that occur in the United States result from ingestion of fecally contaminated, incompletely cooked food such as meat (especially poultry and ground beef), eggs, milk and other dairy products, contaminated vegetables, and even processed foods such as peanut butter. Direct person-to-person spread and spread from common and exotic pets, especially reptiles, occur. Outbreaks from contaminated water have been described.

Salmonella typhimurium and *Salmonella enteritidis* are the most common causes in the United States, but other serotypes may be isolated. Unlike *Shigella* organisms, salmonellae are acid-sensitive; hence, a larger inoculum is required for induction of clinical illness. Reduction of gastric acid secretion through surgery, disease, or pharmacotherapy and prior antibiotic treatment that disrupts the normal intestinal flora reduces the number of organisms required to produce infection. The extremes of age, immunosuppression, and malignancy also predispose to infection. Salmonellae adhere to and invade the intestinal epithelium. They enter macrophages, in which virulent forms can survive and then may disseminate to distant sites.

The clinical features of *Salmonella* gastroenteritis are not distinctive and vary from case to case. After a 12–72-hour incubation period, nausea, vomiting, and fever are common early in the course followed by abdominal cramps and diarrhea, which may be voluminous. Dysentery with bloody stools may occur but is less common than in shigellosis, EHEC, or *Campylobacter* enterocolitis. In most healthy adults, the disease is self-limited, with fever abating within 2–3 days and diarrhea lasting no more than 10 days. Clinical features are often more severe in those with predisposing factors such as immunosuppression, in neonates and the elderly, and in those with other comorbidities. As there are no available tests for rapid diagnosis, confirmation awaits a positive stool culture, which requires 2–3 days. Blood cultures should be obtained in those with severe symptoms and those with conditions predisposing to disseminated or recurrent disease.

There is general agreement that antibiotics are not indicated for individuals in good general health with mild to moderate illness who are not at the extremes of age. There is no convincing evidence that such treatment significantly alters the clinical course, and several studies indicate that antibiotic treatment prolongs fecal shedding of nontyphoidal salmonellae. Thus, supportive care with rehydration forms the basis of treatment. Whether immunocompetent patients with more severe and prolonged illness should be treated is somewhat controversial. Some authorities favor a short course of antibiotics, such as 4–7 days of a fluoroquinolone in that setting. Also controversial is whether infected food handlers and health care workers should be routinely treated.

More definite indications for antibiotic treatment include the immunosuppressed host (AIDS, post-transplant, chemotherapy); those with sickle cell disease or known severe atherosclerotic disease, in whom dissemination may cause osteomyelitis or infection of an atherosclerotic plaque; those with vascular grafts or orthopedic prostheses; infants and the elderly, especially those with additional comorbidities. Most authorities would recommend at least 2 weeks of treatment for these high-risk patients, with a choice of antibiotics guided by the antibiotic resistance pattern of the infecting organism and the patient's comorbidities.

CDC. Antibiotic Resistance Threats in the United States, 2019. Atlanta, GA: U.S. Department of Health and Human Services, CDC; 2019

Hohmann EL. Nontyphoidal salmonellosis. *Clin Infect Dis.* 2001; 15:263–269. [PMID: 11170916]

Tack DM, Ray L, Griffin PM, et al. Preliminary incidence and trends of infections with pathogens transmitted commonly through food - foodborne diseases active surveillance network, 10 U.S. sites, 2016-2019. *MMWR Morb Mortal Wkly Rep.* 2020;69(17):509–514. [PMID: 32352955]; PMCID: PMC7206985.

Onwuezobe IA, Oshun PO, Odigwe CC. Antimicrobials for treating symptomatic non-typhoidal Salmonella infections. *Cochrane Database Syst Rev.* 2012;11:CD001167. [PMID: 23152205]

C. *Campylobacter*

Like nontyphoidal *Salmonella* infections, *Campylobacter* species that infect humans, notably *Campylobacter jejuni* and *Campylobacter coli* as well as some less common species, are carried by a wide array of domestic and wild species. Hence, human *Campylobacter* infections are as common as nontyphoidal *Salmonella* as a cause of foodborne enterocolitis in the United States, with contaminated poultry responsible for approximately 50% of infections. However, beef, lamb, and pork, as well as contaminated vegetables and water or improperly pasteurized milk, have caused major outbreaks. Like *Salmonella* and *Shigella*, *Campylobacter* adhere to and then invade the intestinal epithelium of the small intestine and colon, although the exact mechanisms of adhesion and invasion differ. Like *Salmonella*, *Campylobacter* species are acid-sensitive; as a result, conditions that reduce gastric acid secretion predispose to infection by reducing the number of ingested bacteria required to produce symptomatic disease. The immunosuppressed, especially AIDS patients, and the elderly with comorbid conditions are at risk of more severe *Campylobacter*-induced illness.

The clinical features are not distinctive and often closely resemble those seen with shigellosis or nontyphoidal salmonellosis. After an average 3-day incubation period, a brief prodromal phase with fever and malaise in some patients is rapidly followed by crampy periumbilical abdominal pain and diarrhea. Hematochezia occurs in 15–50% of patients, and the abdominal cramps and diarrhea are often severe. Fever occurs in 70–90% of patients. The disease is usually self-limited, with recovery in 5–9 days, although a minority (~10%) of patients suffer a relapse, usually within a few days following apparent resolution. The abdominal pain in patients with *Campylobacter* infection may be severe and lead to consideration of other diagnoses, such as acute appendicitis, especially in children. As with *Salmonella* and *Shigella* infections, the clinical presentation and gross endoscopic appearance of the colonic mucosa in *Campylobacter* enterocolitis can closely mimic the acute onset or an acute relapse of colitis caused by IBD, especially ulcerative colitis.

Definitive diagnosis requires identification of *Campylobacter* in stool culture. A tentative diagnosis can be made more rapidly with a sensitivity of about 50% by microscopic examination of a stool suspension using phase-contrast or darkfield optics in those instances in which large numbers of *Campylobacter* organisms are excreted in diarrheal stool. The rapidly motile spiral-shaped organisms are characteristic.

Antibiotics may shorten the duration of symptoms if given within 1–2 days of onset. However, as the diagnosis is rarely established that rapidly, and the disease is self-limited in otherwise healthy individuals, routine treatment is not recommended, although this may change as some data now indicate that antibiotic treatment may reduce the incidence of postinfectious irritable bowel syndrome. Supportive therapy with rehydration is recommended. Antibiotic treatment is indicated for patients with prolonged or relapsing illness, the immunosuppressed, those with serious comorbidities, and the elderly. A 3–5-day course of a macrolide such as azithromycin is recommended. Fluoroquinolones are an alternative, although resistance to this group of antibiotics is high, especially in parts of Asia.

Rarely, reactive arthritis or Guillain-Barré syndrome may complicate *C jejuni* infection, with a range of onset of 1 week to 2 months after the presentation with gastrointestinal symptoms.

Kaakoush NO, Castaño-Rodríguez N, Mitchell HM, Man SM. Global epidemiology of Campylobacter infection. *Clin Microbiol Rev.* 2015;28(3):687–720. [PMID: 26062576]

Kirkpatric BD, Tribble DR. Update on human *Campylobacter jejuni* infections. *Curr Opin Gastroenterol.* 2011;27:1–7. [PMID: 21124212]

Ternhag A, Askikainen T, Giesecke J, et al. A meta-analysis on the effects of antibiotic treatment on duration of symptoms caused by infection with *Campylobacter species. Clin Infect Dis.* 2007;44:696–700. [PMID: 17278062]

D. *Yersinia*

Yersinia enterocolitica and *Yersinia pseudotuberculosis* produce enterocolitis with diarrhea in humans. Although *Yersinia* species are widespread throughout the animal kingdom, the strains pathogenic to humans do not produce disease in animals but may be carried by them, especially pigs. Ingestion of contaminated food—especially undercooked pork, but also vegetables grown in contaminated soil, dairy products, and contaminated water—transmits the infection to humans. Both outbreaks and sporadic infections occur in the United States. Between 2015 and 2018, the incidence of yersiniosis has ranged between 0.3 and 0.9 per 100,000. By contrast, the incidence is up to 10-fold greater in some European countries. Individuals with diseases that result in increased iron stores, such as hemochromatosis and thalassemia, appear to be more susceptible to infection. *Yersinia* organisms invade via M cells in the epithelium overlying intestinal lymphoid follicles, which are most abundant as aggregates in the ileum and cecum (Peyer patches) but are present along the length of the alimentary tract. The organisms then proliferate in the lymphoid tissues and can spread to regional mesenteric lymph nodes.

After an incubation period of 1–10 days (median, 4 days), two major patterns of clinical symptoms develop. A typical acute enterocolitis with fever, abdominal cramps, diarrhea (which may be bloody), and in the minority of patients, nausea and vomiting occur. This presentation is nonspecific and indistinguishable from that observed with *Salmonella, Shigella,* or *Campylobacter* enteritis. However, the duration of symptoms among patients with *Yersinia* enterocolitis tends to be longer, averaging 2 weeks in several reported outbreaks. Also, in contrast to gastroenteritis caused by other invasive bacteria, pharyngitis caused by invasion by *Yersinia* of the lymphoid-rich tonsils may accompany *Yersinia* enterocolitis. In the other pattern of illness seen most often in adolescents and young adults, diarrhea may be mild or absent, whereas severe right lower quadrant abdominal pain, fever, and leukocytosis predominate, often mimicking acute appendicitis. If such patients undergo surgery, an acute ileitis and mesenteric adenitis are usually observed.

Diagnosis is best established by culture of *Yersinia* from stool, body fluids, or tissue, if surgical specimens are available. Throat culture may be positive, especially if pharyngitis is present. The laboratory should be alerted when *Yersinia* infection is suspected as screening for *Yersinia* is usually not routine. Serologic tests can be helpful; the presence of immunoglobulin M antibodies to *Yersinia* and a significant rise in antibody titers between acute and convalescent sera support the diagnosis of recent infections, although the latter is of little help during acute illness. In patients in whom symptoms mimic appendicitis, imaging of the right lower quadrant via CT or ultrasound is important; ileitis and mesenteric adenitis are usually present, but the appendix generally appears normal.

Supportive therapy with hydration is the mainstay of treatment. There is no convincing evidence that antibiotic treatment alters the clinical course of uncomplicated *Yersinia* enterocolitis though it does reduce somewhat the duration of fecal shedding of *Yersinia*. Indications for treatment are the immunosuppressed host, complications such as invasive infections and septicemia, and, perhaps, patients with conditions associated with increased iron stores. If oral therapy suffices, in adults fluoroquinolones and in children trimethoprim–sulfamethoxazole are recommended for 5–7 days. If intravenous administration is required, a third-generation cephalosporin is recommended for 2–3 weeks. Complications include reactive arthritis, erythema nodosum, and, rarely, other conditions with autoimmune overtones, including myocarditis, glomerulonephritis, thyroiditis, and hepatitis.

Black RE, Slome S. *Yersinia enterocolitica. Infect Dis Clin North Am.* 1988;2:625–641. [PMID: 3074119]

Long C, Jones TF, Vugia DJ, et al. *Yersinia pseudotuberculosis* and *Y. enterocolitica* infections, FoodNet, 1996-2007. *Emerg Infect Dis.* 2010;16:566–567. [PMID: 20202449]

Tack DM, Marder EP, Griffin PM, et al. Preliminary incidence and trends of infections with pathogens transmitted commonly through food - foodborne diseases active surveillance network, 10 U.S. sites, 2015-2018. *MMWR Morb Mortal Wkly Rep.* 2019;68(16):369–373. [PMID: 31022166]; [PMCID: PMC6483286.

E. Listeriosis

Listeria monocytogenes is an invasive, gram-positive, rod-shaped organism resembling diphtheroids in appearance. *L monocytogenes* is widely found in soil, many animal species, and foodstuffs, most notably cheese, sausage, and other processed delicatessen meats. *L monocytogenes* can proliferate in refrigerated foods. Some infections occur sporadically, but foodborne outbreaks have also been well documented.

In otherwise healthy immunocompetent individuals, the organism invades the intestinal mucosa and causes a self-limited febrile gastroenteritis of relatively short duration, usually 2 days or less. Symptoms are nonspecific and include fever, malaise, muscle aches, nausea, vomiting, and diarrhea. Pregnant patients commonly present with a flu-like illness with or without gastrointestinal symptoms. There is a predilection for invasion of placental tissue, especially during the last trimester, with spread of the organism to the fetus and fetal death or birth of an infected neonate. In infected neonates, immunosuppressed hosts and the elderly, there is a predilection for central nervous system invasion with resulting meningitis, meningoencephalitis, and, rarely, brain abscess. Extraintestinal invasive listeriosis is associated with significant morbidity and mortality.

The diagnosis is usually made by culture of *L monocytogenes* from the blood and cerebrospinal fluid. The significance of isolation of the organism from the stool is unclear as it can be isolated occasionally from asymptomatic individuals. Isolation from stool requires the use of selective media not generally used for routine stool culture. Blood cultures should be obtained from pregnant and immunocompromised patients with fever and constitutional symptoms with or without febrile gastroenteritis.

There is no evidence that antibiotic therapy influences the course of uncomplicated, febrile *Listeria* gastroenteritis in otherwise healthy patients; in many instances, the diagnosis is not established by bacterial isolation and, if it is, symptoms will have resolved. On the other hand, infection in pregnant, elderly, or immunosuppressed patients or in any individual with evidence of spread to other tissues should be treated. Amoxicillin and trimethoprim–sulfamethoxazole have been effective for isolated listerial febrile gastroenteritis.

Jackson KA, Gould LH, Hunter JC, Kucerova Z, Jackson B. Listeriosis outbreaks associated with soft cheeses, United States, 1998-2014. *Emerg Infect Dis*. 2018;24(6):1116–1118. [PMID: 29774843]

Ooi ST, Lorber B. Gastroenteritis due to *Listeria monocytogenes*. *Clin Infect Dis*. 2005;40:1327–1332. [PMID: 15825036]

F. Noncholera *Vibrio*

Several *Vibrio* species distinct from *Vibrio cholerae*, including *Vibrio parahaemolyticus*, can cause diarrheal disease in humans. These organisms thrive in high salt concentrations and are found in saltwater estuaries, especially in the summer and fall, although they also can contaminate fresh water. Most outbreaks and sporadic cases of diarrheal disease result from ingestion of contaminated raw or improperly cooked seafood, especially mollusks (eg, oysters, mussels, or clams) and crustaceans, including crab and shrimp. The number of reported cases in the United States have increased approximately threefold between 1999 and 2014. Most noncholera *Vibrio* species induce diarrhea by producing enterotoxins similar to the heat-labile toxin produced by *V cholerae* or a heat-stable toxin similar to that produced by ETEC. *V parahaemolyticus* produces hemolysins, which appear to correlate with virulence.

The clinical features of noncholera *Vibrio*–induced gastroenteritis are nonspecific and include diarrhea, which may be grossly bloody in a minority of patients, abdominal cramps, fever, and, less commonly, nausea and vomiting. The duration of illness ranges from an average of 3 days for *V parahaemolyticus* to 6 days for the other noncholera *Vibrio* species. Most species may also cause wound infections and, especially in patients who are immunosuppressed or have liver disease, septicemia, the latter with mortality as high as 20%.

Isolation from stool samples requires use of selective media; hence, the laboratory should be alerted that infection with noncholera *Vibrio* is suspected.

Supportive therapy and hydration are the mainstays of treatment. Although controlled trials are lacking and diarrhea is self-limited in immunocompetent individuals, doxycycline or quinolones have been reported to reduce the duration of diarrhea and shedding of *Vibrio* organisms in the stool.

Janda JM, Newton AE, Bopp CA. Vibriosis. *Clin Lab Med*. 2015;35(2):273–288. [PMID: 26004642]

Logar-Henderson C, Ling R, Tuite AR, Fisman DN. Effects of large-scale oceanic phenomena on non-cholera vibriosis incidence in the United States: implications for climate change. *Epidemiol Infect*. 2019;147:e243. [PMID: 31364581]; PMCID: PMC6805737.

G. *Vibrio cholerae*

Cholera is endemic in low-income countries in Asia, Africa, and Central and South America and also causes epidemic outbreaks in these continents largely through contamination of water supplies and, less often, foodstuffs. It has been estimated that there are 3 million cases of cholera and 100,000 deaths per year worldwide. In North America, a few sporadic cases have occurred in recent years, probably through ingestion of contaminated food, largely shellfish. There are more imported infections among travelers than sporadic indigenous infections in the United States. The 2010 cholera epidemic in Haiti was associated with outbreaks in neighboring Mexico, Cuba, and the Dominican Republic. *V cholerae* is acid-sensitive; hence, a large inoculum is required to cause infection in individuals with normal gastric acid secretion. Surviving organisms colonize the small intestine by attaching to the epithelial surface via pili and subsequently elaborate toxins that induce electrolyte and water secretion and alter epithelial permeability in the absence of mucosal inflammation.

Infections range from asymptomatic colonization to devastating, watery diarrhea with fluid losses that can approach 1 L/h. Vomiting may accompany the diarrhea, but a significant fever is uncommon. Massive fecal fluid losses, if not replaced, can rapidly lead to severe dehydration and profound electrolyte disturbances, including hypokalemia and metabolic acidosis, with associated renal failure. The epidemiologic history and clinical picture facilitate diagnosis. *Vibrio* can often be seen in stool examined by phase-contrast or darkfield microscopy and on Gram stain. *V cholerae* is cultured on selective media.

Prompt rehydration is imperative. Oral rehydration solution (see "General Principles" under "Treatment," earlier) is sufficient for most infections and has saved hundreds of thousands of lives and reduced mortality from cholera to fewer than 1% in adults and older children. Ongoing stool fluid losses should be measured to help guide the volume of oral fluid administration. If dehydration is severe or nausea and vomiting preclude adequate oral intake, intravenous hydration is indicated. If facilities or supplies needed for intravenous hydration are unavailable, oral solutions should be administered via nasogastric tube, although aspiration is a hazard. Antibiotics (tetracycline, doxycycline, quinolones, or azithromycin, depending on susceptibility) reduce fluid losses and shorten the duration of diarrhea for those with moderate to severe dehydration. The rBS-WC vaccine, an oral, killed, whole cell vaccine containing the nontoxic cholera toxin B subunit, is approved for use for prophylaxis of traveler's diarrhea (see later) and provides 70–80% protection against *V cholerae* O1 for several years and also protects against ETEC infections. However, it does not provide protection against *V cholerae* O139. The bivalent killed whole-cell vaccine contains whole cells of both *V cholerae* O1 and O139 and provides up to 65% protection for 5 years.

Ali M, Nelson AR, Lopez AL, Sack DA. Updated global burden of cholera in endemic countries. *PLoS Negl Trop Dis.* 2015; 9(6):e0003832. [PMID: 26043000]

Bhattacharya SK, Sur D, Ali M, et al. 5 year efficacy of a bivalent killed whole-cell oral cholera vaccine in Kolkata, India: a cluster-randomised, double-blind, placebo-controlled trial. *Lancet Infect Dis.* 2013;13(12):1050–1056. [PMID: 24140390]

Harris JB, LaRocque RC, Qadri F, et al. Cholera. *Lancet.* 2012;379:2466–2476. [PMID: 22748592]

Khatib AM, Ali M, von Seidlein L, et al. Effectiveness of an oral cholera vaccine in Zanzibar: findings from a mass vaccination campaign and observational cohort study. *Lancet Infect Dis.* 2012;12:837–844. [PMID: 22954655]

Leibovici-Weissman Y, Neuberger A, Bitterman R, Sinclair D, Salam MA, Paul M. Antimicrobial drugs for treating cholera. *Cochrane Database Syst Rev.* 2014;2014(6):CD008625. [PMID: 24944120]

H. *Aeromonas*

Aeromonas species, like noncholera vibrios, thrive in brackish and freshwater environments but also cause disease in fish as well as many land animals. They produce several toxins, adhesins, hemolysins, and proteases, but the exact role of these putative virulence factors in the pathogenesis of disease in humans remains uncertain.

The role of *Aeromonas* species in human diarrheal disease is somewhat controversial. Although small outbreaks among travelers are described and the organisms are sporadically cultured from patients with diarrheal disease, *Aeromonas* have been isolated from 5% to 15% of asymptomatic individuals in low-income countries. An effort to induce disease in normal volunteers by oral challenge was inconclusive. However, there is a general consensus that some *Aeromonas* species can cause diarrheal disease in some individuals.

Symptoms range from watery to dysenteric diarrhea and may be accompanied by nausea and vomiting and, in the minority of patients, fever. Although most cases are self-limited, more protracted diarrhea lasting several weeks has been observed. *Aeromonas*, like noncholera vibrios, can also cause wound infections. Gram-negative sepsis has been reported to occur in the elderly, pediatric, pregnant, and immunosuppressed patients or in patients with liver disease. The diagnosis is made by stool culture, but the laboratory should be alerted that *Aeromonas* species are being sought. Although *Aeromonas* grows readily on conventional media, identifying these organisms is not generally routine.

The disease is self-limited in most patients with *Aeromonas*-associated diarrhea. Anecdotal reports suggest that patients with protracted diarrhea merit antibiotic treatment with trimethoprim–sulfamethoxazole a fluoroquinolone, or a third-generation cephalosporin, depending on the results of susceptibility testing. Controlled trials showing the benefit of antibiotic treatment are not available.

Fernández-Bravo A, Figueras MJ. An update on the genus Aeromonas: taxonomy, epidemiology, and pathogenicity. *Microorganisms.* 2020;8(1):129. [PMID: 31963469]

Parker JL, Shaw JG. Aeromonas spp. Clinical microbiology and disease. *J Infect.* 2011;62:109–118. [PMID: 21163298]

I. *Plesiomonas*

Plesiomonas shigelloides, like *Aeromonas* species, is widely distributed in aquatic environments and among a broad range of sea and land animals. Rare or undercooked shellfish, notably oysters, as well as contaminated brackish water have been incriminated in outbreaks of human diarrheal disease. Unlike *Aeromonas*, the carriage rate among asymptomatic individuals is very low. However, like *Aeromonas*, an attempt to induce disease in volunteers was inconclusive.

The pathogenesis of *Plesiomonas*-induced gastroenteritis is poorly understood, and specific disease-producing virulence factors have not been identified. The clinical features closely resemble those of *Aeromonas*-induced gastroenteritis and range from watery to, in the minority of patients, dysenteric diarrhea. Nausea and vomiting are common, and abdominal cramps may be present. Fever is uncommon.

Although most cases are self-limited with only a few days of symptoms, prolonged diarrhea has been reported. Diagnosis is generally made by culture of *P shigelloides* from the stool, but again, the bacteriology laboratory should be notified that the organism is being sought.

There are no available controlled trials defining the efficacy of treatment with antibiotics. Most cases require no more than supportive treatment. Patients who are immunocompromised and those who have chronic liver disease, bacteremia, extraintestinal infections, or prolonged diarrhea should be treated. Trimethoprim–sulfamethoxazole, quinolones, and cephalosporins are usually effective, but the choice of antibiotic should be guided by sensitivity testing.

Janda JM, Abbott SL, McIver CJ. *Plesiomonas shigelloides* revisited. *Clin Microbiol Rev.* 2016;29(2):349–374. [PMID: 26960939]

J. Enterotoxigenic *E coli*

ETEC have been recognized for years as a major cause of diarrheal disease in infants and children younger than 2 years of age in lower-income nations and, in some series, as the most common cause of traveler's diarrhea at any age. In recent years, large outbreaks in the United States and Europe have also been reported. Transmission generally is via contaminated food or water, and a large inoculum is required. Important virulence factors characterizing ETEC are heat-labile toxin (LT) and a heat-stable toxin (STa). LT closely resembles cholera toxin, stimulating cyclic adenosine monophosphate production, resulting in intestinal crypt chloride and water secretion and reduced sodium chloride absorption by enterocytes. STa stimulates cyclic guanosine monophosphate production, which, much like LT, causes enhanced chloride and water secretion and impaired sodium chloride absorption by the small intestine.

The major clinical manifestation is diarrhea, which ranges from just a few loose stools lasting less than a day to severe, watery diarrhea that may persist for up to five days and result in significant dehydration. Fever is uncommon and, when present, low grade. Nausea and abdominal cramps may accompany the diarrhea, but vomiting is uncommon.

As in cholera, the involved mucosa is not inflamed; hence, fecal leukocytes are absent. ETEC require research techniques (with DNA probes for LT and STa) for identification; they cannot be differentiated from nonpathogenic *E coli* by routine stool culture. In the absence of research facilities, the diagnosis is a clinical one.

Rehydration, again, is the cornerstone of therapy; short courses of antibiotics, including fluoroquinolones, azithromycin, and rifaximin, shorten the duration of illness by a day or so. Lack of a definitive diagnosis in most instances and the self-limited nature of the illness limit their therapeutic use. Prophylaxis is discussed later in the section on traveler's diarrhea.

Beatty ME, Adcock PM, Smith SW, et al. Epidemic diarrhea due to enterotoxigenic *Escherichia coli*. *Clin Infect Dis.* 2006;42: 329–334. [PMID: 16392076]

Fleckenstein JM, Kuhlmann FM. Enterotoxigenic *Escherichia coli* infections. *Curr Infect Dis Rep.* 2019;21(3):9. [PMID: 30830466]

K. Enteropathogenic *E coli*

Enteropathogenic *E coli* (EPEC) primarily cause disease in infants and children younger than 2 years of age. Older children and adults may harbor the causative organism, but overt illness is uncommon. Both outbreaks and sporadic episodes are most common in low-income countries. EPEC attaches to the brush-border surface of enterocytes, activating signal transduction pathways. These activated pathways in turn alter cytoskeletal components, resulting in the effacement of the absorptive surface as well as increased epithelial permeability and altered epithelial barrier function. The resulting diarrhea in neonates and young children can be severe, may be associated with vomiting, and can cause severe dehydration. Most cases are self-limited.

Some commercial laboratories offer a Hep-2 cell adherence assay, but definitive diagnosis usually requires the resources of reference or research laboratories. Rehydration therapy is critical and the cornerstone of treatment. Antibiotics appear effective; trimethoprim–sulfamethoxazole and oral nonabsorbable aminoglycosides have been used.

L. Enteroaggregative *E coli*

Enteroaggregative *E coli* (EAEC) is a relatively recently recognized diarrhea-causing phenotype of *E coli*. EAEC cause disease in all ages and have been identified in both low-income and fully industrialized countries. In one prospective study, EAEC was detected in 4.5% of patients presenting with diarrhea to emergency rooms of two academic centers in Baltimore and New Haven. There is evidence that transmission by contaminated food is a major source of infection. EAEC adhere to cultured Hep-2 cells in a characteristic "stacked brick" fashion; hence, the term *aggregative* has been included in their name. Inflammation-inducing cytotoxin secretion, enterotoxin secretion, and specific adherence factors together with still other virulence factors have been incriminated, but the pathogenesis of diarrhea caused by EAEC is incompletely understood.

Watery diarrhea is a prominent clinical feature and may be accompanied by low-grade fever and abdominal pain. Bloody diarrhea has been reported. Although many episodes of diarrhea are self-limited, EAEC has been identified in stools of children in low-income countries and in adults with AIDS in the United States and Europe with chronic diarrhea.

Identification of EAEC in stools requires use of molecular techniques to identify AggR regulon or the Hep-2 adherence assay, which is not performed in conventional clinical laboratories. Ciprofloxacin, rifaximin, and azithromycin have been reported to be an effective therapy, shortening the duration of diarrhea caused by EAEC, although resistance to all three antibiotics has been reported.

Huang DB, Nataro JP, DuPont HL, et al. Enteroaggregative *Escherichia coli* is a cause of acute diarrheal illness: a meta-analysis. *Clin Infect Dis.* 2006;43:556–563. [PMID: 16886146]

Jenkins C. Enteroaggregative *Escherichia coli. Curr Top Microbiol Immunol.* 2018;416:27–50. [PMID: 30232602]

Nataro JP, Mai V, Johnson J, et al. Diarrheagenic *Escherichia coli* infection in Baltimore, Maryland and New Haven, Connecticut. *Clin Infect Dis.* 2006;43:402–407. [PMID: 16838226]

M. Enteroinvasive *E coli*

Enteroinvasive *E coli* (EIEC) is a relatively uncommon cause of diarrhea found largely in low-income nations and, occasionally, among travelers returning to industrialized nations. It shares virulence factors with *Shigella* strains and invades intestinal epithelial cells, causing mucosal inflammation. The clinical picture is identical to that observed in shigellosis (see earlier discussion), with watery diarrhea often progressing to dysentery accompanied by fever and, in some patients, nausea and vomiting. Diagnosis requires DNA-probe testing by reference or research laboratories. Treatment guidelines follow those for shigellosis; severe cases, especially in children or immunocompromised adults, should be treated with a fluoroquinolone (adults) or azithromycin (children) along with vigorous rehydration as needed.

N. Enterohemorrhagic *E coli*

Since its description over 30 years ago, enterohemorrhagic *E coli* (EHEC) has become recognized as a major health problem. Over 50% of outbreaks are foodborne. EHEC inhabit the intestinal tract of cattle, deer, sheep, and goats, and outbreaks have been traced to undercooked meat, especially ground beef, contaminated vegetables, fruit, and fruit products. Contaminated recreational water sites and direct animal contact, especially at petting zoos, have also been incriminated in outbreaks. Person-to-person contact in venues such as day care centers or nursing homes may also cause outbreaks as only a small inoculum (<100 organisms) can induce disease.

Following ingestion, EHEC adhere to gut epithelial cells and cause epithelial apical surface effacement by mechanisms similar to EPEC. All EHEC strains produce one or more Shiga toxins, which, on entering the systemic circulation, damage endothelial cells, producing vascular damage that may contribute to bloody diarrhea and predispose to HUS, thrombotic thrombocytopenic purpura, and microangiopathic hemolytic anemia. *E coli* O157:H7 is the most common EHEC serotype isolated in the United States, but other Shiga toxin-producing serotypes are being increasingly isolated from outbreaks in the United States and other countries. A particularly virulent strain, *E coli* O104:H4, with adherence genes found in EAEC and genes encoding Shiga

toxin 2 was responsible for a major outbreak in Germany resulting in over 3000 cases traced to contaminated sprouts. Whereas about two-thirds of EHEC cases in the United States occur in children, 89% of cases in the German outbreak were in adults with a preponderance of women and an unusually high 20% incidence of HUS.

After an average incubation period of 3–5 days (a longer median incubation period of 8 days for *E coli* O104:H4 infection), the illness often begins with watery diarrhea for 2–5 days, progressing to bloody diarrhea in up to 90% of patients. Severe cramps and abdominal pain are common, with right lower quadrant tenderness prominent in some patients. Notably, fever is absent in most patients and, if present, is low grade. Peripheral leukocytosis of 10,000–20,000/μL is common. The duration of gastrointestinal symptoms can be only a few days to as long as 2 weeks or more. In some outbreaks, *E coli* O157:H7 has been isolated from patients with much milder or no symptoms, further suggesting a broad range of severity of clinical manifestations.

Endoscopy, if performed, shows a friable, edematous, erythematous colonic mucosa with superficial ulceration. Imaging studies show colonic wall thickening, thumbprinting, and, if contrast is used, mucosal hyperemia, which is often most severe in the right colon. Fecal leukocytes may or may not be present.

The diagnosis can often be suspected from the clinical presentation (bloody stools, abdominal pain, leukocytosis, but little or no fever) and is confirmed by stool cultures using sorbitol-MacConkey agar. An ELISA that detects Shiga toxins in the stool is also available, but occasional false-positive results have been reported.

Treatment is supportive. Rehydration is important. Antimotility agents should be avoided. There is no evidence that antibiotic treatment provides any benefit in EHEC colitis other than possibly reducing the duration of fecal bacterial shedding. Indeed, some series indicate that in children, antibiotic treatment increases the risk of associated HUS by as much as threefold. A trial of administration of a Shiga toxin-binding agent to children with diarrhea and HUS showed no benefit when compared with placebo.

HUS, thrombotic thrombocytopenic purpura, and microangiopathic anemia are the dreaded complications of EHEC infection and occur most often in children younger than 10 years, although older children and adults are not always spared. Details of treatment for these conditions are beyond the scope of this chapter, but treatment is largely supportive, often requiring dialysis for renal disease and, less often, plasma exchange for thrombotic thrombocytopenic purpura.

Frank C, Werber D, Cramer JP, et al. Epidemic profile of Shiga-toxin-producing *Escherichia coli* O104:H4 outbreak in Germany—preliminary report. *N Engl J Med.* 2011;365:1771–1780. [PMID: 21696328]

Pennington H. *Escherichia coli* O157. *Lancet.* 2010;376:1428–1435. [PMID: 20971366]

Wong CS, Mooney JC, Brandt JR, et al. Risk factors for the hemo-lytic uremic syndrome in children infected with *Escherichia coli* O157:H7: a multivariable analysis. *Clin Infect Dis.* 2012;55: 33–41. [PMID: 22431799]

O. *Staphylococcus aureus*

Staphylococcus aureus gastroenteritis is a common cause of food poisoning. The causative food is often contaminated by a food handler. Foods rich in sugar and cream, such as cus-tards, cakes with creamy frostings, salty meats such as ham, and mayonnaise- and cream-containing salads favor *Staphy-lococcus* growth and enterotoxin production at room temper-ature. Within 6 hours of ingestion of foodstuffs containing sufficient toxin, patients develop nausea and vomiting, which may be severe; abdominal cramps; and subsequently, in some, diarrhea. Fever is uncommon. Duration of symptoms rarely exceeds 24 hours, and rapid recovery is the rule.

The diagnosis can best be established by isolating *S aureus* or enterotoxin from the suspected food if an outbreak is sus-pected. Additionally, vomitus or diarrheal stool can be tested for enterotoxin, but this is not routinely done. Treatment is supportive, with hydration and correction of metabolic alka-losis, if present, due to severe vomiting.

P. *Bacillus cereus*

Bacillus cereus, a gram-positive, spore-forming bacillus, can produce two distinct types of food poisoning. Some strains pro-duce a heat-stable toxin in vitro that induces vomiting; other strains produce a heat-labile enterotoxin that causes diarrhea.

The organisms that produce the vomiting syndrome have largely been associated with ingestion of rice, notably fried rice. The vegetative forms are destroyed when rice is boiled, but the spores survive. If the rice is not refrigerated, the spores germinate and toxin is produced that may not be inactivated by flash frying as the fried rice is prepared. A short 2–3-hours incubation period follows toxin ingestion. Then vomiting associated with abdominal cramping develops, which may be associated with mild diarrhea. The illness is self-limited, averaging about 8 hours, and can be treated with antiemetics and, if needed, rehydration. The organisms that produce the diarrheal syndrome have been associated with contaminated meats, sauces, and dairy products. Their longer incubation following ingestion of contaminated food (6–18 hours) sug-gests that the enterotoxin is produced in vivo. Major symp-toms include diarrhea and abdominal cramps; vomiting occurs in fewer than 25% of cases. Symptoms usually clear within 24 hours and should be treated supportively with rehydration, if needed. Antibiotics are not indicated for the treatment of *B cereus* gastroenteritis.

Q. *Clostridium perfringens*

Clostridium perfringens is a gram-positive, anaerobic, spore-forming bacillus widely found in nature in the intestinal flora of many animals and in soil. Type A strains produce a heat-labile enterotoxin that causes intestinal fluid secre-tion and is also cytotoxic to intestinal epithelium. Disease is caused almost exclusively by ingested meat that is inad-equately refrigerated after cooking and is a common cause of foodborne illness in the United States with approximately one million cases annually. After a 12–24-hours incubation, patients develop watery diarrhea and abdominal crampy pain that may be severe, usually in the absence of nausea, vom-iting, or fever. Symptoms generally last less than a day and treatment is supportive; oral rehydration is usually sufficient. Type C strains produce a beta toxin that can result in much more severe illness, which has been termed enteritis necroti-cans or pigbel. It is characterized by intestinal necrosis that may produce perforation requiring surgery. Mortality rates as high as 40% have been reported. This disease has been described largely in South Pacific islands after festive con-sumption of large amounts of improperly cooked pork.

Centers for Disease Control and Prevention (CDC). Fatal foodborne *Clostridium perfringens* illness at a state psychiatric hospital—Louisiana, 2010. *Morb Motal Wkly Rep.* 2012;61:605–608. [PMID: 22895383]

Scallan E, Hoekstra RM, Angulo FJ, et al. Foodborne illness acquired in the United States–major pathogens. *Emerg Infect Dis.* 2011;17(1):7–15. [PMID: 21192848]

Stenfors Arnesen LP, Fagerlund A, Granum PE. From soil to gut: *Bacillus cereus* and its food poisoning toxins. *FEMS Microbiol Rev.* 2008;32(4):579–606. [PMID: 18422617]

R. *Clostridioides difficile*

Clostridioides difficile, a gram-positive, spore-forming bacillus, is the major cause of hospital-acquired infectious diarrhea but also is increasingly recognized as a cause of community-acquired diarrhea. *C difficile* spores are heat and alcohol resistant and can remain infectious in vitro. They may colonize up to 40% of hospitalized patients and 3% of healthy individuals.

Alteration of the normal enterocolonic bacterial flora by prior antibiotic administration is required for the develop-ment of *C difficile* colitis in the large majority of those who develop the disease. Antibiotics most often associated with *C difficile*-induced disease include aminopenicillins, fluoro-quinolones, cephalosporins, and clindamycin, but virtually all antibiotics, even metronidazole, have been incriminated. Cancer chemotherapy or preexisting IBD, especially with colonic involvement, appears to be a risk factor for primary *C difficile* infection. Increasingly, the disease appears to develop in the absence of antecedent antibiotic administra-tion even in otherwise healthy individuals. Other risk factors for development of *C difficile* infection include exposure to any health care facility, debilitating comorbidities, gastrointestinal surgery, and old age. Although still controversial, there is evi-dence that chronic acid suppression with proton pump inhib-itors and, to a lesser degree, H_2-receptor antagonists increase the risk for developing *C difficile* colitis or its recurrence after seemingly effective treatment.

Upon colonizing the intestine, most virulent *C difficile* strains produce toxins A and B. These induce colonic epithelial cytoskeletal damage, mucosal inflammation, and mucosal fluid secretion, resulting in the clinical features described below. The toxin-induced mucosal lesion is characterized by damaged epithelium, mucosal inflammation, and the exudative pseudomembrane, which consists of necrotic debris, inflammatory cells, and mucus adherent to the mucosal surface. Strains that produce only toxin B have been isolated from patients with clinically manifest *C difficile* colitis.

In 2000, the highly virulent strain of *C difficile* (BI/NAP1/027 or PCR ribotype 027) has been identified in North American and subsequently in European outbreaks. This toxinotype III strain has been shown to produce up to 16- and 23-fold greater amounts of toxins A and B, respectively. This has been ascribed to a partial deletion of the *tcdC* gene that normally downregulates toxins A and B production. This highly virulent strain has emerged in concert with the wide use of fluoroquinolones, is frequently resistant to fluoroquinolones, and has been implicated in the increasing frequency and morbidity of *C difficile* enterocolitis in North America and in Europe. Another high toxin-producing hypervirulent strain (PCR ribotype 078, toxinotype V) has been isolated more recently with increasing frequency in Europe and North America.

The clinical features of *C difficile* may range, at the one extreme, from total lack of symptoms in asymptomatic carriers to, at the other extreme, fulminant diarrhea and toxic megacolon requiring emergency surgery. Symptoms usually begin a few days to 2 weeks after initiation of antibiotic treatment, although the latency period may be as long as several months. Malaise, watery diarrhea, lower abdominal pain and tenderness, and low-grade fever are characteristic features. Frank hematochezia is rare, although occult blood loss is common. Mild peripheral leukocytosis is common, and fecal leukocytes are often present, especially in patients with more than mild colitis.

It should be stressed that many of the milder episodes of diarrhea that occur in concert with antibiotic treatment are not infectious in nature. Rather, alterations in the balance of the colonic flora impair salvage carbohydrate digestion and absorption. As a result, the amount of unabsorbed carbohydrates in the colonic lumen is increased, resulting in an osmotic diarrhea.

Demonstration of *C difficile* cytotoxin in diarrheal stool samples is the gold standard for establishing the diagnosis of *C difficile* colitis. Classically this test is performed by culturing fibroblasts in the presence of stool supernate. If toxin is present, the fibroblasts show evidence of cytotoxicity. Sensitivity and specificity of this test range from 95% to 99%, but the assay requires 2–3 days. Available EIAs for *C difficile* toxin are more rapid and less costly, previously felt to be less sensitive. Current recommendations are for a two-step algorithm, initially utilizing either an EIA for GDH. GDH is an enzyme produced by *C difficile* whether or not it is a toxigenic strain, giving the test high sensitivity but low specificity or the highly sensitive PCR assay as a first step. Positive samples are then coupled with an EIA for toxins. Other laboratories will do EIAs for both GDH and *C difficile* toxins and follow with a PCR assay if only one of the EIAs is positive.

In some patients, an immediate, albeit only provisional, diagnosis can be made at anoscopy or sigmoidoscopy if the characteristic pseudomembrane is observed. However, the absence of the pseudomembrane does not exclude *C difficile* colitis as the disease may be confined to the more proximal colon and the rectum and distal colon may be spared. Moreover, not all patients with *C difficile* colitis develop the characteristic pseudomembrane. Imaging studies including abdominal flat films or abdominal CT are nonspecific and may show colonic wall thickening and mucosal contrast enhancement. In patients with fulminant colitis, ileus or toxic megacolon may be evident.

Worrisome signs suggesting severe, potentially life-threatening colitis include florid diarrhea in excess of 10 stools per day; abrupt reduction of diarrhea in the absence of other signs of clinical improvement, which may signal the development of toxic megacolon; increasing abdominal pain and distention; high fever; hypotension, especially if pressors are required; leukocytosis >15,000 cells/mm^3, hypoalbuminemia <3 g/dL; a rising serum creatinine; and colonic dilation on imaging. Patients showing such symptoms and signs must be monitored closely in conjunction with a surgeon and may require potentially lifesaving surgical intervention (see as follows).

Treatment recommendations depend on the severity of clinical illness and host of risk factors. Hospitalized patients should be isolated, and in all cases, caregivers should wash their hands with soap and water after patient contact. Purell and other alcohol-based hand cleaners do not destroy *C difficile* spores. Treatment guidelines have been published by the Society for Healthcare Epidemiology of America and the Infectious Diseases Society of America, the European Society of Clinical Microbiology and by the American College of Gastroenterology. Whenever possible, antibiotics should be discontinued. The most recent guidelines from the Infectious Disease Society of America (IDSA) recommend oral vancomycin (125 mg every 6 hours for 10–14 days) for patients with mild to moderate disease and for patients with severe disease, experiencing their first infection. Fidaxomicin 200 mg twice daily, which appears to have therapeutic equivalence to vancomycin but with a lower incidence of post-treatment recurrence has been approved for treatment of *C difficile* colitis. A course of fidaxomicin costs in excess of eightfold more than a course of vancomycin. Severe disease is defined as a white blood cell count >15,000/mm^3, or a serum creatitine >1.5mg/dL. Fulminant disease also includes hypotension, shock, ileus, or megacolon. Treatment for fulminant disease includes both vancomycin orally or via nasogastric tube (500 mg every 6 hours) and intravenous metronidazole (500 mg every 8 hours) should be begun. In addition, if ileus is present, intracolonic administration of vancomycin (500 mg four to six times daily) should be considered. These very ill patients should be closely monitored with frequent abdominal examinations and daily abdominal flat films to assess for developing megacolon along with serial surgical assessment for the possible need for colectomy. Emergency colectomy may be lifesaving in those few patients who develop progressive fulminant diarrhea, severe ileus, and megacolon with impending perforation or generalized sepsis.

Patients with a new flare of IBD should be tested for *C difficile* infection. Management of patients with *C difficile* infection complicating IBD can be challenging as the clinical presentations of *C difficile* colitis and a flare of IBD can be quite similar. If such a patient fails to improve promptly with treatment for *C difficile* colitis, appropriate concurrent treatment of the coexistent IBD should be implemented or increased.

Relapses after apparent complete resolution occur in approximately 25% of treated patients, most likely caused by reinfection or germination of residual spores remaining in the colon. Retreatment should be with a different therapy than was what used for initial infection. If there is a second relapse, tapering pulsed doses of vancomycin can be tried, starting with 125 mg four times daily and then reducing the dose frequency by 50% every week until 125 mg of vancomycin every 3 days has been administered for 2 weeks. If that fails, fidaxomicin or fecal microbiota transplantation (FMT) should be considered.

For patients with 2 or more relapses, FMT is being used with impressive results. Success rates as reported in several meta-analyses approximate 90% with some initial failures responding to a second FMT. Careful donor screening via history and laboratory tests to exclude the possibility of transmission of an infectious agent is crucial. FMT has been achieved by fecal retention enemas, direct instillation via colonoscopy, fecal infusion via nasoduodenal tube and gelatin capsules containing fecal derived material can be administered orally. Long-term follow-up studies of patients who have received FMT are under way. .

Allegretti JR, Mullish BH, Kelly C, Fischer M. The evolution of the use of faecal microbiota transplantation and emerging therapeutic indications. *Lancet.* 2019;394(10196):420–431. [PMID: 31379333]

Cammarota G, Ianiro G, Kelly CR, et al. International consensus conference on stool banking for faecal microbiota transplantation in clinical practice. *Gut.* 2019;68(12):2111–2121. [PMID: 31563878]; PMCID: PMC6872442.

Crobach MJ, Planche T, Eckert C, et al. European Society of Clinical Microbiology and Infectious Diseases: update of the diagnostic guidance document for *Clostridium difficile* infection. *Clin Microbiol Infect* 2016;22 Suppl 4:S63–S81.

Cohen SH, Gerding DN, Johnson S, et al. Clinical practice guidelines for *Clostridium difficile* infection in adults: 2010 update by the Society for Healthcare Epidemiology of America (SHEA) and the Infectious Diseases Society of America (IDSA). *Infect Control Hosp Epidemiol.* 2010;31:431–455. [PMID: 20307191]

Guh AY, Mu Y, Winston LG, et al. Trends in U.S. burden of *Clostridioides difficile* infection and outcomes. *N Engl J Med* 2020;382:1320–1330. [PMID: 32242357]

Guh AY, Mu Y, Baggs J, et al. Trends in incidence of long-term-care facility onset *Clostridium difficile* infections in 10 US geographic locations during 2011–2015. *Am J Infect Control* 2018;46: 840–842. [PMID: 29329918]

Kassam Z, Lee CH, Yuan Y, Hunt RH. Fecal microbiota transplantation for *Clostridium difficile* infection: systematic review and meta-analysis. *Am J Gastroenterol.* 2013;108:500–508. [PMID: 23511459]

McDonald LC, Gerding DN, Johnson S, et al. Clinical Practice Guidelines for *Clostridium difficile* Infection in Adults and Children: 2017 Update by the Infectious Diseases Society of America (IDSA) and Society for Healthcare Epidemiology of America (SHEA). *Clin Infect Dis* 2018;66:e1–e48. [PMID: 29462280]

S. *Klebsiella oxytoca*

Klebsiella oxytoca causes a relatively uncommon but distinctive antibiotic-associated hemorrhagic colitis. *K oxytoca* has been shown to produce a cytotoxin that has been implicated in the pathogenesis of colitis. Colitis generally occurs during the first week after the introduction of antibiotic therapy, usually with a penicillin, although cases that occurred in concert with administration of other antibiotics, including cephalosporins and quinolones have been described. Most reported patients have been relatively young to middle aged. Bloody diarrhea (uncommon in *C difficile* colitis), abdominal cramps, low-grade fever, and mild to moderate leukocytosis are clinical features. The rectum is often spared, and a patchy hemorrhagic colitis with superficial ulcers but without a pseudomembrane is observed in colonic segments. Mucosal biopsies show an ulcerated mucosa that resembles the lesion observed in patients with EHEC with both inflammatory and ischemic features. The condition is generally self-limited, resolving promptly after the discontinuation of the causative antibiotic and requires only supportive treatment.

Högenauer C, Langner C, Beubler E, et al. *Klebsiella oxytoca* as a causative organism of antibiotic-associated hemorrhagic colitis. *N Engl J Med.* 2006;355:2418–2426. [PMID: 17151365]

Fisher A, Halalau A. A case report and literature review of *Clostridium difficile* negative antibiotic associated hemorrhagic colitis caused by *Klebsiella oxytoca. Case Rep Gastrointest Med.* 2018;2018:7264613. [PMID: 30345122]

3. Protozoal Infections

A. *Giardia lamblia*

Giardia lamblia is the most common protozoal infestation in the United States, where it occurs both endemically and in epidemic outbreaks. It is a common cause of illness worldwide, especially in low-income countries where sanitation is suboptimal and, hence, is a common cause of traveler's diarrhea. *G lamblia* infects other mammals, including beavers, dogs, and cattle. The cyst form of *Giardia* can survive for prolonged periods in most environments. Once cysts are ingested, the distinctive trophozoites are released in the upper small intestine where they multiply by binary fission and colonize the host. The trophozoites attach to the intestinal epithelium but do not invade the mucosa; however, they can produce significant enteritis with mucosal inflammation and architectural changes. Hence, duodenal biopsy specimens can range from those revealing normal mucosal structure to an almost flat mucosa architecturally reminiscent of a lesion of severe celiac disease.

Several factors increase the risk of contracting *G lamblia* infection. These include travel to areas where the water supply may be contaminated, drinking mountain and forest stream or lake water that has not been filtered or boiled, attendance at day care or preschool, and swimming in pools with improperly treated water or in contaminated lakes. The risk of developing giardiasis is higher in patients with immunoglobulin deficiencies and among men who have sex with men. HIV infection by itself is not a known risk factor.

Approximately 50% of individuals infested with *G lamblia* have no symptoms and can be asymptomatic carriers of the parasite for many months. Those that develop symptoms commonly experience diarrhea, flatulence, abdominal cramps, and epigastric pain and nausea. Approximately one-third of symptomatic patients experience vomiting. Significant malabsorption with steatorrhea and weight loss may develop. If left untreated, most symptomatic patients recover spontaneously and eliminate the parasite within 3–4 weeks. However, up to 50% develop chronic infection if untreated, which may result in significant signs and symptoms of intestinal malabsorption (see Chapter 20).

Stool examination for ova and parasites has been used for years to establish the diagnosis, but a single specimen has a yield of only approximately 50%, whereas examination of three separate stool samples increases the yield of positive examinations to 80–90%. The cysts and trophozoites may be seen in diarrheal stools, but only cysts are usually observed in formed stools. Several stool immunoassays with reported sensitivities and specificities approaching 100%, are now being widely used by clinical laboratories including a useful commercial assay that detects both *Giardia* and *Cryptosporidium* antigens. Though rarely needed now, sensitivity and specificity of examining duodenal aspirates and mucosal biopsies for *Giardia* trophozoites also approach 100%. It is wise to exclude the diagnosis among household members of symptomatic patients.

Tinidazole and nitazoxanide are both approved by the US Food and Drug Administration (FDA) for the treatment of giardiasis. A single 2 g dose of tinidazole has been reported to be 90% effective and is approved for patients ≥ 3 years of age. Nitazoxanide (500 mg twice daily for 3 days) is 85% effective and is approved for patients ≥12 months of age. It also treats other protozoa such as *Entamoeba* and *Cryptosporidium*. The effectiveness of albendazole (400 mg daily for 5–10 days) is similar to that of nitroimidazoles. Metronidazole (250 mg three times daily for 5–7 days) is a commonly used treatment and is appropriate for use in infants. Although metronidazole is not approved by the FDA for treatment of giardiasis, reported efficacy rates from a single course of therapy are in the 85–95% range. Paromomycin, which is poorly absorbed can be useful for the treatment of pregnant patients, especially if treatment is required during the first trimester.

Alexander CL, Niebel M, Jones B. The rapid detection of *Cryptosporidium* and *Giardia* species in clinical stools using the Quik Check immunoassay. *Parasitol Int.* 2013;62:552–553. [PMID: 23981506]

Cantey PT, Roy S, Lee B, et al. Study of nonoutbreak giardiasis: novel findings and implications for research. *Am J Med.* 2011;124(12):1175.e1–8. [PMID: 22014792]

Granados CE, Reveiz L, Uribe LG, et al. Drugs for treating giardiasis. *Cochrane Database Syst Rev.* 2012;12:CD007787. [PMID: 23235648]

Zylberberg HM, Green PH, Turner KO, Genta RM, Lebwohl B. Prevalence and predictors of Giardia in the United States. *Dig Dis Sci.* 2017;62(2):432–440. [PMID: 28070825]

B. Cryptosporidiosis

Cryptosporidia are widely found in the animal kingdom. Two coccidial species, *Cryptosporidium hominis* and *Cryptosporidium parvum*, are responsible for most human infections. Cryptosporidiosis is transmitted via contaminated food or water, human-to-human contact, and, occasionally, animal-to-human contact. Major waterborne outbreaks have been well documented. Ingestion of a small number of oocysts can produce colonization and disease. The oocysts release sporozoites, which attach to and invade endodermal epithelia. Ultimately, newly formed oocysts are excreted in large numbers in stools of infected individuals. Both cellular and humoral immune defects predispose to symptomatic disease; indeed, many of the earlier recognized cases of cryptosporidial infection coincided with the recognition of HIV infection.

Although *Cryptosporidium* can cause biliary tract, pancreatic, and respiratory tract disease (see Chapter 10), intestinal infection is the most common manifestation. Infected persons may remain asymptomatic or develop an enteritis characterized by watery diarrhea, abdominal cramps, nausea, and malaise, which usually resolves spontaneously in 2–3 weeks in immunocompetent hosts. The diarrhea can be voluminous, especially in immunosuppressed patients in whom chronic infections with debilitating secretory diarrhea and weight loss may develop.

The diagnosis rests upon identification of cryptosporidia organisms in stool, bile, or tissue samples. A modified acid-fast stain of stool has high specificity but mediocre sensitivity and requires the examination of at least three stool specimens if initial specimens are negative. Several commercially available antigen immunoassay tests for stool examination have specificity and sensitivity approaching 100% (see section on *G lamblia*), as do PCR assays. Intestinal mucosal biopsy samples often reveal cryptosporidia within the extreme apical cytoplasm of the enterocytes.

If treatment is required for immunocompetent patients, nitazoxanide is the drug of choice, although spontaneous resolution of symptoms is the rule. Immunosuppressed patients can also be treated with nitazoxanide, although only some respond. An attempt to restore immunologic competence with highly active antiretroviral therapy (HAART) in HIV-infected patients is crucial. Other agents that have been tried, with generally disappointing results, include paromomycin, metronidazole, clarithromycin, and other antibiotics. Supportive treatment with hydration and antidiarrheal agents is important in the immunosuppressed, and parenteral nutrition may be required. Octreotide has been tried, but few patients respond.

Abubakar I, Aliyu SH, Arumugam C, Hunter PR, Usman NK. Prevention and treatment of cryptosporidiosis in immuno-compromised patients. *Cochrane Database Syst Rev.* 2007 Jan 24;(1):CD004932. [PMID: 17253532]

Smith HV, Corcoran, GD. New drugs for the treatment for cryptosporidiosis. *Curr Opin Infect Dis.* 2004;17:557–564. [PMID: 15640710]

C. Cyclospora cayetanensis

Cyclospora cayetanensis, like *Cryptosporidium* and *Cystoisospora*, is a coccidian that is widely distributed geographically and, hence, a cause of traveler's diarrhea. In immunosuppressed patients, it is a cause of protracted diarrheal illness. The major recognized vectors for human infection in the United States have been imported contaminated fruits and vegetables from regions where cyclosporiasis is endemic, although contaminated water is also likely in low-income countries. Among cases acquired in the United States, the majority occur in the spring or summer.

After a relatively prolonged 1-week incubation period, patients develop watery diarrhea, flatulence, abdominal cramps, and malaise. The illness even in immunocompetent hosts may range from minimal to no symptoms to prolonged illness lasting several weeks and even months if left untreated. In immunosuppressed hosts, especially AIDS patients, prolonged, debilitating illness virtually identical to that caused by other coccidia (*Cryptosporidium* or *Cystoisospora*) may develop. Diagnosis is established by demonstrating oocysts in the stool. It may be necessary to examine several stool samples as shedding of oocysts may be sparse and intermittent. The oocysts are autofluorescent; hence, fluorescence microscopy is useful. Alternatively, modified acid-fast staining is used. A multiplex PCR test to detect *Cyclospora*, *Cystoisospora*, and microsporidia with high sensitivity (87–100%) and high specificity (88–100%) has been described. Biopsies of the intestinal mucosa reveal mucosal inflammation and protozoal epithelial invasion.

Trimethoprim–sulfamethoxazole (160/800 mg twice daily for 7 to 10 days) is an effective treatment for otherwise healthy hosts; larger doses and more prolonged treatment are indicated for immunosuppressed patients. Nitazoxanide or ciprofloxacin can be tried for patients intolerant of trimethoprim–sulfamethoxazole.

D. Cystoisospora belli

Cystoisospora belli, like the other coccidial pathogens, is widely distributed geographically. However, infections occur most commonly in tropical areas. Ingestion of contaminated food or water and person-to-person contact are probably important in transmission. Travelers and immunosuppressed patients are most likely to be infected, but sporadic illness in otherwise healthy hosts occurs in the United States and other developed countries.

Clinical features are not specific and include diarrhea, abdominal discomfort, steatorrhea, weight loss, nausea, vomiting, and malaise. Symptoms are generally self-limited in immunocompetent patients but may wax and wane for months without specific treatment. Among AIDS and other severely immunosuppressed patients, protracted illness with severe diarrhea, malabsorption, and weight loss is the rule without specific therapy.

The diagnosis is established by identifying oocysts in the stool using autofluorescence or modified acid-fast staining. A multiplex PCR test to detect *Cyclospora*, *Cystoisospora*, and microsporidia with high sensitivity (87–100%) and high specificity (88–100%) has been described. Oocysts can also be identified in duodenal aspirates, and examination of mucosal biopsy specimens reveals invasive protozoal forms in the epithelium as well as mild to severe enteritis with mild to marked architectural changes and a mixed inflammatory infiltrate containing many eosinophils. Peripheral eosinophilia may also be present.

Among immunocompetent individuals, treatment is indicated only in those for whom symptoms persist after five to seven days. Treatment with trimethoprim–sulfamethoxazole for 7–10 days is effective in most patients, but more prolonged and even indefinite treatment may be required in AIDS and other immunosuppressed patients to prevent frequent relapses. Quinolones have been used successfully in those intolerant of trimethoprim–sulfamethoxazole. Where possible, immune reconstitution with HAART treatment is important for AIDS patients.

Casillas SM, Hall RL, Herwaldt BL. Cyclosporiasis surveillance - United States, 2011-2015. *MMWR Surveill Summ.* 2019;68(3): 1–16. [PMID: 31002104]

Lequa P, Seas C. *Cystoisospora* and *Cyclospora*. *Curr Opin Infect Dis.* 2013;26:479–483. [PMID: 23982239]

Taniuchi M, Verweij JJ, Sethabutr O, et al. Multiplex polymerase chain reaction method to detect Cyclospora, Cystoisospora, and Microsporidia in stool samples. *Diagn Microbiol Infect Dis.* 2011 Dec;71(4):386–390. [PMID: 21982218]

E. *Entamoeba histolytica*

Entamoeba histolytica infection occurs throughout the world, but the highest prevalence rates are found in low-income countries with suboptimal sanitation in Asia, Africa, and Central and South America. Simply finding amoeba by microscopic examination in stool in the course of epidemiologic studies and clinical evaluation is compromised by the fact that only 10% of *E histolytica* infections are symptomatic and that two noninvasive, nonpathogenic species, *Entamoeba dispar* and *Entamoeba moshkovskii*, colonize humans with far greater frequency than does *E histolytica*.

E histolytica cysts are ingested by consuming contaminated food or water or via fecal-oral contact, often during sexual activity; hence, there is a higher prevalence among homosexuals. Following excystation, trophozoites bind to the colonic epithelial glycocalyx sugars via a trophozoite surface lectin and subsequently invade the colonic mucosa, causing inflammation and ulceration. Systemic dissemination may occur, most often to the liver, resulting in abscess formation.

Clinically, colonic colonization by *E histolytica* produces a wide spectrum of symptoms ranging from no symptoms in the majority of patients to devastating pancolitis with toxic megacolon, requiring emergency colectomy and carrying a mortality rate as high as 50%. In most symptomatic individuals, mild initial diarrhea progresses to dysentery with blood and mucus in the stool and crampy abdominal pain, often with tenesmus. Low-grade fever may be present in the minority of amoebic colitis patients. Anemia and hypoalbuminemia may be present depending on the severity and duration of the colitis. The clinical features can closely mimic ulcerative colitis or Crohn's colitis. Indeed, it is crucial to exclude amoebiasis before administering corticosteroids or other immunosuppressive drugs to presumed ulcerative colitis patients to avoid precipitating fulminant amoebic colitis with toxic megacolon or perforation. Localized infections may produce mass lesions (amoebomas), mimicking colonic malignancy.

Testing for *E histolytica*-specific antigen in the stool is commercially available and has the advantage of selective identification of *E histolytica* and not morphologically identical nonpathogenic strains. Sensitivities and specificities in the range of 90% have been reported. Highly sensitive and specific PCR methods for detecting pathogenic amoeba have also been developed but are used largely in the research setting. Stool microscopy is less sensitive and less specific than stool antigen detection or molecular methods. Using stool concentration techniques and special stains, examination of three specimens results in a sensitivity of approximately 85%. Sigmoidoscopy with collection of mucus from ulcers for microscopy and biopsy samples from the edge of ulcers may supplement antigen testing and stool microscopy. Blood serologic testing is also useful in that absence of antibodies in someone with 7–10 days of symptoms makes the diagnosis less likely. Because antibody levels may persist for prolonged periods after exposure, a positive serologic test does not necessarily indicate acute amoebiasis.

Patients with *E histolytica* colonization should be treated whether symptomatic or not with metronidazole (750 mg three times daily for 10 days) or, alternatively, with tinidazole (2 g daily for 3 days), which may be more effective with fewer side effects. To eliminate residual cysts, treatment with a nitroimidazole should be followed by an intraluminally active drug such as iodoquinol (650 mg three times daily for 20 days) or paromomycin (10 mg three times daily for 7 days). Patients with severe colitis must be observed very closely for the development of surgically emergent toxic megacolon or perforation until a response to metronidazole treatment is evident.

Gonzales MLM, Dans LF, Sio-Aguilar J. Antiamoebic drugs for treating amoebic colitis. *Cochrane Database Syst Rev.* 2019;1(1):CD006085. [PMID: 30624763]

Haque R, Huston CD, Hughes M, et al. Amebiasis. *N Engl J Med.* 2003;348:1565–1573. [PMID: 12700377]

Shirley DT, Farr L, Watanabe K, Moonah S. A review of the global burden, new diagnostics, and current therapeutics for amebiasis. *Open Forum Infect Dis.* 2018;5(7):ofy161. [PMID: 30046644]

4. Fungal Infections: Microsporidia

Previously considered to be protozoa, microsporidia are now classified as fungi. Numerous species infect many life forms, and over 10 species are known to cause disease in humans, with *Enterocytozoon bieneusi* the most common. Involvement of many organs in addition to the intestine has been reported and will not be described here. The majority of clinically significant infections occur in AIDS and other immunosuppressed patients, although infections in travelers and otherwise healthy individuals have been documented.

Ingestion of spores via person-to-person, animal-to-person, foodborne, or waterborne routes has been incriminated as sources of transmission. Microsporidia spores have been isolated from the stools of asymptomatic, healthy, immunocompetent individuals raising questions as to whether the organisms are always the cause of gastrointestinal symptoms ascribed to them. Nevertheless, both self-limited diarrhea and occasionally chronic diarrhea have been reported, especially in travelers and in the elderly.

In immunosuppressed AIDS patients and in some immunosuppressed transplant patients, dehydration and malabsorption clinically indistinguishable from that associated with coccidial infections such as cryptosporidiosis have been noted in association with microsporidial organisms invading intestinal mucosa and with identification of *E bieneusi* or *Enterocytozoon intestinalis* in stool specimens. As in cryptosporidiosis, biliary tract involvement can occur.

Diagnosis is established by stool examination, which is facilitated by using special stains such as a modified trichrome stain or immunofluorescence antibody techniques. Identification of the spores in tissue samples such as intestinal mucosal biopsies by light or electron microscopy also establishes the diagnosis. In addition, several PCR assays have been developed but are not yet widely available.

Albendazole (400 mg twice daily for 2–4 weeks) is the treatment of choice for microsporidiosis but is of limited efficacy in the treatment of E bieneusi infections, the most common form associated with diarrheal disease. Hence, restoration of immunocompetence with HAART in AIDS patients and reduced immunosuppression in transplant patients is desirable if possible. Numerous other antibiotic, antiparasitic, and antifungal agents have been tried without much benefit in immunosuppressed patients with chronic diarrhea who harbor these organisms. Treatment with the antibiotic fumagillin at 60 mg daily for 2 weeks showed promising results in one small placebo-controlled trial and in several uncontrolled reports, although worrisome bone marrow depression was noted in some drug recipients.

Champion L, Durrbach A, Lang P, et al. Fumagillin for treatment of intestinal microsporidiosis in renal transplant recipients. *Am J Transplant*. 2010;10:1925–1930. [PMID: 20636462]

Didier ES, Weiss LM. Microsporidiosis: current status. *Curr Opin Infect Dis*. 2006;19:485–492. [PMID: 16940873]

Heyworth MF. Genetic aspects and environmental sources of microsporidia that infect the human gastrointestinal tract. *Trans R Soc Trop Med Hyg*. 2017;111(1):18–21. [PMID: 28339881]

5. Traveler's Diarrhea

With increasing economic globalization and the increased popularity of tourism to lower-income nations, traveler's diarrhea affects literally millions of travelers each year. A generally accepted definition for traveler's diarrhea is the passage of three or more loose to diarrheal stools in 24 hours often but not invariably associated with other symptoms, including abdominal discomfort, nausea, vomiting, hematochezia, and fever, depending on the cause. Symptoms most often develop 2–10 days after arrival of the traveler but may occur at any time during foreign exposure.

The incidence of traveler's diarrhea varies greatly with geographic region and correlates with the level of sanitation at the travelers' destination. Incidence rates as high as 50% have been noted for selected South and Southeast Asian, Central African, and Central and South American countries, whereas estimated rates are 10–20% in Eastern European countries, the Middle East, the Caribbean Islands, and South Africa, and Central and East Asia. Estimated rates among travelers to and in Northern and Western Europe, the United States, Canada, Australia, New Zealand, Japan, and Singapore are under 10%. Risk factors for the individual traveler other than destination are conditions that interfere with host defenses against enteric infections, as discussed earlier in this chapter. In particular, immunosuppressed patients and patients with hypochlorhydria caused by pharmacologic agents or gastric surgery may be especially vulnerable to developing traveler's diarrhea.

Virtually any of the specific organisms discussed individually in this chapter may be the causative agent for any given case of traveler's diarrhea. Pathogenic bacteria have been estimated to cause up to 90% of traveler's diarrhea in some studies in which an etiologic agent was identified. ETEC and EAEC appear as the most common causes, but invasive bacteria including *Campylobacter*, *Salmonella*, *Shigella* species, and invasive *E coli* predominate among those with dysentery. Both rotaviruses and noroviruses are established causes, the latter being increasingly recognized in outbreaks among cruise passengers. Protozoa such as *Giardia* and cryptosporidia, while less common, have been isolated from a substantial number of travelers with more protracted diarrhea, especially among those who develop malabsorption.

The clinical features will not be belabored here, and the reader is referred to the descriptions of specific infections earlier in the chapter. By far the most common presentation is that associated with ETEC or EAEC infection, with abrupt onset of watery diarrhea lasting a few hours to as long as 5 days. However, the entire spectrum of the clinical features of gastrointestinal infections may be seen, ranging from a few loose stools to severe dysentery with fever or protracted diarrhea with malabsorption, depending on the cause of the infection and the host's immune response capacity.

Because a specific diagnosis is rarely established during travels, treatment is largely empiric. If diarrhea is severe, rehydration is crucial, preferably using an oral rehydration solution with a formula similar to that recommended by the WHO or, if necessary, intravenous hydration. Loperamide (2 mg up to four times daily) can provide symptomatic relief but should not be used in patients with dysentery of unknown cause and should be avoided in patients with possible *C difficile* (those taking prophylactic antibiotics) given the risk of development of toxic megacolon. There is also some evidence, though not conclusive, that antimotility agents can prolong the duration of some enteric infections such as shigellosis. Effective antibiotic therapy reduces the duration of ETEC and EAEC, the most common causes of traveler's diarrhea. Development of antibiotic resistance is a major problem and has reduced the efficacy of trimethoprim–sulfamethoxazole, aminopenicillins, and tetracyclines. Instead, quinolones such as ciprofloxacin or norfloxacin have been widely used in recent years. Azithromycin is now recommended by some as the drug of choice for empiric treatment in areas such as southern Asia, Central and South America, and northern Africa where quinolone-resistant organisms are increasing. The nonabsorbed antibiotic rifaximin is effective against ETEC and, although expensive, may ultimately become the empiric antibiotic treatment of choice for nondysenteric traveler's diarrhea.

Prevention is the most effective approach to reducing the burden of traveler's diarrhea. Patient education is a crucial component of this strategy. Travelers should be instructed not to consume water that has not been thoroughly boiled, filtered with iodine-containing filters, or chemically treated with bleach or tincture of iodine. Drinks, especially those with ice, should be avoided. Teeth should be brushed with bottled or treated water, and ingestion of water while showering should be avoided. Only thoroughly cooked vegetables, fish, shellfish, and meat should be eaten. Sauces and dips such as guacamole are a frequent source of infection. Fruits, unless freshly peeled, should not be eaten. Fruit-, vegetable-, and meat-containing salads should be avoided.

Bismuth subsalicylate (two tablets or 30 mL of the liquid preparation four times daily) can be taken as prophylaxis. However, compliance is generally poor due to the inconvenience, and salicylate toxicity is a small risk especially if intake is prolonged. Antibiotic prophylaxis for the casual, healthy tourist, although often used, is not generally recommended in view of cost and the risk of inducing antibiotic resistance among pathogens. Rather, providing a prescription for an antibiotic for use should the traveler develop diarrhea is more appropriate. Undesirable side effects of antibiotic prophylaxis may include allergic reactions, antibiotic-induced diarrhea, *C difficile* colitis, and yeast infections. Antibiotic prophylaxis can be justified for individuals who are immunocompromised, who have IBD or other significant comorbidities, or for those travelers whose responsibilities and schedule are such that severe traveler's diarrhea would be more than an inconvenience and would potentially negate the purpose of their journey. Quinolones such as ciprofloxacin (500 mg daily) are most widely used, although resistance to these agents is increasing. Rifaximin (200 mg twice daily) is promising, reducing diarrhea up to threefold among travelers to tropical or semitropical regions. The orally administered whole cell vaccine with the nontoxic cholera toxin B subunit (Dukoral) is effective against ETEC, but is not available in the United States. A single-dose live oral vaccine against *V cholerae* (Vaxchora) is FDA approved and recommended for adult travelers up to age 64 visiting areas of high rates of cholera transmission.

Hill DR, Ericsson CD, Pearson RD, et al. The practice of travel medicine: guidelines by the Infectious Diseases Society of America. *Clin Infect Dis.* 2006;43:1499–1539. [PMID: 17109284]

Hu Y, Ren J, Zhan M, Li W, Dai H. Efficacy of rifaximin in prevention of travelers' diarrhea: a meta-analysis of randomized, double-blind, placebo-controlled trials. *J Travel Med.* 2012;19(6):352–356. [PMID: 23379704]

Peltola H, Siitonen A, Kyrönseppä H, et al. Prevention of travellers' diarrhoea by oral B-subunit/whole-cell cholera vaccine. *Lancet.* 1991;338(8778):1285–1289. [PMID: 1682684]

Steffen R, Hill DR, DuPont HL. Traveler's diarrhea: a clinical review. *JAMA.* 2015;313(1):71-80. [PMID: 25562268]

Schlagenhauf P, Weld L, Goorhuis A, et al. Travel-associated infection presenting in Europe (2008-12): an analysis of EuroTravNet longitudinal, surveillance data, and evaluation of the effect of the pre-travel consultation. *Lancet Infect Dis.* 2015;15(1):55–64. [PMID: 25477022]

Wong KK, Burdette E, Mahon BE, Mintz ED, Ryan ET, Reingold AL. Recommendations of the Advisory Committee on immunization practices for use of cholera vaccine. *MMWR Morb Mortal Wkly Rep.* 2017;66(18):482–485. [PMID: 28493859]

6. Medication-Related Diarrhea

Hundreds of medications can produce diarrhea. One only has to peruse the adverse reaction sections related to individual medications in the current *Physician's Desk Reference* to appreciate the scope of the problem. Only a few of the major causes are listed in Table 5–1. To that list could be added antiarrhythmics, cholinergic agents, prokinetics, prostaglandins, and many more. A careful history of all medications, both prescription and nonprescription, as well as herbal remedies and nutritional supplements—*including when they were begun*—must be obtained if unnecessary and costly evaluation seeking the cause of the diarrhea is to be avoided. In the vast majority of cases, though not all, medication-related diarrhea begins within a few days of the initiation of treatment with or a change in dosage of the offending agent.

Mesenteric Vascular Disease

6

Navin L. Kumar, MD

Kunal Jajoo, MD

MESENTERIC ISCHEMIA

ESSENTIAL CONCEPTS

▶ Acute mesenteric ischemia (AMI) is a medical and surgical emergency. Delay in diagnosis is associated with high mortality.

▶ Patients often present with abdominal pain out of proportion to physical examination findings.

▶ Clinical suspicion of AMI necessitates early radiologic evaluation (computed tomographic [CT] angiography, conventional angiography) or exploratory surgery in patients with peritoneal signs.

▶ Chronic mesenteric ischemia (CMI) is a clinical diagnosis. Patients report classic symptoms (eg, intestinal angina) and have radiographic findings showing severe stenoses or occlusion of two or more mesenteric arteries.

▶ Acute colonic ischemia is rarely life threatening and usually resolves with supportive care.

1. Etiology & Pathogenesis

Intestinal ischemia is caused by a reduction in intestinal blood flow, most commonly as a result of occlusion, vasospasm, or hypoperfusion of the mesenteric circulation. It is categorized as acute or chronic, depending on the rapidity and the extent to which blood flow is compromised. Ischemia can involve the small intestine or colon. Acute small intestinal ischemia (ie, AMI) is a medical and surgical emergency that requires prompt diagnosis and a coordinated, interdisciplinary approach. By contrast, acute colonic ischemia (ie, ischemic colitis) is rarely an emergent condition.

Intestinal ischemia can be further categorized as arterial versus venous, embolic versus thrombotic, and occlusive versus nonocclusive. Other causes of bowel ischemia include strangulating obstructions (adhesions, hernias, metastatic malignancy, intussusceptions) and vasculitis (systemic lupus erythematosus, polyarteritis nodosa).

2. Splanchnic Circulation: Anatomy & Physiology

The vascular supply to the intestines includes the celiac artery, the superior mesenteric artery (SMA), and the inferior mesenteric artery (IMA) (Figure 6–1). The celiac axis supplies blood to the stomach and proximal duodenum. The SMA supplies the small bowel from the distal duodenum to the mid-transverse colon. The IMA supplies the mid-transverse colon to the rectum.

When a major artery is occluded, the natural anastomoses or collateral pathways between the major arteries open immediately in response to a fall in arterial pressure distal to the obstruction. The superior and inferior pancreaticoduodenal vessels are collaterals that connect the celiac axis to the SMA. The phrenic artery connects the aorta to the celiac axis. The marginal artery of Drummond and the arc of Riolan are collaterals that connect the SMA and the IMA. The internal iliac arteries provide collaterals to the rectum. Of note, Griffith point in the splenic flexure and Sudeck point in the rectosigmoid area are watershed areas within the colonic blood supply and common locations for acute colonic ischemia.

The splanchnic circulation receives as little as 10% of the cardiac output under basal conditions and as much as 35% postprandially. Approximately 70% of splanchnic inflow goes to the mucosa, which is the most metabolically active area of the gut. The villous tips are the most vulnerable to ischemic injury. Intestinal blood flow is under complex regulation controlled primarily by resistance arterioles and precapillary sphincters. Several vasoactive substances influence intestinal perfusion. Catecholamines, angiotensin II, and vasopressin all can cause vasoconstriction, whereas vasoactive intestinal peptide causes vasodilation. Products of ischemia such as acidosis, hypoxemia, and hyperkalemia have been shown to cause vasodilation. Ischemic damage is caused by both hypoxia and reperfusion injury.

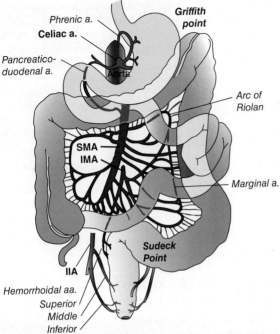

▲ Figure 6–1. Distribution of blood supply to the small intestine and colon from the celiac artery, superior mesenteric artery (SMA), inferior mesenteric artery (IMA), and internal iliac artery (IIA). (Reproduced with permission from Kasper DL, Braunwald E, Fauci AS, et al: *Harrison's Principles of Internal Medicine*, 17th ed. New York, NY: McGraw Hill; 2008.)

Brandt LJ, Feuerstadt P, Longstreth GF, et al. ACG clinical guideline: epidemiology, risk factors, patterns of presentation, diagnosis, and management of colon ischemia (CI). *Am J Gastroenterol* 2015;110:18–44. [PMID: 25559486]

Kirkpatrick ID, Kroeker MA, Greenberg HM. Biphasic CT with mesenteric CT angiography in the evaluation of acute mesenteric ischemia: initial experience. *Radiology*. 2003;229:91–98. [PMID: 12944600]

ACUTE MESENTERIC ISCHEMIA

 ESSENTIALS OF DIAGNOSIS

▶ Maintain a high index of clinical suspicion.

▶ Consider in patients >50 years who present with sudden onset of severe abdominal pain lasting >2 hours, especially if a history of cardiovascular disease or peripheral vascular disease is present.

▶ Consider in patients with abdominal pain out of proportion to physical findings.

▶ Angiography is the diagnostic procedure of choice and is potentially therapeutic.

▶ General Considerations

AMI remains a challenging diagnosis with a mortality rate exceeding 50% for patients requiring surgical intervention. Time to diagnosis and treatment is critical for these patients. The incidence of AMI has increased due to longer life expectancies, increased awareness of ischemic syndromes, and enhanced diagnostic and therapeutic techniques. The various causes of AMI include SMA embolism (50%), SMA thrombosis (15–20%), nonocclusive mesenteric ischemia (NOMI; 20–25%), and mesenteric venous thrombosis (MVT) (5–10%).

1. Mesenteric Artery Embolism & Thrombosis

Embolism to the SMA is most frequently due to a dislodged thrombus originating from the left atrium, left ventricle, left-sided cardiac valves, or the proximal aorta. Risk factors thus include cardiac arrhythmias (eg, atrial fibrillation), cardiac valvular disease including infective endocarditis, recent myocardial infarction, ventricular aneurysm, and aortic atherosclerosis or aneurysm. The emboli usually lodge at sites of normal anatomical narrowing, such as the branching point of an artery. The SMA is most susceptible to embolism due to its narrow takeoff angle and large diameter.

SMA thrombosis usually occurs at the origin of the vessel, which is frequently an area of severe atherosclerotic narrowing. Acute thrombosis usually occurs in a patient with underlying CMI—hence the term acute-on-chronic ischemia. This process is analogous to plaque rupture in acute coronary syndromes. Patients with peripheral arterial disease, advanced age, and decreased cardiac output are at higher risk for this etiology.

▶ Clinical Findings

A. Symptoms & Signs

Patients with AMI present with severe, acute, unremitting abdominal pain strikingly out of proportion to the initial physical findings. On examination, the abdomen may be soft and either nontender or minimally tender. Distention is often the first sign. Later findings may include signs of peritonitis, such as a rigid abdomen or rebound tenderness, especially if infarction or gangrene has occurred. Associated symptoms may include nausea, emesis, and transient nonbloody diarrhea due to urgent bowel evacuation. Occult blood is found in the stool in 50–75% of cases; overt blood in the stool is only seen in advanced ischemia.

B. Laboratory Findings

Laboratory results in patients with AMI are nonspecific and normal values should not delay urgent radiologic evaluation in patients with a high clinical suspicion. Findings in later or more advanced cases include leukocytosis, an elevated hematocrit or hemoglobin secondary to hemoconcentration, and metabolic acidosis due to a rise in serum lactate.

Many investigators have searched for the optimal plasma or serum biomarker to easily identify AMI. Intestinal fatty acid–binding protein (iFABP) levels, glutathione S-transferase, D-lactate, and D-dimer have shown promising but also conflicting results in studies. No single biomarker has achieved sufficient sensitivity, specificity, or accuracy for routine clinical use to diagnose or exclude AMI.

C. Imaging Studies

Historically, standard radiologic imaging has not been useful in diagnosing AMI, because most of the reported "classic" findings (eg, bowel edema, pneumatosis intestinalis, portal venous gas) are not seen until late in the course of the illness. Plain films of the abdomen are usually normal, and the utility of these studies is to exclude other acute abdominal processes such as perforation or obstruction. Mesenteric angiography has been the gold standard for making the diagnosis of AMI; however, high-resolution CT angiography (CTA) has become the initial imaging test of choice due to its noninvasive approach, high diagnostic accuracy, and ability to distinguish embolic from thrombotic mesenteric occlusion. CT findings may be either more specific or nonspecific. More specific findings include thromboembolism in mesenteric arteries, portal venous gas, bowel wall intramural gas or pneumatosis, lack of bowel wall enhancement, and signs of ischemia in other organs. Less specific signs include diffuse bowel wall thickening, striking vascular engorgement, dilated fluid-filled loops of bowel, and mesenteric edema (Figure 6–2). Magnetic resonance angiography (MRA) can produce similar images; however, image acquisition takes longer than for CTA, which limits its use in the setting of an acutely ill patient.

CTA also provides detailed information about the mesenteric vessels and can inform surgical planning. For patients

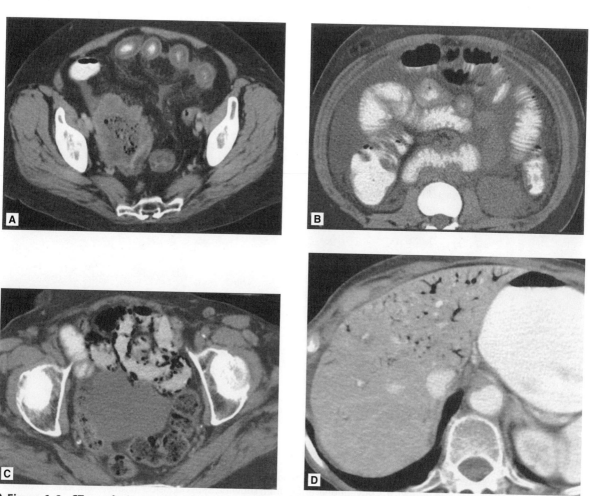

▲ **Figure 6–2.** CT scan findings of intestinal ischemia. **A** and **B.** Small bowel thickening. **C.** Small intestinal pneumatosis. **D.** Portal venous gas. (Reproduced with permission of Koenraad Mortele, MD.)

presenting with more advanced AMI (eg, hemodynamic instability or signs of sepsis or peritonitis), a plain film should be obtained immediately to rule-out perforation.

D. Angiography

Angiography is important in both diagnosis and management of AMI and remains the preferred approach for evaluation of patients with suspected AMI who are hemodynamically stable and do not have signs of advanced intestinal ischemia. Placement of a catheter into the SMA allows visualization of obstructing lesions and facilitates interventions such as infusion of vasodilators into the SMA, percutaneous aspiration of clot or catheter-directed thrombolytic therapy, and/or balloon angioplasty with stent placement (Figure 6–3).

▶ Treatment

The goal of treatment in AMI is to restore intestinal blood flow as rapidly as possible. However, initial management must include hemodynamic resuscitation and correction of precipitating causes of AMI such as arrhythmias, congestive heart failure leading to reduced cardiac output, or volume depletion. Patients require aggressive hemodynamic monitoring and support, correction of fluid and electrolyte abnormalities, and treatment with broad-spectrum antibiotics.

Systemic anti-coagulation should be initiated in most patients with AMI to reduce further thrombus propagation.

Patients with peritoneal signs or clinical suspicion of perforation or gangrene require emergent laparotomy, after hemodynamic stabilization, to immediately restore mesenteric blood flow and resect nonviable bowel. Patients who are hemodynamically stable with no peritoneal signs or evidence of sepsis may alternatively first undergo angiography to confirm the mesenteric arterial occlusion. Once the obstructing lesion is confirmed with angiography, patients can undergo either surgical revascularization (through aortomesenteric bypass grafting, embolectomy, or thromboendarterectomy) or endovascular revascularization (using techniques such as pharmacologic or mechanical thrombectomy, or balloon angioplasty typically with arterial stent placement).

Matsumoto S, Sekine K, Funaoka H, et al. Diagnostic performance of plasma biomarkers in patients with acute intestinal ischaemia. *Br J Surg.* 2014;101:232–238. [PMID: 24402763]

Oldenburg WA, Lau LL, Rodenberg TJ, et al. Acute mesenteric ischemia: a clinical review. *Arch Intern Med.* 2004;164:1054–1062. [PMID: 15159262]

Segatto E, Mortelé K, Ji H, et al. Acute small bowel ischemia: CT imaging findings. *Semin Ultrasound CT MR.* 2003;24:364–376. [PMID: 14620718]

Wiesner W, Khurana B, Ji H, et al. CT of acute bowel ischemia. *Radiology.* 2003;226:635–650. [PMID: 12601205]

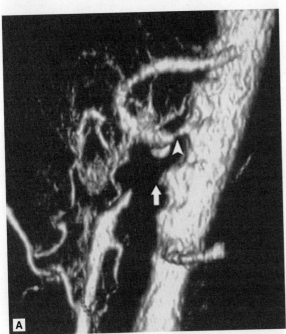
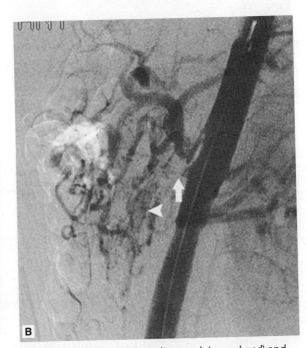

▲ **Figure 6–3.** **A.** Volume-rendered three-dimensional CT scan showing narrowing of the celiac trunk (*arrowhead*) and occlusion of the proximal SMA (*arrow*). **B.** Conventional angiogram showing SMA occlusion (*arrow*). (Reproduced with permission from Kirkpatrick ID, Kroeker MA, Greenberg HM. Biphasic CT with mesenteric CT angiography in the evaluation of acute mesenteric ischemia: initial experience. *Radiology.* 2003;229(1):91–98.)

2. Mesenteric Venous Thrombosis

ESSENTIALS OF DIAGNOSIS

▶ Acute form—maintain a high index of suspicion in patients with recent onset of acute abdominal pain associated with a predisposing condition (ie, heritable or acquired hypercoagulable states).

▶ Diagnosed with 90% sensitivity by contrast CT, MDCT, or vascular angiography.

General Considerations

MVT accounts for 5–10% of all cases of AMI. The conditions responsible for the development of MVT can be identified in over 80% of cases, and risk factors are summarized in Table 6–1. Over 50% of patients with MVT have a personal or family history of deep venous thrombosis or pulmonary embolism. The clinical presentation of MVT can be acute, characterized by a more sudden onset of symptoms; subacute, in which symptoms occur for days or weeks without bowel infarction; or chronic, involving portal or splenic vein thrombosis and stigmata of portal hypertension with or without variceal bleeding.

Pathogenesis

MVT leads to resistance to mesenteric venous blood flow, with resultant bowel wall edema, fluid efflux into the bowel lumen, and systemic hypotension. Due to venous congestion and the relative loss of intravascular volume, arterial inflow is diminished, which can lead to bowel ischemia and, ultimately, infarction. The extent of the venous collateral circulation is a

Table 6-1. Causes of mesenteric venous thrombosis.

1. Hypercoagulable states
  a. Heritable disorder of coagulation
    (1) Factor V Leiden–resistance to activated protein C
    (2) Prothrombin gene mutation-620210A
  b. Acquired hypercoagulable states
    (1) Paroxysmal nocturnal hemoglobinuria
    (2) Myeloproliferative disorders
  c. Deficiencies of anticoagulant proteins
    (1) Protein C and protein S
    (2) Antithrombin
  d. Acquired hypercoagulable states
    (1) Neoplasms
    (2) Oral contraceptives
    (3) Pregnancy
2. Inflammatory disorders
  a. Pancreatitis
  b. Intra-abdominal sepsis
3. Cirrhosis and portal hypertension

key variable influencing whether submucosal hemorrhage or bowel infarction will develop following MVT.

Clinical Findings

A. Symptoms & Signs

As noted, the presentation of MVT can be acute, subacute, or chronic. Symptoms of acute MVT usually begin a few days to a few weeks (mean, 7 days) before presentation and, in 25% of patients, have been present for 30 days before admission. This longer duration of symptoms is in contrast with other forms of AMI, as described above. Nausea, vomiting, and diarrhea are common. Vital sign abnormalities may include fever and hypotension. Abdominal distention with mild to moderate tenderness is often present. Although occult blood is seen in over 50% of patients, the presence of overt blood in the stool usually signifies severe ischemia or bowel infarction and is more rarely encountered. Similarly, peritoneal signs such as guarding and rebound tenderness, lactic acidosis, and increased transaminases are late findings that may be associated with bowel infarction.

In the subacute form of MVT, symptoms such as abdominal pain can be present for several weeks along with an unremarkable physical examination. Patients with chronic MVT are typically asymptomatic and often diagnosed incidentally by imaging studies. Alternatively, these patients may present with sequelae of portal hypertension such as variceal bleeding, ascites, or splenomegaly.

B. Imaging Studies

MVT is diagnosed by cross-sectional imaging that demonstrates thrombosis within the mesenteric veins. CT scan with and without oral and intravenous contrast is the preferred initial study given its widespread availability and timely results. Classical CT findings with a sensitivity of greater than 90% include a dilated superior mesenteric vein with a clot or filling defect in the lumen (Figure 6–4). It should be noted, however, that CT may be less reliable in early thrombosis if small vessels are involved. Portal venous gas, air in the small bowel, or free intraperitoneal air usually indicates intestinal infarction. If an initial CT scan is nondiagnostic and clinical suspicion remains a high, MR venography (MRV) may be pursued.

Treatment

The treatment of acute MVT depends on whether intestinal infarction or perforation has occurred or is strongly suspected. Patients with concerning clinical, radiographic, or laboratory findings should proceed directly to surgery with an open laparotomy and resection of infarcted bowel (see Figure 6–4). Most patients, however, do not have concerns for infarction or perforation and can be managed conservatively with bowel rest, intravenous fluid hydration, prophylactic antibiotics, and anti-coagulation to limit further growth of thrombus and allow for recanalization. Anticoagulation is usually continued for at least 3–6 months and longer if the patient is found to have an underlying hypercoagulable

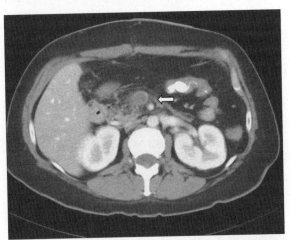

▲ **Figure 6–4.** Acute superior mesenteric vein thrombosis; arrow points to a large thrombus in the proximal superior mesenteric vein. (Reproduced with permission of David Stockwell, MD.)

disorder. Catheter-based techniques with pharmacologic thrombolysis (using streptokinase, urokinase, and tissue plasminogen activator) or mechanical thrombectomy lack large-scale data but are potential options as an adjunct to anti-coagulation in more specialized centers.

Amitrano L, Brancaccio V, Guardascione MA, et al. High prevalence of thrombophilic genotypes in patients with acute mesenteric vein thrombosis. *Am J Gastroenterol.* 2001;96:146–149. [PMID: 11197244]

Harnik IG, Brandt LJ. Mesenteric venous thrombosis. *Vasc Med.* 2010;15:407–418. [PMID: 20926500]

3. Nonocclusive Mesenteric Ischemia

 ESSENTIALS OF DIAGNOSIS

► Accounts for approximately 20% of cases of AMI and results from intense mesenteric vasoconstriction, leading to splanchnic hypoperfusion.

► Suspect in patients with diffuse atherosclerotic disease under conditions of hemodynamic stress (hypotension), in the setting of vasoconstrictive agents (vasopressin, cocaine), and in patients with vasculitis (eg, systemic lupus erythematosus, polyarteritis nodosa).

► Angiography may be both diagnostic and therapeutic.

▶ Clinical Findings

Signs and symptoms of NOMI are similar to those of mesenteric arterial obstruction with acute onset of severe periumbilical abdominal pain out of proportion to exam findings.

The pathogenesis, however, is due to marked constriction of the mesenteric arteries (the SMA is most commonly involved) as opposed to acute thromboembolism. Vasopressin and angiotensin are the most likely mediators of this phenomenon that attempts to maintain cardiac and cerebral blood perfusion at the expense of the splanchnic and peripheral circulation—however, vasospasm can also play a role. Patients who develop NOMI are typically elderly and critically ill with severe cardiovascular disease, but NOMI can also be seen in younger patients with vasculitis or who are on vasoconstricting medications or substances. Predisposing factors include conditions such as cardiogenic or septic shock, cardiac arrythmias, peripheral arterial disease, and dehydration; medications such as diuretics, digoxin, and adrenergic agonists; and therapies such as recent cardiopulmonary bypass and dialysis.

The mortality rate from NOMI is high for several reasons, including advanced patient age, comorbidities, and difficulty in making the diagnosis and reversing ischemia once it has started. As with other causes of AMI, a high index of clinical suspicion is necessary. CTA is typically the first imaging test of choice and helps rule out AMI etiologies such as mesenterial arterial obstruction or venous thrombosis. Given the dynamic and spastic component of NOMI, the diagnosis may be missed on noninvasive imaging and mesenteric angiography must be pursued (Figure 6–5).

▶ Treatment

Treatment of NOMI centers on restoring intestinal blood flow as soon as possible. This goal is achieved by addressing underlying causes such as cardiogenic or septic shock, removing inciting factors such as vasoconstrictive medications, and providing supportive care with fluid resuscitation and broad-spectrum antibiotics. Intra-arterial infusion of vasodilators such as papaverine is a possible adjunctive therapy, although large-scale data is lacking.

Bassiouny HS. Nonocclusive mesenteric ischemia. *Surg Clin North Am.* 1997;97:319–326. [PMID: 9146715]

Brandt LJ, Boley SJ. AGA technical review on intestinal ischemia. American Gastrointestinal Association. *Gastroenterology.* 2000;118:954–968. [PMID: 10784596]

CHRONIC MESENTERIC ISCHEMIA

 ESSENTIALS OF DIAGNOSIS

► Suspect in patients with postprandial abdominal pain, avoidance of eating (which triggers pain), weight loss, and the presence of an abdominal bruit on exam (50% of patients).

► Angiography shows involvement of at least two of three major splanchnic blood vessels.

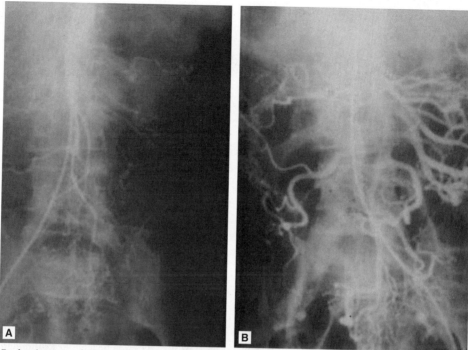

▲ **Figure 6–5.** Angiogram of the superior mesenteric artery in a patient with nonocclusive mesenteric ischemia (NOMI). **A.** Initial angiogram demonstrating diffuse vasoconstriction in setting of hypotensive shock. **B.** Angiogram after 48 hours of papaverine infusion, showing dilation. (Reproduced with permission from Baum S. Abram's Angiography. 4th ed. New York, NY: Little, Brown; 1997.)

General Considerations

CMI is the result of reduced blood flow due to atherosclerotic narrowing of at least two of the three major splanchnic blood vessels (ie, celiac axis, SMA, or IMA). Usually, an adequate collateral circulation has developed between these vessels that prevents intestinal infarction—however, patients remain symptomatic due to the reduced blood supply in the setting of increased demand (fed state). Similarly, stenosis in only one of the three mesenteric arteries does not typically lead to symptoms of CMI due to these extensive collaterals.

Clinical Findings

A. Symptoms & Signs

The classic diagnostic triad for CMI consists of postprandial abdominal pain, weight loss, and an abdominal bruit. This pain from "intestinal angina" is typically recurrent, dull, crampy, and periumbilical, occurring 10–30 minutes after meals and lasting 1–3 hours. Because eating consistently triggers pain, food fear causes patients to eat progressively less, resulting in weight loss and often cachexia. Most patients have a history of cardiovascular or peripheral vascular disease. Of note, some patients with PVD develop symptoms of

CMI after undergoing surgical repair of peripheral vascular lesions due to "steal" physiology (ie, increased blood flow to the extremities and away from the mesenteric circulation).

Physical examination usually reveals a soft abdomen without tenderness during episodes of pain, again consistent with the classic description of pain disproportionate to physical findings. As many as 50% of patients with CMI have an epigastric bruit, especially postprandially; nausea, emesis, and early satiety are commonly associated symptoms. The average duration of symptoms prior to diagnosis is 1 year. Diagnosis is often difficult because of the vague nature of complaints and absence of physical findings.

B. Imaging Studies

CTA is the initial imaging study of choice for CMI; high-grade stenoses in at least two of the three major splanchnic arteries must be demonstrated. Other noninvasive options include MR angiography (less reliable for detecting distal lesions) and duplex ultrasonography (operator-dependent and limited by body habitus). Regardless of imaging study, it is important to correlate angiographic findings with symptoms, because some individuals who have complete occlusion of all three major mesenteric arteries may remain asymptomatic because of collateral blood flow. Although there have been preliminary reports of "stress tests" for intestinal angina, at present there is no functional test with high sensitivity or specificity for confirming a clinical diagnosis of CMI.

Treatment

Once the diagnosis of CMI is made based on symptoms and confirmation of high-grade stenosis or occlusion of two or more mesenteric arteries, the goal is to restore mesenteric arterial flow. Although open surgical revascularization using aortomesenteric grafting was traditionally the optimal approach, recent advances in endovascular therapy have elevated percutaneous angioplasty with or without stenting as first-line therapy given the lower risk of periprocedural morbidity and mortality, albeit with a higher risk of symptom recurrence.

Pecoraro F, Rancic Z, Lachat M, et al. Chronic mesenteric ischemia: critical review and guidelines for management. *Ann Vasc Surg.* 2013;27(1):113–122. [PMID 23088809]

ACUTE COLONIC ISCHEMIA

ESSENTIALS OF DIAGNOSIS

▶ Suspect in patients with sudden onset of crampy, left lower quadrant pain followed by hematochezia within 24 hours.

▶ Diagnosed by colonoscopy or imaging studies (CT).

▶ Bleeding is typically limited and transfusion only rarely required.

General Considerations

Acute colonic ischemia is the most frequent form of mesenteric ischemia, accounting for 75% of all intestinal ischemia and affecting primarily the elderly. It is estimated that colonic ischemia may account for as many as 3 per 1000 hospital admissions. Findings of colonic ischemia are seen in 1 of every 100 colonoscopies and may be misdiagnosed as inflammatory bowel disease or infectious colitis (Plate 3). Colonic ischemia has been described in several clinical settings (Table 6–2), although in many instances, no specific cause can be identified. The risk of colonic ischemia appears to be highest for patients who have recently undergone cardiovascular surgery, and these patients may experience more severe episodes.

Pathogenesis

Ischemic injury to the colon usually occurs due to a sudden and transient reduction in blood flow, resulting in a low-flow state. In the majority of cases (95%), a specific occluding

Table 6-2 Risk factors for colonic Eschernia.

Precipitants of colonic ischemia
Hypotension
Congestive heart failure
Cardiopulmonary bypass
Dialysis
Aortoiliac surgery
Cholesterol emboli
Dehydration
Precipitants in patients < 50 years
Vasculitis (egg, systemic lupus erythematosus)
Hypercoagulable states (factory Leiden), phospholipid antibody syndrome
Sickle cell crisis
Long-distance running
Medications (estrogens, danazol, vasoconstrictors [pseudoephedrine, sumnatriptan], gold, psychotropic drugs, alosetron, antihypertensives, diuretics)
Cocaine
Infections resulting in hemorrhagic colitis (Shigarkr, Escherichia 01571-17, Cofrrprioborter., Kiebsiella oxytoca [especially with use of penicillin derivative], Clostridium difficiiie [10% hemorrhagic colitis])

anatomic lesion cannot be identified. Although it may occur anywhere, colonic ischemia most commonly affects the "watershed" areas of the colon with a limited collateral blood supply, such as the splenic flexure and rectosigmoid colon (Figure 6–6). Ischemia is usually mucosal and rarely transmural; consequently, gangrenous colitis and colonic strictures are infrequent. Eighty-five percent of cases of colonic ischemia resolve spontaneously within 2 weeks.

Clinical Findings

A. Symptoms & Signs

Patients with colonic ischemia usually present with abrupt onset of crampy left lower quadrant abdominal pain, and mild to moderate rectal bleeding or bloody diarrhea within the first 24 hours. Over 90% of patients are older than 60 years. Cardiovascular disease is common, and frequent precipitating factors include hypotension, cardiovascular surgery (coronary artery bypass grafting, aortic aneurysm repair), dialysis, and dehydration (including from extreme exercise). Physical examination reveals mild to moderate abdominal tenderness over the affected bowel, most often left-sided.

In contrast to patients with AMI, those with colonic ischemia do not usually appear acutely ill. Bleeding is usually mild, and patients rarely require blood transfusion. Peritoneal signs, if present, would suggest perforation or peritonitis. Ischemic colitis is usually a singular event, and only 5% of patients develop a recurrence.

The diagnosis is usually established on the basis of clinical history, physical examination, and endoscopic or

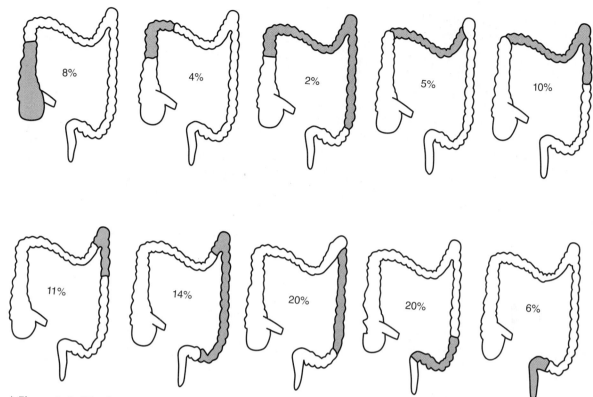

▲ **Figure 6–6.** Distribution of colonic ischemia in 250 cases. (Reproduced with permission from Brandt L, Boley SJ. Colonic ischemia, *Surg Clin North Am* 1992;72(1):203–229.)

radiologic studies. Although most patients who develop colonic ischemia are elderly, the condition can also occur in younger patients. For patients who are younger than 50 years, several precipitants of colonic ischemia should be considered (see Table 6–2). In young women, the triad of smoking, use of oral contraceptives, and carriage of the factor V Leiden mutation may be associated with increased risk of colonic ischemia.

B. Diagnostic Tests

In addition to patient history and physical examination, diagnostic modalities that aid in the evaluation of colonic ischemia include CT scan of the abdomen with intravenous contrast and flexible sigmoidoscopy or colonoscopy. Stool studies should also be performed to exclude infections such as *Escherichia coli* O157:H7, *Campylobacter* enteritis, *Klebsiella oxytoca*, or *Shigella*, which can be associated with hemorrhagic colitis. Of note, plain films of the abdomen are usually nondiagnostic, although thumbprinting representing submucosal hemorrhage and edema may be seen in 20–25% of cases. As the preferred imaging study, CT of the abdomen can demonstrate bowel wall thickening, mucosal and submucosal hemorrhage, pericolic fat stranding, and occasionally bowel wall pneumatosis (Figure 6–7).

Colonoscopy with biopsies makes the definitive diagnosis; however, endoscopy should be avoided in patients with significant abdominal pain or distention because air insufflation may precipitate perforation in cases of severe ischemia. Endoscopic findings frequently include petechial bleeding, pale mucosa, and, in more severe cases, hemorrhagic ulceration (see Plate 3), and biopsy specimens show characteristic findings. Catheter-based angiography is much less useful in the evaluation of colonic ischemia; however, it may be considered if the clinical findings raise concern for concomitant small bowel ischemia or infarction (indicating possible AMI).

▶ Treatment

Most patients with colonic ischemia improve with supportive care including bowel rest, intravenous fluids, and broad-spectrum antibiotics for all but the mildest of cases. Patients should be followed with serial abdominal examinations and monitored for bleeding, fever, leukocytosis, and electrolyte abnormalities. Any medications that can cause vasoconstriction or volume depletion and thereby promote ischemia should be withdrawn (ie, digitalis, glycosides, vasopressin, and diuretics). Marked colonic distention is treated with rectal tubes and nasogastric decompression if necessary. There is no role for anticoagulation given that the majority of

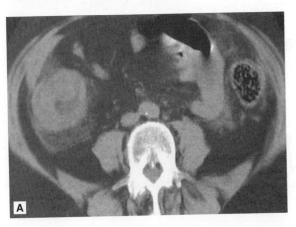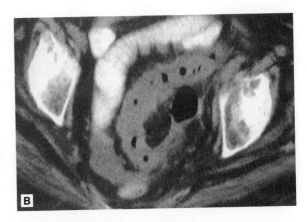

▲ **Figure 6–7.** CT scans demonstrating findings in colonic ischemia. **A.** Colonic thickening. **B.** Pneumatosis. (Reproduced with permission of Koenraad Mortele, MD.)

patients have nonocclusive ischemia. The American Gastro-enterological Association algorithm for diagnosis and manage-ment of acute intestinal ischemia is presented in Figure 6–8.

Patients with evidence of severe colonic ischemia require surgical exploration. Risk factors for severe disease include

peritoneal signs on physical examination; radiographic evi-dence of pneumoperitoneum, pneumatosis, or portal venous gas; and gangrene on colonoscopic examination. In addi-tion, patients who failed to respond to supportive care may also require surgical exploration. Long-term complications,

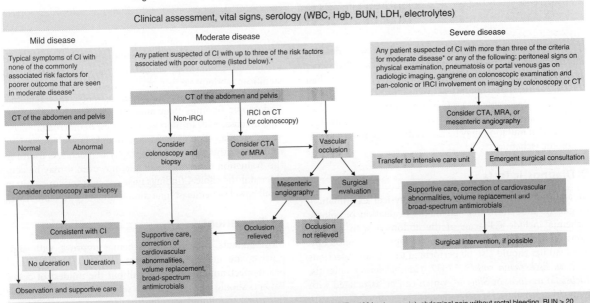

▲ **Figure 6–8.** Algorithm for the management of patients suspected as having colon ischemia. (Reproduced with permis-sion from Brandt LJ, Feuerstadt P, Longstreth GF, et al: ACG clinical guideline: epidemiology, risk factors, patterns of presentation, diagnosis, and management of colon ischemia (CI). *Am J Gastroenterol.* 2015;110(1):18–44.)

including persistent recurrent colitis and colonic structures, are infrequent but may require resection of the affected colonic segment.

In contrast to small bowel ischemia, colonic ischemia is rarely life threatening—particularly for those with nongangrenous disease (<5%). However, some reports suggest that ischemia of the right colon may have a worse prognosis compared with ischemia of other parts of the colon. This higher mortality is likely due to SMA involvement leading to diffuse small intestinal ischemia, which is not present in those with left-sided disease secondary to IMA insufficiency.

Brandt LJ, Feuerstadt P, Blaszka MC. Anatomic patterns, patient characteristics, and clinical outcomes in ischemic colitis: a study of 313 cases supported by histology. *Am J Gastroenterol.* 2010;105:2245–2252. [PMID: 20531399]

Brandt LJ, Feuerstadt P, Longstreth GF, et al. ACG clinical guideline: epidemiology, risk factors, patterns of presentation, diagnosis, and management of colon ischemia (CI). *Am J Gastroenterol.* 2015;110(1):18–45.

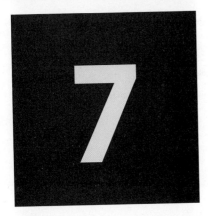

Gastrointestinal & Biliary Complications of Pregnancy

Punyanganie S. de Silva, MBBS, MPH

ESSENTIAL CONCEPTS

▶ Pregnancy can exacerbate many chronic gastrointestinal disorders; the central goal of evaluation is to control symptoms and rule out an urgent need for surgery while minimizing exposure to excessive tests and medications.

▶ Inflammatory bowel disease (IBD) patients should be in remission while trying to conceive, and the majority of IBD medications are safe in pregnancy and breastfeeding.

▶ Appendicitis is the most common indication for surgery during pregnancy.

▶ Gallstones are more common during pregnancy.

▶ Indications for urgent surgery are the same in pregnant as in nonpregnant patients.

▶ Efforts should be made to minimize risk to mother and fetus when performing diagnostic and therapeutic endoscopic and radiologic tests.

▶ General Considerations

The management of gastrointestinal disease during pregnancy poses multiple challenges. First, gastrointestinal diseases are common during pregnancy, and many predisposing gastrointestinal disorders are aggravated by pregnancy. Second, diagnostic options are often limited in pregnancy as there is a need to minimize testing out of concern for both maternal and fetal exposure. Finally, the management of these diseases is more complex due to the need to consider additional risks to both the pregnant mother and the fetus incurred by medications, endoscopic procedures, and surgeries. Data on safety and efficacy of both medications and procedures during pregnancy are often scarce or inadequate; few controlled trials have included pregnant women, and fewer still were designed specifically to study gastrointestinal

disease in this population. Since 2019, the US Food and Drug Administration (FDA) has started to introduce new prescription drug labels. These new labels will replace the old A, B, C, D, and X categories with more helpful information about a medicine's risks during pregnancy and lactation. The new labeling aims to provide more comprehensive risk statement based on human, animal studies, and pharmacological data, enabling the prescriber and consumer to make a more informed decision, rather than referring to the prior pregnancy categories.

Table 7–1 summarizes the prior US FDA categories for medication use in pregnancy.

GASTROESOPHAGEAL REFLUX DISEASE

Gestational reflux is common, affecting up to 80% of pregnant women. The majority of women have no preexisting gastroesophageal reflux disease (GERD), and symptoms often resolve following delivery. Symptoms are more common and more severe during the third trimester. Risk factors for heartburn during pregnancy include a history of heartburn before pregnancy or during previous pregnancies, multiparity, and younger maternal age. Reduced lower esophageal sphincter (LES) pressure and decreased gastric and small bowel motility, possibly mediated by progesterone and to a lesser extent by estrogen, and increased abdominal pressure secondary to the gravid uterus are all implicated in the pathogenesis.

▶ Clinical Findings

Heartburn is the predominant symptom of GERD, and regurgitation may accompany it. Symptoms are exacerbated by reclining and eating, and patients may also report hoarseness, cough, and asthma-like symptoms. Diagnosis is based on symptoms. Esophageal manometry and pH studies are rarely needed, and barium studies should be avoided in pregnancy. If required for severe symptoms, esophagogastroduodenoscopy (EGD) can be performed during pregnancy with

Table 7-1. FDA categories for the use of medications in pregnancy.

FDA Pregnancy Category	Interpretation
A	Controlled studies in animals and women have shown no risk in the first trimester, and possible fetal harm is remote
B	Either animal studies have not demonstrated a fetal risk but there are no controlled studies in pregnant women, or animal studies have shown an adverse effect that was not confirmed in controlled studies in women in the first trimester
C	No controlled studies in humans have been performed, and animal studies have shown adverse events, or studies in humans and animals are not available; should be given if the potential benefit outweighs the risk
D	Positive evidence of fetal risk is available, but the benefits may outweigh the risk if life-threatening or serious disease
X	Studies in animals or humans show fetal abnormalities; drug contraindicated

Reproduced with permission from Mahadevan U, Kane S. American gastroenterological association institute technical review on the use of gastrointestinal medications in pregnancy. *Gastroenterology.* 2006;131(1):283–311.

careful monitoring (see later discussion on endoscopy during pregnancy).

Treatment

Lifestyle modification should be the first line of therapy. This includes avoidance of alcohol, caffeine, mint, chocolate, tobacco, and fatty and spicy foods. Avoiding late night meals and raising the head of the bed can also prevent nighttime symptoms.

Medications used in the treatment of GERD during pregnancy are listed in Table 7-2.

Limited data are available regarding the efficacy and the safety of antacids; however, aluminum- and calcium-containing antacids are considered acceptable in normal therapeutic doses during pregnancy, and limited studies have not shown evidence of teratogenicity in animals. Calcium-based antacids are considered the first line of pharmacologic therapy. All magnesium-containing compounds should be avoided during the last few weeks of pregnancy, as magnesium can slow or arrest labor and may cause convulsions.

Antacids containing alginic acid or magnesium trisilicate should be avoided, as these chemicals have been associated with nephrolithiasis, hypotonia, respiratory distress, and cardiovascular impairment. Antacids containing sodium bicarbonate should not be used because they can cause maternal or fetal metabolic acidosis and fluid overload. Finally, antacids should be taken separately from iron preparations as they can interfere with absorption of iron.

Only a small percentage of relevant drugs are contraindicated for treatment of reflux symptoms in pregnancy. However, not all of these drug agents have been extensively evaluated in pregnant women or during the breastfeeding period.

First line pharmacological agents consist of antacids, alginates, and sucralfate.

Sucralfate, like antacids, is a nonabsorbable medication and has been studied in a randomized controlled trial (RCT) in pregnancy and found to be effective in the treatment of heartburn and regurgitation without presenting any risk to the fetus of pregnant women with normal renal function.

If symptoms persist, most of the histamine-2 receptor blockers (H_2-blockers), can be used except for nizatidine (due to fetal teratogenicity or harm in animal studies). More recently ranitidine has been recalled by the FDA due to concerns of the presence of a probable carcinogenic contaminant known as N-Nitrosodimethylamine (NDMA), which can accumulate over time, resulting in unacceptable consumer levels. Cimetidine is considered safe; however, some authorities recommend avoiding its use in pregnancy because of feminization seen in some animal and human studies. Fewer data are available for famotidine but no contraindications have been recorded. Overall, sucralfate, the above mentioned H_2-blockers and the majority of proton pump inhibitors (PPIs) have been found to be safe in pregnancy even when used in the first trimester.

Although PPIs are more effective than H_2-blockers for controlling symptoms of GERD and healing esophagitis, they are not as well studied in pregnancy. Some investigators suggest documenting failure with H_2-blockers and considering upper endoscopy before empiric trial and reserving for women with intractable symptoms or complicated GERD. Observational studies suggest omeprazole can be used safely during pregnancy; however, increased fetal toxicity in animal studies and some evidence of cardiac malformations in human studies have led to class C categorization by the FDA. Animal studies support the safety of lansoprazole and rabeprazole; pantoprazole and esomeprazole also appear to be safe based on animal data, although studies in humans are limited. More recently a large prospective cohort study failed to find any increase in early childhood fracture risk with maternal antireflux medication use. This suggests that prenatal exposure to antireflux medications does not affect fetal bones to a clinically significant extent. Antireflux surgery during pregnancy should be avoided and is often not necessary as symptoms resolve or improve with delivery.

Table 7–2. Medications used in the treatment of gastroesophageal reflux and peptic ulcer disease.

Drug	FDA Pregnancy Category	Recommendations for Pregnancy	Recommendations for Breast-Feeding
Antacids			
Aluminum containing	None	Most low risk: minimal absorption	Low risk
Calcium containing	None	Most low risk: minimal absorption	Low risk
Magnesium containing	None	Most low risk: minimal absorption	Low risk
Magnesium trisilicates	None	Avoid long-term or high doses	Low risk
Sodium bicarbonate	None	Not safe: alkalosis	Low risk
Mucosal Protectants			
Sucralfate	B	Low risk	No human data: probably compatible
H₂-Receptor Antagonists			
Cimetidine	B	Controlled data: low risk	Compatible
Famotidine	B	Paucity of safety data	Limited human data: probably compatible
Nizatidine	B	Limited human data: low risk in animals	Limited human data: probably compatible
Proton Pump Inhibitors			
Esomeprazole	B	Limited data: low risk	No human data: potential toxicity
Lansoprazole	B	Limited data: low risk	No human data: potential toxicity
Omeprazole	C	Embryonic and fetal toxicity reported, but large data sets suggest low risk	Limited human data: potential toxicity
Pantoprazole	B	Limited data: low risk	No human data: potential toxicity
Rabeprazole	B	Limited data: low risk	No human data: potential toxicity
Promotility Agents			
Cisapride	C	Controlled study: low risk, limited availability	Limited human data: probably compatible
Metoclopramide	B	Low risk	Limited human data: potential toxicity
Treatment of *Helicobacter pylori* Infection			
Amoxicillin	B	Low risk	Compatible
Bismuth	C	Not safe: teratogenicity	No human data: potential toxicity
Clarithromycin	C	Avoid in first trimester	No human data: probably compatible
Metronidazole	B	Low risk: avoid in first trimester	Limited human data: potential toxicity
Tetracycline	D	Not safe: teratogenicity	Compatible

Reproduced with permission from Mahadevan U, Kane S. American gastroenterological association institute technical review on the use of gastrointestinal medications in pregnancy. *Gastroenterology*. 2006;131(1):283–311.

Metoclopramide can be used in very refractory cases and may help treat pregnancy-related bowel hypomotility, which is hypothesized to contribute to pregnancy-related reflux. It has also been shown to increase the LES pressure, which makes it a useful anti reflux agent particularly in refractory cases and in the third trimester. It is used to treat pregnancy-associated nausea and vomiting, and one study shows no association with fetal malformations. For patients who have already undergone antireflux surgery prior to pregnancy, these methods appear to be effective in controlling GERD symptoms during and after pregnancy, and pregnancy does not appear to affect long-term outcomes and failure rates of antireflux surgery.

For patients experiencing symptoms in the postpartum period, antacids and sucralfate are considered safe because of limited maternal absorption. All H_2-blockers are excreted in breast milk; however, cimetidine, and famotidine are felt to be safe during breast-feeding. Nizatidine has been associated with growth retardation in one animal study.

Brygger L, Fristrup CW, Harbo FS, Jørgensen JS. Acute gastric incarceration from thoracic herniation in pregnancy following laparoscopic antireflux surgery. *BMJ Case Rep.* 2013;2013:bcr2012008391. [PMID: 23378556] https://www.fda.gov/drugs/drug-safety-and-availability/fda-updates-and-press-announcements-ndma-zantac-ranitidine

Thélin CS, Richter JE. Review article: the management of heartburn during pregnancy and lactation. *Aliment Pharmacol Ther.* 2020;51(4):421–434. [PMID: 31950535]

Wolfe HL, Wolfe JA, Ranjit A, Banaag A, Pérez Koehlmoos T, Witkop CT. Prenatal use of medications for gastroesophageal reflux disease and early childhood fracture risk. *Birth.* 2019;46(4):656–662. [PMID: 30834583]

NAUSEA & VOMITING

Almost 50% of women experience nausea and vomiting during early pregnancy and an additional 25% have nausea alone. In a prospective study of 160 pregnant women, 80% of the women reporting nausea stated that it lasted all day, suggesting that "morning sickness" may be a misnomer. The onset of nausea is within 4 weeks after the last menstrual period in most patients and typically peaks at 9 weeks of gestation. Sixty percent of cases resolve by the end of the first trimester, and 91% resolve by 20 weeks of gestation. The stimulus for nausea and vomiting is likely produced by the placenta. Recent advances in the genetic study of nausea and vomiting of pregnancy and hyperemesis gravidarum suggest a placental component to the etiology by implicating common variants in genes encoding placental proteins (namely Growth Differentiation Factor 15 [GDF15] and Insulin Like Growth Factor Binding Protein [IGFBP7] and hormone receptors GDNF Family Receptor Alpha Like [GFRAL] and Progesterone receptor PGR]).

Nausea and vomiting are less common in older women, multiparous women, and smokers probably due to smaller placental volumes in these women. Nausea and vomiting during pregnancy are associated with a decreased risk of miscarriage.

The clinical course of nausea and vomiting during pregnancy correlates closely with the level of human chorionic gonadotropin (hCG). It is theorized that hCG may stimulate estrogen production from the ovary; estrogen is known to increase nausea and vomiting. Women with twins or hydatidiform moles, who have higher hCG levels than do other pregnant women, are at a higher risk for these symptoms. Vitamin B deficiency may also contribute since the use of multivitamins containing vitamin B reduces the incidence of nausea and vomiting.

▶ Clinical Findings

A. Symptoms and Signs

A careful evaluation to exclude other disorders and contributing factors is important (Figure 7–1). The presence of heartburn suggests the coexistence of GERD and should prompt treatment with antacid medications (see the earlier discussion of GERD). Although patients can experience soreness of the abdominal muscles and ribs in the setting of recurrent vomiting and retching, abdominal pain is not typically associated with nausea and vomiting during pregnancy.

Epigastric, periumbilical, or right-sided pain can suggest gallstone disease, peptic ulcer disease (PUD), pancreatitis, or appendicitis, and an appropriate workup should be performed to exclude these disorders. Vomitus typically contains recently ingested food or yellow juice. Bilious vomitus or severe periumbilical pain can suggest bowel obstruction.

The patient with uncomplicated pregnancy-associated nausea and vomiting should have normal findings on physical examination. The presence of dehydration or orthostatic hypotension can suggest hyperemesis gravidarum (see later discussion). The presence of abdominal tenderness, rebound, palpable masses, abdominal distention, or a succussion splash should prompt laboratory evaluation and imaging to rule out other causes.

B. Laboratory Findings

An elevated white blood cell count (beyond physiologic leukocytosis of pregnancy or accompanied by a neutrophilia) can suggest the presence of cholecystitis, pancreatitis, appendicitis, or pyelonephritis. A urine specimen for urinalysis and urine culture to exclude urinary tract infection should be obtained. Other relevant testing includes thyroid function testing, liver blood tests (chronic hepatitis C infection can be associated with a high incidence of nausea), hepatitis serologies, and fasting glucose level. Severely abnormal serum

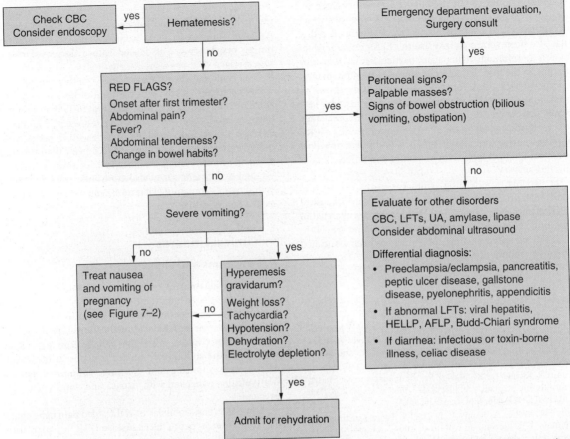

▲ **Figure 7–1.** Evaluation of nausea and vomiting during pregnancy. AFLP, acute fatty liver of pregnancy; CBC, complete blood count; LFT, liver function tests; HELLP, syndrome of hemolysis, elevated liver enzymes, and low platelets; UA, urinalysis.

electrolytes resulting from vomiting suggest the diagnosis of hyperemesis gravidarum.

▶ Treatment

With the majority of pregnant women experiencing nausea and vomiting during pregnancy, the burden of illness can become quite significant if symptoms are under-treated and/or under-diagnosed, thus allowing for progression of the disease. The majority of these women will need at least one visit with a provider to specifically address symptoms, and up to 10% or greater will require pharmacotherapy after failure of conservative measures to adequately control symptoms. Prompt and effective treatment in the outpatient setting is needed once the diagnosis is made. Once treatment has commenced it is important to track symptoms in order to assess for a decrease in or resolution of symptoms as well as an escalation in symptoms requiring additional therapy. Of note, particularly in refractory cases it is important to exclude co-existing GERD, Helicobacter pylori infection, and psychosocial factors.

The medical and nonmedical literature is replete with dietary suggestions for women suffering from this problem. Medical treatment is directed toward control of symptoms (Figure 7–2).

Women should avoid exposure to odors, foods, or supplements that appear to trigger nausea. Typically, fatty foods are avoided because these can delay gastric emptying. Small, frequent meals of bland carbohydrates (starches such as noodles, potatoes, and rice), chicken, and fish are recommended. For patients with severe nausea and vomiting, small sips of salty liquids such as sports beverages or broth are recommended. Juices and creamy or dairy beverages are not advised as these can exacerbate symptoms. Some authors also recommend avoidance of vegetables or high-fiber foods, which can form bezoars. Acupressure is often performed with the use of wrist bands (Seabands) worn continuously for a period of a few days, followed by a hiatus of few days; it is noninvasive, and many women report a reduction in the number of episodes of nausea, although data are equivocal about whether this benefit is actual or partially a placebo effect. Most studies

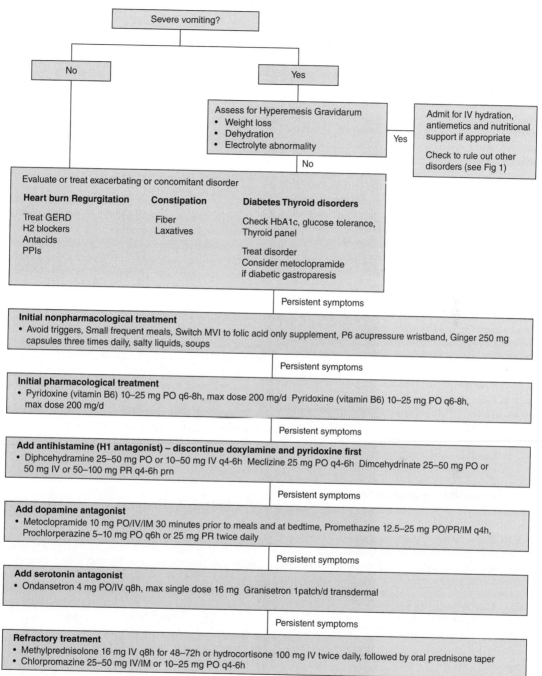

▲ **Figure 7–2.** Approach to treatment of nausea and vomiting during pregnancy. GERD, gastroesophageal reflux disease; IV, intravenous; PPI, proton pump inhibitor.

did not show a significant benefit in the treatment of severe vomiting.

A recent systematic review from 35 RCTs at low risk of bias indicated that ginger, vitamin B6 (pyridoxine), antihistamines, metoclopramide were associated with improved

symptoms compared with placebo. For moderate symptoms, pyridoxine-doxylamine and ondansetron were associated with improved symptoms compared with placebo.

Women who have persistent nausea and vomiting and high concentrations of ketones require intravenous hydration with multivitamins, including thiamine, with follow-up measurement of levels of urinary ketones and electrolytes. Antiemetic agents should be prescribed to these patients. Intravenous fluids help correct dehydration and improve symptoms. Dextrose saline may be more effective at reducing nausea than normal saline

Antihistamines such as meclizine have been used with no reports of teratogenicity. Studies of dimenhydrinate and diphenhydramine during pregnancy have shown conflicting results on safety and efficacy. Phenothiazines such as promethazine, prochlorperazine, and trimethobenzamide are considered low-risk drugs based on studies in pregnant women and also have clinical efficacy in this setting. They are considered more effective than metoclopramide. Metoclopramide is used frequently in Europe for this indication, and one study shows no association with fetal malformations. In a randomized trial, intravenous metoclopramide and intravenous promethazine had similar efficacy in the treatment of hyperemesis, but metoclopramide caused less drowsiness and dizziness. An Israeli cohort study involving 3458 women who were exposed to metoclopramide in the first trimester (in most cases for 1–2 weeks) showed no significant association between exposure and the risk of congenital malformations, low birth weight, preterm delivery, or perinatal death.

In April 2013, the US FDA approved doxylamine succinate 10 mg/pyridoxine hydrochloride 10 mg (Diclegis) as the first medication to specifically treat nausea and vomiting of pregnancy in more than 30 years. It has proven efficacy in randomized, placebo-controlled trials and should be considered a first-line drug.

Other prokinetics such as domperidone (used in Canada), bethanechol, and erythromycin have not been studied. Ondansetron is considered low risk in pregnancy, although its use is typically limited to cases of hyperemesis gravidarum. In a recent 2019 study of 100 Granisetron exposed pregnancies, there was no increased risk for minor or major fetal anomalies.

Three RCTs compared corticosteroids with placebo or promethazine or metoclopramide in women with severe symptoms of nausea and vomiting. Improvements were seen in all corticosteroid groups, but only a significant difference between corticosteroids versus metoclopramide was reported (emesis reduction, 40.9% vs 16.5% at day 2; 71.6% vs 51.2% at day 3; 95.8% vs 76.6% at day 7 [n = 40, P < .001]). For other interventions, evidence was limited.

A summary of therapeutic approach to nausea and vomiting in pregnancy is shown in Figure 7–2.

Clark SM, Dutta E, Hankins GD. The outpatient management and special considerations of nausea and vomiting in pregnancy. *Semin Perinatol.* 2014;38(8):496–502. [PMID: 25267280]

Fejzo MS, Trovik J, Grooten IJ, et al. Nausea and vomiting of pregnancy and hyperemesis gravidarum. *Nat Rev Dis Primers.* 2019;5(1):62. [PMID: 31515515]

McParlin C, O'Donnell A, Robson SC, et al. Treatments for hyperemesis gravidarum and nausea and vomiting in pregnancy: a systematic review. *JAMA.* 2016;316(13):1392–1401. [PMID: 27701665]

Shapira M, Avrahami I, Mazaki-Tovi S, Shai D, Zemet R, Barzilay E. The safety of early pregnancy exposure to granisetron. *Eur J Obstet Gynecol Reprod Biol.* 2020;245:35–38. [PMID: 31841778]

HYPEREMESIS GRAVIDARUM

Hyperemesis gravidarum represents a severe form of nausea and vomiting during pregnancy. It is a clinical diagnosis of exclusion that commonly includes persistent vomiting not attributed to other causes, often with concurrent dehydration (high urine specific gravity), electrolyte abnormalities (hypokalemia), acute starvation with ketonuria, or weight loss often greater than 5% of pre-pregnancy body weight. The incidence of hyperemesis gravidarum is approximately 0.3% to 3% of all pregnancies but varies from study to study given different diagnostic criteria and populations. It remains the most common indication for hospital admission during the first trimester of pregnancy.

Hyperemesis gravidarum is associated with high estrogen levels and is more likely to occur with multiple gestations, gestational trophoblastic disease, and fetal abnormalities such as triploidy, trisomy 21, and hydrops fetalis. It has also been associated with hyperthyroidism, preeclampsia, eclampsia, HELLP syndrome (hemolysis, elevated liver enzymes, and low platelets), and acute fatty liver of pregnancy (AFLP). Although overall, patients with hyperemesis have good fetal outcomes, one study found that patients who experience a loss of 5% or more of body weight have a greater risk of growth retardation or fetal anomalies.

▶ Clinical Findings

A. Symptoms and Signs

Patients may report dry mouth, sialorrhea, hyperolfaction, dysgeusia (altered or metallic taste), and decreased taste sensation. Physical examination may reveal signs of dehydration, including dry mucous membranes and poor skin turgor. The presence of epigastric or right upper quadrant pain, headache, and diplopia can suggest preeclampsia or eclampsia. Blood pressure should be measured and urinalysis performed; hypertension and proteinuria support the diagnosis of preeclampsia. Hyperreflexia and edema may also be present in preeclampsia, and the development of seizures defines eclampsia.

B. Laboratory Findings

Blood chemistries should be evaluated as hypochloremic metabolic alkalosis, hypokalemia, hypomagnesemia, and hyponatremia are common. Complete blood count and liver blood tests should also be checked to evaluate for HELLP syndrome (elevated transaminases without significant elevation of alkaline phosphatase or bilirubin, often with low platelets). AFLP can present with fulminant hepatic failure (elevated prothrombin time, jaundice, and elevated transaminases) and sometimes concurrent renal failure and hypoglycemia. These patients must be transferred to an intensive care unit, and a hepatologist should be consulted immediately. Unlike hyperemesis, HELLP syndrome and AFLP typically occur late in pregnancy, usually in the third trimester. Also, hyperemesis does not typically cause elevation in liver blood tests or renal failure unless severe dehydration is present. Other differential diseases associated with severe vomiting include hepatic vein thrombosis or Budd-Chiari syndrome, which can be diagnosed with a Doppler ultrasound. Celiac sprue can be diagnosed by tissue transglutaminase immunoglobulin A (IgA) and anti-endomysial IgA or endoscopy, or both. *Helicobacter pylori* can be diagnosed by serology, endoscopy, or hydrogen breath test.

Complications

Pregnancies of women with hyperemesis gravidarum can be complicated by low birth weight if the mother has experienced weight loss; however, fetal fatality is rare. Severe vomiting can rarely cause Mallory-Weiss tears or esophageal rupture. Rarely, women can develop peripheral neuropathies due to vitamin B_6 and B_{12} deficiencies. The most serious complication is Wernicke encephalopathy resulting from thiamine deficiency. Poor dietary intake can also result in deficiency of other vitamins and nutrients such as iron, calcium, and folate.

Treatment

Oral and intravenous hydration and repletion of electrolytes is the primary treatment. Thiamine should be administered prior to dextrose to avoid Wernicke encephalopathy. After 24 hours of aggressive intravenous hydration, the infusion should be adjusted to maintain urine output. Once oral hydration is tolerated, broth or salty liquids should be started, followed by small carbohydrate meals such as crackers and noodles. In some cases, nasogastric or nasojejunal feeding may be required. In rare cases, parenteral nutrition has been used, but this should be avoided if possible due to risks of infection, diabetes, cholelithiasis, and risks associated with central line placement. Percutaneous endoscopic gastrostomy tube placement with jejunal extension, during which fetal monitoring and anesthesia support were provided is documented in the literature. Although procedure-related adverse fetal outcomes were not reported, this procedure should be reserved for patients at high nutritional risk, after nasoenteric feeding has failed and parenteral nutrition is contraindicated (hyperglycemia, hypercoagulability, or inadequate venous access). Medications used to control nausea and vomiting are often effective for hyperemesis. One study demonstrated some benefits of powdered root of ginger

(20 mg orally, four times daily) in controlling symptoms. A few case reports describe benefits of erythromycin in controlling hyperemesis. Another study showed some efficacy of methylprednisolone, but steroids can be associated with adverse fetal outcomes. A recent study showed that ondansetron and metoclopramide demonstrated similar antiemetic and antinausea effects, but overall ondansetron was better. Of note however, ondansetron use during the first trimester has been linked to cleft palate and congenital heart defects. Given this, society guidelines recommend that use of ondansetron before 10 weeks of gestation should be individualized. A 2014 preliminary RCT demonstrated the efficacy of transdermal clonidine in the treatment of severe HG, leading to a significant reduction of symptoms and reducing the need for other supportive measures and medications.

Abas MN, Tan PC, Azmi N, Omar SZ. Ondansetron compared with metoclopramide for hyperemesis gravidarum: a randomized controlled trial. *Obstet Gynecol.* 2014;123(6):1272–1279. [PMID: 24807340]

Body C, Christie JA. Gastrointestinal diseases in pregnancy: nausea, vomiting, hyperemesis gravidarum, gastroesophageal reflux disease, constipation, and diarrhea. *Gastroenterol Clin North Am.* 2016;45(2):267–283 [PMID: 27261898]

Maina A, Arrotta M, Cicogna L, et al. Transdermal clonidine in the treatment of severe hyperemesis. A pilot randomised control trial: CLONEMESI. *BJOG.* 2014;121(12):1556–1562. [PMID: 24684734]

CONSTIPATION

New-onset constipation and exacerbation of chronic constipation are common complaints during pregnancy. Constipation occurs in up to 25% of all pregnant women at some point during their pregnancy and may continue for up to three months postpartum. This is in contrast to nonpregnant women of similar age for whom the baseline rate of constipation is only 7%. Increased progesterone during pregnancy decreases colonic smooth muscle contraction to slow motility and may have an inhibitory effect on motilin, a stimulatory gastrointestinal hormone, thereby slowing oro-cecal transit time. In addition, several other physiologic changes are believed to contribute to this problem, including poor fluid intake in the setting of nausea and vomiting, iron supplementation, bed rest, or decreased exercise.

Clinical Findings

A. Symptoms and Signs

Evaluation to exclude other mechanical, hormonal, or systemic etiologies of constipation is important to consider. In uncomplicated constipation, the physical examination should be normal. Physical exam should include a digital rectal exam to assess the anal canal and sphincter tone, as well as observation of the perineum during Valsalva maneuver to identify rectal prolapse. Fever, abdominal pain, tenderness, distention, nausea or vomiting, or obstipation should prompt evaluation for other causes such as bowel obstruction or volvulus.

B. Laboratory Findings

Laboratory testing for thyroid disease, diabetes, and electrolyte abnormalities can be undertaken.

C. Special Tests

Rarely, flexible sigmoidoscopy or anoscopy may be needed to evaluate cases associated with hematochezia.

▶ Treatment

The treatment of constipation during pregnancy is similar to its treatment in nonpregnant patients. First-line therapy consists of dietary fiber, which is the safest and most physiologic way to treat constipation; however, many patients will not respond to dietary fiber alone.

Psyllium, calcium polycarbophil, and methylcellulose are bulk laxatives that can be used as an alternative or adjunct to dietary fiber. These agents should be diluted and taken with food during meals. Fiber increases fecal water content, increases stool weight, decreases colonic transit time, and improves stool consistency. The laxative effect may be delayed for days. Pregnant patients should be warned that fiber can cause bloating and flatulence and instructed to consume sufficient fluids with it. Docusate, a stool softener, can be used alongside fiber supplements and is used routinely in pregnancy; however, there is one case report of neonatal hypomagnesemia associated with maternal oral administration of sodium docusate.

Osmotic laxatives can be used if fiber supplementation fails. Sorbitol and lactulose are poorly absorbed sugars that stimulate fluid accumulation in the colon by an osmotic effect. Lactulose is more expensive and should not be used in diabetic patients because it contains galactose. In addition, it can exacerbate nausea in pregnant patients with this symptom. The American Gastroenterological Association (AGA) suggests polyethylene glycol as a preferred drug for chronic constipation during pregnancy as it causes less abdominal bloating and flatulence than other osmotic laxatives.

Stimulant laxatives are also minimally absorbed and are generally reserved for patients who do not respond to fiber or osmotic laxatives. If used chronically, electrolytes should be monitored as hypokalemia, hypomagnesemia, hyponatremia, and dehydration can result. Senna is generally safe in pregnancy and can be used in combination with bulk laxatives. It can be used at bedtime with fluids up to three times per week. Cascara is milder and is less often associated with abdominal discomfort. Bisacodyl is also safe in pregnancy as tablets or suppository, but can produce some abdominal discomfort when administered orally.

All laxatives should be taken with adequate fluids given their risk of causing electrolyte abnormalities. Fecal impaction should be treated with digital disimpaction. Mineral oil, tap water, or retention enemas can be used to soften stool. Bisacodyl suppository can then be used along with oral agents to treat constipation.

Agents to avoid during pregnancy include castor oil, which can initiate premature uterine contractions; aloe, which has been associated with congenital malformations; and saline hyperosmotic agents such as magnesium laxatives and phosphosoda, which can promote sodium and water retention. Mineral oil is not recommended due to its association with decreased maternal absorption of fat-soluble vitamins. Both castor oil and hyperosmotic saline laxatives cause premature uterine contractions. Prokinetic agents such as lubiprostone and linaclotide have shown adverse events in animal reproduction studies and also not recommended (Table 7–3).

Cartwright R, Johannessen HH. Constipation during and after pregnancy. *BJOG*. 2020;10.1111/1471–0528.16603. [PMID: 33217146]

Kuronen M, Hantunen S, Alanne L, et al. Pregnancy, puerperium and perinatal constipation-an observational hybrid survey on pregnant and postpartum women and their age-matched non-pregnant controls. *BJOG*. 2020;10.1111/1471–0528.16559. [PMID: 33030260]

DIARRHEA

Diarrhea is much less commonly reported than other GI disorders of pregnancy. Acute or chronic diarrhea can occur in pregnant women, and it is believed that pathogenesis and differential diagnosis are similar in pregnant and nonpregnant patients. Most cases of acute diarrhea are caused by viral infections such as rotavirus and Norwalk virus and are associated with large-volume, watery diarrhea that is self-limited. Bacterial illness often produces more frequent stools of small volume, abdominal pain, occasional fever, and blood and leukocytes in the stool.

▶ Clinical Findings

A. Symptoms and Signs

Evaluation of diarrhea is typically warranted only if diarrhea is profuse, leads to dehydration, is bloody, is associated with high fevers, weight loss, malnutrition or if the illness persists for 48 hours without improvement or becomes chronic. Noninfectious causes of acute and chronic diarrhea

Table 7–3. Medications used in the treatment of irritable bowel syndrome.

Drug	FDA Pregnancy Category	Recommendations for Pregnancy	Recommendations for Breast-Feeding
Alosetron	B	Avoid: restricted access	No human data: potential toxicity
Amitriptyline	C	Avoid: no malformations, but worse outcomes	Limited human data: potential toxicity
Bisacodyl	C	Low risk in short-term use	Safety unknown
Bismuth subsalicylate	C	Not safe: teratogenicity	No human data: potential toxicity
Castor oil	X	Uterine contraction and rupture	Possibly unsafe
Cholestyramine	C	Low risk, but can lead to infant coagulopathy	Compatible
Desipramine	C	Avoid: no malformations, but worse outcomes	Limited human data: potential toxicity
Dicyclomine	B	Avoid: possible congenital anomalies	Limited human data: potential toxicity
Diphenoxylate/atropine	C	Teratogenic in animals: no human data	Limited human data: potential toxicity
Docusate	C	Low risk	Compatible
Hyoscyamine	C	No available data	No human data: probably compatible
Imipramine	D	Avoid: no malformations, but worse outcomes	Limited human data: potential toxicity
Kaopectate	C	Unsafe because now contains bismuth	No human data: probably compatible
Lactulose	B	No human studies	No human data: probably compatible
Loperamide	B	Low risk: possible increased cardiovascular defects	Limited human data: probably compatible
Lubiprostone	C	No human studies but pregnancy loss in guinea pigs	Avoid use
Magnesium citrate	B	Avoid long-term use: hypermagnesemia, hyperphosphatemia, dehydration	Compatible
Mineral oil	C	Avoid: neonatal coagulopathy and hemorrhage	Possibly unsafe
Nortriptyline	D	Avoid: no malformations, but worse outcomes	Limited human data: potential toxicity
Paroxetine	D	Avoid: twice as many birth defects as other antidepressants	Potential toxicity
PEG	C	First-choice laxative in pregnancy	Low risk
Senna	C	Low risk in short-term use	Compatible
SSRIs (except paroxetine)	C	Avoid: no malformations, but increased adverse events in fetus	Limited human data: potential toxicity
Simethicone	C	No available data: low risk	No human data: probably compatible
Sodium phosphate		Avoid long-term: hypermagnesemia, hyper-phosphatemia, dehydration	Safety unknown

PEG, polyethylene glycol; SSRI, selective serotonin reuptake inhibitor. Reproduced with permission from Mahadevan U, Kane S. American gastroenterological association institute technical review on the use of gastrointestinal medications in pregnancy. *Gastroenterology.* 2006;131(1):283–311.

include functional diarrhea, food intolerance, use of sugar substitutes such as sorbitol and mannitol, celiac disease and IBD. A careful dietary and family history should be obtained.

B. Laboratory and Imaging Studies

Stool cultures for bacterial pathogens, ova, and parasites, and toxin or enzyme-linked immunosorbent assay (ELISA) for *Clostridium difficile* are the next step in evaluation. Flexible sigmoidoscopy with biopsy is considered safe in pregnancy and can be performed if needed to evaluate bloody or persistent diarrhea.

▶ Treatment

Uncomplicated diarrhea should be treated with oral rehydration using juices, noncaffeinated beverages, and broth. Orange juice and bananas provide potassium, and salted crackers and broth can provide sodium. Small, frequent meals and avoidance of high-fat food, caffeine, dairy, and artificial sweeteners are recommended.

Antibiotics should be used only in the setting of documented infection with bacterial or parasitic microbes. Albendazole is teratogenic in animals, but in the setting of helminthic infections during pregnancy, the benefit is felt to be greater than the theoretical risk. Metronidazole can be used for *C difficile*, *Giardia lamblia*, and *Entamoeba histolytica*, but should be avoided during the first trimester and should not be administered long term because there are no data supporting its use for more than 2–3 weeks at a time. In pregnant women with *C difficile* infection, oral vancomycin is recommended and adverse fetal effects have not been reported following use in the second and third trimesters. Ampicillin and erythromycin stearate have been used for bacterial causes of diarrhea, the latter specifically for *Campylobacter jejuni* infection. Less data are available on vancomycin, but it is also considered a low-risk drug. Azithromycin is not associated with congenital defects but may cause maternal gastrointestinal discomfort during pregnancy. Second-generation cephalosporins such as cefuroxime and cefixime can be used for acute shigellosis. Fluoroquinolones, tetracycline, doxycycline, erythromycin estolate, and trimethoprim–sulfamethoxazole should not be used based on current data available. Rifaximin is a nonabsorbable antibiotic with a wide spectrum of gram-negative and anaerobic coverage that is currently FDA approved for traveler's diarrhea. Although it should eventually be useful during pregnancy, no data are currently available regarding its use in pregnant women.

The medical treatment for diarrhea during pregnancy is limited by the teratogenic side effects of many common drugs, including antidiarrheal agents and cholestyramine, Antidiarrheal agents can be used to control symptoms in severe or persistent disease once active infection has been excluded. Kaolin and pectin are not absorbed and are

Table 7–4. Causes of diarrhea in pregnancy.

Infections
Viruses (norovirus, rotavirus, adenovirus)
Bacteria (*Escherichia coli*, *Salmonella*, *Shigella*, *Campylobacter*, *Clostridium difficile*, *Listeria*)
Protozoa (Entamoeba histolytica, Cryptosporidium, Giardia)
Drug-induced
Increased prostaglandins
Functional bowel disorders
Irritable bowel syndrome – diarrhea predominant, mixed
Functional diarrhea
Inflammatory bowel disease
Malabsorption syndromes
Food intolerance (lactose, fructose, mannitol, sorbitol)
Celiac disease
Small intestinal bacterial overgrowth

probably safe although impairment of iron absorption is a possibility. Loperamide in small doses has been used in and is rated category B during pregnancy. Codeine can also be used in small amounts. Agents to avoid include bismuth subsalicylate (contained in Kaopectate), mainly because of the teratogenicity of salicylates. Diphenoxylate with atropine has also been found to be teratogenic. Alosetron should be avoided as well, because there are few data on its use during pregnancy. Cholestyramine has been used to treat cholestasis of pregnancy safely; however, its use can result in fat-soluble vitamin deficiencies including coagulopathy, which can lead to neonatal intracerebral hemorrhage. (Table 7–4).

Body C, Christie JA. Gastrointestinal diseases in pregnancy: nausea, vomiting, hyperemesis gravidarum, gastroesophageal reflux disease, constipation, and diarrhea. *Gastroenterol Clin North Am.* 2016;45(2):267–283. [PMID: 27261898]

Boers K, Vlasveld T, van der Waart R. Pregnancy and coeliac disease. *BMJ Case Rep.* 2019;12(12):e233226. [PMID: 31888907]

HEMORRHOIDS

Hemorrhoids are common in the US adult population and often become symptomatic or worsen during pregnancy. Two-thirds of pregnant women have anal symptoms during pregnancy and in the postpartum period and the majority suffer from haemorrhoidal complications and anal fissure. The most important risk factor is constipation. In addition poor venous return, increase in circulating blood volume, and extended time in the sitting position are all believed to contribute to this problem.

Clinical Findings

A. Symptoms and Signs

The perianal area should be inspected to rule out other contributions to pain and pruritus such as pinworms, fissures, fistulas, or ulcers. Other causes of rectal bleeding should be investigated, and a flexible sigmoidoscopy performed if needed. Internal hemorrhoids should be graded: first-degree hemorrhoids bleed but do not prolapse and can be visualized by anoscopy; second-degree hemorrhoids protrude during defecation or with straining but revert when straining stops; third-degree hemorrhoids are continuously prolapsed but easily reduced; fourth-degree hemorrhoids cannot be reduced.

Treatment

External hemorrhoids require treatment if they become thrombosed, which often results in pain or discomfort with sitting. A recent study of 495 pregnant women with hemorrhoids revealed that conservative treatment with Sitz bath was more effective than an ano-rectal cream.

If conservative measures such as stool softeners, daily warm sitz baths, and mild analgesics are not effective, surgical excision under local anesthesia is safe during pregnancy and does not affect the fetus. Clot incision and removal is generally only a temporizing measure as thrombosis usually recurs.

Internal hemorrhoids can cause bleeding, pain, or pruritus that may require treatment. Treatment of constipation is essential. Topical therapies such as witch hazel, hydrocortisone cream, and topical anesthetics (eg, benzocaine, dibucaine, or pramoxine) can help treat pruritus. Products containing epinephrine or phenylephrine should be avoided, especially in women with hypertension, diabetes, or fluid overload. If topical measures fail, band ligation for first-, second-, or third-degree internal hemorrhoids or injection sclerotherapy for first- or second-degree hemorrhoids is safe in pregnancy. Band ligation carries the associated risk of acute necrotizing perianal sepsis; however, this complication is rare.

Infrared photocoagulation or laser coagulation of first- and second-degree hemorrhoids is also minimally invasive, although safety in pregnancy has not been demonstrated. For patients who fail office-based procedures or those with fourth-degree lesions, closed excisional hemorrhoidectomy using local anesthesia has been reported to be safe and effective in pregnancy.

Ferdinande K, Dorreman Y, Roelens K, Ceelen W, De Looze D. Anorectal symptoms during pregnancy and postpartum: a prospective cohort study. *Colorectal Dis.* 2018;20(12):1109–1116. [PMID: 29972721]

Shirah BH, Shirah HA, Fallata AH, Alobidy SN, Hawsawi MMA. Hemorrhoids during pregnancy: Sitz bath vs. ano-rectal cream: a comparative prospective study of two conservative treatment protocols. *Women Birth.* 2018;31(4):e272–e277. [PMID: 29055673]

IRRITABLE BOWEL SYNDROME

Irritable bowel syndrome is common in pregnancy, partly because it is a common syndrome in women of childbearing age and partly because pregnancy seems to exacerbate gastrointestinal symptoms associated with the syndrome. Many women experience an increase in constipation, or conversely, an increase in stool frequency. Abdominal pain, bloating, flatulence, and nausea are also exacerbated by pregnancy, it is thought because of the impact of female hormones on gastrointestinal motility.

Clinical Findings

A. Symptoms and Signs

In patients with preexisting irritable bowel syndrome, evaluation mainly consists of ruling out other causes of constipation, irregular stools, and abdominal discomfort. Failure to respond to medical management or alarm symptoms such as bleeding, weight loss, or fever should prompt a search for other causes. In patients who present with irritable bowel syndrome during pregnancy, the diagnosis of irritable bowel syndrome is suggested by the combination of pain, flatulence, irregular defecation, and mucus in stools, and the exacerbation of symptoms by eating and relief by defecation.

Treatment

Dietary measures are the safest way to treat irritable bowel syndrome in pregnancy. Fiber supplementation can be implemented for constipation-predominant, diarrhea-predominant, and alternating irritable bowel syndrome. Patients can add bran to each meal or purchase supplements such as psyllium. Patients should be warned that an increase in bloating and flatulence occurs initially with fiber but may improve with time.

Medications used in the treatment of irritable bowel syndrome are outlined in Table 7–3. For patients with constipation-predominant symptoms who do not respond to bulk laxatives, osmotic laxatives such as polyethylene glycol, sorbitol, or lactulose can be used and are considered low risk in pregnancy. Tap-water enemas can be used to treat fecal impaction. Magnesium citrate and sodium phosphate should be avoided. Linaclotide and lubiprostone are also pregnancy category C drugs. For a full discussion of laxatives that can be used in pregnancy, see the earlier discussion of constipation. For patients with diarrhea-predominant symptoms, a low-fat, nondairy diet should be tried first. After this, loperamide or codeine can be used in small doses after infection is ruled out. For information about antidiarrheal agents for use during pregnancy, see the earlier section on treatment of diarrhea in pregnancy. Alosetron is a 5HT3 receptor antagonist on enteric neurons as well as other peripheral and central neurons that affect the regulation of visceral pain, gastrointestinal secretions, and colonic transit all of which relate to the pathophysiology of IBS. It is currently indicated only in women with severe IBS-D at a dose of 1 mg orally twice daily and is contraindicated in patients with constipation, IBD, diverticulitis, intestinal obstruction, gastrointestinal perforations/adhesions, and ischemic colitis. It can lead to side effects such as constipation, abdominal discomfort, nausea, abdominal distension, regurgitation, reflux, and hemorrhoids. However, it is classed as a pregnancy category B medication.

Antispasmodic agents such as anticholinergics, calcium channel blockers, and direct gut smooth muscle relaxants are used in patients whose irritable bowel syndrome is associated with severe pain, but these agents have not been well studied in pregnancy, and there is a lack of efficacy data to support use. Dicyclomine has been associated with phocomelia in animals and although classified as a category B drug in pregnancy, is rarely used. Most other anticholinergics, such as hyoscyamine, and calcium channel blockers, such as nifedipine, are category C drugs and are not well studied in pregnancy. Antidepressant drugs have been used during pregnancy for treatment of depression, but have not been studied for the treatment of irritable bowel syndrome in pregnancy. Tricyclic antidepressants and selective serotonin reuptake inhibitors (SSRIs) have been associated with short-term neonatal withdrawal symptoms, and cases of neonatal heart failure and electrocardiographic abnormalities have been reported with tricyclic antidepressants. SSRIs such as fluoxetine, paroxetine, sertraline, and citalopram are FDA category C. Paroxetine is associated with increased congenital malformation. The tricyclic agents, nortriptyline and imipramine, are category D drugs, but desipramine and amitriptyline are category C. Narcotics should be avoided because of the risk of tolerance, and benzodiazepines are category D in pregnancy.

Rawla P, Sunkara T, Raj JP. Updated review of current pharmacological and non-pharmacological management of irritable bowel syndrome. *Life Sci.* 2018;212:176–181. [PMID: 3029018]

FECAL INCONTINENCE

Approximately one tenth of pregnant women develop fecal incontinence following childbirth. Fecal incontinence following vaginal delivery can be caused by anal sphincter tears from instrumental delivery or instrumentation, denervation injury, or rectovaginal fistulas. Short ano-vulvar distance, ligamentous hyperlaxity, lack of expulsion control, nonvisualization of the perineum or maneuvers for shoulder dystocia also appear to be risk factors. It is also more common in nulliparous women.

Anal sphincter tears can occur following vaginal delivery with third- or fourth-degree perineal lacerations (those that extend into the muscular layers of the anal sphincter),

incomplete repairs of these lacerations, nerve injury or partial dehiscence following laceration repair, episiotomies (particularly midline episiotomies), a history of anal tears from previous deliveries, and forceps or vacuum delivery. The incidence of anal sphincter tears is lower in elective cesarean deliveries, but fecal incontinence is still common following emergency caesarean deliveries, presumably because some injury to the pelvic floor has already occurred. A recent meta-analysis and systematic review also noted that warm compresses applied during the second stage of labor increase the incidence of intact perineum and lower the risk of episiotomy and severe perineal trauma.

Obstetric fistulas such as genitourinary, anovaginal, and rectovaginal fistulas are more common in pregnant women in underdeveloped countries and are felt to be partly due to prolonged labor leading to pressure necrosis. Fistulas can also be seen after laceration repair or in infected episiotomy sites. Nerve injury, particularly pudendal nerve injury during delivery, has also been implicated in fecal incontinence, but this has not been demonstrated conclusively.

▶ Clinical Findings

A. Symptoms and Signs

Patients can present with pregnancy-related fecal incontinence immediately after or many years following delivery. In most patients, the rectal examination will be normal and rectal tone will be grossly normal; in some cases, it is possible to palpate a defect in the anterior wall.

B. Imaging Studies

The mainstay of evaluation is the endoanal ultrasound (EAUS). Defects in either the external or internal anal sphincter are seen as asymmetries in concentric rings of tissues that surround the anal canal. The internal anal sphincter appears hypoechoic, and defects in this layer appear hyperechoic. The external anal sphincter appears hyperechoic, and defects appear hypoechoic. Typically, pregnancy-related trauma from tears or episiotomies is located anteriorly. Fistulas appear as hypoechoic tracts; air within these tracts appears as focal hyperechoic areas. Findings on EAUS have been validated by anorectal manometry and correlate with anal squeeze pressure and surgical findings and histology. Other studies of EAUS performed before and after surgical repair of sphincter defect show that EAUS documentation of closure of the sphincter defect predicts improvement in fecal incontinence. Anorectal manometry can demonstrate changes in resting and squeeze pressure due to sphincter trauma but is less sensitive in being able to detect tears than anorectal manometry. Pelvic floor magnetic resonance imaging (pelvic MRI) can detect a variety of abnormal static and dynamic pelvic disorders.

Pelvic MRI may be a useful and noninvasive modality but is currently not widely available and has not been well studied for this indication. Pudendal nerve injury can be documented by pudendal nerve terminal motor latency measurements, but the role of pudendal nerve injury in fecal continence is controversial.

▶ Treatment

The treatment of sphincter tears and rectovaginal fistulas is surgical. Sphincteroplasty, when closure of the defect is successful, often leads to improvement in symptoms. A recent Norwegian study assessed effectiveness of 4–6 pelvic floor physiotherapy appointments over a 6 month period in women with fecal incontinence following pregnancy and noted encouraging results.

Durnea CM, Khashan AS, Kenny LC, et al. What is to blame for postnatal pelvic floor dysfunction in primiparous women-Pre-pregnancy or intrapartum risk factors?. *Eur J Obstet Gynecol Reprod Biol.* 2017;214:36–43. [PMID: 28525825]

Johannessen HH, Wibe A, Stordahl A, Sandvik L, Mørkved S. Do pelvic floor muscle exercises reduce postpartum anal incontinence? A randomised controlled trial. *BJOG.* 2017; 124(4):686–694. [PMID: 27272501]

Magoga G, Saccone G, Al-Kouatly HB, et al. Warm perineal compresses during the second stage of labor for reducing perineal trauma: a meta-analysis. *Eur J Obstet Gynecol Reprod Biol.* 2019;240:93–98. [PMID: 31238205]

Melchior C, Bridoux V, Touchais O, Savoye-Collet C, Leroi AM. MRI defaecography in patients with faecal incontinence. *Colorectal Dis.* 2015;17(3):O62–O69. [PMID: 25641440]

Bello OO, Morhason-Bello IO, Ojengbede OA. Nigeria, a high burden state of obstetric fistula: a contextual analysis of key drivers. *Pan Afr Med J.* 2020;36:22. [PMID: 32774599]

INFLAMMATORY BOWEL DISEASE

▶ Clinical Findings

A. Course of IBD during Pregnancy and in the Postpartum Period

Most women with IBD have a normal pregnancy and deliver a healthy baby. Studies have demonstrated that approximately 80% of female patients conceive while their disease is in remission. Pregnancies conceived in remission tend to remain in remission throughout the pregnancy and in the postpartum period. The European Crohn and Colitis organization study group of epidemiology, Epicom, studied the course of IBD in pregnancy and in the postpartum period. This multicenter study assessed the effect of pregnancy on IBD by comparing pregnant IBD patients (92 Crohn's disease [CD] patients, 117 ulcerative colitis [UC]) to nonpregnant IBD patients. Data were collected prospectively during each trimester and up to 6 months postpartum. Demographics including smoking, disease characteristics, IBD medication, disease activity, and pregnancy and newborn outcome were

documented. Disease activity was assessed using the Harvey-Bradshaw Index (HBI) (CD) and the Simple Colitis Clinical Activity Index (SCCAI) (UC). Women with UC had higher risk of flares during pregnancy than women with CD. No significant difference was observed in disease activity between pregnant and nonpregnant CD patients. Of those patients with CD who did flare during pregnancy, factors included use of immunosuppressive therapy and longer duration of disease. Disease flares were significantly higher in patients with UC during pregnancy and in the postpartum period compared to nonpregnant UC patients.

In a more recent study by de Lima-Karagiannis et al, out of a total of 298 pregnancies in 229 IBD patients (157 CD, 66 UC, and 6 IBD unclassified) resulting in 226 live births, active disease at conception was strongly associated with disease relapse during pregnancy (adjusted odds ratio [aOR]=7.66, 95% confidence interval [CI]: 3.77–15.54). This study also noted that pregnant women with UC did relapse more often than women with CD, independent of maternal age, smoking, periconceptional disease activity, previous IBD surgery, and the use of immunosuppressives or anti-tumor necrosis factor (TNF) (aOR=3.71, 95% CI:1.86–7.40).

In addition to disease activity, nonadherence to medication, and more extensive disease in UC have also been shown in other studies to be associated with a higher risk of obstetric complications. Breast-feeding has not been shown to influence risk of postpartum relapse in women with IBD.

B. Pregnancy Outcomes

Patients with unstable UC are also more at risk of adverse fetal outcomes. A large population based study from the US revealed that pregnancy complicated by IBD was associated with increased incidence of small-for-gestational age birth (OR=1.46, 95% confidence interval [CI]=1.14–1.88), spontaneous preterm birth (OR=1.32, 95% CI=1.00–1.76), and preterm premature rupture of membranes (OR=1.95, 95% CI=1.26–3.02). Further stratifying by IBD subtypes, only UC was significantly associated with increased incidence of ischemic placental disease, spontaneous preterm birth and preterm premature rupture of membranes. Crohn's complications during pregnancy are less frequent than that of UC. In a large prospective national Danish cohort study, there was a statistically significant increased risk of ectopic pregnancy in pregnancies of women with CD compared with pregnancies of women without IBD (OR, 1.49; 95% CI, 0.91–2.44). Surgery for IBD before pregnancy increased the risk of ectopic pregnancy, although this increase was not statistically significant.

A meta-analysis of 12 studies including 3907 patients with IBD and 320,531 controls revealed that the incidence of low birth weight (<2500 g) and premature birth (<37 weeks) was increased but the incidence of stillbirth and congenital abnormalities were not. Compared to controls there was a 1.87-fold increase in the incidence of prematurity and nearly double the rate of low birth weight. Rates of caesarean section were 1.5 times higher and the risk of congenital anomalies was 2.37-fold increased. When broken down by subtype women with CD were more likely to deliver by caesarean section and were at higher risk of delivering low-birth-weight infants, women with UC were found to have greater risk of congenital anomalies in two of the studies; this risk was not replicated in the higher quality studies assessed.

The Hungarian Case Control Surveillance of Congenital Abnormalities study found no overall increased risk of congenital abnormalities in children born to 71 women with UC, but a higher risk of limb deficiencies, obstructive urinary congenital abnormalities, and multiple congenital abnormalities was observed. A Danish study of 71 CD patients with active disease during pregnancy compared to 86 with quiescent disease found no increased incidence of low birth weight, low birth weight at term, or congenital abnormalities in either group, but a 3.4-fold increased risk of preterm delivery was reported in those with moderate to severe disease activity. In a recent French national cohort study, pregnancies in women with IBD were associated with increased risks of prematurity (8% vs 5.5%), small for gestational age (11.1% vs 9.8%), and caesarean section (26.1% vs 20.0%), especially among women with active IBD. Disease activity decreased during pregnancy in women with Crohn's disease, but was unchanged in women with UC. In a prior Northern California based study of pregnant IBD and non-IBD women no difference in rates of elective abortions or of congenital anomalies was observed. Furthermore, no difference in rates of congenital anomalies was observed in children born to mothers with UC compared to CD.

Recent data from a prospective US cohort study of 1490 pregnant IBD patients on azathioprine or biologics demonstrated that there were 9% infants with congenital malformations, 3% spontaneous abortions, 7% low birth weights, and 10% on thiopurines preterm births.

There were 4% babies who were small for gestational age, 2% intrauterine growth retardations, 5 (0.30%) stillbirths, 613 (44%) cesarean sections, and 137 (10%) neonatal ICU stays.

These numbers are not significantly higher than that of IBD women not on immunosuppressive or biologic medications. There was also no increased risk of infant infections during the first year of life.

C. Managing IBD Flares during Pregnancy

Active IBD during pregnancy is high risk and should be closely followed by maternal–fetal medicine in a tertiary referral center. High-risk patients are pregnant patients with moderate to severe disease activity, those receiving steroids, biologics, and immunomodulators to control symptoms, patients with perianal disease and with ileoanal pouch anastomosis. Delivery will not cure a flare of IBD but can protect the fetus from adverse outcomes. Strong consideration for delivery should be considered in the case of fulminant UC necessitating colectomy as emergency surgery results in spontaneous abortion or still birth in 50% cases.

Pregnant sick IBD patients are at greater risk of deep vein thrombosis (DVT), venous thromboembolism, antepartum hemorrhage, emergency caesarean delivery, blood transfusions, and malnutrition. In a recent 2020 systematic review and meta-analysis of five studies, DVT risk increased significantly by a RR of 2.74 (95% CI 1.73–4.36) in pregnant women with IBD compared to pregnant women without IBD. We recommend DVT prophylaxis in all hospitalized pregnant IBD patients.

As in nonpregnant patients, new-onset diarrhea should be investigated with stool cultures to rule out an infectious etiology. Hydration, nutrition, and electrolyte maintenance is crucial. Antidiarrheal therapy can be used in pregnancy and loperamide would appear to be safer than diphenoxylate/atropine (category B vs category C). We advise against the use of peptobismol in pregnancy.

Acute flares of IBD can be treated with corticosteroids, although it is considered optimal to use 20mg /day of oral prednisone, in severe disease it is generally accepted that higher doses can be used such as intravenous hydrocortisone, 300 mg/day in divided doses for those with severe disease. Previous reports raised concerns of cleft palates associated with steroid use in the first trimester; however, a prospective study of 311 mothers who received corticosteroids in the first trimester identified no increased risk of congenital malformation, specifically no cases of cleft palate were reported.

While women with IBD often require corticosteroids for treatment of flares, they are also more susceptible to developing gestational diabetes. In a large prospective North American registry, corticosteroid use was associated with gestational diabetes (OR 2.8, 95% CI 1.3–6.0). Of note, in a separate retrospective study this increased risk was not seen with budesonide, therefore, this may be a suitable option to use in women who have milder flares. However, it is also important to note that inadequate control of a flare can lead to significant complications such as fetal distress, premature delivery and miscarriage. Therefore, clinical judgment and close collaboration with obstetricians should be utilized with regards to deciding on an optimal corticosteroid dosage. Other adverse events associated with steroid treatment include pregnancy-induced hypertension and preterm delivery due to premature rupture of membranes.

Remission in severe steroid refractory UC during pregnancy can be effectively induced by biologic induction or dose increased. Additionally, it is acceptable to initiate new biologic therapy during pregnancy if clinically indicated. Postauthorization data by the pregnancy and neonatal outcomes after fetal exposure to biologics and thiopurines in women with IBD (PIANO) study have not demonstrated any increased risk of malformations, spontaneous abortions, preterm birth, low birth weight or infection in the first year of life. Increased maternal IBD activity was however associated with a higher incidence of spontaneous abortions, preterm birth and infant infections.

In addition to anti TNF agents such as infliximab, adalimumab and certolizumab -pegol, golimumab, natalizumab, vedolizumab and ustekinumab exposure in pregnancy was also included in the PIANO cohort. The new oral small molecule therapy, tofacitinib is teratogenic in animal models and is contraindicated in patients attempting pregnancy.

Prior to widespread biologic use, cyclosporine was used for steroid refractory severe UC. There was no association with increased risk of congenital malformations, however there were associated increased rates of prematurity and a higher incidence of small for gestational age infants. However, in these studies was unclear if fetal growth restriction and prematurity were due to cyclosporine or to underlying maternal disease. Nowadays due to the established use of biologics, it is infrequently used.

An acute abdomen in a pregnant patient should be managed aggressively, particularly given the risk of maternal and fetal mortality from intestinal perforation. Indications for surgery during pregnancy include acute refractory colitis, perforation, abscesses, severe hemorrhage, and obstruction. Surgery is technically easier during the second trimester but should be performed if indicated regardless of gestational age, continued illness is more detrimental to the fetus than potential risks of surgery. Risks include preterm labor and spontaneous abortions, due to uterine manipulation. Temporary ileostomy formation is considered safer than primary anastomosis.

Endoscopy is rarely indicated during pregnancy and should only be performed if there is a strong indication and the information obtained is necessary to dictate management if possible endoscopy should be postponed until the second trimester, both colonoscopy and sigmoidoscopy appear to be safe in the second trimester. Risks to the fetus can be minimized by using no/minimal endoscopic medications and anesthesiologist's presence during endoscopy. This is discussed in more detail later in this chapter.

In a recent study, fecal calprotectin significantly correlated with increased clinical activity through all stages of pregnancy. These findings were further supported in a systematic review, thereby inferring that fecal calprotectin is perhaps the most optimal noninvasive option to monitor disease activity in pregnancy. Other noninvasive tests such as serum CRP, hemoglobin, and albumin did not demonstrate similar correlation, therefore are less useful.

D. Imaging and Endoscopic Studies

1. Diagnostic radiology during pregnancy—Various imaging modalities are available for diagnostic use in IBD patients during pregnancy. These include x-ray, ultrasonography, MRI in the second and third trimesters, and computed tomography (CT) after 25 weeks of gestation. In humans, growth retardation, microcephaly, and mental retardation are the most common adverse effects from high-dose radiation. Based on data from atomic bomb survivors, it appears that the risk of central nervous system effects is greatest with

exposure at 8–15 weeks of gestation, with no proven risk at less than 8 weeks of gestation or greater than 25 weeks of gestation. Thus, at 8–15 weeks of gestation, the fetus is at greatest risk for radiation-induced mental retardation, and the risk appears to be at doses of at least 20 rad. For example, the risk of severe mental retardation in fetuses exposed to ionizing radiation is approximately 40% at 100 rad of exposure and as high as 60% at 150 rad of exposure. Even multiple diagnostic x-ray procedures rarely result in ionizing radiation exposure to this degree. Fetal risks of anomalies, growth restriction, or abortions are not increased with radiation exposure of less than 5 rad, a level above the range of exposure of most diagnostic procedures. The risk of carcinogenesis as a result of in utero exposure to ionizing radiation is unclear but is probably very small. It is estimated that a 1–2 rad fetal exposure may increase the risk of leukemia by a factor of 1.2–2.0 over natural incidence and that an estimated 1 in 2000 children exposed to ionizing radiation in utero will develop childhood leukemia. This is increased from a background rate of 1 in 3000.

With MRI, magnets that alter the energy state of hydrogen protons are used instead of ionizing radiation. MRI is somewhat useful in establishing the diagnosis or evaluating the activity of CD in the second and third trimesters. Ultrasonography involves the use of sound waves and is not a form of ionizing radiation. Although previously thought to be less useful in evaluating CD, it is being increasingly used during pregnancy, but remains operator dependent.

Most intravenous contrast agents used with CT contain derivatives of iodine and have not been studied in humans; however, many have been studied in animals and do not appear to be teratogenic. Neonatal hypothyroidism has been associated with some iodinated contrast agents taken during pregnancy, and for this reason, these compounds are avoided unless essential for the correct diagnosis. Neonatal thyroid function should be checked during the first week if iodinated contrast media has been given during pregnancy. Paramagnetic contrast agents used during MRI have not been studied in pregnant women. Animal studies have demonstrated increased rates of spontaneous abortion, skeletal abnormalities, and visceral abnormalities when given at two to seven times the recommended human dose. The agents should be used only if the potential benefit justifies the potential risk. Only a tiny amount of iodinated or gadolinium-based contrast medium given to the lactating mother reaches the milk and only a minute proportion is absorbed.

2. Endoscopy during pregnancy—Flexible sigmoidoscopy is generally safe during pregnancy and can be performed if needed to evaluate the severity of a flare or to rule out hematochezia or diarrhea from another source. Colonoscopy is generally avoided in pregnancy (see later discussion of endoscopy during pregnancy). The indications for performing sigmoidoscopy in pregnant patients are similar to indications in nonpregnant patients and include evaluation of diarrhea, hematochezia, and abdominal pain or mass. In one study, 15 of 17 patients with IBD who underwent sigmoidoscopy during pregnancy had a change in management based on findings. A recent 2020 study of 48 patients did not find any adverse obstetric events or hospitalizations associated with sigmoidoscopy for IBD. Sigmoidoscopy findings led to a change in management in over three quarters of women. It is therefore considered preferable to colonoscopy which poses a higher risk.

Treatment

Treatment of IBD during pregnancy is similar to that of non-pregnant patients.

A. Pharmacotherapy

Tables 7–5 to 7–7 outline considerations relating to medication use in pregnant and breast-feeding women.

B. Medications

There are no RCTs examining the effect of medications on pregnancy and breast-feeding; evidence is derived from case series and observational studies. In general, the benefits of continuing medical treatment for IBD in pregnancy outweigh the risks; however, thalidomide and methotrexate are absolutely contraindicated. Treatment with 5-aminosalicylic acid preparations, glucocorticoids, thiopurines, TNF inhibitors, ustekinumab and vedolizumab are acceptable during pregnancy and lactation.

Table 7–5. Inflammatory bowel disease medications and pregnancy.

May be Used	Data Insufficient for Substance Recommendation	Not Recommended
Adalimumab	[a]Golimumab	Methotrexate
Azathioprine/ 6-mercaptopurine	[a]Ustekinumab	Mycophenolate
Certolizumab Pegol	[a]Vedolizumab	Tofacitinib
Cyclosoprine A	[a]Budesonide	
Inflizimab		
Loperamide		
Mesalamine		
Prednisone/ prednisolone		
Sulfasalazine		
Tacrolimus		

[a]Studies in women with IBD and rheumatoid arthritis have shown that these medications are relatively safe during pregnancy (see text discussion).

Table 7–6. Inflammatory bowel disease medications and breastfeeding.

May be Used	Data Insufficient for Substance Recommendation	Not Recommended
Adalimumab	[a]Golimumab	Methotrexate
Azathioprine/ 6-mercaptopurine	[a]Ustekinumab	Mycophenolate
Balsalazide	[a]Vedolizumab	Tofacitinib
Certolizumab Pegol	[a]Budesonide	
Cyclosoprine A	Metronidazole	
Inflizimab	Ciprofloxacin	
Loperamide		
Mesalamine		
Prednisone/ prednisolone		
Sulfasalazine		
Tacrolimus		

[a]Studies in women with IBD and rheumatoid arthritis have shown that these medications are relatively safe during pregnancy (see text discussion).

In a 20 year large study of 1703 children of mothers aged 15–45 years with IBD, the risks of congenital malformations following in-utero exposure to 5-aminosalicylates (5-ASAs), thiopurines, and corticosteroids during the first trimester were studied. The risk of a major congenital anomaly was 2.7% and 2.8% in 384,811 children of mothers with and without IBD. No association between medication use and congenital abnormalities was found; the adjusted odds ratio of a major congenital anomaly associated with 5-ASAs was 0.82 (95% CI, 0.42–1.61) with corticosteroids 0.48 (95% CI, 0.15–1.50) and 1.27 (95% CI, 0.48–3.39) for thiopurines.

Mesalamine at doses up to 4.8 g/day has been shown to be safe in pregnancy. A meta-analysis of seven studies with a total of 2200 pregnant women with IBD reported that 642 received 5-ASA drugs (mesalazine, sulfasalazine, or olsalazine) and 1158 received no medication and there was no more than 1.16-fold increase in congenital malformations, 2.38-fold increase in still births, 1.14-fold increase in spontaneous abortions, 1.35-fold increase in preterm delivery, and 0.93-fold increase in low birth weight. Sulfasalazine influences folic acid metabolism and folate supplementation is recommended (2 mg daily).

Because corticosteroids can increase the risk of gestational diabetes and adverse pregnancy outcomes, they should not be used as maintenance therapy during pregnancy. Methotrexate needs to be stopped at least 3 months prior to conception due to its teratogenic effects. If an alternate medication is

Table 7–7. Frequently used medications in pregnant IBD women.

Drug	Cat	Usual Dosage	Additional Comments
Corticosteroids	C/D	Variable	Prednisone and prednisolone oral solution, immediate-release prednisone tablets, and methylprednisolone (C); prednisone oral delayed release tablets (D). Has been associated with cleft lip with or without cleft palate and deceased infant birth weight. Effective in inducing but not maintaining remission.
Budesonide	C	9 mg qd	Likely safe for use in patients with ileocolonic Crohn's disease and UC but no controlled studies available in pregnant women.
Infliximab Adalimumab Certolizumab pegol Golimumab Vedolizumab Ustekinumab	B	Based on retail brand	Appear safe – see text
6 Mercaptopurine/ azathioprine	D	Starting at 50 mg	Use is justified if patient has active disease refractory to other oral or topical agents. Possibly minimal teratogenicity in human fetuses. See text.
Cyclosporine C	C	Weight-based dosing	Use is justified if patient has active disease refractory other oral or topical agents. Can cause small-for-gestational-age births
Metronidazole	B	750–1500 mg daily in divided doses	Appears safe during pregnancy but use in limited to second and third trimesters because of potential mutagenicity in the first trimester
Fluoroquinolones	C	Based on retail brand	Limited safety data; usually avoided during pregnancy because of possible effects on collagen development
Loperamide	B	2 mg after each unformed stool	Anti-diarrheal agent of choice during pregnancy
Diphenoxylate/atropine sulfate	C	10 mL 4 times a day	Should be avoided during pregnancy.

needed, stability on the new medication for at least 3 months should be achieved before attempting conception.

The CCFA funded PIANO Registry (A Multicenter National Prospective Study of Pregnancy and Neonatal Outcomes in Women with Inflammatory Bowel Disease) followed 1490 women with IBD during pregnancy. Of the 1490 women, 869 had exposure to biologics (642 as monotherapy), and 242 had exposure to 6-mercaptopurine/azathioprine as monotherapy. In all, 227 women had combination therapy with anti-TNF medications, vedolizumab and thiopurines. Exposure to biologics and thiopurines was not associated with increased rates of congenital abnormalities, infant height and weight, overall infection rates or delay in milestone development at 4, 9, and 12 months. Adjusting for disease activity, mothers exposed to combination therapy had marginally higher rates of preterm birth (relative risk [RR] = 1.8; 1.0–3.3). Controlling for disease activity, infants whose mothers used combination therapy had no increased risk of NICU stay (RR = 1.5; 0.8–2.8). The rate of spontaneous abortion was lower in the PIANO cohort than documented in the general population, and a history of prior spontaneous abortion and increased maternal disease activities were identified as risk factors spontaneous abortion. Increased maternal IBD activity was associated with increased risk of preterm birth and pre-term birth associated with increased infant infections. The UC patients had more disease activity than those with CD during each trimester.

Data from the prospectively maintained TREAT Registry of more than 6200 CD patient report outcomes of 168 pregnancies, 117 of which were exposed to infliximab, with no difference in rates of miscarriage (10% vs 6.7%) or neonatal complications (6.9% vs 10%) between those exposed and not exposed to infliximab during pregnancy. Reports from the Infliximab Safety Database describe no differences in adverse fetal outcomes in those 96 women (82 CD, 1 UC, 10 rheumatoid arthritis) exposed to infliximab at conception and during early pregnancy compared to nonexposed.

A retrospective, multicenter study of thiopurine and anti-TNF-α safety during pregnancy analyzed 571 pregnancies. One hundred and eighty-seven pregnancies were exposed to thiopurines, 66 to anti-TNF-α agents, and 318 had no drug exposure. Unfavorable global pregnancy outcomes occurred in 31.8% exposed to no medications, 21.9% exposed to thiopurines, and 34.8% exposed to biologics. Rates of pregnancy complications were similar across all groups (27.7%, 20.9%, and 30.3%). Neonatal complications were lowest in those exposed to thiopurines (13.9%) compared to nonexposed (23.3%) and those exposed to anti-TNF agents (21.2%).

Infliximab and adalimumab are immunoglobulin G1 (IgG1) antibodies that can cross the placenta during the second and third trimesters, are detectable in the cord blood at delivery and can be detected in the infant for up to 6 months, raising the possibility of potential adverse effects in the offspring include infection, risks of vaccination, and impaired immune development.

Infants exposed to these two biologics in-utero are advised to avoid the first dose of the rotavirus vaccine which is a live vaccine, but may have all other immunizations as per schedule. A 2020 systematic review and meta-analysis did not find an increased use of infantile antibiotics (OR 0.91, 95% CI 0.73–1.14) or infection-related hospitalizations (OR 1.57, 95% CI 1.02–2.40) in infants exposed to biologics. However in a sub-group analysis, there was an increased association with infantile upper respiratory tract infections (OR 1.57, 95% CI 1.02–2.40, I = 4%).

Furthermore, in a Large Danish cohort study on long term health outcomes of 1048 children exposed to biologics and thiopurines in-utero, no increased risk of infections, psychiatric diagnoses/ASD/ADHD, or malignancies during childhood/adolescence were found following thiopurine exposure. Following in-utero exposure to anti-TNFs, the risk of respiratory, urological/gynaecological infections, and other infections was increased during the first year of life. HR 1.34 (95% CI 1.03–1.74), 2.36 (95% CI 1.15–4.81) and 1.61 (95% CI 1.21–2.13), respectively.

Studies have shown that discontinuation of anti-TNF therapy before 30 weeks' gestation can still result in detectable cord blood samples. Thirty-one pregnancies in 28 women (18 infliximab and 13 adalimumab) were studied, 12 (71%) of the patients taking infliximab and all patients taking adalimumab discontinued treatment before gestational week 30. Of those who discontinued adalimumab, two patients experienced a relapse of IBD. There were 28 live births, three miscarriages (one in an infliximab-treated patient and two in adalimumab-treated patients). The mean cord blood level of infliximab was significantly lower among women who received the drug 10 weeks or more before delivery (2.8–1 mg/mL) compared to those who received infliximab closer to delivery (10–2.3 mg/mL). Adalimumab was detected in five samples of cord blood (mean concentration 1.7–0.4 mg/mL) and was undetectable in one patient who discontinued the treatment at gestational week 22.

A further study of 31 pregnant women on biologics (11 IFX, 10 ADA, and 10 CZP) measured serum concentrations of drugs at birth in the mother, infant, and cord blood at delivery and monthly in infants until the drug was undetectable. IFX and ADA concentrations were higher in infant and cord blood than the mother, but the levels of CZP were significantly lower (median level cord IFX 160% greater than mother, ADA 153% greater than mother, CZP 3.9% of maternal level). ADA and IFX were detectable for up to 6 months in the infants. No adverse pregnancy events or congenital malformations were reported. We advise against switching pregnant women over to certolizumab over placental transfer concerns if they are well on infliximab or adalimumab.

In summary, multiple studies from the IBD literature have demonstrated the safety of biologics during pregnancy. The American College of Gastroenterology (AGA) recently published guidelines for management of IBD during pregnancy. In summary:

- Monotherapy is preferred for maintenance therapy.
- Continuation of biologic therapy in pregnancy has been associated with reduced flares, decreased disease activity, and fewer postpartum flares, with a lower incidence of adverse pregnancy outcomes.
- While most biologics, aside from certolizumab, actively cross the placenta, safety data from prospective trials and large nationwide cohorts of women who continued taking biologics in pregnancy have not shown an increase in adverse fetal outcomes.
- Generally, combination therapy with both biologics and immunomodulatory thiopurines is discouraged due to increased risk of infection in the infant per current AGA guidelines, though this has not been consistently shown. It is an individual decision whether to stop the based on indication for combination therapy and severity of the patient's disease. However, physicians are advised to avoid starting thiopurine therapy for the first time in pregnancy due to the risk of pancreatitis, leukopenia, and the delayed time to effect.

Although the AGA guidelines on therapeutic drug monitoring did not include a recommendation on prophylactic monitoring of anti-TNF levels in patients in remission, it may be worthwhile to monitor it prior to and during a pregnancy.

This is because a subtherapeutic level may lead to flares in pregnant women, and supratherapeutic levels may lead to increased transfer of biologics across the placenta.

During the third trimester, the AGA recommends that appropriate IBD medications including biologics should be continued without interruption. Since biologic drug level exposure to the fetus may increase towards the end of the pregnancy term, dosing can be adjusted in order to achieve lowest serum concentrations at the time of confinement.

Current recommendations are that one should plan for the final pregnancy injection of adalimumab 2–3 weeks before expected date of confinement and resume 1–2 weeks postpartum.

With infliximab one should plan the final pregnancy infusion 6–10 weeks before expected date of conception and resume postpartum if on an eight week dosing schedule. If dosing is every 4 weeks then plan to discontinue 4–5 weeks before expected conception date.

Ustekinumab and vedolizumab should follow a similar schedule.

The dose should be based on pre-pregnancy weight during pregnancy and in the immediate postpartum period. Since certolizumab -pegol does not cross the placenta this can be used uninterrupted during pregnancy.

Since tofacitinib is potentially teratogenic, a washout period of one week is recommended before attempting conception.

Adalimumab, infliximab, and certolizumab pegol are all safe during breast feeding.

Ciprofloxacin and metronidazole are antibiotics commonly used in the management of IBD. A meta-analysis did not find any relationship between metronidazole exposure during the first trimester of pregnancy and birth defects; it appears to be safe in short courses but long-term use in pregnancy is not recommended. The use of ciprofloxacin is not recommended in pregnant women due to effects on cartilage growth; however, among 200 pregnancies exposed to fluoroquinolones (including ciprofloxacin) there was no increased incidence of clinically significant musculoskeletal dysfunctions.

Altogether these recent studies suggest that thiopurines and anti-TNF-α agents' use during pregnancy does not increase the risk of birth defects; however, more large prospective trials with longer follow-up periods are required to assess the impact of these medications on the developing immune system.

C. Nursing

Therapy with 5-aminosalicylic acid preparations, glucocorticoids, thiopurines, and TNF inhibitors are acceptable during lactation. Breast-feeding is also discouraged while on treatment with cyclosporine, metronidazole, and ciprofloxacin and is contraindicated in women using methotrexate, which is excreted into breast milk, accumulates in neonatal tissues. Low levels of corticosteroids are found in breast milk and are of no clinical significance. To minimize exposure, a 4-hour delay after oral dosing might be recommended. Minimal amounts of infliximab and (1/200 of serum levels) adalimumab levels (1/100 of serum) have been detected in breast milk 2–3 days after IFX infusion and 3–8 days after ADA injection. In a recent US study of 824 women who had enrolled in the PIANO cohort, 310 were breast feeding while on biologic or combination therapy. 72 women provided samples of breast milk (29 IFX, 21 ADA, 13 certolizumab, 1 golimumab, 6 ustekinumab, and 2 natalizumab). Only 29 women demonstrated detectable drug levels. In a peak time range of 12–24 hours, the concentration of biologic in the milk was very low (0.15–1.57 ug/mL) These levels are thought to be clinically insignificant. Breast-fed infants of mothers on biologic medications demonstrated similar rates of milestone achievement and risk of infection as breastfed infants of mothers not on biologic medications and nonbreastfed infants. They were also not more likely to have an infection in the first 12 months of life compared with unexposed infants or infants who were not breastfed. The study authors concluded that biologic medications are compatible with breastfeeding, and there is no increased risk of infection or negative impact on infants exposed to low levels of biologic

medications transferred through breast milk. With regards to other GI medications, Loperamide is also compatible with nursing. Sulfasalazine and 5-ASAs are found in low concentrations in breast milk and infants whose mothers are using these agents should be observed for the development of diarrhea.

D. Surgery

Indications for surgery during pregnancy include uncontrollable bleeding, obstruction, perforation, fulminant disease refractory to medical management, or intra-abdominal abscess that cannot be drained by other methods. A systematic review of surgical management of complicated IBD in pregnant patients noted 86 cases over a 60 year period and noted that a free or contained small bowel perforation was the commonest reason for surgery in CD and medically refractory or fulminant UC or toxic megacolon was the main indication for surgery in UC. Surgery during the second trimester carries a lower rate of miscarriage than during the first trimester and is technically less complicated than during the third trimester. Laparoscopic surgery is often the preferred approach in the first and second trimesters, due to its diagnostic and therapeutic role, smaller incision, likelihood of less adhesion formation and quicker recovery. A study using the Danish National Registries of 1,202,870 pregnancies, including 4490 (0.4%) women who had nonobstetric abdominal surgery during pregnancy showed increased risk of small for gestational age, very preterm births, preterm birth and miscarriage among women who underwent surgery during pregnancy; the greatest risk for these outcomes occurred within 14 days after surgery. Total colectomy for fulminant UC has a 50–60% fetal mortality rate, and if possible, biologic therapy, or early delivery is preferable.

E. Delivery

In general, the method of the delivery should be dictated by obstetric indication. Vaginal delivery and cesarean delivery are safe for patients with an ileal pouch–anal anastomosis, and episiotomy is not contraindicated in IBD unless perianal disease is present. Caesarian section should also be considered here to avoid future pouch dysfunction in IPAA patients and maintain sphincter functionality. Patients with perianal disease can proceed with vaginal delivery unless their disease is active as this can precipitate a flare in disease activity. Patients with fulminant UC should also undergo cesarean delivery. Women in remission or with mild disease without perianal activity generally deliver vaginally unless the circumstances of pregnancy dictate otherwise. In general, it is best to avoid an operative vaginal delivery (ie, forceps or vacuum delivery) as these patients have the most long-term complications such as rectovaginal fistulas. (Figure 7–3).

de Lima-Karagiannis A, Zelinkova-Detkova Z, van der Woude CJ. The effects of active IBD during pregnancy in the era of novel IBD therapies. *Am J Gastroenterol.* 2016;111(9):1305–1312 [PMID: 27349339]

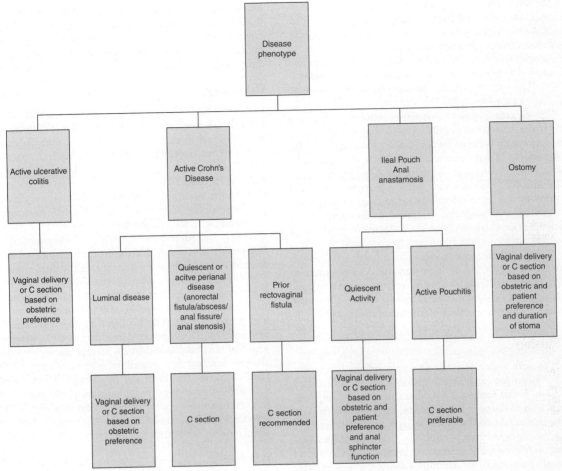

▲ **Figure 7–3.** Mode of delivery in IBD patients.

de Silva PS, Hansen HH, Wehberg S, Friedman S, Nørgård BM. Risk of ectopic pregnancy in women with inflammatory bowel disease: a 22-year Nationwide Cohort Study. *Clin Gastroenterol Hepatol.* 2018;16(1):83–89. [PMID: 28694133]

Friedman S, Nielsen J, Nøhr EA, Jølving LR, Nørgård BM. Comparison of time to pregnancy in women with and without inflammatory bowel diseases. *Clin Gastroenterol Hepatol.* 2020;18(7):1537–1544. [PMID: 31446182]

Getahun D, Fassett MJ, Longstreth G et al. Association between maternal inflammatory bowel disease and adverse perinatal outcomes. *J Perinatol.* 2014;34(6):435–440. [PMID: 24651735]

Killeen S, Gunn J, Hartley J. Surgical management of complicated and medically refractory inflammatory bowel disease during pregnancy. *Colorectal Dis.* 2017;19(2):123–138. [PMID: 27317641]

Kim YH, Pfaller B, Marson A, Yim HW, Huang V, Ito S. The risk of venous thromboembolism in women with inflammatory bowel disease during pregnancy and the postpartum period: a systematic review and meta-analysis. *Medicine (Baltimore).* 2019;98(38):e17309. [PMID: 31568016]

Leung YP, Kaplan GG, Coward S, et al. Intrapartum corticosteroid use significantly increases the risk of gestational diabetes in women with inflammatory bowel disease. *J Crohns Colitis.* 2015;9:223–230. [PMID: 25576754]

Lin K, Martin CF, Dassopoulos T, et al. Pregnancy outcomes amongst mothers with inflammatory bowel disease exposed to systemic cortico- steroids: results of the PIANO registry. *Gastroenterology.* 2014;146:S-1.

Shannahan SE, Erlich JM, Peppercorn MA. Insights into the treatment of inflammatory bowel disease in pregnancy. *Therap Adv Gastroenterol.* 2019;12:1756284819852231. [PMID: 31191713]

Mahadevan U, Robinson C, Bernasko N, et al. Inflammatory bowel disease in pregnancy clinical care pathway: a report from the American Gastroenterological Association IBD parenthood project working group. American Journal of Obstetrics and Gynecology. 2019;220(4):308–323. [PMID: 30948039]

Nørgård BM, Nielsen J, Friedman S. In utero exposure to thiopurines/anti-TNF agents and long-term health outcomes during childhood and adolescence in Denmark. *Aliment Pharmacol Ther.* 2020;52(5):829–842. [PMID: 32677731]

Gubatan J, Nielsen OH, Levitte S, et al. Biologics during pregnancy in women with inflammatory bowel disease and risk of infantile infections: a systematic review and meta-analysis. *Am J Gastroenterol.* 2020;10.14309/ajg.0000000000000910. [PMID: 33110017]

Picardo S, Seow CH. A pharmacological approach to managing inflammatory bowel disease during conception, pregnancy and breastfeeding: biologic and oral small molecule therapy. *Drugs.* 2019;79(10):1053–1063. [PMID: 31183768]

Puri A, Bharadwaj V, Sachdeva S. Extent of disease is a major outcome predictor in patients with ulcerative colitis and pregnancy. *Indian J Gastroenterol.* 2015;34(2):108–111. [PMID: 25895048]

Tandon P, Leung K, Yusuf A, Huang VW. Noninvasive methods for assessing inflammatory bowel disease activity in pregnancy: a systematic review. *J Clin Gastroenterol.* 2019;53(8):574–581. [PMID: 31306343]

Rasmussen AS, Christiansen CF, Ulrichsen SP, Uldbjerg N, Nørgaard M. Non-obstetric abdominal surgery during pregnancy and birth outcomes: a Danish registry-based cohort study. *Acta Obstet Gynecol Scand.* 2020;99(4):469–476. [PMID: 31774546]

Watanabe C, Nagahori M, Fujii T, et al. Non-adherence to medications in pregnant ulcerative colitis patients contributes to disease flares and adverse pregnancy outcomes. *Dig Dis Sci.* 2020 Apr 6. [PMID: 32249373]

Yu A, Friedman S, Ananthakrishnan AN. Characteristics and long-term outcomes of pregnancy-onset inflammatory bowel disease: a case-control study. *Inflamm Bowel Dis.* 2021;27(4):476–481. [PMID: 32426824]

Meyer A, Drouin J, Weill A, Carbonnel F, Dray-Spira R. Pregnancy in women with inflammatory bowel disease: a French nationwide study 2010-2018. *Aliment Pharmacol Ther.* 2020;52(9):1480–1490. [PMID: 33095502]

Mahadevan U, Long MD, Kane SV, et al. Pregnancy and neonatal outcomes after fetal exposure to biologics and thiopurines among women with inflammatory bowel disease. *Gastroenterology.* 2021;160(4):1131–1139. [PMID: 33227283]

Kammerlander H, Nielsen J, Kjeldsen J, et al. Fecal calprotectin during pregnancy in women with moderate-severe inflammatory bowel disease. *Inflamm Bowel Dis.* 2018;24(4):839–848. [PMID: 29506137]

Ko MS, Rudrapatna VA, Avila P, Mahadevan U. Safety of flexible sigmoidoscopy in pregnant patients with known or suspected inflammatory bowel disease. *Dig Dis Sci.* 2020;65(10):2979–2985. [PMID: 32034603]

Matro R, Martin CF, Wolf D, Shah SA, Mahadevan U. Exposure concentrations of infants breastfed by women receiving biologic therapies for inflammatory bowel diseases and effects of breastfeeding on infections and development. *Gastroenterology.* 2018;155(3):696–704. [PMID: 29857090]

ABDOMINAL PAIN

The differential diagnosis of abdominal pain in pregnant patients, just as in nonpregnant patients, is extensive and deserves careful evaluation. Because imaging tests are often avoided during pregnancy, there is often heavy reliance on the history, physical examination, and laboratory testing. Location and severity of pain are critical to evaluation. (Figure 7–4) Diffuse pain can suggest intestinal obstruction; peritoneal inflammation from pancreatitis, appendicitis, or intra-abdominal abscess; or metabolic abnormalities such as uremia, porphyria, and diabetes. Upper abdominal pain can suggest biliary disease, PUD, or mediastinal pathology such as esophageal rupture, pneumonia, rib fracture, pulmonary embolism, Mallory-Weiss tear, esophageal stricture, and myocardial infarction. In addition, some diseases may present with epigastric pain or localize to the left side, such as PUD, splenic infarcts or abscess, splenic artery aneurysm (more common in pregnancy), gastric volvulus, and incarcerated paraesophageal hernia. Right upper quadrant pain can suggest hepatitis, hepatic vascular engorgement, hepatic hematoma, hepatic malignancy, preeclampsia, or HELLP syndrome. Biliary diseases such as biliary colic, choledocholithiasis, cholangitis, and cholecystitis may also present with epigastric discomfort or localize to the right side. Right lower quadrant pain can indicate appendicitis, ruptured Meckel diverticulum, CD, intussusception, bowel infection or perforation, or colon cancer. Left lower quadrant pain can indicate diverticulitis, sigmoid volvulus, colon cancer, bowel infection or perforation, IBD, and irritable bowel syndrome. Any lower abdominal discomfort can suggest gynecologic or obstetric causes such as ruptured ectopic pregnancy (severe pain), ovarian cyst rupture, pelvic inflammatory disease, tubo-ovarian abscess, uterine fibroids, impending abortion, adnexal mass, salpingitis, endometriosis, ruptured corpus luteum, or cervical or ovarian cancer. Nephrolithiasis and pyelonephritis can manifest right- or left-sided, upper or lower abdominal pain.

Vascular causes such as mesenteric ischemia and abdominal aortic aneurysm can cause diffuse or localized pain and should always be considered in the differential as they may present as medical or surgical emergencies. Spontaneous hepatic rupture is an abdominal emergency unique to pregnancy. It typically occurs late in pregnancy; is associated with subcapsular hematoma, preeclampsia, and HELLP syndrome; and presents with severe right-sided or epigastric pain, sometimes radiating to the right shoulder. It can be diagnosed with ultrasound, and when signs of rupture or expanding subcapsular hematoma are seen, the patient should undergo immediate cesarean delivery; intraoperative packing, hepatic resection, or hepatic artery ligation are often needed to control bleeding.

▶ Clinical Findings

A. Symptoms and Signs

A careful history of pain onset, character, severity, and location is critical. Important signs on physical examination include the presence of fever, hypotension, and tachycardia; these findings should prompt a search for causes of

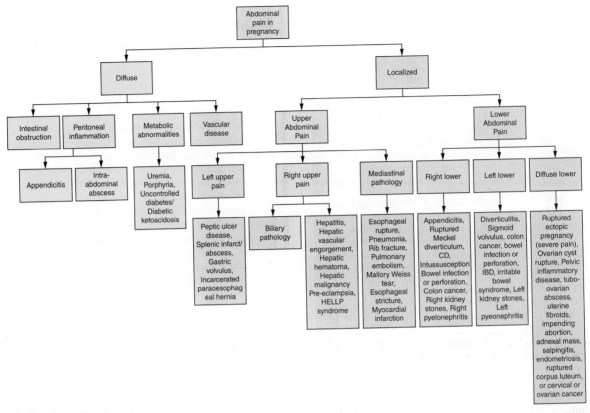

▲ **Figure 7–4.** Approach to abdominal pain during pregnancy.

abdominal infection or acute abdomen. Classic physical examination findings of peritonitis may be absent due to abdominal wall laxity in pregnancy; however, the presence of a rigid abdomen is a likely indicator of peritonitis.

B. Laboratory and Imaging Studies

Any patient presenting with significant abdominal pain should undergo laboratory tests, including complete blood count and differential, serum electrolytes, liver function tests, coagulation profile, and amylase and lipase levels. Physiologic changes in these values that occur normally during pregnancy, such as elevation in white blood cell count, anemia, elevated alkaline phosphate, elevated erythrocyte sedimentation rate, and mild hyponatremia, all should be kept in mind during evaluation.

Ultrasound is considered low risk and should be the imaging study of choice if needed. Abdominal radiographs are avoided if possible due to radiation exposure to the fetus, but may be indicated when bowel perforation or obstruction is suspected. MRI is preferable to CT scanning to avoid ionizing radiation, but gadolinium should be avoided during the

first trimester if possible. Any radiologic testing should be preceded by counseling of the patient.

▶ Treatment

Treatment is based on the disorder. Evaluation and treatment of common gastrointestinal problems in pregnancy are discussed in later sections of this chapter. Biliary and liver diseases of pregnancy are discussed in another Chapter.

Kunovsky L, Hemmelova B, Kala Z, Dolina J, Konecny S, Penka I. Crohn's disease and pregnancy: a case report of an acute abdomen. *Int J Colorectal Dis.* 2016;31(8):1493–1494. [PMID: 26992730]

Makhijani R, Bhagat VH, Fayek M. Colon cancer presenting as pseudo-obstruction during pregnancy - a case report. *Obstet Med.* 2017;10(4):198–200. [PMID: 29225684]

Wang QY, Ye XH, Ding J, Wu XK. Segmental small bowel necrosis associated with antiphospholipid syndrome: a case report. *World J Gastroenterol.* 2015;21(13):4096–4100. [PMID: 25852299]

Zhao Q, Zhang S, Dong A. An Unusual Case of Abdominal Pain. *Gastroenterology.* 2018;154(8):e1-e2. [PMID: 28870529]

PEPTIC ULCER DISEASE

There is no evidence to support an increased incidence of PUD during pregnancy, and in fact, many studies suggest a decreased incidence. However, in a recent nationwide retrospective cohorts study between 1999 and 2015, prevalence of PUD in pregnancy increased from 4/100,000 to 11/100,000, respectively. Pregnant women with PUD are usually older and more likely to have increased comorbidity.

Both gastric and duodenal ulcers do occur and detection is difficult, as avoidance of invasive testing is desirable during pregnancy. Despite the lower incidence of invasive testing in pregnant women, a recent large national database study did not find increased adverse peptic ulcer related outcomes in pregnant women diagnosed with PUD. In contrast, women with PUD during pregnancy were more likely to have an increased risk of pregnancy related outcomes such as intrauterine growth restriction, pre-term birth and congenital anomalies.

Clinical Findings

A. Symptoms and Signs

The symptoms of PUD are the same in pregnant as in nonpregnant patients and include epigastric pain, abdominal distention, eructation, postprandial nausea and vomiting, anorexia, and rarely, hematemesis, melena, hematochezia, or peritonitis. Differentiating ulcer disease from other conditions that present with similar symptoms is an important part of evaluation. Nausea and vomiting associated with pregnancy are often most pronounced in the first trimester, whereas PUD worsens during the third trimester. The physical examination may reveal signs of complications from PUD; such as fever, infection, sepsis and shock.

Heme-positive stool or visible blood on rectal examination may suggest bleeding from an ulcer. Peritoneal signs should prompt surgical consultation for possible perforated ulcer. In a large US cohort it was noted that transfusion was less likely to occur in pregnant women as compared to nonpregnant women. Pregnant women also experienced shorter hospital stays.

B. Laboratory, Imaging, and Endoscopic Studies

Liver blood tests and an ultrasound scan should be obtained to evaluate for cholelithiasis, choledocholithiasis, viral hepatitis, AFLP, and HELLP syndrome. Right upper quadrant tenderness, a history of fatty food intolerance, fever, and leukocytosis can suggest cholecystitis, which can also be diagnosed by ultrasound. Pancreatitis can be suggested by pain that is exacerbated with eating, pain radiating to the back, a history of alcoholism, gallstones, prior pancreatitis, leukocytosis, and fever; amylase and lipase levels should be checked. An electrocardiogram should be obtained to exclude myocardial ischemia. Urinalysis and urine culture should also be obtained to exclude urinary tract infection.

Abdominal radiographs are avoided in pregnancy but should be obtained in suspected perforation. Barium studies are also avoided, but upper endoscopy should be performed when symptoms are severe and refractory to intensive medical therapy, when complications including hemorrhage and gastric outlet obstruction occur, or when gastric adenocarcinoma or lymphoma is suspected. The safety of endoscopy in pregnancy is discussed separately, later in this chapter.

Treatment

The symptoms of PUD are difficult to distinguish from GERD; however, the medical treatment for both is identical and should be attempted first unless indications for endoscopy, discussed earlier, are present. Medical treatment for suspected PUD and GERD includes antacids, sucralfate, H_2-blockers, and if needed PPIs (see earlier discussion of treatment of GERD in pregnancy). Misoprostol is contraindicated in pregnancy. Triple-drug therapy for treatment of H pylori should be deferred if possible until after delivery due to the low risk of complications from PUD and possible fetal risk from antibiotics. Treatment of H pylori associated with mucosa-associated lymphoid tissue tumor is indicated, however, and should not be deferred. Amoxicillin (class B), metronidazole (class B), and clarithromycin (class C) can be used, although treatment during the first trimester should be avoided if possible. Both tetracycline and bismuth subsalicylate are relatively contraindicated during pregnancy.

Endoscopy is indicated in patients with gastrointestinal bleeding suspected to be from PUD. Very little is known about the risks of therapeutic endoscopic therapy for PUD or hemostasis for other disorders such as variceal bleeding or Mallory-Weiss tear. However, one study did find that pregnant women who underwent EGD were more likely to experience a venous thromboembolism than nonpregnant women.

Therapeutic endoscopy is currently an experimental procedure during pregnancy but is justifiable when the only alternative is surgery. The indications for surgery for PUD are the same in pregnant as in nonpregnant patients and include uncontrollable hemorrhage, perforation, and gastric outlet obstruction.

Rosen C, Czuzoj-Shulman N, Mishkin DS, Abenhaim HA. Pregnancy outcomes among women with peptic ulcer disease. *J Perinat Med.* 2020;48(3):209–216. [PMID: 32083450]

Rosen C, Czuzoj-Shulman N, Mishkin DS, Abenhaim HA. Management and outcomes of peptic ulcer disease in pregnancy. *J Matern Fetal Neonatal Med.* 2021;34(9):1368–1374. [PMID: 31242793]

BILIARY DISEASE

Cholelithiasis is common in pregnancy with the incidence reported to be between 2.5% and 12.5%. However, most patients with gallstones remain asymptomatic. Pregnancy predisposes to gallstone formation through the following mechanisms: increased bile lithogenicity mediated by estrogen and decreased gallbladder contractility mediated by progesterone are implicated in the causality. Obesity, pre-pregnancy weight gain, Hispanic ethnicity, and maternal age are risk factors for gallstone disease during pregnancy.

▶ Clinical Findings

A. Symptoms and Signs

Symptomatic patients may present with anorexia, nausea, vomiting, right upper quadrant or epigastric pain, and a history of symptoms exacerbated by fatty foods. The pain can radiate to the back or right shoulder. Although termed "biliary colic," severe pain from gallstones can last several hours. The presence of fever, tachycardia, leukocytosis, elevated neutrophil count, right upper quadrant tenderness, and Murphy sign may indicate the presence of cholecystitis.

B. Laboratory and Imaging Studies

Abnormal liver blood tests may indicate the presence of choledocholithiasis (keeping in mind physiologic elevation of alkaline phosphatase in pregnancy). Elevated amylase and lipase can indicate pancreatitis. A right upper quadrant ultrasound is safe in pregnancy and has a high degree of accuracy in detecting gallstones. The presence of sonographic Murphy sign, gallbladder wall thickening, pericholecystic fluid, or stranding can suggest cholecystitis. Common bile duct or intrahepatic duct dilation can suggest choledocholithiasis. The ultrasonographer should evaluate for liver and pancreatic disease as well.

▶ Treatment

The management of gallstones in the absence of cholecystitis or choledocholithiasis is medical, including avoidance of fatty foods and a brief period of bowel rest and pain control if needed. For patients who do not respond to medical therapy or who develop recurrent symptoms, early operative management is advocated as there is a high rate of recurrence and risk of complications during pregnancy. For those patients who do not undergo intervention, and have conservative treatment, the majority require surgical intervention within two years of delivery.

When cholecystitis is present, intravenous antibiotics should be started. Intravenous cefazolin and extended-spectrum penicillin are effective and generally considered safe in pregnancy. Because of the risk of fetal loss, teratogenesis, and preterm labor during the first trimester, and the risk of preterm labor, premature delivery, and technical difficulties due to the gravid uterus during the third trimester, surgery is often delayed until the second trimester or after delivery if possible.

Recent improvements in less-invasive surgical techniques may lead to improved surgical outcomes. A recent study showed that conservative management of cholelithiasis and its complications during pregnancy is associated with recurrent biliary symptoms and frequent emergency department visits.

Gallstone pancreatitis, choledocholithiasis, or acute cholecystitis that fails to resolve is an indication for early surgery. Typically, laparoscopic surgery is performed during the first two trimesters, but open procedures are often required in the third trimester. Laparoscopic surgery is associated with fewer complications.

Routine intraoperative cholangiography is not recommended during pregnancy due to radiation exposure; however, bile duct exploration and intraoperative ultrasound are alternatives. Successful laparoscopic common bile duct exploration during acute gallstone pancreatitis has been reported in the first and second trimesters. If performed, cholangiography should be undertaken with a fetal shield to minimize radiation.

Choledocholithiasis is rare in pregnancy, but endoscopic retrograde cholangiopancreatography (ERCP) with stone extraction, sphincterotomy, or stent insertion can all be performed and is indicated for common bile duct stones and cholangitis.

Lammert F, Gurusamy K, Ko CW, et al. Gallstones. *Nat Rev Dis Primers*. 2016;2:16024. [PMID: 27121416]

Sedaghat N, Cao AM, Eslick GD, Cox MR. Laparoscopic versus open cholecystectomy in pregnancy: a systematic review and meta-analysis. *Surg Endosc*. 2017;31(2):673–679. [PMID: 27324332]

Hedström J, Nilsson J, Andersson R, Andersson B. Changing management of gallstone-related disease in pregnancy - a retrospective cohort analysis. *Scand J Gastroenterol*. 2017;52(9):1016–1021. [PMID: 28599581]

PANCREATITIS

Acute pancreatitis in pregnancy (APIP) is a rare but severe condition with the incidence of approximately 1 out of 1000–12,000 pregnant women. It is most common during the third trimester and postpartum. Gallstones are the cause in the vast majority of pregnant patients with pancreatitis; however, the typical differential diagnosis of pregnancy still applies, and alcoholism, hypercalcemia, hypertriglyceridemia, infections, trauma, and medication-induced causes should be ruled out.

▶ Clinical Findings

Clinical presentation and elevated amylase and lipase levels are typically diagnostic, as pancreatic enzyme levels are not affected by pregnancy. Ultrasound can diagnose gallstones and choledocholithiasis (bile duct dilation) and can also sometimes visualize pancreatic inflammation. CT scan is reserved for severe, refractory pancreatitis to evaluate for areas of pancreatitis necrosis, and MRI may be a safer alternative during pregnancy.

Treatment

Medical management includes stopping oral intake, aggressive intravenous fluids, histamine blockers, and PPI. Laboratory values such as calcium, blood urea nitrogen, creatinine, white blood cell count, and hematocrit should be monitored carefully. Meperidine is typically chosen for pain control and is a category B drug; it appears to be safe for use in pregnancy. For severe pancreatitis, surgical debridement or endoscopic or percutaneous drainage of abscesses or pseudocysts should not be delayed. Severe pancreatitis may in rare cases require antibiotics and parenteral nutrition. Although endoscopic procedures and tests involving radiation are generally avoided during pregnancy, one study noted a significant relapse rate in patients with gallstone pancreatitis. These findings argue for ERCP, cholecystectomy, or both. Currently, acute gallstone pancreatitis complicated by evidence of persistent biliary obstruction is one of the indications for ERCP with sphincterotomy during all stages of pregnancy. Cholecystectomy is often deferred until the second trimester or postpartum period. One study revealed that there is an increased incidence of postpartum acute pancreatitis secondary to gallstones in the first two years following delivery. Pancreatitis is associated with fetal wastage in the first trimester and premature labor in the third trimester. Despite advances in medical treatment maternal and perinal mortality rates are still as high as 3.3–18.7%. However, this is considerably lower if pancreatitis improves quickly with medical management.

Ducarme G, Maire F, Chatel P, et al. Acute pancreatitis during pregnancy: a review. J Perinatol. 2014;34:87–94. [PMID: 24355941]

Jin D, Tan J, Jiang J, Philips D, Liu L. The early predictive value of routine laboratory tests on the severity of acute pancreatitis patients in pregnancy: a retrospective study. *Sci Rep.* 2020;10(1):10087. [PMID: 32572085]

Maringhini A, Dardanoni G, Fantaci G, Patti R, Maringhini M. Acute Pancreatitis during and after pregnancy: incidence, risk factors, and prognosis. *Dig Dis Sci.* 2020;10.1007/s10620-020-06608-5. [PMID: 33085013]

APPENDICITIS

Acute appendicitis is the most common gastrointestinal disorder requiring surgery during pregnancy. The key to management is prompt diagnosis.

Clinical Findings

A. Symptoms and Signs

Patients typically present with anorexia, nausea, vomiting, and abdominal pain; however, in pregnancy, this presentation needs to be distinguished from conditions such as nausea and vomiting of pregnancy, particularly in the first trimester. Abdominal pain associated with appendicitis can be located in nontraditional places. During the first trimester, the appendix has the usual right lower quadrant location, and patients typically present with periumbilical pain that migrates to the right lower quadrant. During the second and third trimesters, however, the appendix gradually moves upward and laterally until by the third trimester, it is located in the right upper quadrant (Figure 7–5). This

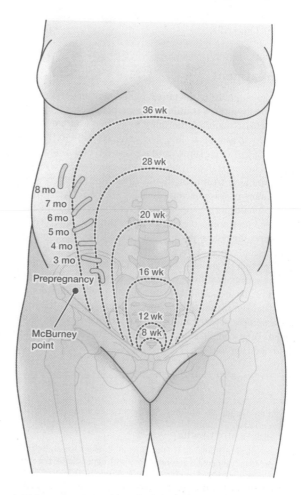

▲ **Figure 7–5.** Changes in location and direction of the appendix during pregnancy in relationship to the McBurney point and the height of the fundus at various weeks of gestation.

changes the presentation of appendicitis and can delay diagnosis and management. Fever, tachycardia, abdominal tenderness, and peritoneal signs can be clues to an inflamed appendix, but their absence does not rule out appendicitis.

B. Laboratory and Imaging Studies

Although pregnancy can elevate the white blood cell count, a finding of more than 80% neutrophils on the differential is suggestive of an acute disorder. Abdominal ultrasound can be diagnostic during the first trimester but less helpful when the appendix migrates. Abdominal CT scan can be used to diagnose appendicitis; however, this exposes the fetus to radiation teratogenicity. Diagnostic laparoscopy can also be performed if there is diagnostic uncertainty. If there is any suspicion of appendicitis, surgical consultation should be obtained immediately.

▶ Treatment

Once appendicitis is diagnosed, either clinically or by imaging, usually surgery is indicated, as appendiceal perforation can increase maternal mortality to as high as 4% and fetal mortality to as high as 20%. The only exception to this is in the setting of active labor, in which case it is undertaken after vaginal or cesarean delivery if labor is prolonged. Perioperative antibiotic treatment should cover both Gram negative and Gram-positive bacteria (usually with a second generation cephalosporin) and coverage for anaerobes (clindamycin or metronidazole). Delaying surgical intervention increases the risk of perforation. In the first two trimesters, laparoscopic appendectomy can be done safely; previously it was felt that laparotomy is indicated in the third trimester or in the setting of diffuse peritonitis. However, a recent large study of laparoscopic appendectomy in all trimesters did not find significant third trimester complications following laparoscopic surgery and length of hospital stay was shortened. Fetal complications are similar between laparoscopic and open approaches.

Aptilon Duque G, Mohney S. Appendicitis in pregnancy. In: *StatPearls*. Treasure Island (FL): StatPearls Publishing; July 10, 2020. [PMID: 31869106]

Mantoglu B, Altintoprak F, Firat N, et al. Reasons for undesirable pregnancy outcomes among women with appendicitis: the experience of a tertiary center. *Emerg Med Int.* 2020;2020:6039862. [PMID: 33014470]

Tumati A, Yang J, Zhang X, et al. Pregnant patients requiring appendectomy: comparison between open and laparoscopic approaches in NY State. *Surg Endosc.* 2020;10.1007/s00464-020-07911-y. [PMID: 32926252]

INTESTINAL OBSTRUCTION, PSEUDO-OBSTRUCTION, & GASTROINTESTINAL CANCER

Pregnancy complicated by intestinal obstruction is very rare, with an incidence of between approximately 1/5000 and 1/66,000. The commonest cause for intestinal obstruction is intestinal volvulus. Other important causes in pregnancy include adhesions. Most cases of volvulus during pregnancy occur during the third trimester because of the sigmoid colon being displaced by the gravid uterus out of the pelvis, leading the colon to twist around its fixation points. Other causes of intestinal obstruction include intussusception, hernia, acute appendicitis, slow transit constipation and gastric and colorectal cancer (CRC). Incarcerated diaphragmatic hernias are rare but more common during pregnancy and have a high rate of complications.

▶ Clinical Findings

Prompt recognition and treatment of obstruction and pseudo-obstruction are critical. Sigmoid volvulus during pregnancy is associated with high maternal (6%) and fetal mortality (26%) even with appropriate intervention. Patients present with constipation, progressive abdominal pain, and abdominal distention. Later on, bilious vomiting and obstipation can be present. Abdominal radiographs and CT scans may be required for evaluation and are typically diagnostic of this condition. Flexible sigmoidoscopy or colonoscopy may be required for diagnosis or decompression. Pseudo-obstruction or colonic distention without obstruction can occur following delivery; symptoms are similar to those of intestinal obstruction. Pseudo-obstruction is typically diagnosed with abdominal radiographs. Colon and gastric cancer are the most common gastrointestinal malignancies during pregnancy and can cause bleeding, anemia, abdominal pain, or obstruction.

▶ Treatment

Conservative management includes nasogastric decompression, fluid resuscitation, monitoring of electrolytes, bowel rest, and careful use of analgesia. Prophylactic antibiotics should be considered. Pseudo-obstruction and some cases of volvulus or adhesion-induced small bowel obstruction will resolve with conservative management. Suspected intestinal ischemia, perforation, persistent tachycardia, fever, abdominal tenderness, and failure to resolve with conservative management are indications for surgery.

Patients with postpartum pseudo-obstruction should be followed radiographically if required. A colonic diameter greater than 10–12 cm increases the risk of colonic perforation. Neostigmine or colonic decompression can be performed for pseudo-obstruction if required to avoid surgery.

In the absence of peritonitis or bowel perforation, endoscopic decompression is safe for mother and fetus even in the third trimester. Volvulus during pregnancy may be treated by decompression with colonoscopy, flexible sigmoidoscopy, or rectal tube; however, surgery may be required if the condition is recurrent or persistent. Hernias frequently require surgical repair, and an incidental incarcerated diaphragmatic hernia should be repaired during surgery due to risk of strangulation. Mortality can be high for volvulus or intestinal ischemia, and preterm delivery is common in patients who require surgery.

CRC during pregnancy is rare, with an incidence ranging from 0.0008% to 0.008%. With the rising age of child-bearing age, it is likely that there will be a corresponding rise in incidence of cancer diagnosis. Diagnosis can be extremely challenging as symptoms can often mimic pregnancy symptoms leading to diagnostic delays. Patients with gastrointestinal cancer diagnosed during pregnancy should undergo colonoscopy for biopsy and for evaluation of synchronous lesions. Carcinoembryonic antigen (CEA) during pregnancy may be elevated in the presence of a CRC, but usually is within the normal range, and thus is not a good screening tool for CRC in pregnancy.

Resections can be performed during the first half of pregnancy but are often deferred until after delivery. There is no contraindication to vaginal delivery as long as the birth canal is not obstructed. All options should be discussed with the patient. A multi-disciplinary approach is essential. Chemotherapy is typically delayed until the second trimester, and pelvic radiation is often delayed until after delivery to protect the fetus. Maternal outcome in CRC diagnosed during pregnancy is similar to that of the general population; however, pregnant women with gastric cancer often present with advanced disease and have a worse survival rate than non-pregnant women.

Cao S, Okekpe CC, Dombrovsky I, Valenzuela GJ, Roloff K. Colorectal cancer diagnosed during pregnancy with delayed treatment. *Cureus*. 2020;12(5):e8261. [PMID: 32596079]

Rottenstreich M, Mosmar K, Ehrlich Z, Kitroser E, Grisaru-Granovsky S. Flexible endoscopic decompression for treatment of sigmoid volvulus in pregnancy. *Eur J Obstet Gynecol Reprod Biol*. 2019;242:184–185. [PMID: 31570177]

Zhao XY, Wang X, Li CQ, Zhang Q, He AQ, Liu G. Intestinal obstruction in pregnancy with reverse rotation of the midgut: a case report. *World J Clin Cases*. 2020;8(16):3553–3559. [PMID: 32913863]

ENDOSCOPY IN PREGNANCY

Although endoscopy is routine in the evaluation of many gastrointestinal disorders, it is typically only performed when absolutely needed in pregnancy due to the risk to the fetus of sedative medications, particularly in the first trimester, and technical complexity during the third trimester leading to

Table 7–8. Indications for endoscopy in pregnancy.

Severe or refractory nausea and vomiting or abdominal pain
Dysphagia or odynophagia
Strong suspicion of colon mass
Severe diarrhea with negative evaluation
Biliary pancreatitis, symptomatic choledocholithiasis, or cholangitis
Biliary or pancreatic ductal injury

premature labor. All gastrointestinal endoscopic procedures in pregnant patients should be performed in hospitals by expert endoscopists and an obstetrician should be informed (Table 7–8). EGD and flexible sigmoidoscopy may be safe for the fetus and pregnant patient in any trimester, however colonoscopy should be limited to the second trimester.

Procedural sedative and analgesic medications can cause overdosage, allergic reaction, teratogenesis, and hemodynamic instability of the mother leading to hypoxia and hypotension of the fetus.

To prevent hypotension and subsequent maternal hypoxia, patients should be positioned in the left lateral position and given intravenous hydration with normal saline or high osmolar solutions. Patients with gastrointestinal bleeding should be resuscitated with packed erythrocytes and fluid as needed before the procedure. Antihypertensives prior to the procedure and colonic overdistention during the procedure should be avoided, and minimal sedation and analgesia should be used. Patients should not be placed or moved to the supine position (because the gravid uterus compresses the vena cava and can lead to hypotension). If procedural hypotension occurs intravenous fluids should be given and the patient's position changed to drain blood from the lower extremities to the vital organs. Consideration should be given to terminating the procedure. Premature uterine contractions during endoscopy may require tocolytics such as magnesium sulfate or terbutaline. Consultation with an obstetrician is important, and anesthesiologic assistance with the procedure should always be considered. The risks of medications used during endoscopy and considerations relating to specific procedures are outlined below.

1. Medications Used During Endoscopy

A. Meperidine

Meperidine is an opiate analgesic and a category B drug in pregnancy; it has a rating of D when used in high doses and for a prolonged period of time at term. Although it is rapidly transferred across the placenta, it has been used extensively in pregnancy and, with the exception of one study that noted a higher rate of congenital inguinal hernias, teratogenicity has not been observed even with exposure during the first trimester. Repeated administration of meperidine at high doses may cause progressive accumulation of normeperidine, maternal respiratory depression, and maternal seizures.

The drug can cause diminished fetal beat-to-beat cardiac variability that can last 1 hour after administration; however, this is generally transient and not considered a poor prognostic sign. Dose should be restricted to 50 or 75 mg intravenously during routine endoscopy. It used to be preferred over benzodiazepines for endoscopic procedures. But now has been overtaken by short-acting analgesics. It is approved by the American Academy of Pediatrics in single dose administration for breast-feeding women. Dosage should be restricted to 50 or 75 mg intravenously during routine endoscopy (Table 7–9).

Table 7–9. Medications used for endoscopy.

Drug	FDA Pregnancy Category	Recommendations for Pregnancy	Recommendations for Breast-Feeding
Ampicillin	B	Low risk to use when prophylaxis required	Compatible
Diatrizoate	D	Minimal use for therapeutic ERCP	Limited human data: probably compatible
Diazepam	D	Avoid if possible. Some congenital malformations and mental retardation may be associated	Limited human data: potential toxicity
Electricity	—	Use for therapeutic ERCP	No human data
Epinephrine	C	Avoid unless for hemostasis	No human data: potential toxicity
Fentanyl	C	Safe in low doses	Compatible
Flumazenil	C	Fetal risks are unknown, but it should be given carefully in small dose. Only for significant benzodiazepine overdose	No human data: probably compatible
Gentamicin	C	Short courses low risk, check serum levels if used for >48 hours	Compatible
Glucagon	B	Avoid except for ERCP	No human data
Ketamine	B	Low doses throughout pregnancy	No human data
Lidocaine	B	Gargle and spit	Limited human data: probably compatible
Meperidine	B but D at term	Use in low doses. Repeated high and prolonged doses can cause respiratory depression	Compatible
Midazolam	D	Use in low doses. Limit especially in first trimester	Limited human data: potential toxicity
Nitrous oxide	C	Short duration exposure poses no significant risk but do not use as first line agent	No human data: probably compatible
Naloxone	B	Only for severe narcotic overdoses. It is probably safe but should be used only in respiratory depression, systemic hypotension, or unresponsiveness in a closely monitored pregnant woman after endoscopy	No human data: probably compatible
PEG electrolyte	C	No human studies available	Probably low risk
Propofol	B	Can be used in any trimester but avoid higher doses closer to term	Limited human data: probably compatible
Simethicone	C	Can be avoided, but low risk	No human data: probably compatible
Sodium glycol electrolyte	C	Low risk one-time use	No human data

ERCP, endoscopic retrograde cholangiopancreatography; PEG, polyethylene glycol. Reproduced with permission from Mahadevan U, Kane S. American gastroenterological association institute technical review on the use of gastrointestinal medications in pregnancy. *Gastroenterology.* 2006;131(1):283–311.

B. Diazepam and Midazolam

Benzodiazepines are commonly used before gastrointestinal endoscopy to reduce anxiety, induce brief amnesia, and produce muscle relaxation.

Diazepam is categorized as a class D drug during pregnancy due to earlier studies suggesting an association between use during early pregnancy and cleft palates in animals and humans, as well as other congenital malformations and neonatal neurobehavioral abnormalities, cardiac defects and Mobius syndrome.

There is limited information about the effects of midazolam exposure in utero. Exposure during parturition suggests transient respiratory depression and abnormal neurobehavioral responsiveness, but little is known about the effects of fetal exposure during the first or second trimester. Because of its similarity to diazepam, midazolam is classified as category D during pregnancy; in general, however, it is preferable to diazepam if one of these agents is required during endoscopy and meperidine cannot be used.

C. Propofol

Propofol is a category B drug used by anesthesiologists for sedation during endoscopy. It is a short acting anesthetic agent with a quick recovery period. Nowadays, it is the sedation of choice among anesthesiologists during pregnancy. The advantages include a greater depth of sedation, quicker onset, and shorter duration of action than the benzodiazepines. It is considered safe for use during parturition, but at this time, there is inadequate experience to recommend its use during the first trimester.

D. Fentanyl

Fentanyl is a pregnancy category C drug. Studies in rats showed injury to embryos, but some human studies of use during labor found no evidence of neonatal toxicity. It is used in low doses for endoscopy during pregnancy despite some case reports describing respiratory depression and muscle rigidity in neonates. Frequent use has been associated with neonatal withdrawal in a mother with opiate addiction.

E. Ketamine

Ketamine is used by anesthesiologists during endoscopy because of its rapid action of onset, short duration of effects, and ability to sedate people who experience insufficient sedation from propofol. Ketamine has been used during labor and delivery, and although some neonatal respiratory depression may occur, it is often less than that of other sedatives. It has not been associated with teratogenicity and is classified as pregnancy category B; however, it is relatively unstudied during the first trimester.

F. Reversal Agents

Naloxone (pregnancy category B) is an opioid reversal agent. It is appropriate for administration in pregnant patients with signs of narcotic toxicity from sedation, such as respiratory depression, hypotension, or unresponsiveness. It should not be used in patients who are opiate dependent, however, due to the risk of maternal and fetal withdrawal. Naloxone should be used only when necessary and carefully administered in small, titrated doses. Overdose can cause maternal myocardial infarction, pulmonary edema, or severe hypertension.

Flumazenil (Category C) is a benzodiazepine reversal agent used during or following endoscopy procedures. Little is known about fetal risk. Overdose can cause maternal seizures and maternal and neonatal withdrawal, especially in patients who chronically use benzodiazepines. It should be used only if absolutely needed for benzodiazepine toxicity. There are no data regarding either reversal agent during breast-feeding. The risk of benzodiazepine overdose may be minimized by careful and slow titration of minimal doses of benzodiazepines required for endoscopy.

G. Lidocaine

Lidocaine is classed as a pregnancy category B drug based on studies showing no harm in rats and safety during parturition and appears safe for use as a numbing agent for the oropharynx during upper endoscopy. It is recommended that the patient gargle and spit it out rather than swallow it to minimize systemic absorption.

H. Simethicone

Simethicone is used to coalesce gastric bubbles during endoscopy and is a pregnancy category C drug. When used during endoscopy, however, it is unlikely to be absorbed and therefore unlikely to be a risk during either pregnancy or breast-feeding.

I. Glucagon

Glucagon is a pregnancy category B drug. Although there is no evidence of harm in rats, it is uncharacterized in pregnant humans. The AGA supports its use in decreasing motility in endoscopy with the goal of decreasing procedure time, particularly during therapeutic ERCP.

J. Contrast Agents

Diatrizoate contrast is used during ERCP and is classified as pregnancy category D because of the risk to fetal thyroid function during amniography. However, it has been used in diagnostic and therapeutic endoscopy without fetal harm and in the setting of maternal cholangitis, the benefits likely outweigh the risks.

Mahadevan U, Kane S. American Gastroenterological Association Institute position statement on the use of gastrointestinal medications in pregnancy. *Gastroenterology*. 2006;131:278–282. [PMID: 17261292]

Mahadevan U, Kane S. American Gastroenterological Association Institute technical review on the use of gastrointestinal medications in pregnancy. *Gastroenterology*. 2006;131:283–311. [PMID: 16831610]

ASGE Standard of Practice Committee, Shergill AK, Ben-Menachem T, et al. Guidelines for endoscopy in pregnant and lactating women [published correction appears in Gastrointest Endosc. 2013 May;77(5):833]. *Gastrointest Endosc*. 2012;76(1):18–24. [PMID: 22579258]

2. Endoscopic Retrograde Cholangiopancreatography

Pregnancy is associated with an increased risk of gallstone formation. The incidence of cholelithiasis has been reported to be 10% in the general population, whereas the incidence of cholelithiasis and biliary sludge in pregnancy has been reported to be up to 12% and 30%, respectively

Choledocholithiasis occurs in one out of every 1200 deliveries and is the most common indication for ERCP during pregnancy. Other indications for ERCP include severe acute gallstone pancreatitis, cholangitis, bile duct injury, and pancreatic duct disruption. Untreated gall stone pancreatitis during pregnancy has a high fetal and maternal mortality rate between 30% and 40%. The major concerns regarding ERCP in pregnancy is due to radiation exposure to the fetus and the risk of the procedure on the outcome of pregnancy. To minimize risk in pregnancy, less-invasive testing should be considered to confirm the presence of gallstones in the bile duct in the setting of choledocholithiasis, cholangitis, and gallstone pancreatitis. Endoscopic ultrasound has been used with high diagnostic accuracy to confirm or exclude choledocholithiasis. However, this technique has some negative aspects such as a long procedure time, increased costs, and expertise requirements.

There are a few reports of the use of ultrasound-guided or endoscopic needle-knife papillotomy for choledocholithiasis without exposure to fluoroscopy. Magnetic resonance cholangiopancreatography (MRCP) has been reported in numerous case studies without any significant reported side effects, however, the safety of MRI, especially in the first trimester, has not been rigorously tested.

A recent study of 7787 hospitalizations for acute biliary pancreatitis in pregnant women revealed that they were less likely to undergo timely endoscopic biliary decompression and cholecystectomy leading to more frequent readmission.

In the literature after ERCP, preterm birth has been reported in 4.6% of patients, and the other procedure-related complications included post-ERCP pancreatitis (4.6%), spontaneous abortion (0.9%), and fetal distress (0.6%). The risk of post- ERCP pancreatitis appears to be higher with repeated papillary cannulation and thermal injury of electrocautery during sphincterotomy.

Postsphincterotomy bleeding or stent placement, or both, is usually necessary to prevent future recurrence.

If possible ERCP should be avoided in the first trimester. The second trimester is felt to be the safest time to perform ERCP but it can be performed throughout gestation if there is an emergency indication. Although a growing body of data supports the safety of ERCP during pregnancy, precautions to minimize radiation risk to the fetus should be taken, particularly during the first trimester. By taking appropriate precautions, fetal radiation exposure can be well below the 50–100 mSv level that is associated with teratogenicity. ERCP in pregnant patients should be carried out in a safe, quick, and effective manner, and the complication rate must be low. Although nonradiation ERCP with the bile aspiration technique appears to be a favorable method in this group of patients, sufficient definition of the biliary system cannot be obtained with this technique, and residual stones may be left in the common bile duct that may lead to recurrent pancreatitis or cholangitis.

Limiting fluoroscopy time, using the anterior–posterior beam projection, lead apron shielding of patient, increased experience of endoscopist and avoiding hard copy radiographs can reduce radiation exposure. ERCP can also be performed without fluoroscopy by using a wire-guided cannulation technique. Bile duct cannulation can be confirmed by bile aspiration or visualization of bile around the guidewire. After biliary sphincterotomy and balloon sweeping, stone extraction can be confirmed by normalization of laboratory indices44 or by inspection of the bile duct with choledochoscopy or endoscopic ultrasound.

The patient should be in the left lateral recumbent position, facilitating both the procedure and blood flow to the fetus. The grounding pad should be placed so that the uterus is not between the pad and the sphincterotome.

If antibiotics are required, penicillins or cephalosporins are preferred. Clindamycin is generally safe in patients with allergies to penicillin. Tetracycline, quinolones, and streptomycin should be avoided. Metronidazole should be avoided during the first trimester, and sulfonamides and nitrofurantoin should be avoided in the third trimester.

De Lima A, Galjart B, Wisse PH, Bramer WM, van der Woude CJ. Does lower gastrointestinal endoscopy during pregnancy pose a risk for mother and child? – a systematic review. *BMC Gastroenterol*. 2015;15:15. [PMID: 25849032]

Konduk BT, Bayraktar O. Efficacy and safety of endoscopic retrograde cholangiopancreatography in pregnancy: a high-volume study with long-term follow-up. *Turk J Gastroenterol*. 2019;30(9):811–816. [PMID: 31258133]

Luthra AK, Patel KP, Li F, et al. Endoscopic intervention and cholecystectomy in pregnant women with acute biliary pancreatitis decrease early readmissions [published correction appears in Gastrointest Endosc. 2019 Aug;90(2):323]. *Gastrointest Endosc*. 2019;89(6):1169–1177. [PMID: 30503844]

Savas N. Gastrointestinal endoscopy in pregnancy. *World J Gastroenterol*. 2014;20(41):15241–15252. [PMID: 25386072]

Schwarzman P, Baumfeld Y, Bar-Niv Z, et al. The effect of non-obstetric invasive procedures during pregnancy on perinatal outcomes. *Arch Gynecol Obstet*. 2015;292(3):603–608. [PMID: 25804519]

3. Esophagogastroduodenoscopy

The most common indications for EGD in pregnant patients include major or continued GI hemorrhage, dysphagia, and refractory nausea and vomiting (see Table 7–8). The EGD procedure is reasonably safe for the fetus and may be performed when strongly indicated during pregnancy.

Informed consent should still involve a discussion of possible fetal risks related to sedation and the procedure. An obstetrician should be involved to determine if fetal monitoring is needed. The American Society for Gastrointestinal Endoscopy (ASGE) also recommends that patients not lie in the supine position during recovery due to the risk of inferior vena cava compression. During the procedure the patient should be placed in the left lateral position with the head elevated due to an increased risk of regurgitation of gastric contents in pregnant patients. Aspiration should be avoided by aggressive perioral suctioning, elevation of the head of the patient, nasogastric aspiration in patients with upper gastrointestinal bleeding before EGD, and aspiration of the gastric lake during the procedure. For patients with gastrointestinal bleeding, resuscitation should be performed before the procedure to the extent possible.

Cappell MS. Risks versus benefits of gastrointestinal endoscopy during pregnancy. *Nat Rev Gastroenterol Hepatol.* 2011;8(11):610–634. [PMID: 21970872]

ASGE Standard of Practice Committee, Shergill AK, Ben-Menachem T, et al. Guidelines for endoscopy in pregnant and lactating women. *Gastrointest Endosc.* 2012;76(1):18–24. [PMID: 22579258]

4. Flexible Sigmoidoscopy & Colonoscopy

The most common symptom leading to the use of lower endoscopy during pregnancy is hematochezia. Severe diarrhea, abdominal pain, colonoscopic decompression of volvulus, and evaluation of a mass lesion are other possible indications. Another indication for lower endoscopy during pregnancy is incarceration of the gravid uterus; in this condition, the uterus becomes lodged beneath the inferior margin of the sacral promontory. One report has described five patients who underwent successful colonoscopic release by intubating the sigmoid colon to apply pressure to the anterior wall of the rectum after manual reduction had failed. No adverse fetal outcomes were observed, and the alternative would have been surgery, which carries a much higher risk.

A recent systematic review of three retrospective cohort studies of the safety of lower gastrointestinal endoscopy during pregnancy found that there was no difference in birth outcomes and adverse events between the study and the control group. However it was not clear in which trimester the procedures were undertaken. In contrast a 2017 Swedish study using registry data from 100 Swedish hospitals combined 1109 sigmoidoscopies and colonoscopies. In this study the authors concluded that endoscopy during pregnancy is associated with increased risk of preterm birth or small for gestational age, but not of congenital malformation or stillbirth. However, these risks are small and likely due to intrafamilial factors or disease activity. In a more recent study of sigmoidoscopy in pregnant women with IBD it was concluded that sigmoidoscopy may be safer than colonoscopy during pregnancy due to its lesser invasiveness, reduced need for anesthesia or sedation, and simpler endoscopic technique.

Flexible sigmoidoscopy has been performed without adverse outcome in all three trimesters of pregnancy. Most procedures are done with minimal bowel preparation (tap-water enemas) and without sedation to minimize adverse effects. Although hemodynamic monitoring of the mother should always be a part of the procedure, most reported cases did not involve any fetal monitoring, though this may be considered, especially in cases of maternal hemodynamic instability.

Colonoscopy is rarely indicated during pregnancy. The second trimester is generally considered the safest time to perform colonoscopy during pregnancy. The theoretical risks of colonoscopy include premature labor, uterine rupture, placental abruption, and fetal compression.

Patients should be placed in the left or right lateral decubitus position, minimal external compression away from the uterus should be used, and maternal and fetal monitoring should be utilized. Trauma to the uterus from compression or colonoscope looping should be avoided.

The safety of polyethylene glycol electrolyte isotonic cathartic solutions has not been studied in pregnancy. Polyethylene glycol solutions are classified as pregnancy category C. Sodium phosphate preparations (category C) may cause fluid and electrolyte abnormalities and should be used with caution.

Cappell MS. Improving the safety of endoscopy in pregnancy: approaching gravidity with gravitas. *Dig Dis Sci.* 2020;65(10):2745–2748. [PMID: 32840706]

De Lima A, Galjart B, Wisse PH, Bramer WM, van der Woude CJ. Does lower gastrointestinal endoscopy during pregnancy pose a risk for mother and child? – a systematic review. *BMC Gastroenterol.* 2015;15:15. [PMID: 25849032]

Ko MS, Rudrapatna VA, Avila P, Mahadevan U. Safety of flexible sigmoidoscopy in pregnant patients with known or suspected inflammatory bowel disease. *Dig Dis Sci.* 2020;65(10):2979–2985. [PMID: 32034603]

Ludvigsson JF, Lebwohl B, Ekbom A, et al. Outcomes of pregnancies for women undergoing endoscopy while they were pregnant: n Nationwide cohort study. *Gastroenterology.* 2017;152(3):554–563. [PMID: 27773807]

5. Gastrointestinal Bleeding & Endoscopic Therapy

There are very few data on the risks related to endoscopic therapy in pregnancy. Because endoscopy is often performed for the indication of gastrointestinal bleeding, endoscopic hemostasis may be required to maintain hemodynamic stability of the mother and fetus and to avoid the greater risks of persistent bleeding or surgery. No adverse events related to the use of thermocoagulation in pregnancy have been reported in case reports and small studies; however, electric current can cross the amniotic fluid, and the risk of fetal exposure remains. The ASGE recommends that bipolar cautery should be used rather than monopolar to reduce the risk of fetal exposure to stray current. The patient should be positioned so that the uterus is not between the electrical catheter and the grounding pad.

Epinephrine is a category C drug during pregnancy because of the theoretical risk of decreasing placental perfusion. Although no adverse outcomes have been reported in pregnancy when used during endoscopy, the drug should be used sparingly, to avoid systemic effects on both the mother and the fetus. Hemoclips have not been studied but may be safer than methods that involve injection of substances or electric current.

In the case of lower endoscopy, lesions such as polyps may be identified. If there is no urgent need to remove or biopsy the lesion, many endoscopists will defer intervention until after delivery to avoid exposure to bleeding risks or risks of electrocautery. In these situations, tattooing the lesion can be considered; India ink is generally felt to be safe in nonpregnant patients, although there are no existing studies examining its use in pregnant patients. Methylene blue is labeled as a teratogen and should be avoided during pregnancy.

Patients with cirrhosis and portal hypertension are at increased risk for variceal bleeding during pregnancy due to physiologic rises in portal pressure and increased volume in the splanchnic vessels during pregnancy. Variceal bleeding is associated with poor fetal outcomes, and effective hemostasis is critical. Case reports of esophageal banding and sclerotherapy have shown effectiveness in controlling variceal hemorrhage without any reports of fetal harm. Because there is a theoretical risk of the sclerosant entering the fetal circulation, many authors recommend banding as the preferred method, and some suggest that it may be more effective. Somatostatin and octreotide have not been studied in pregnancy but are thought to be relatively safe. Vasopressin is not recommended due to the risk of placental ischemia. Additionally, a reported series of cases has described the control of gastric varices with cyanoacrylate glue during pregnancy. Recent case reports suggest transjugular intrahepatic portosystemic shunt (TIPS) creation to be a safe procedure during pregnancy in preventing variceal bleeding complications; however, it is not typically employed in severely decompensated cirrhosis.

Keepanasseril A, Gupta A, Ramesh D, Kothandaraman K, Jeganathan YS, Maurya DK. Maternal-fetal outcome in pregnancies complicated with non-cirrhotic portal hypertension: experience from a Tertiary Centre in South India. *Hepatol Int.* 2020;14(5):842–849. [PMID: 32588317]

Park C, Patel YA, Suhocki P, et al. High-risk third trimester pregnancy with decompensated cirrhosis safely delivered following emergent preoperative interventional radiology for mitigation of variceal bleeding. *Clin Imaging.* 2020;68:143–147. [PMID: 32615516]

6. Video Capsule Endoscopy

Video capsule endoscopy (VCE) is relatively contraindicated in pregnancy. It may be a useful alternative or adjunct to endoscopy during pregnancy as it does not require sedation and does not exert mechanical pressure on the uterus. Theoretically the gravid uterus and effect of pregnancy on motility may retard the passage of the capsule, but these factors should not predispose to retention in the absence of strictures or bowel obstruction. On the other hand, radiographs to confirm passage, and surgery in the event of retention, would involve risks to the mother and the fetus. The safety of this method has not been evaluated in pregnancy, but it is theoretically promising as a less-invasive diagnostic approach to luminal disease.

Bandorski D, Kurniawan N, Baltes P, et al. Contraindications for video capsule endoscopy. *World J Gastroenterol.* 2016;22(45):9898–9908. [PMID: 28018097]

Mustafa BF, Samaan M, Langmead L, Khasraw M. Small bowel video capsule endoscopy: an overview. *Expert Rev Gastroenterol Hepatol.* 2013;7(4):323–329. [PMID: 23639090]

A summary of approach to endoscopy in pregnancy is detailed in Table 7–10.

7. Alternatives to Diagnostic Endoscopic Procedures

Upper gastrointestinal series, barium enemas, abdominal radiographs, angiography, and CT are generally avoided in pregnancy due to radiation teratogenicity. Fetal malformations, growth restriction, or abortion have not been reported with radiation exposure of less than 50 mGy.

Bleeding scans are also contraindicated due to ionizing radiation. MRI, on the other hand, is believed to be safer in pregnancy than CT scans; short-term exposure to electromagnetic radiation from MRI does not appear to produce harmful fetal effects. Noncontrast MRI is considered safe by the American College of Radiology and the American College of Obstetricians and Gynaecologists. MRCP may be an alternative to diagnostic ERCP during pregnancy. The contrast used for MRI scans—gadolinium—is water-soluble and can cross the placenta into the fetal circulation and amniotic fluid. Free gadolinium is toxic and is therefore given in a chelated (bound) form. Gadolinium has been found to be teratogenic in animal studies in high and repeated doses.

Table 7–10. Summary of approach to endoscopy in pregnancy.

Pre – procedural considerations:
Preoperative consultation with an obstetrician, regardless of fetal gestational age.
Strong indication for endoscopic procedure should always be present, particularly in high-risk pregnancies.
Whenever possible defer procedures to second trimester.

Intra-procedural considerations:
Minimize procedure time.
Position patient in left pelvic tilt or left lateral position to avoid vena cava or aortic compression.

Medication considerations:
Use lowest effective dose of sedative medications.
Use category B drugs whenever possible.

Fetal safety and monitoring during procedures:
Whenever possible monitor fetal heart rate.
Procedures should always be performed in a hospital, ideally in an institution with obstetric, neonatal and pediatric services.
Ideally procedures should be performed.
Prior to 24 weeks of fetal gestation: confirm the presence of the fetal heart rate by Doppler before sedation is administered and on completion of the endoscopic procedure.
After 24 weeks of fetal gestation: simultaneous electronic fetal heart and uterine contraction monitoring should be performed before and after the procedure.

In IBD patients' intestinal ultrasonography can provide a useful adjunctive, noninvasive assessment to evaluate disease activity and complications and have been shown to have similar diagnostic accuracy when compared to CT and MRI.

Committee on Obstetric Practice. Committee Opinion No. 723: Guidelines for Diagnostic Imaging During Pregnancy and Lactation [published correction appears in Obstet Gynecol. 2018;132(3):786]. *Obstet Gynecol.* 2017;130(4):e210–e216. [PMID: 28937575]

Flanagan E, Bell S. Abdominal Imaging in pregnancy (maternal and foetal risks). *Best Pract Res Clin Gastroenterol.* 2020;44–45:101664. [PMID: 32359678]

Liver Disease in Pregnancy

Rachel Placzek, PA-C

Anna Rutherford, MD, MPH

ESSENTIAL CONCEPTS

▶ Most liver biochemical tests are unchanged during pregnancy.

▶ Exceptions are serum albumin, total protein, bilirubin (decreased), alkaline phosphatase and cholesterol (increased).

▶ Several conditions unique to pregnancy may lead to liver test abnormalities or hepatic impairment:

  ▶ Hyperemesis gravidarum (HG), often in the first trimester, invariably before the 20th week of pregnancy.

  ▶ Intrahepatic cholestasis of pregnancy (ICP), often in the second or third trimester (pruritus and mild liver test abnormalities).

  ▶ Acute fatty liver disease of pregnancy (AFLP) in the third trimester (nausea and vomiting, abdominal pain, jaundice, oliguria, hypertransaminasemia, hyperbilirubinemia, coagulopathy, thrombocytopenia, renal failure, and hypoglycemia).

  ▶ Preeclampsia (classic triad of hypertension, proteinuria, and edema) and eclampsia (preeclamptic triad plus seizures and coma) in the second or third trimester.

  ▶ HELLP syndrome (hemolysis, elevated liver enzymes, and low platelets), between the start of the third trimester and the immediate postpartum period, often manifesting as weight gain, right upper quadrant pain, edema, and hypertension.

▶ Initial assessment of liver enzyme abnormalities in pregnancy should begin with noninvasive testing, including laboratory and radiographic studies. Ultrasound is the preferred initial imaging modality in pregnancy.

▶ General Considerations

Various hepatic conditions may occur in pregnancy, and the interpretation of common liver biochemical tests in women who are pregnant can sometimes be challenging. Among the specific conditions unique to pregnancy that may manifest with altered liver tests are HG, ICP, AFLP, preeclampsia/eclampsia, and HELLP syndrome. Other common hepatic conditions, such as viral hepatitis and cirrhosis, are not unique to but can manifest during pregnancy.

Brady CW. Liver disease in pregnancy: what's new. *Hepatol Commun.* 2020;4:145–156. [PMID: 32035601]

Sarkar M, Brady CW, Fleckenstein J, et al. Reproductive health & liver disease: practice guidance by the American Association for the Study of Liver Disease. *Hepatology.* 2021;73(1):318–365. [PMID: 32946672]

INTERPRETATION OF LIVER BIOCHEMICAL TESTS DURING PREGNANCY

The pregnant state is accompanied by a 30–50% increase in blood volume. As a result, several biochemical values are reduced during pregnancy. These include serum albumin, total protein, and bilirubin (Table 8–1).

The most significant change is noted during the second trimester. The serum alkaline phosphatase level is elevated because of the presence of placental-derived alkaline phosphatase. The biliary-derived alkaline phosphatase remains within the normal range as illustrated by normal levels of γ-glutamyl transpeptidase (GGT) and 5'-nucleotidase (5' NT). Serum cholesterol also increases to approximately twice its prepregnancy level. Lastly, the hepatic markers of inflammation, alanine aminotransferase (ALT), and aspartate aminotransferase (AST), are typically unchanged or slightly decreased.

Pathologic conditions that result in abnormal biochemical tests during pregnancy tend to be divided into three broad categories: (1) those that lead to a mild increase in transaminases, (2) those that lead to marked increase in transaminases,

Table 8–1. Liver biochemical test findings in pregnancy.

Biochemical Test	Value During Pregnancy
Albumin	Decreased
Total protein	Decreased
Bilirubin	Normal/Decreased
Alkaline phosphatase	Increased
ALT	Normal/Decreased
AST	Normal/Decreased
GGT	Normal/Decreased
5′ NT	Normal
Cholesterol	Increased
Platelets	Normal
Prothrombin time	Normal
AFP	Increased

AFP, alpha-fetoprotein; ALT, alanine aminotransferase; AST, aspartate aminotransferase; GGT, γ-glutamyl transpeptidase; 5′ NT, 5′-nucleotidase;.

and (3) those that result in predominantly cholestatic biochemical abnormalities. Conditions that lead to mild increase in transaminases include preeclampsia, eclampsia, HELLP syndrome, Budd-Chiari syndrome, ICP, drug-induced hepatitis, and chronic liver diseases. Those that result in marked increase in ALT and AST also include preeclampsia and eclampsia, especially in the setting of hepatic infarct, AFLP, Budd-Chiari syndrome with portal vein thrombosis, hepatic rupture, acute viral or autoimmune hepatitis (AIH), drug-induced hepatitis, and ischemic hepatopathy ("shock liver"). Lastly, conditions that result predominantly in cholestasis include ICP, choledocholithiasis, or drug-induced cholestasis.

Evaluation of abnormal biochemical tests during pregnancy should begin with noninvasive testing, which may include laboratory or radiographic studies. Ultrasound is the preferred initial imaging modality in pregnancy. Magnetic resonance imaging (MRI) without contrast is also considered safe in the setting of pregnancy. However, gadolinium should be avoided given associated teratogenicity and transplacental transfer. Invasive testing, such as liver biopsy and endoscopy can be performed in pregnancy when needed. When able, endoscopy should be delayed until the second trimester.

HEPATIC CONDITIONS UNIQUE TO PREGNANCY

Hyperemesis Gravidarum

HG occurs in 0.3–2% of pregnancies, usually within the first trimester, and is defined as excessive and intractable nausea and vomiting. Severe forms are associated with metabolic derangements such as carbohydrate depletion, dehydration, electrolyte disturbance, and weight loss greater than or equal to 5% of prepregnancy body weight. Risk factors for HG include multiple gestations, molar pregnancies, and fetal anomalies such as hydrops fetalis and trisomy 21. Liver biochemical abnormalities, specifically elevations in aminotransferases, are seen in more than 50% of patients hospitalized for HG. The level of aminotransferase elevation is typically two to three times the upper limit of normal, but can be elevated up to 20 times the upper limit of normal. It appears that the severity of nausea and vomiting correlates well with the degree of liver enzyme elevations. Fulminant liver failure has not been reported. Jaundice is rare (Table 8–2).

The cause of hepatic dysfunction in HG is unclear. Current investigations underscore the potential roles of starvation injury, release of inflammatory cytokines by the placenta, and impairment of fatty acid oxidation in the pathogenesis of the liver disease in HG.

Treatment is symptom management-based with intravenous hydration, correction of electrolyte abnormalities, nutrition and antiemetics. In the most severe cases, parenteral feeding may be necessary. Liver function abnormalities usually return to normal levels within a few days of volume expansion and the cessation of vomiting and no long-term sequelae of liver dysfunction have been described.

Ahmed KT, Almashhrawi AA, Rahman RN, et al. Liver diseases in pregnancy: diseases unique to pregnancy. *World J Gastroenterol.* 2013;19:7639-7646. [PMID: 25288051]

Ryan JM, Heneghan MA. Pregnancy and the liver. *Clin Liver Dis.* 2014;4:51–54.

Intrahepatic Cholestasis of Pregnancy

ICP is characterized by pruritus and increased serum bile acids and/or transaminases and usually occurs in the second and third trimester of pregnancy and resolves with delivery. Incidence varies considerably with country and ethnicity, the highest rates reported in Chile and Bolivia in the 1970s. The incidence ranges from 0.3% to 5.6% (in a predominantly Latina population in Los Angeles) in the United States and 0.5–1.5% in Europe. Risk factors for ICP include multiparity, advanced maternal age, metabolic syndrome, chronic hepatitis C infection, personal or family history of ICP, and previous cholestasis while on oral contraceptives.

Mutations of genes encoding several proteins involved in hepatobiliary transport have been associated with ICP. Mutations in the *ABCB4* (adenosine triphosphate–binding cassette, subfamily B, member 4) gene which encodes the hepatic phospholipid transporter *MDR3* (multidrug resistance 3), the bile salt export pump (ABCB11) and ATP8B1, have been found in patients with ICP.

Pruritus is the most common symptom, occurring in 80% of patients, is most severe at night and occurs most reliably in the palms and soles without a rash. In fewer than 10% of

CHAPTER 8

Table 8–2. Clinical features of liver disorders unique to pregnancy.

Disorder	Onset	Symptoms and Signs	Laboratory and Imaging Findings
Hyperemesis gravidarum	Mostly first trimester (unusual after 20 weeks)	Nausea and vomiting	ALT/AST 1–2× Bilirubin <5 mg/dL Positive urinary ketone
ICP	Second and third trimester	Pruritus and jaundice	ALT/AST 1–4× Bilirubin < 5mg/dL Bile acids 30–100x
AFLP	Third trimester	RUQ pain, jaundice, nonspecific symptoms	ALT/AST 1–10× Bilirubin >10× Hypoglycemia PT/PTT increased Platelets decreased CT/US—fatty infiltration Liver biopsy—microvesicular steatosis
Preeclampsia/eclampsia	Second and third trimesters (20 weeks prior to delivery)	Hypertension, edema	ALT/AST 1–10× Bilirubin <5 PT/PTT increased Proteinuria Platelets decreased
HELLP syndrome	Third trimester	Nonspecific RUQ pain ± hypertension	ALT/AST 1–10×
			Bilirubin <5 mg/dL
			PT/PTT increased
			Platelets decreased
			Hemolysis
Hepatic rupture	Late second to third trimester	Acute abdominal pain	ALT/AST 2–100×
		Hypotension	PT/PTT increased
		Nausea	Platelets decreased
		Vomiting	CT/US—hematoma, hemoperitoneum

AFLP, acute fatty liver disease of pregnancy; ALT, alanine aminotransferase; AST, aspartate aminotransferase; CT, computed tomography; HELLP, hemolysis, elevated liver enzymes, and low platelets; ICP, intrahepatic cholestasis of pregnancy; PT, prothrombin time; PTT, partial thromboplastin time; RUQ, right upper quadrant; US, ultrasound.
Adapted with permission from Wolf JL. Liver disease in pregnancy. *Med Clin North Am*. 1996;80(5):1167–1187.

patients with pruritus, jaundice may occur. Jaundice without pruritus is very rare in ICP. The diagnosis is often made by clinical history, although liver enzymes may be elevated. ALT is especially a very sensitive test for the diagnosis of ICP and may be significantly elevated, mimicking acute viral hepatitis. Serum levels of bile acids are usually elevated and a cutoff value of 10 μmol/L is usually used to diagnose ICP. Bile acid elevations may precede liver test abnormalities, and the levels correlate with fetal distress in severe ICP, defined as bile acid concentration above 40 μmol/L. Serum bile acid and ALT decrease rapidly after delivery and normalize within a few weeks. Alkaline phosphatase is not a useful test to diagnose cholestasis in pregnancy, as it is increased during the second and third trimester in normal pregnancy as a result of production by the placenta. Importantly, serum GGT is normal or only slightly increased in ICP. Ultrasound may show gallstones, but there should be no evidence of biliary obstruction.

The recommended treatment for ICP is ursodeoxycholic acid (UDCA), a hydrophilic bile acid which improves the hepatobiliary bile acid transport. UDCA is typically prescribed at a dose of 10–15 mg/kg/day, and has been shown to reduce pruritus as well as ALT and both maternal and fetal bile acid levels. There are no adverse effects for the mother or the fetus. Although meta-analyses suggest that UDCA may reduce risk of fetal complications, a more recent randomized, placebo controlled study has shown no improvement in fetal outcomes, including perinatal death, preterm delivery, or admission to neonatal unit, with UDCA versus placebo.

Sudden intrauterine fetal death (IUFD) is a rare event (1–2%) but is unpredictable and remains the most feared complication of ICP. Routine deliveries at 36–37 weeks of gestation is recommended to prevent IUFD. The timing of delivery should be discussed on an individual basis, balancing the risk of sudden IUFD against prematurity. From week 37 of gestation, serum bile acid above 40 µmol/L should lead to prompt delivery. Maternal prognosis is usually good. Cholestasis frequently recurs in subsequent pregnancies (60–70%). ICP is not a contraindication for oral contraceptives and may be started once the liver tests have normalized after delivery.

Arrese M, Macias RI, Briz O, Perez MJ, Marin JJ. Molecular pathogenesis of intrahepatic cholestasis of pregnancy. Expert Rev Mol Med. 2008;10:e9. [PMID: 18371245]

Bacq Y, Sentilhes L. Intrahepatic cholestasis of pregnancy: diagnosis and management. Clin Liver Dis. 2014;14:58–60. [PMID: 30992922]

Bacq Y, Sentilhes L, Glantz A, et al. Efficacy of ursodeoxycholic acid in treating intrahepatic cholestasis of pregnancy: a meta-analysis. Gastroenterology. 2012;143:1492–1501. [PMID: 22892336]

Chappell LC, Bell JL, Smith A, et al. PITCHES Study Group. Ursodeoxycholic acid versus placebo in women with intrahepatic cholestasis of pregnancy (PITCHES): a randomized controlled trial. Lancet 2019;394:849–860. [PMID: 31378395]

Marschall HU, Wilkstrom Shemer E, Ludvigsson JF, Stephansson O. Intrahepatic cholestasis of pregnancy and associated hepatobiliary disease: a population-based cohort study. Hepatology. 2013;58:1385–1391. [PMID: 23564560]

Acute Fatty Liver of Pregnancy

AFLP is a rare obstetric emergency that occurs most often in the third trimester with an incidence of 1 in 7000-15,000 deliveries. Maternal mortality is estimated at around 10–15%. The pathogenesis of AFLP is related to a defect in β-oxidation of long chain fatty acids in the fetus. The most commonly invoked molecular defect is a mutation in the long chain-3 hydroxyacyl CoA dehydrogenase (LCHAD). Mothers who are heterozygotes for LCHAD are at risk. This deficiency is related to a common G1528C mutation. The disorder arises from excess unmetabolized long chain fatty acids, generated by a fetus homozygous for an LCHAD mutation, which passes to the mother who is an LCHAD mutation heterozygote, leading to subsequent hepatotoxicity. Although LCHAD is implicated in the disease, other disorders of β-oxidation of long chain fatty acid have been associated with AFLP. There is at least one case report of a deficiency in palmitoyl transferase leading to AFLP. About 20% of women who develop AFLP carry LCHAD-deficient fetuses. Therefore, screening the newborn of AFLP mothers for this mutation can be lifesaving. Newborns with LCHAD deficiency present with a

metabolic crisis in the first year of life and can experience sudden death at a few months of age. LCHAD-deficient newborns can be treated with dietary modifications, with dramatic reduction in morbidity and mortality.

The clinical presentation may be nonspecific and include fatigue, nausea and vomiting, abdominal pain, and jaundice. Laboratory evaluation may show elevated transaminases (typically 300–500 units/L but could be >1000 units/L), hyperbilirubinemia, coagulopathy, elevated blood urea nitrogen (BUN) and creatinine, hyperuricemia, thrombocytopenia, and hypoglycemia. About 10% of patients will have DIC. Hypertension, ascites, and edema may be present. Half of the patients may have associated preeclampsia. Hepatic encephalopathy occurs later and should immediately alert the physician to the possibility of AFLP. In severe untreated cases, rapid progression over a few hours to days to acute liver failure with coma, hypoglycemia, renal failure, and coagulopathy ensue, with a high risk of maternal and fetal death. Ultrasound and computed tomography (CT) scans often show fatty infiltration of the liver. Liver biopsy examination shows microvesicular steatosis, although widespread inflammation or necrosis is not typically seen.

Management includes prompt delivery. Laboratory and clinical abnormalities may persist for up to a week postpartum. Liver transplantation is an option if liver failure does not improve after delivery. Fetal mortality is estimated at 20%; developmental delay, hypoglycemia, and striated muscle dysfunction are all potential complications. Therapy with medium chain fatty acids is often necessary for infants with homozygous LCHAD deficiency.

Liu J, Ghaziani T, Wolf J. Acute fatty liver of pregnancy: an update on pathogenesis, diagnosis, and management. Am J Gastroenterol. 2017;112(6):838–846 [PMID: 28291236]

Newson DB, Byrne JJ, Cunningham FG. Acute fatty liver of pregnancy. Clin Obstet Gynecol. 2019;63:152–164.

Hypertensive Disorders of Pregnancy

Hypertensive disorders of pregnancy which affect the liver include preeclampsia, eclampsia, and HELLP syndrome. Preeclampsia occurs in 2–8% of pregnancies globally. It is characterized by new onset or worsening hypertension, frequently with proteinuria >300 mg/day, or end organ involvement after 20 weeks gestation. Hypertension is defined in pregnancy as a blood pressure >140/90 in a previously normotensive woman. Pregnant women with systolic blood pressure of >160 mmHg or diastolic blood pressure >110 mmHg and/or evidence of organ involvement are considered to have preeclampsia with severe features. Preeclampsia with severe features is associated with an increased risk of morbidity and mortality. Eclampsia is characterized by the development of generalized seizures in the setting of preeclampsia, occurring in 1.9% of women with preeclampsia and 3.2% of women with severe preeclampsia.

HELLP syndrome is considered a variant of severe preeclampsia, and is characterized by hemolysis, elevated liver enzymes, and low platelet count. It occurs in 0.2–0.6% of all pregnancies and in 10–20% of patients with severe preeclampsia. While HELLP syndrome most commonly presents in the third trimester, 20-30% of cases arise in the early postpartum period. Although HELLP syndrome shows symptoms similar to preeclampsia and is one of the criteria that can define severe disease, it can develop in women without any signs or symptoms of preeclampsia.

Inadequate vascular placental perfusion is the leading hypothesis in the etiology of preeclampsia, eclampsia, and HELLP syndrome. Uteroplacental ischemia leads to oxidative stress and release of antiangiogenic factors leading to generalized endothelial dysfunction and thrombotic microangiopathy with subsequent microangiopathic hemolytic anemia and liver damage in patients with HELLP.

Presenting symptoms are nonspecific and may include weight gain, right upper quadrant pain (90%), nausea or vomiting (50%), jaundice (40%), and nonspecific viral-like illness. Signs and symptoms of preeclampsia may or may not be present. Signs of other organ involvement including pulmonary edema, renal insufficiency, and cerebral or visual symptoms may be present. Elevation of transaminases (two- to threefold) is seen in up to 10% of patients with severe preeclampsia. The frequency and degree of elevated transaminases are much higher in HELLP syndrome than in severe preeclampsia. Transaminases are typically >500 IU/L. Hemolysis is the hallmark of the HELLP syndrome triad. The trends in platelet count and serum lactate dehydrogenase (LDH) levels predict the speed of recovery. The diagnosis is often made on clinical grounds and exclusion of other conditions with similar symptoms including acute viral hepatitis, hemolytic uremic syndrome (HUS), thrombotic thrombocytopenic purpura (TTP), and AFLP. The classic hepatic lesion associated with HELLP syndrome is periportal or focal parenchymal necrosis.

Administration of low dose aspirin has shown a reduction in the development of preeclampsia and fetal growth restriction. This should be initiated between 12 and 28 weeks gestation in women with any high-risk factor for preeclampsia or more than one moderate-risk factor. High-risk factors include previous pregnancy with preeclampsia, multiple gestations, renal disease, autoimmune disease, diabetes, and chronic hypertension. Moderate-risk factors include nulliparity, advanced maternal age, obesity, and family history of preeclampsia.

For women with preeclampsia without severe features, delivery is recommended for those presenting at or beyond 37 weeks gestation. For those who present earlier in pregnancy, expectant management with close monitoring is appropriate. However, prompt delivery is warranted at any gestational age for those with severe hypertension, end-organ dysfunction, or concerns about fetal status. Antenatal corticosteroids should be considered in women who are <34 weeks gestation to promote fetal lung maturity. All women with HELLP syndrome should be managed by bed rest and control of hypertension. All women with preeclampsia and HELLP syndrome should receive intravenous magnesium sulfate to prevent seizures and cerebral changes during the intrapartum and postpartum period.

Hepatic rupture is a rare but catastrophic complication of HELLP syndrome and management with hepatic artery ligation, hepatic packing or lobectomy, arterial embolization, and liver transplantation have been described.

HELLP syndrome can recur in subsequent pregnancies and is associated with high risk of complications including fetal prematurity and intrauterine growth retardation.

ACOG Committee on Practice Bulletins. Gestational hypertension and preeclampsia: ACOG Practice Bulletin, Number 222. *Obstet Gynecol.* 2020;135(6):237–260. [PMID: 32443079]

Hammoud GM, Ibdah JA. Preeclampsia-induced liver dysfunction, HELLP syndrome, and acute fatty liver of pregnancy. *Clin Liver Dis.* 2014;4:69–73. [PMID: 30992924]

Kia L, Rinella ME. Interpretation and management of hepatic abnormalities in pregnancy. *Clin Gastroenterol Hepatol.* 2013;11:1392–1398. [PMID: 23707777]

▶ Liver Hematoma & Rupture

Hepatic rupture most often occurs in the setting of HELLP syndrome. Other causes are preeclampsia, AFLP, cocaine abuse, neoplasms, sickle cell disease, polyarteritis nodosa, and rupture of hepatic adenoma during pregnancy. Intraparenchymal hemorrhage typically precedes the rupture. Imaging is required for the diagnosis, which should be suspected in any pregnant woman with right upper quadrant pain, preeclampsia, and shock. Intact hematomas are managed conservatively. Cases of rupture should be managed by a team skilled in liver trauma. After relative stability is achieved, angiography may be attempted. Surgical options include hepatic artery ligation, packing, or resection of the affected part of the liver. Hepatic hemorrhage or rupture carries a high risk of mortality for mother and fetus.

CONDITIONS NOT UNIQUE TO PREGNANCY

1. Viral Hepatitis

Acute viral hepatitis from hepatitis A, B, C, D, and E can occur in pregnant women as in nonpregnant patients. Nonhepatotropic viruses such as cytomegalovirus, Epstein-Barr virus, and herpes simplex virus (HSV) can also cause hepatic injury in pregnant women. The risk of vertical transmission of hepatitis viruses is higher in pregnant women with acute versus chronic infection. In general, the risk is not increased with vaginal delivery and cesarean section should not be recommended to prevent transmission of hepatitis viruses.

Considerations in managing pregnant patients with some of these hepatitides are presented here. For additional information about acute and chronic hepatitis, see Chapters 41 and 42.

A. Hepatitis A

The incidence and management of hepatitis A are the same in pregnant as in nonpregnant individuals (see Chapter 41). The management of hepatitis A is conservative. Perinatal transmission is rare, but there may be horizontal transmission at the time of delivery. Hepatitis A vaccine and immunoglobulin are safe during pregnancy.

B. Hepatitis B

Flares of chronic hepatitis B virus (HBV) have been reported during pregnancy and the postpartum period. These are usually mild and may sometimes lead to spontaneous loss of hepatitis e antigen (HBeAg). In the absence of prophylaxis, the risk of vertical transmission to the fetus is as high as 90% and is higher in the mothers who are HBeAg-positive or who have high serum HBV DNA levels. Screening of all pregnant women for hepatitis B surface antigen (HBsAg) at the first antenatal visit is critical, because perinatal transmission of HBV leads to chronic infection in 90% of infants. All children born to hepatitis B surface antigen-positive mothers should receive hepatitis B immunoglobulin (HBIG) at the time of birth and the first dose of their hepatitis B vaccination within 12 hours of birth. Subsequent doses of hepatitis B vaccination should be administered at 1–2 months of age and again at 6 months of age.

Prophylaxis with the combination of HBIG and hepatitis B vaccination decreases the vertical transmission rate to 5–10%. The residual failure rate appears to occur in newborns of mothers with very high viral loads often greater than 200,000 IU/mL. Oral antiviral therapy in mothers with high HBV DNA during the third trimester of pregnancy has been shown to reduce the rate of prophylaxis failure. Tenofovir disoproxil fumarate (TDF) is the preferred choice for antiviral treatment in pregnancy. Treatment should be considered when maternal HBV DNA is greater than 200,000 IU/mL and started at week 28–32 of pregnancy to allow adequate time for viral suppression. Treatment can be stopped after delivery if the goal is only to reduce the risk of perinatal transmission. Mothers should be closely monitored for 6 months after treatment is stopped, as HBV flares may occur after treatment discontinuation. Breast-feeding is safe for women with chronic HBV, including women on antiviral therapy.

C. Hepatitis C

Hepatitis C virus (HCV) infection is not a contraindication to pregnancy, but vertical transmission is around 5% in mothers who are positive for HCV RNA. The risk is higher if the mother is coinfected with HIV (10%) or high level of HCV viremia. Breast-feeding is safe. Currently, there is no means to prevent maternal-infant transmission of HCV. Treatment during pregnancy is not recommended as there is limited data on safety of direct acting antivirals (DAAs) in pregnant women. Children born to HCV infected mothers should be screened for HCV with HCV antibody at age 18 months. If negative, the child is not infected. If positive, a HCV RNA should be obtained to confirm infection.

D. Hepatitis E

Acute hepatitis E during pregnancy can cause severe hepatitis and acute liver failure, especially in the third trimester, with a maternal mortality rate of 16–20%.

E. Herpes Simplex

HSV infection during pregnancy is rare, but can cause hepatitis and acute liver failure, especially in the third trimester. Both primary and latent infection with HSV-1 or HSV-2 can cause hepatitis. Presentation is usually with fever and significantly elevated transaminases. Oropharyngeal or genital lesions, or both, are seen in roughly 50% of infected persons; thus, their absence does not eliminate this as a possible etiology.

Factors associated with possible diagnosis include low bilirubin in the presence of elevated transaminases (anicteric hepatitis), AST greater than ALT, third trimester of pregnancy, and immunocompromised state. Diagnosis can be made through polymerase chain reaction (PCR) testing for HSV DNA or liver biopsy, which is the gold standard. The biopsy sample often shows minimal inflammatory infiltrate and is characterized by zonal necrosis of hepatocytes.

Untreated patients have a higher rate of death or liver transplantation compared to treated patients (88% vs 55%). Because the results of PCR testing and biopsy examination are often not available for several days, clinical decision making in the absence of these findings is important. If suspicion is high, therapy with acyclovir or valacyclovir (pregnancy class B drugs) should be started immediately while awaiting diagnostic results.

Brown RS, McMahon BR, Lok ASF, et al. Antiviral therapy in chronic hepatitis B viral infection during pregnancy: a systematic review and meta-analysis. *Hepatology*, 2016:63:319–333. [PMID 26565396]

Chappell C, Hillier S, Crowe D, et al. Hepatitis C virus screening among children exposed during pregnancy. *Pediatrics*. 2018:141(6):e20173273. [PMID 29720535]

Kwon H, Lok AS. Viral hepatitis and pregnancy. *Clin Liver Dis*. 2014;4:55–57.

Ly KN, Jiles RB, Teshale EH, et al. Hepatitis C virus infection among reproductive-aged women and children in the United States 2006 to 2014. *Ann Intern Med* 2017;166:775–782. [PMID: 28492929]

McCormack Al, Rabie N, Whittemore B, et al. HSV hepatitis in pregnancy: a review of the literature. *Obstet Gynecol Surv* 2019;74:93–98. [PMID: 30756123]

Pan CQ, Duan Z, Dai E, et al. Tenofovir to prevent hepatitis B transmission in mothers with high viral load. *N Engl J Med* 2016;374:2324–2334. [PMID: 27305192]

2. Budd-Chiari Syndrome

This syndrome results from an obstruction of the hepatic vein or the supra-hepatic portion of the vena cava. The most common reason is thrombosis. Because of increased risk of thrombotic events in pregnancy, this disorder should be considered in any pregnant woman with right upper quadrant pain, rapid weight gain, and ascites.

Diagnosis is made with Doppler imaging.

Treatment is anticoagulation with heparin and transjugular intrahepatic portosystemic shunting, or liver transplantation in severe cases. Warfarin cannot be used during pregnancy.

Horton JD, San Miguel FL, Ortiz JA. Budd-Chiari syndrome: illustrated review of current management. *Liver Int.* 2008;28:455–466. [PMID: 18339072]

3. Wilson Disease

Wilson disease is a disorder of copper metabolism that results in systemic manifestations, with hepatic and neurologic symptoms as the most prominent components (see Chapter 42). The disease is often diagnosed in the first four decades of life; thus issues related to disease management become a concern during their childbearing years.

In general, patients whose disease is well controlled during pregnancy do well. Therapy should continue throughout pregnancy as fulminant liver failure has been reported in patients who discontinue therapy. Limited data exist regarding the safety of chelators (penicillamine, trientine) in pregnancy. Reduction of the dose in the third trimester is required to maintain adequate copper supply to the fetus. Zinc is considered the first-line treatment in pregnancy and for women wishing to conceive.

Malik A, Khawaja A, Sheik L. Wilson's disease in pregnancy: case series and review of the literature. *BMC Res Notes.* 2013;6:421. [PMID: 24139602]

Pfeiffenberger J. Pregnancy in Wilson's disease: management and outcome. *Hepatology.* 2018;67:1261–1269. [PMID: 28859232]

4. Autoimmune Hepatitis

AIH is a chronic heterogeneous hepatic disorder characterized by the presence of autoantibodies and elevated γ-globulins (see Chapter 42). It is more common in women than in men and often presents in women of childbearing age. Therefore, AIH in pregnancy is a common condition.

There have been reports of cases of spontaneous remission during pregnancy, as well as liver decompensation. Poor outcome has been associated with poor disease control prior to conception. Patients should be closely monitored for disease flare throughout pregnancy and postpartum. The mainstay of treatment is immunosuppression, usually with prednisone and/or azathioprine. Mycophenolic acid products are contraindicated in pregnancy and lactation. Therapy should be continued during pregnancy because relapse is associated with disease progression. Although azathioprine is a pregnancy class D agent based on congenital malformation in rodents, there has been no evidence of increased teratogenicity among children born to mothers receiving azathioprine or any adverse effects of breast-feeding in this population. Regardless, counseling is recommended prior to conception in women actively treated with azathioprine. Overall pregnancy is well tolerated, and pregnancy outcomes in patients with AIH, with regard to fetal loss, cesarean sectioning, and stillbirths, are similar to that of the general population.

Czaja AJ. Autoimmune hepatitis in special patient populations. *Best Pract Res Clin Gastroenterol.* 2011;25:689–700. [PMID: 22117635]

Llovet LP, Horta D, Eliz MG, et al. Presentation and outcomes of pregnancy in patients with autoimmune hepatitis. *Clin Gastroenterol Hepatol* 2019;17:2819–2821. [PMID: 30616023]

Westbrook RH, Yeoman AD, Kriese S, Heneghan MA. Outcomes of pregnancy in women with autoimmune hepatitis. *J Autoimmun.* 2012;38:J239–J244. [PMID: 22261501]

5. Cirrhosis

Rates of pregnancy in women with cirrhosis are increasing. The overall fertility rate in this population is unknown, and is affected by the hypothalamic-pituitary dysfunction in cirrhosis which can lead to amenorrhea or anovulation. Fertility may be influenced by the etiology of the underlying liver disease, and is maintained in patients with AIH, primary biliary cirrhosis, and primary sclerosing cholangitis.

Pregnancy in the cirrhotic patient is associated with increased maternal morbidity and mortality. These rates vary widely, reflecting the heterogeneity of subjects in retrospective studies and case series. In a US retrospective study of 339 pregnant cirrhotic patients, maternal mortality rate was 1.8%. However, in another prospective study, maternal mortality was reported as high as 7.8%. The major cause of maternal morbidity and mortality in pregnant cirrhotics is increased portal hypertension and variceal bleeding. This occurs as a result of plasma volume expansion and compression of the inferior vena cava in late pregnancy. Previous studies have estimated the risk of esophageal variceal bleeding as high as 30–50%. However, more recent data from the United States Nationwide Inpatient Sample database have reported a rate of esophageal variceal bleed of 5%. A recent review of the Swedish Medical Birth Register and Swedish National Patient Register looked at 103 pregnancies in women with cirrhosis and identified only one case of variceal bleeding. The efficacy of primary prophylaxis of variceal bleeding is not supported by evidence, but it is recommended given the high maternal mortality associated with acute bleeding. Esophageal variceal screening with endoscopy is recommended in the second trimester for all pregnant women with cirrhosis, unless endoscopy has been performed within one year prior to conception. Management of esophageal varices in pregnancy is similar to that of a nonpregnant patient. High-grade varices should be treated with esophageal variceal ligation, which is preferred over nonselective β-blockers, as they have been reported to cause intrauterine growth retardation, neonatal bradycardia, and hypoglycemia. There are no reliable data to show superiority of cesarean delivery over vaginal delivery; thus, decisions should be made guided by obstetric indications.

Advanced liver disease is also associated with increased risk of obstetrical complications including premature labor, intrauterine growth restriction, placental abruption, and cesarean section. A recent retrospective review of pregnant patients with cirrhosis showed that the live birth rate was 75%.

Multiple recent studies have looked at whether noninvasive markers can predict pregnancy outcomes in women with chronic liver disease. A retrospective study showed a correlation between the model for end-stage liver disease (MELD) score greater than 10 at conception and poor pregnancy outcome. Another study found that albumin-bilirubin score was predictive of live birth while AST to platelet ratio index was predictive of ability to proceed beyond 37 weeks gestation.

6. Liver Transplantation

The American Society of Transplantation suggests liver transplant (LT) recipients wait at least 1 year after LT before conceiving, with careful consideration of history of rejection, infections, stability of graft function, and immunosuppressive regimen. Maternal mortality and fetal survival are similar in LT recipients to that of general U.S. population, however maternal complications including hypertensive diseases of pregnancy, gestational diabetes, cesarean delivery, and preterm delivery occur at a higher rate in LT recipients.

Gonsalkorala E, Cannon MD, Lim TY. Non-invasive markers (ALBI and APRI) predict pregnancy outcomes in women with chronic liver disease. Am J Gastroenterol. 2019;114:267–275. [PMID: 29973705]

Hagstrom H, Hojer J, Hanns-Ulrich M. Outcomes of pregnancy in mothers with cirrhosis: a national population study of 1.3 million pregnancies. Hepatol Commun. 2018;2:1299–1305. [PMID: 30411076]

Palatnik A, Rinella ME. Medical and obstetric complications among pregnant women with liver cirrhosis. Obstet Gynecol 2017;129:1118–1123. [PMID: 28486373]

Rahim MN, Long L, Penna L, et al. Pregnancy in liver transplantation. Liver Transpl. 2020;26:564–581. [PMID: 31950556]

Shaheen AA, Myers RP. The outcomes of pregnancy in patients with cirrhosis: a population-based study. Liver Int. 2010;30:275–283. [PMID: 19874491]

Westbrook RH, Yeoman AD, O'Grady JG, Harrison PM, Devlin J, Heneghan MA. Model for end-stage liver disease predicts outcome in cirrhotic patients during pregnancy. Clin Gastroenterol Hepatol. 2011;9:694–699. [PMID: 21570482]

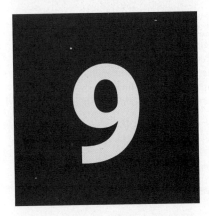

State-of-the-Art Imaging of the Gastrointestinal System

Francesco Alessandrino, MD

Alan J. Cubre, MD

General Considerations

Since the advent of computerized tomography (CT) and magnetic resonance imaging (MRI), many imaging modalities have been integrated into the diagnosis and management of gastrointestinal (GI) disease. Significant developments in CT, magnetic resonance (MR), and positron emission tomography (PET) technology, make radiologists essential consultants in the diagnosis and evaluation of a vast array of diseases involving the GI system.

Multidetector-row CT (MDCT) is readily available and with recent advances in machine components, hardware, and software, the modality has fast image acquisition, short processing times, and excellent spatial resolution. An additional benefit to the advances in hardware and software has also reduced radiation dose with maintenance, if not improvement, in image quality. The uses for CT diagnosis in GI imaging are vast, both as primary means to diagnose disease and to complement or concurrently diagnose complications of GI disease. Some specific accepted indications for CT of the GI system include staging and resectability assessment of pancreatic cancer, diagnosis and treatment monitoring for hepatocellular carcinoma (HCC).

MRI uses radio waves in a large superconducting magnet to create images with superior contrast resolution relative to CT. In recent years, software, hardware, and machine components have also allowed for faster image acquisition, better contrast resolution, and improved spatial and temporal resolution. MRI plays an indispensable role in the diagnosis and evaluation of hepatobiliary and pancreas pathology and has an important role in evaluation of GI tract disease. When imaging modalities are compared, MRI results, in a vast array of abdominal diseases, provide a more accurate delineation of the extent of disease, improved disease characterization, and improved disease detection compared to CT or ultrasound (US). Within the imaging exams created for MRI, there are also more specialized MRI exams that are uniquely tailored to evaluate a specific disease, complications of a disease, or an organ. As an example, MR enterography is tailored to evaluate the lower GI tract in inflammatory bowel disease and secondary complications in additional organs. Often, MRI is a cost-effective imaging technique in the evaluation of a vast array of liver function abnormalities, exocrine pancreatic diseases, and biliary disorders. Currently, some accepted indications for MRI of the GI system include: HCC screening, liver lesion characterization, pancreatic cyst diagnosis and evaluation, inflammatory bowel disease, rectal cancer staging, perianal disease, and abnormal placenta implantation. Coupling MRIs superior contrast resolution, improved spatial resolution, and improved temporal resolution with a lack of ionizing radiation, MRI also is an indispensable tool in the acute pregnant abdomen.

PET is another rapidly evolving technique with increasing applications in GI diseases, mostly for initial staging in GI cancer and restaging after therapy. The majority of PET are performed with the 18F-fluorodeoxyglucose (FDG), a glucose analog which relies on the preferential use of anaerobic glycolysis and increased glucose uptake in neoplastic and inflammatory cells compared to normal glucose uptake and aerobic respiration in healthy normal cells, thereby permitting differentiation between the cell types. New radiotracers have also been approved for use for GI diseases, including gallium 68-DOTATATE for neuroendocrine tumors (NET). PET is conjointly done with CT for anatomical localization while PET in conjunction with MR has been increasingly used in recent years.

Coupled with these recent innovations in cross-sectional imaging and optical endoscopy, there has been a steady decline in the utilization of more traditional diagnostic imaging methods used in the past to evaluate the GI system, particularly fluoroscopy. Upper and lower tract fluoroscopic examinations are now used in very specific indications as CT, CT/MR enterography, and CT colonography have largely replaced common fluoroscopic exams. Despite this, esophagrams and upper GI studies remain cost-effective and minimally invasive exams that can be used to ascertain multiple cause of dysphagia in the evaluation of the upper GI tract.

US, on the other hand, is still used for many indications, including evaluation of right upper quadrant pain, screening of HCC, and evaluation of gallbladder polyps. Furthermore, contrast-enhanced US can aid in the evaluation of focal liver lesions in adults and pediatric patients, given the recent approval of an intravenous US contrast agent.

This chapter details current imaging algorithms and key imaging features of various diseases involving the GI system with a special emphasis on the most commonly used imaging techniques in clinical practice.

GASTROINTESTINAL TRACT IMAGING

1. Esophagus

A. Imaging Algorithm

Fluoroscopic examination of the esophagus after contrast administration has a high yield to detect esophageal pathology, motility, and anatomy. In this regard, a fluoroscopy examination is useful in detecting functional and pathologic disorders. Despite this, optical endoscopy and manometry has largely replaced fluoroscopic examination particularly since endoscopy can provide both a diagnosis and tissue sampling.

The standard fluoroscopic study of the esophagus is a double contrast esophagram involving air contrast images to evaluate the mucosa and contrast only images to provide a functional assessment of motility, reflux, and luminal narrowing or rings. The double contrast esophagram is invaluable in the evaluation of dysphagia, atypical chest pain, gastroesophageal reflux disease (GERD), esophageal foreign bodies, motility disorders, esophagitis; and postoperative assessment of the integrity of the esophagus following local surgery or invasive procedures. Cross sectional imaging such as CT and PET/CT, has little use in the role of diagnosis of primary esophageal disorders, but the imaging modalities are used in esophageal cancer staging for both locoregional disease and distant metastasis. An exception is the CT esophagram which is performed before and after the administration of a specialized oral contrast solution involving contrast, water, and sodium bicarbonate (CO_2 gas). The CT esophagram has become increasingly used for the evaluation of esophageal leak in postsurgical patients with a higher sensitivity (100% vs 67%) compared to a fluoroscopic examination.

American College of Radiology. ACR Appropriateness Criteria Dysphagia. https://acsearch.acr.org/docs/69471/Narrative/ Accessed April 10, 2020.

American College of Radiology. ACR Practice parameter for the performance of esophagrams and upper gastrointestinal examinations in adults. https://www.acr.org/-/media/ACR/Files/Practice-Parameters/UpperGIAdults.pdf Accessed April 10, 2020.

Levine MS, Rubesin SE, Laufer I. Barium esophagography: a study for all seasons. *Clin Gastroenterol Hepatol.* 2008;6:11–25. [PMID: 18083069]

Upponi S, Ganeshan A, D'Costa H, et al. Radiological detection of post-oesophagectomy anastomotic leak – a comparison between multidetector CT and fluoroscopy. *Br J Radiol.* 2008;81(967):545–548. [PMID: 18559902]

B. Inflammation & Infection

Gastroesophageal reflux disease (see Chapter 12). Barium studies have proved invaluable in patients with GERD to document the presence of a hiatal hernia, gastroesophageal reflux, reflux esophagitis, and to detect reflux complications, such as ulcerations, strictures, metaplasia, and neoplasms. Barium studies are also helpful in assessing patients prior to antireflux surgery and in patients after antireflux surgery with new or recurrent symptoms.

When the GERD is untreated and diagnosed fluoroscopically, air contrast images of the mucosa demonstrate a fine nodular or granular appearance with small well-defined radiolucencies caused by mucosal edema. In more advanced disease, contrast-filled ulcers may be present near the gastroesophageal junction on the posterior esophageal wall. An additional manifestation of GERD in the presence of a hiatal hernia often includes a peptic stricture (Figure 9–1). As the inflammation from GERD becomes more chronic

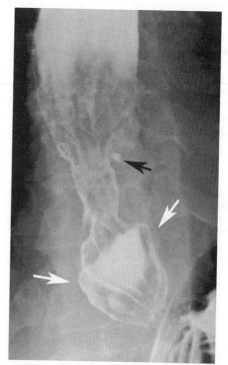

▲ **Figure 9–1.** Peptic stricture and ulceration. Upright double-contrast esophagram shows a smooth, tapered stricture in the distal esophagus above a hiatal hernia (*white arrows*). Also note a small barium-filled ulceration (*black arrow*) on the left lateral wall.

and untreated, Barrett's esophagus may develop. On the air contrast component of an esophagram, the classic imaging manifestations of Barrett's esophagus is a high, midesophageal stricture, peptic stricture, ulcer, or a mucosal reticular pattern (see Chapter 13).

Infectious esophagitis is most frequently encountered in patients who are immunocompromised. *Candida albicans*, herpes simplex virus, cytomegalovirus (CMV), and HIV are often the infectious agents. On a double contrast esophagram, *Candida* esophagitis is typified as discrete, linear, plaque-like lesions separated by normal intervening mucosa, with a predilection for the upper and mid-esophagus. In contradistinction, Herpes esophagitis shows small barium-filled ulcers on a normal background mucosa. CMV and HIV esophagitis, on the other hand present with giant, flat ulcerations that are typically several centimeters in length.

C. Neoplasia

Esophageal carcinoma. The double-contrast esophagram has a reported sensitivity of approximately 95% in the detection of esophageal cancer compared to endoscopy. However, the sensitivity for detection of small and early carcinomas may be significantly lower.

The vast majority of esophageal neoplasms are squamous cell carcinomas, arising from the middle and upper esophagus, and adenocarcinomas, arising in distal third or esophagogastric junction, with the incidence of the two subtypes varying regionally.

The appearance of esophageal cancers on barium studies is variable and has been described as infiltrating, polypoid, ulcerative, or varicoid (Figure 9–2). Once a carcinoma is detected, PET/CT imaging is increasingly used for clinical staging, particularly detecting nonregional lymphadenopathy or distant metastases (Plate 4).

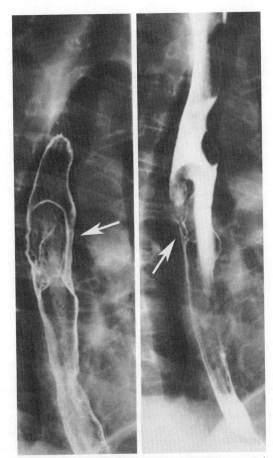

▲ **Figure 9–2.** Polypoid esophageal carcinoma. Upright double-contrast esophagram shows a thick, polypoid, and irregular tumor (*arrows*) in the midesophagus.

Baker ME, Einstein DM. Barium esophagram: does it have a role in gastroesophageal reflux disease? *Gastroenterol Clin North Am.* 2014;43:47–68. [PMID: 24503359]

Foley KG, Fielding P, Lewis WG, et al. Prognostic significance of novel 18F-FDG PET/CT defined tumour variables in patients with oesophageal cancer. *Eur J Radiol.* 2014;83:1069–1073. [PMID: 24794862]

Gage-White L. Incidence of Zenker's diverticulum with hiatus hernia. *Laryngoscope.* 1988;98(5):527–530. [PMID: 3129629]

Levine MS, Chu P, Furth EE, Rubesin SE, Laufer I, Herlinger H. Carcinoma of the esophagus and esophagogastric junction: sensitivity of radiographic diagnosis. *AJR Am J Roentgenol.* 1997;168:1423–1426. [PMID: 9168701]

Schweigert M, Dubecz A, Stein HJ. Oesophageal cancer–an overview. *Nat Rev Gastroenterol Hepatol.* 2013;10(4):230–244. [PMID: 23296250]

D. Functional Disorders (See Chapter 14)

Functional disorders of the esophagus are commonly due to problems with motility such as achalasia and diffuse esophageal spasm (DES) which will be briefly discussed here due to their classic imaging appearance.

Achalasia can be categorized as primary or secondary. Patients with primary, or idiopathic, achalasia are typically young, and lack esophageal peristalsis and have incomplete relaxation of the lower esophageal sphincter. Secondary achalasia, or pseudoachalasia, is most commonly caused by tumors at the gastroesophageal junction or other causes, including Chagas disease.

On barium studies, the esophagus appears patulous, flaccid, and obstructed by a tapered, bird beak-like narrowing at the gastroesophageal junction. Radiographically it can sometimes be difficult to distinguish primary from secondary causes of achalasia. In patients with secondary achalasia, a small retrospective study demonstrated that the length of the narrowed segment is often greater than 3.5 cm and may appear nodular or ulcerated.

A timed barium esophagram can be used to identify achalasia and to assess esophageal emptying before and after minimally invasive therapy for achalasia. With this technique, patients ingest a 250 mL low-density barium sulfate suspension within 30–45 seconds and upright spot images obtained at 1, 2, and 5 minutes after the last swallow of barium. The images obtained are meant to detect a column of barium proximal to the achalasia. In treatment naive patients, a barium column of 2 cm in height at 5 minutes from administration of contrast, identifies achalasia with a sensitivity of 85% and specificity of 86%. After treatment for achalasia such as a myotomy, the timed barium esophagram will show no retention of contrast in the esophagus, or a significant decrease in the height of the barium column at the timed exposures.

DES is characterized by intermittent, abnormal esophageal peristalsis with presence of multiple, simultaneous nonperistaltic contractions. In approximately 15% of patients with DES, lumen-obliterating nonperistaltic contractions can be seen that compartmentalize the esophagus, producing a classic "corkscrew" esophagus on barium studies.

Zenker diverticulum (see Chapter 14) is an acquired mucosal herniation between the horizontal and oblique fibers of the cricopharyngeus muscle. On barium studies, a contrast-filled midline sac is seen posterior to the pharyngoesophageal junction, commonly observed at C5–C6 level (Figure 9–3) proximal to a prominent cricopharyngeal muscle is commonly identified. When a Zenker's diverticulum

is clinically suspected, diagnosing the diverticulum prior to endoscopy may prevent an iatrogenic perforation. A Zenker's diverticulum is also associated with hiatal hernia, and any assessment of the esophagus and stomach should carefully scrutinize the distal esophagus.

Killian-Jamieson diverticulum is an acquired esophageal mucosal diverticulum herniating through a muscular defect of the cervical esophagus located just below the cricopharyngeus muscle. On barium studies, a left-sided, anterior outpouching of the cervical esophagus is observed, although sometimes it can be bilateral.

Blonski W, Kumar A, Feldman J, Richter JE. Timed barium swallow: diagnostic role and predictive value in untreated achalasia, esophagogastric junction outflow obstruction, and non-achalasia dysphagia. *Am J Gastroenterol.* 2018;113(2):196–203. [PMID: 29257145]

Kostic SV, Rice TW, Baker ME et al. Timed barium esophagogram: a simple physiologic assessment for achalasia. *J Thorac Cardiovasc Surg.* 2000;120:935–946 [PMID: 11044320]

Woodfield CA, Levine MS, Rubesin SE, Langlotz CP, Laufer I. Diagnosis of primary versus secondary achalasia: reassessment of clinical and radiographic criteria. *AJR Am J Roentgenol.* 2000;175(3):727–731. [PMID: 10954457]

2. Stomach

A. Imaging Algorithm

Upper endoscopy has essentially replaced fluoroscopic studies as the primary investigation in patients with suspected gastric or duodenal pathology. When endoscopy is contraindicated or unsuccessful, a well-performed upper GI study utilizing an air contrast technique is the next preferred diagnostic test. Upper GI studies can readily detect mucosal and submucosal abnormalities that distort the gastric wall with high sensitivity. Additionally, an upper GI study displays the upper GI tract anatomy prior to bariatric surgery, depicts gastric volvulus, and gastric outlet obstruction. An upper GI study is also indispensable in the immediate postbariatric patient in the evaluation of leaks, or in diagnosing delayed postoperative bariatric surgery complications such as gastrojejunal strictures or marginal ulcers. MDCT with neutral contrast material, such as water, has been proposed as an excellent imaging test to evaluate the gastric wall, especially in the evaluation of gastric neoplasms. Other diagnostic methods utilized to diagnose and stage gastric neoplasms include endoscopic US (EUS), MRI, and PET/CT scan.

Rubesin SE, Levine MS, Laufer I. Double-contrast upper gastrointestinal radiography: a pattern approach for diseases of the stomach. *Radiology.* 2008;246:33–48. [PMID: 18096527]

B. Neoplasms

Adenocarcinoma is the most common gastric malignancy representing approximately 90% of all gastric malignancies.

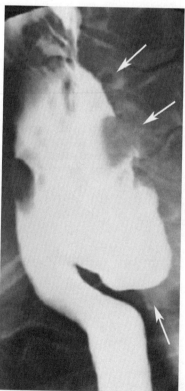

▲ **Figure 9–3.** Zenker diverticulum. Lateral view from a single-contrast esophagram shows a barium-filled diverticulum (*arrows*) posterior to the cervical esophagus.

Other primary gastric malignancies occur much less frequently and include lymphoma (<5%), GI stromal tumors (GISTs) (<2%), and malignant carcinoid (<1%). Gastric malignancy diagnosis is typically made by endoscopy. Gastric cancer staging is based on endoscopy, EUS, CT, and PET/CT. EUS has a role in local staging and should be combined with CT or PET/CT to identify locoregional or distant metastasis as CT and PET/CT detect distant metastasis with a reported sensitivity of 90%.

National Comprehensive Cancer Network Clinical Practice Guidelines in Oncology. Pancreatic adenocarcinoma Version 3.2020. https://www.nccn.org/professionals/physician_gls/PDF/pancreatic.pdf. Published August 14, 2020. Accessed September 8, 2020.

Spolverato G, Ejaz A, Kim Y, et al. Use of endoscopic ultrasound in the preoperative staging of gastric cancer: a multi-institutional study of the US gastric cancer collaborative. *J Am Coll Surg.* 2015;220:48–56. [PMID: 25283742]

In particular, CT, currently the staging modality of choice, can identify the primary tumor, assess for local spread, and detect nodal involvement, peritoneal carcinomatosis, and distant metastases. When identifying the primary gastric tumor, masses larger than 5 mm may present as a focal enhancing soft tissue mass or as diffuse thickening of the gastric wall on CT or MRI (Figure 9–4). Classic imaging features of gastric cancer include the presence of a lobulated or nodular mass with irregular ulceration (Figure 9–5). For a scirrhous adenocarcinomas, the stomach demonstrates long segment circumferential narrowing and focal mucosal nodularity.

The next most common gastric malignancy is gastric lymphoma. Gastric lymphoma typically appears as segmental or diffuse gastric wall thickening. In contrast to gastric adenocarcinoma, lymphoma typically involves more than one anatomic region of the stomach, is unlikely to cause gastric outlet obstruction, and may be associated with lymphadenopathy below the renal hila.

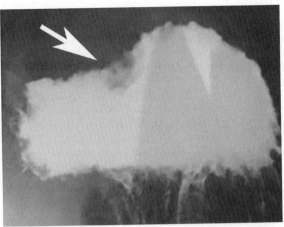

▲ **Figure 9–5.** Gastric adenocarcinoma. Upright double-contrast upper GI image shows a large irregular mass (*arrow*) arising from the fundus.

The third most common gastric malignancy is gastrointestinal stromal tumor (GIST). Gastric GISTs most often originate in the muscularis propria and therefore are extra mucosal in origin and exophytic. The most common location for a gastric GIST is the gastric fundus or body. Often an upper GI examination may be negative. When GISTs are diagnosed with cross sectional imaging, small masses appear as intra-mural hypervascular lesions on CT or MRI. Larger GISTs tend to necrose, hemorrhage, or ulcerate (Figure 9–6).

The genomic expression profile of GISTs plays an important role in metastatic potential and response to treatment. GISTs that metastasize to lymph nodes are often succinate dehydrogenase deficient while GISTs with cKIT mutations, which comprise the majority of GISTs (95%), do not

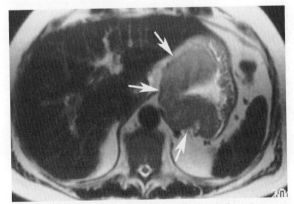

▲ **Figure 9–4.** Gastric adenocarcinoma. Axial T2-weighted MR image shows a thick hyperintense mass (*arrows*) arising from the gastric cardia.

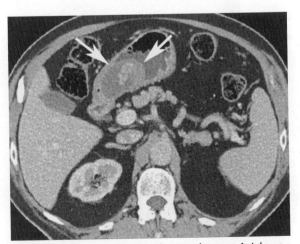

▲ **Figure 9–6.** Gastrointestinal stromal tumor. Axial MDCT image shows a well-defined hypervascular mass (*arrows*) in the gastric body.

metastasize to lymph nodes. The genomic expression profile of GIST's has also been linked to the tumors' morphology with wild-type weak or negative KIT expression GISTs appearing as heterogeneous masses containing cystic regions and soft tissue elements.

Imaging, particularly cross-sectional imaging with contrast enhanced CT, PET/CT, and MRI with diffusion weighted imaging plays an important role in evaluating a GIST's response to therapy. When GISTs are treated with imatinib, a tyrosine kinase inhibitor, a successful treatment response is typically tumor vascularity regression with decreased internal enhancement, but variable tumor size regression.

Alessandrino F, Tirumani SH, Jagannathan JP, Ramaiya NH. Imaging surveillance of gastrointestinal stromal tumour: current recommendation by National Comprehensive Cancer Network and European Society of Medical Oncology-European Reference Network for rare adult solid cancers. *Clin Radiol.* 2019;74(10):746–755. [PMID: 31345555]

Choi H, Charnsangavej C, Faria SC, et al. Correlation of computed tomography and positron emission tomography in patients with metastatic gastrointestinal stromal tumour treated at a single institution with imatinib mesylate: proposal of new computed tomography response criteria. *J Clin Oncol.* 2007;25:1753–1759. [PMID: 17470865]

Oppelt PJ, Hirbe AC, Van Tine BA. Gastrointestinal stromal tumors (GISTs): point mutations matter in management, a review. *J Gastrointest Oncol.* 2017;8(3):466–473. [PMID: 28736634]

Tang L, Zhang XP, Sun YS, et al. Gastrointestinal stromal tumours treated with imatinib mesylate: apparent diffusion coefficient in the evaluation of therapy response in patients. *Radiology.* 2011;258:729–738. [PMID: 21193597]

Tateishi U, Miyake M, Maeda T, Arai Y, Seki K, Hasegawa T. CT and MRI findings in KIT-weak or KIT-negative atypical gastrointestinal stromal tumors. *Eur Radiol.* 2006;16:1537–1543. [PMID: 16397744]

C. Infection & Inflammation

Focal injury. Peptic ulcer disease (see Chapter 16) is most commonly caused by infection by *Helicobacter pylori* or by nonsteroidal anti-inflammatory drugs (NSAIDs). Most duodenal ulcers are caused by *H pylori,* while most gastric ulcers are caused by NSAIDs. A true ulcer extends through the muscularis mucosa into the deeper layers of the gastric wall while an erosion is focal necrosis confined to the epithelium or lamina propria. On upper GI studies, a depressed lesion greater than several millimeters in depth is called an ulcer. Most peptic ulcers appear as round or ovoid collections of barium filling the ulcer crater with smooth, straight folds radiating to the ulcer's edge (Figure 9–7). The presence of a Hampton line (a thin radiolucent line traversing the base of the crater due to undermining of the submucosa) is diagnostic of a benign gastric ulcer. CT does not detect most peptic ulcers because they affect only the superficial layers of the gastric wall. However, deep peptic ulcers manifesting as focal wall thickening or

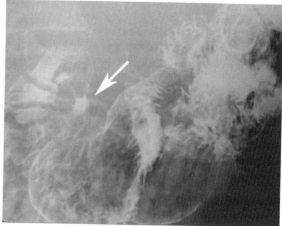

▲ **Figure 9–7.** Gastric benign ulcer. Double-contrast upper GI study shows a small ulcer (*arrow*) with radiating folds surrounding it.

undulation with inflammatory changes in the adjacent soft tissues may be readily detected by CT.

Diffuse Injury. More extensive and diffuse inflammation manifests as gastritis. When gastritis is due to *H pylori,* it typically appears on barium studies as thickened, scalloped folds that have a longitudinal or transverse orientation. On CT, the most common manifestation of gastritis is thickening of the gastric folds (Figure 9–8). In severe gastritis, the gastric wall appears stratified due to extensive submucosal edema and mucosal hyperenhancement. This striated appearance helps to distinguish gastritis from gastric cancers. *H pylori* gastritis is by far the most likely cause of focally or diffusely thickened folds, especially involving the body and antrum. A life-threatening form of gastritis is emphysematous gastritis in which gastric pneumatosis (gas in the stomach wall) is depicted. When the etiology of the emphysematous gastritis is thought to be infectious, *Escherichia coli* may be the cause.

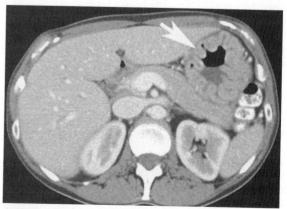

▲ **Figure 9–8.** Gastritis. Axial MDCT image shows severe thickening of the gastric folds (*arrow*).

An additional inflammatory condition with a pathogno-monic imaging appearance is Ménétrier disease. Typically, Ménétrier disease causes massive enlargement of the rugal folds involving the gastric fundus and body with sparing of the antrum. An additional cause of marked gastric wall thickening is Zollinger Ellison syndrome which is discussed later in the chapter.

Rubesin SE, Levine MS, Laufer I. Double-contrast upper gastrointestinal radiography: a pattern approach for diseases of the stomach. *Radiology*. 2008;246(1):33–48. [PMID:18096527]

3. Small Bowel

A. Imaging Algorithm

Prior to CT enterography, MRI enterography, capsule endoscopy, and push enteroscopy, the small bowel was studied with fluoroscopic imaging techniques, such as small bowel follow-through (SBFT) or enteroclysis. The latter technique would use an air contrast technique or contrast and laxative to evaluate for small bowel mucosal pathology. However, the accuracy of SBFT and enteroclysis for detecting and characterizing small bowel pathology depends on operator experience and institutional imaging practice patterns. Moreover, in contrast to additional cross-sectional imaging techniques apart from optical evaluation of the small bowel, a SBFT or enteroclysis only directly evaluates the small bowel mucosa.

Traditionally, a SBFT is performed after an upper GI study. After the completion of the upper GI study, the patient drinks an additional 0.5L of barium contrast, and multiple spot radiographs are performed every 15–45 minutes until the contrast opacifies the proximal right colon or cecum. In enteroclysis, contrast is administered via an enteric tube in the mid duodenum or proximal jejunum. Gas (either air or CO_2) can be insufflated through the enteric tube to produce a double contrast evaluation of the small bowel. In both techniques, paddle compression is performed during fluoroscopic examination of the bowel to evaluate small bowel peristalsis, and isolate loops of bowel with mucosal pathology.

The modalities replacing SBFT and enteroclysis are CT and MRI enterorrhaphy (CTE, MRE); these techniques are accurate for detecting small bowel pathology, particularly active Crohn's disease (CD). CTE and MRE use a neutral oral contrast agent to distend the bowel, while simultaneously evaluating inner wall or mucosal enhancement with the use of an intravenous contrast agent. MRE is performed with increasing frequency due to the lack of ionizing radiation, especially in young patients with CD who need repeat imaging to monitor therapeutic response.

CT has supplanted abdominal radiography in the evaluation of the acute abdomen. Abdominal radiographs are still widely used for specific clinical indications. Those clinical indications include: detection and evaluation of adynamic ileus, small bowel perforation, small bowel obstruction, positioning of nasoenteric tubes, gastric tubes, jejunostomy tubes, and foreign bodies.

B. CT Enterography Technique

CT enterography is preferably performed using an MDCT scanner after the oral administration of barium sulfate 0.1% w/v suspension prior to the exam. In the evaluation of inflammatory bowel disease, specifically Crohn's disease, a single CT acquisition is performed after the administration of intravenous nonionic contrast during enteric to portal venous phase (image acquisition 50–70 seconds after beginning of the injection).

Elsayes KM, Al-Hawary MM, Jagdish J, Ganesh HS, Platt JF. CT enterography: principles, trends, and interpretation of findings. *Radiographics*. 2010;30(7):1955–1970. [PMID: 21057129]

Patak MA, Mortele KJ, Ros PR. Multidetector row CT of the small bowel. *Radiol Clin North Am*. 2005;43:1063–1077. [PMID: 16253662]

C. MR Enterography Technique

MRE should be performed with a 1.5 or 3T scanner 60 minutes after oral administration of an enteric contrast agent. Antiperistalsis medications, such as intravenous glucagon, can be administered before the study. Images are acquired before contrast media injection with a gadolinium chelate contrast media, during enteric phase (between 45 and 70 seconds after contrast media injection), and during two additional postcontrast phases acquired consecutively after the enteric phase sequence. The different sequences in MR enterography allow identification of active inflammation (inner wall enhancement and bowel wall edema).

D. Crohn's Disease

CTE and MRE are invaluable tools to identify the extent of inflammatory bowel disease, active inflammation versus prior inflammation, complications, extraintestinal manifestations of disease, and response to therapy. Studies have shown that MRE and CTE may detect small bowel inflammation not seen at ileocolonoscopy and MRE findings correlate with the severity of endoscopic inflammation.

CTE and MRE findings in Crohn's disease can be divided into: findings related to inflammation, findings related to penetrating disease and findings involving the mesentery. In some patients, there may be overlapping findings.

Mural stratification, inner wall or transmural hyperenhancement along the mesenteric border, wall edema, seen as hyperintense wall on T2-weighted fat-saturated images, engorged vasa recta ("comb sign") (Figure 9–9) and edema of the mesenteric fat all correlate with active inflammation. Hyperenhancing mesenteric adenopathy can also be observed in active inflammation.

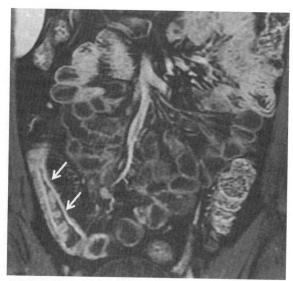

▲ **Figure 9–9.** Crohn's disease. Coronal fat-suppressed postcontrast T1-weighted MR image shows mucosal hyperenhancement of the wall of the terminal ileum (*arrows*) with engorgement of the vasa recta (comb sign).

While MRE and CTE are both highly accurate to assess disease extent in CD, MRE is particularly valuable to assess disease activity, assess response to medical treatment, assess for perianal fistula and abscesses, and assess extra intestinal manifestations such as primary sclerosing cholangitis. Both MRE and CTE techniques are designed to help screen for extraintestinal manifestations of inflammatory bowel disease but cannot fully characterize certain manifestations. In the specific instance of perianal disease or primary sclerosing cholangitis contemporaneous with inflammatory bowel disease, a dedicated pelvic MRI and liver MRI/MRCP should be obtained to fully evaluate the perianal fistula/abscess or the extent of biliary structuring, respectively.

Baker ME, Hara AK, Platt JF, Maglinte DD, Fletcher JG. CT enterography for Crohn's disease: optimal technique and imaging issues. *Abdom Imaging.* 2015;40(5):938–952. [PMID: 25637126]

Bruining DH, Zimmermann EM, Loftus EV Jr, et al. Consensus recommendations for evaluation, interpretation, and utilization of computed tomography and magnetic resonance enterography in patients with small bowel Crohn's disease. *Radiology.* 2018;286(3):776–799. [PMID: 29319414]

Gee MS, Nimkin K, Hsu M, et al. Prospective evaluation of MR enterography as the primary imaging modality for pediatric Crohn's disease assessment. *AJR Am J Roentgenol.* 2011; 197:224–231. [PMID: 21701034]

Grand DJ, Guglielmo FF, Al-Hawary MM. MR enterography in Crohn's disease: current consensus on optimal imaging technique and future advances from the SAR Crohn's disease-focused panel. *Abdom Imaging.* 2015;40(5):953–964. [PMID: 25666967]

Guglielmo FF, Anupindi SA, Fletcher JG, et al. Small bowel Crohn's disease at CT and MR enterography: imaging atlas and glossary of terms. *Radiographics.* 2020;40(2):354–375. [PMID: 31951512]

Nehra AK, Sheedy SP, Wells ML, et al. Imaging findings of ileal inflammation at computed tomography and magnetic resonance enterography: what do they mean when ileoscopy and biopsy are negative? *J Crohns Colitis.* 2020;14(4):455–464.

Samuel S, Bruining DH, Loftus EV Jr, et al. . Endoscopic skipping of the distal terminal ileum in Crohn's disease can lead to negative results from ileocolonoscopy. *Clin Gastroenterol Hepatol* 2012;10:1253–1259.

Tolan DJ, Greenhalgh R, Zealley IA, Halligan S, Taylor SA. MR enterographic manifestations of small bowel Crohn's disease. *Radiographics.* 2010;30(2):367–384. [PMID: 20228323]

E. Small Bowel Obstruction

The early diagnosis of bowel obstruction is critical in preventing complications, particularly ischemia and perforation. The sensitivity and specificity of conventional radiography in diagnosing obstruction ranges from 53% to 90% and from 77% to 89% respectively and are highly dependent on the experience of the radiologist (Figure 9–10). While abdominal radiography may be the initial radiologic examination, MDCT is the single best imaging tool for suspected small bowel obstruction as it can be effectively used to reveal the site and cause of obstruction. Sensitivity and specificity of MDCT for small bowel obstruction exceeds 90% and can

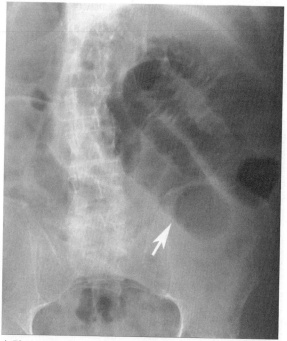

▲ **Figure 9–10.** Small bowel obstruction. Abdominal radiograph image shows severe dilation of jejunal small bowel loops with acute transition (*arrow*).

accurately identify the cause of obstruction in 95%, 70%, and 82%, for adhesions, hernia, and tumor, respectively.

More than 60% of all small bowel obstructions are caused by adhesions followed by hernias and extrinsic compression from neoplasm. MDCT also depicts signs of threatened bowel viability with accuracy greater than 90%. MDCT is also excellent for detecting external hernias and for characterizing the bowel and mesentery in the hernia sac in patients with internal herniation.

Jaffe TA, Martin LC, Thomas J, et al. Small-bowel obstruction: coronal reformations from isotropic voxels at 16-section multidetector row CT. *Radiology*. 2006;238:135–142. [PMID: 16293807]

Li Z, Zhang L, Liu X, Yuan F, Song B. Diagnostic utility of CT for small bowel obstruction: systematic review and meta-analysis. *PLoS One*. 2019;14(12):e0226740. [PMID: 31887146]

Thompson WM, Kilani RK, Smith BB, et al. Accuracy of abdominal radiography in acute small-bowel obstruction: does reviewer experience matter? *AJR Am J Roentgenol*. 2007;188:W233–W238. [PMID: 17312028]

F. Mesenteric Ischemia (See Chapter 6)

MDCT obtained with intravenous contrast during arterial and portal venous phase is the most accurate diagnostic tool for mesenteric ischemia and should be used as the first-line imaging modality. CT is invaluable for accurately identifying ischemic bowel segments and complications, determining the primary causes of ischemia, and excluding other causes of acute abdominal pain. CT findings in acute bowel ischemia consist of various morphologic changes, including wall thickening, dilation, abnormal or absent wall enhancement, mesenteric stranding, vascular engorgement, ascites, pneumatosis, and portal venous gas (Figure 9–11). Maximum intensity projections (MIP) and angiographic 3D reconstructed images are crucial to visualize the distal branches of

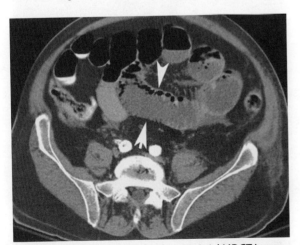

▲ **Figure 9–11.** Mesenteric ischemia. Axial MDCT image shows lack of enhancement of the small bowel wall (*arrow*) and presence of pneumatosis (*arrowhead*).

the mesenteric arteries and veins, which sometimes are not easily visualized on axial images. MDCT imaging also can be used in the follow-up of patients after surgery, particularly in the assessment of bypass graft patency which is well documented by MIP and 3D images.

Kanasaki S, Furukawa A, Fumoto K, et al. Acute mesenteric ischemia: multidetector CT findings and endovascular management. *Radiographics*. 2018;38(3):945–961. [PMID: 29757725]

G. Neoplasms

Diagnosis of small bowel tumors is challenging because they are uncommon, often small and associated with nonspecific clinical prodromes. MDCT plays an important role in ruling out alternative diagnoses. In patients with clinically suspected small bowel tumor with normal findings on abdominopelvic MDCT, MRE should be performed, given the higher sensitivity in detecting intraluminal lesions of the small bowel relative to CTE.

Masselli G, Casciani E, Polettini E, Laghi F, Gualdi G. Magnetic resonance imaging of small bowel neoplasms. *Cancer Imaging*. 2013;13:92–99. [PMID: 23524074]

Masselli G, Gualdi G. MR imaging of the small bowel. *Radiology*. 2012;264:333–348. [PMID: 22821694]

Masselli G, Di Tola M, Casciani E, et al. Diagnosis of small-bowel diseases: prospective comparison of multi-detector row CT enterography with MR enterography. *Radiology*. 2016;279(2):420–431 [PMID: 26599801]

Benign small bowel tumors are uncommon and are typically detected on CT or MR as incidental findings. The most common benign tumors are lipomas and leiomyomas. Lipomas are easily recognized by their internal fat (–90 to –120 Hounsfield units [HU]) while leiomyomas are characterized as a homogenous enhancing submucosal mass with a well-circumscribed border.

Malignant tumors of the small intestine include adenocarcinoma, carcinoid, lymphoma, and GIST. Adenocarcinoma is the most common malignant small bowel tumor accounting for approximately 40% of all primary small bowel neoplasms. Most adenocarcinomas are located in the duodenum (Figure 9–12). Adenocarcinomas are often visualized as a focal area of wall thickening encasing the lumen. The second most common primary small bowel neoplasm is carcinoid, representing approximately 25% of all primary small bowel neoplasms. Carcinoid tumors usually present as small bowel enhancing nodules. Carcinoids may metastasize to the mesentery (Figure 9–13) which on imaging is often seen as a spiculated mesenteric mass containing calcifications in approximately 70% of the cases. Non-Hodgkin lymphoma is the third most common malignant small bowel tumor, accounting for approximately 10–15% of all primary small bowel neoplasms. Primary small bowel lymphomas often appear as a focally thickened, aneurysmally dilated

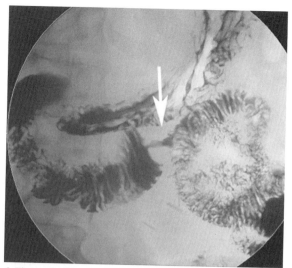

▲ **Figure 9–12.** Duodenal adenocarcinoma. Upright double-contrast upper GI image shows an apple-core lesion (*arrow*) at the level of the third portion of the duodenum.

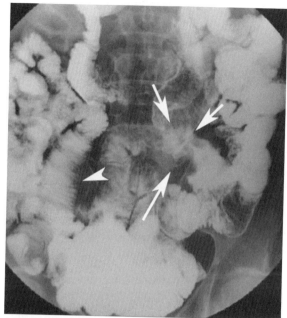

▲ **Figure 9–14.** Small bowel lymphoma in celiac sprue. SBFT image shows an irregular mass in the distal jejunum (*arrows*), mild dilation of small bowel loops, and jejunization of the ileum (*arrowhead*).

loop (Figure 9–14). Primary small bowel lymphoma can be detected with small bowel contrast studies and CT; however, CT offers the advantage of simultaneously detecting adenopathy and the extraluminal extent of disease. GISTs the next most common small bowel neoplasm, and account for approximately 9% of all primary small bowel neoplasms. Like elsewhere in the bowel, GISTs appear as large, bulky masses. Central necrosis and ulceration are common. MDCT and MR imaging are especially helpful in defining the exact site of origin and help for surgical resection.

Sailer J, Zacherl J, Schima W. MDCT of small bowel tumours. *Cancer Imaging.* 2007;17:224–233. [PMID: 18083648]

H. Miscellaneous Conditions

Several additional uncommon small bowel abnormalities can be divided into two broad categories: inflammation, and malpositioning. Uncommon inflammatory small bowel conditions include graft-versus-host disease, diverticulitis, and radiation enteritis while uncommon small bowel malpositions include intussusception, hernias, and volvulus. These conditions typically have a distinct imaging appearance and are often easily diagnosed using multiplanar MDCT.

For the inflammatory group, findings of graft-versus-host-disease are nonspecific and include gastric and bowel wall thickening, bowel dilation, mucosal enhancement, and engorgement of the vasa recta adjacent to the affected vessels

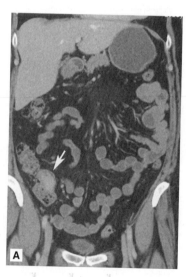

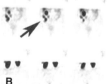

▲ **Figure 9–13.** Ileal carcinoid. **A.** Coronal CT enterography image shows a hypervascular mass (*arrow*) in the wall of the terminal ileum. **B.** Selected images from an octreotide nuclear medicine study show increased uptake of the tracer in the terminal ileum (*arrow*).

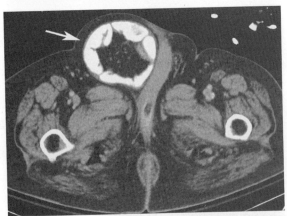

▲ **Figure 9–15.** Inguinal hernia. Axial MDCT image shows the presence of nonobstructed small bowel loops (*arrow*) in a right-sided inguinal hernia.

on MDCT. Diverticulitis appear as focal eccentric bowel wall thickening and/or focal stranding surrounding a diverticulum. On MDCT, the key to the diagnosis of radiation enteritis is the presence of abnormal findings only in the bowel loops in the region of the radiation port.

For the mispositioned category, intussusception on MDCT shows the "bowel-within-bowel configuration" in which the layers of the bowel are duplicated forming concentric rings, when observed perpendicularly to the bowel lumen. Different types of abdominal hernias can be reliably diagnosed with MDCT, including inguinal hernias (Figure 9–15). Inguinal hernias can be either direct or indirect. Indirect hernias are the most common and occur predominantly in males when the peritoneal sac enters the inguinal canal and exits at the external ring. On imaging an indirect inguinal hernia will have fat or peritoneal contents lateral to the inferior epigastric vessels. Due to their long course, indirect hernias can become incarcerated, leading to bowel obstruction and infarction. Direct hernias are less common and occur when the hernia enters the inguinal canal medial to the inferior epigastric vessels.

In cases of volvulus on MDCT, besides signs of small bowel obstruction, the whirlpool sign can also be observed, with rotation of the bowel around its mesentery, leading to twisting of the mesenteric vessels.

4. Appendix

A. Imaging Algorithm

Choosing an imaging modality to evaluate the appendix depends on the patient's age and body habitus. In children and young adults, US has proven to be a reliable technique to diagnose acute appendicitis provided there is an ideal acoustic window and the appendix can be visualized. Graded-compression US, performed with increasing transducer pressure over the site of maximal tenderness to displace

normal overlying bowel gas, has variable accuracy depending on the patient's body habitus and on the experience of the sonographer. In a meta-analysis comparing US with CT for the diagnosis of appendicitis, sensitivity and specificity of graded-compression US were 78% and 83%, respectively. In contrast CT has a sensitivity ranging between 87% and 100%, and a specificity between 89% and 99% in diagnosing appendicitis. Furthermore, CT allows for diagnosis of even early appendicitis and can lead to alternative diagnoses that mimic the clinical presentation of appendicitis. For the aforementioned reasons, CT is often favored as the imaging modality for evaluating the appendix in obese and older patients.

MRI of the appendix is used in specific clinical scenarios, specifically, young patients and pregnant patients with excellent diagnostic accuracy. A recent prospective study on 198 nonpregnant patients older than 12 years of age with suspected appendicitis showed that the diagnostic performance of MRI is exceptionally high and similar to the performance of CT.

Coursey CA, Nelson RC, Patel MB, et al. Making the diagnosis of acute appendicitis: do more preoperative CT scans mean fewer negative appendectomies? A 10-year study. *Radiology.* 2010;254(2):460–468. [PMID: 20093517]

Duke E, Kalb B, Arif-Tiwari H, et al. A systematic review and meta-analysis of diagnostic performance of MRI for evaluation of acute appendicitis. *AJR Am J Roentgenol.* 2016;206(3):508–517. [PMID: 27504714]

Keller C, Wang NE, Imler DL, Vasanawala SS, Bruzoni M, Quinn JV. Predictors of nondiagnostic ultrasound for appendicitis. *J Emerg Med.* 2017;52(3):318–323. [PMID: 27692650]

Leeuwenburgh MM, Wiarda BM, Wiezer MJ, et al. Comparison of imaging strategies with conditional contrast-enhanced CT and unenhanced MR imaging in patients suspected of having appendicitis: a multicenter diagnostic performance study. *Radiology.* 2013;268:135–143. [PMID: 23481162]

Repplinger MD, Pickhardt PJ, Robbins JB, et al. Prospective comparison of the diagnostic accuracy of MR imaging versus CT for acute appendicitis. *Radiology.* 2018;288(2):467–475. [PMID: 29688158]

van Randen A, Bipat S, Zwinderman AH, Ubbink DT, Stoker J, Boermeester MA. Acute appendicitis: meta-analysis of diagnostic performance of CT and graded compression US related to prevalence of disease. *Radiology.* 2008;249(1):97–106. [PMID: 18682583]

B. Appendicitis

On US, an aperistaltic noncompressible thickened (>6 mm) appendix with thickened walls (>3 mm) surrounded by free fluid, with increased echogenicity of the adjacent fat with or without appendicoliths within the lumen is diagnostic of appendicitis. The target sign is also frequently observed, with a hypoechoic lumen of the appendix surrounded by hyperechoic inner layer and hypoechoic muscularis layer when the appendix is imaged transversely (Figure 9–16).

On CT, an appendix with a diameter of more than 6 mm, with an edematous or hyperenhancing wall, stranding of the surrounding mesenteric fat, and, sometimes, inflammatory

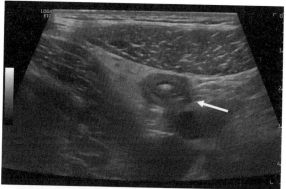

▲ **Figure 9–16.** Appendicitis. Ultrasound image obtained perpendicular to the long axis of the appendix shows the "target sign" with the hypoechoic lumen of the appendix (arrow), containing a phlebolith, surrounded by hyperechoic inner layer and hypoechoic muscularis layer.

changes in the adjacent cecum is diagnostic of appendicitis (Figure 9–17). Given the significant overlap between noninflamed and inflamed appendix using a diameter size threshold of >6 mm, a stricter size threshold of >8 mm has been proposed, yielding a sensitivity and specificity of 90.2% and 91.5% for diagnosis of appendicitis. The presence of inflammation (fat stranding) in the periappendiceal fat is reported to have a sensitivity of 100% and a specificity of 80% for appendicitis. If an appendicolith is present on CT, along with pericecal inflammation, the scan is virtually diagnostic for appendicitis.

Perforation is one of the serious complications that may occur in acute appendicitis, and CT often confirms the diagnosis. Perforated appendix is suspected in the presence of a nonenhancing segment or segmental defect in the appendiceal wall. If signs of a wall defect are not present, secondary signs of perforation include peri-appendiceal fluid

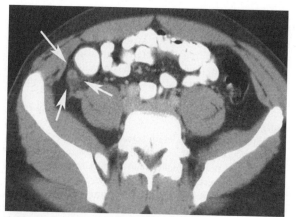

▲ **Figure 9–17.** Appendicitis. Axial MDCT image shows hyperenhancement of the wall of the appendix and peri-appendiceal fat stranding (arrows).

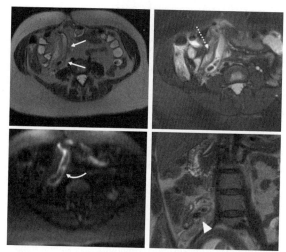

▲ **Figure 9–18.** Appendicitis. MRI images obtained in axial and coronal planes show the fluid-filled appendix (arrow), wall edema (T2 bright signal) (dashed arrow), wall restriction (curved arrow), containing phleboliths (arrowhead).

collections, or extraluminal gas. When the peri-appendiceal fluid collections have thick enhancing walls, the collection is typically an abscess, thereby confirming appendiceal perforation. An advantage of CT relative to US, is that CT can diagnose pylephlebitis (infectious thrombosis of the portal vein or any of its branches) or a pylephlebitic liver abscesses. CT-guided abscess drainage is used in cases in which surgeons elect to operate electively after appendiceal perforation.

On MRI, a dilated (>7 mm), fluid filled appendix with wall thickening, wall edema (T2 bright signal), and wall restriction is diagnostic of appendicitis (Figure 9–18). A halo of T2-hyperintense signal adjacent to the appendix represents inflammation and edema.

Expert Panel on Gastrointestinal Imaging:, Garcia EM, Camacho MA, Karolyi DR, et al. ACR Appropriateness Criteria® right lower quadrant pain-suspected appendicitis. *J Am Coll Radiol.* 2018;15(11S):S373–S387. [PMID: 30392606]

Mervak BM, Wilson SB, Handly BD, Altun E, Burke LM. MRI of acute appendicitis. *J Magn Reson Imaging.* 2019;50(5): 1367–1376. [PMID: 30883988]

Nitta N, Takahashi M, Furukawa A, et al. MR imaging of the normal appendix and acute appendicitis. *J Magn Reson Imaging.* 2005;21:156–165. [PMID: 15666398]

5. Large Bowel

A. Imaging Algorithm

Among the various imaging modalities available, CT is almost universally accepted as the primary modality for the evaluation of patients suspected of having various conditions involving the large bowel. Key advantages of CT over other imaging modalities include the fact that CT not only allows accurate demonstration of the colonic wall but also outlines the pericolonic tissues and adjacent structures. CT can help assess infectious and inflammatory conditions, facilitate diagnosis and staging of colonic neoplasms, and screen for colorectal cancer. The latter is typically performed using a dedicated CT method, known as CT colonography or virtual colonoscopy.

CT colonography has several advantages, similarities, and disadvantages to optical colonoscopy. Advantages for CT colonography relative to optical colonoscopy include: no sedation, a minimally invasive exam, and short image acquisition time relative to procedural time. Similarities to optical colonoscopy include: the patient must undergo a bowel preparation prior to the exam, and the exam requires colonic insufflation with carbon dioxide to distend the colonic lumen. Disadvantages for CT colonography include radiation exposure, and polyp/adenoma/carcinoma diagnosis without tissue sampling. Currently, CT colonography is recommended every 5 years. Often CT colonography is used for a failed optical colonoscopy or a medical contraindication for colonoscopy.

Additional modalities to evaluate the colon lumen and mucosa include MR colonography or a barium enema. MR colonography is performed using contrast within the colonic lumen, resulting in increased and decreased signal intensity accordingly to the contrast used. A double contrast barium enema for colon cancer screening is now rarely performed and has been replaced by CT colonography. A single- contrast barium enema is still performed and reserved for specifical clinical indications such as evaluation of postoperative strictures, anastomotic leaks and colonic fistulae.

Wolf AMD, Fontham ETH, Church TR, et al. Colorectal cancer screening for average-risk adults: 2018 guideline update from the American Cancer Society. *CA Cancer J Clin.* 2018;68(4): 250–281. [PMID: 29846947]

B. CT Colonography Technique

Optimal CT colonography technique requires careful preparation of the colon. Residual colonic stool can simulate polyps or masses; thus any preparation that clears the colon of fecal matter will suffice. Stool markers (mostly barium, eg, Tagitol) or iodine can be administered orally 24–48 hours before CT to improve differentiation between polyps, adenomas, carcinoma, and retained stool. This technique is called fecal tagging. When diagnostic CT colonography is performed as an alternative to failed optical colonoscopy or there is a medical contraindication for colonoscopy, the CT examination is performed with intravenous contrast media.

Once the CT colonography is performed, most radiologists use a primary two-dimensional (2D) interpretation with so-called lumen tracking, starting from the rectum and following the course of the bowel from slice to slice to the cecum

for image analysis. Primary 3D endoluminal assessment of the colon (endoluminal "fly-through") is less often performed as it is more time consuming and more susceptible to pitfalls. However, three-dimensional endoluminal images are useful to confirm the presence of a lesion and to improve diagnostic confidence. It is imperative that the 2D images are reviewed by using colon window settings (approximately W: 1500, L: −150). In addition, soft tissue windows must be used for further characterization of suspected lesions and when searching for extracolonic abnormalities.

C. MR Colonography Technique

As with CT colonography, in MR colonography the patient undergoes a bowel preparation and careful distention of the colon. The colon is instilled with a 1.5–2.5 L of a warm water enema solution. Just before instillation of water, an anti-peristaltic agent (scopolamine, glucagon) is administered. Sequences are obtained with patient in a supine position before and 75 seconds after intravenous gadolinium-based contrast media.

Rimola J, Rodríguez S, García-Bosch O, et al. Role of 3.0-T MR colonography in the evaluation of inflammatory bowel disease. *Radiographics.* 2009;29:701–719. [PMID:19448111]

Santillan CS. MR imaging techniques of the bowel. *Magn Reson Imaging Clin N Am.* 2014;22:1–11. [PMID: 24238128]

Thornton E, Morrin MM, Yee J. Current status of MR colonography. *Radiographics.* 2010;30:201–218. [PMID: 20083594]

D. Polyps & Malignancies

The majority of colorectal cancers arise within benign adenomatous polyps and follow the well-studied adenoma-carcinoma pathway. Colonic carcinoma develops over approximately 10 years.

Colorectal imaging and screening is designed to detect early stage malignancies or premalignant lesions (see Chapter 24). Colorectal polyps appear as round, oval, or lobulated intraluminal lesions and are homogeneous in attenuation (Figure 9–19). Most large colorectal carcinomas are fungating and often luminal-narrowing conspicuous masses (Figure 9–20). In contradistinction, sessile colorectal adenomas and carcinomas are relatively inconspicuous, not only on 3D endoluminal images, but also on thin 2D images due to their relatively flat, minimally raised morphology.

When patients undergo screening, the prevalence of malignancy is directly correlated with the size of the polyp or lesion: for polyps smaller than 10 mm, the prevalence of malignancy is very low (only 1%). Furthermore, the differential for diminutive filling defects (<5 mm) includes normal mucosal protrusion, adherent fecal material, hyperplastic polyps, or small adenomatous polyps. However, for patients with polyps or lesion larger than 10 mm in which the risk of malignancy is increased, the polyp or lesion is excised.

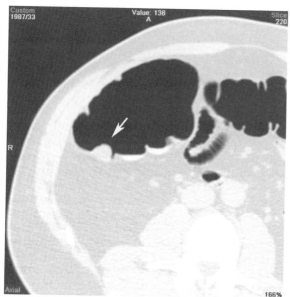

▲ **Figure 9–19.** Colonic polyp. Axial MDCT image displayed in a "colon" window shows a 1.2-cm polyp (*arrow*) in the ascending colon. (For corresponding 3D endoluminal reconstructed image, see Plate 5).

When patients undergo a virtual colonoscopy with CT or MR, the clinical significance of missing a diminutive adenoma is likely minimal, particularly since most patients undergoing repeat virtual colonoscopy at 5-year intervals. For polyps or lesions ranging in size from 5 mm to 9 mm, current recommendations suggest removing these lesions if visualized endoscopically. For polyps or lesion that are very small (<5 mm), there is debate as to whether these polyps should be reported at all.

Pickhardt PJ, Choi JR, Hwang I, et al. Computed tomographic virtual colonoscopy to screen for colorectal neoplasia in asymptomatic adults. *N Engl J Med.* 2003;349(23):2191–2200. [PMID: 14657426]

Zalis ME, Barish MA, Choi JR, et al. CT colonography reporting and data system: a consensus proposal. *Radiology.* 2005;236:3–9. [PMID: 15987959]

E. Inflammatory Bowel Disease

Patients with inflammatory bowel disease, either Crohn's Disease or Ulcerative Colitis, may have isolated colonic disease. Many of the imaging features used to diagnose inflammatory bowel disease on CT are derived from the appearance of the colon on barium enema examinations. While double-contrast enemas and optical colonoscopy are superior to CT for demonstrating superficial changes in the mucosa, CT is advantageous in identifying extra-colonic complications, such as penetrating disease, perforation or abscess formation (Figure 9–21).

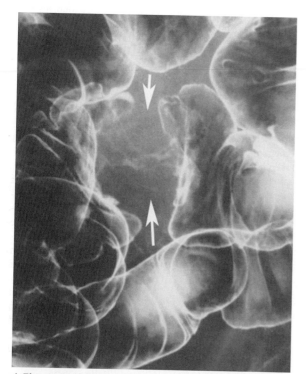

▲ **Figure 9–20.** Colon cancer. Double-contrast barium enema image shows an apple-core lesion in the sigmoid colon with irregularity of the mucosa (*arrows*).

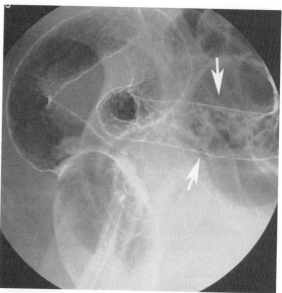

▲ **Figure 9–21.** Ulcerative colitis. Double-contrast barium enema image shows numerous contrast-filled superficial ulcerations (*arrows*) with loss of normal colonic haustrations.

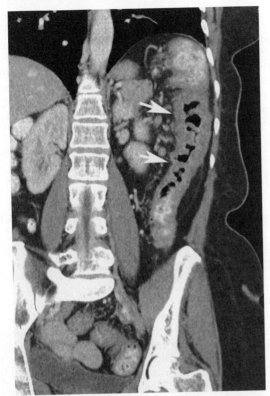

▲ **Figure 9–22.** Ulcerative colitis. Coronal MDCT image shows mild symmetric wall thickening (*arrows*) of the left colon with associated lymphadenopathy in the mesocolon.

On CT, both Crohn's disease and ulcerative colitis have inflammatory changes of the bowel, but have distinct imaging patterns. Distinguishing features of Crohn's disease include: eccentric or asymmetric wall thickening, typically along the mesenteric border; the rectum is typically spared from disease; the distribution of disease is typically discontinuous and involves mainly the right-sided colon; the wall thickening is usually greater than 10 mm; and common sings of penetrating disease are seen such as a pericolonic inflammatory mass (phlegmon), sinus tracts, or fistulas. In contradistinction, ulcerative colitis, typically has a symmetrically thickened colonic wall; the wall measures less than 10 mm; the rectum is always involved, and the distribution of disease is continuous and mainly involves the left colon. Secondary signs of pericolonic inflammation, including the proliferation of perirectal fat and the presence of pericolic adenopathy are nonspecific (Figure 9–22). Similar disease features of Crohn's disease and ulcerative colitis are found with MR colonography.

Both CT and MR are useful for diagnosing inflammatory bowel complications such as fistula, abscess, inflammatory stenosis, fibrofatty proliferation, or colorectal cancer.

Andersen K, Vogt C, Blondin D, et al. Multi-detector CT-colonography in inflammatory bowel disease: prospective analysis of CT-findings to high-resolution video colonoscopy. *Eur J Radiol.* 2006;58(1):140–146. [PMID: 16337356]

Rimola J, Ordás I. MR colonography in inflammatory bowel disease. *Magn Reson Imaging Clin N Am.* 2014;22:23–33. [PMID: 24238130]

F. Infectious Conditions

Pseudomembranous colitis is a toxin-mediated disease without microbial invasion into the bowel wall. *Clostridium difficile* is responsible for the disease which typically occurs after antibiotic use. On CT, pseudomembranous colitis usually manifests as marked bowel wall thickening measuring on average 10–15 mm. The edematous wall thickening is homogeneously low in attenuation on CT. In addition to severe wall thickening, two imaging features can be seen with disease. The first, a relatively specific sign for the disease, is the "accordion" sign, which can be observed when intravenous contrast material is trapped between the large pseudomembranes of *C. difficile* colitis. Second, swollen nodular projections ("wall nodularity") protruding into the lumen (the CT equivalent to "thumbprinting" classically seen in barium enema) is often seen, particularly in severe disease. The feared complication of *Pseudomembranous colitis* is *toxic megacolon*. As the colitis progresses to toxic megacolon, the colon enlarges on serial imaging with loss of haustral markings, pseudopolyps and thumbprinting from mucosal edema. If the *Pseudomembranous colitis* remains unabated, colonic perforation may occur.

Typhlitis, also termed neutropenic colitis, is seen in neutropenic and immunosuppressed patients. The underlying etiology for typhlitis includes CMV infection, neoplastic infiltration, ischemia, and mucosal hemorrhage. The disease usually presents acutely with right lower quadrant pain, fever, and bloody diarrhea. On imaging, typhlitis is characterized by circumferential cecal wall edema/thickening (hypoattenuating bowel wall on CT), frequently also involving the ascending colon and terminal ileum. There is also pericolonic inflammatory stranding within the mesentery or retroperitoneum. CT is the imaging modality of choice for the diagnosis, since barium enema or colonoscopy carry a high risk of bowel perforation. Complications that require surgical or percutaneous intervention include intramural perforation with pneumatosis, transmural necrosis with pneumoperitoneum, and pericolic abscesses.

Boland GW, Lee MJ, Cats AM, Ferraro MJ, Matthia AR, Mueller PR. *Clostridium difficile* colitis: correlation of CT findings with severity of clinical disease. *Clin Radiol.* 1995;50:153–156. [PMID: 7889703]

Guerri S, Danti G, Frezzetti G, Lucarelli E, Pradella S, Miele V. *Clostridium difficile* colitis: CT findings and differential diagnosis. *Radiol Med.* 2019;124(12):1185–1198. [PMID: 31302848]

Thoeni RF, Cello JP. CT imaging of colitis. *Radiology.* 2006;250:623–638. [PMID: 16926320]

G. Ischemic Colitis (See Chapter 6)

There are a spectrum of ischemic changes in the colon that include mild, superficial necrosis and mucosal hemorrhage, to transmural infarction. The latter may or may not result in perforation. The etiology for colonic ischemia is acute mesenteric vessel occlusion due to thromboembolism, dissection, or arteriosclerosis. While the aforementioned vasculopathies are due to partial or total intrinsic vascular occlusion; ischemic colitis is most commonly caused by decreased perfusion. If the colonic perfusion pressure falls in hypovolemic shock, cardiogenic shock, or septic shock, systemic and local regulatory mechanisms preserve blood supply to the brain, heart, and muscles by reducing splanchnic perfusion. When colonic ischemia develops, the distribution of ischemia depends on the etiology and may also depend on the patients age. In older patients with shock, colonic ischemia may develop around the watershed areas at the splenic flexure or in the rectosigmoid colon. Rarely in younger patients ischemic colitis may involve the cecum and ascending colon, usually related to hemorrhagic shock in the setting of penetrating or blunt trauma. When patients develop colonic ischemia after cocaine use, the ischemia can be seen in the right colon or in the rectosigmoid colon.

On CT, the distribution of colonic ischemia may be diffuse, localized, segmental, or focal depending of the pathophysiology of the ischemia. Imaging findings, in part, depend on whether intravenous contrast is administered. Imaging findings independent of contrast administration include wall thickening, fold enlargement, or loss of haustra in the affected bowel segments. In the case of wall thickening, the bowel wall can be enlarged due to edema or hemorrhage. When edema is the predominant sign of ischemia, the ischemic bowel wall is hypodense with a shaggy inner wall. When hemorrhage is the predominant sign of ischemia, the ischemic bowel will be hyperdense due to mucosal and submucosal hemorrhage.

Following the administration of iodinated contrast material, the ischemic bowel wall may show heterogeneous enhancement, absent wall enhancement, or regions of decreased enhancement. Pericolic stranding in the surrounding mesenteric/retroperitoneal fat is also commonly observed although wall thickening is the most common finding in ischemia, decreased or even absent wall enhancement is the most specific CT finding for bowel ischemia, with reported specificity of 96%, compared to 67% for bowel wall thickening (Figure 9–23).

Plastaras L, Vuitton L, Badet N, Koch S, Di Martino V, Delabrousse E. Acute colitis: differential diagnosis using multidetector CT. *Clin Radiol.* 2015;70(3):262–269. [PMID: 25522900]

6. Anorectum

A. Imaging Algorithm

MRI is the imaging modality of choice in the diagnosis of perianal fistulas, rectal cancer, and pelvic floor dysfunction.

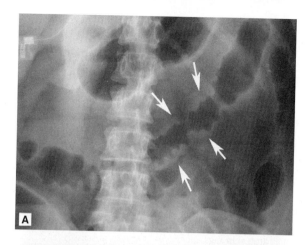

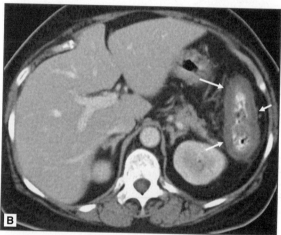

▲ **Figure 9–23.** Ischemic colitis. **A.** KUB (kidney, ureter, bladder) image shows wall thickening (*arrows*) of the transverse colon with thumbprinting. **B.** Axial MDCT image shows thickening of the wall of the left colon (*arrows*) with lack of wall enhancement.

MRI is used in these select diseases due to tissue contrast resolution and delineation of pelvic floor anatomy.

For perianal fistulas, clinical history and physical examination under anesthesia often are sufficient for diagnosis. MRI assessment of perianal fistula provides important anatomic and pathologic information required to guide surgical management, as imaging establishes the relation of the fistula to the anal sphincteric complex and identifies peri-rectal abscesses.

As the spatial resolution of MRI has improved, rectal MRI is now invaluable in the local staging of rectal cancer, and can identify patients who are candidates for surgical resection, patients who require neoadjuvant therapy, or patients with unresectable disease.

In the evaluation of pelvic floor dysfunction, pelvic floor weakness is characterized by abnormal and symptomatic displacement of pelvic organs. It represents a complex clinical problem most commonly seen in middle-aged and elderly parous women. Both fluoroscopic colpocystodefecography and MR defecography surpass physical examination in the detection and characterization of functional abnormalities of the anorectum and surrounding pelvic structures. The advantage of MR defecography relative to fluoroscopic colpocystodefecography includes the lack of ionizing radiation, as well as depiction of the pelvic floor musculature and soft tissues in relationship to the dynamic movement of pelvic floor compartments during defecation. The latter is particularly useful in patients who may undergo surgery.

B. Perianal Fistula

Perianal disease encompasses a wide range of conditions including skin tags, ulceration, fissures, abscesses, and fistulas. Fistulas associated with Crohn's disease tend to be complex, with secondary extensions and abscesses; as a result, their diagnosis and treatment can be particularly challenging. Accurate anatomic mapping of the fistulas and the identification of abscesses are critical in determining medical versus surgical management. The method of diagnostic investigation for perianal disease depends in part on local expertise, available facilities, and patient tolerance. High soft tissue contrast resolution, multiplanar capability, and lack of ionizing radiation make MRI a well-suited imaging modality for the diagnosis of perianal disease, particularly in CD. T1-weighted images delineate the sphincter complex anatomy while T2 weighted images and postgadolinium T1 weighted images determine if a fistula has active inflammation. Active inflammation is demonstrated by high T2 signal in the fistula track with early enhancement. (Figure 9–24). A fistula's conspicuity can be further accentuated by fat suppression techniques,

which suppresses fat signal in the pelvis thus maximizing fluid signal contrast.

There are two classification systems for perianal fistulas: the Parks classification, a surgically based classification, to minimize operative trauma to the anal sphincters and prevent recurrence and the St James's University Hospital MRI-based classification. After intervention, MRI is used to evaluate the fistula. A favorable treatment response is typically seen with a smaller fistula track diameter, resolution of prior abscesses, enhancing granulation tissue in the track, and decreased inflammatory changes in the rectum and perineum. A healed fibrotic fistula track has intrinsic low T2 signal and progressive enhancement.

Thipphavong S, Costa AF, Ali HA, Wang DC, Brar MS, Jhaveri KS. Structured reporting of MRI for perianal fistula. Abdom Radiol (NY). 2019;44(4):1295–1305. [PMID: 30474723]

Wise PE, Schwartz DA. The evaluation and treatment of Crohn's perianal fistulae: EUA, EUS, MRI, and other imaging modalities. *Gastroenterol Clin North Am.* 2012;41:379–391. [PMID: 22500524]

C. Neoplasms

Rectal MRI is the preferred modality for rectal cancer in pretreatment staging, in restaging after chemoradiation, and in diagnosing local recurrence.

Rectal MRI has largely replaced transrectal US (TRUS) in rectal cancer staging for many reasons. When TRUS was used, its strength was in depicting different layers of the rectal wall. Despite this strength, the primary failure of TRUS was the over staging of T2 tumors due to the extensive peritumoral fibrosis/tissue reaction surrounding the primary tumor. TRUS has other limitations, such as operator dependency, limitation to tumors located 8–10 cm from the anal verge when a rigid probe is used, and inability to assess stenotic tumors or the tumor mesorectal fascia relationship. Given these limitations of TRUS, rectal MRI has supplanting TRUS for local rectal cancer staging.

MRI for local rectal cancer staging can be used with or without an endorectal coil. There are both advantages and disadvantages to endorectal coil use. The primary benefit of an endorectal coil is that it can increase image spatial resolution. However, the benefit is negated in the evaluation of high rectal cancers which are superior to the coil. The disadvantages of an endorectal coil include patient discomfort and a stenotic cancer prevents endorectal coil placement. As MR field strength and image quality have improved, pelvic MRI without endorectal coil has become the standard of care for rectal cancer staging prior to treatment. Rectal MRI has a sensitivity, and specificity of 87%, and 75% for main tumor (T) staging and 77% and 71% for nodal (N) staging respectively.

The optimal imaging sequences for rectal MRI comprises high spatial resolution multiplanar T2-weighted thin (<3 mm) section sequences obtained on high-field-strength (3 Tesla)

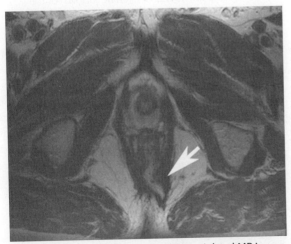

▲ **Figure 9–24.** Anal fistula. Axial T2-weighted MR image shows the presence of a fluid-filled hyperintense fistula (*arrow*) that transgresses the external anal sphincter.

MRI centered axially and coronally along the long axis of the tumor. These T2-weighted images permit differentiation of rectal wall layers, tumoral extent into the mesorectal fat, or extramural vascular invasion (invasion into a peri-rectal vessel). Additional acquired MRI sequences complement the primary anatomic T2 weighted sequences that define the T stage. Large field of view pelvic sequences are used for evaluation of distant lymph node chains. While diffusion weighted images with high b value (≥ 800 sec/mm^2) and T1-weighted sequences with intravenous contrast can often help with localization and extent of the primary tumor.

To determine the best treatment options for rectal cancer as well as prognosis, MRI reports should describe the tumor location (low, mid, and high rectum, and position within the rectal wall with a clock face), morphology (polypoid, ulcerating, circumferential, or semicircumferential pattern), mucinous content (presence of very T2 hyperintense signal), T category, anal sphincter complex involvement, circumferential resection margins status, involvement of the pelvic sidewall, extramural vascular invasion, and nodal status (Figure 9–25).

Al-Sukhni E, Milot L, Fruitman M, et al. Diagnostic accuracy of MRI for assessment of T category, lymph node metastases, and circumferential resection margin involvement in patients with rectal cancer: a systematic review and meta-analysis. *Ann Surg Oncol.* 2012;19(7):2212–2223. [PMID: 22271205]

Bipat S, Glas AS, Slors FJ, et al. Rectal cancer: local staging and assessment of lymph node involvement with endoluminal US, CT, and MR imaging—a meta-analysis. *Radiology.* 2004;232:773–783. [PMID: 15273331]

Horvat N, Carlos Tavares Rocha C, Clemente Oliveira B, Petkovska I, Gollub MJ. MRI of rectal cancer: tumor staging, imaging techniques, and management. *Radiographics.* 2019;39(2):367–387. [PMID: 30768361]

Kosinski L, Habr-Gama A, Ludwig K, Perez R. Shifting concepts in rectal cancer management: a review of contemporary primary rectal cancer treatment strategies. *CA Cancer J Clin.* 2012;62:173–202. [PMID: 22488575]

Muthusamy VR, Chang KJ. Optimal methods for staging rectal cancer. *Clin Cancer Res.* 2007;13:S6877–S6884. [PMID: 18006793]

Tapan U, Ozbayrak M, Tatlı S. MRI in local staging of rectal cancer: an update. *Diagn Interv Radiol.* 2014;20(5):390–398. [PMID: 25010367]

D. Pelvic Floor Dysfunction

At present, functional pelvic floor abnormalities represent a common health care problem. These abnormalities result in more than 300,000 surgeries in the United States annually, and it is estimated that approximately 15% of older multiparous women suffer from some sort of pelvic floor support defect. These conditions often have a significant impact on quality of life and result in a variety of symptoms, including chronic pelvic pain, urinary or fecal incontinence, and constipation. Because physical examination is not a reliable method for evaluating these symptoms, an objective assessment of rectal evacuation that is reproducible and allows quantification is extremely valuable. Fluoroscopic defecography is conventionally used to evaluate functional and anatomic anorectal disorders (Figure 9–26). MRI defecography provides a new and better alternative to study all pelvic visceral movements in a dynamic fashion.

Mortele KJ, Fairhurst J. Dynamic MR defecography of the posterior compartment: indications, techniques, and MRI features. *Eur J Radiol.* 2007;61:462–472. [PMID: 17145152]

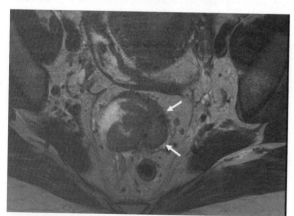

▲ **Figure 9–25.** Rectal cancer. Axial T2-weighted MR image shows a T3 rectal cancer arising from the left lateral wall of the rectum with extension beyond the muscularis propria (*arrows*).

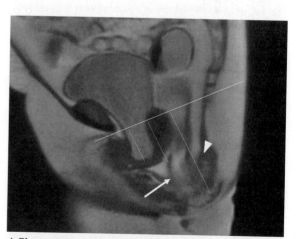

▲ **Figure 9–26.** Pelvic floor prolapse. Sagittal MR image from a dynamic defecography study shows tricompartimental pelvic floor prolapse with intra-anal rectal intussusception (*arrowhead*) and the presence of an anterior rectocele (*arrow*).

LIVER IMAGING

1. Diffuse Liver Diseases

A. Imaging Algorithm

During the last decade, the role of the radiologist in evaluating patients with diffuse liver disease has expanded. In some cases, such as fatty liver and iron overload, MRI imaging plays an important role in diagnosis and quantification. In other liver diseases, such as hepatitis and cirrhosis, imaging is crucial in imaging surveillance for HCC.

de Souza DA, Parente DB, de Araújo AL, Mortelé KJ. Modern imaging evaluation of the liver: emerging MR imaging techniques and indications. *Magn Reson Imaging Clin N Am.* 2013;21:337–363. [PMID: 23642557]

Mortele KJ, Ros PR. Imaging of diffuse liver disease. *Semin Liver Dis.* 2001;21:195–212. [PMID: 11436572]

B. Cirrhosis

Cirrhosis is the diffuse, progressive process of liver fibrosis, pathologically characterized by architectural distortion and nodular regenerative change. The presence of intrahepatic and extrahepatic imaging findings of cirrhosis depends on the severity of the cirrhosis (Figure 9–27). Enlargement of the hilar periportal space, in the absence of other conventional signs, has been described as a helpful sign in the diagnosis of early cirrhosis. More pronounced lobar or segmental changes of hepatic morphology such as atrophy of the right hepatic lobe and left medial segment, enlargement of the caudate lobe and left lateral segment, and the expanded gallbladder fossa sign are seen in advanced cirrhosis.

Recent advances in MR technology allow for identification and severity of liver fibrosis. The MRI is coupled with

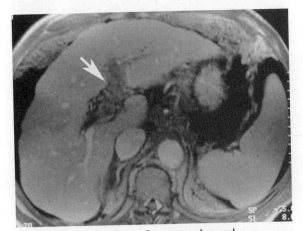

▲ **Figure 9–27.** Cirrhosis. Contrast-enhanced T1-weighted axial MR image shows a nodular contour of the liver, splenomegaly, and ascites. Note portal vein thrombosis (*arrow*).

a device that generates mechanical waves and special MRI sequences measure the displacement of the liver which is a direct measure of liver stiffness, which in turn correlates with the degree of fibrosis. This MRI technique is termed MR elastography. Currently, liver MR elastography is the most accurate imaging technique to identify and stage liver fibrosis, with accuracy comparable to liver biopsy in advanced fibrosis.

Guglielmo FF, Venkatesh SK, Mitchell DG. Liver MR elastography technique and image interpretation: pearls and pitfalls. *Radiographics.* 2019;39(7):1983–2002. [PMID: 31626569]

Morisaka H, Motosugi U, Ichikawa S, et al. Magnetic resonance elastography is as accurate as liver biopsy for liver fibrosis staging. *J Magn Reson Imaging.* 2018;47(5):1268–1275. [PMID: 29030995]

Accurate identification of benign and malignant hepatocellular nodules arising in the cirrhotic liver is crucial. Nowadays, MRI is by far the most specific imaging technique for differentiating those nodules based on characteristic signal intensity and enhancement pattern. *Regenerative nodules*, like normal liver, invariably have a portal venous blood supply with minimal blood supply from the hepatic artery. As a consequence, they are usually isointense with background liver on both T1- and T2-weighted images, and they show no predominant enhancement following gadolinium administration. *Dysplastic nodules* are premalignant nodules found in approximately 25% of cirrhotic livers. Similar to regenerative nodules, the main blood supply to dysplastic nodules is from the portal venous system. A dysplastic nodule is typically homogeneously hyperintense on T1-weighted images, hypointense on T2-weighted images, shows a portal-venous phase enhancement, is smaller than 3 cm, and has no capsule. In cases of dysplastic nodules with foci of HCC, the classic appearance is that of a "nodule within a nodule," consisting of a high signal intensity focus of HCC within a low signal intensity dysplastic nodule on T2-weighted images. For contrast enhanced MRIs using gadoxetate disodium, a specific contrast agent with approximately 50% biliary excretion, there is a specific delayed hepatobiliary phase, that allows for detection of specific liver lesions. In the case of dysplastic nodules dedifferentiating to HCC, a progressive reduction in uptake of gadoxetate disodium is observed on delayed phase imaging.

Extrahepatic signs of cirrhosis include features of portal hypertension, such as splenomegaly, portosystemic collateral vessels, combined with findings that can be partially attributed to intrinsic hepatocellular dysfunction including ascites, bowel wall edema, and gallbladder wall thickening. MR angiography provides useful information regarding the presence, location, and flow pattern in portosystemic shunts. These findings are useful both for diagnostic purposes (eg, detection of bleeding varices) and for treatment planning (eg, prior to transjugular intrahepatic portosystemic shunt placement or shunt surgery). Lately, time-resolved 3D phase-contrast MRI with three-directional flow encoding, also referred to as "4D flow MRI," has become a valuable tool to investigate not only vascular anatomy but also portal vein system hemodynamics.

Hanna RF, Aguirre DA, Kased N, Emery SC, Peterson MR, Sirlin CB. Cirrhosis-associated hepatocellular nodules: correlation of histopathologic and MR imaging features. *Radiographics.* 2008;28:747–769. [PMID: 18480482]

Quaia E, De Paoli L, Pizzolato R, et al. Predictors of dysplastic nodule diagnosis in patients with liver cirrhosis on unenhanced and gadobenate dimeglumine-enhanced MRI with dynamic and hepatobiliary phase. *AJR Am J Roentgenol.* 2013;200:553–562. [PMID: 23436844]

Roldán-Alzate A, Francois CJ, Wieben O, Reeder SB. Emerging applications of abdominal 4D flow MRI. *AJR Am J Roentgenol.* 2016;207(1):58–66. [PMID: 27187681]

C. Storage Diseases

The two primary storage diseases of the liver are hepatic steatosis and iron deposition. *Hepatic steatosis* results from a variety of abnormal metabolic processes. The distribution of steatosis can be variable, ranging from focal, regional, or diffuse (Figure 9–28). Undoubtedly the most sensitive imaging technique to detect fatty change of the liver is the use of a specific type of MR pulse sequences termed in and out phase, which allows the detection of microscopic/intravoxel fat. On out-of-phase images, areas with a significant amount of intravoxel fat will show lower signal intensity than on the corresponding in-phase images, and this loss of signal intensity between the two types of images allows the radiologist to establish the diagnosis of fatty liver (Figure 9–29). On imaging, several morphological and geographic features enable correct identification of focal fat deposition or focal fat sparring: typically periligamentous and periportal location, lack

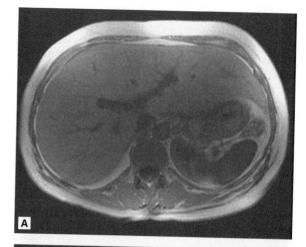

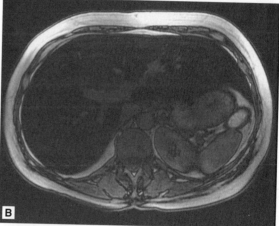

▲ **Figure 9–29.** Steatosis. **A.** Axial in-phase unenhanced T1-weighted MR image shows a normal hyperintense appearance of the liver parenchyma. **B.** Axial out-of-phase unenhanced T1-weighted MR image shows a significant drop in signal of the liver compatible with steatosis.

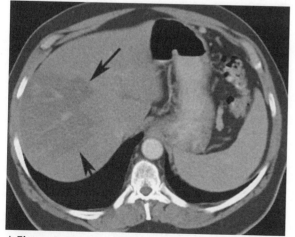

▲ **Figure 9–28.** Steatosis. Axial MDCT image shows a wedge-shaped area of low attenuation (*arrows*) in the right lobe of the liver with vessels coursing through it.

of mass effect, sharply angulated boundaries of the area, non-spherical shape, lack of vascular displacement or distortion, and lobar or segmental distribution. Fatty changes can also be detected on CT and US, with diffuse or focal hypodensity and echogenicity of the liver, respectively. Compared to CT and US, however, MRI shows higher sensitivity and specificity for evaluation of hepatic steatosis: a metanalysis comparing US, CT, and MRI, using biopsy as a reference standard, showed that mean sensitivity for US was 73.3–90.5%, for CT was 46.1–72.0%, and for MRI was 82.0–97.4%; while mean specificity for US was 69.6–85.2%, for CT was 88.1–94.6%, and for MRI was 76.1–95.3%. In the last years, MRI derived proton density fat fraction (MRI-PDFF) has emerged as an accurate quantification method of liver fat content. A longitudinal study on 50 patients who underwent serial evaluations with liver biopsy and MRI-PDFF, showed that the latter is more sensitive than histology to determine grade of steatosis and to quantify changes in the liver fat content.

Iron deposition in the liver can either be primary (hereditary) or secondary. Primary iron deposition or, *Hereditary hemochromatosis*, is characterized by excessive deposition of iron into the hepatocytes, pancreatic acinar cells, myocardium, joints, endocrine glands, and skin. The liver represents the ideal organ to quantify iron for three reasons: one, the liver is the primary storage organ for iron, second, iron overload first appears in the liver, and third, the concentration of iron in the liver has a linear relationship to total body iron. MRI is far more specific than any other imaging modality for the characterization and quantification of iron overload due to the unique magnetic susceptibility effect of iron. Accumulated iron in the hepatocytes results in significant reduction of signal intensity of the liver parenchyma on T2-weighted images, particularly T2*-weighted gradient-echo sequences. Different MR imaging–based noninvasive techniques exists for quantitative assessment of liver iron overload, which are now considered the standard of care in diagnosis, quantification, and monitoring of iron overload. One technique for determining liver iron concentration involves comparing the signal intensity of liver with that of paraspinal muscles, which are normally less intense than liver and not prone to excessive iron accumulation on multiple GRE sequences.

In patients with secondary iron deposition, *hemosiderosis or siderosis*, either due to transfusional iron overload states or dyserythropoiesis, the excessive iron is processed and accumulates in organs containing reticuloendothelial cells, including liver, spleen, and bone marrow. As a result, although the distribution of iron in patients with siderosis is demonstrated in the liver as diffuse low signal intensity changes similar to those seen in primary hemochromatosis. The distinguishing diagnostic feature between primary and secondary iron deposition is the extrahepatic signal intensity changes in the spleen and bone marrow which enable MRI to distinguish primary hemochromatosis from hemosiderosis. In cases of intravascular hemolysis, seen in patients with heart valves due to mechanical stress, or in patients with paroxysmal nocturnal hemoglobinuria, or in patients with hemolytic crises of sickle cell disease, iron deposition can also be observed in the kidneys.

D. Diffuse Vascular Disorders

Budd-Chiari syndrome is defined as obstruction of the large hepatic venous outflow pathways, typically at the level of the hepatic veins or inferior vena cava (IVC). Imaging findings associated with Budd-Chiari syndrome include direct findings of hepatic venous obstruction, secondary morphologic changes of the liver, and extrahepatic features. Direct diagnostic features are the visualization of intraluminal material (web, tumor, thrombus) within the hepatic veins or IVC. The absence of hepatic vein flow or presence of flow disturbances, including reversed flow in hepatic veins, on Doppler US is

also diagnostic. Additional features supporting the diagnosis include presence of intrahepatic venous collaterals, nonvisualization of the hepatic veins or IVC, and dilation of the azygos venous system. Indirect morphologic changes in the liver result from the tremendous venous congestion produced by the outflow obstruction. In the acute setting, the peripheral portion of the liver becomes congested and swollen and appears hypoechoic on sonography, hypodense on CT, and hyperintense on T2-weighted images. In contrast, the central portions of the liver, because of the direct drainage into the IVC, show increased enhancement on contrast-enhanced imaging studies. Over time, as the disease enters a chronic phase, these central portions of the liver hypertrophies while the liver periphery atrophies (Figure 9–30).

Sinusoidal obstruction syndrome (SOS), also known as *Veno-occlusive disease* is another cause of hepatic outflow obstruction but differs from Budd-Chiari syndrome in that SOS involves inflammation and obstruction of the postsinusoidal venules. SOS is usually associated with prior full body chemoradiation in leukemia patients or certain herbal medications and tea ("bush tea" disease). There are no direct imaging signs diagnostic of SOS, as this entity is a pathologic diagnosis. Indirect imaging signs which may suggestive of the disease include hepatomegaly, and heterogenous parenchymal enhancement (mosaic-like) due to congestion. The hepatic veins and IVC, although narrowed due to the hepatic edema, are patent. The portal vein can appear dilated and with reduced or hepatofugal flow. Additional secondary signs include an elevated hepatic artery resistive index (>0.8) splenomegaly, ascites, and gallbladder wall thickening can also be observed.

Passive hepatic congestion is typically caused by right-sided heart failure. The liver shows a heterogeneous mosaic-like enhancement, similar to Budd-Chiari syndrome and

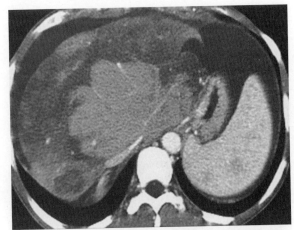

▲ **Figure 9–30.** Budd-Chiari syndrome. Axial MDCT image shows enlargement and hyperenhancement of the caudate lobe with congestion and atrophy of the periphery of the liver. Note the presence of ascites.

SOS, but in passive hepatic congestion the IVC and hepatic veins are enlarged due to increased right heart pressures.

Bohte AE, van Werven JR, Bipat S, Stoker J. The diagnostic accuracy of US, CT, MRI and 1H-MRS for the evaluation of hepatic steatosis compared with liver biopsy: a meta-analysis. *Eur Radiol.* 2011;21(1):87–97. [PMID: 20680289]

Caussy C, Reeder SB, Sirlin CB, Loomba R. Noninvasive, quantitative assessment of liver fat by MRI-PDFF as an endpoint in NASH trials. *Hepatology.* 2018;68(2):763–772. [PMID: 29356032]; PMCID: PMC6054824.

Labranche R, Gilbert G, Cerny M, et al. Liver iron quantification with MR imaging: a primer for radiologists. *Radiographics.* 2018;38(2):392–412. [PMID: 29528818]

Noureddin M, Lam J, Peterson MR, et al. Utility of magnetic resonance imaging versus histology for quantifying changes in liver fat in nonalcoholic fatty liver disease trials. *Hepatology.* 2013;58(6):1930–1940. [PMID: 23696515]

Virmani V, Ramanathan S, Virmani VS, Kielar A, Sheikh A, Ryan J. Non-neoplastic hepatic vascular diseases: spectrum of CT and MRI appearances. *Clin Radiol.* 2014;69:538–548. [PMID: 24581966]

2. Focal Liver Lesions

A. Imaging Algorithm

Because the clinical implications and therapeutic strategies of focal liver lesions vary tremendously depending on their pathology, the ability to differentiate focal hepatic lesions is extremely important. The development of both dynamic multiphasic CT and fast multiphasic MRI coupled with the ability to use tailored MR techniques (such as fat-suppression sequences and in/out phase imaging) have facilitated assessment of the morphologic and hemodynamic features of liver tumors thus allowing differentiation between benign and malignant liver lesions. In the majority of cases, familiarity with the most relevant CT and MRI features, in combination with additional clinical information, provides enough information for lesion characterization and in certain cases obviates the need for a liver biopsy.

In the next sections we will discuss benign liver lesions, including hepatic cysts, hemangiomas, and focal nodular hyperplasias (FNHs), hepatic adenomas and malignant liver lesions, including HCCs, intrahepatic cholangiocarcinomas (ICC) and metastases.

B. Benign Liver Lesions (See Chapter 51)

Hepatic cysts are developmental anomalies present in 2.5% of the population. They can be either solitary or multiple in hepatorenal polycystic disease. Hepatic cysts are well defined and anechoic on US, homogeneously hypodense on nonenhanced CT scans, and show no enhancement following administration of contrast. On MRI, hepatic cysts have very low signal intensity on T1-weighted and very high signal intensity on T2-weighted images. They are typically round or ovoid shaped, well margined, do not have a capsule, and lack enhancement following gadolinium contrast administration.

Hemangioma is the most common benign hepatic tumor. Hemangiomas are usually solitary (80%), measure less than 4 cm in diameter, and are most often peripherally located. A giant hemangioma is larger than 10 cm in diameter and often contains central cleft-like areas of fibrosis or cystic degeneration. Hemangiomas typically appear homogeneously hyperechoic on US with posterior acoustic enhancement. The classic appearance on CT is that of a well-defined hypodense lesion showing peripheral globular discontinuous enhancement during early phase imaging after contrast administration. On delayed images, the mass usually shows a centripetal fill-in with persistent delayed enhancement. MRI findings in hemangiomas mirror the CT imaging appearance on post-contrast images. On intrinsic T1- and T2-weighted images, the lesions show decreased and markedly increased signal intensity, respectively. Dynamic T1-weighted postcontrast imaging parallels dynamic contrast CT showing a peripheral nodular discontinuous enhancement pattern progressing to homogeneity. In 94% of the large hemangiomas, however, a persistent hypointense center is present on delayed images due to variable degree of fibrosis and cystic degeneration (Figure 9–31). With liver-specific contrast media (Gd-BOPTA, Gd-EOB) hemangiomas appear hypointense at hepatocellular phase images since lesional enhancement parallels the blood pool.

FNH is a rare (3%) benign tumor predominantly diagnosed in asymptomatic women during the third to fifth decades of life. Multiple FNHs are observed in 20% of cases. On CT, FNH is classically seen as a solitary hypo- or isodense area with early arterial phase enhancement related to its vascular supply derived from the hepatic artery- and isodensity to liver on portal venous and delayed phase after contrast injection. The presence of a central scar has been reported to occur in less than 50% of cases (Figure 9–32A), which demonstrates delayed enhancement. Typical MRI features of FNH are isointensity on T1- weighted images, iso- to faint hyperintensity on T2-weighted images, homogeneity, hypervascularity (96%) with enhancing characteristic similar to the ones described for CT, and the presence of a central scar, which is hyperintense on T2-weighted images due to its vascular, biliary, and myxoid stroma components (Figure 9–32B). With liver specific contrast media (Gd-BOPTA, Gd-EOB) is administered, most FNH will appear hyperintense at hepatocellular phase imaging sequences. When the FNH is not hyperintense on hepatocellular phase imaging, the remaining FNH's may be hypointense, inhomogeneously hyperintense, isointense, or hypointense with a hyperintense ring. The central scar appears hypointense on hepatocellular phase images.

Hepatic adenoma is a rare benign neoplasm historically associated with oral contraceptive use and younger women. The relative incidence of adenomas has remained relatively constant despite dose changes in oral contraceptives, likely

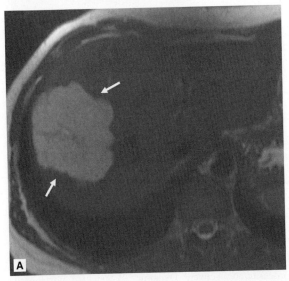
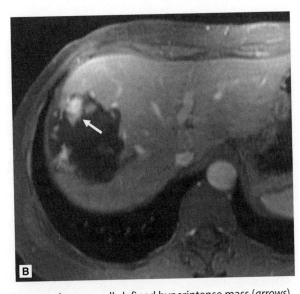

▲ **Figure 9–31.** Hepatic hemangioma. **A.** T2-weighted axial MR image shows a well-defined hyperintense mass (*arrows*) in the right lobe of the liver. **B.** Contrast-enhanced T1-weighted axial MR image shows peripheral nodular incomplete enhancement (*arrow*) of the lesion.

offset by the increase in obesity and liver steatosis. Given the potential complications associated with adenomas, including hemorrhage and dedifferentiation to HCC, confidently diagnosing an adenoma is crucial and, in many cases, can be confidently done by imaging.

In 2006 adenomas were classified into four pathological types based upon each adenoma's molecular profile. Recently in 2017 that classification was revised into eight unique subtypes with the newly designated adenomas originating from adenomas previously lumped into the unclassified category. The eight subtypes include Hepatocyte nuclear factor 1 alpha (HNF1α) mutated adenoma (HNF1α-A),

Inflammatory adenoma (IA), previously named telangiectatic FNH, β-catenin activated adenomas (β-A), β-catenin activated adenoma exon 7/8, β-catenin activated inflammatory adenomas exon 3, β-catenin activated inflammatory adenomas exon 7/8 (βI-A), sonic hedgehog adenoma (SH-A), and unclassified adenomas. In some cases identifying the subtype is critical for clinical management as β-A are more likely to undergo malignant degeneration and SH-A are more likely to hemorrhage.

The molecular pathogenesis of some adenoma subtypes have different cellular characteristics that manifest with unique imaging characteristics. Adenomas demonstrate

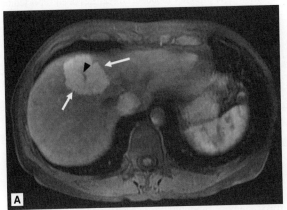
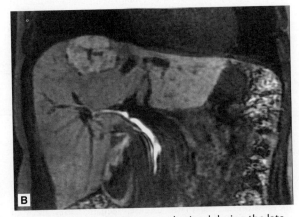

▲ **Figure 9–32.** Focal nodular hyperplasia. **A.** Contrast-enhanced T1-weighted axial MR image obtained during the late arterial phase shows a homogeneous hypervascular mass (*arrows*) with the presence of a small central scar (*black arrowhead*). **B.** Coronal MR image obtained 20 minutes after administration of hepatospecific contrast agent shows retention of the contrast in the FNH.

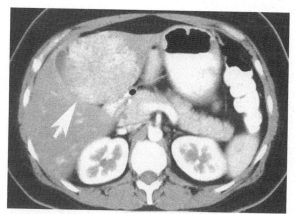

▲ **Figure 9–33.** Hepatic adenoma. Axial MDCT image shows a large heterogeneously hyperenhancing mass (*arrow*) in segment IV of the liver.

arterial enhancement due to the lack of portal blood supply. The degree of intralesional hemorrhage or fat content vary, leading to different appearances on US and CT. On US adenomas may appear as well demarcated hypo- (due to hemorrhage) or hyperechoic (due to fat) lesions, sometimes with a hypoechoic halo of focal fatty sparing. On CT, adenomas may appear as hypo- iso- or hyperattenuating on unenhanced CT. Following contrast administration, they usually enhance early and homogenously since they have an arterial blood supply (Figure 9–33) but are isodense on portal venous and delayed phase.

MRI is the diagnostic modality of choice for identifying and characterizing adenomas due to the ability to confidently identify fat, hemorrhage, and enhancement characteristics. Some of the unique imaging characteristics are directly attributable to the cellular histology of the adenoma such as in I-A and HNF1α-A. The most common adenoma is the I-A. Histologically, I-A has inflammatory reaction, intralesional neutrophils, and marked sinusoidal congestion which can manifest as diffuse hyperintense T2 signal. When the T2 signal is peripherally band like, the "atoll sign" is present. Increased T1 signal in I-A correlations directly with the degree intralesional hemorrhage content, while arterial enhancement is moderate to marked with persistent delayed enhancement. On hepatobiliary phase imaging, the I-A can have intermediate signal intensity due to retained contrast in the dilated sinusoids. HNF1α-A is the second most common adenoma, and histologically defined by fat globules and balloon degeneration. Due to the fat globules, HNF1α-A will have intravoxel signal drop out on opposed phase MRI sequences which is indicative of intralesional fat in the adenoma. HNF1α-A adenomas also will have moderate arterial enhancement with persistent delayed enhancement. HNF1α-A are hypointense on heptobiliary phase imaging. The third most common adenoma is the β-A. Histologically, these adenomas have cellular atypia, pseudoglandular formation and varying degrees of necrosis and

hemorrhage. The lesion may have hyperintense patchy T2 signal. If intravoxel fat is present, the fat is often heterogenous or patchy. β-A demonstrates arterial homogenous or heterogenous hyperenhancement, washout, and a capsule. On hepatobiliary phase imaging the β-A can be isointense to hyperintense in contrast to the background liver parenchyma due to β-catenin upregulation of the organic anion transporting protein (OATP) receptors that are responsible for intracellular hepatobiliary contrast uptake. For simplicity, the remaining adenomas do not have pathognomonic imaging characteristics although as indicated by the name, βI-A can overlapping MRI signal characteristics with β-A and I-A. Of note, the SH-A do not have well defined imaging characteristics on MRI, although the adenomas are at increased risk of bleeding.

Frydrychowicz A, Lubner MG, Brown JJ, et al. Hepatobiliary MR imaging with gadolinium-based contrast agents. *J Magn Reson Imaging*. 2012;35:492–511. [PMID: 22334493]

Mortele KJ, Ros PR. Benign liver neoplasms. *Clin Liver Dis*. 2002;6:119–145. [PMID: 11933585]

Tekath M, Klotz T, Montoriol PF, Joubert-Zakeyh J, Garcier JM, Da Ines D. Fat-containing lesions of the liver: a pictorial essay. *Diagn Interv Imaging*. 2015;96(2):201–211. [PMID: 24388602]

Zulfiqar M, Sirlin CB, Yoneda N, et al. Hepatocellular adenomas, understanding the pathomolecular lexicon, MRI features, terminology, and pitfalls to inform a standardized approach. *J. Magn. Reson. Imaging*. 2020;51:1630–1640. [PMID: 31418986]

C. Malignant Liver Lesions (See Chapter 51)

HCC comprises the vast majority of primary malignant liver lesions and typically arises in patients with cirrhosis. The current paradigm for screening includes US or CT and MRI in selected patients. In patients with an abnormal screening exam or a high clinical suspicion of HCC, diagnostic imaging with multiphase CT or MRI is recommended.

Unlike other carcinomas, HCC is largely diagnosed by imaging and not by histology. To help standardize imaging reporting, The Liver Imaging Reporting and Data System (LI-RADS) was created for standardizing the terminology, technique, interpretation, reporting, and data collection of liver imaging. LI-RADS was originally developed in 2011 by the American College of Radiology, and now is integrated with the American Association for the Study of Liver Disease (AASLD) practice guidelines.

In LI-RADS, visible lesions (termed observations), are categorized based on major and ancillary imaging features, into different categories reflecting their relative probability of being HCC, ranging from LR1 (definitely benign) to LR5 (definitely HCC). Additional categories are also present in LI-RADS v2018, including LR-NC (noncategorizable due to image omission) and LR-TIV (tumor in vein), and other hepatic malignant neoplasms labeled as LR-M. In addition, categories for treated observations are also included, such as LR-TR Nonviable, LR-TR Equivocal or LR-TR Viable,

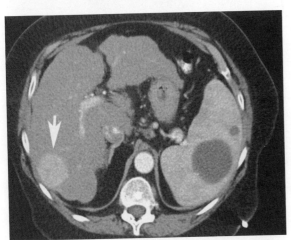

▲ **Figure 9–34.** Hepatocellular carcinoma. Axial MDCT image shows a round homogeneous and hypervascular mass in the right lobe of the liver (*arrow*) in a patient with underlying cirrhosis.

depending on characteristic enhancement patterns after treatment.

Major imaging features for HCC which help stratify a lesions probability for HCC comprise nonrim arterial hyperenhancement; nonperipheral "washout" (reduction in enhancement in whole or in part relative to composite liver tissue from earlier to later phase resulting in hypoenhancement in portal venous or delayed phases); presence of an enhancing capsule; threshold growth (increase in size of the observation by ≥50% in ≤6 months). A ≥20 mm observation with nonrim arterial hyperenhancement and ≥1 major feature is categorized as LR-5 (definitely HCC) (Figures 9–34 and 9–35). Ancillary features, which include fat sparing in solid mass (which favor malignancy), presence of a nodule-in nodule (which favor HCC), or marked T2 hyperintensity

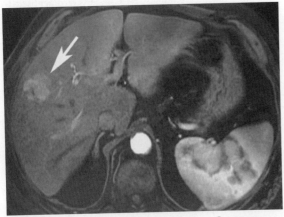

▲ **Figure 9–35.** Hepatocellular carcinoma. Contrast-enhanced T1-weighted axial MR image shows a homogeneous hypervascular mass (*arrow*).

(which favor benignity), may be used at radiologist discretion. These ancillary features are used for improved characterization of malignant and nonmalignant lesions and increased confidence in the probability assessment of HCC by imaging. The ancillary features also allow a radiologist to either upgrade or downgrade a LI-RADS score for a lesion with one exception: an ancillary feature cannot be used to upgrade a lesion to LR-5 (definite HCC).

The Organ Procurement and Transplantation Network (OPTN) classification which defines the imaging requisites for liver transplantation, is applied in the United States in transplant candidates. Besides outlining minimal technical recommendations for imaging of the liver, mandatory diagnostic criteria for HCC, reporting requirements and requirements for imaging interpretations, the OPTN classification defines five categories to describe observations, with category five reserved for definitive HCC. Since the inception of LI-RADS, efforts have been made to increase congruence between the two classification systems.

The infiltrative or diffuse variant or HCC can be difficult to distinguish from morphologic features and imaging features of cirrhosis, and detection relies on primary and secondary imaging signs, such as the presence of tumor in vein, the presence of heterogeneous enhancing ill-defined diffusion restricting nodules, and the presence of architectural distortion.

American College of Radiology: Liver Imaging Reporting and Data System. https://www.acr.org/-/media/ACR/Files/Clinical-Resources/LIRADS/LI-RADS-2018-Manual-5Dec18.pdf?la=en Accessed May 17, 2020.

Marrero JA, Kulik LM, Sirlin CB, et al. Diagnosis, staging, and management of hepatocellular carcinoma: 2018 Practice Guidance by the American Association for the Study of Liver Diseases. *Hepatology*. 2018;68(2):723–750. [PMID: 29624699]

ICC is relatively uncommon, but the second most common primary hepatic malignant neoplasm. Several risk factors for ICC include Caroli disease, primary sclerosing cholangitis, and clonorchiasis. Because of the peripheral localization of ICC relative to the bile ducts, jaundice is seldom present at presentation. On CT, ICC usually presents as a large hypoattenuating mass (6–10 cm), irregularly delineated, with satellite nodules (62%), and sometimes a central scar. Other MRI features of ICC are encasement of the portal vein, usually without evidence of thrombus (25–75%), focal liver atrophy (43%), dilation of peripheral intrahepatic bile ducts (29%), capsular retraction (21%), small calcifications, and gradual centripetal contrast enhancement. Cholangiocarcinoma can be hypointense or less commonly can show isointense/hyperintense internal areas during hepatobiliary phase imaging, due to contrast agent pooling in the fibrous stroma.

Three subtypes, with different macroscopic and imaging characteristics have been described. One type, mass-forming cholangiocarcinoma, presents as a homogeneous mass with heterogeneous gradual centripetal enhancement, possible associated capsular retraction and dilation of the bile ducts distal to the mass. The second type, periductal infiltrating: cholangiocarcinoma, presents with areas of enhancing duct wall thickening with narrowing the involved duct, most commonly occurring at the hepatic hilum, with dilatation of the upstream bile ducts. The third type, intraductal cholangiocarcinoma presents with ductal ectasia with or without an evident mass.

Metastases. Secondary liver lesions are due to metastasis from other primary malignancies. CT appearances of hepatic metastases depend on the vascularity of the lesions compared with the normal liver parenchyma. Hypovascular lesions, such as colorectal adenocarcinoma metastases, show a lower attenuation compared with normal liver and are best detected on portal venous phase contrast-enhanced images (Figure 9–36). Hypervascular metastases, including those from endocrine tumors, melanoma, sarcoma, renal cell carcinoma, and certain subtypes of breast and lung carcinoma, enhance more rapidly than normal liver and require arterial phase imaging for accurate depiction. Infrequently, metastases are indiscrete and only detectable through indirect features, such as diffuse parenchymal heterogeneity, vascular and architectural distortion, or alterations of the liver contour such as capsular retraction. In cases where there is often diffuse liver metastasis, especially in breast cancer patients treated with gemcitabine or other types of systemic chemotherapies, the liver will have a nodular border and atrophy, imaging features often seen with cirrhosis, but due to the underlying breast metastasis and is termed "pseudocirrhosis." Other indirect signs that may be seen with both small and large metastases include central amorphous calcifications in mucinous primary malignancies, peripheral washout during the delayed phase, and biliary or vascular invasion.

On MRI, hepatic metastases are typically mildly hyperintense on T2-weighted images, are hypointense on T1-weighted images, and appear hypointense or hyper-intense following

gadolinium administration, depending on their vascularity. Hepatospecific contrast agents, such as Gd-EOB or Gd-BOPTA, are useful in the detection of hepatic metastatic disease; as liver metastasis are markedly hypointense to the liver parenchyma on delayed phase imaging, and thus significantly more conspicuous. In some cases, such as breast metastases or adenocarcinoma, a rim enhancement, or "target sign" in the hepatobiliary phase has been described.

Ha S, Lee CH, Kim BH, et al. Paradoxical uptake of Gd-EOB-DTPA on the hepatobiliary phase in the evaluation of hepatic metastasis from breast cancer: is the "target sign" a common finding? *Magn Reson Imaging.* 2012;30:1083–1090. [PMID: 22578929]

Seo N, Kim DY, Choi JY. Cross-sectional imaging of intrahepatic cholangiocarcinoma: development, growth, spread, and prognosis. *AJR Am J Roentgenol.* 2017;209(2):W64–W75. [PMID: 28570102]

BILIARY IMAGING

1. Stone Disease (See Chapter 52)

A. Imaging Algorithm

US is still the modality of choice for the evaluation of the gallbladder and biliary ductal system. US is fast, readily available, noninvasive, and does not use ionizing radiation. US, however, has some inherent limitations; these include the dependence of diagnostic accuracy on the skill of the operator, body habitus, an acoustic window without bowel gas, and patient cooperation.

Many biliary stones do not contain a sufficient calcium for CT detection. Hence the sensitivity of CT to detect gallstones is low, ranging from 39% to 75%. While CT may not diagnose noncalcified biliary stones, with the aid of CT multiplanar images, CT can identify indirect signs of biliary stones such as biliary duct enlargement. CT can also localize the level of biliary obstruction and associated complications. In some cases, thin-section unenhanced CT imaging may be useful in detecting partially calcified ductal stones. Furthermore, dual-energy CT which enables the concurrent acquisition of data with use of two different x-ray energy spectra, allows detection of noncalcified stones with significantly increased sensitivity for detection of gallstones and choledocholithiasis, particularly compared to conventional CT.

MRI has an increasing role in the routine workup of patients with suspected choledocholithiasis when compared with US or CT. Today, MRCP has replaced endoscopic retrograde cholangiopancreatography (ERCP) in many institutions in the initial diagnostic workup of choledocholithiasis, especially in patients with low and intermediate probability of having common bile duct stones (CBD). Compared with ERCP, MRCP has the following advantages: noninvasive, short exam time without sedation, avoids possible complications of ERCP, including pancreatitis and hemorrhage. MRCP can also be performed in patients in whom ERCP is difficult

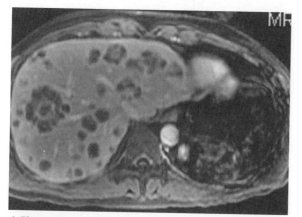

▲ **Figure 9–36.** Colorectal cancer metastases. Contrast-enhanced T1-weighted axial MR image shows numerous hypovascular masses scattered throughout the liver.

due to anatomic alterations of the upper intestinal tract from previous surgery, such as in patients with Roux-en-Y Gastric Bypass. The primary advantage of ERCP is its diagnostic and interventional potential.

Benarroch-Gampel J, Boyd CA, Sheffield KM, Townsend CM Jr, Riall TS. Overuse of CT in patients with complicated gallstone disease. *J Am Coll Surg.* 2011;213(4):524–530. [PMID: 21862355]

Kiewiet JJ, Leeuwenburgh MM, Bipat S, Bossuyt PM, Stoker J, Boermeester MA. A systematic review and meta-analysis of diagnostic performance of imaging in acute cholecystitis. *Radiology.* 2012;264:708–720. [PMID: 22798223]

Levy AD, Murakata LA, Abbott RM, et al. From the archives of the AFIP. Benign tumors and tumorlike lesions of the gallbladder and extrahepatic bile ducts: radiologic-pathologic correlation. Armed Forces Institute of Pathology. *Radiographics.* 2002;22:387–413. [PMID: 11896229]

Mortele KJ, Wiesner W, Cantisani V, et al. Usual and unusual causes of extrahepatic cholestasis: assessment with magnetic resonance cholangiography and fast MRI. *Abdom Imaging.* 2004;29:87–99. [PMID: 15160760]

Patel NB, Oto A, Thomas S. Multidetector CT of emergent biliary pathologic conditions. *Radiographics.* 2013;33:1867–1888. [PMID: 24224584]

Ratanaprasatporn L, Uyeda JW, Wortman JR, Richardson I, Sodickson AD. Multimodality imaging, including dual-energy CT, in the evaluation of gallbladder disease. *Radiographics.* 2018;38(1):75–89. [PMID: 29320323]

B. Cholelithiasis & Choledocholithiasis

Gallstones. Only approximately 15–20% of gallstones contain enough calcium to be depicted on plain radiographs. US has >95% sensitivity for the detection of cholelithiasis. A gallstone can be diagnosed with certainty on US when a mobile hyperechoic intraluminal filling defect is identified along with acoustic shadowing (Figure 9–37). CT detects only approximately 80% of gallstones seen sonographically. In depicting cholelithiasis, MRCP with conventional MRI has sensitivity comparable to sonography. MRCP is especially useful when sonography results are equivocal for cholelithaisis or there is clinical suspicion for additional pathology, such as pancreastitis. Furthermore, CBD stones can be detected with much greater sensitivity with MRCP than with ultrasonography.

Choledocholithiasis is the most common cause of biliary obstruction. US is not as capable of detecting CBD stones as gallstone and has a reported sensitivity of 13% to 75% for choledocholithiasis. The major difficulty of US is detecting distal CBD stones, especially when there is no associated acoustic shadowing or ductal dilation (30% of cases). CT with multiplanar reformations, has sensitivity of 69–87% and specificity of 83–92% for the detection of choledocholithiasis. MRCP is the most accurate imaging modality in the detection and characterization of CBD stones, with sensitivity of 89–95% and specificity of 95–100% for the detection of choledocholithiasis. CBD stones are usually hypointense on both

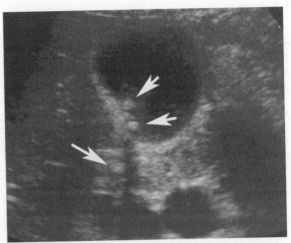

▲ **Figure 9–37.** Gallstones. Sagittal ultrasound image shows hyperechoic stones in the gallbladder along with shadowing (*short arrows*). Also note a nonshadowing stone in the cystic duct (*long arrow*).

T1- and T2-weighted images and are typically surrounded by bile (Figure 9–38). On axial images, the stone typically reveals a dependent position in the duct, thus differentiating it from pneumobilia (gas is in the nondependent position of the duct) and T2 flow /bile artifacts (typically centrally located).

2. Inflammatory Conditions

A. Imaging Algorithm

For simplification, the biliary tree can be divided into the bile ducts and the gallbladder when discussing biliary

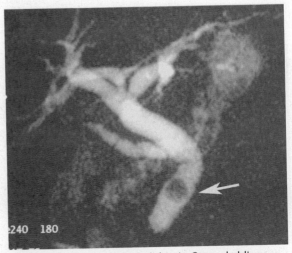

▲ **Figure 9–38.** Choledocholithiasis. Coronal oblique thick-slab MRCP image shows a round filling defect (*arrow*) in the distal common bile duct.

inflammation. This allows for a simple inflammation dichotomy; inflammation of the gallbladder, cholecystitis, and inflammation of the biliary tree, cholangitis. For suspected cholecystitis, US is the initial imaging modality in the diagnostic work up. CT and MRI are typically reserved for cases in which US results are equivocal or an alternative diagnosis is considered while hepatobiliary scintigraphy has greater sensitivity and specificity than US and can also be used in equivocal cases. For cholangitis, MRI with MRCP has proven to be as sensitive ERCP.

B. Acute Cholecystitis (See Chapter 52)

Sonographic findings supportive of the diagnosis of acute cholecystitis include the presence of gallstones, gallbladder wall thickening greater than 3 mm, pericholecystic fluid, and the detection of tenderness directly over the gallbladder (sonographic Murphy sign). When all these findings are present, the sensitivity for the diagnosis of acute cholecystitis with US is more than 90%. Other ancillary signs in acute cholecystitis include, gallbladder distention and sludge. CT features of acute cholecystitis include the presence of gallstones, gallbladder wall thickening greater than 3 mm, pericholecystic fluid and fat stranding, hydrops, and hyperenhancement of segment IV of the liver due to hyperemia (Figure 9–39). On T2-weighted unenhanced MR images, inflammatory pericholecystic changes are visualized as linear and strandlike structures of high signal intensity around the gallbladder fossa and pericholecystic fat. MRI features of acute cholecystitis show a thickened gallbladder wall, which has increased signal intensity on T2-weighted images. Gadolinium-enhanced T1-weighted images are useful in depicting inflammatory changes of the gallbladder wall, pericholecystic fat, and intrahepatic periportal tissues. Contrast enhancement of the gallbladder wall is increased, and on dynamic imaging, there is a transient enhancement of liver segments adjacent to the gallbladder on early images. The role of MRCP in the diagnostic workup of acute cholecystitis is mainly to detect small cystic duct and gallbladder neck calculi. Impacted cystic duct or gallbladder neck calculi can be demonstrated with MRCP accurately to a resolution as low as 2 mm. Hepatobiliary scintigraphy (HIDA scan), being the most sensitive test for acute cholecystitis, should be reserved for patients with equivocal US findings, and will demonstrate nonvisualization of the gallbladder. It should be noted however that false negative may occur in certain conditions, such as in patients with prior sphincterotomy or severe liver disease. Intravenous morphine, which can be administered before the study or 60 minutes after the hepatobiliary scintigraphy shows nonvisualization of the gallbladder, increases the specificity for acute cholecystitis.

C. Chronic Cholecystitis (See Chapter 52)

Chronic cholecystitis may be asymptomatic or may present as acute inflammation on a background of chronic inflammation. Other manifestations of this entity may be

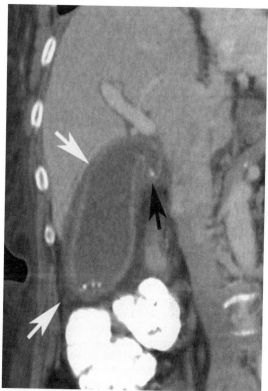

▲ **Figure 9–39.** Acute cholecystitis. Coronal MDCT image shows hydrops of the gallbladder (*white arrows*), pericholecystic fluid, and gallstones. Note a stone in the neck of the gallbladder (*black arrow*).

biliary colic, fistula formation, hydrops of the gallbladder, or perforation. Deposition of calcium within the gallbladder wall, a condition termed porcelain gallbladder, is an uncommon manifestation of chronic cholecystitis and is associated with an increased prevalence of gallbladder carcinoma (Figure 9–40).

On imaging studies, chronic cholecystitis may have findings similar to those of acute cholecystitis, such as wall thickening and stones. However, the gallbladder is typically contracted around the stones rather than distended. Furthermore, on contrast-enhanced images, the degree of contrast enhancement of the gallbladder wall is significantly lower in comparison with acute cholecystitis. The transient pericholecystic liver enhancement on early postcontrast images, which is described with acute cholecystitis, is also not evident in chronic cholecystitis. Secondary signs of malignancy, such as local invasion, distant metastases, and bile duct dilation, are helpful in distinguishing chronic cholecystitis from gallbladder carcinoma.

D. Cholangitis

Cholangitis can be categorized as bacterial cholangitis, primary sclerosing cholangitis, and secondary sclerosing

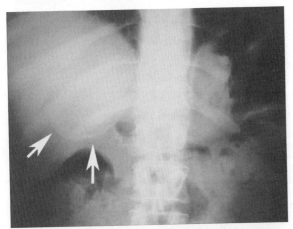

▲ **Figure 9–40.** Porcelain gallbladder. KUB (kidney, ureter, bladder) image shows linear calcifications in the wall of the gallbladder (*arrows*).

cholangitis or chronic pyogenic (obstructive) cholangitis. Primary sclerosing cholangitis is an autoimmune disorder characterized by obliterative fibrotic inflammation of the bile ducts and, typically, both intrahepatic and extrahepatic bile ducts are involved simultaneously. On MRCP, the characteristic appearance is marked by the presence of multiple stenoses, minor dilation of the proximal segments (due to periductal fibrosis), a beaded appearance of intrahepatic bile ducts, presence of sacculations resembling diverticula, enhancing bile duct wall, and intrahepatic lithiasis. The use of a hepatocyte-specific contrast agent allows performing simultaneous functional and morphologic imaging of the biliary tract.

Katabathina VS, Dasyam AK, Dasyam N, Hosseinzadeh K. Adult bile duct strictures: role of MR imaging and MR cholangiopancreatography in characterization. *Radiographics.* 2014;34:565–586. [PMID: 24819781]

3. Neoplastic Processes

A. Imaging Algorithm

MRCP is very valuable in the evaluation of the patient with jaundice caused by malignant biliary obstruction. The accuracy of MRCP in assessing the level and the morphology of the malignant obstruction is comparable to that of ERCP or percutaneous transhepatic cholangiography. However, compared with ERCP, MRCP may more accurately depict suprahilar tumor extension in cases of severe confluence stricturing (because in such cases the accuracy of ERCP will be impaired due to insufficient contrast filling). Another advantage of MRCP is its ability to visualize an undrained bile duct without injection of contrast material, thus potentially avoiding secondary cholangitis. In addition, portal venous invasion and hepatic metastases in patients can be detected

accurately with dynamic contrast-enhanced MRI sequences coupled to a MRCP protocol. MRI and MRCP offers significant advantages in the preoperative staging of hilar cholangiocarcinoma, because the bile duct, vascular structures, and liver parenchyma are all assessed simultaneously.

B. Gallbladder Carcinoma

Adenocarcinoma is the most common malignancy of the gallbladder and represents over 90% of gallbladder neoplasms. Other gallbladder neoplasms include squamous cell carcinoma, anaplastic carcinoma, and sarcoma. Gallstones are detected concurrently with gallbladder carcinoma in more than 70% of the cases. Three common imaging appearances for gallbladder carcinoma are seen. The most common appearance is a mass replacing the gallbladder fossa (55%) (Figure 9–41). The second most common appearance is either focal or diffuse gallbladder wall thickening (25%); this pattern is the most difficult to diagnose because of the small size of early masses. In addition, diffuse wall thickening is also caused by a wide variety of other pathologic conditions, such as acute and chronic cholecystitis, adenomyomatosis, and hypoproteinemia. The third most common appearance is an intraluminal polypoid mass. Unfortunately, gallbladder carcinoma usually presents with advanced disease as metastases are seen in 75% of the cases at the time of initial diagnosis.

C. Extrahepatic Cholangiocarcinoma

Extrahepatic cholangiocarcinomas (ECC) are biliary adenocarcinomas located at the bifurcation, proximal hepatic duct (Klatskin tumors), or distal bile ducts. ECC patients are older, presenting with painless jaundice, weight loss, and cholangitis. Once the diagnosis has been established, accurate local staging of the tumor is essential for clinical management, because few patients are eligible for surgery at the time of diagnosis.

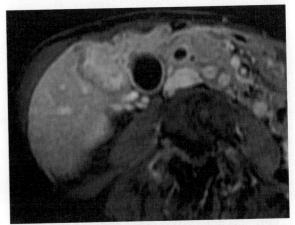

▲ **Figure 9–41.** Gallbladder carcinoma. Axial fat-suppressed contrast-enhanced T1-weighted image shows large mass arising from the gallbladder wall with extension into the adjacent liver parenchyma.

The Bismuth-Corlette classification, which is based on the extent of ductal infiltration, is a widely accepted classification system for perihilar cholangiocarcinomas.

On cross sectional imaging, these tumors typically present as a mass located at the liver hilum causing intrahepatic biliary dilation. On MRI, they are usually hypointense on T1-weighted images and slightly hyperintense on T2-weighted images with heterogeneous and variable enhancement following gadolinium administration. MRCP images typically reveal a malignant stricture at the bifurcation, with proximal biliary dilation; nodular intraductal tumor components are occasionally seen (Figure 9–42). Hilar ECC can involve the distal common hepatic duct alone (Bismuth type I), the confluence of the left and right hepatic duct (Bismuth type II), the confluence and either the right (Bismuth type IIIa) or the left (Bismuth type IIIb) hepatic duct, or both the left and right secondary confluence (Bismuth type IV).

4. Developmental Disorders

A. Imaging Algorithm

Congenital biliary anomalies are commonly encountered on imaging studies and can be accurately diagnosed, with increasing level of specificity, by US, CT, MRCP, and ERCP.

B. Choledochal Cysts

Choledochal cysts are rare congenital biliary tract anomalies characterized by biliary ductal dilation. The five subtypes, as described by Todani, have different pathophysiologies but are classified by the anatomic distribution of bile ducts cystic changes.

A *type I choledochal cyst* (Figure 9–43), the most common type, is a choledochal cyst confined to the extrahepatic bile duct.

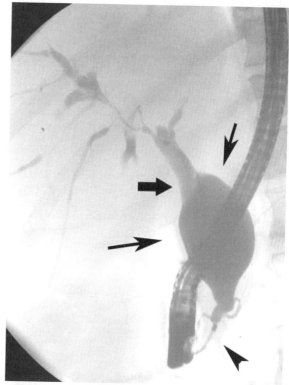

▲ **Figure 9–43.** Type I choledochal cyst. ERCP image shows saccular dilation of the extrahepatic bile duct (*arrows*) with presence of a long common channel (*arrowhead*) and mass cholangiocarcinoma (*thick arrow*) arising from the cranial aspect of the cyst.

This cyst results from an anomalous pancreaticobiliary union characterized by formation of a long, frequently ectatic common channel. This type has been subclassified into three types: type Ia shows dilatation of the entire extrahepatic biliary tract. Type Ib shows dilatation of a focal segment of the extrahepatic biliary tract. Type Ic, which shows dilatation of the common bile duct portion of the extrahepatic biliary tract.

A *type II choledochal cyst* represents a true diverticulum of the extrahepatic bile duct.

The *type III choledochal cyst* (Figure 9–44), also known as a choledochocele, is formed by ectasia of the intramural (intraduodenal segment) CBD. It is not embryologically related to the other cystic dilations of the choledochal cysts.

The *type IV choledochal cysts* are, by definition, multiple and can have both intrahepatic and extrahepatic components.

Caroli disease (Todani type V choledochal cyst) is a rare congenital cystic dilation of the intrahepatic bile ducts. It is an autosomal-recessive disorder resulting from the arrest of or derangement in the normal embryologic remodeling of ducts that, in turn, causes varying degrees of destructive inflammation and segmental dilation. If the large intrahepatic

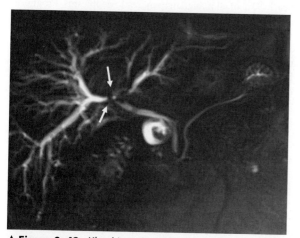

▲ **Figure 9–42.** Klatskin tumor. Thick slab oblique coronal MRCP image shows intrahepatic biliary ductal dilation with the presence of an obstructing mass (*arrows*) at the level of the porta hepatis.

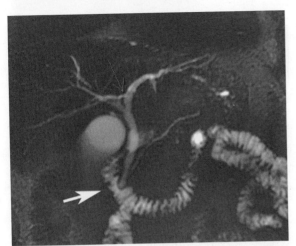

▲ **Figure 9–44.** Type III choledochal cyst. Oblique coronal MRCP image shows telescoping of the distal common bile duct (*arrow*) in the duodenum.

bile ducts are affected, the result is Caroli disease, whereas abnormal development of the small interlobular bile ducts results in congenital hepatic fibrosis. If all levels of the intrahepatic biliary tree are involved, features of both congenital hepatic fibrosis and Caroli disease are present; this condition has been termed Caroli syndrome. Imaging methods show intrahepatic saccular or fusiform dilated cystic structures of varying sizes that communicate with the biliary tree. The presence of tiny dots with contrast enhancement within the dilated intrahepatic bile duct ("central dot sign") is considered very suggestive of Caroli disease. The "central dot sign" represents the portal branches surrounded by cystic alterations of the intrahepatic biliary ducts.

Mortelé KJ, Rocha TC, Streeter JL, Taylor AJ. Multimodality imaging of pancreatic and biliary congenital anomalies. *Radiographics*. 2006;26:715–731. [PMID: 16702450]

PANCREATIC IMAGING

1. Pancreatic Neoplasms (See Chapter 31)

A. Imaging Algorithm

With the introduction of MDCT, the visualization of the pancreas has dramatically improved. Therefore, MDCT is a superb tool for detection of solid neoplasms, with an >90% overall diagnostic accuracy to assess resectability. Recent studies have compared the accuracy of MRI in staging pancreatic carcinoma with CT. With breath-hold imaging and the use of phased array coils, dynamic MRI was shown to be superior to CT in detection of small tumors (<2 cm), while both modalities performed equally well in establishing the degree of vascular involvement. Other studies indicate that the two modalities perform comparably in the global assessment of resectability. PET/CT may be helpful in accurately staging pancreatic cancer by detecting distant metastatic disease.

Given MRI's sensitivity to detect fluid, it is not surprising that this modality has great potential to accurately assess cystic pancreatic neoplasms. The cyst fluid improves intralesional contrast resolution, often rendering subtle irregularities of the cyst wall that aid in differential diagnosis between benign and malignant neoplasms. When MRI and MRCP are combined with MR pancreatography, the duct system can be visualized and the relation of these lesions to the main and branch ducts may be predicted. MRCP has been shown to be more sensitive than CT and ERCP in the depiction of these lesions.

Koelblinger C, Ba-Ssalamah A, Goetzinger P, et al. Gadobenate dimeglumine-enhanced 3.0-T MR imaging versus multiphasic 64-detector row CT: prospective evaluation in patients suspected of having pancreatic cancer. *Radiology*. 2011;259(3):757–766.

Mortele KJ, Ji H, Ros PR. CT and magnetic resonance imaging in pancreatic and biliary tract malignancies. *Gastrointest Endosc*. 2002;56(suppl):S206–S212. [PMID: 12447269]

Park HS, Lee JM, Choi HK, Hong SH, Han JK, Choi BI. Preoperative evaluation of pancreatic cancer: comparison of gadolinium-enhanced dynamic MRI with MR cholangiopancreatography versus MDCT. *J Magn Reson Imaging*. 2009;30(3):586–595.

Shah S, Mortele KJ. Uncommon solid pancreatic neoplasms: ultrasound, computed tomography, and magnetic resonance imaging features. *Semin Ultrasound CT MR*. 2007;28:357–370. [PMID: 17970552]

B. Ductal Adenocarcinoma

Pancreatic ductal adenocarcinoma (PDAC) accounts for nearly 95% of all malignant pancreatic neoplasms. Prognosis is poor, with a 5-year survival rate ranging from 1% to 5%; at the time of clinical presentation, 66% of patients have an advanced tumor stage, with metastatic disease present in 85% of cases. The majority of tumors are located in the pancreatic head, and because of the involvement of the CBD, they present earlier than tumors arising in the body or tail of pancreas.

CT is the imaging modality of choice for the detection and preoperative staging of pancreatic cancer according to the National Comprehensive Cancer Network guidelines version 1.2020. Modern CT scanners provide enormous capabilities for fast data acquisition and narrow collimation, resulting in accuracies of 96% for detecting pancreatic tumors. Preoperative assessment of resectability for pancreatic cancer is obtained with a dedicated pancreatic protocol which includes a late arterial phase, for evaluation of arterial contact and presence of arterial variants, a portal venous phase, for evaluation of venous contact. Patients with borderline resectable pancreatic cancer, can be restaged with CT obtained during pancreatic and portal venous phase, which will suffice for local restaging as well as for preoperative restaging of the disease.

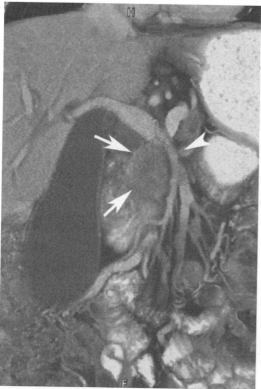

▲ **Figure 9–45.** Pancreatic adenocarcinoma. Curved, reformatted CT image shows a low-density pancreatic mass (*arrows*) with invasion of the superior mesenteric vein (*arrowhead*).

On contrast-enhanced MDCT images, most PDAC present as hypoattenuating lesions with respect to the surrounding normal pancreatic parenchyma (Figure 9–45). Indirect CT signs of an isoattenuating pancreatic cancer relative to the pancreatic parenchyma include dilation of the CBD and pancreatic duct without calculi, dilation of the pancreatic duct in the body and tail but not in the head, a homogenous zone in a heterogeneous atrophic gland, bulging of the uncinate process, and atrophy of the pancreatic tail.

The primary goal of initial staging by imaging is to determine whether PDAC is surgically resectable with the intent to get a curative surgical margin, or R0 resection. R0 is defined as no gross macroscopic or microscopic disease. On imaging, PDAC can be classified as resectable, borderline resectable, and locally advanced, based on the degree of vascular invasion by CT or MRI. Per the National Comprehensive Cancer Network version 1.2020 guidelines, a pancreatic adenocarcinoma is considered locally advanced, thus unresectable in the following scenarios: 1) greater than 180 degree solid tumor contact with the superior mesenteric artery or the celiac axis for pancreatic head or uncinate process; tumor 2) greater than 180 degree solid tumor contact with the celiac

artery or aorta for pancreatic body or tail tumor; 3) unreconstructible portal vein or superior mesenteric vein due to tumoral involvement or occlusion.

The detection of hepatic metastases is also critical in the preoperative staging of the patients, because distant metastasis makes PDAC treatment nonoperative. While MDCT scanners have the ability to identify very small lesions (<5 mm) due to the spatial resolution, MRI, has improved detection of hepatic metastases. The National Comprehensive Cancer Network guidelines version 1.2020 recommend the use of MRI in patients with small or indeterminate hepatic lesions seen on preoperative CT. On MRI, detection of pancreatic adenocarcinoma is based on noncontrast T1-weighted fat-suppressed images and postgadolinium T1-weighted images, obtained in arterial, pancreatic, and portal venous phase. On T1-weighted fat-suppressed images, pancreatic cancer appears as a low signal intensity mass relative to the mild to high signal intensity normal pancreatic tissue (Figure 9–46). MRCP as an adjunct to MRI has also proven an accurate means of evaluating the level and causes of pancreatic ductal obstruction. A major advantage of MRCP is that the visualization of the duct is based on the signal features in the pancreatic secretions. Thus, one can visualize the duct before and after an obstructing lesion.

PET with F-18 fluorodeoxyglucose (F-18 FDG PET) has a limited role in pancreatic imaging. In a comparison between CT and F-18 PET, F-18 PET was more sensitive than CT for detecting malignancy (92% vs 65%), as well as more specific (85% vs 61%). However, vascular invasion could not be assessed on PET/CT and thus has limited utility in the preoperative assessment of pancreatic adenocarcinoma.

Al-Hawary MM, Francis IR, Chari ST, et al. Pancreatic ductal adenocarcinoma radiology reporting template: consensus statement of the Society of Abdominal Radiology and the American Pancreatic Association. *Radiology*. 2014;270(1): 248–260. [PMID: 24354378]

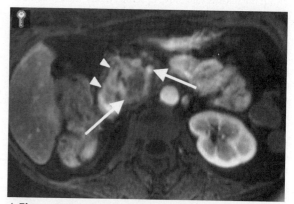

▲ **Figure 9–46.** Pancreatic adenocarcinoma. Contrast-enhanced T1-weighted axial MR image shows a hypovascular pancreatic mass (*arrows*). Note the normal enhancing residual pancreas (*arrowhead*).

Kauhanen SP, Komar G, Seppänen MP, et al. A prospective diagnostic accuracy study of 18F-fluorodeoxyglucose positron emission tomography/computed tomography, multidetector row computed tomography, and magnetic resonance imaging in primary diagnosis and staging of pancreatic cancer. *Ann Surg.* 2009;250:957–963. [PMID: 19687736]

National Comprehensive Cancer Network Clinical Practice Guidelines in Oncology. Pancreatic adenocarcinoma Version 1.2020. https://www.nccn.org/professionals/physician_gls/PDF/pancreatic.pdf. Published November 26, 2019. Accessed May 25, 2020.

Yoon SH, Lee JM, Cho JY, et al. Small (≤20 mm) pancreatic adenocarcinomas: analysis of enhancement patterns and secondary signs with multiphasic multidetector CT. *Radiology.* 2011;259:442–452. [PMID: 21406627]

Zaky AM, Wolfgang CL, Weiss MJ, Javed AA, Fishman EK, Zaheer A. Tumor-vessel relationships in pancreatic ductal adenocarcinoma at multidetector CT: different classification systems and their influence on treatment planning. *Radiographics.* 2017;37(1):93–112. [PMID: 27885893]

Zins M, Matos C, Cassinotto C. Pancreatic adenocarcinoma staging in the era of preoperative chemotherapy and radiation therapy. *Radiology.* 2018;287(2):374–390. [PMID: 29668413]

C. Cystic Pancreatic Tumors (See Chapter 31)

Cystic pancreatic tumors comprise are a diverse group of lesions, ranging from benign to malignant lesions, which can often be differentiated solely based of their characteristic imaging features.

Serous cystadenoma is a benign neoplasm that occurs most frequently in the pancreatic head of elderly female patients. This well-circumscribed tumor is often lobulated and contains a central, stellate, calcified scar in addition to multiple small cysts divided by thin septations. The tumor is hypervascular secondary to its rich subepithelial capillary network. On imaging this tumor may be homogeneously solid, or, more commonly, a predominantly cystic mass with multiple small cysts. The presence of six or more small cysts within the mass is suggestive of serous rather than mucinous cystic neoplasm. On unenhanced MDCT scans, serous cystic tumors are low-density, solid, or, more commonly, multiple cyst-containing lesions with attenuation similar to water. The appearance of a *serous cystadenoma* can range from an irregular heterogeneously enhancing mass, when it contains innumerable tiny cysts, to a homogenous mass on postcontrast images, when it contains dominant fibrous stroma. Serous cystic tumors are usually markedly hyperintense on T2-weighted MR images, although some central areas of low signal intensity may occasionally be seen related to the presence of a fibrous scar (Figure 9–47). On T1-weighted MR images, the tumor has low signal intensity, except in cases in which hemorrhage is present.

Mucinous cystic tumors range from tumors with malignant potential to frankly malignant mucinous cystadenocarcinomas. In 95% of cases, they occur in women during their fourth to sixth decades. Most commonly, mucinous cystic tumors are located in the tail or body of the pancreas.

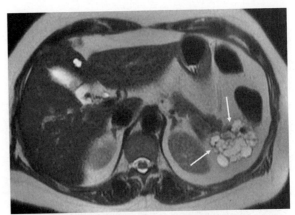

▲ **Figure 9–47.** Serous microcystic cystadenoma. Axial T2-weighted image shows a lobulated cystic mass (*arrows*) composed of numerous small cysts.

These encapsulated hypovascular tumors are most frequently multilocular. They may contain internal septations, solid papillary excretions, and occasionally peripheral calcifications. Unenhanced MDCT shows a round mass, which is well delineated and has smooth external margins. Attenuation values are usually similar to that of water. Contrast enhanced CT may demonstrate enhancement of the wall and the presence of thin septations; on the internal surface of the tumor, nodularities representing papillary projections may also be observed. MRI studies depict the unilocular or multilocular cystic nature of this mass. If a mucinous cystic neoplasm appears unilocular without septations on imaging, differentiation from a pseudocyst may not be possible. MR is also advantageous in that it can show internal septations, mural nodules, and solid excrescences in the tumor wall.

Intraductal papillary mucinous neoplasms (IPMN) are often classified into main and branch duct types. The branch duct type mostly presents in the uncinate process or pancreatic head, but it can also involve the body or tail. On unenhanced CT, branch-duct tumor appears as clusters of multiple small cysts or as a single cystic lesion with irregular, lobulated margins and septations (Figure 9–48). Diffuse or segmental dilation of the main pancreatic duct is typical for main-duct type tumors. Contrast-enhanced thin-section CT images may demonstrate communications between dilated cystic segments and the main pancreatic duct. MDCT may also depict the papilla bulging into the duodenal lumen and hyperdense filling defects secondary to mucin in the dilated duct. On MRCP, a dilated main pancreatic duct with a unilocular or multilocular cystic lesion is typical (Figure 9–49); communication between the main pancreatic duct and the cystic lesion may be depicted.

When certain defined imaging findings are present, the IPMNs should be further evaluated with EUS or should undergo surgical resection. The presence of an enhancing solid component >5 mm, a main pancreatic duct caliber ≥10 mm, or obstructive jaundice represent "high-risk stigmata,"

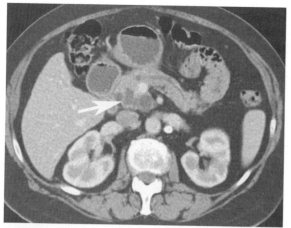

▲ **Figure 9–48.** Intraductal papillary mucinous neoplasm-branch duct. Axial CT image shows a dilated pancreatic side-branch duct (*arrow*) in the uncinate process.

for which surgical resection is recommended. Additional "worrisome features" that should prompt at least evaluation with EUS include: cyst ≥3 cm, enhancing mural nodule <5 mm, thickened enhancing cyst walls, diameter of the main pancreatic duct of 5–9 mm, abrupt change in the main pancreatic duct caliber with distal pancreatic atrophy, lymphadenopathy, an elevated serum level of carbohydrate antigen (CA)19-9 and a rapid rate of cyst growth >5 mm/2 years.

Mortelé KJ. Cystic pancreatic neoplasms: imaging features and management strategy. *Semin Roentgenol.* 2013;48:253–263. [PMID: 23796376]

Tanaka M, Fernández-Del Castillo C, Kamisawa T, et al. Revisions of international consensus Fukuoka guidelines for the management of IPMN of the pancreas. *Pancreatology.* 2017;17(5): 738–753. [PMID: 28735806]

D. Neuroendocrine Tumors

Pancreatic NETs, physiologically, are defined whether they procedure functioning hormones. The pancreatic NETs are commonly classified as functioning and nonfunctioning. For functioning NETs, there are five hormonal subtypes: insulinoma, gastrinoma, glucagonomas, vipomas, and somatostatinomas. *Insulinoma* is the most common and, at the time of diagnosis, is usually smaller than 1.5 cm with only 5–10% are malignant. *Gastrinoma* (see Chapter 15) is the second most common endocrine tumor of the pancreas. *Glucagonomas* and *vipomas* represent fewer than 10% of endocrine pancreatic tumors, and the majority of them are malignant. These latter tumors are found predominantly in the pancreatic body and tail and tend to be larger than insulinomas or gastrinomas. *Somatostatinoma* is the rarest endocrine pancreatic tumor (<1%), and frequently malignant at the time of diagnosis (75%).

On multiphasic contrast-enhanced MDCT, both functioning and nonfunctioning NETs present as hypervascular lesions, best seen in the early phases of pancreatic enhancement (Figure 9–50). Using optimized thin-slice CT scans, small tumors can be visualized. These tumors can present with metastases to liver, mesenteric lymph nodes, peritoneum, and bones.

On MRI, insulinomas and gastrinomas appear as lesions with low signal intensity on T1-weighted and high signal intensity on T2-weighted imaging and have avid enhancement since they are hypervascular. Ring-like enhancement in the periphery of the tumor is typically seen, while the center may remain hypointense secondary to fibrosis. The more uncommon but generally larger hyperfunctioning and nonhyperfunctioning tumors present with slightly low signal intensity on T1-weighted and bright signal intensity on T2-weighted MRI.

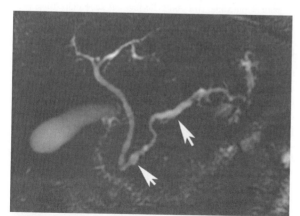

▲ **Figure 9–49.** Intraductal papillary mucinous neoplasm-main duct. Oblique coronal MRCP image shows irregular segmental dilation (*arrows*) of the main pancreatic duct.

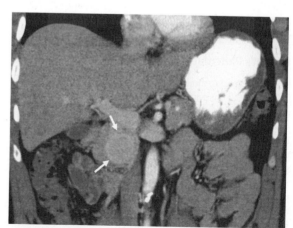

▲ **Figure 9–50.** Islet cell tumor. Coronal MDCT image shows a heterogeneously enhancing hypervascular mass in the pancreatic head (*arrows*).

Apart from anatomical imaging, functional imaging isotopes can also be used for detection, staging, and restaging of pancreatic NETs. Among the isotopes used for detection, which include 111In-pentetreotide SPECT/CT and 23I-Tyr3-octreotide paired with gamma camera, gallium 68 DOTATATE-PET/CT has higher sensitivity for detecting NETs. Thus, Gallium 68 DOTATATE-PET/CT has a role in detection, staging, evaluation for recurrence after surgical resection. The functional isotopes can also be used for identification of an unknown primary in patients with metastatic NETs. Dual imaging with FDG PET/CT and gallium 68 DOTATATE PET allows whole-body tumor grading and assessment of tumor heterogeneity, and can be used in selected cases, especially in patients with poorly differentiated NETs, in which DOTATATE PET may not depict the entire metastatic burden.

Humphrey PE, Alessandrino F, Bellizzi AM, Mortele KJ. Non-hyperfunctioning pancreatic endocrine tumors: multimodality imaging features with histopathological correlation. *Abdom Imaging*. 2015;40(7):2398–2410. [PMID: 25989932]

Sanli Y, Garg I, Kandathil A, et al. Neuroendocrine tumor diagnosis and management: 68Ga-DOTATATE PET/CT. *AJR Am J Roentgenol*. 2018;211(2):267–277. [PMID: 29975116]

2. Pancreatic Inflammation

A. Imaging Algorithm

The role of imaging in patients with suspected pancreatitis is to help diagnose pancreatitis, try to establish the cause of the disease, assess disease severity, and detect complications. In assessment of acute pancreatitis, MRI, as well as CT, can depict the presence and extent of necrosis and peripancreatic fluid collections. MRI is used instead of routine CT in some cases because mild pancreatitis cannot be well visualized by CT. MRI is better in defining the internal composition of peripancreatic fluid collections and is capable of detecting underlying causes of pancreatitis (eg, pancreas divisum, choledocholithiasis).

B. Acute Pancreatitis (See Chapter 28)

Of all the imaging modalities, CT is the most commonly used to evaluate acute pancreatitis. Contrast-enhanced CT plays a critical role in establishing necrosis in acute pancreatitis. CT features in mild acute pancreatitis consist of normal findings or focal or diffuse enlargement of the pancreas, normal pancreatic enhancement with or without peripancreatic fat stranding. In more severe cases, pancreatic parenchymal necrosis develops with acute necrotic fluid collections that occur mostly around the pancreas, in the anterior pararenal space, posterior pararenal space, and lesser sac (Figure 9–51). CT is also used for staging of pancreatitis severity; follow-up, and monitoring of established local pancreatic complications; for demonstrating other nonpancreatic sequelae, such

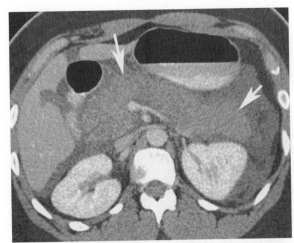

▲ **Figure 9–51.** Acute pancreatitis. Axial MDCT image shows a diffusely enlarged pancreatic gland (*arrows*). Note the lack of normal enhancement and presence of acute fluid collections in the retroperitoneum.

as renal, splenic, vascular, and GI complications; and for interventional procedural guidance.

In the assessment of acute pancreatitis, MRI can depict the presence and extent of necrosis and peripancreatic fluid collections and hemorrhage. Gadolinium-enhanced MRI is particularly useful for the assessment of pancreatic parenchymal perfusion and the presence of necrosis. T2-weighted sequences are the most sensitive for demonstrating fluid collections. Furthermore, by using additional MRCP or MR angiography sequences, MRI enables accurate diagnosis of underlying etiologies for pancreatitis, such as choledocholithiasis, or pancreas divisum, and vascular complications, respectively.

Mortele KJ, Wiesner W, Intriere L, et al. A modified CT severity index for evaluating acute pancreatitis: improved correlation with patient outcome. *AJR Am J Roentgenol*. 2004;183:1261–1265. [PMID: 15505289]

C. Chronic Pancreatitis (See Chapter 29)

Chronic pancreatitis is a progressive, irreversible inflammatory, and fibrosing disease of the pancreas. CT findings of chronic pancreatitis include dilation of the main pancreatic duct, parenchymal atrophy, pancreatic calcifications, and pseudocysts (Figure 9–52). In chronic pancreatitis, optimal MRI examination should include T1- and T2-weighted images and MRCP sequences. The role of MRCP in chronic pancreatitis is still controversial but evolving. Comparisons between MRCP and ERCP in cases of chronic pancreatitis have revealed agreement of 83–100% for identification of ductal dilation, 70–92% for identification of narrowing, and 92–100% for identification of filling defects, respectively. A prospective study on 99 subjects compared the accuracy of

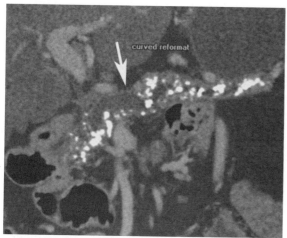

▲ **Figure 9–52.** Chronic pancreatitis. Curved, reformatted CT image shows an atrophic pancreas with numerous calcifications and irregular ductal dilation (*arrow*).

EUS and MRCP with a composite gold standard using ERCP, surgical pathology, and/or long-term clinical follow-up for the diagnosis of chronic pancreatitis. EUS showed 93% sensitivity and 93% specificity while MRCP showed 65% sensitivity and 90% specificity for diagnosis of chronic pancreatitis.

Several centers have investigated functional imaging of the pancreas with MRI in evaluation of chronic pancreatitis by obtaining MRCP images before and after intravenous secretin administration, showing improved visualization of the pancreatic duct and its side branches. Furthermore, the volume of effluent into the duodenal lumen can be graded, allowing a relative estimation of the exocrine function. In particular, secretin-enhanced MRCP has proven useful in ruling out chronic pancreatitis given that ductal changes may precede parenchymal changes in chronic pancreatitis and thus secretin MRCP may have a role in early chronic pancreatitis detection. Nonetheless, given its significant cost and relative unavailability, its use in clinical practice is limited.

Conwell DL, Lee LS, Yadav D, et al. American Pancreatic Association practice guidelines in chronic pancreatitis: evidence-based report on diagnostic guidelines. *Pancreas.* 2014;43:1143–1162. [PMID: 25333398]

Ketwaroo G, Brown A, Young B, et al. Defining the accuracy of secretin pancreatic function testing in patients with suspected early chronic pancreatitis. *Am J Gastroenterol.* 2013;108: 1360–1366. [PMID: 23711627]

Pungpapong S, Wallace MB, Woodward TA, Noh KW, Raimondo M. Accuracy of endoscopic ultrasonography and magnetic resonance cholangiopancreatography for the diagnosis of chronic pancreatitis: a prospective comparison study. *J Clin Gastroenterol.* 2007;41(1):88–93. [PMID: 17198070]

Souza D, Alessandrino F, Ketwaroo GA, Sawhney M, Mortele KJ. Accuracy of a novel noninvasive secretin-enhanced MRCP severity index scoring system for diagnosis of chronic pancreatitis: correlation with EUS-based Rosemont criteria. *Radiol Med.* 2020;125(9):816–826. [PMID: 32266691]

3. Developmental Disorders

A. Imaging Algorithm

The definitive diagnosis of the two most important pancreatic developmental variants, pancreas divisum and annular pancreas, is made with ERCP. MDCT and MRI, however, may depict both pancreas divisum and annular pancreas. MRCP has been shown to be extremely sensitive and specific for depicting pancreas divisum.

B. Congenital Anomalies

Pancreas divisum is the most common congenital anomaly of the pancreatic ductal system, being reported in up to 10% of the population. The ventral duct (duct of Wirsung) drains only the ventral pancreatic anlage through the major papilla while the majority of the gland empties into the minor papilla through the dorsal duct or duct of Santorini. Pancreas divisum is usually asymptomatic but is found more frequently in patients with chronic abdominal pain, elevated pancreatic function tests, and idiopathic pancreatitis than in the general population. MRCP easily demonstrates the noncommunicating dorsal and ventral ducts in pancreatic divisum.

Annular pancreas is a rare congenital anomaly in which incomplete rotation of the ventral anlage leads to a segment of the pancreas encircling the second part of the duodenum. The incidence of annular pancreas is 1 in 2000. Annular pancreas can be diagnosed on the basis of CT, MRI, and ERCP findings that reveal pancreatic tissue and an annular duct encircling the descending duodenum.

Mortele KJ, Rocha TC, Streeter JL, et al. Multimodality imaging of pancreatic and biliary congenital anomalies. *Radiographics.* 2006;26:715–731. [PMID: 16702450]

Mortele KJ, Wiesner W, Zou K, et al. Asymptomatic nonspecific serum hyperamylasemia and hyperlipasemia: spectrum of MRCP findings and clinical implications. *Abdom Imaging.* 2004;29:109–114. [PMID: 15160763]

SUMMARY OF CURRENT RECOMMENDATIONS

Developments in imaging technology in recent years have led to many improvements in the field of diagnostic GI radiology. Many semi-invasive diagnostic methods are being replaced by noninvasive imaging technologies. MRCP has widely replaced ERCP in the diagnosis and staging of pancreatobiliary disorders; virtual colonoscopy is an efficient screening method for colon cancer; and MRI enterography is becoming the standard imaging technique for many small bowel disorders. As a result, there has been a significant decline in the use of fluoroscopic imaging techniques. While CT continues to be the most effective modality for the initial evaluation of patients with many diseases involving the GI system particularly the acute abdomen. MRI and MRCP are reserved for specific diseases and clinical indications, such as diagnosis of HCC, inflammatory bowel disease, and cystic pancreatic lesions. PET/CT, on the other hand, is primarily used on oncologic imaging and reserved for staging of selected GI cancers.

Acute and Chronic Gastrointestinal Toxicities of Oncologic Therapy

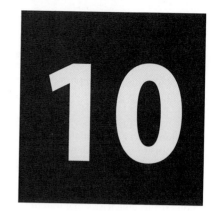

Lawrence Kogan, MD

Shilpa Grover, MD, MPH

ESSENTIAL CONCEPTS

▶ The incidence of acute gastrointestinal complications of antineoplastic treatment is high. However, symptoms may be mild and the presentation delayed.

▶ Nausea, vomiting, and diarrhea are highly prevalent in cancer patients while on antineoplastic therapy. However, their management varies based on the underlying etiology, which can frequently be multifactorial.

▶ Molecular targeted agents and immune checkpoint inhibitors (ICIs) can cause several other gastrointestinal complications in addition to diarrhea/colitis. These include hepatitis, gastrointestinal bleeding, perforation, and rarely pancreatitis.

▶ Early evaluation and management of gastrointestinal toxicities are essential to avoid serious complications.

▶ Cancer survivors who are not on active treatment require monitoring and intervention for the long-term sequelae of cancer and its treatment.

Gastrointestinal toxicity from antineoplastic therapy can cause significant morbidity and adversely impact ongoing oncologic care. With advances in cancer care, it is also important to address long-term sequela of antineoplastic therapy which can impact quality of life.

ACUTE COMPLICATIONS

1. Diarrhea

General Considerations

Diarrhea is a frequent side effect of antineoplastic therapy. However, the incidence and mechanisms by which diarrhea occurs vary with chemotherapy, molecular targeted therapy, and in patients on immunotherapy for cancer.

A. Chemotherapy

Cytotoxic chemotherapy that targets rapidly dividing cells was the first treatment class for cancer and remains the standard of care for many types of malignancy. Although effective at killing cancer cells, they can cause significant systemic side effects. Chemotherapy induced diarrhea is common amongst multiple different regimens, but is most frequently reported with fluoropyrimidines (5- fluorouracil), their prodrugs (eg, capecitabine), and irinotecan. Approximately 50–90% of patients on these agents have diarrhea, and in 5–20% of patients' symptoms are severe.

B. Molecular Targeted Therapy

Aberrant activation of kinases is an important step in oncogenesis. Tyrosine kinase inhibitors (TKIs) include intravenously administered monoclonal antibodies that target the ligand or receptor and orally administered small molecule inhibitors which target one or more intracellular kinases. Diarrhea is a common adverse effect of kinase inhibitors, with 50–95% of patients having some diarrhea and an eight-fold greater risk of developing high-grade diarrhea compared to placebo. Kinase inhibitors targeting epidermal growth factor receptor (EGFR) and vascular epithelial growth factor receptor (VEGF) are frequent causes of diarrhea that can be more severe when used in conjunction with chemotherapy. EGFR inhibitors are frequently associated with more severe diarrhea that occurs early in the course of treatment. Human epidermal growth factor receptor 2 (HER2) inhibitors such as trastuzumab and newer HER2 inhibitors such as neratinib can cause diarrhea in almost all patients and severe symptoms in up to 40%. Aside from TKIs, other targeted therapies can also cause diarrhea. Mild to moderate diarrhea has been observed in approximately 80% of patients treated with anaplastic lymphoma kinase (ALK) inhibitors such as ceritinib or oral inhibitors of cyclin-dependent kinases (CDK) 4 and 6 such as abemaciclib and in half the patients treated with combinations of MEK and BRAF inhibitors (trametinib/dabrafenib, binimetinib/encorafenib).

C. Immune Checkpoint Inhibitors

Cytotoxic T-lymphocyte-associated antigen 4 and pro-grammed cell death protein 1 and its ligand (PD-1/PD-L1) are inhibitory immune receptors (immune checkpoints) that are broadly considered as physiologic brakes to an unregu-lated immune response which is triggered by the presence of tumor antigenic material. ICIs are monoclonal antibodies that inactivate these brakes and thereby facilitate immune activation and an anti-tumor response. However, activated T-cells can cross-react with host antigens and cause a variety of immune-related adverse events (irAE), particularly in the gastrointestinal tract.

Gastrointestinal toxicity, and more specifically colitis, is among the leading irAE's that lead to withdrawal or discon-tinuation of ICIs. In clinical trials of patients treated with CTLA-4 inhibitor, ipilimumab, diarrhea is reported in 23–33% of which 3–6% is severe (Grade 3 or 4 by com-mon terminology criteria for adverse events; CTCAE) (Table 10–1). Patients treated with PD-1/PD-L1 blockade monotherapy have a lower incidence of diarrhea (11–19%) and symptoms are usually milder, with severe diarrhea seen in 1–3%. The use of anti-CTLA-4 and anti-PD-1/PD-L1 anti-bodies in combination has the highest incidence of colitis (44%, Grade 3–4 in 9%).

Nonsteroidal anti-inflammatory drug use, pre-existing inflammatory bowel disease or microscopic colitis, and low serum vitamin D levels have been implicated as risk factors for the development of ICI colitis. The incidence of ICI diar-rhea and colitis also appears to be dose related in patients treated with CTLA-4 inhibitor ipilimumab. Increased fecal Bacteroidetes phylum and its families (Bacteroida-ceae, Rikenellaceae, and Barnesiellaceae), as well as micro-bial genetic pathways involved in polyamine transport and B vitamin biosynthesis, are correlated with resistance to the development of colitis following CTLA-4 blockade. Serum markers, such as interleukin-17 and absolute eosinophil count correlate with severe colitis and overall irAE's. It is unclear if the underlying tumor histology is a risk factor for ICI colitis or whether apparent differences in rates of ICI coli-tis in patients with melanoma are due to higher use of ipilim-umab and increased physician awareness.

▶ Pathogenesis

Mechanisms for chemotherapy-induced diarrhea include increased secretion of electrolytes by luminal secretagogues, a decrease in intestinal absorptive capacity due to direct epi-thelial injury or surgery, an increase in intraluminal osmotic substances leading to watery diarrhea and enhanced gastro-intestinal motility from surgery.

The mechanism of diarrhea due to TKIs is unknown, but it is likely multifactorial. Tyrosine kinase receptors are overexpressed in gut epithelia and it is suspected that secre-tory diarrhea can result from activation of intestinal chlo-ride secretory pathways. Pancreatic atrophy from epithelial hypoxia can result in steatorrhea. Inhibition of EGFR which has stimulatory effects on enterocyte proliferation can lead to mucosal atrophy and secondary malabsorption. Agents that target KIT, which is also expressed on the interstitial cells of Cajal, the pacemakers of the GI tract, can alter GI tract motility.

Diarrhea caused by checkpoint inhibitor immunotherapy with CTLA-4 and PD-1/PD-L1 inhibitors is immune medi-ated. Antineoplastic activity of ICIs results from their effect on immune checkpoints that normally serve to dampen the immune response and protect against detrimental inflamma-tion and autoimmunity. However, the mechanism of check-point blockade toxicity is unclear. Patients with CTLA-4 haploinsufficiency have severe inflammatory disease of the colon and phenotypic similarities to CTLA-4 blockade. The increase in incidence of toxicity due to ipilimumab with higher doses suggests that toxicity may arise after a thresh-old level of CTLA-4 is inhibited. Differences in the extent of receptor occupancy are hypothesized as a possible expla-nation for why some individuals are more susceptible to

Table 10–1. Common terminology criteria for adverse events grading for diarrhea & enterocolitis.

	Grade 1	Grade 2	Grade 3	Grade 4	Grade 5
Diarrhea	• Increase of <4 stools/day from baseline • Mild increase in ostomy output	• Increase in 4–6 stools/day from baseline • Moderate increase in ostomy output. • Limiting instrumental ADL	• Increase in ≥7 stools/day from baseline • Hospitalization indicated • Severe increase in ostomy output. • Limiting self-care ADL	• Life-threatening conse-quences or urgent inter-vention indicated	• Death
Enterocolitis	• Asymptomatic; clinical or diagnos-tic observation only; no intervention indicated	• Abdominal pain; mucus or blood in stool	• Severe abdominal pain; peritoneal signs	• Life-threatening consequences • Urgent intervention indicated	• Death

Data from Common Terminology Criteria for Adverse Events (CTCAE v5), November 17, 2017, U.S. Department of Health and Human Services, National Institutes of Health, National Cancer Institute.

developing toxicities than others. It has also been hypothesized that an infectious trigger may lead to inflammatory toxicities when downregulation of T-cell responses through immune checkpoints is inhibited.

Clinical Presentation

Diarrhea associated with VEGF inhibitors is usually mild to moderate in severity but can be severe when used in conjunction with chemotherapy or radiotherapy. EGFR inhibitors are frequently associated with more severe diarrhea that occurs early in the course of treatment (within 1 week). Immune-related diarrhea secondary to ICIs is usually a consequence of underlying colonic inflammation. Patients with diarrhea/colitis usually present with frequent nonbloody stools associated with urgency, although bloody diarrhea can occur. Approximately 25% of patients with ICI related diarrhea have concomitant enteritis, but in rare cases, patients may present with diarrhea due to enteritis alone. The median onset of diarrhea in patients treated with ipilimumab or nivolumab is approximately 6–8 weeks after initiation of therapy whereas the onset appears to be later in patients treated with anti-PD-1/PD-L1 therapy. In patients with concurrent upper gastrointestinal tract involvement, other symptoms include nausea, vomiting, early satiety, and bloating.

Diagnostic Evaluation

The evaluation of diarrhea is based on the duration, severity, and presence of alarm features that may warrant hospitalization.

A. Laboratory Studies

Laboratory evaluation should include a complete blood count, and comprehensive metabolic panel for associated electrolyte derangements and hepatotoxicity (Table 10–2). Routine evaluation should include stool testing for *Clostridioides difficile* in those with recent antibiotic exposure and stool culture for bacterial pathogens such as *Escherichia coli*, *Salmonella*, *Shigella* and *Campylobacter*, *Yersinia*, *Vibrio* or *Aeromomas*. In addition, patients with risk factors or recent travel to endemic areas additional testing should be considered. An elevated fecal calprotectin level may be indicative of intestinal inflammation secondary to ICI colitis, but it has limitations in sensitivity and may not be elevated in patients with ICI enteritis.

Table 10–2. Evaluation of diarrhea in patients with cancer on antineoplastic therapy.

Evaluation	Indication	Test
Stool tests	• All patients with ≥1 Grade 1[a] diarrhea	• Stool bacterial cultures (*Salmonella*, *Shigella*, *Campylobacter*) and testing for Shiga toxin • Fecal calprotectin • *Clostridioides* (previously *Clostridium*) difficile • Fecal calprotectin • Rotavirus stool antigen[b] • Norovirus PCR[b]
	• Patients with ≥1 Grade 1 diarrhea and additional risk factors (travel, ongoing outbreak, seafood or shellfish exposure)	• Vibrio • Aeromonas • Listeria • Yersinia • Stool ova and parasite smear (for Giardia and cryptosporidium)
Blood tests	• All patients with ≥1 Grade 1 diarrhea	• Complete metabolic panel • Complete blood count • Thyroid stimulating hormone • Celiac serologies

Imaging	• Grade 3 or 4 diarrhea
	• Diarrhea of any grade with any one of the following:
	  • Fever
	  • Abdominal pain
	  • Concerning abdominal examination findings (ie, severe tenderness, or peritoneal signs)
	  • Concern for toxic megacolon
		• Abdominal computed tomography scan

[a]Common terminology criteria for adverse events grading of diarrhea.
[b]Diagnostic tests for norovirus and rotavirus must be interpreted together with epidemiologic and clinical factors. Norovirus can cause a prolonged diarrheal illness in immunocompromised patients.
PCR: Polymerase chain reaction.

B. Abdominal Imaging

Abdominal computed tomography (CT) findings in patients with ICI colitis are not specific and include mesenteric vessel engorgement, marked thickening of the bowel wall, mucosal hyperenhancement, and a fluid-filled colon. Colitis on imaging may be diffuse or segmental. A segmental colitis associated with diverticulosis and isolated rectosigmoid colitis without diverticulosis have been associated with ICI colitis.

C. Endoscopy

All patients with bloody diarrhea, and those with persistent nonbloody diarrhea should undergo endoscopic evaluation. Endoscopic evaluation serves to rule out cytomegalovirus infection, can support a specific diagnosis (eg, ICI colitis) and can guide therapy. In patients on ICIs, a flexible sigmoidoscopy with biopsies of the left colon can be diagnostic in approximately 95% of patients. However, sigmoidoscopy risks missing the most severe colitis, if present, as it may be located in the proximal colon.

Ipilimumab-induced colitis can result in continuous inflammation from the anus to the cecum. This inflammation is characterized by edema, erythema, and friability, with diffuse shallow ulceration. There may be isolated inflammation of the small bowel or colon that appears normal or with mild abnormalities. On histopathology, a neutrophilic inflammation with increased intraepithelial lymphocytes, and crypt epithelial cell apoptosis may be seen. Granulomas are rare and features of chronicity may be limited or absent. In a minority of patients, chronic changes to the epithelial architecture may be seen on initial presentation. Lymphocytic colitis and collagenous colitis have been reported in approximately 12% of cases with increased lymphoplasmacytic infiltrate in the lamina propria and intraepithelial lymphocytosis in the surface epithelium with scattered crypt apoptosis. The severity of endoscopic findings and the presence of pancolitis have been associated with the need for infliximab.

▶ Management

A. General Measures in All Patients

Volume depletion in patients with grade 1 or 2 diarrhea can usually be managed with oral hydration. Most patients with grade 3 or 4 diarrhea or those with alarm signs (abdominal pain, hematochezia, fever), require hospitalization for intravenous fluids and close monitoring and correction of electrolyte derangements. Dietary recommendations in this setting have not been extensively evaluated. Patients should be advised to restrict dietary lactose as secondary lactose malabsorption can develop due to concomitant enteritis. Dietary supplements with high-osmolality and medications that exacerbate diarrhea should be avoided.

B. Specific Measures Based on Severity and Oncologic Therapy

1. Cytotoxic chemotherapy and targeted therapy—In patients with diarrhea due to cytotoxic chemotherapy or targeted therapy, the decision to continue treatment varies according to the specific drug, and prescribing information generally includes recommendations for dose modification for individual drugs. Antidiarrheal medication may be used once an infection has been ruled out. Octreotide is indicated in patients with persistent diarrhea despite loperamide.

2. Immune checkpoint inhibitors—Once an infectious etiology has been excluded with appropriate laboratory testing, patients with mild symptoms (CTCAE grade 1 diarrhea or less than 4 bowel movements per day) that persists for more than 2 weeks, or ≥ grade 2 symptoms (4–7 bowel movements per day), should be treated with glucocorticoid therapy. Patients may be initially treated with budesonide (9 mg/day for at least 8 weeks) which is then tapered by 3 mg increments for a total of 4–6 weeks of therapy. Patients with persistent grade 1 diarrhea who do not respond to budesonide or patients with grade 2 diarrhea for more than 3 days require treatment with prednisone (0.5–1 mg/kg/day). In patients who respond, prednisone is gradually tapered by 5–10 mg/week with the goal of discontinuing prednisone over 6–8 weeks (Table 10–3).

Patients with alarm symptoms or severe enterocolitis (grade 3 or 4 diarrhea) require high doses of intravenous corticosteroids (methylprednisolone 1–2 mg/kg/day). Bowel rest is not recommended in patients with severe symptoms in the absence of fulminant disease. In patients who respond, intravenous glucocorticoids should be converted to equivalent dose of oral glucocorticoids in 3 to 5 days. Oral glucocorticoids should be tapered over 6 weeks by decreasing the dose by 5–10 mg every week.

Patients who do not improve with intravenous corticosteroids after approximately 3 days should be considered steroid refractory and treated with tumor necrosis factor (anti-TNF)-alpha inhibitor infliximab (5–10 mg/kg). Vedolizumab, a humanized anti-alpha-4-beta-7 integrin monoclonal antibody is an alternative in patients with steroid-dependent or steroid-refractory enterocolitis, particularly if colitis is infliximab refractory.

▶ Prognosis & Implications for Oncologic Treatment

Diarrhea related to TKI drug toxicity has been correlated with clinical benefit or a predictive factor of tumor response. It has also been associated with increased time to progression.

Data are conflicting for the association between the incidence of irAEs and the antitumor efficacy of immunotherapy. Development of diarrhea and/or colitis during use

Table 10–3. Evaluation & management of ICI colitis.

	Testing	Treatment	Management of ICI
Grade 1	Stool and blood tests[a]	• Oral rehydration • Budesonide for progressing or persistent symptoms >2 weeks	• Continue ICI
Grade 1 with persistent symptoms or Grade 2	Above, plus • Abdominal CT in selected patients • Endoscopic evaluation	• Oral rehydration • Oral prednisone (0.5–1 mg/kg)	• Discontinue CTLA-4 agent • Hold PD-1/PDL-1 agent till symptoms improve to ≤ grade 1 • Taper prednisone over 4–6 weeks • Worsening symptoms, manage as Grade 3

Alarm signs and/or Grade 3/4 diarrhea	Above, with
	• Abdominal CT
	• Urgent endoscopic evaluation
		• Consider hospitalization
		• IV steroids (methylprednisolone 1–2mg/kg, or equivalent)
		• Biologic agents (infliximab, vedolizumab) for steroid refractory symptoms or steroid dependent colitis.
			• Discontinue CTLA-4 agent
			• PD-1/PDL-1 agent:
			  • Grade 3- Hold PD-1/PDL-1 agent till symptoms improve to ≤ grade 1
			  • Grade 4: Discontinue CTLA-4 agent

[a]Table 10–1.

Alarm signs: severe abdominal pain, fever/sepsis, bloody diarrhea, hypovolemia, moderate/severe nausea or vomiting.

of one checkpoint inhibitor does not necessarily prohibit the use of another. The decision to rechallenge after prior toxicity is based on the severity of colitis, the immunotherapy regimen (CTLA-4, PD-1/PD-L1, or combination), the response to systemic immunosuppression/need for biologic therapy, and from an oncologic standpoint, both the tumor response to the initial immunotherapy regimen and the presence of alternative treatment options.

Andreyev J, Ross P, Donnellan C, et al. Guidance on the management of diarrhea during cancer chemotherapy. *Lancet Oncol.* 2014;15(10):e447–e460. [PMID: 25186048]

Bossi P, Antonuzzo A, Cherny NI, et al. Diarrhoea in adult cancer patients: ESMO Clinical Practice Guidelines. *Ann Oncol.* 2018;29(suppl 4):iv126–iv142. [PMID: 29931177]

Brahmer JR, Lacchetti C, Schneider BJ, et al., Management of immune-related adverse events in patients treated with immune checkpoint inhibitor therapy: American Society of Clinical Oncology Clinical Practice Guideline. *J Clin Oncol.* 2018;36(17):1714–1768. [PMID: 29442540]

Dougan M, Wang Y, Rubio-Tapia A, et al. AGA clinical practice update on diagnosis and management of immune checkpoint inhibitor (ICI) colitis and hepatitis: expert review. *Gastroenterology.* 2021;160(4):1384–1393. [PMID: 33080231]

Dubin K, Callahan MK, Ren B, et al. Intestinal microbiome analyses identify melanoma patients at risk for checkpoint-blockade-induced colitis. *Nat Commun.* 2016;7:10391. [PMID: 26837003]

Grover S, Dougan M, Tyan K, et al. Vitamin D intake is associated with decreased risk of immune checkpoint inhibitor-induced colitis. *Cancer.* 2020;126(16):3758–3767. [PMID: 32567084]

Grover S, Ruan AB, Srivoleti P, et al. Safety of immune checkpoint inhibitors in patients with pre-existing inflammatory bowel disease and microscopic colitis. *JCO Oncol Pract.* 2020;16(9):e933–e942. [PMID: 32401685]

Li J, Gu J. Diarrhea with epidermal growth factor receptor tyrosine kinase inhibitors in cancer patients: a meta-analysis of randomized controlled trials. *Crit Rev Oncol Hematol.* 2019;134:31–38. [PMID: 30771871]

Marthey L, Mateus C, Mussini C, et al. Cancer immunotherapy with anti-CTLA-4 monoclonal antibodies induces an inflammatory bowel disease. *J Crohns Colitis.* 2016;10(4):395–401. [PMID: 26783344]

Naidoo J, Page DB, Li BT, et al. Toxicities of the anti-PD-1 and anti-PD-L1 immune checkpoint antibodies [published correction appears in Ann Oncol. 2016 Jul;27(7):1362]. *Ann Oncol.* 2015;26(12):2375–2391. [PMID: 26371282]

1. Gastrointestinal Bleeding

General Considerations

Gastrointestinal bleeding in patients with cancer may result from a direct complication of the underlying cancer or as a consequence of treatment. Bleeding can also result from other benign minor lesions such as erosive gastropathy and duodenopathy from cytotoxic chemotherapy, particularly in the setting of anticoagulant use. Bleeding may also be more difficult to control due to coexisting coagulopathies, thrombocytopenia or hepatic dysfunction. In a cohort of 451 patients with acute and chronic leukemias and other myeloproliferative disorders, the incidence of gastrointestinal bleeding was approximately 7%. The most prevalent causes of upper gastrointestinal bleeding were erosive gastritis, duodenal ulcers, and neutropenic enterocolitis. These disorders were frequently complicated by thrombocytopenia. Patients with cancer on emetogenic chemotherapy can present with hematemesis from a Mallory Weiss tear. Variceal bleeding may result from noncirrhotic portal hypertension due to neoplastic occlusion of the intrahepatic portal vein or oncologic therapy (eg, trastuzumab, oxaliplatin or doxorubicin).

Although rare, the most likely infectious causes of bleeding in immunocompromised patients are Herpes Simplex Virus (HSV) and cytomegalovirus (CMV). While HSV tends to cause shallow ulcers in the esophagus, CMV usually leads to intestinal ulcers. This bleeding is typically slow and self-limited.

Radiotherapy (RT) can cause microvascular injury leading to tissue ischemia. Risk factors of RT induced gastrointestinal toxicity include the cumulative dose, dose per fraction irradiated volume, specific area of exposure, and RT technique employed. In patients with prostate cancer, the use of three-dimensional conformal RT techniques of intensity-modulated RT and image-guided RT may minimize the dose delivered to the anal canal and inferior rectum, decreasing the risk of radiation proctitis.

Hemobilia is a rare cause of acute gastrointestinal bleeding but should be considered in any patient with acute upper gastrointestinal bleed and a recent history of hepatic parenchymal or biliary tract instrumentation and/or injury (eg, liver biopsy, endoscopic biliary biopsies or stenting) and in patients with hepatic or bile duct tumors

Clinical Presentation

Patients with acute upper gastrointestinal bleeding may present with hematemesis, melena, or hematochezia; those with lower gastrointestinal bleeding may present with hematochezia or melena. Symptoms in patients with radiation proctitis following pelvic RT include diarrhea, urgency, tenesmus, and gastrointestinal bleeding which can range from mild self-limited hematochezia to severe symptomatic gastrointestinal bleeding. Radiation effects or direct extension of tumor can cause fistula development to the aorta and other vascular structures resulting in massive upper gastrointestinal bleed. Bleeding can result from diffuse mucosal ulceration or from erosion into an underlying vessel. More commonly however, patients may have chronic GI bleeding manifested by iron deficiency anemia.

Diagnostic Evaluation & Management Considerations

The diagnostic and initial therapeutic approach to patients with GI bleeding for benign etiologies of gastrointestinal bleeding are similar in patients with cancer as those without cancer.

However, it is important to consider that chemotherapy-induced platelet dysfunction may affect normal homeostatic

mechanisms. There are no robust data as to the minimal safe platelet count for safe therapeutic endoscopy. However, platelet transfusions should be readily available when performing therapeutic endoscopy in patients with a platelet count below a threshold of 50–80,000/µl. The management of gastrointestinal bleeding either from a primary tumor or metastatic disease is endoscopically challenging. Endoscopic hemostasis with contact thermal therapy has low to modest rates of achieving immediate hemostasis but has high recurrent bleeding rates. Argon plasma coagulation has the advantage of ease of application, rapid and wide treatment of multiple lesions related to tumor bleeding, and reduced depth of penetration, thereby limiting the risk of perforation. However, data on the use of APC in the management of endoluminal tumor bleeding are limited to small retrospective studies. Small retrospective series that have evaluated the efficacy of hemostatic powder in upper GI-tumor related bleeding have reported successful hemostasis rates of up to 93%, but with rebleeding as early as 3 days after initial treatment. In addition, if initial application is unsuccessful in controlling bleeding, the use of hemostatic spray precludes tumor visualization and makes the use of other methods of hemostasis more challenging. Embolization for tumor related bleeding also has some notable challenges and limitations. The arterial supply to the tumor independent of the bowel mucosa is rarely visualized. The risk of bowel ischemia must therefore be balanced with the extent of embolization. Embolization may not result in complete cessation of bleeding which may be venous in nature but reduces blood flow to allow for hemostasis. Endoscopic measures and embolization are temporizing measures until more definitive oncologic therapy can be undertaken.

Arena M, Masci E, Eusebi LH, et al. Hemospray for treatment of acute bleeding due to upper gastrointestinal tumours. *Dig Liver Dis.* 2017;49(5):514–517. [PMID: 28065526]

Soylu AR, Buyukasik Y, Cetiner D, et al. Overt gastrointestinal bleeding in haematologic neoplasms. *Dig Liver Dis.* 2005;37(12):917–922. [PMID: 16243010]

Torres HA, Kontoyiannis DP, Bodey GP, et al. Gastrointestinal cytomegalovirus disease in patients with cancer: a two decade experience in a tertiary care cancer center. *Eur J Cancer.* 2005;41(15):2268–2279. [PMID: 16143517]

Yu T, Zhang Q, Zheng T, et al. The effectiveness of intensity modulated radiation therapy versus three-dimensional radiation therapy in prostate cancer: a meta-analysis of the literatures. *PLoS One.* 2016;11(5):e0154499. [PMID: 27171271]

2. Gastrointestinal Perforation

General Considerations

Gastrointestinal perforation may result from tumor necrosis, obstruction, or as a result of ischemic injury following chemotherapy or RT. VEGF targeted therapies in particular have been associated with an increased risk of gastrointestinal bleeding and perforation. This risk has been most widely noted with bevacizumab, a humanized anti-VEGF monoclonal antibody which may cause ulceration, fistulation or free perforation in 0.9% of patients within 1 year of treatment. Proposed mechanisms for bevacizumab induced bleeding include ulceration in areas of tumor necrosis, ulceration from disturbed platelet-endothelial cell homeostasis in the submucosa, impaired healing of pathologic or surgical bowel injury, and mesenteric ischemia from thrombosis and/or vasoconstriction. In a meta-analysis of 34 trials, bevacizumab therapy significantly increased the risk of fatal adverse events especially when combined with chemotherapeutic agents such as platinum (cisplatin, carboplatin, or oxaliplatin) and taxanes (paclitaxel or docetaxel). Other risk factors for gastrointestinal perforation include concurrent radiation, corticosteroid use, the presence of tumor in situ, peritoneal carcinomatosis, and surgery. However, gastrointestinal bleeding and perforation can occur in the absence of risk factors, at sites distant to the tumor, and in the absence of disease in the peritoneal cavity. Gastrointestinal perforation has also been reported in patients treated with small-molecule EGFR inhibitors (ie, erlotinib and gefitinib), phosphoinositide 3-kinase (PI3K) delta inhibitors (idelalisib), and in 1% of patients treated with an MEK inhibitor, trametinib.

Clinical Presentation

Unlike immunocompetent patients who present with sudden or severe pain spontaneously or following endoscopy or surgery, patients on immunosuppressive therapy may have an impaired inflammatory response, and little pain or tenderness on physical examination. They may also present after the development of an abscess, or fistula. Signs and symptoms of early sepsis can also be nonspecific and include chills, malaise, and headache until they develop fulminant sepsis.

Diagnostic Evaluation

Gastrointestinal perforation may be suspected based upon history and physical examination findings, but the diagnosis is established by imaging. Abdominal CT scan can identify extraluminal gas and the site of the perforation.

Management

Initial management of the patient with gastrointestinal perforation includes intravenous fluids and broad-spectrum antibiotic therapy. Surgical consultation should be sought early in patients with suspected gastrointestinal perforation. Indications for surgical intervention include the presence of abdominal sepsis, worsening or continuing abdominal pain, and diffuse peritonitis. However, the decision to undergo surgery should take into consideration the patient's overall prognosis and goals of oncologic care.

Prevention

This risk of gastrointestinal perforation is the basis for present recommendations to hold VEGF-inhibitor therapy for 6 weeks before and 4 weeks after surgery. In patients undergoing endoscopic procedures, management should be based on the inherent risk of perforation associated with the procedure. Data suggest that low-risk endoscopic procedures may be performed without an increased risk of complications. However, for elective high-risk procedures, VEGF-inhibitor therapy should be avoided within 6 weeks of the last VEGF-inhibitor dose.

Huang H, Zheng Y, Zhu J, Zhang J, Chen H, Chen X. An updated meta-analysis of fatal adverse events caused by bevacizumab therapy in cancer patients. *PLoS One.* 2014;9(3):e89960. [PMID: 24599121]

Krajewski KM, Braschi-Amirfarzan M, DiPiro PJ, Jagannathan JP, Shinagare AB. Molecular targeted therapy in modern oncology: imaging assessment of treatment response and toxicities. *Korean J Radiol.* 2017;18(1):28–41. [PMID: 28096716]

Mourad N, Lourenço N, Delyon J, et al. Severe gastrointestinal toxicity of MEK inhibitors. *Melanoma Res.* 2019;29(5):556–559. [PMID: 31095035]

3. Nausea & Vomiting
General Considerations

Nausea and vomiting are highly prevalent symptoms in patients with cancer and can cause significant morbidity. These symptoms may be secondary to a variety of causes, including:

- side effects from emetogenic antineoplastic therapy, concurrent medications (ie, opioid analgesics),
- gastroparesis,
- iatrogenic (ie, postsurgical or celiac plexus nerve block),
- radiation therapy,
- metabolic abnormalities (ie, hypercalcemia, adrenal insufficiency),
- bowel obstruction secondary to intrinsic or extrinsic compression, adhesions, or postradiation fibrosis and
- increased intracranial pressure from primary brain tumors or metastatic disease.

The incidence of nausea or vomiting associated with antineoplastic therapy varies widely based on the treatment regimen. Overall, nausea and vomiting are most commonly seen in patients treated with cytotoxic chemotherapy, followed by TKIs and ICIs.

A. Cytotoxic Chemotherapy

Chemotherapeutic agents vary widely in their risk of emetogenicity which can range from minimal to high (>90%).

The use of highly emetogenic cytotoxic chemotherapy include high dose cyclophosphamide, cyclophosphamide-anthracycline combination and cisplatin. Although overall less emetogenic than cytotoxic chemotherapy, TKIs are generally in the medium emetogenic risk category, with a risk of 30–90%. Overall, ICIs carry the lowest of emetogenic risk. Ipilimumab is considered low risk (10–30%), while nivolumab and pembrolizumab are considered minimal risk, with a probability <10%.

Pathogenesis

The pathogenesis of emesis is complex, multifactorial and incompletely understood. The strongest evidence supports a hormonally mediated response to free radicals that is then propagated through the central and peripheral nervous systems. For acute chemotherapy-induced nausea and vomiting serotonin is released by enterochromaffin cells in the small intestine, which then binds to 5-HT3 receptors on vagal afferent nerves and send signals back to the vomiting centers of the brain. Delayed chemotherapy-induced nausea and vomiting is felt to be a result of chemotherapy acting directly on the area postrema of the brainstem, which then releases substance P leading to neurokinin-1 receptor activation, triggering nausea and vomiting. This centrally mediated response presents at least 24 hours after treatment.

Clinical Presentation

Nausea and vomiting following chemotherapy may be acute, delayed, or anticipatory emesis.

- *Acute emesis:* Usually presents 1–2 hours after a chemotherapy treatment, with severity peaking about 6 hours and improvement after 24 hours.
- *Delayed emesis:* Usually presents 24–120 hours after a chemotherapy treatment, but is not as severe as acute emesis.
- *Anticipatory emesis:* Triggered by external stimuli such as smells or images prior to the delivery of cancer treatment.

Diagnostic Evaluation

Historical clues and concurrent symptoms may be indicative of a specific etiology and can guide evaluation. The presence of concurrent pain and new abdominal distension is suggestive of an intestinal obstruction. Vomiting of food several hours after a meal and a succussion splash on physical examination are suggestive of a gastric outlet obstruction or gastroparesis, particularly if nausea is relieved after emesis. Projectile vomiting suggests an intracranial etiology for nausea and vomiting, and the presence of associated vertigo and nystagmus suggest underlying vestibular dysfunction. Gastroesophageal reflux disease and constipation are two common etiologies for nausea in patients with cancer.

Constipation may be secondary to one of several etiologies including autonomic dysfunction, the use of opioid medications and 5-HT$_3$ antagonists, and primary gastrointestinal tumor or metastatic disease.

Laboratory Evaluation

Initial workup of nausea and vomiting includes laboratory studies including serum sodium, calcium, albumin, potassium, creatinine, and blood urea nitrogen/creatinine. Additional evaluation is based on the suspected etiology includes an abdominal imaging (abdominal CT or plain radiographs). However, CT has a low sensitivity for peritoneal implants particularly when deposits are small (<1 cm) in size. Upper endoscopy serves to rule out gastric outlet obstruction, infiltrative (ie, amyloidosis secondary to plasma cell dyscrasia), and inflammatory (immune mediated gastritis in patients on ICIs) etiologies. Magnetic resonance imaging of the brain should be considered in patients with neurogenic vomiting.

Management

Management of nausea and vomiting is based on the underlying etiology. As examples, corticosteroids are indicated for patients with intracerebral edema and in those with adrenal insufficiency. In patients with gastroparesis, initial management is with dietary modification and prokinetics like metoclopramide with the addition of antiemetics for patients (eg, phenothiazine, prochlorperazine) with persistent symptoms. In selected patients with refractory symptoms, drainage gastrostomy tube and feeding jejunostomy tube can provide symptom palliation by decompression and nutritional support, respectively. For patients with severe constipation secondary to opioid medication, these medications should be avoided and laxative therapy is indicated. Of note, methylnaltrexone should be used with caution in patients with advanced cancer given the concern for perforation. In patients with nausea and vomiting that is secondary to antitumor therapy, medication classes for management include 5-HT3 antagonists, neurokinin-1 (NK1) inhibitors, corticosteroids and atypical antipsychotics (eg, olanzapine). Prophylactic use of one or more classes is recommended based on the emetic risk of the chemotherapy regimen. Many of these medications, as well as benzodiazepines (eg, lorazepam) are used for management of breakthrough symptoms. Special care should be taken to monitor patients' QT intervals, which can be prolonged with antiemetic medications and can cause cardiac dysrhythmias if not controlled. Although synthetic oral cannabinoids (eg, dronabinol) are approved for the treatment of breakthrough nausea or vomiting, they have modest efficacy and side-effects which have limited their use. The management of anticipatory nausea and vomiting is largely comprised of behavioral therapy and and/or benzodiazepines.

Dranitsaris G, Bouganim N, Milano C, et al. Prospective validation of a prediction tool for identifying patients at high risk for chemotherapy-induced nausea and vomiting. *J Support Oncol.* 2013;11(1):14–21. [PMID: 22763232]

Hesketh PJ, Kris MG, Basch E, et al. Antiemetics: ASCO Guideline Update [published correction appears in *J Clin Oncol.* 2020 Nov 10;38(32):3825]. *J Clin Oncol.* 2020;38(24):2782–2797. [PMID: 32658626]

Rapoport BL. Delayed chemotherapy-induced nausea and vomiting: pathogenesis, incidence, and current management. *Front Pharmacol.* 2017;8:19. [PMID: 28194109]

Razvi Y, Chan S, McFarlane T, et al. ASCO, NCCN, MASCC/ ESMO: a comparison of antiemetic guidelines for the treatment of chemotherapy-induced nausea and vomiting in adult patients. *Support Care Cancer.* 2019;27(1):87–95. [PMID: 30284039]

4. Pancreatic Toxicity

Clinical Presentation

Patients may be asymptomatic and present with elevated pancreatic enzymes in the absence of pancreatitis on CT can be seen in patients on ICIs and in patients on TKIs (eg, sorafenib, sunitinib and pazopanib). In one study of patients on sorafenib, the incidence of asymptomatic elevations in pancreatic enzymes was 56%, however acute pancreatitis was rare. Pancreatic atrophy in the absence of elevations in amylase or lipase has also been noted in patients treated with sunitinib and sorafenib. While the etiology of this phenomenon is unclear, the antiangiogenic effects of TKI leading to microvascular insufficiency have been implicated. In retrospective studies, the presence of pancreatic atrophy has been associated with poor prognosis and shorter survival. Prospective studies are needed to validate these findings.

A wide range of cytotoxic chemotherapy can be associated with acute pancreatitis, including platinum agents, antimetabolites, and taxanes. In patients on ICIs, the incidence of acute pancreatitis is low. Patients usually present with asymptomatic elevations in pancreatic lipase. In a systematic review and meta-analysis of clinical trials the incidence of asymptomatic lipase elevation after ICI use and grade 2 pancreatitis were 2.7% and 1.9%, respectively. No pancreatitis related mortality has been reported in these clinical trials. Patients treated with CTLA-4 inhibitors had a higher incidence of pancreatitis as compared to patients treated with PD-1 inhibitors (4% vs 1%). Patients treated with a combination of CTLA4 and PD-1 inhibitors had a 10 fold higher risk of acute pancreatitis as compared with CTLA-4 or PD-1 inhibitors alone. Patients treated with ICIs for melanoma had an increased incidence of pancreatitis as compared to nonmelanoma cancers.

Diagnostic Evaluation

Patients on ICIs with pancreatic enzyme elevations and vague abdominal pain, should be evaluated for nonpancreatic etiologies for abdominal pain. These may include coexisting immunotherapy gastritis or enterocolitis and in such cases, endoscopic evaluation with mucosal biopsies should be pursued to evaluate for inflammation. In asymptomatic patients, it is important to consider that elevations in pancreatic enzymes may not be due to underlying pancreatic inflammation, but due to T cell mediated inflammation of other organs that produce these enzymes. Other nonimmune mediated causes for pancreatic enzyme elevation should also be considered. This should include laboratory evaluation for renal failure (which can delay clearance of these enzymes). Abdominal imaging with pancreatic protocol CT or MRCP can rule out pancreatic duct obstruction from metastatic disease.

Management

Patients with pancreatic enzyme elevations without abdominal pain or evidence of acute pancreatitis on abdominal imaging can be monitored clinically without the need for immunosuppressive therapy. While subclinical pancreatic inflammation has been associated with pancreatic exocrine insufficiency and diabetes, the risk of these in patients with asymptomatic pancreatic enzyme elevations is unclear. Routine assessment of these enzymes in asymptomatic patients should not be performed. Immunosuppression with corticosteroids for patients on ICIs should be reserved for patients with symptomatic acute pancreatitis.

George J, Bajaj D, Sankaramangalam K, et al. Incidence of pancreatitis with the use of immune checkpoint inhibitors (ICI) in advanced cancers: a systematic review and meta-analysis. *Pancreatology.* 2019;19(4):587–594. [PMID: 31076344]

Shinagare AB, Steele E, Braschi-Amirfarzan M, Tirumani SH, Ramaiya NH. Sunitinib-associated pancreatic atrophy in patients with gastrointestinal stromal tumor: a toxicity with prognostic implications detected at imaging. *Radiology.* 2016; 281(1):140–149. [PMID: 27643769]

5. Pneumatosis Intestinalis

General Considerations

Although rare, the presence of air in the bowel wall, otherwise known as pneumatosis intestinalis, has been observed in patients on TKIs (erlotinib, crizotinib, cetuximab), and less so in patients receiving cytotoxic chemotherapy.

Clinical Presentation

Patients are usually asymptomatic and the presence of pneumatosis is often discovered incidentally. Complications including intestinal obstruction, volvulus, intussusception, hematochezia, and pneumoperitoneum due to cyst rupture, are rare.

Diagnostic Evaluation

Characteristic findings of pneumatosis intestinalis on abdominal CT scan include circumferential (cystic) collections of air adjacent to the lumen of the bowel that run in parallel with the wall of the bowel or linear collections without the air-contrast or air-fluid levels characteristically seen with intraluminal air.

Management

The management of pneumatosis intestinalis due to cancer treatment does not differ from that of individuals with pneumatosis intestinalis due to other etiologies. The presence of portal venous gas or decreased mural contrast-enhancement on CT scan, peritoneal signs, metabolic acidosis or an elevated lactate level should raise the suspicion for bowel infarction and warrant surgical evaluation. However, in the absence of these features or symptoms, patients can be managed conservatively with withdrawal of TKI treatment. Limited data suggest that pneumatosis intestinalis can recur with reinitiation of TKIs.

Abu-Sbeih H, Ali FS, Chen E, et al. Neutropenic enterocolitis: clinical features and outcomes. *Dis Colon Rectum.* 2020;63(3):381–388. [PMID: 31842164]

Gray EJ, Darvishzadeh A, Sharma A, Ganeshan D, Faria SC, Lall C. Cancer therapy-related complications in the bowel and mesentery: an imaging perspective. *Abdom Radiol (NY).* 2016; 41(10):2031–2047. [PMID: 27277528]

6. Biliary Tract Toxicity

Biliary complications associated with the use of molecular targeted therapy are rare but include acalculous cholecystitis, gallbladder perforation, and sclerosing cholangitis. Certain TKIs such as lenvatinib may present a higher risk for gallbladder disease, but this risk needs to be evaluated with additional studies. The management remains the same as for other patients with symptomatic gallbladder pathology, with surgical resection as curative treatment.

Nervo A, Ragni A, Gallo M, et al. Symptomatic biliary disorders during lenvatinib treatment for thyroid cancer: an underestimated problem. *Thyroid.* 2020;30(2):229–236. [PMID: 31854230]

Ngo D, Jia JB, Green CS, Gulati AT, Lall C. Cancer therapy related complications in the liver, pancreas, and biliary system: an imaging perspective. *Insights Imaging.* 2015;6(6):665–677. [PMID: 26443452]

CHRONIC GASTROINTESTINAL COMPLICATIONS

Chronic gastrointestinal complications of antineoplastic can significantly impact quality of life. These complications may arise months or years after completion of treatment, particularly in patients treated with RT. As examples, chronic enteritis, can cause diarrhea/steatorrhea due to carbohydrate malabsorption, small intestinal bacterial overgrowth, and bile acid malabsorption. Strictures can cause abdominal pain and bowel obstruction, and iron deficiency anemia from chronic bleeding. In addition to screening for cancer recurrence, patients with a history of cancer require careful follow-up for these gastrointestinal complications.

Andreyev HJ. GI consequences of cancer treatment: a clinical perspective. *Radiat Res.* 2016;185(4):341–348. [PMID: 27018776]

Numico G, Longo V, Courthod G, Silvestris N. Cancer survivorship: long-term side-effects of anticancer treatments of gastrointestinal cancer. *Curr Opin Oncol.* 2015;27(4):351–357. [PMID: 26049277]

Mast Cell Disorders

11

Matthew J. Hamilton, MD

Mariana Castells, MD, PhD

ESSENTIALS OF DIAGNOSIS FOR MAST CELL ACTIVATION SYNDROME

▶ Signs and symptoms of mast cell activation that involve at least two organ systems and may include abdominal pain, diarrhea, flushing, headache, and concentration difficulties.

▶ No other medical disorder better explains these signs and symptoms.

▶ Objective evidence of mast cell activation while symptomatic including increased levels of tryptase on a blood test, and/or elevated levels of mast cell metabolites including histamine and/or prostaglandin in a 24-hour urine specimen.

▶ Reduced symptoms with medications that block mast cell mediators such as antihistamines, cromolyn, ketotifen, and leukotriene antagonists.

ESSENTIALS OF DIAGNOSIS FOR SYSTEMIC MASTOCYTOSIS

▶ Symptoms of mast cell activation as stated previously as well as specific clinical manifestations such as anaphylaxis and evidence of organ dysfunction, organ enlargement, and/or unexplained bone disease in more aggressive forms.

▶ Characteristic physical examination findings particularly urticaria pigmentosa.

▶ Serum tryptase >20 ng/mL or >11.4 ng/mL in patients with characteristic signs and symptoms of mastocytosis including anaphylaxis.

▶ Documentation of abnormal clustering of 15 or more mast cells in aggregates or sheets on a bone marrow or extracutaneous biopsy (eg, liver, intestine).

▶ Demonstration of a clonal mast cell population such as abnormal cell morphology (eg, spindle forms), specific cell surface marker expression (eg, CD2, CD25), and/or positive mutational analysis (eg, *D816V* mutation on the mast cell *KIT* gene).

General Considerations

Mast cell disorders are increasingly recognized as a cause of chronic abdominal symptoms. Interestingly, the presenting signs and symptoms of mast cell activation are seen in all the types of mast cell disorders including disorders where abnormal clonal mast cells can be identified (eg, systemic mastocytosis) and disorders where the mast cells are believed to be nonclonal but with abnormal activation (eg, mast cell activation syndrome) (see Classification section for more details). These patients may complain of abdominal pain, diarrhea, nausea and vomiting, reflux, and bloating. Patients with systemic mastocytosis may additionally be at risk for peptic ulcer disease, and in the more aggressive stage portal hypertension and intestinal malabsorption.

A thorough history and physical examination is necessary to illicit the signs and symptoms of mast cell activation (see Clinical Findings section). Objective evidence of mast cell activation can be obtained with various laboratory tests and further testing should be performed to further differentiate between the various disorders that present with mast cell activation. Once the diagnosis is suspected and other medical disorders have been ruled out, patients should undergo a trial of anti-mast cell mediator and mast cell stabilizer medications with a plan to carefully assess treatment response. Depending on the type of mast cell disorder, specific treatments, and further testing may be warranted. The correct diagnosis of a mast cell disorder may lead to specific treatment with excellent symptom relief, improved quality of life, and prevention of unnecessary tests and procedures.

Classifications of Mast Cell Disorders

Once a mast cell disorder is suspected, it is important to try to classify the patient into the appropriate group of disorders. Although the underlying treatment of mast cell activation symptoms is not different (see Treatment section), there may be specific management strategies to consider for each subtype.

A. Clonal Mast Cell Disorders

1. Systemic mastocytosis—These patients present with the signs and symptoms of mast cell activation and may have characteristic skin lesions such as urticaria pigmentosa and a history of anaphylaxis. The hallmark is an accumulation of clonal forms of mast cells in clusters or sheets in the bone marrow and extracutaneous sites including the liver and intestine. The clonal population of mast cells may be identified by abnormal cell surface expression, morphology, or mutational analysis of the KIT gene. The serum tryptase is elevated on baseline testing >20 ng/mL or >11.4 ng/mL with coexisting anaphylaxis or high clinical suspicion of mastocytosis.

There are several subclassifications of systemic mastocytosis. The majority of adult patients have indolent mastocytosis with the features described earlier. A smaller minority will present with or progress to smoldering mastocytosis or aggressive mastocytosis. In the smoldering subclass, patients will display two or more "B" findings that are characteristic of an increased mast cell burden in the tissues but they maintain normal organ function. These may include a serum tryptase >200 ng/mL, a bone marrow biopsy that has >30% mast cells, and/or enlargement of the liver, spleen, and/or lymph nodes. In aggressive mastocytosis, patients may harbor at least one "C" finding that suggests that the mast cell burden is causing organ dysfunction. Patients with this subclass may therefore have cytopenias with an absolute neutrophil count <1000 cells/μL, hemoglobin <10 g/dL, and platelets <100,000 cells/μL, organ dysfunction including portal hypertension and associated complications, hypersplenism, intestinal malabsorption, and severe bone disease such as osteoporosis with pathologic fractures.

When classifying adult patients with systemic mastocytosis, a co-existing clonal non–mast cell hematologic lineage disorder needs to be ruled out with a bone marrow biopsy. The presence of a myeloproliferative, myelodysplastic, or lymphoproliferative hematologic disorder in a patient who also has systemic mastocytosis typifies the fourth subclass. Finally, a fifth type is mast cell leukemia. This subclass is the least common but carries the highest mortality. It is characterized by abnormal mast cells identified in the peripheral circulation where mast cells are usually not detected. They may comprise >10% of the total circulating cells and appear as blasts, have a high nucleus to cytoplasm ratio, and/or contain mitotic figures. Mast cell leukemia is also suspected when >20% of a bone marrow aspirate has these abnormal features.

2. Monoclonal mast cell activation syndrome—Patients with this classification of clonal mast cell disorder also present with signs and symptoms of mast cell activation and may be at increased risk for anaphylactic episodes. Mast cells in the bone marrow in these patients may express the surface marker CD25 the D816V mutation in the mast cell surface receptor KIT, but are not found in aggregates of 15 or more mast cells. Baseline tryptase levels in this clonal mast cell disorder are generally normal.

3. Maculopapular cutaneous mastocytosis—Patients with skin lesions, signs and symptoms of mast cell activation, and abnormal populations of mast cells confined to the skin have cutaneous mastocytosis. This will not be discussed in detail in this chapter.

B. Nonclonal Mast Cell Disorders

1. Mast cell activation syndrome—Although the clinical presentation and treatment of systemic mastocytosis has been well appreciated and studied, mast cell activation syndrome has only recently been characterized. In this mast cell disorder, patients present with signs and symptoms of mast cell activation but generally have normal numbers of mast cells in the bone marrow and tissues and no evidence of clonal forms that are seen in the clonal mast cell disorders. These patients may present with anaphylaxis but current expert consensus opinion is that patients who present with anaphylaxis without mastocytosis may be better characterized as having idiopathic anaphylaxis. The treatment and prognosis is described in the following section. Patients with mast cell activation syndrome may respond well to treatments and are not thought to have any complications related specifically to the abnormal mast cell activation. These patients are not known to progress to systemic mastocytosis.

2. Hereditary alpha tryptasemia—Patients who have similar clinical manifestations to mast cell activation syndrome and other features such as hypermobile joints and a baseline serum tryptase >8 ng/mL may be evaluated for hereditary alpha tryptasemia. It was recently discovered that these patients have increased copies of the TPSAB1 gene that encodes for alpha tryptase. Although the mechanisms of disease pathogenesis are currently being evaluated, the clinical management is similar to mast cell activation syndrome.

3. Diseases that cause secondary mast cell activation—Signs and symptoms of mast cell activation may be seen in primary IgE-mediated allergic disorders and idiopathic anaphylaxis. Various autoimmune and chronic inflammatory conditions such as rheumatoid arthritis, lupus, and inflammatory bowel disease may also present with mast cell activation.

Akin C. Mast cell activation syndromes. *J Allergy Clin Immunol.* 2017;140(2):349–355. [PMID: 28780942]

Akin C, Scott LM, Kocabas CN, et al. Demonstration of an aberrant mast-cell population with clonal markers in a subset of patients with "idiopathic" anaphylaxis. *Blood.* 2007;110:2331–2333. [PMID: 17638853]

Hamilton MJ, Hornick JL, Akin C, Castells MC, Greenberger NJ. Mast cell activation syndrome: a newly recognized disorder with systemic clinical manifestations. *J Allergy Clin Immunol.* 2011;128:147–152. [PMID: 21621255]

Lyons JJ. Hereditary alpha tryptasemia: genotyping and associated clinical features. *Immunol Allergy Clin North Am.* 2018;38(3):483–495. [PMID: 30007465]

Lyons JJ, Yu X, Hughes JD, et al. Elevated basal serum tryptase identifies a multisystem disorder associated with increased TPSAB1 copy number. *Nat Genet.* 2016;48(12):1564–1569. [PMID: 27749843]

Pardanani A, Pardanani A. Systemic mastocytosis in adults: 2019 update on diagnosis, risk stratification and management. *Am J Hematol.* 2019;94(3):363–377. [PMID: 30536695]

Picard M, Giavina-Bianchi P, Mezzano V, et al. Expanding spectrum of mast cell activation disorders: Monoclonal and idiopathic mast cell activation syndromes. *Clin Therapeut.* 2013;35(5):548–562. [PMID: 23642289]

Valent P, Akin C, Arock M, et al. Definitions, criteria and global classification of mast cell disorders with special reference to mast cell activation syndromes: a consensus proposal. *Int Arch Allergy Immunol.* 2012;157:215–225. [PMID: 22041891]

▶ Pathogenesis of Mast Cell Disorders

A. Systemic Mastocytosis

Signs and symptoms may be related to the mast cell mediators themselves or infiltration of the mast cells in the various tissues. On a molecular basis, mutations have been identified in the gene that encodes *KIT* which is a cell surface receptor for stem cell factor (SCF). SCF is a growth factor important for the development, proliferation, and survival of mast cells. The mutations that have been identified in *KIT* are thought to contribute to the marked expansion of clonal mast cells. *KIT* mutations arise in about 95% of patients with systemic mastocytosis and the most common mutation is the *Asp816Val* mutation on exon 17. In general, the identified mutations in *KIT* are somatic and the common forms of mastocytosis that are due in part to these mutations and are not hereditary.

Mast cells have well-formed granules in the cytoplasm that allow for quick release of the mediators housed within these granules upon mast cell activation. These mediators may be released from the granules all at once (eg, when activated by the IgE receptor to cause "degranulation" as is seen in anaphylaxis) or by the more "piecemeal" release of the mediators that may be seen when mast cells are activated by their IgG, complement, or toll-like receptors. Upon activation, mediators that are released into the extracellular environment from the granules in seconds to minutes include histamine, neutral proteases including tryptase, and proteoglycans such as heparin. These mediators affect vascular permeability, bronchoconstriction, and edema and are responsible for many of the symptoms of allergy and anaphylaxis. Specific actions on the intestine include increased acid production (histamine), increased epithelial permeability (histamine, proteases), chemotaxis of inflammatory cells such as neutrophils and eosinophils (proteases), and gut motility.

In the next phase of mast cell activation, mast cells release mediators that have been "newly generated" from phospholipid membranes and include the leukotrienes, prostaglandins, and platelet activating factor. These mediators in the gut may also affect epithelial membrane permeability and immune cell chemotaxis.

Finally, mast cells may produce and release a vast array of chemokines and cytokines that contribute to inflammatory responses in the tissue microenvironment. Mast cells may release a T helper 2 (Th2) set of cytokines but may also release tumor necrosis factor α (TNF-α), TGF-β, and many more. The profile of cytokines and chemokines released may depend on the phenotype of an individual mast cell within a various tissue compartment that is dictated by a certain inflammatory condition.

B. Mast Cell Activation Syndrome

The signs and symptoms are thought to be directly related to the actions of the mast cell mediators. While the numbers and gross morphology of the mast cells appear to be normal in this disorder, the mast cells inappropriately release the mediators. Although patients have been found to harbor many point mutations in the *KIT* gene, there has not been any distinct abnormality at the molecular level to account for the signs and symptoms observed in these patients. It is unclear whether mast cells in this disorder are responding to abnormal extracellular signals (eg, too much STM), or an intrinsic cellular defect that lowers the mast cell threshold for activation, or some combination thereof. Furthermore, mast cells express an array of cell surface receptors including MRGPRX2 which has recently been shown to cause non-IgE-allergic type reactions driven by basic secretagogues and may account for many of the adverse side effects of medications that these patients experience.

Patients with mast cell activation present heterogeneously which may reflect different underlying mast cell pathologies. While one patient may have predominant gastrointestinal (GI) symptoms with intermittent abdominal pain and diarrhea and elevated urine histamine levels, another may have more predominant flushing of the skin, bone pain, and concentration difficulties and an elevated urine prostaglandin level. There has been no observed correlation between the profile of symptoms in a mast cell activation syndrome patient and the pattern of mast cell mediators on laboratory testing.

Clinical Findings

The overall clinical features of the mast cell disorders are similar. Several unique manifestations may distinguish and differentiate them from other medical disorders with similar presentations.

A. Signs & Symptoms

Patients with mast cell disorders may be readily identified after a thorough history and physical examination. The signs and symptoms are predominately due to the release of the mast cell mediators in the tissues where mast cells reside. Mast cells are found in all layers of the intestine from the upper tract to the lower colon. Patients undergoing mast cell activation therefore present with upper GI symptoms such as gastroesophageal reflux, dyspepsia, bloating, and nausea. Lower GI symptoms include chronic, intermittent loose stools and cramping abdominal pain. Patients with systemic mastocytosis may be at risk for peptic ulcer disease and bleeding due to excessive histamine release and its action on gastric acid production.

The key to the diagnosis of mast cell disorders is identifying a pattern of signs and symptoms in multiple organ systems. Therefore, patients may manifest mast cell activation in the skin (flushing, pruritis, sweating, and dermatographism), nose and ocular areas (rhinitis, and itchy eyes), lungs (wheezing), heart (tachycardia and palpitations), and nervous system (numbness and tingling of the extremities, poor concentration, and memory). Patients may also present with psychiatric conditions such as anxiety and depression, and complain of bone pain and fatigue. The symptoms may be intermittent or more chronic and persistent.

A clinical manifestation that has been observed in patients with mast cell activation syndrome is an association with dysautonomia and most often the postural orthostatic tachycardia syndrome (ie, "POTS"). Patients with this manifestation may present with feelings of light-headedness, nausea, anxiety, and fatigue particularly with prolonged sitting or standing. On physical examination, an increase in heart rate of 30 beats/min with standing or sitting that persists up to 10 minutes should raise suspicion of this associated disorder. More specific tests and treatments are then warranted by a specialist. Many of these patients may also have hypermobile joints and meet criteria for Ehlers-Danlos Syndrome.

Several manifestations are specific for patients with mastocytosis and are important to identify to support this diagnosis. In the skin, the finding of urticaria pigmentosa is seen in 90% of adult patients with systemic mastocytosis and therefore should be assessed in any patient with a suspected mast cell disorder. The urticaria appears as lesions that are yellow-tan to reddish-brown in color and may be macular and/or papular. They are most often found on the extremities followed by the trunk and rarely on the palms, soles, and face. If a suspected lesion is rubbed a local reaction of increased erythema and warmth at the site might develop and is known as Darier's sign. Patients with systemic mastocytosis may rarely have mastocytomas which are raised nodular lesions millimeters to centimeters in size. The signs and symptoms that suggest smoldering and aggressive mastocytosis include hepatomegaly with manifestations of portal hypertension, splenomegaly with signs of hypersplenism, intestinal malabsorption due to mast cell infiltration in the mucosal compartment of the intestines, lymphadenopathy, and bone marrow failure presenting with various combinations of the cytopenias.

B. Endoscopy

Patients with a suspected mast cell disorder who have intermittent and/or chronic GI symptoms should undergo upper endoscopy and/or colonoscopy determined by the location of the predominant symptoms. Patients with abdominal pain and diarrhea should have both procedures done while the patient with reflux symptoms and nausea may only need an upper endoscopy. Endoscopy is generally safe in this population of patients. However, appropriate precautions and consultation with an anesthesiologist are recommended given the high rate of medication intolerances and allergies in these patients.

Conscious sedation medications that are considered to be safe are propofol, versed, fentanyl, and ketamine as they are thought not to precipitate mast cell activation. If a patient has a history of hypotensive episodes, anaphylaxis, or an active mast cell activation flare, it is advised to premedicate with diphenhydramine 25–50 mg intravenously (IV) 1 hour before or at the time of the procedure, and optionally corticosteroid (prednisone 25–50 mg) orally 12 and 2 hours before the procedure in addition to their normal regimen of morning medications. Providers should be aware of the risk of anaphylaxis and be prepared to treat with epinephrine for hypotension or respiratory compromise.

The endoscopy and colonoscopy are generally normal in mast cell disorders and the most important reason to carry out these tests is to rule out other causes for the patient's clinical presentation. In the upper GI tract, biopsies should be obtained to evaluate for other inflammatory conditions such as celiac disease and eosinophilic disorders. In the lower GI tract, systematic biopsies in the colon and terminal ileum can help identify inflammatory bowel disease or microscopic colitis. The GI tract should be surveyed for anatomic lesions that may lead to symptoms such as strictures, tumors, and peptic ulcer disease. While there are no specific endoscopic features that suggest mast cell activation syndrome, patients with systemic mastocytosis with intestinal involvement may have areas that appear mildly inflamed with loss of the vascular markings, and an edematous and/or erythematous appearance. Patients with smoldering or aggressive mastocytosis may have erosive disease or raised lesions such as nodules or polyps in the mucosa.

C. Intestinal Histopathology

When biopsies are taken in a patient known or suspected to have a mast cell disorder, a special request should be sent to the pathologist to evaluate for mast cells because routine hematoxylin and eosin staining will not readily identify them. Standard immunohistochemistry using antibodies directed against *KIT* and/or tryptase have been traditionally used. The number of mast cells that may be detected on mucosal biopsy in patients with mast cell activation syndrome is within the range of what is considered normal (10–25 mast cells per high-power field [HPF]). Patients who have mastocytosis however, may have a striking increase of mast cells per HPF (50–100). These mast cells may be seen in sheets near the basement membrane of the surface epithelium or in clusters throughout the mucosal layer. When systemic mastocytosis is suspected based on the clinical presentation or clustering of mast cells in the mucosal layer, a special stain for the cell surface marker CD25 is sensitive to detect the clonal mast cells and if detected is a minor criterion to establish this diagnosis.

D. Diagnostic Criteria

1. Systemic mastocytosis—The criteria established by the World Health Organization should be applied and a definitive diagnosis of systemic mastocytosis is made with a combination of one major and one minor criterion or three minor criteria.

a. Major criterion—Presence of multifocal dense aggregates containing at least 15 mast cells in the bone marrow or extracutaneous sites.

b. Minor criterion 1—Atypical morphology of mast cells including elongated or spindle forms in >25% of the total observed mast cells in the bone marrow or extracutaneous sites.

c. Minor criterion 2—Positive mutational analysis revealing the *Asp816Val* mutation for *KIT* in the bone marrow, blood, or extracutaneous site.

d. Minor criterion 3—Mast cells in the bone marrow or extracutaneous site express the cell surface markers CD2 or CD25 characteristic of the clonal mast cell population.

e. Minor criterion 4—Baseline serum tryptase is >20 ng/mL or >11.4 ng/mL in patients with coexisting anaphylaxis or other features associated with a high pretest probability for mastocytosis.

2. Mast cell activation syndrome

a. Patients have typical signs and symptoms of mast cell activation that affect two or more organ systems.

b. Patients have objective evidence that signs and symptoms are attributed to mast cell activation. Ideally, tests for serum tryptase, and 24-hour urine metabolites of mast cell mediators including histamine, prostaglandin, and leukotriene are elevated beyond their baseline levels on at least two different occasions during a period of symptoms.

c. Patients exhibit a symptom response to medications that block the action of mast cell mediators or inhibit mast cell mediator release.

d. No other medical condition better explains the patient's signs, symptoms, and clinical test results.

▶ Differential Diagnosis

Many of the signs and symptoms of mast cell activation are individually nonspecific and may be characteristic of other medical disorders. Given the multisystem nature of mast cell disorders, providers should consider autoimmune conditions, endocrinopathies, malignancies, and chronic infections. Patients with flushing and diarrhea should be evaluated for carcinoid syndrome and vasoactive intestinal peptide-secreting tumors. Patients with flushing and episodic hypertension should be assessed for pheochromocytoma. Flushing can also be a manifestation of patients with medullary thyroid cancer. Patients with angioedema of the skin, larynx, and intestine should be evaluated for hereditary or acquired angioedema. Patients who are found to have sclerotic lesions of the bone should be assessed for metastatic cancer.

As mentioned earlier, patients with signs and symptoms of mast cell activation but with documented episodes of anaphylaxis may be better classified as having idiopathic anaphylaxis. Patients with primary IgE-mediated allergic disease may present with mast cell symptoms such as hives, rash, wheezing, and naso-ocular symptoms. More specific treatments targeting allergy would be more appropriate and consultation with an allergist is recommended to distinguish between these disorders. As mentioned, several inflammatory and autoimmune conditions may present with secondary mast cell activation and treatment should be directed at the underlying primary disorder.

Bonamichi-Santos R, Yoshimi-Kanamori K, Giavina-Bianchi P, et al. Association of postural tachycardia syndrome and Ehlers-Danlos Syndrome with mast cell activation disorders. *Immunol Allergy Clin North Am.* 2018;38(3):497–504. [PMID: 30007466]

Castells M, Austen KF. Mastocytosis: mediator-related signs and symptoms. *Int Arch Allergy Immunol.* 2002;127:147–152. [PMID: 11919427]

Doyle LA, Sepehr GJ, Hamilton MJ, et al. A clinicopathologic study of 24 cases of systemic mastocytosis involving the gastrointestinal tract and assessment of mucosal mast cell density in irritable bowel syndrome and asymptomatic patients. *Am J Surg Pathol.* 2014;38:832–843. [PMID: 24618605]

McNeil BD, Pundir P, Meeker S, et al. Identification of a mast cell-specific receptor crucial for pseudo-allergic drug reactions. *Nature.* 2015;519(7542):237–241. [PMID: 25517090]

Orsolini G, Viapiana O, Rossini M, et al. Bone disease in masto-cytosis. *Immunol Allergy Clin North Am.* 2018;38(3):443–454. [PMID: 30007462]

Valent P, Akin C, Bonadonna P, et al. Proposed diagnostic algo-rithm for patients with suspected mast cell activation syndrome. *J Allergy Clin Immunol Pract.* 2019;7(4):1125–1133. [PMID: 30737190]

Valent P, Akin C, Metcalfe DD. Mastocytosis: 2016 updated WHO classification and novel emerging treatment concepts. *Blood* 2017;129(11):1420–1427. [PMID: 28031180]

▶ Treatment

A. For Mast Cell Activation

1. Antihistamines—These are the mainstay of medical treatment for patients who exhibit signs and symptoms of mast cell activation. Short-acting on-demand sublingual loratadine (a non-sedating type 1 antihistamine) can be con-sidered around the time of diagnosis to establish whether or not a patient's symptoms appropriately respond. Alter-natively, diphenhydramine and hydroxyzine (sedating type 1 antihistamines) can also be considered in this capacity. If a patient has a symptomatic response and has other clini-cal manifestations of mast cell activation, then a combina-tion of non-sedating type 1 and type 2 antihistamines can be used on a daily basis. A baseline regimen should include once- to twice-daily dosing that provides adequate control of symptoms and is tolerated well. During periods of increased symptoms, this regimen can be titrated to 2–3× the baseline dosage in order to achieve control of symptoms with the plan to de-escalate once symptoms are improved. Prolonged use of daily antihistamines may lead to diminished response, so this strategy of maintaining the dosage at the lowest possible level to control symptoms is optimal. As needed, diphen-hydramine can be reserved for breakthrough symptoms.

2. Mast cell stabilizers—Cromolyn is an effective medical treatment to treat mast cell specific symptoms when antihis-tamines alone are not sufficient. Although the exact mecha-nisms of action are not known, cromolyn is thought to act on the mast cell membrane to inhibit release of mast cell media-tors upon activation. Although the systemic absorption is poor, cromolyn has been found to be effective for the treat-ment of skin, respiratory, and cardiac symptoms in addition to GI symptoms. A limiting side effect may be osmotic-type diarrhea or other reactions at higher doses and so cromolyn is generally started at half the recommended total daily dose and then increased slowly over several weeks to the standard dose (200 mg four times a day 30 minutes before meals). Similar to antihistamines, the maintenance dose should be the lowest dose that controls symptoms and this may be increased during a time of increased symptoms. Oral ketotifen is thought to have type 1 antihistamine properties as well as mast cell stabilizing properties and may be used in patients with mast cell activa-tion and particularly those who cannot tolerate cromolyn. It is dosed twice a day and may have the side effect of sedation.

3. Leukotriene and prostaglandin inhibitors—Third-line agents for the treatment of mast cell activation include drugs that are designed to block the leukotriene and prosta-glandin mediators. Once- to twice-daily montelukast, once-daily zafirlukast, and twice-daily zileuton can be prescribed and may be effective for pulmonary symptoms such as wheezing, as well as flushing, pruritis, and abdominal cramp-ing. Aspirin has been shown to be an effective treatment in patients with mast cell activation, elevated prostaglandin lev-els, and flushing. Optimal dosing is 650–1300 mg in divided doses. Because many of these patients may have adverse reac-tions to aspirin and NSAIDs, it is advisable to have patients take their first doses in a monitored setting. It is also recom-mended that these patients take a concomitant proton pump inhibitor in order to protect against aspirin-induced peptic ulcer disease. This is particularly important in patients with mastocytosis who may be at risk for peptic ulcers at baseline.

4. Other treatments—Patients with a history of anaphy-laxis must have at all times two epinephrine injector pens and the appropriate knowledge about how and when to use them. Anti-IgE therapy (omalizumab) has been found to effectively prevent provoked and unprovoked anaphylaxis in mastocy-tosis patients but natural forms of mast cell stabilizers (eg, luteolin, quercitin) are investigational at this time. Opiate use should be avoided due to the chronic nature of symptoms and the potential to exacerbate mast cell mediator release and further complicate abdominal symptoms.

B. Specific Systemic Mastocytosis Therapy

The medical therapy for patients with indolent systemic mas-tocytosis is generally the same as that for mast cell activation syndrome (see later) and mast cell activation in general. These patients are often advised to take a proton pump inhibitor to combat the histamine-induced gastric acid production that can lead to peptic ulcer disease and diarrhea. Due to the risk of degenerative bone disease, it is recommended that these patients take daily vitamin D and calcium and a bisphospho-nate if osteoporosis is detected. The treatment of osteopenia or osteoporosis may be best directed by a bone specialist. The specific treatment for patients with aggressive mastocytosis is beyond the scope of this chapter but includes cytoreductive agents and tyrosine kinase inhibitors, including midostaurin and avapritinib. Although aggressive mastocytosis cannot be cured, the mast cell burden can be reduced to restore organ function. Mast cell leukemia is treated with chemotherapeu-tic agents.

C. Specific Mast Cell Activation Syndrome Therapy

In addition to targeting the symptoms associated with mast cell activation (detailed earlier), it is important to approach systematically the patients' symptoms by system to try to achieve optimal control. With regards to GI symptoms, the treatment strategy adopted for patients with irritable bowel syndrome (where the pathophysiology is thought to be due in part to mast cell activation) can be employed. In these patients as in patients with mast cell activation syndrome, treatment is directed at the most prominent symptoms. If these symptoms are not optimally controlled after treatment with anti–mast cell mediator therapy, then additional medications can be considered for abdominal pain (eg, low-dose anticholinergics, selective serotonin reuptake inhibitors), bloating and gas, and diarrhea (eg, antidiarrheals such as Imodium, Lomotil, and bile acid sequestrants). Similar adjunct therapies should be considered for symptoms in other organ systems.

In order to optimally treat these patients, mental health should be addressed. Patients should be encouraged to remain physically active with walking, stretching, yoga, and similar activities. These patients should be evaluated for depression and anxiety and evaluated and treated by the appropriate providers. Patients should have appropriate coping strategies and support systems in place. Relaxation strategies to alleviate stress and anxiety such as meditation can be offered.

Patients with mast cell activation syndrome should have their diets routinely assessed to ensure that they are getting the proper balance of the major food groups, as well as vitamins and minerals. Diets can also be reviewed to see what may be contributing to the GI symptoms. Patients with mast cell activation may have multiple food intolerances and patients should be encouraged to keep a food diary to identify them. Patients with diarrhea can be educated about the proper fiber balance (limiting the irritable fibers) and those with bloating and gas can be instructed to avoid the high gas-forming foods. Consultation with a nutritionist is helpful to ensure a balanced diet that addresses the patient's symptoms and nutritional needs.

Clinical Course & Prognosis

Patients with mast cell disorders generally have a good overall prognosis and normal mortality. Prompt and proper diagnosis can reduce the substantial morbidity that may be associated with mast cell activation. Patients may become debilitated due to the chronic and severe nature of the symptoms. Many patients with anaphylaxis suffer from a type of post-traumatic stress syndrome due to the life-threatening nature of this manifestation. It is also noted that many patients with mast cell disorders may suffer from concomitant psychiatric disorders such as anxiety and depression. It is unclear whether this is related to the disorder itself or from having a chronic medical condition. Whichever the case, it is clear that the successful management of mast cell disorders must address these issues. Patients with indolent systemic mastocytosis generally have a good prognosis as long as symptoms are managed well and complications such as peptic ulcer disease and osteoporosis are prevented. These patients should be routinely assessed by specialists for the progression to aggressive systemic mastocytosis where organ dysfunction can lead to significant morbidity and mortality. As discussed earlier, the rare mast cell leukemia carries a grave prognosis.

Unresolved Issues

There are many unresolved issues with regards to the diagnosis and treatment of mast cell disorders. Although the GI tract is a primary location of mast cells and likely contains the highest number of mast cell progenitors in the body, little has been published regarding the GI manifestations of these disorders. Taking into account the increased recognition of mast cell disorders, the overall prevalence is thought to be increasing in western societies. It is likely that factors such as antibiotics, vaccinations, and lack of microbes that affect the microbial composition lining mucosal surfaces have led to changes in the composition and number of mast cells. Treatment to restore the richness and diversity of the intestinal microbiome may therefore prove to be effective such as with the use of prebiotics and probiotics. For mast cell activation syndrome, biomarkers are needed to diagnose this disorder and well-tolerated and efficacious treatments will increase the chances of symptom remission. For patients with mastocytosis, a curative medical treatment is needed that targets and eliminates the clonal mast cells.

Castells M, Butterfield J. Mast cell activation syndrome and mastocytosis: initial treatment options and long-term management. *J Allergy Clin Immunol Pract.* 2019;7(4):1097–1106. [PMID: 30961835]

Gotlib J, Kluin-Nelemans HC, George TI, et al. Efficacy and safety of midostaurin in advanced systemic mastocytosis. *N Engl J Med.* 2016;374(26):2530–2541. [PMID: 27355533]

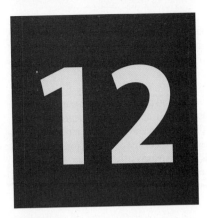

Gastroesophageal Reflux Disease

Walter W. Chan, MD, MPH

▶ Heartburn, regurgitation, and dysphagia.

▶ "Alarm signs"—dysphagia, odynophagia, weight loss, family history of upper gastrointestinal (GI) tract cancers, persistent nausea and emesis, long duration of symptoms (>10 years), and incomplete response to treatment.

▶ Atypical manifestations (eg, asthma) are common.

General Considerations

Gastroesophageal reflux disease (GERD) is the most common and costly digestive disease. It accounts for over 8 million outpatient visits in the United States each year, and annual prescriptions for proton pump inhibitors (PPIs) to diagnose and manage GERD are estimated to exceed 8.2 billion, totaling over 10 billion in cost. GERD is a chronic disorder resulting from the retrograde flow of gastroduodenal contents into the esophagus or adjacent organs, and producing a variable spectrum of symptoms, with or without tissue damage. Transient inappropriate relaxation of the lower esophageal sphincter (LES) is the predominant pathophysiologic mechanism in the majority of GERD patients. Hiatal hernia, reduced LES pressure, or delayed gastric emptying may also play a role in patients with moderate to severe disease.

Peery AF, Dellen ES, Lund J, et al. Burden of gastrointestinal disease in the United States: 2012 update. *Gastroenterology.* 2012;143:1179–1187. [PMID: 22885331]

Shaheen NJ, Hansen RA, Morgan DR, et al. The burden of gastrointestinal and liver diseases. *Am J Gastroenterol.* 2006;101: 2128–2138.

A. Epidemiology

The prevalence of GERD in the United States appears to be increasing. In Western populations, 25% of people report having heartburn at least once a month, 12% at least once per week, and 5% describe having symptoms on a daily basis. There appears to be no gender predominance of heartburn symptoms; men and women are affected equally. The relationship of age and reflux is unclear. One study has suggested an association between advancing age and fewer reflux symptoms but the presence of more severe esophagitis. There is an unequivocal positive association between body mass index and reflux symptoms, and the increasing rate of obesity has been proposed as a cause of growth in GERD incidence. Inappropriate relaxation of the LES can be exacerbated by obesity. Even moderate weight gain among persons of normal weight is thought to cause or exacerbate reflux symptoms. These epidemiologic characteristics should be considered when evaluating a patient with typical and atypical GERD.

Johnson DA, Fennerty MB. Heartburn severity underestimates erosive esophagitis severity in elderly patients with gastroesophageal reflux disease. *Gastroenterology.* 2004;126:660–664. [PMID: 14988819]

Moayyedi P, Axon AT. Review article: gastroesophageal reflux disease: the extent of the problem. *Aliment Pharmacol Ther.* 2005;22(suppl 1):11–19. [PMID: 16042655]

B. Pathogenesis

Pathologic reflux of gastric contents occurs when the refluxate overcomes the antireflux barriers of the gastroesophageal junction, often in a postprandial state. The antireflux barrier of the gastroesophageal junction is anatomically and physiologically complex and vulnerable to a number of potential mechanisms of reflux. The primary antireflux mechanism is the LES, a segment of smooth muscle in the lower esophagus that is chronically contracted to maintain a pressure that is approximately 15 mm Hg above intragastric pressure. The

Table 12–1. Medications that can cause GERD or esophagitis.

Decrease LES Pressure	Cause Direct Mucosal Injury
β-Adrenergic agonists, including inhalers	
α-Adrenergic antagonists	Alendronate
Anticholinergics	Aspirin
Calcium channel blockers	Iron salts
Diazepam	Nonsteroidal anti-inflammatory drugs
Estrogens	
Narcotics	Potassium chloride tablets
Progesterone	Quinidine
Theophylline	Tetracycline
Tricyclic antidepressants	

LES, lower esophageal sphincter.

crural diaphragm, composed of striated muscles and forming the esophageal hiatus, also contributes to the antireflux barrier at the gastroesophageal junction. The two main patterns of LES dysfunction associated with GERD are (1) a hypotensive LES and (2) pathologic transient LES relaxations. Anatomic disruption of the gastroesophageal junction, commonly associated with a hiatal hernia and proximal migration of the LES, contributes to the pathogenesis of reflux disease through disruption of the antireflux barrier. Transient LES relaxations in the absence of swallowing account for the majority of reflux events in individuals with normal LES pressure and clinically mild reflux disease. Chronically low LES pressure is the predominant GERD mechanism in patients with severe reflux disease, such as in patients with scleroderma.

Gastric factors can play a significant role in producing GERD. Gastric factors that promote GERD include increased gastric volume after meals, increased gastric pressure due to obesity, recumbency after meals, and delayed gastric emptying or gastroparesis, which can be idiopathic or drug induced. Increased gastric distention can cause an increase

Table 12–2. Factors that can precipitate or exacerbate GERD symptoms.

Medications (see Table 12–1)
Foods
  Caffeine
  Chocolate
  Peppermint
  Alcohol (red wine pH = 3.25)
  Carbonated beverages (cola pH = 2.75)
  Citrus fruits (orange juice pH = 3.25)
  Tomato-based products (tomato juice pH = 3.25)
  Vinegar (pH = 3.00)
Lifestyle factors
  Weight gain
  Smoking
  Eating prior to recumbency

in transient LES relaxations and the volume of refluxate, particularly in GERD patients with large hiatal hernias. Delayed gastric emptying, or gastroparesis, may be present in approximately 15% of patients with GERD and is frequently underdiagnosed.

Other factors that decrease LES pressure and contribute to GERD are medications, lifestyle behaviors, and the ingestion of certain foods. Certain medicines can exacerbate GERD by lowering LES pressure; others can cause esophagitis by direct mucosal injury (Table 12–1). Certain foods, beverages, and behaviors will cause heartburn by reducing LES pressure (Table 12–2). Fatty foods, peppermint, chocolate, caffeinated beverages, alcohol, and smoking can all decrease LES pressure.

El-Serag HB, Ergun GA, Pandolfino J, et al. Obesity increases oesophageal acid exposure. *Gut.* 2007;56:749–755. [PMID: 17127706]

Horowitz M, Su YG, Rayner CK, et al. Gastroparesis: prevalence, clinical significance and treatment. *Can J Gastroenterol.* 2001;15:805–813. [PMID: 11773947]

Jacobson BC, Somers SC, Fuchs CS, et al. Body-mass index and symptoms of gastroesophageal reflux in women. *N Engl J Med.* 2006;354:2340–2348. [PMID: 16738270]

Jones MP, Sloan SS, Rabine JC, et al. Hiatal hernia size is the dominant determinant of esophagitis presence and severity in gastroesophageal reflux disease. *Am J Gastroenterol.* 2001;96:1711–1717. [PMID: 11419819]

Kahrilas PJ. GERD pathogenesis, pathophysiology and clinical manifestations. *Cleve Clin J Med.* 2003;70(suppl 5):S4–S19. [PMID: 14705378]

Clinical Findings

A. Symptoms & Signs

GERD is defined as symptoms or mucosal damage produced by the abnormal reflux of gastric contents into the esophagus. The typical manifestations of GERD are heartburn, regurgitation, and dysphagia. Other symptoms associated with GERD include water brash, a globus (lump in the throat) sensation, odynophagia, and nausea. Heartburn (pyrosis) is defined as a retrosternal burning discomfort located in the epigastric area that may radiate up toward the neck and typically occurs in the postprandial period, especially after a high-fat or a large-volume meal. Postural changes such as bending over often exacerbate patients' symptoms. Symptoms can also be aggravated by ingestion of certain foods or beverages, such as tomato sauce, peppermint, chocolate, coffee, tea, and alcohol. When assessing a patient with GERD symptoms, the duration and severity of symptoms should be investigated. Patients who present with typical symptoms with a minimum frequency of twice a week for 4–8 weeks or more should be considered as having GERD. At initial presentation, it is important to consider a patient's age and the presence of "alarm signs" (Table 12–3). New-onset symptoms

Table 12–3. "Alarm" signs that necessitate further evaluation of GERD.

Dysphagia
Odynophagia
Weight loss
Gastrointestinal (GI) bleeding
Family history of upper GI tract cancer
Anemia
Advanced age

at older age or the presence of any alarm signs necessitates the evaluation of GERD symptoms with an upper endoscopy or imaging modality to rule out any signs of underlying malignancy.

Atypical manifestations of GERD refer to symptoms that are extraesophageal, including pulmonary and otolaryngoloic manifestations, as well as noncardiac chest pain (Table 12–4). According to published studies in the literature, pathologic GERD can be found in 30–80% of adult patients with asthma, although their causal relationship is not completely clear. GERD may serve as a trigger for asthma via microaspiration of gastric acid with subsequent airway irritation or vagally mediated effects of acid on the upper airway. However, changes in the thoracoabdominal pressure gradient from asthma-induced pulmonary hyperinflation may disrupt the antireflux barrier and the use of bronchodilators may also lower the LES tone, thus promoting reflux. While GERD should be considered as a possible etiology in adults with new-onset asthma, prior studies did not show significant benefits in routine use of acid-suppressing agents for management of all asthma patients. Expert opinion guidelines suggest empiric acid-suppression therapy for asthma patients with typical esophageal symptoms of GERD. In the absence of concomitant esophageal symptoms, the empiric use of acid-suppressing agents among asthmatics remains controversial. An increasing incidence of GERD has also been associated with other pulmonary disorders such as idiopathic pulmonary fibrosis or chronic obstructive pulmonary disease. GERD has also been linked to injury and rejection of allografts in lung transplant patients. Similarly, the causal relationship and the role of reflux therapy in the management

of these pulmonary disorders need further investigation. In laryngopharyngeal reflux, the regurgitated gastric contents reach the upper aerodigestive tract, leading to ear, nose, and throat symptoms such as chronic cough, hoarseness, sore throat, globus sensation, and otitis media.

Patients with gastroparesis and GERD may present with concomitant nausea, vomiting, or early satiety. These patients may not respond to antisecretory agents alone, as the refluxate contains bile and digestive enzymes in addition to gastric acid. Gastroparesis should be suspected in patients with an acute or subacute onset of GERD, particularly after an episode of viral upper respiratory infection or gastroenteritis. The natural history of GERD with acute gastroparesis is that the majority of patients will achieve symptomatic resolution, although some may need treatment with prokinetic agents. Antisecretory agents may offer some symptomatic relief and reduce gastric volume. Dietary changes such as low-fat, frequent, small meals may also be helpful in controlling symptoms.

Chan WW, Ahuja N, Fisichella PM, et al. Extraesophageal syndrome of gastroesophageal reflux: relationships with lung disease and transplantation outcome. *Ann N Y Acad Sci.* 2020;1482(1):95–105. [PMID: 32808313]

Chan WW, Chiou E, Obstein KL, et al. The efficacy of proton pump inhibitors for the treatment of asthma in adults: a meta-analysis. *Arch Intern Med.* 2011;171(7):620–629. [PMID: 21482834]

Horowitz M, Su YG, Rayner CK, et al. Gastroparesis: prevalence, clinical significance and treatment. *Can J Gastroenterol.* 2001;15:805–813. [PMID: 11773947]

Vakil N, van Zanten SV, Kahrilas P, et al. The Montreal definition and classification of gastroesophageal reflux disease: a global evidence-based consensus. *Am J Gastroenterol* 2006; 101:1900–1920. [PMID: 16928254]

B. Diagnosis

Classic GERD can be diagnosed by taking a thorough symptom history and confirmed by a complete response to medical therapy (a "PPI test"). In general, diagnostic testing is reserved for patients who fail to respond to a trial of adequate medical therapy or for patients who have alarm symptoms with GERD (Figure 12–1). Available tests include upper GI series, upper endoscopy, ambulatory reflux monitoring (ARM), and esophageal manometry.

PPI therapy is very effective in healing reflux esophagitis. Patients who have no symptom response to PPI therapy are unlikely to have GERD. A meta-analysis that assessed the accuracy of normal or high-dose PPI for 1–4 weeks in the diagnosis of GERD found a pooled sensitivity of 78% (95% confidence interval [CI] 66–86%) and a specificity of 54% (44–65%) when ambulatory pH monitoring was used as a gold standard. Diagnostic testing for GERD patients is indicated in those who fail a PPI trial or have alarm signs.

Radiologic studies are of limited use in the management of GERD due to poor sensitivity in milder forms of GERD,

Table 12–4. Extraesophageal manifestations of GERD.

Otitis medi	Frequent throat clearing
Asthma	Globus
Chronic sinusitis	Tracheobronchitis
Dental erosions	Chronic cough
Aphthous ulcers	Aspiration pneumonia
Halitosis	Pulmonary fibrosis
Pharyngitis	Chronic bronchitis
Laryngitis	Bronchiectasis
Laryngospasm	Noncardiac chest pain
Postnasal drip	Sleep apnea

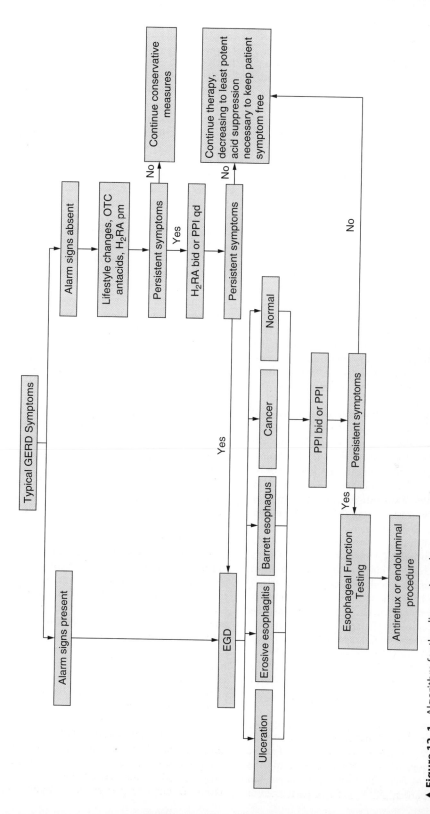

▲ **Figure 12–1.** Algorithm for the diagnosis and treatment of gastroesophageal reflux (GERD). bid, twice daily; EGD, esophagogastroduodenoscopy; H₂RA, H₂-receptor antagonist; OTC, over-the-counter; prn, as needed; qd, daily.

but they may detect moderate to severe esophagitis, strictures, hiatal hernias, and tumors. The studies that are most commonly used are the barium swallow, which only examines the esophagus, and the upper GI series, which examines the esophagus, stomach, and upper small intestine. The primary utility of radiographic studies in GERD is to rule out other conditions in patients in whom there is a low clinical suspicion for significant disease, or to assess for complications of GERD such as peptic strictures. These studies can help evaluate peptic ulcer disease and tumors as a cause of a patient's symptoms. In addition, radiographic studies can be helpful in the evaluation of a patient with dysphagia to rule out peptic rings, which can sometimes be difficult to visualize on upper endoscopy. Compared with endoscopy, radiologic studies are noninvasive, widely available, and relatively inexpensive. However, they are less sensitive and specific than upper endoscopy, and require an operator skill that may be becoming scarcer in the era of cross-sectional imaging.

Upper endoscopy, in addition to excluding the presence of other diseases such as tumors and peptic ulcers, can detect and grade the severity of GERD-induced esophagitis (Plate 6). Upper endoscopy is highly specific (90–95%) for GERD but has limited sensitivity (~50%). The extent and severity of mucosal injury can be assessed endoscopically. The Los Angeles classification of esophagitis quantifies the length and circumference of mucosal breaks. Upper endoscopy also allows the evaluation of any complications of the disease, such as strictures or Barrett esophagus. According to the most recent expert consensus (the Lyon Consensus), the presence of high-grade esophagitis (LA grade C or D), long-segment Barrett's esophagus, or peptic strictures on upper endoscopy serves as conclusive evidence for pathologic reflux, while lower grade esophagitis (LA grade A or B) is considered borderline or inconclusive evidence. If a patient has dysphagia and a stricture is detected, dilation of the stricture can be performed during the same procedure. Esophageal biopsy can also be obtained in those eosinophilic esophagitis is suspected. Upper endoscopy is, therefore, the initial test of choice in evaluating complicated GERD patients and symptoms refractory to medical therapy. The most recently published clinical guidelines from the American College of Physician recommend upper endoscopy in reflux patients with alarm symptoms, persistent symptoms despite 4–8 weeks of twice-daily PPI therapy, severe esophagitis (to assess healing after treatment and rule out Barrett esophagus), and recurrent dysphagia in the setting of a history of stricture. They also suggest that upper endoscopy may be indicated in men aged 50 or above with chronic reflux symptoms and additional risk factors, such as nocturnal reflux, hiatal hernia, tobacco use, or elevated body mass index.

ARM studies allow objective quantification of overall reflux burden and the assessment of the correlation between patient-reported symptoms and reflux events. One type of ARM is pH monitoring, which continuously records the distal esophageal pH to determine whether a patient has increased acid reflux burden. The test can be performed in two ways: (1) a probe that is passed transnasally to localize the pH sensor at 5 cm above the manometrically determined LES and (2) an endoscopically-placed pill-sized capsule (the Bravo wireless capsule) that is attached to the distal esophagus. The study may be performed for 24 hours for probe-based studies and 48–96 hours for capsule-based studies. The data are collected by a battery-powered device carried by the patient, who also records when meals are eaten and symptoms are experienced. This technique allows for correlation between symptoms and reflux episodes. Ambulatory esophageal pH monitoring records the timing, duration, and number of reflux episodes. Acid reflux episodes are defined as an esophageal pH below 4. Reflux burden is most commonly expressed by acid exposure time (AET), defined as the proportion of time throughout the analyzed study during which the esophagus has a pH of 4 or less. Per the Lyon consensus on the diagnosis of GERD, AET>6% is considered conclusive evidence for GERD, while AET<4% is evidence against pathologic reflux. An AET between 4% and 6% is borderline or inconclusive for GERD.

Multichannel intraluminal impedance testing is a newer ARM technology that detects changes in the resistance of electrical current on a catheter placed within the esophagus. Liquid, which has higher conductance and thus lower resistance than air, would lead to a drop in measured impedance when flowing by various sensing electrodes located throughout the catheter. Therefore, an impedance catheter can detect antegrade and retrograde transit of liquid boluses in the esophagus, regardless of acidity. With a combined pH and impedance catheter, it is possible to identify not only acid reflux episodes (pH <4), but also weakly acidic (4< pH <7) or nonacidic reflux (pH >7). This test may be helpful in patients who have suspected GERD or extraesophageal symptoms of GERD but inadequate response to high-dose PPI therapy or negative esophageal pH tests. It can help identify conditions with symptoms that may be similar to GERD, such as supragastric belching. While impedance testing provides tremendous potential in management of patients with refractory or atypical reflux symptoms, further studies correlating impedance measures of reflux and clinical outcomes such as response to antireflux surgery are needed to better define its role in reflux care, particularly when there is no increase in acid exposure. Per current expert consensus guidelines, the total number of reflux episodes identified by impedance represents a supportive measure of reflux. Total reflux episodes <40 on impedance serves as evidence against pathologic reflux, while reflux episodes >80 is considered an adjunctive evidence for GERD.

The indications for ARM can be divided into two main categories: (1) to determine if a patient's typical or atypical symptoms are related to GERD, and (2) to assess the reasons for persistent symptoms refractory to therapy among patients with previously proven GERD. ARM is also important in the preoperative assessment of patients presenting for antireflux surgery, as it has been shown to help prognosticate response. The study may be performed while the patient remains on- or off-acid suppression therapy, depending on the indication and pretest probability for GERD. For patients with low pretest probability (ie, no or low-grade esophagitis on endoscopy, atypical symptoms, lack of response to acid suppression), ARM should be performed off therapy to determine whether the patient has pathologic reflux. Preoperative evaluations for antireflux surgery should also be completed off acid suppression, as it has been shown to predict postoperative outcomes. On the other hand, among patients with high pretest probability for or previously proven GERD (ie, prior high-grade esophagitis, long segment Barrett's, peptic stricture, or abnormal ARM), testing should be performed on medication to assess whether the persistent symptoms are due to inadequate acid suppression, nonacidic reflux, visceral hypersensitivity, or functional causes.

Esophageal manometry measures esophageal body peristalsis and upper/LES function utilizing a transnasally-placed catheter with pressure sensors. The role of esophageal manometry in the evaluation of GERD includes the assessment of primary esophageal dysmotility and anatomical landmarks, identification of supportive evidence of GERD (hiatal hernia, hypomotility, hypotensive gastroesophageal junction), and assistance in ARM probe placement. It also evaluates for contraindications to antireflux surgery (eg, achalasia) and has been shown to help prognosticate surgical outcomes.

The overall summary of the interpretation of esophageal testing for the diagnosis of GERD per the expert guidelines from the most recent Lyon Consensus is shown in Table 12–5.

Chan WW, Haroian LR, Gyawali CP. Value of preoperative esophageal function studies before laparoscopic antireflux surgery. *Surg Endosc.* 2011;25(9):2943–2949. [PMID: 21424193]

Gyawali CP, Carlson DA, Chen JW, et al. ACG Clinical Guidelines: clinical use of esophageal physiologic testing. *Am J Gastroenterol.* 2020;115(9):1412–1428. [PMID: 32769426]

Gyawali CP, Kahrilas PJ, Savarino E, et al. Modern diagnosis of GERD: the Lyon Consensus. *Gut.* 2018;67(7):1351–1362. [PMID: 29437910]

Katz PO, Gerson LB, Vela MF. ACG Clinical Guidelines for the diagnosis and management of gastroesophageal reflux disease. *Am J Gastroenterol.* 2013;108(3):308–328. [PMID: 23419381]

Numans ME, Lau J, de Wit NJ, et al. Short-term treatment with proton pump inhibitors as a test for gastroesophageal reflux disease: a meta-analysis of diagnostic test characteristics. *Ann Intern Med.* 2004;140:518–527. [PMID: 15068979]

Patel A, Sayuk GS, Kushnir VM, et al. GERD phenotypes from pH-impedance monitoring predict symptomatic outcomes on prospective evaluation. *Neurogastroenterol Motil.* 201628(4):513–521. [PMID: 26686239]

Pritchett JM, Aslam M, Slaughter JC, et al. Efficacy of esophageal impedance/pH monitoring in patients with refractory gastroesophageal reflux disease, on and off therapy. *Clin Gastroenterol Hepatol.* 2009;7:743–748. [PMID: 19281866]

Shaheen NJ, Weinberg DS, Denberg TD, et al. Upper endoscopy for gastroesophageal reflux disease: best practice advice from the clinical guidelines committee of the American College of Physicians. *Ann Intern Med.* 2012;157:808–816. [PMID: 23208168]

Complications

Complications from chronic GERD include bleeding from esophageal erosions or ulceration, stricture formation, and Barrett esophagus.

A. Esophageal Ulcers

Although somewhat counterintuitive, the severity and duration of GERD symptoms poorly correlates with the presence or severity of esophagitis. Esophageal ulcers due to

Table 12–5. Interpretation of esophageal testing for GERD per Lyon Consensus.

Evidence of GERD	Endoscopy	pH or pH-Impedance	HRM
Conclusive evidence for pathologic reflux	LA grades C & D esophagitis Long segment Barrett's Peptic esophageal stricture	AET >6%	
Borderline or inconclusive evidence	LA grades A & B esophagitis	AET 4–6% Reflux episodes 40–80	
Adjunctive or supportive evidence	Histopathology (score) Electron microscopy (DIS) Low mucosal impedance	Reflux-symptom association Reflux episodes >80 Low MNBI Low PSPWI	Hypotensive EGJ Hiatus hernia Esophageal hypomotility
Evidence against pathology reflux		AET <4% Reflux episodes <40	

DIS, dilated intercellular spaces; EGJ, esophagogastric junction; HRM, high-resolution esophageal manometry; MNBI, mean nocturnal baseline impedance; PSPWI, postreflux swallow-induced peristaltic wave index, AET, acid exposure time.
Data from Gyawali CP, Kahrilas PJ, Savarino E, et al: Modern diagnosis of GERD: the Lyon Consensus. *Gut.* 2018;67(7):1351–1362.

esophagitis account for approximately 2% of all upper GI bleeding. The vast majority of esophageal peptic ulcers heal completely with acid-suppression therapy using PPIs.

B. Peptic Esophageal Strictures

Peptic esophageal strictures have been described in 10% of patients who seek medical attention for GERD symptoms. When questioned, most patients with esophageal strictures report dysphagia for an average of 4–6 years, and up to 25% deny any prior GERD. Weight loss, a cardinal symptom of esophageal cancer, is uncommon with peptic strictures because patients gradually learn to change their dietary habits to avoid foods that cause dysphagia.

C. Esophageal Carcinoma

Although the severity and duration of GERD symptoms appear to have little correlation with the presence of esophagitis, there is increasing evidence that frequent, severe GERD, particularly nocturnal, is a major risk factor for the development of esophageal adenocarcinoma. The incidence of esophageal adenocarcinoma is increasing in the United States and Europe at a very rapid rate. Esophageal adenocarcinoma and its predisposing risk factor, Barrett esophagus, are discussed in Chapter 14.

▶ Treatment

The goals of treatment for GERD are to resolve symptoms, heal esophagitis, and prevent complications of GERD. Once a patient is in remission, the goal is to maintain remission from symptoms and prevent further tissue injury.

A. Lifestyle, Medical, & Mechanical Therapies

A cornerstone of the treatment of GERD is lifestyle modifications. Patients are instructed to avoid foods and acid-containing beverages that can exacerbate their symptoms of GERD (see Table 12–2). Patients should avoid lying down for 3 hours after eating as ingested food may remain in the stomach and contribute to reflux. This practice is a frequent trigger of GERD symptoms and one of the most effective lifestyle changes a patient can institute to control symptoms. Smaller and frequent meals are also recommended for GERD patients. Elevation of the head of the bed by 6 in (by placing blocks underneath the feet at the head of the bed or using a wedge) can also reduce symptoms by using gravity to prevent reflux. It is recommended that patients avoid wearing tight-fitting clothing. Patients should be instructed to stop smoking and lose weight, which can be critical to reducing or eliminating symptoms. The current epidemic of obesity is a major contributing factor to increasing prevalence of GERD. Lifestyle modifications aimed at weight loss among patients with obesity including diet and exercise may also help reduce GERD symptoms.

Medical treatment is characterized mainly by antacid and antisecretory agents. Over-the-counter antacids are taken at least twice a month by more than one-fourth of the US population. Antacids provide symptom relief by neutralizing refluxed gastric acid thereby increasing esophageal pH and inactivating pepsin. Antacids are inexpensive, readily available, convenient, and effective. Short-term use of antacids for occasional symptoms is safe.

Histamine-2 (H_2)-receptor antagonists inhibit the secretion of gastric acid by competitively blocking the H_2-receptors located on gastric parietal cells. H_2-blockers have an excellent safety record and have been approved by the US Food and Drug Administration (FDA) for over-the-counter sales. Low-dose H_2-receptor antagonists not only prevent heartburn symptoms when taken before meals but also relieve meal-induced heartburn symptoms in 15–40 minutes when taken after meals. H_2-receptor antagonists should be given twice daily to be most effective in patients with frequent GERD. While these drugs are approximately 75% effective in patients with mild to moderate degrees of esophagitis, they are only 50% effective in healing moderate to severe esophagitis. Therefore, H_2-receptor antagonists are appropriate for patients with mild to moderate GERD and remain a major treatment modality for reflux symptoms.

PPIs act by blocking the hydrogen–potassium ATPase on the apical surface of the parietal cell. PPIs are more effective than H_2-receptor antagonists because they act on the final common pathway of acid secretion rather than one of its three receptors (histamine, acetylcholine, and gastrin). The timing of PPI use is important as these drugs are most effective when taken in a fasting state 15–30 minutes before meals, as proton pumps are then activated by meals and become available for blocking by the medication. Recent studies have shown that inappropriate timing of PPI use is common among patients with inadequate response to the drug.

Side effects of PPI can occur in up to 3% of patients and can include headaches and diarrhea. Rare side effects include hepatitis and interstitial nephritis. PPIs induce the cytochrome P450 system, necessitating dosage adjustments of warfarin, phenytoin, and diazepam. There was controversy about the effect of PPIs on clopidogrel, which is a prodrug that is converted to its active form via the cytochrome P450 system (CYP2C19). PPIs are both a substrate and an inhibitor of CYP2C19, which may potentially reduce clopidogrel's inhibitory effect on platelet P2Y12. Early observational clinical studies on the influence of PPIs on the effectiveness of clopidogrel have shown conflicting results. However, a large prospective randomized trial in clopidogrel users of omeprazole versus placebo showed no significant difference in cardiovascular events, along with a significant reduction in GI events. Therefore, current evidence does not justify a conclusion that PPI use is associated with clinical cardiovascular events among clopidogrel users.

PPIs are indicated as initial therapy in patients with moderate to severe GERD and in patients with complications of GERD such as bleeding and strictures. A study reviewing 26 trials involving 4064 patients that compared PPIs with H_2-receptor antagonists showed that PPI therapy was

Table 12–6. Efficacy of proton pump inhibitors in decreasing intragastric pH.

Therapy	% Time pH >4.0[a]	No. Hours pH >4.0[b]	Mean pH
Esomeprazole, 40 mg	58.43	14.0	4.04
Rabeprazole, 20 mg	50.53	12.1	3.70
Omeprazole, 20 mg	49.16	11.8	3.54
Lansoprazole, 30 mg	47.98	11.5	3.56
Pantoprazole, 40 mg	41.94	10.1	3.33

[a]Percentage of time that intragastric pH was 4.0.
[b]Mean 24-hour intragastric pH on day 5 by treatment group (n = 34).
Adapted with permission from Miner P Jr, Katz PO, Chen Y, et al: Gastric acid control with esomeprazole, lansoprazole, omeprazole, pantoprazole, and rabeprazole: a five-way crossover study. *Am J Gastroenterol.* 2003;98(12):2616–2620.

significantly better than H_2-receptor antagonist therapy in treatment of esophagitis at 4–8 weeks. Independent comparisons of the currently available PPIs have consistently shown first-generation PPIs (all except esomeprazole) to be essentially equal in esophagitis healing rates and intragastric profiles. There have been several reports that rabeprazole has a faster onset of action than the others; however, the clinical significance of this is debatable. A comparison of all five available PPIs in controlling 24-hour intragastric pH showed a statistically significant advantage for esomeprazole on day 5 of therapy (Table 12–6).

The safety of long-term PPI therapy has been demonstrated by the treatment of millions of patients over the past 20 years and the approval by the FDA for the over-the-counter availability of several of these drugs. During the initial testing of these medicines, gastric carcinoids were seen in animal models. This complication has not been demonstrated to occur in humans. There is also a theoretical concern about interference with nutrient absorption (especially magnesium, calcium, iron, and protein) due to a significant decrease in gastric acid production. However, there has only been a demonstrable reduction in absorption of magnesium. A modest reduction of vitamin B_{12} levels has been seen with long-term PPI use, which may be due to a decrease in protein-bound vitamin B_{12} absorption. Therefore, vitamin B_{12} levels should be periodically monitored in patients who are on continuous PPI therapy for more than 5 years. Increased positive breath test for bacterial overgrowth of the small bowel has been noted to occur in patients on chronic PPIs, although the clinical significance is not clear. The use of PPIs has also been associated with increased rates of community-acquired pneumonias, *Clostridium difficile* infection, and hip fractures in observational studies. However, in a large randomized, placebo-controlled trial, pantoprazole use for 3 years was not associated with any adverse event other than an increased risk of enteric infection. Overall, current clinical evidence suggests that use of PPIs, even for long-term management, is safe and should not be avoided when clinically indicated. Nevertheless, dose reduction or discontinuation should be

attempted when symptoms are under control to maintain patients on the lowest possible dose.

Although most patients with GERD are successfully managed with lifestyle modifications and antisecretory therapy, some patients may have persistent symptoms despite treatment. Antireflux therapies aiming to enhance the mechanical barrier at the LES may be needed in this population to reduce nonacidic reflux or provide further symptom relief. Baclofen has been shown to be effective in increasing basal LES tone and inhibiting transient LES relaxation, thereby decreasing reflux. However, the use of baclofen has been limited by its short half-life and poor patient tolerability. Surgery remains the mainstay of antireflux therapies and may be employed in patients with a good clinical response to medical treatments who wish to discontinue medications or in patients who have failed medical therapy.

Reflux hypersensitivity or a functional cause may play a role in esophageal symptoms, particularly among patients with persistent symptoms refractory to antisecretory therapy. ARM may help identify these patients with reflux hypersensitivity (normal reflux burden, significant symptom-reflux association) or functional disorder (normal reflux burden, negative symptom-reflux association). Neuromodulator therapy, such as tricyclic antidepressant, and behavioral therapy, such as diaphragmatic breathing or cognitive behavioral therapy, may be effective in treatment of these patients.

B. Surgical Considerations

Antireflux surgery has been performed since the early 1950s. The goal of antireflux surgery is to narrow the lower esophageal luminal diameter to prevent the reflux of gastroduodenal contents. In a prospective, randomized trial of medical versus surgical treatment for patients with reflux-related refractory heartburn, antireflux surgery was associated with significantly higher rate of symptom improvement than continued medical therapy. The most widely performed procedure is the Nissen fundoplication, which involves wrapping of the fundus around the bottom of the esophagus to enhance the antireflux barrier. Several studies have reported a symptomatic response of 80–90% in patients undergoing this fundoplication procedure. A review of six randomized controlled trials comparing open and laparoscopic fundoplications found no difference in the GERD recurrence rate between the two procedures, but demonstrated a lower operative morbidity and shorter postoperative hospital stay with the laparoscopic approach. However, up to 62% of patients may again require medications 10 years after their antireflux surgery.

Complications of fundoplication include dysphagia, chest pain, gas-bloat syndrome, postoperative flatulence, and vagal nerve injuries leading to gastroparesis and diarrhea. The prevalence of these complications ranges between 5% and 20%. Postoperative dysphagia occurs in up to 18% of patients, with early dysphagia occurring in approximately 20% of patients and late dysphagia occurring in 6% of patients at 2 years. Toupet fundoplication is an alternate form of the surgery that involves a partial (270°) wrap, rather than the full (360°) wrap of a Nissen. In a head-to-head randomized clinical trial, both types of fundoplication resulted in comparable improvement in acid exposure, symptoms, and health-related quality of life, although Toupet was associated with less solid food dysphagia postoperatively.

A new surgical antireflux therapy approved in recent years involves the placement of a bracelet with magnetic beads at the gastroesophageal junction. Approximation of these beads by magnetic force creates a barrier at the gastroesophageal junction to prevent refluxing of gastric contents. During swallowing, the propulsive force from esophageal peristalsis leads to separation of these magnetic beads and opening of the bracelet, allowing passage of the food bolus through the gastroesophageal junction. This procedure has been found to be effective in selected patients, particularly those without a large hiatal hernia or significant esophageal dysmotility, and may be considered as an alternative to traditional fundoplication. Further studies are needed to assess the long-term efficacy and safety of this procedure.

As discussed above, obesity has been associated with increased prevalence of GERD. For patients with obesity and significant GERD symptoms, bariatric surgery may be more effective for reflux than traditional antireflux procedures and should be considered as a strategy for management of GERD. Among the bariatric surgical options, Roux-en-Y gastric bypass may be most preferable, as other strategies such as adjustable gastric band and sleeve gastrectomy may be associated with increased reflux.

C. Endoscopic Antireflux Procedures

Various endoscopic techniques have been developed for the treatment of GERD. The two types of endoscopic therapies currently available are (1) transoral incisionless fundoplication (TIF), which involves endoscopically wrapping part of the fundus around the gastroesophageal junction using suturing techniques, and (2) radiofrequency ablation to the lower esophageal region to enhance the barrier function. Most studies of endoscopic therapy have reported limited follow-up information for a relatively small number of patients or are without controlled data.

Although some studies demonstrated a decrease in 24-hour intraesophageal acid exposure, normalization of acid exposure was the exception rather than the rule for these techniques. In addition, while improvement in symptoms has been shown, they were either not significantly different from sham control or not compared to a control arm. Complications associated with these endoscopic antireflux procedures include bleeding, aspiration pneumonia, perforation, mediastinitis, and rarely, death. Future studies are needed to better understand the mechanism of these treatments and improve the efficacy and durability of these endoscopic procedures.

Bhatt DL, Cryer BL, Contant CF, et al. COGENT Investigators. Clopidogrel with or without omeprazole in coronary artery disease. N Engl J Med. 2010;363:1909–1917. [PMID: 20925534]

Bytzer P, Morocutti A, Kennerly P, et al. ROSE Trial Investigators. Effect of rabeprazole and omeprazole on the onset of gastroesophageal reflux disease symptom relief during the first seven days of treatment. Scand J Gastroenterol. 2006;41:1132–1140. [PMID: 15990197]

Catarci M, Gentileschi P, Papi C, et al. Evidence-based appraisal of antireflux fundoplication. Ann Surg. 2004;239:325–337. [PMID: 15075649]

Corley DA, Kubo A, Zhao W, et al. Proton pump inhibitors and histamine-2 receptor antagonists are associated with hip fractures among at-risk patients. Gastroenterology. 2010;139:93–101. [PMID: 20353792]

Cundy T, Mackay J. Proton pump inhibitors and severe hypomagnesemia. Curr Opin Gastroenterol 2011;27:180–185. [PMID: 20856115]

Finlayson SR, Laycock WS, Birkmeyer JD. National trends in utilization and outcomes of antireflux surgery. Surg Endosc. 2003;17:864–867. [PMID: 12632134]

Flum DR, Koepsell T, Heagerty P, et al. The nationwide frequency of major adverse outcomes in antireflux surgery and the role of surgeon experience, 1992–1997. J Am Coll Surg. 2002;195:611–618. [PMID: 12437246]

Ganz RA, Peters JH, Horgan S, et al. Esophageal sphincter device for gastroesophageal reflux disease. N Engl J Med. 2013;368(8):719–727. [PMID: 23425164]

Hunter JG, Kahrilas PJ, Bell RC, et al. Efficacy of transoral fundoplication vs omeprazole for treatment of regurgitation in a randomized controlled trial. Gastroenterology. 2015;148(2):324–333.e5. [PMID: 25448925]

Kaltenbach T, Crockett S, Gerson LB. Are lifestyle measures effective in patients with gastroesophageal reflux disease? An evidence-based approach. Arch Intern Med. 2006;166:965–971. [PMID: 16682569]

Klinkenberg-Knol EC, Nelis F, Dent J. Long-term omeprazole treatment in resistant gastroesophageal reflux disease: efficacy, safety, and influence on gastric mucosa. Gastroenterology. 2000;118:661–669. [PMID: 10734017]

Klok RM, Postma MJ, van Hout BA, et al. Meta-analysis: comparing the efficacy of proton pump inhibitors in short-term use. Aliment Pharmacol Therapeut. 2003;17:1237–1245. [PMID: 12755827]

Laheij RJ, Sturkenboom MC, Hassing RJ, et al. Risk of community-acquired pneumonia and use of gastric acid-suppressive drugs. *JAMA*. 2004;292:1955–1960. [PMID: 15507580]

Linsky A, Gupta K, Lawler EV, et al. Proton pump inhibitors and risk for recurrent *Clostridium difficile* infection. *Arch Intern Med*. 2010;170:772–778. [PMID: 20458084]

Lo WK, Chan WW. Proton pump inhibitor use and the risk of small intestinal bacterial overgrowth: a meta-analysis. *Clin Gastroenterol Hepatol*. 2013;11:483–490. [PMID: 23270866]

Moayyedi P, Eikelboom JW, Bosch J, et al. Safety of proton pump inhibitors based on a large, multi-year, randomized trial of patients receiving rivaroxaban or aspirin. *Gastroenterology*. 2019;157(3):682–691.e2. [PMID: 31152740]

Pallati PK, Shaligram A, Shostrom VK, et al. Improvement in gastroesophageal reflux disease symptoms after various bariatric procedures: review of the Bariatric Outcomes Longitudinal Database. *Surg Obes Relat Dis*. 2014;10(3):502–507. [PMID: 24238733]

Spechler SJ, Lee E, Ahnen D, et al. Long-term outcome of medical and surgical therapies for gastroesophageal reflux disease: follow-up of a randomized controlled trial. *JAMA*. 2001; 285:2331–2338. [PMID: 11343480]

Spechler SJ, Hunter JG, Jones KM, et al. Randomized trial of medical versus surgical treatment for refractory heartburn. *N Engl J Med*. 2019;381(16):1513–1523. [PMID: 31618539]

Targownik LE, Lix LM, Leung S, et al. Proton-pump inhibitor use is not associated with osteoporosis or accelerated bone mineral density loss. *Gastroenterology*. 2010;138:896–904. [PMID: 19931262]

Yang YX, Lewis JD, Epstein S, et al. Long-term proton pump inhibitor therapy and risk of hip fracture. *JAMA*. 2006;296:2947–2953. [PMID: 17190895]

Zhang Q, Lehmann A, Rigda R, et al. Control of transient lower oesophageal sphincter relaxations and reflux by the GABA(B) agonist baclofen in patients with gastro-oesophageal reflux disease. *Gut*. 2002;50:19–24. [PMID: 11772961]

E. Management of Peptic Esophageal Strictures

1. Esophageal dilation—Peptic strictures of the esophagus due to GERD account for nearly 80% of esophageal strictures, although this may be decreasing due to the use of PPIs. The primary indication for esophageal dilation is to relieve dysphagia; empiric dilatation with large-bore dilators cannot be recommended if no structural abnormalities are seen endoscopically.

Three general types of dilators are currently in use. These are (1) mercury or tungsten-filled bougies (Maloney or Hurst), (2) wire-guided polyvinyl dilators (Savary-Gilliard or American), and (3) TTS ("through the scope") balloon dilators. Maloney bougies have a tapered tip and can be passed blindly or under fluoroscopic control. Savary and American dilators are passed over a guidewire that has been positioned in the antrum, with or without fluoroscopic guidance. TTS dilating balloons are available in either single or multiple diameters that may be passed with or without wire guidance.

In preparation for endoscopic dilation, anticoagulants should be discontinued. Routine antibiotic coverage is not recommended; however, endocarditis prophylaxis should be followed. Patients should be informed of the risks associated with esophageal dilation; the principal complications are perforation, bleeding, and aspiration. The perforation rate for esophageal strictures after dilation has been reported to be 0.1–0.4%. Perforation is more common in radiation-induced strictures, malignant strictures, complex strictures due to lye ingestion, and in patients with achalasia.

The degree of dilation within an endoscopic session should be based on the severity of the luminal narrowing (Plates 7 and 8). A "rule of three" has been described for esophageal dilation using bougie dilators. After moderate resistance is encountered, no more than three consecutive dilators in increments of 1 mm should be passed in a single session. This rule does not appear to directly apply to balloon dilators in simple esophageal strictures, which may be incrementally dilated greater than 3 mm. No data exist on the optimal time the balloon should remain inflated. Dilation therapy for a symptomatic Schatzki ring should be directed toward achieving rupture of the ring.

No clear advantage has been demonstrated between bougie and TTS dilators. In patients with benign peptic strictures, the long-term benefits of dilation appear greatest when a luminal diameter of more than 12 mm is achieved. For peptic strictures, smaller lumen diameter, presence of a hiatal hernia greater than 5 cm, persistence of heartburn after dilation, and number of dilations needed for initial dysphagia relief were significant predictors of early symptomatic recurrence.

2. Proton pump inhibitors—Patients with peptic strictures should be treated with PPI therapy. Patients with peptic strictures complicated by food impactions should undergo treatment with PPIs prior to dilation of the peptic stricture. PPI use decreases stricture recurrence and the need for repeat stricture dilation.

Hernandez LV, Jacobson JW, Harris MS. Comparison among the perforation rates of Maloney, balloon and Savary dilation of esophageal strictures. *Gastrointest Endosc*. 2000;51:460–462. [PMID: 10744819]

Said A, Brust DJ, Gaumnitz EA, et al. Predictors of early recurrence of benign esophageal strictures. *Am J Gastroenterol*. 2003;98:1252–1256. [PMID: 12818265]

Standards of Practice Committee, Egan JV, Baron TH, Adler DG, et al. Esophageal dilatation. *Gastrointest Endosc*. 2006;63: 755–760. [PMID: 16650533]

Course & Prognosis

Once patients without esophagitis have responded to lifestyle changes and medical therapy, and achieved remission from clinical symptoms, most should have a trial of medication tapering. Symptom relief should be sustained for 2–3 months before attempting to withdraw medications. PPI therapy can be tapered to an every-other-day regimen or to a reduced dose (if possible), or switched to a H_2-blocker. Most patients who are treated with H_2-blockers are on twice-daily medications, and the initial tapering should be to a once-a-day regimen. If a patient tolerates a taper for 2–4 weeks without an increase in symptoms, the dosage can be further decreased or the medication discontinued. The goal of long-term treatment is to step down management to the lowest level of medical therapy that controls symptoms. However, if a patient experiences recurrent symptoms, the medication regimen should be increased until symptom resolution is achieved.

If GERD patients on long-term PPI therapy are abruptly withdrawn (not tapered) from their medicine, many will experience symptoms that are worse than their initial presenting complaints. This phenomenon of "rebound hypersecretion" occurs when parietal cells secrete elevated amounts of acid after a prolonged blockade. A prolonged tapering of PPI therapy helps improve these symptoms. Eradication of corpus predominant *Helicobacter pylori* infection has been found to worsen rebound gastric hypersecretion, as corpus predominant gastritis normally leads to a decrease in acid production. On the other hand, antral predominant *H pylori* infection is associated with acid hypersecretion, and eradication may lead to improvement in acid-related symptoms.

Therapy for GERD is frequently chronic and long-term in most patients as the underlying disorder is dysfunction of the LES, which is usually not directly affected by medical therapy. Among patients with erosive esophagitis, more than 80% will relapse if their therapy is stopped. The same medication that induces remission is usually required in the same dosage to maintain remission. In those with nonerosive GERD, on-demand therapy is a cost-effective alternative to maintenance treatment.

Long-term GERD treatment can be challenging, but empowering patients to recognize the dietary and lifestyle choices that produce symptoms enables the majority of motivated patients to wean themselves off medical therapy. For those patients who are unable to discontinue acid-suppression therapy due to symptom recurrence, the medical therapies available are fortunately very effective and generally safe.

Inadomi JM, Jamal R, Murata GH, et al. Step-down management of gastroesophageal reflux disease. *Gastroenterology.* 2001;121:1095–1100. [PMID: 11677201]

Inadomi JM, McIntyre L, Bernard L, et al. Step-down from multiple-to single-dose proton pump inhibitors (PPIs): a prospective study of patients with heartburn or acid regurgitation completely relieved with PPIs. *Am J Gastroenterol.* 2003; 98:1940–1944. [PMID: 14499769]

Barrett Esophagus

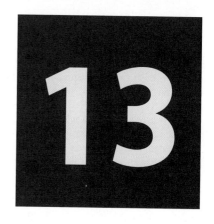

Kunal Jajoo, MD

ESSENTIALS OF DIAGNOSIS

▶ Replacement of normal squamous epithelium of the distal esophagus with specialized intestinal metaplasia (SIM).

▶ Endoscopy and biopsy are essential for an accurate diagnosis.

▶ Presence of high-grade dysplasia should be confirmed by two expert gastrointestinal pathologists.

▶ Risk factors for progression to adenocarcinoma include presence of dysplasia, long segment of Barrett esophagus, and mucosal abnormalities (nodules, ulcerations, or strictures).

General Considerations

Barrett esophagus is the replacement of the normal squamous epithelium of the distal esophagus with SIM. It is thought to be caused by chronic gastroesophageal reflux disease (GERD), which leads to esophagitis and subsequent metaplastic change of the esophageal lining. SIM may be protective against further injury by gastric acid; however, this metaplastic epithelium is also associated with an increased risk for esophageal adenocarcinoma. There is considerable ongoing debate regarding various aspects of Barrett esophagus, such as the exact neoplastic risk it confers as well as its management if it has become dysplastic.

Sharma P. Clinical practice. Barrett's esophagus. *N Engl J Med.* 2009;361:2548–2556. [PMID: 20032324]

A. Epidemiology

The overall prevalence of Barrett esophagus in the adult population of the United States is estimated to be 5.6% (although estimates have varied from 0.9% to more than 20% depending on the population studied). In patients with GERD, the prevalence of Barrett esophagus is higher, approximately 5–10%. In patients with severe GERD, such as those with erosive esophagitis, the prevalence is approximately 10%; in patients with peptic strictures of the esophagus, the prevalence is almost 30%. Barrett esophagus affects males more than females by a ratio of approximately 3:1. The typical patient is a Caucasian, middle-aged male. In certain studies, alcohol and smoking have been found to be risk factors for the presence of Barrett esophagus. The conclusion that Barrett esophagus is an acquired complication of chronic GERD is supported by the fact that Barrett esophagus is exceedingly rare in children with competent lower esophageal sphincters (LES).

Hayeck TJ, Kong CY, Spechler SJ, et al. The prevalence of Barrett's esophagus in the US: estimates from a simulation model confirmed by SEER data. *Dis Esophagus.* 2010;23:451–457. [PMID: 20353441]

Spechler SJ, Fitzgerald RC, Prasad GA, et al. History, molecular mechanisms, and endoscopic treatment of Barrett's esophagus. *Gastroenterology.* 2010;138:854–869. [PMID: 20080098]

B. Pathogenesis

The components of the refluxate in GERD (both gastric acid and bile salts) are important etiologic factors in the development of Barrett esophagus. Esophageal pH monitoring studies have shown that patients with Barrett esophagus have more esophageal acid exposure than healthy controls or even patients with mild heartburn. The greater acid exposure in Barrett esophagus results from longer periods of acid reflux, rather than from a greater number of reflux episodes. Patients with Barrett esophagus may be predisposed to more severe acid reflux episodes due to mechanical dysfunction of the LES as well as the decreased amplitude of distal esophageal contractions.

Helicobacter pylori infection of the stomach causes chronic inflammation that can result in gastric intestinal metaplasia and cancer. However, there is no clear association between *H pylori* infection and GERD, and the organism does not infect the esophagus. In fact, *H pylori* infection of the stomach may actually protect the esophagus from GERD and Barrett esophagus.

The role of bile salts in refluxed gastric acid in the development of Barrett esophagus continues to be debated and investigated. Increased levels of refluxed bile acid concentrations have been found in patients with Barrett esophagus. Acid and bile have been shown to induce a class of homeobox genes (*Cdx*), which are regulators of cell differentiation, and this has been postulated to result in metaplasia. Some clinicians argue that the increased reflux of bile salts in these patients necessitates a mechanical treatment for their GERD, such as a fundoplication. Finally, the genetic and environmental factors that also play a role in the development of Barrett esophagus are continuing to be understood.

Rubenstein JH, Inadomi JM, Scheiman J, et al. Association between *Helicobacter pylori* and Barrett's esophagus, erosive esophagitis, and gastroesophageal reflux symptoms. *Clin Gastroenterol Hepatol.* 2014;12:239–245. [PMID: 23988686]

Souza RF, Krishnan K, Spechler SJ. Acid, bile and CDX: the ABCs of making Barrett's metaplasia. *Am J Physiol Gastrointest Liver Physiol.* 2008;295:G211–G218. [PMID: 18556417]

▶ Clinical Findings

Barrett esophagus cannot be detected on clinical assessment alone, as there are no specific symptoms that distinguish this condition from GERD without Barrett esophagus. The gold standard for the diagnosis of Barrett esophagus is upper endoscopy with biopsy of the distal esophagus.

A. Endoscopic & Biopsy Findings

Barrett esophagus is diagnosed when mucosal biopsies confirm the presence of SIM in a columnar-lined distal esophagus. In normal individuals, the squamocolumnar junction (SCJ), demarcated as the Z-line, coincides with the gastroesophageal junction (GEJ). The SCJ is the transition from the pale squamous mucosa of the esophagus to the salmon-colored gastric mucosa. Endoscopically, the GEJ is best defined as the top of the gastric folds. If there is proximal displacement of the SCJ above the top of the gastric folds into the tubular esophagus, a columnar-lined esophagus is present and biopsies should be taken (Plate 9).

Early studies defined the diagnosis of Barrett esophagus as the presence of 3 cm of columnar-lined distal esophagus with SIM (Plate 10). Subsequent work deemed the presence of less than 3 cm of SIM as "short-segment" Barrett esophagus. The significance of intestinal metaplasia at the SCJ is debatable, and at present, it is not recommended that a normal-appearing SCJ, including irregular Z-line, be biopsied.

It is important to note that intestinal metaplasia of the cardia cannot be distinguished from intestinal metaplasia of the esophagus. Therefore, the proximal displacement of the SCJ into the tubular esophagus must be documented endoscopically in order to diagnose a patient with Barrett esophagus.

The clinical significance of Barrett esophagus length is important as studies have confirmed that longer segments have higher risks of progression to adenocarcinoma. To maintain consistency across studies of Barrett esophagus, the Prague criteria were established to determine the extent of disease. By these criteria, the extent of circumferential (C) and maximal (M) visualized Barrett esophagus is measured, and standard definitions of endoscopic landmarks are used. These criteria have good interobserver reliability for Barrett esophagus ≥1 cm in length. It remains to be determined whether these criteria will become adopted broadly.

Biopsy specimens of Barrett esophagus are classified as nondysplastic, indefinite for dysplasia, low-grade dysplasia, or high-grade dysplasia. The diagnosis of dysplasia is typically reserved for lesions in which nuclear atypia is present on the mucosal surface.

Avidan B, Sonnenberg A, Schnell T, et al. Hiatal hernia size, Barrett's length and severity of acid reflux are all risk factors for esophageal adenocarcinoma. *Am J Gastroenterol.* 2002;97:1930–1936. [PMID: 12190156]

Sharma P, Dent J, Armstrong D, et al. The development and validation of an endoscopic grading system for Barrett's esophagus: the Prague C & M criteria. *Gastroenterology.* 2006;131:1392–1399. [PMID: 17101315]

Sharma P, McQuaid K, Dent J, et al. A critical review of the diagnosis and management of Barrett's esophagus: the AGA Chicago workshop. *Gastroenterology.* 2004;127:310–330. [PMID: 15236196]

Wang KE, Sampliner RE. Practice Parameters Committee of the American College of Gastroenterology. Updated guidelines for the diagnosis, surveillance and therapy of Barrett's esophagus. *Am J Gastroenterol.* 2008;103:788–797. [PMID: 18341497]

B. Screening

Screening refers to performing a test on a large asymptomatic sample of the population to identify a disease. The role of screening upper endoscopy for Barrett esophagus is unclear, and the major gastroenterologic societies are not unanimous in their recommendations. Patients with chronic GERD are at increased risk for Barrett esophagus, and the prevalence of Barrett esophagus is higher in middle-aged white males, suggesting that screening should be reserved for this higher risk subgroup. The American College of Gastroenterology guideline acknowledges the controversy in screening for Barrett esophagus and only states that the highest yield is achieved in screening patients over age 50 with chronic GERD symptoms.

Decision analysis studies that have examined the cost-effectiveness of screening for Barrett esophagus have shown conflicting results. In addition, a significant proportion of patients with esophageal adenocarcinoma report no prior symptoms of reflux. What cannot be debated, however, is that the majority of patients newly diagnosed with esophageal cancer have not had a previous diagnosis of Barrett esophagus, emphasizing a need for more effective screening strategies. As the cost of esophageal visualization decreases with newer techniques such as transnasal and video capsule endoscopy, these issues will need to be readdressed.

Shaheen NJ, Falk GW, Iyer PG, et al. ACG Clinical Guideline: Diagnosis and Management of Barrett's Esophagus. *Am J Gastroenterol.* 2016;111:30–50. [PMID: 26526079]

Taylor JB, Rubenstein JH. Meta-analyses of the effect of symptoms of gastroesophageal reflux on the risk of Barrett's esophagus. *Am J Gastroenterol.* 2010;105:1730–1737. [PMID: 20485283]

C. Surveillance

Surveillance in patients with Barrett esophagus refers to the performance of serial endoscopies at regular intervals with the goal of detecting dysplasia and early cancer at a curable stage. If the incidence of cancer in patients with Barrett esophagus was high, surveillance would be cost-effective; however, if the incidence was low, an extremely small proportion of the at-risk population would benefit. The overall risk of cancer in Barrett esophagus patients is estimated to be approximately 0.5% per year. Stated another way, the risk of any given patient with Barrett esophagus developing cancer is approximately 1 in 200 per year.

As with screening, the cost-effectiveness of surveillance in Barrett esophagus is debated. Retrospective data have shown that cancers detected during Barrett esophagus surveillance are more likely to be found at an early stage and are associated with better survival compared with those not detected during surveillance. Such retrospective studies are subject to both lead-time and length of time bias. A few studies have demonstrated no difference in overall survival between patients with Barrett esophagus and the general population, calling into question the utility of Barrett esophagus endoscopic surveillance. Barrett esophagus patients more frequently die from causes other than esophageal adenocarcinoma, suggesting that surveillance is of no benefit to the vast majority of these patients. It is not clear which patients who are known to have Barrett esophagus benefit from surveillance.

At present, until better markers of risk stratification are found, the surveillance interval of upper endoscopy is determined by the degree of dysplasia found in a Barrett esophagus segment. Barrett esophagus biomarkers are being actively investigated because the diagnosis and detection of dysplasia have significant limitations. There is a high rate of interobserver variability in the reading of dysplasia, particularly among community pathologists as it can be difficult to distinguish between inflammatory changes and dysplasia. In addition, random biopsy surveillance introduces the possibility

of sampling error given that the distribution of dysplasia throughout a Barrett esophagus segment can be patchy. At present, the presence of dysplasia in a Barrett esophagus segment remains the best method of cancer risk stratification. It is strongly recommended that when a diagnosis of dysplastic Barrett esophagus is being considered, the histopathologic slides be reviewed by two pathologists with expertise in this area.

Currently, upper endoscopy with four-quadrant "jumbo" biopsies at 2-cm intervals remains the best method for obtaining surveillance biopsies once esophageal inflammation related to GERD has been well controlled with antisecretory therapy. Biopsy specimens should be obtained in four quadrants at 2-cm intervals beginning at the end of the tubular esophagus (top of the gastric folds) and continuing proximally to the SCJ. Any mucosal abnormalities such as ulcerations, strictures, or nodules should be extensively sampled, ideally by endoscopic mucosal resection (EMR). At present, chromoendoscopy and other "optical biopsy" techniques have not been validated on a large scale and are not recommended for standard use.

The recommendations of the major gastroenterologic societies differ slightly regarding the time interval between surveillance endoscopies in Barrett esophagus (Table 13–1). If a patient is found to have Barrett esophagus without dysplasia on incident endoscopy, it is generally recommended that a repeat esophagogastroduodenoscopy (EGD) be performed in 3–5 years. The previous recommendation for a 1-year follow-up examination has been eliminated given the low-risk of progression, as long as complete visual inspection and biopsies were performed at the incident endoscopy. A large trial of over 1200 patients demonstrated that 98.6% of patients with nondysplastic Barrett esophagus were cancer free at the 5-year follow-up. It is important to note that in a recent retrospective study of patients with Barrett esophagus, 53% of patients who developed high-grade dysplasia or cancer had two consecutive initial endoscopies with biopsies that revealed nondysplastic mucosa.

Shaheen NJ, Falk GW, Iyer PG, et al. ACG Clinical Guideline: diagnosis and management of Barrett's esophagus. *Am J Gastroenterol.* 2016;111:30–50. [PMID: 26526079]

Wani S, Falk G, Hall M, et al. Patients with non-dysplastic Barrett's esophagus have low risks for developing dysplasia or esophageal adenocarcinoma. *Clin Gastroenterol Hepatol.* 2011;9:220–227. [PMID: 21115133]

D. Risk Factors for Progression to Adenocarcinoma

Many studies have assessed risk factors for the development of adenocarcinoma in patients with Barrett esophagus (Table 13–2). Dysplasia is the primary risk factor for progression to adenocarcinoma. Dysplastic transformation of Barrett esophagus epithelium is thought to precede the development of adenocarcinoma, although whether this

Table 13–1. Summary of recommendations for surveillance endoscopies in Barrett esophagus.

	ASGE	ACG	AGA
Screening	Insufficient evidence on the effectiveness of screening. If screening is performed, strategy should identify at-risk patients	Screening is controversial; consider screening for those with multiple risk factors	Screening suggested for those with multiple risk factors
No dysplasia	Repeat EGD every 3–5 years	Repeat EGD every 3–5 years	Repeat EGD every 3–5 years
Low-grade dysplasia	Confirm pathology Endoscopic therapy preferred; annual surveillance for patients who wish to avoid adverse events	Confirm pathology Endoscopic therapy is preferred, annual surveillance is an acceptable alternative	Confirm pathology Repeat EGD in 3–6 months to rule out a visible lesion Endoscopic therapy or surveillance are both reasonable options
High-grade dysplasia	Confirm pathology Endoscopic therapy preferred over surgery, resect all visible lesions, ablate any remaining Barrett	Confirm pathology Repeat EGD to exclude cancer; if mucosal irregularity, then EMR Treat with ablative therapies	Confirm pathology Endoscopic therapy preferred, otherwise 3 month surveillance

ACG, American College of Gastroenterology; AGA, American Gastroenterological Association; ASGE, American Society for Gastrointestinal Endoscopy; EGD, esophagogastroduodenoscopy; EMR, endoscopic mucosal resection; GERD, gastroesophageal reflux disease.

progression occurs without interruption from nondysplastic Barrett esophagus to low-grade dysplasia to high-grade dysplasia is unclear. Patients with short-segment Barrett esophagus appear to have a lower incidence of dysplasia since less mucosa is involved (6–8% in short-segment Barrett esophagus vs 15–24% in long-segment Barrett esophagus). Furthermore, the risk of adenocarcinoma has been estimated to be 2–15 times higher with long-segment Barrett esophagus compared to short-segment Barrett esophagus. Biomarkers for the development of adenocarcinoma in Barrett esophagus patients, such as aneuploidy and p53 loss of heterozygosity as determined by flow cytometry, immunohistochemistry, and fluorescence in situ hybridization (FISH) to aid in the detection of dysplasia, are still experimental.

Cooper BT, Chapman W, Neumann CS, et al. Continuous treatment of Barrett's oesophagus patients with proton pump inhibitors up to 13 years: observations on regression and cancer incidence. *Aliment Pharm Ther.* 2006;23:727–733. [PMID: 16556174]

Prasad GA, Bansal A, Sharma P, et al. Predictors of progression in Barrett's esophagus: current knowledge and future directions. *Am J Gastroenterol.* 2010;105:1490–1502. [PMID: 20104216]

Qumseya, B, Sultan S, Bain P, et al. ASGE guideline on screening and surveillance of Barrett's esophagus. *Gastrointest Endosc.* 2019;90:335–359.e2. [PMID: 31439127]

Sharma P, Shaheen NJ, Katzk D, et al. AGA clinical practice update on endoscopic treatment of Barrett's esophagus with dysplasia and/or early cancer: expert review. *Gastroenterology.* 2020;158:760–769. [PMID: 31730766]

Wongsurawat VJ, Finley JC, Galipeau PC, et al. Genetic mechanisms of TP53 loss of heterozygosity in Barrett's esophagus: implications for biomarker validation. *Cancer Epidemiol Biomarkers Prev.* 2006;15:509–516. [PMID: 16537709]

Table 13–2. Risk factors for esophageal adenocarcinoma in patients with Barrett esophagus.

Clinical factors	Diet low in fruits and vegetables High body mass index Male gender Older age Tobacco smoking Heavy alcohol use Working in a stooped posture Less use of proton pump inhibitors Fewer heartburn symptoms Use of medicines that relax the lower esophageal sphincter
Endoscopic factors	Long segment of Barrett esophagus Mucosal abnormalities Nodularity Ulceration Strictures
Histologic factors	High-grade dysplasia
Biomarkers	Aneuploidy p53 loss of heterozygosity

▶ Treatment

A. Nondysplastic Barrett Esophagus

Patients with Barrett esophagus should be placed on once daily proton pump inhibitor (PPI) therapy indefinitely. There are data demonstrating that patients on PPIs have a lower rate of progression to dysplasia and adenocarcinoma than patients not taking PPIs. In one study, the cumulative incidence of dysplasia was significantly lower among patients who received PPI after Barrett esophagus diagnosis than in those who received no therapy or histamine receptor antagonists. Furthermore, among those on PPIs, a longer duration of use was associated with a less frequent occurrence of dysplasia. Every patient diagnosed with Barrett esophagus should be treated with a PPI whether or not symptomatic GERD is present.

At present, there are not enough data to support ablative therapies for nondysplastic Barrett esophagus. In the future, biomarkers may provide better risk stratification justifying endoscopic ablation of nondysplastic Barrett esophagus in high-risk patients. However, given that the vast majority of patients with Barrett esophagus do not progress to adenocarcinoma, the use of these methods for this indication cannot currently be recommended.

Data suggest that, despite long-term antisecretory therapy, long segments of Barrett esophagus do not regress. Normalization of SIM has been described in cases of "ultra-short" Barrett esophagus and short-segment Barrett esophagus. Patients with long segments of Barrett esophagus should be informed that their Barrett esophagus will not regress and that they should remain on PPI therapy indefinitely and undergo surveillance endoscopies.

Cyclooxygenase (COX)-2 inhibitors (both aspirin and nonsteroidal anti-inflammatory drugs [NSAIDs]) have been studied as chemoprevention of Barrett esophagus progression. A study of esophagectomy specimens correlating COX-2 immunopositivity and clinical course demonstrated that tumors expressing higher levels of COX-2 were more likely to be associated with distant metastases, local recurrence, and reduced survival. A meta-analysis of cohort studies estimated that aspirin use was inversely associated with esophageal adenocarcinoma (odds ratio [OR] 0.64, 95% confidence interval [CI] 0.52–0.79) with a similar reduction in risk observed for NSAIDs (OR 0.65, 95% CI 0.50–0.85). Statin medications have also been proposed as chemopreventive agents for esophageal carcinoma. A recent large case-control study demonstrated that patients with Barrett esophagus on antisecretory therapy who filled prescriptions for either NSAID medications or statin medications had a reduced risk of developing esophageal adenocarcinoma. In the future, chemoprevention of Barrett esophagus progression may become the standard of care if further human clinical studies can substantiate these findings.

Abnet CC, Freedman ND, Kamangar F, et al. Non-steroidal anti-inflammatory drugs and risk of gastric and oesophageal adenocarcinomas: results from a cohort study and a meta-analysis. *Br J Cancer*. 2009;100:551–557. [PMID: 19156150]

Nguyen DM, Richardson P, El-Serag HB. Medications (NSAIDs, statins, proton pump inhibitors) and the risk of esophageal adenocarcinoma in patients with Barrett's esophagus. *Gastroenterology*. 2010;138:2260–2266. [PMID: 20188100]

Singh S, Garg SK, Singh PP, et al. Acid-suppressive medications and risk of oesophageal adenocarcinoma in patients with Barrett's oesophagus: a systematic review and meta-analysis. *Gut*. 2014;63:1229–37. [PMID: 24221456]

B. Indefinite-Grade Dysplasia

In indefinite-grade dysplasia, nuclear enlargement, crowding, hyperchromatism, prominence of the nucleoli, and mild stratification can be seen but are confined to the lower portion of the glands, whereas the upper portion of the glands and surface epithelium show less abnormality or are normal. The diagnosis of dysplasia should be made with caution when atypical changes do not involve the mucosal surface.

Active inflammation due to GERD may cause nuclear changes that mimic both low-grade and high-grade dysplasia. If a biopsy specimen is obtained adjacent to an ulcer and numerous neutrophils infiltrate the epithelium, the diagnosis of dysplasia may not be possible and the diagnosis of "indefinite for dysplasia" may be assigned.

If Barrett esophagus surveillance biopsy specimens are obtained and indefinite-grade dysplasia is the highest-grade lesion found, aggressive antisecretory therapy should be instituted and repeat surveillance biopsies should be performed in 3 months.

C. Low-Grade Dysplasia

Low-grade dysplasia is characterized by mucosal cells with nuclei that are larger and hyperchromatic, with irregular contours that are basally located in the cell with minimal or no stratification (Plate 11). As with other grades of dysplasia, the interpretations of low-grade dysplasia biopsy specimens should be considered for review by experts in esophageal pathology. Extensive surveillance biopsies should be done to confirm that low-grade dysplasia is the highest grade lesion in a Barrett esophagus segment.

Several clinical studies have not demonstrated a significantly increased malignant potential of Barrett esophagus with low-grade dysplasia. In these studies, the risk of progression to esophageal adenocarcinoma was not significantly higher in patients with low-grade dysplasia than in those without dysplasia. In addition, some case series have demonstrated a transient nature to low-grade dysplasia, which can regress and revert to nondysplastic Barrett esophagus on subsequent biopsies. More recent data suggest that the extent of low-grade dysplasia measured as the mean proportion of low-grade dysplastic crypts may be a more significant predictor of esophageal adenocarcinoma outcome than the presence of low-grade dysplasia alone.

The natural history of low-grade dysplasia is variable; it can persist for long periods of time or even revert to nondysplastic Barrett esophagus. A repeat EGD with surveillance biopsies should be performed within 3–6 months after low-grade dysplasia is detected to confirm it is the highest grade lesion present and then annually as long as low-grade dysplasia persists. Given the emerging data regarding the implications of a large dysplastic burden, a shorter interval may be considered if multiple biopsies reveal a large number of low-grade crypts.

Sharma P. Low-grade dysplasia in Barrett's esophagus. *Gastroenterology.* 2004;127:1233–1238. [PMID: 15481000]

Srivastava A, Hornick JL, Li X, et al. Extent of low-grade dysplasia is a risk factor for the development of esophageal adenocarcinoma in Barrett's esophagus. *Am J Gastroenterol.* 2006;102:483–493. [PMID: 17338734]

D. High-Grade Dysplasia

The accurate pathologic diagnosis of high-grade dysplasia is critically important because therapeutic intervention may be initiated based on its diagnosis. Histopathologically, at low magnification power, distortion of the glandular architecture is usually present and may be marked. The glands are composed of branching and lateral budding of crypts and a villiform configuration of the mucosal surface. Most importantly, the diagnosis of high-grade dysplasia requires that the dysplastic epithelium on the mucosal surface demonstrate loss of nuclear polarity and the absence of a consistent relationship of nuclei to each other (Plate 12).

The clinical implications of the presence of high-grade dysplasia in Barrett esophagus remain somewhat controversial. Owing to the risk of occult, coincident malignancy in a Barrett esophagus segment as well as the higher risk of progression to malignancy, the previous standard recommendation was that all patients diagnosed with high-grade dysplasia undergo esophagectomy once the diagnosis was confirmed by two experienced GI pathologists. Esophagectomy is a very invasive surgery and is associated with 3–10% mortality and up to 45% morbidity. Subsequent studies found that the rate of progression to esophageal adenocarcinoma in patients with high-grade dysplasia can vary widely from 15% to 60% and, in a subset of patients, may not occur at all. A retrospective review of patients referred for esophagectomy for Barrett esophagus with high-grade dysplasia or intramucosal carcinoma found that only 6.7% had submucosal invasion, suggesting that endoscopic therapies could have been considered. Therefore, the recommendations regarding the management of high-grade dysplasia have evolved toward endoscopic therapy.

It is imperative that the diagnosis of high-grade dysplasia be confirmed by two expert GI pathologists prior to formulating a treatment plan. Extensive surveillance biopsies must be performed every 1 cm in all four quadrants of the Barrett esophagus segment and any suspicious nodules or ulcerations must be sampled in order to rule out the presence of any malignancy. An assessment of the patient's operative risk should be performed. After the preceding information has been obtained, a treatment plan can be formulated with the patient's input regarding the risks and benefits of each course of action.

If a patient is found to have high-grade dysplasia in a nodule or a focal, discrete lesion, EMR should be considered. This is a method of endoscopically resecting the mucosal layer of the esophagus after separating it from the muscular layer with a submucosal injection of saline (Plates 13 and 14) or band ligation. The main risks of EMR include bleeding and perforation. An endoscopic ultrasound should be performed prior to considering EMR to confirm that the stage of the lesion is superficial and appropriate for endoscopic resection. If the resected specimen is removed en bloc, the completeness of cancer resection may be assessed pathologically. Frequently EMR is combined with an endoscopic ablative technique, such as radiofrequency ablation, to treat high-grade dysplasia and intramucosal carcinoma.

Radiofrequency ablation is a mucosal eradication technique whereby bipolar energy is applied to abnormal mucosa through a catheter or balloon under endoscopic guidance. (Plates 15, 16, and 17.) The lining of the esophagus is ablated with a superficial burn of approximately 500–1000 μm. The risks of radiofrequency ablation include post-treatment strictures in about 5% of patients, chest pain, and bleeding. A meta-analysis reviewing the outcomes of endoscopic therapy versus surgical therapy for high-grade dysplasia or intramucosal carcinoma found no significant difference in neoplastic remission rate or survival rate at 5 years, but the endoscopic therapy groups had significantly lower complication rates and higher recurrence rates of neoplastic.

Various other endoscopic ablative techniques have been developed to treat dysplastic Barrett esophagus epithelium, including photodynamic therapy, focal thermal, and cryoablation methods. Long-term comparative studies are needed to determine which method is the safest and most effective; however, it appears that radiofrequency ablation holds significant promise, with multiple studies demonstrating a ≥90% eradication rate for high-grade dysplasia.

The treatment of high-grade dysplasia has evolved over time from a standard recommendation of esophagectomy for all patients to a primarily endoscopic approach. Once two expert GI pathologists have confirmed the diagnosis, the patient's co-morbid risk and the local endoscopic expertise should be considered before deciding between endoscopic eradication therapy or intensive surveillance.

Prasad GA, Wang KK, Buttar NS, et al. Long-term survival following endoscopic and surgical treatment of high-grade dysplasia in Barrett's esophagus. *Gastroenterology.* 2007;132:1226–1233. [PMID: 17408660]

Shaheen NJ, Sharma P, Overholt BF, et al. Radiofrequency ablation in Barrett's esophagus with dysplasia. *N Engl J Med.* 2009;360:2277–2288. [PMID: 19474425]

Wang VS, Hornick JL, Sepulveda JA, et al. Low prevalence of submucosal invasive carcinoma at esophagectomy for high-grade dysplasia or intramucosal adenocarcinoma in Barrett's esophagus: a 20-year experience. *Gastrointest Endosc.* 2009;69:777–783. [PMID: 19136106]

Wani S, Qumseya B, Sultan S, et al. Endoscopic eradication therapy for patients with Barrett's esophagus-associated dysplasia and intramucosal cancer. *Gastrointest Endosc.* 2018;87:907–931. [PMID: 29397943]

Wu J, Pan YM, Wang TT, et al. Endotherapy versus surgery for early neoplasia in Barrett's esophagus: a meta-analysis. *Gastrointest Endosc.* 2014;79:233–241. [PMID: 24079410]

▶ Course & Prognosis

The vast majority of patients with Barrett esophagus have no long-term sequelae from the presence of metaplastic esophageal epithelium other than the inconvenience of undergoing surveillance endoscopy. Patients should be reassured that despite the increased risk of progression to adenocarcinoma, the number of patients who progress is very small. Surveillance protocols result in detection of earlier stage adenocarcinoma. The goal of treatment of patients with Barrett esophagus is to adequately control their GERD, which empiric evidence suggests may prevent progression to malignancy. If patients require antireflux surgery to control their GERD, the risk of adenocarcinoma is not reduced and continued surveillance is required, even if the patient is asymptomatic.

For the minority of patients who have more advanced disease, the treatment of Barrett esophagus has evolved to primarily endoscopic therapy. Endoscopic ablation and endoscopic resection techniques are the mainstays of therapy for Barrett with dysplasia. This is based upon high quality evidence demonstrating a reduction in progression to adenocarcinoma as a result of these therapies.

The course and prognosis for the majority of patients with Barrett esophagus are benign, and despite the anxiety that this diagnosis can provoke in patients, the disease can be managed effectively by appropriate surveillance, acid-suppression therapy, and patient reassurance.

Hvid-Jensen F, Pedersen L, Drewes AM, et al. Incidence of adenocarcinoma among patients with Barrett's esophagus. *N Engl J Med.* 2011;365:1375–1383. [PMID: 21995385]

Wani S, Qumseya B, Sultan S, et al. Endoscopic eradication therapy for patients with Barrett's esophagus-associated dysplasia and intramucosal cancer. *Gastrointest Endosc.* 2018;87:907–931. [PMID: 29397943]

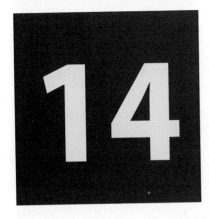

Oropharyngeal & Esophageal Motility Disorders

Hiroshi Mashimo, MD, PhD

▶ General Considerations

Oropharyngeal and esophageal motility disorders can have a significant impact on patients' quality of life. Diagnosis and management can be challenging because mechanical and functional problems may interact to cause patients' symptoms.

Dysphagia (difficulty swallowing) must be distinguished from odynophagia (pain on swallowing) and acute aphagia (inability to swallow, most commonly from food impaction eg, due to stricture, Schatski ring, and eosinophilic esophagitis in adults). Symptoms that do not necessarily correlate with the immediate process of swallowing, such as rumination and globus sensation, should also be discerned.

Dysphagia can be considered as arising from disorders in three anatomic phases of a normal swallow (Table 14–1): (1) oral (also called preparatory) phase, (2) oropharyngeal phase (also called transfer dysphagia) involving the oropharynx, larynx, and upper esophageal sphincter (UES), and (3) esophageal phase, involving the esophageal body, lower esophageal sphincter (LES), and gastroesophageal junction (GEJ). The causes of dysphagia are many, and some may overlap these phases of swallow. Specific entities are considered here.

Allen J, Dewan K, Herbert H, Randall DR, Starmer H, Stein E. Aspects of the assessment and management of pharyngoesophageal dysphagia. *Ann N Y Acad Sci.* 2020;1482(1):5–15. [PMID: 32794195]

Kim JP, Kahrilas PJ. How I approach dysphagia. *Curr Gastroenterol Rep.* 2019;21(10):49. [PMID: 31432250]

▼ OROPHARYNGEAL MOTILITY DISORDERS

OROPHARYNGEAL DYSPHAGIA

 ESSENTIALS OF DIAGNOSIS

- ▶ History of poor oral bolus preparation and control (manifest by drooling, food spillage, piecemeal swallows, or dysarthria) or pharyngeal dysfunction (manifest by difficulty in initiating a swallow, nasal and oral regurgitation, dysphonia, aspiration and coughing with swallowing, or food sticking at the level of the throat immediately after swallows).

- ▶ Evidence of a generalized neuromuscular disorder.

- ▶ Documentation by videofluoroscopic swallowing study (VFSS) or fiberoptic endoscopic evaluation of swallowing (FEES).

▶ General Considerations

Many neuromuscular and structural disorders can cause oropharyngeal dysphagia (Table 14–2). Among these are cortical lesions, supranuclear, nuclear, and cranial nerve lesions, defects of neurotransmission at the motor end plates, muscular diseases, and obstructive lesions from luminal defects or from extrinsic compression. Esophageal lesions may also exacerbate oropharyngeal dysfunction, including achalasia.

Many patients with dysphagia are elderly and develop symptoms secondary to other disorders, especially diseases of the central nervous system such as strokes. In older patients, dysphagia is more often the result of head and neck

Table 14–1. Phases of swallow.

Oral phase
Food enters mouth
Chewing and mixture with saliva
Bolus formation
Oropharyngeal phase
Tongue elevation and bolus delivery to pharynx
Soft palate elevation, sealing nasopharynx
Anterior and upward elevation of larynx and hyoid
Posteriorly and downward closure by epiglottis
Stopping respiration
Shortening of pharynx
Esophageal phase
Quick relaxation of UES
More prolonged relaxation of LES
Bolus passage into esophagus
Peristaltic contraction of esophagus
Bolus enters stomach

Data from Langmore SE. Endoscopic evaluation of oral and pharyngeal phases of swallowing. GI Motility Online.

Table 14–2. Disorders causing oropharyngeal dysphagia.

1. **Diseases of central nervous system**
   - Brain injury: cerebrovascular accidents, cerebrovascular disease, cerebral palsy
   - Brain tumors
   - Dementias, including Alzheimer disease
   - Parkinson disease and other extrapyramidal lesions
   - Infections: rabies, tetanus, neurosyphilis, Lyme disease
   - Metabolic encephalopathy, encephalitis, meningitis
   - Multiple sclerosis (bulbar and pseudobulbar palsy)
   - Amyotrophic lateral sclerosis (motor neuron disease)
   - Poliomyelitis and postpoliomyelitis syndrome
2. **Diseases of cranial nerves (V, VII, IX, X, XII)**
   - Basilar meningitis (chronic inflammatory, neoplastic)
   - Nerve injury
   - Neuropathy (Guillain-Barré syndrome, Huntington disease, familial dysautonomia, sarcoid, diabetic, and other causes)
3. **Neuromuscular**
   - Myasthenia gravis
   - Lambert-Eaton myasthenic or paraneoplastic syndromes
   - Botulinum toxin, diphtheria
   - Aminoglycosides and other drugs
4. **Muscle disorders**
   - Myositis (polymyositis, dermatomyositis, sarcoidosis)
   - Metabolic myopathy (mitochondrial myopathy, thyroid myopathy, Cushing syndrome, Wilson disease)
   - Primary myopathies (myotonic dystrophy, oculopharyngeal muscular dystrophy)
5. **Structural disorders**
   - Intrinsic obstruction (oropharyngeal tumors, cricopharyngeal bar, cervical webs)
   - Zenker diverticulum
   - Osteophytes
   - Congenital defects (eg, cleft palate, diverticulas)
   - Poor dentition
   - Mucositis (eg, *Candida*, herpes, cytomegalovirus), oral ulcers, xerostomia
6. **Iatrogenic causes**
   - Surgical complications
   - Radiation (acute or chronic)
   - Corrosive injury (caustic, pill induced)
   - Medication side effects (eg, neuroleptics, chemotherapy, long-term penicillamine)

Adapted with permission from Kasper DL, Braunwald E, Fauci AS, et al: *Harrison's Principles of Internal Medicine*, 17th ed. New York, NY: McGraw Hill; 2008.

injuries or cancers of the mouth or throat. Evidence of neurologic illnesses, nasal regurgitation and frequent coughing immediately upon swallowing, and poor oral coordination of bolus formation or dysphonia may help suggest the greater likelihood of oropharyngeal dysphagia over esophageal dysmotility. Diagnosis, assessment of severity, and optimal therapeutic intervention are generally guided by VFSS.

▶ Clinical Findings

A. Symptoms & Signs

History and physical examination provide valuable information for identifying the etiology of the oropharyngeal dysphagia. Defects in different phases of oropharyngeal swallowing (see Table 14–1) should be identified by careful analysis of symptoms and signs.

Defects in the oral preparatory phase of swallowing manifest as chewing problems, oral stasis of food, inability to form a bolus, and coughing, choking, or aspiration pneumonia from regurgitation and aspiration. Poor dentition and inadequate saliva can aggravate underlying motility disorders. These symptoms occur during or immediately after the onset of swallowing and are usually more problematic with liquids than solids in causing symptoms of misdirection. However, patients after a stroke are prone to "silent aspiration," that is, without cough or other outward signs of difficulty. Aspiration should be considered in mentally altered and debilitated patients with recurrent pneumonia, chronic congestion, and low-grade fever or leukocytosis, particularly if they have weak cough or voice, or a gurgled-hoarse voice

after swallows. The presence or absence of a gag reflex poorly distinguishes patients at higher risk for aspiration.

Generally, problems in the pharyngeal phase result in dysphagia, which the patient may localize to the throat. Often the patient makes repeated attempts to clear the throat of food or saliva. Halitosis can occur with large Zenker diverticulum, but could also be seen in esophageal causes such as advanced achalasia or long-term obstruction leading to decomposing food.

Abnormalities of the UES phase have no distinctive symptoms, but impaired UES opening further impairs pharyngeal transport and may aggravate the symptoms of pharyngeal stasis. On the other hand, a hypotonic UES may lead to esophagopharyngeal reflux and aspiration not related to swallowing.

Because many neuromuscular structures involved in swallowing are also involved in speech, dysarthria and dysphonia are common in these patients. Moreover, patients usually have evidence of neuromuscular defects in other parts of the body. Many patients with oropharyngeal dysphagia have impaired consciousness and cognitive functions that make evaluation difficult.

B. Videofluoroscopic Swallowing Study

VFSS allows slow-motion replay of lateral and anteroposterior views of the oral and pharyngeal phases of swallow, which normally takes less than a second to complete. As performed by a speech pathologist, it is the study of choice for evaluating the severity and mechanism of oropharyngeal dysphagia and overt or silent aspiration (Figure 14–1). VFSS can reveal disorder of UES opening and estimate pharyngeal strength based on a validated pharyngeal constriction ratio which, when elevated, portends a higher aspiration risk. VFSS, using different consistencies of the bolus and various head-positioning and glottis maneuvers, can also identify conditions to reduce aspiration. In comparison, barium swallow or an upper gastrointestinal series is generally not useful in evaluating oropharyngeal dysphagia, but should be considered if history is suggestive of esophageal pathology. However, plain radiographs and computed tomography (CT) scan of the neck may reveal structural lesions such as tumors and cysts, and imaging studies may be obtained before upper endoscopy because pharyngeal and upper esophageal abnormalities such as diverticula and malignant strictures may perforate in this poorly visualized region, although there are reports refuting this potentially increased endoscopic risk without prior imaging.

C. Pharyngoesophageal Manometry

Because of the complex anatomy and radial asymmetry of the oral and pharyngeal passages, the speed of coordinated contractions, and common displacement of the catheter during the swallow, intraluminal manometry has not been usually helpful. With the advent of high resolution solid-state transducers, manometry may be useful in the evaluation of UES relaxation and timing expressed as integrated UES relaxation pressure and resistance to flow across the UES (intrabolus pressure or admittance). However, these measures are variable with age, gender, and viscosity of bolus, and UES basal pressure varies greatly from emotional stress, wakefulness, and respiration. Normal values are being further defined to guide therapy such as the need for myotomy, and identify patients at risk for aspiration, while real-time evaluation may have role in biofeedback and retraining.

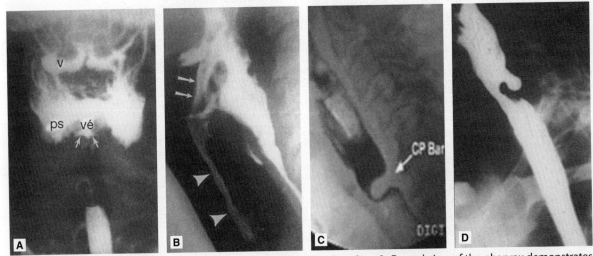

▲ **Figure 14–1.** Radiologic appearance of oropharyngeal motility disorders. **A.** Frontal view of the pharynx demonstrates aspiration of retained bolus. Note that there is retention of contrast in the valleculas (v) and piriform sinuses (ps). No swallow is taking place, yet there is entry of contrast into the laryngeal vestibule (ve) and between the vocal folds and in the ventricle *(arrows)*. **B.** A stop-frame print from a cinepharyngogram in the lateral position shows incomplete laryngeal closure during swallowing with laryngeal penetration *(arrows)* and aspiration *(arrowheads)* down into the trachea. The bolus is passing through the open cricopharyngeus into the cervical esophagus. Degenerative change is noted in the cervical spine. **C.** Cricopharyngeal bar. **D.** Zenker diverticulum. ((A) Reproduced with permission from Jones B: *Normal and Abnormal Swallowing: Imaging in Diagnosis and Therapy,* 2nd ed. New York, NY: Springer-Verlag; 2003. (B) Reproduced with permission from Jones B, Donner MW: *Normal and Abnormal Swallowing: Imaging in Diagnosis and Therapy.* New York, NY: Springer-Verlag; 1991.)

D. Videoendoscopy

Regular upper endoscopy is generally not helpful in the evaluation of oropharyngeal dysphagia; however, videoendoscopy, available at some specialized centers, can provide information, particularly about structural causes of oropharyngeal dysphagia such as tumors and Zenker diverticulum that may provide complementary information to VFSS. Narrow-caliber transnasal esophagoscopy can be performed in the office setting and, if available, is the most expedient study to guide management.

Ahuja NK, Chan WW. Assessing upper esophageal sphincter function in clinical practice: a primer. *Curr Gastroenterol Rep.* 2016;18(2):7. [PMID: 26768897]

Espitalier F, Fanous A, Aviv J, et al. International consensus (ICON) on assessment of oropharyngeal dysphagia. *Eur Ann Otorhinolaryngol Head Neck Dis.* 2018;135(1S):S17–S21. [PMID: 29396225]

Omari TI, Ciucci M, Gozdzikowska K, et al. High-resolution pharyngeal manometry and impedance: protocols and metrics-recommendations of a high-resolution pharyngeal manometry international working group. *Dysphagia.* 2020;35(2):281–295. [PMID: 31168756]

Romero-Gangonellis E, Virgili-Casas MN, Dominguez-Rubio R, et al. Evaluation of dysphagia in motor neuron disease. *Dysphagia* 2020;36(4):558–573. [PMID: 32797289]

Watts S, Gaziano J, Jacobs J, Richter J. Improving the diagnostic capability of the modified barium swallow study through standardization of an esophageal sweep protocol. *Dysphagia.* 2019;34(1):34–42. [PMID: 30635777]

Differential Diagnosis

Figure 14–2 is an algorithm outlining an approach to the patient with oropharyngeal dysphagia.

Complications

The major complications of oropharyngeal dysphagia are fatal pulmonary aspiration and pneumonia, malnutrition, and weight loss.

Treatment

Evaluation and management by a deglutition team consisting of a deglutitionist (speech and swallow therapist), radiologist, gastroenterologist, otolaryngologist, and neurologist provide the best outcome in the care of these patients. Deglutitionists assess the risk of aspiration, type of food, and patient posture that is most likely to prevent aspiration and facilitate safe swallowing. Certain rehabilitative exercises to strengthen swallowing muscles may be helpful. Electrical stimulation of muscles is also being explored as newer avenues of therapy for oropharyngeal dysphagia. Investigations are performed to find the underlying cause of the disorder

and appropriate therapy, if available, is initiated. If oral feeding cannot be undertaken safely, a percutaneous endoscopic gastrostomy (PEG) tube is placed by a gastroenterologist. The overall management of the patient, rather than focused treatment of the swallowing difficulty, is essential for effective management.

Course & Prognosis

Prognosis depends on the underlying cause, compliance with therapy, and prevention of acute pulmonary complications. Patients with cerebrovascular accidents may regain their swallowing function after 6–8 weeks. Those with diseases such as myasthenia gravis, metabolic myopathies such as thyroid disorders, polymyositis, and Parkinson disease usually respond to appropriate treatment. Other patients, such as those with muscular dystrophy, amyotrophic lateral sclerosis, and multiple sclerosis, sometimes develop recurrent aspiration pneumonia that may prove fatal.

Bulat RS, Orlando RC. Oropharyngeal dysphagia. *Curr Treat Options Gastroenterol.* 2005;8(4):269–274. [PMID: 16009027]

Panebianco M, Marchese-Ragona R, Masiero S, Restivo DA. Dysphagia in neurological diseases: a literature review. *Neurol Sci.* 2020;41(11):3067–3073. [PMID: 7567719]

IMPAIRED UES RELAXATION, CRICOPHARYNGEAL SPASMS, & CRICOPHARYNGEAL BAR

UES dysfunction has been variably defined and described. Cricopharyngeal "achalasia" is a confused and often misused term since the diagnosis is rarely made by manometric or electromyographic evidence, but historically used upon radiographic evidence for impaired opening of the UES. Thus, more precise terms should be used such as impaired UES relaxation, cricopharyngeal spasms, and cricopharyngeal bar. The clinical presentation of these entities comprising UES dysfunction is variable, but most patients complain of food sticking in the lower third of the neck. Patients may also experience heartburn, choking, odynophagia, and less commonly dysphonia or globus sensation during swallows. The dysfunction is primary if confined to the cricopharyngeus muscle without neurologic or systemic cause, and secondary if produced by another disease process. Primary UES dysfunction, in turn, is subdivided into idiopathic and intrinsic myopathies (eg, polymyositis, inclusion body myositis, muscular dystrophy, and hypothyroidism). Secondary causes include strokes, amyotrophic lateral sclerosis, polio, oculopharyngeal dysphagia (which may accompany strokes, or from late manifestation of a rare inherited oculopharyngeal muscular dystrophy), and peripheral nerve disorders such as myasthenia gravis and diabetic neuropathy. Gastroesophageal reflux disorder (GERD) has also been suggested to cause cricopharyngeal spasm.

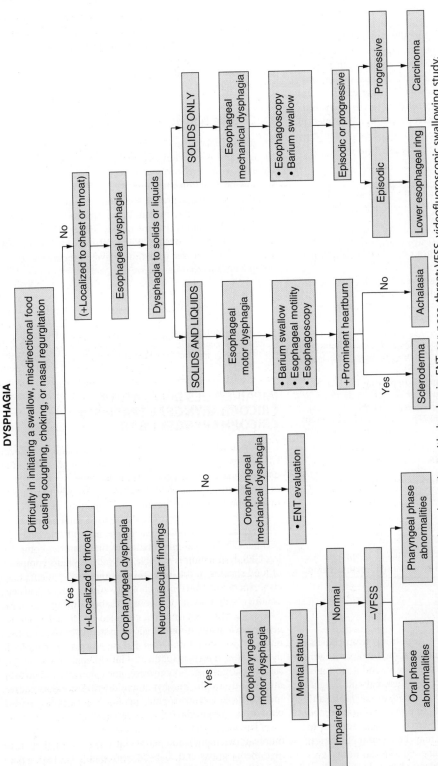

▲ **Figure 14–2.** Algorithm outlining an approach to the patient with dysphagia. ENT, ear, nose, throat; VFSS, videofluoroscopic swallowing study.

The diagnostic criteria for UES dysfunction remain controversial. The plain radiographic appearance is not reliable in making this diagnosis, and some experts advocate highly specialized radiologic (VFSS) and solid-state manometric probe studies, as failed UES relaxation has been implicated in increased risk for aspiration. However, lack of data and standardization in manometric measurements (eg, in antero-posterior, lateral, or circumferential pressures), and the possibility of the manometric catheter eliciting cricopharyngeal spasms have thwarted their standard use. Many clinicians base their diagnosis simply on symptoms. Thus, the true incidence is unknown but may involve 5–25% of patients being evaluated for dysphagia.

A classic radiographic finding is a cricopharyngeal "bar," or prominent projection on the posterior pharyngeal wall at the level of the larynx upon swallowing but with normal forward movement of the larynx on swallowing (see Figure 14–1C). This has been equated with UES "achalasia," but manometric studies of patients with cricopharyngeal bars generally reveal normal UES pressure and relaxation, thus are not associated with impaired UES relaxation or UES spasms. Indeed, a transient cricopharyngeal bar is seen in up to 5% of individuals without dysphagia undergoing upper gastrointestinal studies and can be produced in normal individuals during a Valsalva maneuver. A persistent cricopharyngeal bar may be caused by fibrosis or frank myositis in the cricopharyngeus. Some cases have been reported with dermatomyositis or inclusion body myositis. However, muscle biopsies are not routinely taken.

UES dysfunction is poorly responsive to medical therapy including muscle relaxants. Cricopharyngeal myotomy is usually not helpful unless obstruction at the cricopharyngeus is demonstrated by videofluoroscopy in a severely symptomatic patient, such as those with significant aspiration or weight loss. Similarly, local injection of botulinum toxin A for cricopharyngeal achalasia is falling out of favor with recognition that the injection is rarely well localized to the affected muscles, leakage outside the cricopharyngeus may result in temporary dysphonia or aspiration, and effects appear to be short lived with Cochrane review showing insufficient evidence to support its use. However, a trial injection may be considered to aid in making the diagnosis, or for patients who are poor surgical candidates. These procedures are contraindicated in patients with cervical tumors, and relatively contraindicated in those with a fibrotic lesion after neck irradiation, or with a progressive neurologic disorder such as bulbar palsy. One exception appears to be patients with oculopharyngeal dysphagia, who appear to do well with myotomy either by traditional open transcervical surgery or increasingly by endoscopic laser operation. Particularly in the elderly, repeated dilations using a balloon dilator or rigid Savary dilator may be performed, generally with wire guidance. Myotomy is also contraindicated in the presence of severe GERD because it may lead to pharyngeal and pulmonary aspiration. In patients with GERD, aggressive therapy with proton pump inhibitors (PPIs) is warranted in addition to management of the underlying disorder. The classic surgical approach is external cricopharyngeal myotomy.

Lee T, Park JH, Sohn C, et al. Failed deglutitive upper esophageal sphincter relaxation is a risk factor for aspiration in stroke patients with oropharyngeal dysphagia. *J Neurogastroenterol Motil.* 2017;23(1):34–40. [PMID: 5216632]

Wang AY, Kadkade R, Kahrilas PJ, Hirano I. Effectiveness of esophageal dilation for symptomatic cricopharyngeal bar. *Gastrointest Endosc.* 2005;61(1):148–152. [PMID: 15672078]

ZENKER DIVERTICULUM

Zenker diverticulum arises in the posterior wall of the hypopharynx, just above the cricopharyngeus muscle. The pathogenesis of Zenker diverticulum is not fully understood. It may form due to natural weakness of the pharynx (Killian triangle) associated with impaired opening of the cricopharyngeus muscle. Barium swallow or VFSS shows characteristic findings that allow easy diagnosis (see Figure 14–1D). With time, the diverticulum may become very large. Zenker diverticulum may retain food and secretions and classically leads to halitosis, delayed regurgitation, recurrent aspiration, and pneumonia. Dysphagia is usually due to compression of a food-filled diverticulum of the esophagus. Treatment is diverticulectomy with cricopharyngeal myotomy, and transoral approaches have also been introduced as an alternative and minimally invasive treatment.

Haddad N, Agarwal P, Levi JR, Tracy JC, Tracy LF. Presentation and management of Killian Jamieson diverticulum: a comprehensive literature review. *Ann Otol Rhinol Laryngol.* 2020;129(4):394–400. [PMID: 31707793]

GLOBUS PHARYNGEUS

Globus pharyngeus is considered a functional disorder characterized by the persistent or intermittent nonpainful sensation of a lump or foreign body in the throat, but without any difficulty in swallowing or pain on swallowing. This disorder is equally prevalent in men and women, although women may be more health care-seeking. Its cause is unknown, but is likely multifactorial including direct irritation by retrograde flow of gastric contents, known as laryngopharyngeal reflux (LPR, covered in Chapter 12), or a vagovagal reflex from distention or acid-exposure of the distal esophagus causing UES hypertonicity. Smoking, alcohol, high salt, stress, and anxiety have been described as risk factors, and symptoms may be associated with an underlying psychiatric disorder or experienced during an emotional event. Over half of these patients also have GERD or LPR, and empiric 3-month trial of high-dose acid suppression such as a PPI taken twice daily

30–60 minutes before breakfast and dinner is often recommended for chronic globus, which improves symptoms in a third of the patients. Sodium alginate may be added at bedtime for refractory patients, although given the paucity of controlled treatment studies, evidence-based treatment guidelines for globus are presently unavailable. Those unresponsive to acid suppression may warrant further workup including ambulatory impedance/pH monitoring, manometry, endoscopy, and or radiological imaging studies. Esophageal manometry may reveal nonspecific motility disorders in about half of the patients, but achalasia has been reported in patients with these symptoms, even devoid of dysphagia. Findings on barium swallow are generally normal, but may discern pharyngeal dysfunction or possible cricopharyngeal bar in patients with these symptoms. Videofluoroscopy performed by speech and language therapists has been reported to reveal various abnormalities in about a third of cases. Given the prevalence of these abnormalities, along with such findings as cervical osteophytes, reflux, and hiatal hernia in the general population, their causal link to globus remains unclear. The routine use of nasolaryngoscopy in patients with typical globus remains controversial and results, when performed, are generally normal but may reveal rare laryngopharyngeal tumors or pharyngeal inflammation from LPR. Prompt flexible endoscopy by ENT and/or gastroenterologist is recommended in patients with "red flags" for example, unexpected weight loss, bleeding/anemia, odynophagia, dysphagia, change in voice, throat pain, and lateralization and has better detection of upper digestive tract malignancies over radiological imaging. One observational report describes improvement after ablation of cervical inlet patches by upper endoscopy. In most cases, treatment consists of reassurance. Patients with concurrent psychiatric disorders such as depression, panic, and somatization may benefit from tricyclic antidepressant therapy. Relaxation therapy has also been reported as helpful in refractory patients.

Hamilton NJI, Wilcock J, Hannan SA. A lump in the throat: laryngopharyngeal reflux. *BMJ.* 2020;371:m4091. [PMID: 33139245]

Jarvenpaa P, Arkkila P, Aaltonen LM. Globus pharyngeus: a review of etiology, diagnostics, and treatment. *Eur Arch Otorhinolaryngol.* 2018;275(8):1945–1953. [PMID: 29943257]

Selleslagh M, van Oudenhove L, Pauwels A, Tack J, Rommel N. The complexity of globus: a multidisciplinary perspective. *Nat Rev Gastroenterol Hepatol.* 2014;11(4):220–233. [PMID: 24296583]

Zerbib F, Rommel N, Pandolfino J, Gyawali CP. ESNM/ANMS review. Diagnosis and management of globus sensation: a clinical challenge. *Neurogastroenterol Motil.* 2020;32(9):e13850. [PMID: 32329203]

ESOPHAGEAL MOTILITY DISORDERS

Three esophageal motility disorders commonly seen in clinical practice are esophageal motor dysphagia, GERD, and esophageal chest pain. In these disorders, symptoms result from dysfunction of one or more of the mechanisms necessary for normal esophageal function.

Esophageal motility disorders are classified, depending on the involvement of one or more of the three components of esophageal peristalsis, as disorders of inhibitory innervation, excitatory innervation, or smooth muscles (Figure 14–3).

The inhibitory innervation to the esophagus consists of vagal preganglionic neurons and the postganglionic neurons in the myenteric plexus, which release vasoactive intestinal peptide (VIP) and nitric oxide. The inhibitory pathway is responsible for relaxation of the LES and the gradient of

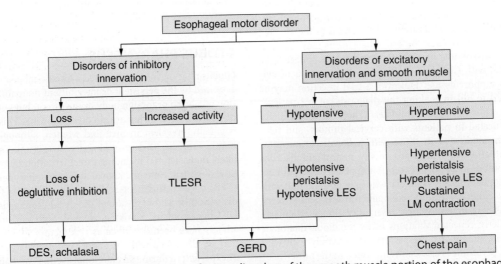

▲ **Figure 14–3.** Pathophysiologic classification of motor disorders of the smooth muscle portion of the esophagus. DES, diffuse esophageal spasm; GERD, gastroesophageal reflux disease; LES, lower esophageal sphincter; LM, longitudinal muscle; TLESR, transient lower esophageal sphincter relaxation.

peristaltic contraction in the esophageal body. Deficiency of inhibitory innervation results in achalasia and diffuse esophageal spasm. In achalasia, both the LES and esophageal body are affected, whereas in diffuse esophageal spasm, the esophageal body is primarily affected. Increased inhibitory nerve activity is responsible for so-called transient LES relaxation (TLESR).

The excitatory innervation consists of vagal preganglionic neurons and postganglionic neurons that release acetylcholine and substance P. The excitatory nerves contribute to basal LES hypertension, hypertensive contraction, and the force of peristaltic contraction. Deficiency of the excitatory nerves causes hypotensive LES and hypotensive peristaltic contractions. The esophageal body and LES consist of phasic and tonic muscles, respectively. Phasic muscles of the esophageal body contract during peristalsis, and tonic muscles of LES are responsible for tonic contraction. Muscle disorders may lead to hypotensive LES and hypotensive peristalsis.

In most conditions outlined below, a combination of imaging studies and intraluminal pressure measurements directs toward obtaining an accurate clinical diagnosis. High-resolution esophageal manometry (HRM) has also allowed a hierarchical analysis of esophageal motility disorders. impedance planimetry

Dogan I, Mittal RK. Esophageal motor disorders: recent advances. *Curr Opin Gastroenterol.* 2006;22(4):417–422. [PMID: 16760760]

Nikaki K, Sawada A, Ustaoglu A, Sifrim D. Neuronal control of esophageal peristalsis and its role in esophageal disease. *Curr Gastroenterol Rep.* 2019;21(11):59. [PMID: 31760496]

ESOPHAGEAL MOTOR DYSPHAGIA

 ESSENTIALS OF DIAGNOSIS

▶ Dysphagia to solids and liquids, localized to the chest or throat, not during but generally seconds to minutes after swallows.

▶ Associated symptoms of chest pain and regurgitation.

▶ Coughing and choking spells at night and unrelated to swallowing.

▶ Symptoms of GERD.

▶ Upper endoscopy to rule out structural abnormalities (eg, malignancy, narrowing) and obtain biopsies to rule out eosinophilic esophagitis

▶ Confirmation of abnormal motility by barium study and esophageal manometry.

▶ General Considerations

Dysphagia must be distinguished from odynophagia (pain on swallowing), which suggests a breach in mucosal integrity eg, by trauma, infection, inflammation, or irradiation, and from acute aphagia (inability to swallow), which suggests either central nervous system injury especially when accompanied by dysarthria or other neurological deficits, or an acute food impaction that may necessitate glucagon or endoscopic evaluation and therapy. The role of upper endoscopy is to rule out mucosal abnormalities such as strictures, webs, malignancies, infections, and eosinophilic esophagitis. The latter (see Chapter 15) has emerged as a major entity found in up to 15% of patients undergoing endoscopy for dysphagia, and is the most common cause of acute food impaction in the emergency room. Thus it is standard practice to obtain endoscopic biopsies in patients with dysphagia, even in absence of its often characteristic mucosal rings, furrows, and exudates. Additionally, full-column barium swallow may reveal muscular rings, which are often missed on endoscopy. Manometric studies differentiate specific motility disorders.

▶ Pathogenesis

Motor dysphagia in the thoracic esophagus occurs when deglutitive inhibition is lacking due to loss of nitrergic nerve function rendering peristaltic contractions nonperistaltic; when the LES does not relax properly in response to swallow; or when the peristaltic contractions are weak due to muscle weakness. Causes of esophageal motor dysphagia are listed in Table 14–3.

▶ Clinical Findings

A. Symptoms & Signs

Dysphagia resulting from dysfunction of the esophageal body is described as a feeling that the bolus becomes "stuck" or "hung up" on the way down. This may be accompanied by pain or discomfort. The patient typically describes difficulty in swallowing both solids and liquids. Although most patients feel as though the bolus stops at the level of the suprasternal notch, the area of obstruction may be well below this. Many patients have associated symptoms of regurgitation and chest pain.

B. Radiography

Chest radiographs may show mediastinal widening and air-fluid level when a food-filled dilated esophagus is present as in long-standing achalasia. Barium swallow may show the characteristic appearance of achalasia or diffuse esophageal spasm (Figure 14–4). Radiographic studies also help in excluding mechanical causes of dysphagia and may better discern extrinsic compression, such as from an aberrant right subclavian artery (dysphagia lusoria). A 13 mm barium tablet or solid bolus may also demonstrate subtle lesions in

Table 14–3. Causes of esophageal dysphagia.

1. **Disorders of cervical esophagus**
   (see "Oropharyngeal Motility Disorders" in text)
2. **Disorders of thoracic esophagus**
   a. **Structural disorders**
      (1) Intrinsic (mucosal) diseases narrowing lumen (inflammation, fibrosis, tumor)
         • Peptic strictures from GERD
         • Esophageal rings and webs (eg, Plummer-Vinson syndrome)
         • Esophageal tumors
         • Esophageal injury (caustic, pill associated, sclerotherapy for varices, radiation)
         • Infectious esophagitis
         • Eosinophilic esophagitis
      (2) Extrinsic (mediastinal) diseases obstructing by direct invasion or enlarged lymph nodes
         • Mediastinal tumors (lung cancers, lymphoma)
         • Pulmonary infections (tuberculosis, histoplasmosis)
         • Cardiovascular (dilated atrium, vascular compression)
      (3) Postsurgical (eg, postfundoplication, antireflux devices)
   b. **Disease of smooth muscle or excitatory nerves**
      (1) Weak muscle contraction or LES tone
         • Idiopathic
         • Scleroderma and related collagen vascular diseases
         • Hollow visceral myopathy
         • Myotonic dystrophy
         • Metabolic neuromyopathy (amyloid, alcohol, diabetes)
         • Drugs—anticholinergics, smooth muscle relaxants
      (2) Enhanced muscle contraction
         • Hypertensive peristalsis (nutcracker esophagus)
         • Hypertensive LES, hypercontractile LES
   c. **Disorders of inhibitory innervation**
      (1) Diffuse esophageal spasm
      (2) Achalasia
         • Primary
         • Secondary (Chagas disease, carcinoma, lymphoma, neuropathic intestinal pseudo-obstruction syndrome)
         • Contractile (muscular) lower esophageal ring

LES, lower esophageal sphincter.
Adapted with permission from Kasper DL, Braunwald E, Fauci AS, et al: *Harrison's Principles of Internal Medicine*, 17th ed. New York, NY: McGraw Hill; 2008.

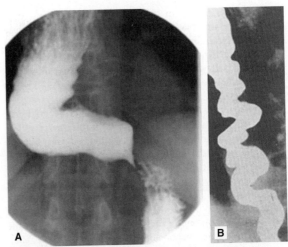

▲ **Figure 14–4.** Radiologic appearance of motor disorders of the smooth muscle portion of the esophagus. **A.** Note the sigmoid-shaped esophagus and "bird-beaking" of the lower end in achalasia. **B.** Corkscrew appearance in diffuse esophageal spasm. (B: Reproduced with permission of Dr. Harvey Goldstein.)

incorporate paired rings of electrodes for multiple intraluminal impedance (MII) to evaluate additionally the esophageal transit and clearance of the swallowed bolus. The MII/HRM involves nasal passage of the catheter into the esophagus and stomach. Figure 14–5 summarizes patterns of esophageal motility in normal subjects and in a variety of esophageal motility disorders. Introduction of the Chicago Classification has allowed a diagnostic algorithm for interpreting HRM in the diagnosis of esophageal motility disorders (Figure 14–6). Clinical indications for manometry are to evaluate dysphagia for the diagnosis of primary motility disorders of the esophagus, assess patients with persistent reflux since motility disorders such as achalasia and scleroderma may mimic reflux symptoms, and to study candidates for fundoplication to minimize postsurgical dysphagia. Manometry may also be used to determine the location of the LES prior to placement of multi-channel impedance and pH catheters.

D. Endoscopy

Endoscopy is required in most patients with esophageal motility disorders that cause dysphagia and is generally the initial test for evaluating dysphagia. This step is necessary to exclude mechanical causes of dysphagia, mechanical lesions such as peptic stricture and other complications of an erosive esophagitis, and lesions such as adenocarcinoma at the GEJ that may produce secondary achalasia. Biopsies at multiple levels of the esophageal body are generally obtained to rule out eosinophilic esophagitis, even in the presence of normal-appearing mucosa.

patients with dysphagia, although rarely obviates the need for a subsequent endoscopy. Videofluoroscopic examination of the esophagus may identify abnormalities in peristaltic sequence and in the force of peristaltic contractions, and a timed barium esophagram may help assess patients before and after treatment of achalasia, for example.

C. Manometry

Esophageal manometry can be used to measure the strength (amplitude), duration, and sequential nature of the contractions of the esophageal body, as well as the resting pressure and relaxation of the LES. The flexible catheter has an array of pressure sensors allowing for HRM, and current catheters

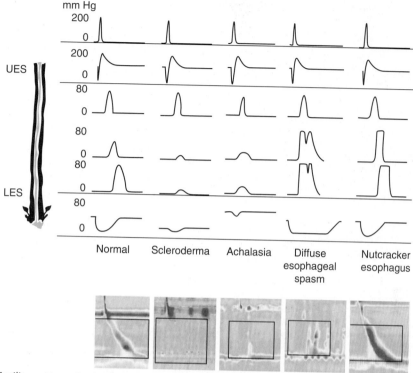

▲ **Figure 14–5.** Motility patterns in esophageal smooth muscle disorders. LES, lower esophageal sphincter; UES, upper esophageal sphincter. (Reproduced with permission from Kasper DL, Braunwald E, Fauci AS, et al: *Harrison's Principles of Internal Medicine,* 17th ed. New York, NY: McGraw Hill; 2008.)

E. Functional Luminal Imaging Probe (FLIP)

FLIP is a balloon-based impedance planimetry introduced as a diagnostic and therapeutic tool that may be performed during a sedated upper endoscopy to assess movement of esophageal body contour, and distensibility index (ratio of cross sectional area to intraballoon pressure) of the GEJ. Reduced distensibility index has been correlated with food impaction and need for dilation in eosinophilic esophagitis, and may also play a role in the management of achalasia (below).

▶ Differential Diagnosis

Refer to Figure 14–2, which outlines an approach to the patient with dysphagia.

▶ Treatment

Management of esophageal motility disorders depends on the type of the disorder and its clinical consequences. (For details, see "Disorders of Inhibitory Innervation" and "Disorders of Excitatory Nerves and Smooth Muscles" later in this chapter.)

Kahrilas PJ, Bredenoord AJ, Carlson DA, Pandolfino JE. Advances in management of esophageal motility disorders. *Clin Gastroenterol Hepatol.* 2018;16(11):1692–1700. [PMID: 29702296]

Malagelada JR, Bazzoli F, Boeckxstaens G, et al. World gastroenterology organisation global guidelines: dysphagia—global guidelines and cascades update September 2014. *J Clin Gastroenterol.* 2015;49:370–378. [PMID: 25853874]

Savarino E, di Pietro M, Bredenoord AJ, et al. Use of the functional lumen imaging probe in clinical esophagology. *Am J Gastroenterol.* 2020;115(11):1786–1796. [PMID: 33156096]

Triggs J, Pandolfino J. Recent advances in dysphagia management. *F1000 Res.* 2019;8:1–9. [PMID: 6719674]

GASTROESOPHAGEAL REFLUX DISEASE

GERD (see Chapter 12) is the most common manifestation of impaired esophageal motility and one of the most common disorders seen in clinical practice. The basic cause of GERD is incompetent antireflux neuromechanical barriers at the GEJ, which normally prevents backflow of gastric acid into the stomach. Competence of the gastroesophageal barrier is the result of the intra-abdominal location of the LES, mucosal folds at the GEJ, LES closure, reflex LES contraction, and the diaphragmatic crura. Factors such as increased

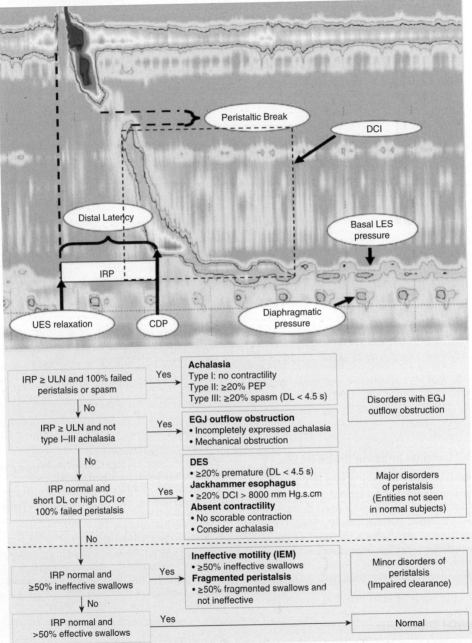

▲ Figure 14–6. Chicago Classification of high resolution manometry based on software analysis of indicated regions of the swallow pattern: Contractile Deceleration Point (CDP), Integrated Relaxation Pressure (the minimal averaged pressure spanning a 4 second relaxation period at the esophagogastric junction [EGJ]), Distal Latency (the interval between UES relaxation and CDP), Peristaltic break (any break in the 20mmHg isobaric contour, often normally seen at the transition zone between striated and smooth muscle portions of the esophagus), and Distal Contractile Integral (DCI, representing the length, strength and persistence of swallow-induced contraction wave in distal esophagus) are analyzed by software to identify disorders of EGJ outflow obstruction, and major and minor peristaltic disorders.

intra-abdominal pressure that may arise from a multitude of conditions including obesity and gastric stasis resulting from conditions like diabetic gastroparesis increase the likelihood of developing GERD.

The pathogenesis of GERD is complicated and multifactorial. Important esophageal motor abnormalities underlying GERD are hypotensive LES, TLESR, or both. Hypotensive esophageal contractions are commonly associated with hypotensive LES and contribute to reflux-associated esophageal mucosal damage.

Although the main clinical manifestations of GERD are heartburn and regurgitation, other manifestations, including development of chronic cough and the premalignant condition Barrett esophagus, may occur. Moreover, the majority of patients with GERD do not have symptoms. Manifestations and complications of GERD are discussed in detail in Chapter 12.

Lin S, Li H, Fang X. Esophageal motor dysfunctions in gastroesophageal reflux disease and therapeutic perspectives. *J Neurogastroenterol Motil.* 30 2019;25(4):499–507. [PMID: 31760496]

ESOPHAGEAL CHEST PAIN

 ### ESSENTIALS OF DIAGNOSIS

▶ Chronic symptoms.

▶ Rule out life-threatening conditions (eg, ischemic heart disease, vascular abnormalities).

▶ Rule out panic disorder, related psychiatric disorders, and musculoskeletal disorders.

▶ Well-accepted causes are reflux esophagitis, achalasia, and diffuse esophageal spasm.

▶ Probable causes are hypertensive esophageal motor disorders, sustained longitudinal muscle contraction, and esophageal hypersensitivity.

▶ General Considerations

Heartburn and odynophagia are classical symptoms of esophageal disease. However, some patients with esophageal disorders present with chest pain that is neither typical heartburn nor odynophagia. Esophageal chest pain may resemble cardiac chest pain and life-threatening cardiac and rarer vascular abnormalities need to be ruled out. This overlap is due to the spinal primary sensory afferent that carries cardiac and esophageal nociceptive information and also innervates common cutaneous segments.

▶ Pathogenesis

For practical purposes, causes of chronic esophageal chest pain can be divided into well-accepted and possible causes.

A. Well-Accepted Causes of Esophageal Chest Pain

Well-established causes of chest pain are reflux esophagitis and motility disorders such as achalasia and diffuse esophageal spasm. Overall, reflux esophagitis is the most common cause of noncardiac chest pain.

B. Probable Causes of Esophageal Chest Pain

Esophageal disorders that have been proposed as causes of chest pain are hypertensive esophageal motility disorders, sustained longitudinal muscle contraction, esophageal hypersensitivity, and esophageal sensory neuropathy.

1. Hypertensive esophageal motility disorders—Some esophageal motility disorders, particularly those associated with hypertensive esophageal peristaltic contractions (so-called "nutcracker" or "jackhammer" esophagus), hypertensive LES, and hypercontracting LES, have been identified during manometric evaluation of patients with unexplained chest pain. Therefore, these manometric diagnoses were proposed as causing chest pain. However, a causal relationship has not been established. Moreover, a temporal association between these conditions and chest pain has not been documented, and treatment of the hypercontractile states with smooth muscle relaxants has not proved to be effective in the relief of chest pain.

2. Sustained longitudinal muscle contraction—Dynamic high-resolution endoscopic ultrasound has shown that episodes of chest pain are associated with sustained contraction of the esophageal longitudinal muscle. The longitudinal muscle contraction remains undetected by intraluminal manometry. Therefore, sustained esophageal longitudinal muscle contraction has been proposed as a cause of chest pain in patients with normal esophageal manometry. Further studies are needed to fully establish this sustained contraction as the cause of unexplained chest pain, since esophageal shortening in response to intraluminal acid appears not to correlate with symptoms.

3. Defects in sensory nerves and pain perception—Several studies suggest that the esophagus may develop sensory hypersensitivity, in which stimuli that do not normally produce pain are perceived as painful. Esophageal hypersensitivity may be a part of generalized visceral hypersensitivity. The pathophysiology of visceral hypersensitivity is not fully understood but may occur peripherally in the esophageal afferent nerves or centrally in the central nervous system. Esophageal hypersensitivity is demonstrated by showing a reduced threshold to esophageal balloon distention. Esophageal mucosal hypersensitivity can also be tested by the esophageal acid perfusion test (Bernstein test), discussed later.

▶ Clinical Findings

Chest pain is a common and alarming symptom. Acute chest pain syndromes may be due to life-threatening conditions such as myocardial infarction, aortic dissection, pulmonary embolism, esophageal perforation, acute bolus obstruction, or penetrating esophageal ulcer. Patients with these conditions require emergent care.

Patients presenting with chronic chest pain should undergo careful clinical evaluation to classify them into the following broad groups: cardiac chest pain, musculoskeletal chest pain, psychosomatic chest pain, esophageal chest pain, and miscellaneous causes of chest pain. In the majority of patients, the origin of chest pain is easily identified and treated. However, in some patients, the origin of chest pain remains obscure.

▶ Differential Diagnosis & Treatment

An algorithm outlining an approach to the patient with chest pain of unknown origin (CPUO) is presented in Figure 14–7. A working definition of CPUO has not been developed.

However, it is clear that this diagnosis should be used only after careful initial evaluation. For example, cardiac evaluation and treatment should be performed for patients with ischemic heart disease and typical symptoms of cardiac ischemia; a trial of a PPI should be initiated for patients suspected of having heartburn and GERD; a trial of nonsteroidal anti-inflammatory drugs (NSAIDs) and possibly skeletal muscle relaxants should be used for those with musculoskeletal disorders; and a therapeutic trial should be started for those with panic disorder.

A. Chest Pain of Unknown Origin

Patients in whom the initial evaluation does not yield a cause are identified as having CPUO. The first step in the evaluation

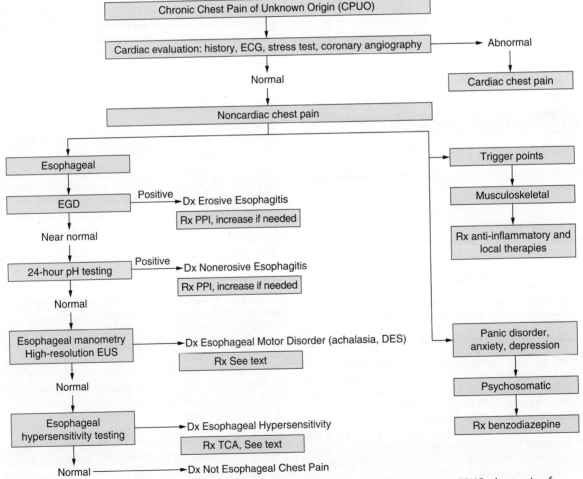

▲ **Figure 14–7.** Algorithm outlining an approach to the patient with unexplained chest pain. CPUO, chest pain of unknown origin; DES, diffuse esophageal spasm; Dx, diagnosis; ECG, electrocardiogram; EGD, esophagogastroduodenoscopy; EUS, esophageal ultrasound; PPI, proton pump inhibitor; Rx, prescription; TCA, tricyclic antidepressant. (Reproduced with permission from Fang J, Bjorkman D. A critical approach to noncardiac chest pain: pathophysiology, diagnosis, and treatment. *Am J Gastroenterol.* 2001;96(4):958–968.)

of a patient with CPUO is to carefully exclude coronary artery disease because of the life-threatening nature of cardiac chest pain. This may require coronary angiography, which remains the gold standard, apart from careful consideration of cardiac causes of chest pain. The speculative cardiac causes of chest pain include microvascular angina or syndrome X. This diagnosis is sometimes considered in patients with atypical anginal symptoms and normal coronary arteries, especially when abnormalities are present on noninvasive tests of cardiac function such as exercise radionuclide angiography or exercise thallium scintigraphy. Similarly, mitral valve prolapse is frequently present in patients with chest pain of undetermined etiology; however, most investigators agree that it does not cause chest pain. CPUO patients in whom cardiac causes of chest pain have been excluded are identified as having noncardiac chest pain. These patients require careful screening for esophageal, musculoskeletal, psychosomatic, and miscellaneous causes of chest pain.

B. Reflux Esophagitis

Reflux esophagitis is one of the most common causes of esophageal chest pain. Among patients with reflux, 10–20% will have chest pain alone, and reflux esophagitis remains the most common cause of unexplained chest pain. Therefore, the first step is to prescribe a therapeutic trial of a PPI if this therapy has not already been initiated. If there is no satisfactory response, the patient should undergo endoscopic examination. Esophageal erosions, ulcers, and peptic strictures provide evidence of GERD, which should be treated with a PPI, including high-dose therapy if needed. If no or minimal mucosal abnormalities are found, high-magnification endoscopy or narrow band image endoscopy may be performed to look for microerosions. Mucosal biopsies should be obtained in patients with negative endoscopic results. These patients should undergo pH monitoring by placement of a pH capsule in the distal esophagus. If capsule monitoring is not available, 24-hour ambulatory esophageal pH testing should be performed. Mucosal biopsy specimens may show enlarged intercellular spaces, which are thought to represent very early mucosal damage in reflux esophagitis. Patients having abnormal mucosal biopsy and esophageal pH findings are diagnosed as having nonerosive reflux disease and treated aggressively with PPI therapy.

C. Esophageal Motility Problems & Esophageal Hypersensitivity

In patients showing no evidence of esophagitis, intraluminal manometry should be performed to evaluate for the presence of motility disorders such as early achalasia, diffuse esophageal spasm, and hypertensive esophageal motility. These disorders comprise only a small number of cases of unexplained chest pain. Patients who have normal esophageal motility should be evaluated for esophageal hypersensitivity by determining the threshold to esophageal distention

by intraesophageal balloon inflation. Mucosal sensitivity may be determined by the acid perfusion test (also called the Bernstein test), in which 0.1% hydrochloric acid is perfused by catheter into the distal esophagus.

The antidepressant trazodone (100–150 mg/day), which has no direct effect on esophageal motility, has been effective in decreasing the distress of esophageal symptoms in patients with motility disorders. This suggests that underlying psychiatric problems may play a role in patients with esophageal motility abnormalities. Use of trazodone in men is limited by the side effect of priapism. Surgical myotomy has no role in the management of patients with chest pain and motility disorders other than achalasia.

D. Musculoskeletal Chest Pain

The diagnosis of musculoskeletal chest pain may be overlooked in the initial evaluation of the patient with CPUO. Careful history and physical examination are required. Several musculoskeletal disorders may cause chest pain. Localized myofascial pain, ankylosing spondylitis, fibromyalgia, Tietze syndrome, rheumatoid arthritis, thoracic outlet syndrome, and "slipping rib" syndrome should be considered in the differential diagnosis. The diagnosis of fibromyalgia is based on at least a 3-month history of widespread pain, with more than 10–18 trigger points of tenderness on digital palpation. Patients with musculoskeletal chest pain are treated with reassurance, application of local heat, NSAIDs, and corticosteroid–lidocaine injection when appropriate. Patients with fibromyalgia may benefit from cyclobenzaprine (2.5–10 mg four times daily) or amitriptyline (10–50 mg at bedtime).

E. Psychiatric Disorders

Psychiatric disorders, including depression, anxiety, and panic disorder, may not be recognized initially as a cause of chest pain, in part because these disorders are very common in clinical practice, affecting approximately 5% of the US population. Patients with symptoms of panic and anxiety should be referred to a psychiatric specialist for diagnostic evaluation and treatment. Treatment of these disorders includes antidepressants, anxiolytics, and cognitive-behavioral therapy. Many patients with these disorders require education about their disease, and gentle persuasion and reassurance that effective treatment exists, before they will accept these recommendations.

F. More Than One Cause of Chest Pain

It is important to recognize the various disorders that cause chest pain as they are very common and more than one cause may be present concurrently. For example, the incidence of GERD is markedly increased in patients with ischemic heart disease because of the overlapping risk factors for the two diseases and also because smooth muscle relaxants that are used in the treatment of coronary angina aggravate GERD.

Similarly, patients with unexplained chest pain may be diagnosed with esophageal motility disorder, panic disorder, and microvascular angina. Moreover, many of these patients complain of characteristic chest pain during catheterization with right ventricular stimulation, suggesting a heightened visceral nociception.

Course & Prognosis

Patients with CPUO have a normal survival rate. However, their quality of life and functional status are markedly impaired. Most patients continue to experience chest pain and functional impairment even after a diagnosis of CPUO has been made, resulting in high utilization of health care resources and associated medical costs.

Barret M, Herregods TV, Oors JM, Smout AJ, Bredenoord AJ. Diagnostic yield of 24-hour esophageal manometry in non-cardiac chest pain. *Neurogastroenterol Motil.* 2016;28(8):1186–1193. [PMID: 27018150]

Fass R, Shibli F, Tawil J. Diagnosis and management of functional chest pain in the Rome IV era. *J Neurogastroenterol Motil.* 2019;25(4):487–498. [PMID: 31587539]

Heinrich H, Sweis R. The role of oesophageal physiological testing in the assessment of noncardiac chest pain. *Ther Adv Chronic Dis.* 2018;9(12):257-267. [PMID: 30719270]

McIntosh K, Paterson WG. Sustained esophageal longitudinal smooth muscle contraction may not be a cause of noncardiac chest pain. *Neurogastroenterol Motil.* 2018;30(11):e13428. [PMID: 30069979]

Yamasaki T, Fass R. Noncardiac chest pain: diagnosis and management. *Curr Opin Gastroenterol.* 2017;33(4):293–300. [PMID: 28463855]

DISORDERS OF INHIBITORY INNERVATION

1. Achalasia

 ESSENTIALS OF DIAGNOSIS

▶ Slowly progressive esophageal dysphagia to both solids and liquids.

▶ Absence of acid reflux.

▶ Regurgitation of undigested food without acid or bile; episodes of pneumonia.

▶ Chest radiograph may show a mediastinal mass with air-fluid levels.

▶ Barium esophagogram shows a dilated esophagus without peristalsis and a "bird beak" in the distal esophagus.

▶ Esophageal manometry shows nonperistaltic esophageal contractions and failure of LES relaxation on swallowing.

General Considerations

Achalasia is a disorder of the thoracic esophagus characterized by nonperistaltic esophageal contractions and impaired relaxation of the LES in response to swallowing. It results primarily from degeneration of nitrergic inhibitory neurons in the myenteric plexus. Achalasia is an important but uncommon clinical disorder with an incidence of approximately 1.6 in 100,000 persons, but is increasing possibly from increased detection. It most often manifests between the ages of 25 and 50 but affects patients of all ages, and both sexes. Diagnosis is generally established on the basis of radiologic findings and manometric studies, and by ruling out secondary causes such as cancer. Definitive therapy is surgical or endoscopic myotomy, but various medical and endoscopic treatments have been employed for symptomatic relief.

Pathogenesis

Achalasia is associated with degeneration of postganglionic inhibitory neurons, which release nitric oxide and VIP. Postganglionic excitatory neurons may also be affected in advanced disease. Preganglionic vagal fibers and vagal nuclei may also be involved.

Most cases in the United States are of no known cause and are classified as idiopathic achalasia. A viral etiology for the inflammation has also been proposed, but no clear association has been found with adenovirus, human papilloma virus, measles, varicella zoster, or herpes simplex virus-1. Autoimmunity has been proposed as contributing to the etiology based on observation of T-lymphocyte infiltration in the myenteric plexus, a higher prevalence of the disorder in patients with certain HLA types, and genomic analysis demonstrating single-nucleotide polymorphisms specifically in the HLA-DQ region conferring increased risk for achalasia. Autoantibodies to neurons are also found in many patients with achalasia.

Familial achalasia comprises about 2–5% of all cases and generally involves an autosomal-recessive mode of inheritance, particularly in children younger than 4 years. In children, this may be part of the Allgrove (or AAA) syndrome (achalasia, alacrima, achlorhydria), which may also be associated with adrenocorticotropic hormone insensitivity, microcephaly, and nerve deafness. Additionally, a small percentage of patients have associated neurodegenerative diseases such as Parkinson disease and hereditary cerebellar ataxia.

Secondary achalasia refers to inhibitory neuronal degeneration caused by a known etiologic agent such as *Trypanosoma cruzi* (the causative organism in Chagas disease) and carcinoma.

Although the cause of primary achalasia is largely unknown, degenerative changes have been noted in the dorsal motor nucleus (Lewy bodies), along with degeneration of vagal fibers and loss of ganglion cells in the esophageal body and LES. In particular, there may be an inflammatory response, predominantly of T-cell lymphocytes. However, these changes are not consistent and may be secondary to an enteric nervous system disease involving loss of nitrergic and VIP-containing neurons (the main relaxatory mediators of the esophageal smooth muscle) and a decrease in the number of interstitial cells of Cajal. Muscular hypertrophy, possibly secondary to the denervation, and variable extent of muscle degeneration have also been described. However, these muscular and neuronal changes cannot be assessed by evaluation of mucosal biopsies obtained during endoscopy. Newer approaches are being assessed for obtaining full-thickness biopsies to facilitate evaluation of neuromuscular pathology.

Furuzawa-Carballeda J, Torres-Landa S, Valdovinos MA, Coss-Adame E, Martin Del Campo LA, Torres-Villalobos G. New insights into the pathophysiology of achalasia and implications for future treatment. *World J Gastroenterol.* 2016; 22(35):7892–7907. [PMID: 27672286]

Samo S, Carlson DA, Gregory DL, Gawel SH, Pandolfino JE, Kahrilas PJ. Incidence and prevalence of achalasia in Central Chicago, 2004-2014, since the widespread use of high-resolution manometry. *Clin Gastroenterol Hepatol.* 2017;15(3):366–373. [PMID: 27581064]

▶ Clinical Features

A. Symptoms & Signs

Dysphagia is the most common presenting symptom of achalasia and is present in nearly all patients. Dysphagia to both liquids and solids is characteristic of this disease; however, symptoms may initially involve primarily solids, followed by liquids. Dysphagia is mainly localized to the lower chest, although it may be localized to the neck. Generally, it is worsened by emotional stress or hurried eating. Patients often complain of taking longer to eat a meal, or of drinking a large amount of liquid to clear the food from the esophagus. They may even describe having to stand up, perform the Valsalva maneuver, or arch their backs to help clear food from the esophagus.

The second most frequent presenting symptom is regurgitation of food, which is generally undigested, nonbilious, and nonacidic. Patients may wake in the middle of the night as a result of coughing or choking after regurgitation, the content of which is often described as white and foamy, arising from an inability to clear saliva from the esophagus. Chest pain and heartburn occur in approximately 40% of patients and can be misdiagnosed as GERD. However, the heartburn is generally not postprandial or responsive to antacids.

Mild weight loss is noted in approximately 85% of patients and may even mimic cancer when profound. However, the interval from the presenting symptom to the point at which the patient seeks medical attention is quite variable, sometimes extending beyond a decade.

B. Laboratory Findings

Some patients with idiopathic achalasia have increased antineuronal antibodies, including anti–Hu-1 antineuronal antibodies. Enzyme-linked immunosorbent assay (ELISA) tests, agglutination tests, and confirmatory assays, including immunofluorescence, immunoblot, Western blot, and radio-immunoprecipitation tests, may aid in identifying *T cruzi* in patients with achalasia caused by Chagas disease.

C. Radiographic Imaging Studies

Barium esophagogram, the preferred initial method of evaluation in patients with dysphagia, may reveal characteristically smooth, symmetric narrowing or "bird-beaking" of the distal esophagus, and often a dilated esophagus with no peristaltic activity and poor esophageal emptying. In severe achalasia, chest radiographs may reveal a dilated esophagus containing food, possibly air-fluid level within the esophagus in the upright position, absence of gastric air bubble, and sometimes a tubular mediastinal mass beside the aorta. Administration of a smooth muscle relaxant such as sublingual nitroglycerin or inhaled amyl nitrate may cause relaxation of the LES and distinguish achalasia from pseudoachalasia arising from mechanical causes. Severe cases may reveal a markedly dilated and tortuous esophagus, called a sigmoid esophagus (see Figure 14–4).

D. Endoscopy

Esophagogastroduodenoscopy is not sensitive in the diagnosis of esophageal motility disorders. However, it is very useful in excluding mechanical disorders by allowing dilation of rings and ruling out other causes of the motility disorder (eg, infiltration by GEJ cancer, causing secondary achalasia), and inflammatory conditions such as eosinophilic esophagitis that may present with dysphagia.

E. Manometry & FLIP

Even while advanced achalasia may be strongly suspected based on the characteristic radiological appearances, the diagnosis should be confirmed by esophageal manometry, which typically reveals complete absence of peristalsis, incomplete LES relaxation (<50% of baseline pressure), and often but not necessarily increased lower esophageal basal tone (>30 mm Hg). Weak contractions may be noted in the esophageal body, which are simultaneous or appear simultaneous but identical if the esophageal body becomes a single lumen (common cavity effect) (see Figure 14–5). Esophageal pressures may also exceed gastric pressures when the esophagus is filled with food or fluid. Three subtypes have been described: type 1, or classic subtype, with absent peristalsis and absent pressurization; type 2, or esophageal compression subtype, with aperistalsis and panesophageal pressurization in greater than 20% of swallows; and type 3, or spastic subtype, with high-amplitude spastic contractions of the esophagus in greater than 20% of swallows with or without preservation of distal peristalsis. Treatment outcomes have been shown to differ among these manometric subtypes (see later). FLIP is a complementary diagnostic tool when manometry or barium studies are inconclusive, or to assess the adequacy of GEJ disruption during and after myotomy or pneumatic dilation.

Differential Diagnosis

The differential diagnosis of achalasia begins with the broad differential diagnosis of dysphagia and exclusion of mechanical causes of dysphagia. A major concern is to exclude malignancy, which is more likely in patients with dysphagia of shorter duration (<4 months), disease progression, dysphagia predominantly for solids rather than liquids, and weight loss. In contrast, achalasia and other primary motility disorders are more likely if the dysphagia is for both solids and liquids (in contrast to dysphagia mainly to solids for structural abnormalities such as benign or malignant strictures), has existed for several months to years, and is not associated with weight loss. However, strictures, neoplasms, vascular rings, webs, foreign bodies, and severe esophagitis (peptic, infectious, chemical, drug induced, eosinophilic) are also among frequently encountered entities.

Achalasia must also be distinguished from other motility disorders such as diffuse esophageal spasm and scleroderma that has been complicated by a peptic stricture. The next step is to determine whether it is due to an identifiable cause. These cases, termed secondary achalasia, may be due to infection with *T cruzi* (Chagas disease) or neural degeneration as a paraneoplastic syndrome associated with many malignancies. GEJ carcinoma may produce myenteric plexus degeneration by local tumor invasion, resulting in achalasia. The term *pseudoachalasia* is used when there is no functional cause of achalasia but the GEJ is narrowed due to outside compression or fibrosis and the esophageal body is dilated due to obstruction. Patients with secondary achalasia due to tumor at the GEJ present with more recent and progressive onset of dysphagia or with progressive weight loss. Careful retroflexed inspection of the cardia and GEJ by upper endoscopy is necessary.

Treatment

Current options for treatment of achalasia are directed at removing the functional obstruction caused by the nonrelaxing LES. However, these therapeutic modalities do not restore peristalsis. Treatment includes pharmacologic therapy, pneumatic dilation of the LES, surgical or endoscopic myotomy, and botulinum toxin injection therapy. Treatment outcome differs in the three manometric subclasses of achalasia: type 2 is most responsive to pneumatic dilation or Heller myotomy, type 3 is less responsive, and type 1 is least responsive to either treatment.

A. Pharmacologic Therapy

Sublingual nitroglycerin, calcium channel blockers, phosphodiesterase inhibitors, and anticholinergics are used to relieve the symptoms in the subset of patients who have mild symptoms without esophageal dilation, or are unable to undergo dilations or surgery.

B. Pneumatic Dilation

The disruption of muscle requires far larger diameters compared with disruption of mucosal lesions such as strictures. A 3-cm diameter balloon is used initially. Based on patient's response, successive dilations of up to 4 cm can be applied. At each session, a balloon is placed under fluoroscopic guidance to stretch the area of the GEJ. In less than 4% of dilations, perforations occur that may require surgical repair, although most can be managed conservatively. In experienced hands, the efficacy of pneumatic dilation and laparoscopic surgery are nearly equal, and dilation appears to be the more cost-effective initial approach. FLIP with a 3-cm diameter balloon may also allow more controlled dilation without fluoroscopy and appears promising although larger diameter balloons are currently not available. These balloon dilations are relatively contraindicated in patients with large epiphrenic diverticulum and those with significant cardiac or pulmonary disease considering their morbidity or mortality in case of a perforation.

C. Surgical Myotomy

A modified Heller cardiomyotomy of the LES and cardia results in good to excellent symptomatic relief in over 85% of patients. GERD is expected to ensue in up to 20% of patients. Myotomy can also be performed using a laparoscopic approach; this is less invasive, reduces postoperative complications, and allows a shorter hospital stay. The success of surgery does not appear to be compromised by prior botulinum or pneumatic dilation treatments.

D. Endoscopic Myotomy

Peroral endoscopic myotomy (POEM) is a form of natural orifice transluminal endoscopic surgery (NOTES) which performs incisionless surgery using flexible endoscopes. NOTES generally involves making a submucosal tunneling to exit the gastrointestinal tract distal from the mucosal incision to allow a protective mucosal flap that can be closed with endoscopic clips. In a refined POEM, the dysfunctional circular muscle of the LES is divided, leaving the longitudinal muscle layer intact, thereby adding, at least theoretically, additional margin of safety against perforation while retaining the efficacy of surgical myotomy. However, the incidence of pneumoperitoneum or pneumothorax (40%), including need for decompression/chest drainage (20%) may be high, in part owing to learning curve at various institutions, and shorter length myotomy has been advocated by some investigators, although long-term efficacies of various POEMs have not been compared. Over the past decade, POEM has become the primary treatment for the majority of patients at some high-volume centers. While the incidence of post-POEM GERD symptoms ranges from 30% to 40%, most could be medically managed without the need for antireflux surgery.

E. Botulinum Toxin Injection

Botulinum toxin A is injected directly into the LES using an endoscope. Approximately 20–25 units of the toxin are used per injection into four quadrants in the LES. This results in reduction of lower esophageal pressures in 85% of patients. However, approximately 50% of patients relapse with symptoms over the next 6–9 months. Approximately 25% have a sustained response lasting more than 1 year. Approximately 75% of initial responders who relapse have improvement with repeat injection therapy. Because of the lower efficacy and sustained response compared with surgical myotomy, this method is often reserved for elderly patients with life expectancy under 2 years, and those with multiple medical problems with high surgical risks.

F. Esophageal Stents

Long-term placement of esophageal stents as primary treatment of achalasia had fallen out of favor owing to frequent complications of stent migration and serious erosions. However, a specifically-designed 30 mm stent has shown promise with low migration (6%) and high remission rate (>80%) on 2-year follow-up.

▶ Course & Prognosis

Untreated, achalasia can lead to severe weight loss mimicking cancer, and respiratory complications such as stridor. Patients may develop distal esophageal diverticulum and bezoars. After surgery, patients may develop GERD, strictures, and Barrett esophagus. Achalasia is also associated with increased risk of esophageal cancer, but screening protocol has not been established in this population.

Arora Z, Thota PN, Sanaka MR. Achalasia: current therapeutic options. *Ther Adv Chronic Dis.* 2017;8(6–7):101–108. [PMID: 5502956]

Gunasingam N, Perczuk A, Talbot M, Kaffes A, Saxena P. Update on therapeutic interventions for the management of achalasia. *J Gastroenterol Hepatol.* 2016;31(8):1422–1428. [PMID: 27060999]

Moran RA, Brewer Gutierrez OI, Rahden B, et al. Impedance planimetry values for predicting clinical response following peroral endoscopic myotomy. *Endoscopy.* 2020. [PMID: 33147642]

Schlottmann F, Neto RML, Herbella FAM, Patti MG. Esophageal achalasia: pathophysiology, clinical presentation, and diagnostic evaluation. *Am Surg.* 2018;84(4):467–472. [PMID: 29712590]

Vaezi MF, Pandolfino JE, Yadlapati RH, Greer KB, Kavitt RT. ACG clinical guidelines: diagnosis and management of achalasia. *Am J Gastroenterol.* 2020;115(9):1393–1411. [PMID: 32773454]

2. Diffuse Esophageal Spasm

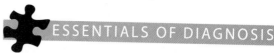

ESSENTIALS OF DIAGNOSIS

▶ Nonperistaltic simultaneous contractions of the esophagus.

▶ Dysphagia to solids and liquids and chest pain are common presenting symptoms.

▶ Some patients may progress to achalasia.

▶ General Considerations

The reported incidence of diffuse esophageal spasm depends on the diagnostic criteria used. When large amplitude of contractions is considered in the diagnosis, only 3–5% of patients undergoing manometry for suspected esophageal motility disorders fit the diagnostic criteria. Diffuse esophageal spasm is a disorder of the thoracic esophagus resulting from impairment of inhibitory innervation. It involves the esophagus but spares the LES, leading to nonperistaltic contractions but normal LES relaxation, as evidenced on manometry. The amplitude of the contractions may be normal, increased, or decreased. Acid suppression and other medical and endoscopic treatments may alleviate symptoms. A subset of patients may progress to achalasia.

▶ Pathogenesis

Nonperistaltic contractions are due to loss of deglutitive inhibition associated with impaired inhibitory nerve function in the esophageal body. The amplitude of contractions involves many components, including the rebound contraction, which is dependent on the inhibitory nerves, cholinergic excitatory nerves, and myogenic factors. Loss of inhibitory nerves alone would be expected to reduce the force of contraction whereas compensatory cholinergic and myogenic factors may lead to increased force of contraction. However, little is known about the pathology of diffuse esophageal spasm. There appears to be patchy neural degeneration localized to nerve processes rather than degeneration of nerve cell bodies, as evidenced in achalasia. Hypertrophy of the muscularis propria and associated development of distal esophageal diverticula also occur.

▶ Clinical Features

A. Symptoms & Signs

Chest pain, dysphagia, and regurgitation are the main presenting symptoms. Chest pain may be particularly prominent in patients with high-amplitude and protracted contractions and can occur at rest, with swallowing, or with emotional stress. The pain is generally retrosternal but can radiate to the back, sides of the chest, both arms, or the jaw. Pain can last from seconds to several minutes and can mimic that of cardiac angina. Dysphagia for solids and liquids can be present. Regurgitation of food that fails to move into the stomach may occur.

B. Imaging Studies

Findings on barium swallow may be normal or show non-propagated contractions (called tertiary contractions), particularly below the aortic arch, with the appearance of curling or multiple ripples in the wall, sacculations, and pseudodiverticula, leading to the appearance of a "corkscrew" esophagus in severe cases.

C. Manometry

The diagnosis is generally made by esophageal manometry, which reveals more than 20% of wet swallows as simultaneous contractions. However, because the disorder is episodic, manometric findings can be entirely normal at the time of study. Simultaneous contractions must be distinguished from identical contraction patterns suggestive of a common cavity effect from functional or mechanical obstruction in the esophagus during the study. Moreover, occasional nonperistaltic contractions can occur normally. The amplitude of the nonperistaltic contractions can be increased, normal, or even decreased, and sometimes the contractions are multipeaked. However, LES relaxation is normal, and normally conducted peristaltic contraction must be evidenced in at least one swallow.

Methods to provoke esophageal spasm, including cold swallows and edrophonium, can induce chest pain but may not necessarily correlate with motility changes. Thus, provocation tests have limited utility.

▶ Differential Diagnosis

Diffuse esophageal spasm must be distinguished from other causes of chest pain, especially cardiac ischemia. Esophageal motility disorders are an uncommon cause of noncardiac chest pain, which is more commonly caused by reflux esophagitis or visceral hypersensitivity.

▶ Treatment

The mainstay of therapy is reassurance, control of esophageal acidification by PPIs or histamine receptor antagonists, and use of smooth muscle relaxants such as nitrates and calcium channel blockers. There are no controlled studies to substantiate any particular treatment modality, although smooth muscle relaxants or anticholinergic agents used for achalasia may be helpful for improving symptoms. Some studies suggest that low-dose tricyclic antidepressant therapy may be a better option for treating chest pain. Empiric bougienage

has been advocated, but studies comparing large versus small caliber bougies showed no differences in response rate, suggestive of a placebo effect. Similarly, there have been no controlled studies to validate the use of botulinum toxin either into the LES or at intervals along the esophageal body. Long esophageal myotomy is rarely used to treat intractable dysphagia and chest pain, particularly when associated with pulsion diverticula, and there are early reports of success with POEM.

▶ Course & Prognosis

Patients may have intermittent dysphagia and chest pain for many years without progression. A small subset of these patients (~5%) develops vigorous or classic achalasia, which should be suspected if patients develop regurgitation with worsening dysphagia.

Khalaf M, Chowdhary S, Elias PS, Castell D. Distal esophageal spasm: a review. *Am J Med.* 2018;131(9):1034–1040. [PMID: 29605413]

Roman S, Kahrilas PJ. Distal esophageal spasm. *Curr Opin Gastroenterol.* 2015;31(4):328–333. [PMID: 26039725]

Sugihara Y, Sakae H, Hamada K, Okada H. Peroral endoscopic myotomy is an effective treatment for diffuse esophageal spasm. *Clin Case Rep.* 2020;8(5):927–928. [PMID: 32477548]

3. Inappropriate Transient Lower Esophageal Sphincter Relaxation

LES relaxation normally occurs on swallowing, belching, or vomiting reflexes. When it occurs in the absence of such activities, it has been called inappropriate transient LES relaxation or simply transient LES relaxation (TLESR). TLESR is vagovagal inhibitory reflex that is mediated via the nitrergic inhibitory nerves to the LES. The frequency of TLESR is increased by gastric distention. Increased frequency of TLESR has been shown to be an important cause of GERD. Diagnosis of TLESR can only be made by long-term manometric recordings, which are employed mainly in research but not in common clinical practice.

Basal LES pressure is dependent on the myogenic tone of the sphincter muscle, and superimposed, counterbalancing influence of inhibitory and excitatory nerves. The force of peristaltic contraction is dependent on the contractile ability of the smooth muscle and influence of the excitatory as well as the inhibitory nerves. The inhibitory nerves are responsible not only for inhibition but also for the rebound contraction that follows the inhibition. Therefore, loss of rebound contraction can only occur if the preceding deglutitive inhibition is also lost. Disorders of TLESR that involve normal deglutitive inhibition and peristaltic sequence can be classified into hypotensive and hypertensive esophageal motility disorders and are described in the following sections.

DISORDERS OF EXCITATORY NERVES AND SMOOTH MUSCLES

1. Hypotensive Esophageal Disorders

ESSENTIALS OF DIAGNOSIS

▶ GERD and dysphagia.

▶ Hypotensive LES (LES pressure <10 mm Hg).

▶ Hypotensive peristaltic contractions (<30 mm Hg).

General Considerations

Hypotensive esophageal disorders include hypotensive LES, hypotensive peristaltic contraction, or both. Hypotensive LES may lead to GERD, and hypotensive peristaltic contractions manifest manometrically as ineffective esophageal motility (IEM, defined by 50% ineffective peristaltic sequence with DCI<450 mm Hg cm s but normal LES relaxation), may lead to dysphagia, impaired esophageal clearing of refluxed material, and accentuation of GERD, although can be identified in asymptomatic individuals and may represent a normal variant. A multiple rapid swallow sequence assessed during manometry may assess esophageal contraction reserve and may predict individuals who develop dysphagia after fundoplication.

Pathogenesis

Hypotensive esophageal disorders are due to either impaired excitatory innervation or impaired muscle contractility. Most cases are idiopathic, but a few are secondary to known causes, which include anticholinergic agents, smooth muscle relaxants, estrogens, progesterone, and pregnancy. Other important causes are connective tissue disorders, particularly scleroderma and intestinal pseudo-obstruction syndrome. The latter may be caused by muscular atrophy, disease or impairment of the cholinergic neurons, or both. Most cases of hypotensive LES are idiopathic in nature.

Clinical Findings

Refer to GERD and scleroderma esophagus elsewhere in this chapter.

Treatment

Refer to GERD and scleroderma esophagus elsewhere in this chapter.

Balko RA, Codipilly DC, Ravi K. Minor esophageal functional disorders: are they relevant? *Curr Treat Options Gastroenterol.* 2020. [PMID: 31953604]

Gyawali CP, Sifrim D, Carlson DA, et al. Ineffective esophageal motility: concepts, future directions, and conclusions from the Stanford 2018 symposium. *Neurogastroenterol Motil.* 2019;31(9):e13584. [PMID: 30974032]

Reddy CA, Baker JR, Lau J, Chen JW. High-resolution manometry diagnosis of ineffective esophageal motility is associated with higher reflux burden. *Dig Dis Sci.* 2019;64(8):2199–2205. [PMID: 31041641]

2. Hypertensive Esophageal Disorders

ESSENTIALS OF DIAGNOSIS

▶ Hypertensive LES, hypercontracting LES, and hypertensive peristalsis identified on intraluminal manometry.

▶ Sustained longitudinal muscle contraction diagnosed by high-frequency endoscopic ultrasound.

▶ Usually noted in patients being evaluated for noncardiac chest pain or dysphagia.

General Considerations

Hypercontractile syndromes include entities such as hypertensive and hypercontracting LES that may lead to esophagogastric junction outlet obstruction, hypertensive peristalsis (nutcracker esophagus), and sustained contraction of the esophageal longitudinal muscle.

Pathogenesis

These hypercontractile states may result from overactive excitatory nerves or stress. The cause is unknown, but patients may have esophageal hypersensitivity.

Clinical Findings

A. Symptoms & Signs

When hypertensive peristalsis or nutcracker esophagus was initially described, it was a common manometric abnormality found in patients with noncardiac chest pain. However, it is now appreciated that these episodes of high-amplitude contraction coincide poorly with chest pain and may be an epiphenomenon or perhaps a marker for hypersensitivity or a hyperreactive esophagus. Dysphagia has been reported by some patients with manometric findings of hypercontractile esophagus.

There are no physical findings specific for hypercontractile esophagus.

B. Laboratory, Imaging, & Manometric Studies

Hypertensive peristalsis is the most common manometric finding in patients referred for evaluation of noncardiac angina-like chest pain. Generally, barium studies show normal peristalsis, normal esophageal transit, and no structural esophageal disease. Esophagoscopy is also normal.

Prolonged ambulatory manometric studies reveal that some patients with hypertensive peristalsis have nonperistaltic contractions during mealtime, but not during standard wet swallows of a standard manometric study.

A subset of these patients may have inappropriate contractions of the esophageal longitudinal muscles that are poorly transduced on standard manometric evaluations but may be revealed on esophageal ultrasonography.

Specimens are rarely available for pathologic examination of these hypercontractile states, although a single report has described loss of intramural neurons in the LES of patients with isolated hypertensive LES.

As the names imply, hypertensive peristalsis, hypertensive LES, and hypercontracting LES are diagnosed manometrically. In hypertensive peristalsis, the amplitude of the peristaltic contractions exceeds 180 mm Hg or the duration of contraction exceeds 7.5 seconds. In hypertensive LES, the basal pressure of the LES exceeds 40 mm Hg. Similarly, hypercontracting LES shows prolonged and high-amplitude postrelaxation (rebound) contraction.

Differential Diagnosis

As with achalasia, ischemic heart disease must be excluded in patients presenting with chest pain. GERD is the most common cause of atypical noncardiac chest pain and should be excluded, either with an empiric trial of PPI therapy or through ambulatory pH testing. Findings may be confounded by chronic opiate use. Other causes of chest pain include chest wall origin, pericarditis, atelectasis, and panic attacks.

Treatment

Anticholinergic drugs and smooth muscle relaxants (nitrates and calcium channel blockers) are often used but have unproven value. Low-dose tricyclic antidepressants may improve chest pain in some patients, perhaps because of their modulation of visceral hypersensitivity. Cognitive-behavioral therapy has also been employed with benefit to some patients.

Patcharatrakul T, Alkaddour A, Pitisuttithum P, et al. How to approach esophagogastric junction outflow obstruction? *Ann N Y Acad Sci.* 2020;1481(1):210–223. [PMID: 32557701]

Samo S, Qayed E. Esophagogastric junction outflow obstruction: where are we now in diagnosis and management? *World J Gastroenterol.* 2019;25(4):411–417. [PMID: 30700938]

3. Scleroderma Esophagus

ESSENTIALS OF DIAGNOSIS

▶ Absent LES tone and esophageal peristalsis.

▶ Symptoms of GERD or dysphagia, or both, may experience chest pain and odynophagia

▶ Respiratory compromise from aspiration or direct lung involvement.

General Considerations

Esophageal scleroderma occurs as part of a connective tissue disorder and leads to atrophy of esophageal smooth muscle with consequent loss of LES tone and force of esophageal peristalsis. The condition occurs in 75–85% of patients with scleroderma and affects particularly women in the age group of 30–50. Patients with Raynaud phenomenon frequently have esophageal motor abnormalities.

Pathogenesis

The cause of scleroderma is unknown, but it is thought to involve an autoimmune response. Progressive atrophy and sclerosis of the esophageal smooth muscles lead to poor peristaltic contractions in the distal esophagus and to LES incompetence. Microvessel disease in scleroderma may lead to intramural neuronal dysfunction early in the disease. Subsequently, fibrosis and atrophy of esophageal smooth muscle develop, leading to a markedly hypotensive LES and loss of peristaltic contractions in the smooth muscle segment of the esophagus.

Clinical Findings

Diagnosis is confirmed by the presence of Raynaud phenomenon and cutaneous manifestations of scleroderma along with symptoms of dysphagia and GERD. Physiologic changes in the esophagus contribute to poor esophageal clearance and marked gastroesophageal reflux. This can result in reflux esophagitis and strictures (17–29%) in advanced cases. Pulmonary interstitial fibrosis can result from either direct involvement of the disease, or from aspiration of refluxate.

A. Symptoms & Signs

Owing to LES incompetence and lack of esophageal acid clearance from lack of esophageal peristalsis, patients often have severe GERD, leading to heartburn, regurgitation, dysphagia, and chest pain. However, symptoms can be relatively mild despite severe mucosal disease, and esophageal disease correlates better with degree of pulmonary involvement rather than disease in the stomach or intestine. Dysphagia may occur even in the absence of obvious skin and joint involvement, although Raynaud phenomenon is usually present.

B. Laboratory Findings

Certain autoimmune markers such as the antiendonuclear antigens and anti–ScL-70 and anticentromere antibodies may be present.

C. Imaging Studies

In advanced disease, barium swallow reveals a dilated esophagus with poor esophageal clearance and weak contractions.

D. Manometry & FLIP

Since the use of HRM, manometry has been the preferred study of patients with systemic sclerosis, with findings of absent or ineffective peristalsis of the distal esophagus in combination with a hypotensive LES. Sometimes, swallow-induced contractions are nonperistaltic, suggesting additional impairment of the nitrergic inhibitory nerves. FLIP has been shown in a small study of esophageal scleroderma patients to discern lower EGJ yield pressure and higher esophageal distensibility compared to healthy controls.

► Differential Diagnosis

In the absence of other features of a connective tissue disorder, scleroderma can be confused with primary GERD. Cutaneous manifestations of scleroderma may be absent in up to 5% of patients. History of Raynaud phenomenon may be very useful in the diagnosis. Pulmonary fibrosis may even be attributed to repeated aspiration from GERD. In patients presenting with dysphagia, eosinophilic esophagitis should be excluded by multiple mucosal biopsies obtained at different levels of the esophagus. Scleroderma esophagus may sometimes be confused with achalasia, particularly in patients with a dilated esophagus on barium swallow and poor peristaltic contractions in the thoracic esophagus on barium swallow or esophageal manometry. However, patulous and hypotensive LES on endoscopic and manometric findings can distinguish the two. In scleroderma, LES is usually patulous unless complicating peptic stricture is present.

► Treatment

There is no specific treatment for esophageal scleroderma. Severe reflux, which is generally the source of the patient's predominant symptoms, is treated with PPIs, often requiring double-dose, twice-daily administration. Prokinetic drugs including metoclopramide and erythromycin may increase LES pressure, but with variable results, and buspirone has been reported to increase LES and peristaltic pressure with improvement in heartburn and regurgitation. However, these drugs must be used with caution regarding potential central nervous system and cardiovascular side effects. Esophageal bougienage may be required for strictures. Generally, antireflux surgery should be avoided because of the risk of severe postoperative dysphagia. Otherwise, a partial fundoplication, generally with a Collis procedure and esophageal lengthening, is performed. More recently a Roux-en-Y gastric bypass has been forwarded as a potential surgical alternative, although caution has been raised in setting of small intestinal dysmotility and bacterial overgrowth prevalent in systemic sclerosis.

Denaxas K, Ladas SD, Karamanolis GP. Evaluation and management of esophageal manifestations in systemic sclerosis. *Ann Gastroenterol.* 2018;31(2):165–170. [PMID: 29507463]

Laique S, Singh T, Dornblaser D, et al. Clinical characteristics and associated systemic diseases in patients with esophageal "Absent Contractility"-a clinical algorithm. *J Clin Gastroenterol.* 2019;53(3):184–190. [PMID: 29356781]

Tetreault MP, Kahrilas P. GI manifestations with a focus on the esophagus: recent progress in understanding pathogenesis. *Curr Rheumatol Rep.* 2019;21(8):42. [PMID: 31270707]

Eosinophilic Esophagitis

Wai-Kit Lo, MD

Matthew J. Hamilton, MD

ESSENTIALS OF DIAGNOSIS

▶ In adults, a major symptom is recurrent dysphagia, often with food impaction; mean age at diagnosis is 34 and mean duration of symptoms before treatment is 4.5 years.

▶ Esophageal biopsy shows dense eosinophilic infiltration (≥15 eosinophils per high-power field [HPF]), often in the distal and mid-esophagus.

▶ Diagnostic criteria include: (1) clinical symptoms of esophageal dysfunction; (2) increased eosinophils in esophageal mucosal biopsies; (3) secondary causes of esophageal eosinophilia have been excluded.

▶ Resolution of eosinophilia with medical anti-reflux treatment may suggest a proton pump inhibitor (PPI)-responsive subset of eosinophilic esophagitis (EoE) patients, although PPI alone is not sufficient to manage the majority of patients with EoE.

General Considerations

EoE is a chronic and increasingly recognized inflammatory disorder of the esophagitis characterized by abnormal infiltration of eosinophils of the esophageal mucosa, often resulting in dysphagia and food impaction. The disorder is being diagnosed with much greater frequency by virtue of increased endoscopy volume and disease recognition. Studies have indicated that the incidence has increased more than fourfold in the last 5–10 years. More than 80% of patients diagnosed with EoE complain of dysphagia, and between 5% and 16% of patients undergoing endoscopic evaluation for dysphagia are found to have EoE. Further, more than 50% of patients presenting with frank food impaction are diagnosed with EoE. By contrast, in children and adolescents, gastro-esophageal reflux symptoms are as common as food impaction and dysphagia.

Epidemiology

EoE occurs in both the pediatric age group and adults. About 70–75% of the patients are male, and the most common age of presentation is in the 20s and 30s. In older case series, the mean age at diagnosis was 34 years. In addition, in the older literature, symptom duration prior to diagnosis averaged 4.5 years, though in a recent systematic review, the time between symptom onset and diagnosis was more pronounced in adults (3–8 years) compared to children (1.2–3.5 years). For reasons that are not clear, the disease is more common in Whites. The increased incidence appears to be due not only to increased recognition of the disorder, but perhaps other factors as well. This is evidenced by a population-based study that documented incidence of EoE in Olmsted County, Minnesota, where the incidence was 9.5 per 100,000 patients per year, and the prevalence was 55 patients per 100,000. Similar population-based studies around the world have also concluded that the incidence of EoE is increasing over time and may actually be approaching that of inflammatory bowel disease.

Shaheen NJ, Mukkada V, Eichinger CS, et al. Natural history of eosinophilic esophagitis: a systematic review of epidemiology and disease course. *Dis Esophagus.* 2018;31(8):doy015. [PMID: 29617744]

Pathogenesis

The pathogenesis of EoE is incompletely defined. However, considerable evidence suggests that EoE is an allergic disorder induced by antigen sensitization either through foods or/and environmental allergens, resulting in epithelial barrier dysfunction.

A majority of patients have evidence of food allergies and a concurrent history of respiratory allergies. A seasonal variation has been documented in the diagnosis of EoE that correlated with pollen counts. By contrast, IgE-mediated food anaphylaxis is uncommon, occurring in less than 15% of pediatric patients with EoE.

The recruitment of eosinophils occurs in several inflammatory or infectious conditions and after exposure to inhaled or ingested allergens. Eosinophils also release chemoattractants, such as interleukins, which can perpetuate an inflammatory response. The latter phenomenon has led to trials of interleukin inhibitors in the treatment of EoE although there are none that are currently approved.

Inage E, Furuta GT, Menard-Katcher C, Masterson JC. Eosinophilic esophagitis: pathophysiology and its clinical implications. *Am J Physiol Gastrointest Liver Physiol.* 2018;315(5):G879–G886. [PMID: 30212252]

O'Shea KM, Aceves SS, Dellon ES, et al. Pathophysiology of eosinophilic esophagitis. *Gastroenterology.* 2018;154(2):333–345. [PMID: 28757265]

Clinical Findings

A. Symptoms & Signs

The leading symptom in adults is recurrent episodes of dysphagia. Mean duration of symptoms before diagnosis and initiation of treatment in one large series was 4.5 years. Recurrent dysphagia is present in the majority of patients, as is the history of food impaction. A personal history of allergic diseases (ie, airway, food, or skin allergies) is frequently present. Serum immunoglobulin E (IgE) elevations have been documented in one series in two-thirds of the patients. However, it should be emphasized that there is no difference in symptoms, endoscopic findings, or histology in patients with increased serum IgE levels versus those with normal IgE levels. Symptoms appear to be more pronounced in patients with peripheral blood eosinophilia. Another clinical feature is the presence of symptoms of GERD, dyspepsia, and xiphosternal and retrosternal discomfort that are seemingly refractory to medical management. In children and adolescents, symptoms include vomiting, regurgitation, GERD symptoms not responding to medical management, upper abdominal pain, and food impaction in the esophagus.

B. Endoscopy

Endoscopic features associated with EoE are highly variable and may include a normal appearance. Other more frequent findings include trachea-like circular rings that can be transient or fixed, white exudates, white nodules with granularity, linear furrowing, and vertical lines on the esophageal mucosa. In addition, the passage of the endoscope may lead to localized, contact trauma. Finally, strictures in the proximal, middle, or distal esophagitis are sometimes encountered. Examples of typical endoscopic findings in EoE are shown in Plates 18 and 19.

Other disorders also may be associated with increased eosinophilic infiltration of the esophagus (see below).

Accordingly, biopsies should be taken in both the distal and mid-esophagus in patients with suspected EoE. Characteristic histologic findings in eosinophilic EoE are shown in Plate 20.

The wide variance in disease severity from an endoscopic and histologic standpoint has revealed three pathogenically distinct subtypes including a mild inflammatory subtype with a normal-appearing esophagus, a more severe inflammatory type that may be steroid unresponsive, and a fibrostenotic subtype. However, it is unknown to what extent one subtype may progress to a more severe subtype, and it remains unclear how these phenotypic differences should guide further evaluation and management.

Ruffner MA, Cianferoni A. Phenotypes and endotypes in eosinophilic esophagitis. *Ann Allergy Asthma Immunol.* 2020;124(3):233–239. [PMID: 31862435]

Shoda T, Wen T, Aceves SS, et al. Eosinophilic esophagitis endotype classification by molecular, clinical, and histopathological analyses: a cross-sectional study. *Lancet Gastroenterol Hepatol.* 2018;3(7):477–488. [PMID: 29730081]

Warners MJ, Oude Nijhuis RAB, de Wijkerslooth LRH, et al. The natural course of eosinophilic esophagitis and long-term consequences of undiagnosed disease in a large cohort. *Am J Gastroenterol.* 2018;113(6):836–844. [PMID: 29700481]

C. Diagnostic Criteria

The usual criteria for the diagnosis of EoE include the following:

1. Clinical symptoms of esophageal dysfunction, especially dysphagia and a history of food impaction.

2. Biopsies of the esophageal mucosa reveal a dense inflammatory cell infiltration (ie, >15 eosinophils/HPF).

3. Secondary causes of esophageal eosinophilia have been excluded.

Previously, persistent eosinophilia following a 2-month trial of PPI was used as a diagnostic criterion. However, it is now believed that patients with PPI-responsive disease may be a subset of EoE patients, rather than a distinct entity, as some patients with initial response to PPI therapy may require additional EoE-targeted treatment in the future.

As noted below under treatment considerations, responses to treatment such as dietary elimination and topical corticosteroids support are not required for diagnosis. With regards to esophageal biopsies, two to four biopsies should be obtained from the proximal or mid-esophagus, as well as the distal esophagus to maximize the likelihood of detecting esophageal eosinophilia in all patients. Further, at the time of diagnosis, additional biopsies from the stomach and/or duodenum may be considered to rule out other causes of eosinophilia, especially if the patient experiences additional clinical symptoms such as abdominal pain, diarrhea, or weight loss.

Differential Diagnosis

It may be difficult to distinguish between EoE and GERD in clinical practice. Data from one study included 151 patients with EoE and 126 with GERD. Features that independently predicted EoE included younger age; symptoms of dysphagia; documented food allergies; observation of esophageal rings, linear furrows, white plaques, or exudates by upper endoscopy; absence of a hiatal hernia; and a higher maximum eosinophil count. The Endoscopic Reference Score (EREFS), a validated scoring system to predict EoE based on endoscopic assessment of Exudate, Rings, Edema, Furrows, and Strictures may be helpful to describe endoscopic disease severity, particularly for research purposes. However, there remains variability in endoscopist reporting of the scoring components, and there is poor correlation between endoscopy findings and clinical severity and histology in adults, which may limit its clinical applicability.

Although increased eosinophilic infiltration in the esophagus is characteristic of EoE, this finding is not specific. Other disorders that may be associated with increased eosinophilic infiltration of the esophagitis include GERD, Crohn's disease, hypereosinophilic syndrome, cardiovascular disease, drug-induced esophagitis, and infectious esophagitis (ie, herpes or *Candida*). Increased eosinophils may be found in the distal esophagus in reflux esophagitis, but usually the proximal or mid-esophagus are spared.

Dellon ES, Gibbs WB, Fritchie KJ, et al. Clinical, endoscopic, and histologic findings distinguish eosinophilic esophagitis from gastroesophageal reflux disease. *Clin Gastroenterol Hepatol.* 2009;7:1305–1313. [PMID: 19733260]

Dellon ES, Gonsalves N, Hirano I, et al. ACG clinical guideline: evidenced based approach to the diagnosis and management of esophageal eosinophilia and eosinophilic esophagitis (EoE). *Am J Gastroenterol.* 2013;108():679–692. [PMID: 23567357]

Rodrigo S, Abboud G, Oh D, et al. High intraepithelial eosinophil counts in esophageal squamous epithelium are not specific for eosinophilic esophagitis in adults. *Am J Gastroenterol.* 2008;103:435–442. [PMID: 18289205]

Rodriguez-Sanchez J, Barrio-Andres J, Nantes Castillejo O, et al. The Endoscopic Reference Score shows modest accuracy to predict either clinical or histological activity in adult patients with eosinophilic oesophagitis. *Aliment Pharmacol Ther.* 2017;45(2):300–309. [PMID: 27868216]

Straumann A, Katzka DA. Diagnosis and treatment of eosinophilic esophagitis. *Gastroenterology.* 2018;154(2):346–359. [PMID: 28756235]

Treatment

A. Topical Corticosteroids

Several studies that have employed topical fluticasone in doses ranging from 220 to 440 µg two to four times daily have demonstrated symptom improvement and complete resolution of symptoms in up to 75% of cases. In contrast to its use in the treatment of pulmonary disease and asthma, patients are generally instructed to swallow rather than inhale the fluticasone and not use a spacer. Twice-daily fluticasone is usually administered for 6–12 weeks, and during this interval, clinical and histologic symptoms are improved in the vast majority of patients. Patients receiving the higher dose of fluticasone are more likely to develop esophageal candidiasis. Furthermore, higher doses of fluticasone (ie, >440 µg/day) have been associated with systemic side effects, including cataracts and adrenal suppression. Although the use of swallowed corticosteroids is effective in relieving symptoms for a short period of time (4 months or less), long-term efficacy remains controversial. It should be emphasized that symptoms are more likely to recur in a period of 4–18 months after therapy has been discontinued in approximately half of the patients.

An alternative to swallowed fluticasone is the use of a suspension of budesonide. Pulmicort Respules are a liquid-based formulation of budesonide containing 0.5 mg of budesonide, and 2 mL of Pulmicort Respules mixed with five packets of sucralose will make a dose of 10–15 mL slurry that can be swallowed twice daily. Although data are limited, this preparation may be a viable alternative to using swallowed fluticasone. This preparation was well-tolerated in adolescent and adult patients with active disease, and led to histologic and symptomatic improvement after a 15-day treatment course compared to placebo. More recently, the budesonide orodispersible tablet formulation, which dissolves in the mouth and is slowly swallowed, given at a dose of 1 mg twice a day for six weeks, was shown to be more effective than placebo in inducing histologic and clinical remission of EoE.

B. Systemic Corticosteroids

Systemic corticosteroids are effective in EoE, but side effects limit their use, especially for periods longer than 4 weeks. They may be indicated when urgent symptom relief is required as with patients experiencing severe dysphagia, dehydration, and significant weight loss or esophageal strictures.

C. Esophageal Dilation

Esophageal dilation may be necessary in patients with strictures, but it must be done carefully as it has been associated with deep mucosal tears, esophageal perforation, increased postendoscopic analgesia, and difficulty in inserting the endoscope. A recent pooled meta-analysis demonstrated that a majority of patients experienced clinical improvement after endoscopic dilation. Of the studies included, no deaths were noted, and the most common adverse events were a small mucosal tear in 22% of patients, followed by deep mucosal tear in 4% of patients.

D. Leukotriene Receptor Antagonists

The leukotriene receptor antagonist montelukast has been studied in a small number of patients with EoE; eight patients showed a complete resolution of symptoms with a dosage of

20–40 mg/day and maintained this response for a median of 14 months. However, once the medication was discontinued, six of the eight patients had a recurrence of their symptoms. Data are insufficient to recommend leukotriene receptor antagonists for the treatment of EoE.

E. Cromolyn Sodium

Despite the perceived importance of mast cells in EoE pathogenesis, Cromolyn sodium, a mast cell stabilizer, has not shown any apparent benefit for patients with EoE although it has no significant adverse effects.

F. Dietary Therapy

Dietary therapy is an important emerging form of therapy for EoE. Three different dietary approaches have been examined.

1. Elemental (amino-based formula diets)—Peterson et al. (2013) assessed the efficacy of an elemental diet in adults with EoE. Eighteen adults with EoE were given an elemental diet for 4 weeks or just 2 weeks if their response was complete. Symptoms and histologic findings, based on biweekly biopsies, were monitored. Six subjects were rebiopsied 2–7 days after resuming a normal diet. There was a complete or nearly complete response, that is, <10 eosinophils/HPF in 72% of the subjects. There was substantial histologic improvement after 4 weeks on the elemental diet. These findings support the concept that EoE in adults is substantially triggered by food. It should be noted that while elemental diets are effective in alleviating symptoms and affecting objective evidence of improvement, these diets are not well tolerated in some patients.

2. Specific food elimination diets—This can be difficult because patients are typically sensitive to multiple food groups that include common and uncommon foods. Efficacy of specific food elimination diets remains controversial. Several studies have demonstrated poor correlation of diagnostic skin testing, radioallergosorbent (RAST) testing, and IgE skin prick tests for specific food allergens, with clinical symptoms or tissue inflammation.

3. Empiric elimination diet with removal of common food allergens—One center reported a significant improvement in patients on a specific six-food elimination diet. Kagalwalla and colleagues demonstrated that eliminating the six most common allergenic foods (cow's milk dairy, eggs, wheat, soy, peanuts, and fish/shellfish) resulted in significant improvement in 74% of the 35 EoE patients who received the six-food elimination diet. In another study by Molina-Infante, a "2-4-6" elimination diet was tested where the two most common allergens (cow's milk and wheat) were eliminated and patients were assessed for response before removing eggs and soy/legumes, and then nuts and seafood. Response was assessed by endoscopy and biopsy, and 76% of those who participated achieved remission after the first step, with another 13% responding after the second step.

G. Treatment of Gastroesophageal Reflux Disease

Patients in the PPI-responsive subset of EoE may have a robust response to antireflux therapy with PPI, particularly twice-a-day dosing applied for at least 8 weeks. Patients with overlapping GERD and EoE may also benefit from antireflux treatment. However, in most cases of primary EoE, PPI alone is usually not successful or achieves only a partial response.

Greuter T, Hirano I, Dellon ES. Emerging therapies for eosinophilic esophagitis. *J Allergy Clin Immunol.* 2020;145(1):38–45. [PMID: 31705907]

Kagalwalla AF, Sentongo TA, Ritz S, et al. Effects of six-food elimination diet on clinical and histologic outcomes in eosinophilic esophagitis. *Clin Gastroenterol.* 2006;4:1097–1102. [PMID: 16860614]

Konikoff MR, Noel RJ, Blanchard C, et al. Randomized, double-blind, placebo-controlled trial of fluticasone propionate for pediatric eosinophilic esophagitis. *Gastroenterology.* 2006;131:1381–1391. [PMID: 17101314]

Lucendo AJ, Miehlke S, Schlag C, et al. Efficacy of budesonide orodispersible tablets as induction therapy for eosinophilic esophagitis in a randomized placebo-controlled trial. *Gastroenterology.* 2019;157(1):74–86. [PMID: 30922997]

Molina-Infante J, Arias A, Alcedo J, et al. Step-up empiric elimination diet for pediatric and adult eosinophilic esophagitis: The 2-4-6 study. *J Allergy Clin Immunol.* 2018;141(4):1365–1372. [PMID: 29074457]

Molina-Infante J, Lucendo AJ. Dietary therapy for eosinophilic esophagitis. *J Allergy Clin Immunol.* 2018;142(1):41–47. [PMID: 29522850]

Moole H, Jacob K, Duvvuri A, et al. Role of endoscopic esophageal dilation in managing eosinophilic esophagitis: a systematic review and meta-analysis. *Medicine (Baltimore).* 2017;96(14):e5877. [PMID: 28383396]

Peterson KA, Byrne KR, Vinson LA, et al. Elemental diet induces histologic response in adult eosinophilic esophagitis. *Am J Gastroenterol.* 2013;108:759–766. [PMID: 23381017]

▶ Course & Prognosis

Straumann and coworkers described 30 patients followed for a mean of 7.2 years (range, 1.4–11.5 years); 23% of the patients reported increased dysphagia and 36.7% reported stable symptoms. Mean duration of symptoms before treatment was 4.6 years. Recurrent episodes of dysphagia were documented in 29 of 30 patients, and the symptoms were more pronounced in patients with peripheral eosinophilia. EoE does not seem to be associated with esophageal metaplasia (ie, Barrett esophagus or cardiac metaplasia or esophageal neoplasms). There are no standard guidelines for endoscopic monitoring after diagnosis, and the clinical practice at our institution ranges from annual screening endoscopy with biopsies, to early endoscopic evaluation with symptom recurrence.

Straumann A, Spichtin HP, Grize L, et al. Natural history of primary eosinophilic esophagitis: a follow-up of 30 adult patients for 11.5 years. *Gastroenterology*. 2003;125:1660–1669. [PMID: 14724818]

▶ Unresolved Issues

There are several unresolved issues with regard to the natural history and treatment of EoE. Treatment end points and maintenance medical management remain incompletely defined. We generally recommend repeating an upper endoscopy with mid- and distal-esophageal biopsies approximately 8 weeks after initiation of a new therapy, to evaluate histologic response. Treatment initiatives are aimed at relieving symptoms, which may or may not be accompanied by histologic resolution of EoE.

In this regard, after treatment, esophageal eosinophilia can persist, and such patients may be asymptomatic or only have minimal symptoms. There is no consensus on how to define histologic remission in response to treatment. It may be necessary to continue treatment in patients with documented EoE and persistent esophageal symptoms in the absence of esophageal abnormalities. As mentioned in the prior section, a schedule for disease surveillance with endoscopy remains poorly defined. The disease frequently recurs when therapy is discontinued (ie, glucocorticosteroids) or dietary modifications are discontinued. In these patients and in those who are considered to have moderate to severe disease, there is a pipeline of biologic treatments targeting Th2 inflammatory pathways and eosinophil recruitment that hold promise for an expanded armamentarium for the treatment of EoE.

Peptic Ulcer Disease

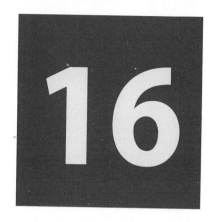

Edward Lew, MD, MPH

ESSENTIALS OF DIAGNOSIS

▶ Peptic ulcers are mucosal defects in the stomach or small intestine.

▶ *Helicobacter pylori* infection, nonsteroidal anti-inflammatory drugs (NSAIDs), and aspirin use are the most common causes.

▶ Patients may have epigastric pain or complications such as gastrointestinal (GI) bleeding, perforation, and obstruction.

▶ Diagnosis is often made by endoscopy or radiologic studies.

General Considerations

Peptic ulcers are defects or breaks in the gastric or small intestinal mucosa that have depth and extend through the muscularis mucosae. In contrast to erosions, which are small and superficial mucosal lesions, peptic ulcers can vary in size from 5 mm to several centimeters and may lead to complications such as GI bleeding, obstruction, penetration, and perforation.

The pathogenesis of peptic ulcers is multifactorial and arises from an imbalance of protective and aggressive factors such as when GI mucosal defense mechanisms are impaired in the presence of gastric acid and pepsin. Peptic ulcer disease was long considered an idiopathic and lifelong disorder. This paradigm changed dramatically in 1984 when Marshall and Warren reported that a curved bacillus, initially named *Campylobacter pyloridis* and subsequently classified as *H pylori*, was linked to ulcers. Multiple studies have since shown that eradication of *H pylori* significantly reduces the rate of ulcer recurrence. Another major risk factor for peptic ulcers is the use of NSAIDs and aspirin. These medications generally exert their therapeutic and toxic effects by inhibiting the enzymes cyclooxygenase-1 (COX-1) and cyclooxygenase-2

(COX-2), which, in turn, impair mucosal protection and promote ulcers. The treatment of ulcer patients has been revolutionized since the development of the acid-suppressive medications such as the histamine-2 (H_2)-receptor blockers and proton pump inhibitors (PPIs), the synthetic prostaglandin misoprostol, and the selective COX-2 inhibitors. Only a small fraction of ulcers is associated with neoplasia or caused by acid hyper-secretory states such as Zollinger-Ellison syndrome and other rare disorders.

The incidence of both gastric and duodenal ulcers in developed countries rapidly increased throughout the 19th century and peaked during the first half of the 20th century. Since the 1950s, however, the incidence and prevalence of both ulcers have steadily declined. There has also been a decrease in the prevalence of *H pylori* over recent decades, attributed to improved hygiene and widespread use of antibiotics in developed countries. Hospital discharge data for the general U.S. population showed that the age-adjusted hospitalization rates for peptic ulcer disease and *H pylori* were highest among adults age 65 years and older and decreased with each subsequent age group. These trends are thought to reflect an underlying birth cohort effect with a decrease in *H pylori* incidence among younger generations.

The lifetime prevalence of peptic ulcers in the general population is estimated to be about 5–10% with an incidence of 0.1–0.3% per year. The development of peptic ulcer increases with age, with most ulcers occurring between 25 and 64 years of age. A systematic review of the literature on the epidemiology of peptic ulcer disease estimated an annual incidence ranging from 0.10% to 0.19% for physician-diagnosed peptic ulcers and from 0.03% to 0.17% for peptic ulcers diagnosed during hospitalization. However, more current estimates are likely to be lower especially in developed countries because of a declining incidence of peptic ulcers during the past 20 to 30 years along with a decline in *H pylori* infection. GI bleeding, perforation, and gastric outlet obstruction are the main complications of peptic ulcers. The incidence of bleeding ulcers in the general population ranges from 0.27 and 1.06 per 1000 person-years, while that of perforated ulcers is 0.03 to 0.30 per 1000 person-years. Although hospital admissions for peptic ulcer bleeding have steadily declined, the case fatality rate remains as high as 5–10%. Peptic ulcer complications can also adversely affect functional status and quality of life.

Gurusamy KS, Pallari E. Medical versus surgical treatment for refractory or recurrent peptic ulcer. *Cochrane Database Syst Rev.* 2016;3(3): CD011523. [PMID: 27025289]

Lanas A, Chan FKL. Peptic ulcer disease. *Lancet.* 2017; 390:613–624. [PMID: 28242110]

Malmi H, Kautiainen H, Virta LJ, Färkkilä N, Koskenpato J, Färkkilä MA. Incidence and complications of peptic ulcer disease requiring hospitalisation have markedly decreased in Finland. *Aliment Pharmacol Ther.* 2014;39(5):496–506 [PMID: 24461085]

Sverdén E, Agréus L, Dunn JM, Lagergren J. Peptic ulcer disease. *BMJ.* 2019;367:l5495. [PMID: 31578179]

▶ Pathogenesis

A. Causes of Peptic Ulcers

H pylori infection and the use of NSAIDs and aspirin have numerous effects on the GI tract and are the most common causes of peptic ulcers (Table 16–1). In general, both factors disrupt normal mucosal defenses and repair, making the mucosa more susceptible to acid. Suppression of gastric acid secretion using pharmacologic agents heals ulcers and reduces future complications. Only a few patients have an underlying acid hypersecretory state causing ulcers. For example, less than 1% of patients with duodenal ulcers have a gastrin-secreting tumor causing profound acid secretion as part of the Zollinger-Ellison syndrome. Approximately 3–5% of gastric ulcers represent malignancy including adenocarcinoma, lymphoma, or metastatic lesions. Other infections

and conditions that increase ulcer formation include cytomegalovirus or herpes simplex (especially among immunosuppressed patients), tuberculosis, Crohn's disease, the use of other non-NSAID medications, hyperparathyroidism, sarcoidosis, myeloproliferative disorder, and systemic mastocytosis.

Cigarette smoking also promotes the development of ulcers and may interact with *H pylori* and NSAIDs to increase mucosal injury. Smoking also impairs ulcer healing and increases ulcer recurrence. Several studies suggest that alcohol use and diet do not appear to increase ulcer formation, whereas emotional stress may predispose some individuals to ulcers. Critically ill patients with severe burns, physical trauma, or multiple organ failure also have an increased risk of developing gastroduodenal ulcers and associated complications. There is also an association of peptic ulcers with medical conditions such as chronic obstructive lung disease and chronic renal failure, but the mechanisms are unclear. A genetic susceptibility has been reported but is thought to stem mainly from intra familial infection with *H pylori*. Recent studies suggest that an increasing proportion of ulcers are idiopathic, as they are not related to *H pylori*, NSAIDs, aspirin, acid hypersecretion, or any other known cause. In a pooled analysis of six clinical trials, for example, 27% of duodenal ulcers had no etiologic cause identified. In other studies, the proportion of idiopathic ulcers that is *H pylori* negative and NSAID negative without any other detectable causes ranges from 20% to 44%. Patients who develop bleeding from *H pylori* negative and non-NSAID idiopathic ulcers have also been shown to have a nearly four-fold increased risk of recurrent GI bleeding and higher mortality as compared to patients with bleeding from *H pylori* associated ulcers. These idiopathic ulcers appear to be more common in older people with comorbid conditions and have a high rate of relapse.

Emma S, Lars A, Jason MD, Jesper L. Peptic ulcer disease *BMJ.* 2019;367:l5495. [PMID: 31578179]

Kavitt RT, Lipowska AM, Anyane-Yeboa A, Gralnek IM. Diagnosis and treatment of peptic ulcer disease. *Am J Med.* 2019;132(4):447–456. [PMID: 30611829]

Crooks CJ1, West J, Card TR. Comorbidities affect risk of nonvariceal upper gastrointestinal bleeding. *Gastroenterology.* 2013;144:1384–1393. [PMID: 23470619]

B. *Helicobacter pylori* Infection

H pylori is a spiral gram-negative urease-producing bacterium that can be found in the mucus coating the gastric mucosa or between the mucus layer and gastric epithelium. Multiple factors enable the bacterium to live in the hostile stomach acid environment, including its ability to produce urease, which helps alkalinize the surrounding pH. *H pylori* infection is most commonly acquired in childhood and results in a chronic active gastritis that is usually lifelong without specific treatment. Risk factors for acquiring *H pylori* include low socioeconomic status, household crowding, and country

Table 16–1. Risk factors for peptic ulcers.

Helicobacter pylori infection
NSAIDs and aspirin use
Other medications (eg, potassium chloride, concomitant use of corticosteroids with NSAIDs, bisphosphonates, selective serotonin reuptake inhibitors, sirolimus, mycophenolate mofetil, 5-fluorouracil)
Neoplasia
Acid hypersecretory disorders (eg, Zollinger-Ellison syndrome)
Hyperparathyroidism
Crohn's disease
Sarcoidosis
Myeloproliferative disorder
Systemic mastocytosis
Other rare infections (eg, cytomegalovirus, herpes simplex, tuberculosis)
Critically ill patients with severe burns, head injury, physical trauma, or multiple organ failure

NSAIDs, nonsteroidal anti-inflammatory drugs.

of origin. In most regions, the main mechanism of spread is intrafamilial transmission. The prevalence of *H pylori* varies among different countries and remains high in most developing countries and is generally related to socioeconomic status and levels of hygiene. Most infected persons remain asymptomatic, but approximately 10–15% develop peptic ulcer disease during their lifetime. In addition to causing chronic gastritis and peptic ulcers, *H pylori* has been associated with the development of gastric adenocarcinoma and gastric mucosa-associated lymphoid tissue (MALT) lymphoma. A study from Japan with a mean follow-up of 7.8 years reported that gastric cancer developed in 2.9% of patients with peptic ulcer, dyspepsia, and gastric hyperplasia who had *H pylori* infection but in none of the uninfected patients with these conditions. There is an increased incidence of gastric cancer associated with *H pylori* in other areas including the Middle East, Southeast Asia, the Mediterranean, Eastern Europe, Central America, and South America. In 1994, the International Agency for Research on Cancer classified *H pylori* as a group 1 carcinogen and a definite cause of gastric cancer in humans.

Infection with *H pylori* increases the risk of peptic ulcers and GI bleeding from threefold to sevenfold. Depending on the population, *H pylori* is present in up to 70–90% of patients with duodenal ulcers and up to 30–60% of gastric ulcers. Multiple clinical studies show that *H pylori* eradication reduces ulcer recurrence to less than 10% as compared with recurrences of 70% with acid suppression alone. *H pylori* generally causes mucosal injury and ulcer complications through inflammation and cytokines. Despite a vigorous systemic and mucosal humoral response, antibody production does not lead to eradication of the infection.

H pylori is a highly heterogeneous bacterium. A combination of microbial and host factors determines the outcome of *H pylori* infection. The virulence of the organism, host genetics, and environmental factors affect the distribution and severity of gastric inflammation and level of acid secretion. The ability of *H pylori* strains to produce different proteins has been linked to their virulence and affects the host immune response. Several *H pylori* virulence factors have been associated with gastric atrophy, intestinal metaplasia, and risk of disease. For example, the presence of *H pylori* virulence factors that affect the induction of proinflammatory cytokine release or adhesion to the epithelial cell partly explain geographic differences in the incidence of gastric cancer. Several of these bacterial virulence factors include the *Cag* patho-genicity island (*cag*PAI), PicB, and the vacuolating cytotoxin (VacA). *H pylori* also expresses adhesins such as blood group antigen-binding adhesin (BabA) and outer inflammatory protein adhesion (OipA) which facilitate attachment of the bacteria to gastric epithelium. *H pylori* that express the cytotoxin-associated gene A (*CagA*-positive strains) reportedly represent virulent strains having greater interactions with humans. Several genes in a genomic fragment that make up a Cag pathogenicity island encode components of a type IV secretion island that translocates CagA

in host cells and affects cell growth and cytokine production. CagA is a highly antigenic protein that is associated with a prominent inflammatory response by eliciting interleukin-8 production. *H pylori* strains that also express active forms of VacA or the outer membrane proteins BabA and OipA are similarly associated with a higher risk of diseases than are strains that lack these factors.

Blaser MJ. Heterogeneity of *Helicobacter pylori. Eur J Gastroenterol Hepatol.* 2012;9(suppl 1):S3–S6. [PMID: 22498905]

Hooi JKY, Lai WY, Ng WK, et al. Global prevalence of *Helicobacter pylori* infection: systematic review and meta-analysis. *Gastroenterology.* 2017;153:420–429. [PMID: 28456631]

Robinson K, John C Atherton JC. The spectrum of Helicobacter-mediated diseases. *Annu Rev Pathol.* 2021;16:123–144. [PMID: 33197219]

Sheila EC. *Helicobacter pylori* infection. *N Engl J Med.* 2019; 380(12):1158–1165. [PMID: 30893536]

C. Aspirin & NSAIDS

Aspirin and NSAIDs are among the most frequently used drugs worldwide. NSAIDs are used to treat pain and inflammation, whereas aspirin is being increasingly used for primary and secondary prevention of cardiovascular events. Unfortunately, these drugs have substantial GI toxicity and are associated with the development of peptic ulcers and life-threatening GI bleeding. Endoscopic studies have shown that up to 15–30% of patients on NSAIDs develop gastric and duodenal ulcers. Epidemiologic studies also suggest that the risks of ulcer complications and death among regular NSAID users are 3–10 times higher as compared with those not taking these drugs. The elderly are at particularly increased risk, and one study found that the adjusted hospitalization rate for ulcer complications was 16.7 per 1000 person-years among elderly Medicaid patients on NSAIDs, in contrast to a rate of 4.2 among nonusers, with an attributable rate of 12.5 excess hospitalizations for ulcer disease per 1000 person-years among users.

Aspirin and other NSAIDs generally exert their therapeutic and toxic effects by inhibiting COX-1 and COX-2 isoenzymes, which, in turn, decrease prostaglandin synthesis. COX-1 is the rate-limiting enzyme for GI prostaglandins that normally help maintain mucosal blood flow and increase secretion of mucus and bicarbonate. Inhibition of COX-1 impairs mucosal protection and leads to ulcers. The risks of peptic ulcers and GI bleeding are dependent on the dose, duration, and type of NSAID. Older age and a previous history of GI bleeding or ulcers significantly increase the development of peptic ulcers among NSAID users. In a meta-analysis, the pooled relative risks for ulcer complications ranged from 1.6 to 9.2, according to the individual NSAID, with a pooled relative risk of 1.6 for aspirin. Even very low doses of aspirin have been associated with ulcers and GI bleeding, suggesting that there are no true safe doses of aspirin. A case-control study, for example, found that low-dose aspirin and nonaspirin NSAIDs both significantly increased the risk of ulcer bleeding with odds ratios of 2.4 and 7.4, respectively. Concomitant use of NSAIDs or aspirin with corticosteroids, selective serotonin-reuptake inhibitors, aldosterone antagonists, or anticoagulants significantly increase the risk of upper GI bleeding.

Laine L, Curtis SP, Cryer B, et al. Risk factors for NSAID-associated upper GI clinical events in a long-term prospective study of 34 701 arthritis patients. *Aliment Pharmacol Ther.* 2010;32:1240–1248. [PMID: 20955443]

Lanas A, Chan FKL. Peptic ulcer disease. *Lancet.* 2017;390:613–624. [PMID: 28242110]

Masclee GM, Valkhoff VE, Coloma PM, et al. Risk of upper gastrointestinal bleeding from different drug combinations. *Gastroenterology.* 2014;147(4):784–792. [PMID: 24937265]

▶ Clinical Findings

A. Symptoms & Signs

Epigastric pain is the classic symptom associated with peptic ulcer disease. The pain is often described as a gnawing, dull, aching, "empty," or "hunger-like" sensation. The classic pain associated with duodenal ulcer is sometimes relieved with ingestion of milk, food, or antacids but recurs 2–4 hours after eating and may also awaken the patient at night. In contrast, most patients with gastric ulcers report that eating exacerbates the pain. During fasting, they may have relief of their symptoms, which then recur shortly after eating. As a result, some gastric ulcer patients experience nausea, avoidance of food/anorexia, and even weight loss.

Peptic ulcer symptoms tend to recur at intervals of weeks or months due to healing and relapse while patients continue to have H pylori infection or use NSAIDs. An acute worsening or change in the pain characteristic such as generalized pain may arise from ulcer penetration or perforation. Alarm symptoms such as melena, hematemesis, guaiac-positive stools, and unexplained anemia suggest possible ulcer bleeding, while persistent vomiting may represent obstruction. Early satiety, anorexia, and unexplained weight loss may arise from cancer. Patients with upper abdominal pain with radiation to the back may have penetration, while those with severe or worsening abdominal pain may have perforation. However, many ulcer patients present with few or no symptoms until the development of complications such as GI bleeding, perforation, penetration, and obstruction. In one study, abdominal pain was absent in over 30% of older patients with peptic ulcers seen on upper endoscopy. Less common symptoms such as nausea and vomiting may arise from a gastric outlet obstruction with ulcer edema or scarring.

The physical examination is unreliable and often normal, although some ulcer patients have epigastric tenderness to deep palpation. Occult or gross blood may be detected in the setting of bleeding ulcers. Tachycardia and orthostasis may be found in patients with significant bleeding or dehydration, while a rigid abdomen with diffuse rebound tenderness may reflect ulcer perforation with peritonitis. Rarely, a distended abdomen or a succession splash can be noted in patients with an ulcer that is complicated by outlet obstruction.

Most duodenal ulcers develop in the bulb or pylori channel. Patients with duodenal ulcers tend to have a younger age of onset, often between 30 and 55 years of age on average. These duodenal ulcer patients also have an increased parietal cell mass and acid secretion (with increased average basal and nocturnal gastric acid secretion). Bicarbonate secretion has been reported to be impaired among patients with active duodenal ulcers. It is thought that the imbalance between duodenal acid load and buffering capacity leads to the development of small islands of gastric metaplasia in the duodenal bulb. Colonization of these islands by H pylori subsequently leads to duodenitis and duodenal ulcer.

In the stomach, most benign ulcers are found in the antrum and lesser curvature of the stomach at the junction of the body and antrum. Gastric ulcers often occur later in life, usually among patients between the ages of 55 and 70 years with a peak incidence in the sixth decade. Patients with gastric ulcers often have normal or decreased acid secretion. A few patients present with both gastric and duodenal ulcers are found to have increased acid secretion. The gastric ulcers in these patients tend to be in the distal antrum or pyloric channel.

B. Endoscopy

Definitive diagnosis of peptic ulcers can be made using upper endoscopy. Endoscopy has a much higher diagnostic yield than barium contrast radiology and enables biopsy specimens to be obtained for evaluation of H pylori infection and underlying malignancy. Because up to 5% of gastric ulcers are malignant, it is generally recommended that biopsy samples be taken from the ulcer margin or that a follow-up endoscopy be scheduled 12 weeks after starting acid-suppressive medications to document complete healing. Ulcers greater than 3 cm in size and those that are associated with a mass are more likely to be malignant. In contrast, the incidence of malignant duodenal ulcers is extremely low; thus, they do not routinely require biopsy. Actively bleeding ulcers or ulcers at high risk for rebleeding can also be treated during endoscopy with hemostasis therapy.

Patients suspected of having an ulcer who present with alarm symptoms, such as GI bleeding, early satiety, and unexplained weight loss, and those who are elderly should undergo prompt evaluation with endoscopy. Patients who are found to have multiple ulcers, refractory ulcers, or ulcers in unusual locations, such as postbulbar or jejunum, or who have diarrhea and weight loss should also be considered for evaluation of Zollinger-Ellison syndrome.

In contrast, there is some controversy as to the best approach for initial evaluation and treatment of young patients under the age of 50–55 years who present with ulcer-like symptoms or dyspepsia without alarm symptoms, in an area with a low incidence of gastric cancer and a prevalence of *H pylori* over 20%. Possible options include (1) testing and treating for *H pylori*, (2) treating with acid-suppressive medications and monitoring response, or (3) making a direct referral for evaluation with upper endoscopy. Prompt endoscopy potentially offers a small benefit in terms of finding a specific diagnosis and directing treatment but is not cost effective for the initial management of dyspepsia as compared to the other strategies. Instead, several other studies recommend that young patients with undifferentiated dyspepsia initially undergo noninvasive testing for *H pylori* followed by treatment if this infection is present. Successful cure of *H pylori* potentially reduces the need for endoscopy as well as ulcer recurrence, and clinical studies suggest that this strategy does not adversely affect outcomes. Further evaluation with endoscopy is recommended for patients with persistent symptoms despite therapy. Alternatively, young patients with a presentation suggestive of uncomplicated ulcers may first be given empiric treatment with acid-suppressive medications. Further evaluation is recommended if these patients continue to have persistent or recurrent symptoms 2–4 weeks later. All patients should discontinue aspirin and NSAIDs if possible, as well as stop alcohol, smoking, and use of illicit drugs. In one large clinical trial, patients having dyspepsia without alarm symptoms were randomized to testing and treating for *H pylori* versus empiric PPI therapy. After 1 year of follow-up, patients in the two groups had a similar rate of persistent dyspeptic symptoms, and both strategies were found to be equally cost effective in the initial management of dyspepsia. It is notable that over 80% of these patients continued to experience dyspeptic symptoms despite eradication of *H pylori* (82%) or acid-suppressive therapy (83%).

Delaney BC, Qume M, Moayyedi P, et al. *Helicobacter pylori* test and treat versus proton pump inhibitor in initial management of dyspepsia in primary care: multicentre randomized controlled trial (MRC-CUBE trial). *BMJ.* 2008;336:651–654. [PMID: 18310262]

Eusebi LH, Black CJ, Howden CW, et al. Effectiveness of management strategies for uninvestigated dyspepsia: systematic review and network meta-analysis. *BMJ.* 2019;367:l6483s. [PMID: 31826881]

C. Barium Studies

Barium upper GI studies are safer and cheaper than endoscopy, but they have limited accuracy for detecting ulcers and other mucosal lesions. In contrast to endoscopy, barium upper GI studies do not permit biopsy and other specimens to be obtained for histologic evaluation or allow immediate treatment of bleeding ulcers.

D. Tests to Diagnose *Helicobacter pylori* Infection

Several methods are available to detect *H pylori* infection (Table 16–2). The noninvasive tests include serologic testing, urea breath test, and stool antigen test. Infection can also be detected during endoscopy in which a biopsy sample is

Table 16–2. Diagnostic tests for *Helicobacter pylori*.

Test	Sensitivity (%)	Specificity (%)	Comments
Noninvasive			
Urea breath test	95–100	91–98	Recommended for both screening and confirming cure; recent use of antibiotics, bismuth, and PPIs can increase false-negative results
H pylori stool antigen test	91–96	93–97	Can be used for initial diagnosis and to confirm successful cure; recent use of antibiotics, bismuth, and PPIs can decrease antigen load in stool
Serologic ELISA	85–92	79–83	Detects exposure to *H pylori* but cannot be used to confirm successful cure after treatment. May remain positive for years after eradication of *H. pylori* infection. However, test not influenced by recent use of PPI or antibiotics.
Invasive			
Endoscopy with biopsy			
• Histology	>95	>95–98	Widely used method of diagnosis during endoscopy; sensitivity is improved by taking at least 2 biopsies from antrum and 1 from body of stomach
• Rapid urease test (CLO test)	93–97	95–100	Reduced accuracy reported among patients with GI bleeding
• Culture	70–80	100	Technically demanding; sensitivity varies among laboratories

CLO, *Campylobacter*-like organism; ELISA, enzyme-linked immunosorbent assay; GI, gastrointestinal; PPI, proton pump inhibitor.
Note: Patients are recommended to stop bismuth, antibiotics, and proton pump inhibitors at least 4 weeks before *H. pylori* testing for active infection using either urea breath test, stool antigen test, and histology.

obtained for a rapid urease testing, histologic study, or even culture. Serum immunoassays for immunoglobulin G (IgG) antibodies to *H pylori* are inexpensive but have a reported sensitivity of 85% and specificity of 79%. As a result, the positive predictive value of serologic testing is limited in populations with a low pretest probability of having the infection such as areas in which the prevalence is 30% or less. The prevalence of *H pylori* in the United States is estimated to be 30%. Moreover, serologic testing should not be used to determine the success of *H pylori* cure after treatment since antibody titers can persist for years and do not always become negative. The urea breath test or the stool antigen test can be used for both the initial diagnosis and follow-up of eradication therapy because they have excellent sensitivities and specificities. Urea breath testing is based on detecting *H pylori*-derived urease activity in the stomach (with a sensitivity and specificity exceeding 95%), whereas the stool antigen test uses polyclonal anti-*H pylori* capture antibody adsorbed to microwells (with sensitivity and specificity exceeding 92%). It is generally recommended to wait at least 4 weeks or more after completing eradication therapy to confirm successful cure. To help minimize false-negative results, PPIs should be withheld for at least 2–4 weeks and antibiotics and bismuth compounds for 4 weeks prior to testing, as these drugs have suppressive effects on *H pylori*. Since the use of H2-receptor blockers does not need to be restricted, they may be used to help manage heartburn and other GI symptoms prior to *H pylori* testing.

In patients who undergo endoscopy, an antral biopsy can be obtained for rapid urease testing, which has a sensitivity of 89–100% and specificity of 92–100%. Biopsies can also be performed, and specimens sent for histologic examination using routine hematoxylin and eosin staining. The presence of polymorphonuclear leukocytes in inflamed gastric tissue is suggestive of *H pylori* gastritis. In biopsy specimens in which *H pylori* cannot be found, the use of modified Giemsa, Warthin-Starry, Genta, and other stains may be helpful. Culture of *H pylori* from biopsy samples has a specificity of 100% if results are positive, but it is not routinely performed. Because culture is difficult to perform and expensive, it is usually reserved to determine antibiotic susceptibilities for patients who fail to respond to second-line eradication therapy.

Differential Diagnosis

In some studies, only half of patients with peptic ulcer present with classic symptoms. Unfortunately, the history and physical examination are neither sensitive nor specific enough to accurately diagnose peptic ulcers or distinguish between duodenal and gastric ulcers. A diagnosis of a peptic ulcer may be suspected in selected patients presenting with epigastric pain, but the differential is broad and includes gastroesophageal reflux disease, biliary tract disease, hepatitis, pancreatitis, abdominal aortic aneurysm, gastroparesis, functional dyspepsia, neoplasia, mesenteric ischemia, and myocardial ischemic pain, among others.

Although peptic ulcers can be diagnosed during upper endoscopy, laboratory and radiologic tests may help narrow the differential diagnosis. Some ulcer patients are anemic due to acute bleeding or chronic blood loss from benign or malignant ulcers. Liver function tests and levels of amylase and lipase should be checked to help evaluate for hepatitis and pancreatitis. An abdominal ultrasound may show gallstone disease or an abdominal aortic aneurysm. An electrocardiogram and measurement of cardiac enzymes help evaluate myocardial causes of pain. Finally, an acute abdominal series with upright and lateral decubitus views showing free air suggests perforation.

Complications

The most common complication associated with peptic ulcers is the development of GI hemorrhage. Up to 15% of peptic ulcers bleed, and affected patients have a mortality rate of 4.5–8.5%. Patients older than 60 years of age have a higher incidence of bleeding ulcers and mortality. Those who also have a large initial bleed, continued or recurrent bleeding, or severe comorbid illnesses have the greatest risk of death. Patients with bleeding ulcers can present with hematemesis or coffee ground emesis, passage of black tarry stool, and rarely, hematochezia.

Up to 7% of ulcer patients have perforation with severe abdominal pain and a rigid abdomen from peritonitis. Owing to the widespread use of NSAIDs among the elderly, they are at increased risk, and many do not present with antecedent ulcer pain or peritoneal findings. Penetration occurs when the ulcer crater erodes into an adjacent organ as, for example, when a duodenal ulcer penetrates the pancreas leading to pancreatitis or a gastric ulcer penetrates the left hepatic lobe.

Gastric outlet obstruction occurs in less than 2% of ulcer patients and may arise from ulcer inflammation and edema in the prepyloric area. Chronic ulcer scarring in the prepyloric area can also lead to a fixed mechanical obstruction that may require endoscopic balloon dilation or surgical therapy. This diagnosis should be suspected in patients who complain of nausea, vomiting, early satiety, and weight loss, especially if they also have dehydration and electrolyte imbalances.

Treatment
A. General Principles

Treatment of peptic ulcers consists of healing the ulcer and preventing ulcer recurrences and future complications. All ulcer patients should be tested and treated for *H pylori* even if they have a clear history of NSAID or aspirin use. It is not clinically possible to determine whether ulcers arise directly from *H pylori*, NSAID/aspirin use, or a combination of these factors. Although *H pylori* and NSAID use cause most ulcers, the level of acid secretion still plays a role in pathogenesis and healing. Multiple studies show that the administration of acid-suppressive medications promotes active ulcer healing.

Bleeding peptic ulcers account for 40–60% of patients presenting with acute upper GI bleeding. Please refer to Chapter 20 for further details on the diagnosis and management of these patients. In summary, patients suspected of having significant ulcer bleeding should be started on an intravenous PPI followed by prompt endoscopy within 24 hours of presentation. Patients with tachycardia (heart rate ≥100 beats per minute), hypotension (systolic blood pressure ≤100 mm Hg), age older than 60 years, and major coexisting conditions are at increased risk for further bleeding and death. There are several risk-assessment tools such as the Glasgow-Blatchford score that help stratify low- and high-risk patients. Using a restrictive blood transfusion strategy to target a hemoglobin >7 g/dL has been associated with a lower risk of further bleeding and all cause mortality. However, a higher hemoglobin threshold may be considered for symptomatic patients or those with underlying cardiovascular disease. The administration of intravenous PPIs before endoscopy downstages the ulcer lesion and the need for hemostasis therapy as compared to placebo. After endoscopic hemostasis, PPIs have also been shown to significantly reduce rebleeding, the need for repeat endoscopic therapy, and surgery. Intravenous therapy also reduced mortality in Asian trials and in a subgroup of ulcer patients having active bleeding or a nonbleeding visible vessel. Intravenous PPI therapy should be maintained for the first 72 hours in high-risk patients since most rebleeding occurs during this time. Other meta-analyses suggest that intermittent or twice daily dosing of an intravenous PPI is not inferior to a high dose continuous infusion. The promotility agent, erythromycin at 250 mg given intravenously 30 minutes prior to endoscopy increases gastric motility and visualization of the mucosa, which may reduce the need for blood transfusions and repeat endoscopy.

A recent randomized clinical trial reported no outcome differences between urgent versus early endoscopy (defined as endoscopy within 6 hours versus 6–24 hours after GI consultation, respectively) for 30-day all-cause mortality, recurrent bleeding, transfusion requirement, or length of hospital stay. In multiple studies, endoscopic hemostasis has been shown to significantly reduce rebleeding, surgery, and mortality and is recommended for high-risk ulcers, based on their endoscopic appearance and likelihood of further bleeding. High-risk ulcers include those that are actively spurting or oozing blood, those that have a nonbleeding visible vessel, or those that have an adherent clot. Please refer to Chapter 20: Acute Upper Gastrointestinal Bleeding for more details on the various hemostasis strategies, which may include a combination of thermocoagulation therapy (using bipolar electrocoagulation probes or heater probes), placement of hemoclips (mechanical therapy), and injection of epinephrine, alcohol, or a sclerosant (injection therapy). Thermocoagulation or clip placement, either alone or with epinephrine injection, are effective, but epinephrine injection alone is not recommended. Instead, adding a second modality to epinephrine injection is superior to epinephrine injection alone in reducing recurrent bleeding, surgery, and mortality. Endoscopic therapy should be repeated if bleeding recurs. Surgery or transcatheter arterial embolization can be performed if repeat endoscopic therapy fails. Complications of bleeding or perforation occur in about 0.5% of patients undergoing endoscopic therapy. Second-look endoscopy may be useful in selected patients but is not routinely recommended. Nonhealing gastric ulcers should be biopsied or closely followed to exclude underlying neoplasia. After discharge, patients having high-risk ulcers and clinical factors such as tachycardia and hypotension, older age, or major coexisting conditions should receive PPI therapy twice daily for 2 weeks followed by once daily dosing. In contrast, patients having erosions or ulcers without high-risk endoscopic findings and no hemodynamic instability or major coexisting conditions can be given once daily PPI therapy.

Barkun AN, Almadi M, Kuipers EJ, et al. Management of nonvariceal upper gastrointestinal bleeding: guideline recommendations from the International Consensus Group. *Ann Intern Med.* 2019;171:805–822.

Laine L. Upper gastrointestinal bleeding due to a peptic ulcer. *N Engl J Med.* 2016;375(12):1198. [PMID: 27653581]

Lau JY, Yu Y, Tang RS, et al. Timing of endoscopy for acute upper gastrointestinal bleeding. *N Engl J Med.* 2020;382:1299–1308.

Sung JJ, Chiu PW, Chan FKL, et al. Asia-Pacific working group consensus on non-variceal upper gastrointestinal bleeding: an update 2018. *Gut.* 2018;67(10):1757–1768. [PMID: 29691276]

B. Peptic Ulcers in Patients Requiring Chronic NSAIDs

Patients who develop peptic ulcers while using NSAIDs should be tested and treated for *H pylori* and the NSAID should be discontinued if possible. *H pylori* eradication alone is insufficient to completely prevent recurrent GI complications among ulcer patients who continue to take NSAIDs. Acid-suppressive medication, usually with a PPI, should also be administered to help the ulcer. PPIs block acid secretion by irreversibly binding and inhibiting the hydrogen-potassium ATPase that resides on the luminal surface of the parietal cell. Commonly used PPIs include omeprazole, lansoprazole, pantoprazole, rabeprazole, and esomeprazole. Potassium-competitive acid blockers such as vonoprazan are also now being developed that reportedly have a more rapid onset of action, longer duration and more effective acid suppression than the PPIs. Among different patients, there may be less pharmacokinetic variation than the PPI since clinical efficacy is not altered by CYP2C19 polymorphisms.

If patients cannot switch to acetaminophen and require chronic NSAIDs, they should consider taking the lowest effective NSAID dose along with co-therapy with either a PPI or a prostaglandin analog called misoprostol. These drugs have been shown to significantly reduce recurrent ulcer complications among chronic NSAID users. Unfortunately, misoprostol at 200 mcg four times daily is often associated with cramps, diarrhea, and poor patient compliance.

Drugs that selectively inhibit COX-2 were developed to have similar analgesic and anti-inflammatory effects as traditional NSAIDs but with a reduced risk of GI complications. Several studies have suggested that COX-2 inhibitors help treat musculoskeletal as well as arthritic conditions with fewer ulcer complications because they do not inhibit the gastric mucosal prostaglandins. Among healed ulcer patients, the use of a COX-2 inhibitor had a lower rate of adverse upper and lower GI events as compared to the strategy of providing a traditional NSAID with PPI co-therapy. Another trial has also shown that combining a selective COX-2 inhibitor with a PPI was even more effective in preventing recurrent ulcer bleeding than taking a COX-2 inhibitor alone. However, COX-2 inhibitors have been also associated with an increased risk of cardiovascular and thrombotic events. The exact mechanisms for this are not clear but may be related to the fact that thromboxane A2 is a COX-1-mediated product that causes irreversible platelet aggregation, vasoconstriction, and smooth muscle proliferation. In contrast, prostacyclin is synthesized from COX-2 and is an inhibitor of platelet aggregation while causing vasodilation and inhibition of smooth muscle proliferation. Selective inhibition of COX-2 may lead to an imbalance in these products that promotes thrombosis. Thus, clinicians must be judicious when prescribing these drugs. COX-2 inhibitors should be considered for chronic NSAID patients who have a substantial risk of ulcer complications but a low risk of cardiovascular disease. The addition of low-dose aspirin to a COX-2 inhibitor increases the ulcer rate to that seen with nonselective NSAIDs. A recent randomized clinical trial found that among patients with cardio-thrombotic diseases and a history of upper GI bleeding combining a COX-2 inhibitor plus proton-pump inhibitor is superior to using a nonselective NSAIDs plus proton-pump inhibitor for prevention of recurrent upper GI bleeding. As a result, this strategy should be considered for patients at high risk of both cardiovascular and GI events who require aspirin and NSAID for cardiovascular and anti-inflammatory therapies.

Barkun AN, Almadi M, Kuipers EJ, et al. Management of nonvariceal upper gastrointestinal bleeding: guideline recommendations from the International Consensus Group. Ann Intern Med. 2019;171:805–822. [PMID: 31634917]

Chan FKL, Ching JYL, Tse YK, et al. Gastrointestinal safety of celecoxib versus naproxen in patients with cardiothrombotic diseases and arthritis after upper gastrointestinal bleeding (concern): an industry-independent, double-blind, double-dummy, randomised trial. The Lancet. 2017;389:2375–2382. [PMID: 31924632]

Laine L, Jensen DM. Management of patients with ulcer bleeding. Am J Gastroenterol. 2012;107(3):345–360. [PMID: 22310222]

C. Peptic Ulcers in Patients Requiring Chronic Antiplatelet Therapy or Antithrombotic Therapy

The use of enteric-coated or buffered aspirin does not substantially reduce the risk of ulcer complications compared to noncoated aspirin due to the systemic effects of these drugs. There are also other widely used antiplatelet drugs such as clopidogrel that selectively and irreversibly block the adenosine diphosphate receptor on platelets. Clopidogrel, with or without aspirin, has been shown to be beneficial in the treatment of acute coronary syndrome and in the prevention of ischemic events among patients with atherosclerotic diseases. As expected, the combined use of clopidogrel with aspirin causes a greater increase in GI bleeding risk compared to aspirin alone.

Patients who are taking aspirin and present with potential ulcer complications such as GI bleeding should receive intravenous PPI therapy and undergo upper endoscopy. Ulcers that are found to have high-risk bleeding stigmata are then treated with hemostasis therapy. Testing and treating for H pylori as well as providing secondary prophylaxis with a PPI have been shown to be effective in reducing recurrent aspirin-induced GI complications. The coadministration of an acid lowering medication such as a PPI with aspirin greatly reduces recurrent ulcer bleeding as compared to switching patients to clopidogrel alone. One randomized trial reported that PPIs were superior to high-dose H_2-receptor antagonists in preventing recurrent aspirin-related ulcers and erosions. However, another randomized clinical trial of high-risk aspirin users found no significant difference in using a H_2-receptor antagonist versus a PPI to prevent recurrent upper GI bleeding and ulcers. In this study, a slightly lower proportion of patients receiving a PPI along with aspirin developing recurrent bleeding or ulcer than did patients receiving a H2-receptor antagonist with aspirin, but this difference was not statistically significant.

Among patients requiring chronic aspirin therapy who suffer an acute ulcer bleed, it had been unclear when to safely resume aspirin. Restarting aspirin before the ulcer has adequately healed potentially increases recurrent bleeding, but delayed administration of aspirin may also lead to greater cardiovascular or ischemic events in high-risk patients. This issue has been addressed in a large study of aspirin patients with a bleeding ulcer who underwent endoscopic hemostasis followed by maintenance therapy with a PPI. These patients were then randomized to promptly resuming aspirin versus withholding aspirin for 8 weeks after endoscopy. Patients who continued taking aspirin had no significant increase in rebleeding but had significantly lower mortality at 30 days (1% vs 9%) and 8 weeks (1% vs 13%). The protective effects of aspirin appear to outweigh its potential for further short-term GI complications that mainly occurred within 5 days after the index bleed. Aspirin should thus be restarted as soon as the risk for cardiovascular events outweighs the risk for recurrent ulcer complications. Current recommendations include resuming aspirin 1–7 days after the bleeding stops and providing co-therapy with a PPI to reduce rebleeding.

The management of patients requiring other antiplatelet or antithrombotic therapy who develop peptic ulcers and GI bleeding should be tailored to individual patients based on the severity of bleeding and risk of thromboembolism. For example, patients receiving dual antiplatelet therapy for a drug-eluding stent should not stop both antiplatelet drugs because of a high rate of stent thrombosis. Patients receiving warfarin but develop severe ulcer bleeding exacerbated by coagulopathy may be managed using various approaches that include vitamin K, fresh frozen plasma, prothrombin complex concentrates, or recombinant factor VIIa, and each have different advantages and disadvantages for the individual patient. Warfarin should be resumed once adequate hemostasis has been achieved. The use of direct oral anticoagulants (DOACs) has been shown to be more effective than warfarin in reducing thromboembolism risk, however, DOACs cannot be reversed by vitamin K and some agents have a higher risk of major GI bleeding than warfarin. Decisions regarding management of acute GI bleeding from DOACs depends on the severity of bleeding, timing of the last dose, creatinine clearance and hepatic function. DOACs have a rapid onset of action and restarting these drugs should be delayed until adequate hemostasis has been achieved. For example, the Asian Pacific Association of Gastroenterology and the Asian Pacific Society for Digestive Endoscopy recommend resuming DOACs by day 3 once hemostasis is achieved, and without bridging therapy. The following guidelines are also from an international consensus group for the management of upper GI bleeding that are conditional recommendations based on low-quality evidence: 1) In patients with previous ulcer bleeding receiving cardiovascular prophylaxis with single- or dual-antiplatelet therapy, the use of PPI therapy is recommended over no therapy. 2) In patients with previous ulcer bleeding requiring continued cardiovascular prophylaxis with anticoagulant therapy (vitamin K antagonists, DOACs), the use of PPI therapy is recommended over no therapy. This international consensus group also commented on weighing the risks and benefits of PPI therapy. They acknowledged that meta-analyses of primarily observational studies have suggested possible associations between PPI therapy and adverse effects, including community-acquired pneumonia, hip fracture, colorectal cancer, chronic kidney disease, community-acquired enteric infection, and *Clostridium difficile* infection. However, their analysis of factors, such as consistency, specificity, temporality, and biological plausibility, as well as confounding factors, showed that the evidence for causality is very weak. The consensus group felt that for high-risk patients with an ongoing need for anticoagulants, the evidence suggests that the benefits of secondary prophylaxis outweigh the risks. They concluded that the unproven potential and rare safety concerns should not prevent treatment for patients at risk for life-threatening consequences.

Barkun AN, Almadi M, Kuipers EJ, et al. Management of nonvariceal upper gastrointestinal bleeding: guideline recommendations from the International Consensus Group. *Ann Intern Med.* 2019;171:805–822.

Chan FKL, Goh KL, Reddy N, et al. Management of patients on antithrombotic agents undergoing emergency and elective endoscopy: joint Asian Pacific Association of Gastroenterology (APAGE) and Asian Pacific Society for Digestive Endoscopy (APSDE) practice guidelines. *Gut.* 2018;67:405–417 [PMID: 29331946]

Chan FK, Kyaw M, Tanigawa T, et al. Similar efficacy of proton-pump inhibitors vs H2-receptor antagonists in reducing risk of upper gastrointestinal bleeding or ulcers in high-risk users of low-dose aspirin. *Gastroenterology.* 2017;152(1):105–110. [PMID: 27641510]

Lanas A, Chan FKL. Peptic ulcer disease. *Lancet.* 2017;390: 613–624. [PMID: 28242110]

Sengupta N, Marshall AL, Jones BA, et al. Rebleeding vs thromboembolism after hospitalization for gastrointestinal bleeding in patients on direct oral anticoagulants. *Clin Gastroenterol Hepatol.* 2018;16(12):1893–1900. [PMID: 29775794]

D. Eradication Therapy for *Helicobacter pylori* Infection

Patients with active duodenal or gastric ulcers and those with a prior ulcer history should be tested and treated for *H pylori*. The number of patients who would need to be treated for *H pylori* infection to prevent a recurrent duodenal ulcer is two and for recurrent gastric ulcer is three. After successful cure, reinfection with *H pylori* is considered rare. In the United States, the estimated incidence is approximately 1 reinfection per 100 patients per year. Patients with early stage MALT lymphoma (type I or II) should also be tested and treated for *H pylori* since eradication of this infection can induce remission in many patients when the tumor is limited to the stomach. However, the treatment of more advanced stages of MALToma may also involve chemotherapy, radiation, and surgery. There are several GI consensus groups, including the Maastricht V Consensus Report that recommend testing and treating several other groups of patients for *H pylori*, but there is limited evidence of benefit. This includes patients diagnosed with gastric adenocarcinoma, especially those with early-stage disease undergoing resection. In a randomized clinical trial among patients with early gastric cancer or high grade adenoma who underwent endoscopic resection, those who received *H pylori* treatment had a lower incidence of metachronous gastric cancer and improvement from baseline in the grade of gastric glandular atrophy at the corpus than did patients who received placebo. Other groups who should be considered for *H pylori* testing and treating include patients found to have atrophic gastritis or intestinal metaplasia, and first-degree relatives of patients with gastric adenocarcinoma since the relatives themselves are at increased risk of gastric cancer partly due to the intra familial transmission of *H pylori*. Although the mechanisms are unknown, a few studies suggest that *H pylori* may play a role in autoimmune disorders such as idiopathic thrombocytopenic purpura. Eradication of *H pylori* has been shown to increase the platelet count in these patients. It is also recommended to consider testing and treating for *H pylori* among patients with vitamin B12 deficiency and otherwise unexplained iron deficiency anemia. Successful *H. pylori* eradication among patients with unexplained iron deficiency anemia may reverse the anemia and improve iron absorption. Some studies also suggest that screening and treating for *H pylori* among patients who are starting or taking long-term NSAID therapy or those taking long-term aspirin may reduce the risk of peptic ulcer disease or ulcer bleeding. To date, it remains controversial whether to test and treat all patients with functional dyspepsia, gastroesophageal reflux disease, or other non-GI disorders as well as asymptomatic individuals.

The success of *H pylori* eradication depends on bacterial factors as well as the type and duration of therapy, and patient compliance. Patients most often fail to respond to initial *H pylori* therapy because of antibiotic resistance and/or noncompliance with taking the prescribed regimen. The appropriate treatment regimen for eradication of *H. pylori* should be tailored according to local prevalence of antibiotic resistance if available. Antibiotic resistance to *H pylori* is categorized as primary if there has not been any previous eradication therapy, or as secondary if resistance was acquired as a result of ineffective eradication attempts. A careful patient history including any penicillin allergies and inquiry about prior use of specific antibiotics such as macrolide antibiotics (eg, clarithromycin, azithromycin, and erythromycin) should be obtained to assess for possible resistance. Prior to initiating eradication therapy, patients should also be given careful instructions not to arbitrarily miss any doses.

There are multiple treatment regimens for *H pylori* eradication and most include a PPI combined with 2 or more antibiotics for 7–14 days (Table 16–3). Some commonly prescribed antibiotics include amoxicillin, clarithromycin, metronidazole, tetracycline, and levofloxacin; studies often report cure rates ranging from 70% to 90% with these agents. Meta-analyses suggest that a 14-day treatment regimen has higher eradication rates and is more cost effective compared with 7-day therapy. Due to regional antibiotic resistance differences, a 14-day regimen is more effective in the United States and is recommended by the U.S. Food and Drug Administration. Triple therapy was previously a commonly prescribed regimen that uses a PPI (given twice daily) along with clarithromycin (500 mg twice daily) and amoxicillin (1 g twice daily) or metronidazole (500 mg twice daily, for penicillin-allergic patients). Unfortunately, *H pylori* is becoming increasingly resistant to clarithromycin, metronidazole, and levofloxacin in many areas of the world. A clarithromycin-based regimen should not be used in areas where the resistance rate is known to be greater than 15%. In contrast to metronidazole, *H pylori* resistance to clarithromycin cannot be easily overcome by increasing the dose of the drug. Clarithromycin-resistance has been reported to be as high as 30% in Southern Europe and even 50% in China.

The clarithromycin resistance rates in many different geographic regions in the United States are not known and thus many authorities have advocated for surveillance registries for *H pylori* resistance and local therapy success rates.

The best strategy is to achieve successful cure of *H pylori* on the first attempt to minimize costs and to avoid retreating, retesting, and potential adverse effects on other gut microbiota. The use of antibiotic susceptibility data would help limit inappropriate antibiotic use, prevent widespread resistance in other organisms and reduce costs, but these data are typically not available in the US or many other parts of the world. Several experts and consensus groups have reviewed the best available evidence and published treatment guidelines including the American College of Gastroenterology (ACG), the European Helicobacter and Microbiota Study Group (Maastricht V/Florence report), and the Canadian Association of Gastroenterology/Canadian Helicobacter Study Group (Toronto Consensus). To maximize successful eradication on the first attempt, most experts agree that quadruple therapy should have a more prominent role and most treatments should be given for 14 days.

For first line therapy, bismuth quadruple therapy is recommended especially in areas with resistance to clarithromycin and metronidazole while concomitant therapy is useful for patients from areas of low resistance to clarithromycin where bismuth is not available. Bismuth quadruple therapy, for example, includes a PPI twice daily and four-times-daily dosing of antibiotics with tetracycline (500 mg) and metronidazole (250–500 mg), along with bismuth subsalicylate or subcitrate. Patients with a true penicillin allergy should use the bismuth quadruple therapy or the clarithromycin based triple therapy with metronidazole if there is no prior use of macrolides and the patient is from an area of low clarithromycin resistance.

If a patient fails an initial treatment for *H pylori* eradication, it is generally recommended to avoid re-using the antibiotics in that failed regimen, especially if it included clarithromycin and levofloxacin. However, it is reasonable to consider re-using metronidazole in a bismuth regimen due to a synergistic effect as well as re-using amoxicillin and tetracycline because resistance to these agents is rare. Depending on what agents were used, an acceptable second line therapy includes the bismuth quadruple therapy or levofloxacin triple therapy. After failure of a second attempt or subsequent attempts, it is then highly recommended to consider culture with susceptibility testing if possible. If this is not available, then again depending on the prior regimens, it is acceptable to consider bismuth quadruple therapy (if patients were on clarithromycin triple therapy and then levofloxacin-based therapy), as well as concomitant therapy. There are also recommendations for a high-dose dual therapy with amoxicillin (750 mg qid) and a PPI (20 mg qid) as well as regimens using rifabutin as salvage treatment for *H pylori*. Unfortunately, rifabutin has been associated with 2% incidence of myelotoxicity among patients being treated for *H pylori* which appears to be reversible and does not appear to increase

Table 16-3. Common treatment regimens for *Helicobacter pylori*.

Treatment Regimen	Duration	Comments
Quadruple bismuth therapy		
PPI twice daily Tetracycline, 500 mg four times daily Metronidazole, 250-500 mg four times daily or 500 mg three times daily Bismuth four times daily: -Bismuth subcitrate 120-300 mg or 420 mg -Bismuth subsalicylate 300 or 524 mg	14 days	Recommended for first line therapy as well as for second line or rescue therapy, especially in areas with high resistance to clarithromycin.
Concomitant therapy nonbismuth quadruple therapy		
PPI twice daily Amoxicillin 1000 mg twice daily Metronidazole 500 mg or Tinidazole 500 mg twice daily Clarithromycin 500 mg twice daily	14 days	First line therapy in areas with low primary resistance to clarithromycin. Also recommended for rescue therapy.
Triple therapy		
PPI twice daily Clarithromycin 500 mg twice daily, or Metronidazole, 500 mg twice daily Amoxicillin 1000 mg twice daily	14 days	Restricted use for first line therapy if the clarithromycin resistance rate is less than 15% in the community.
PPI twice daily Clarithromycin 500 mg twice daily Metronidazole 500 mg twice daily	14 days	Restricted use for first-line therapy in penicillin-allergic patients if the clarithromycin resistance rate is less than 15% in the community.
Levofloxacin-based triple therapy		
PPI twice daily Levofloxacin 250 mg twice daily or 500 mg once daily Amoxicillin 1000 mg twice daily for 10 days	10–14 days	Recommended for second-line or rescue therapy but ACG states may also consider for first line.
Sequential nonbismuth quadruple		
PPI twice daily Amoxicillin 1000 mg twice daily for the first half only Metronidazole 500 mg + Clarithromycin 500 mg twice daily for the second half of therapy only	10–14 days	ACG states may consider for first line therapy. The efficacy of clarithromycin sequential therapy may be suboptimal in areas with a high rate of triple therapy failure.
Hybrid nonbismuth quadruple therapy		
PPI twice daily Amoxicillin 1000 mg twice daily Metronidazole 500 mg + Clarithromycin 500 mg twice daily for the second half of therapy only	14 days	Hybrid therapy is not widely endorsed for first line therapy.
High-dose dual therapy		
Rabeprazole 20 mg four times daily Amoxicillin 75 mg four times daily	14 days	Recommended option for second-line or rescue therapy.
Rifabutin therapy		
PPI twice daily Amoxicillin, 1000 mg twice daily Rifabutin 150 mg twice daily or 300 mg daily	10 days	Recommended option for third or fourth-line rescue therapy if susceptibility testing is not available.

ACG, American College of Gastroenterology; PPI, proton pump inhibitor. The dose of PPI will depend on brand used.
In many regimens, metronidazole can be substituted by tinidazole.
The eradication rate is significantly affected by the regional variation in *H. pylori* resistance patterns.

susceptibility to infections. However, because of this risk, the ACG recommends prescribing the rifabutin regimen for 10 days. Otherwise, most authorities recommend 14 days for all salvage therapies. To date, the evidence for any benefit in using adjunct probiotics to improve eradication rates or reduce treatment-associated side effects remains low but is still being studied.

Chey WD, Leontiadis GI, Howden CW, Moss SF. ACG Clinical Guideline: treatment of *Helicobacter pylori* infection. *Am J Gastroenterol*. 2017;112(2):212–239. [PMID: 28071659]

Choi IJ, Kook MC, Kim YI, et al. *Helicobacter pylori* therapy for the prevention of metachronous gastric cancer. *N Engl J Med*. 2018;378(12):1085–1095. [PMID: 29562147]Malfertheiner P, Megraud F, O'Morain CA, et al. Management of *Helicobacter pylori* infection-the Maastricht V/Florence Consensus Report. *Gut*. 2017;66(1):6–30. [PMID: 27707777]

Fallone CA, Chiba N, van Zanten SV, et al. The Toronto consensus for the treatment of *Helicobacter pylori* infection in adults. *Gastroenterology*. 2016;151(1):51–69. [PMID: 27102658]

Fallone CA, Moss SF, Malfertheiner P. Reconciliation of recent *Helicobacter pylori* treatment guidelines in a time of increasing resistance to antibiotics. *Gastroenterology*. 2019;157(1):44–53. [PMID: 30998990]

E. *Helicobacter pylori* & Gastric Adenocarcinoma

Up to 5% of gastric ulcers represent underlying neoplasia in some countries. Although the incidence of gastric cancer has steadily declined over the past few decades, it remains a major cause of cancer death worldwide. There is wide regional variation in the incidence of gastric cancer. High incidence rates have been reported in Japan, Eastern Asia, Eastern Europe, and parts of Latin America, while low incidence rates have been reported in the United States and Western Europe. Gastric carcinogenesis, especially for intestinal type gastric cancer is a multistep process, starting from chronic gastritis and progressing over many years to atrophy, intestinal metaplasia, dysplasia, and eventually adenocarcinoma. In animal studies, long-term infection with *H pylori* in Mongolian gerbils has been shown to induce gastric adenocarcinoma. Three meta-analyses of case-control and cohort studies report summary odds ratios for *H pylori* and gastric adenocarcinoma of 1.92 (95% confidence interval [CI], 1.32–2.78), 2.5 (95% CI, 1.90–3.40), and 2.04 (95% CI, 1.69–2.45). It is believed that the chronic gastric inflammation from *H pylori* infection can promote gastric carcinogenesis and progress to the precancerous changes of atrophic gastritis and intestinal metaplasia. The risk of gastric cancer increases in relation to the severity and extent of those precancerous changes. Chronic *H pylori* infection also contributes to gastric mucosal genetic instability by reducing gastric acid secretion, which can promote the growth of gastric microbiome that processes dietary components into carcinogens. Studies show that eradicating *H pylori* can resolve the gastric inflammation. This can potentially stop further gastric mucosal damage, prevent

further *H pylori* induced DNA damage, improve gastric acid secretion, and restore the microbiome toward normal.

Early data supporting a direct association of *H pylori* and gastric cancer in humans comes from a long-term cohort study from Japan by Uemura and colleagues. In this study, 1526 patients with various GI disorders, including duodenal ulcers, gastric ulcers, gastric hyperplasia, and nonulcer dyspepsia, underwent endoscopy with biopsy at enrollment and then 1–3 years after enrollment. There were 1246 *H pylori*-infected and 280 uninfected patients followed for a mean duration of 7.8 years. Among the *H pylori* patients, 253 received eradication therapy at an early stage of follow-up. Gastric cancer developed in approximately 3% of the infected patients but in none of the uninfected patients. In addition, none of the *H pylori* patients who received eradication therapy developed gastric cancer. *H pylori* patients with severe gastric atrophy, corpus-predominant gastritis, and intestinal metaplasia were at significantly higher risk for gastric cancer. The risk was also increased in almost all subgroups of *H pylori*-infected patients (those with gastric ulcers, gastric hyperplastic polyps, or nonulcer dyspepsia) but not in those with duodenal ulcers. It is noteworthy that infected patients who received eradication therapy did not develop gastric cancer. These results support the notion that eradication of *H pylori* may potentially prevent or delay the development of cancer.

In a systematic review and meta-analysis of 24 studies, eradication of *H pylori* infection reduced the incidence of gastric cancer. After adjustment for baseline gastric cancer incidence, individuals with eradication of *H pylori* infection had a lower incidence of gastric cancer than those who did not receive eradication therapy (pooled incidence rate ratio = 0.53; 95% CI: 0.44–0.64). Eradication provided significant benefit for asymptomatic infected individuals (pooled incidence rate ratio, 0.62; 95% CI: 0.49–0.79) and individuals after endoscopic resection of gastric cancers (pooled incidence rate ratio, 0.46; 95% CI: 0.35–0.60).

It is known that the risk of gastric cancer is greater in patients with low gastric acidity such as those with severe atrophic gastritis with intestinal metaplasia and pernicious anemia. Patients who have had a partial gastrectomy are also at risk for gastric cancer after a long latency period, but their risk appears greater after an additional acid-reducing procedure such as vagotomy. Low acid secretion has been hypothesized to predispose to gastric cancer by affecting vitamin C absorption and overgrowth of salivary and intestinal bacteria in the stomach, which potentially promote the formation of carcinogenic nitrosamines. Chronic inflammation with alterations to DNA or changes in expression of cytokines and chemokines may also affect early progression. Host genetics also play a key role, and studies have shown how human genetic polymorphisms profoundly affect gastric carcinogenesis. For example, interleukin-1β is an important proinflammatory cytokine and a powerful inhibitor of acid secretion. Levels of interleukin-1β within the gastric mucosa are increased by *H pylori* infection. Genetic polymorphisms that promote high expression of interleukin-1β help explain why some *H pylori*–infected patients develop gastric cancer while others do not.

Cover TL, Blaser MJ. *Helicobacter pylori* in health and disease. *Gastroenterology.* 2009;136:1863–1873. [PMID: 19457415]

Lee YC, Chiang TH, Chou CK, et al. Association between *Helicobacter pylori* eradication and gastric cancer incidence: a systematic review and meta-analysis. *Gastroenterology.* 2016;150(5):1113–1124. [PMID: 26836587]

Sheila EC. *Helicobacter pylori* infection. *N Engl J Med.* 2019;380(12):1158–1165. [PMID: 30893536]

Uemura N, Okamoto S, Yamamoto S, et al. *Helicobacter pylori* infection and the development of gastric cancer. *N Engl J Med.* 2001;345(11):784–9.

F. *Helicobacter pylori* & Gastric MALT Lymphoma

Gastric MALT lymphoma is a clonal B-cell neoplasm arising from postgerminal center B-cells in the marginal zone of lymphoid follicles. There is strong evidence supporting a causative role of *H pylori* infection in the development of gastric low-grade B-cell lymphoma from MALT. Epidemiologic studies have shown that significantly more patients with gastric MALT lymphomas than matched controls have had *H pylori* infection. In addition, *H pylori* gastritis has been associated with the induction of gastric lymphoid follicles. It is thought that the *H pylori*–generated immune responses leads to lymphoid hyperplasia, which along with genetic aberrations activates intracellular survival pathways.

The disease can then progress due to proliferation and resistance to apoptosis, and the emergence of a malignant clone. A proliferation-inducing ligand (APRIL) produced by macrophages in the *H pylori*–infected gastric mucosa also plays an important role in promoting the survival and proliferation of neoplastic B cells. Several investigators have even been able to detect the lymphoma B-cell clone in the chronic *H pylori* gastritis that preceded the lymphoma. Nevertheless, the strongest evidence of a causal association is that *H pylori* eradication can induce remission in these patients. Several studies suggested that eradication of *H pylori* leads to a complete remission of the lymphoma in 60–90% of cases and a pooled data analysis of 34 studies showed that successful cure of *H pylori* infection was associated with remission of gastric MALT lymphoma in 78% of patients. Many of these patients remain in remission for years.

Filip PV, Cuciureanu D, Laura Sorina Diaconu LS, et al. MALT lymphoma: epidemiology, clinical diagnosis and treatment. *J Med Life.* 2018;11(3):187–193. [PMID: 30364585]

Nakamura S, Matsumoto T. Treatment strategy for gastric mucosa-associated lymphoid tissue lymphoma. *Gastroenterol Clin North Am.* 2015;44(3):649–660. [PMID: 26314674]

Munari F, Lonardi S, Cassatella MA, et al. Tumor-associated macrophages as major source of APRIL in gastric MALT lymphoma. *Blood.* 2011;117:6612–6616. [PMID: 21527528]

Zullo A, Hassan C, Ridola L, et al. Gastric MALT lymphoma: old and new insights. *Ann Gastroenterol.* 2014;27:27–33. [PMID: 24714739]

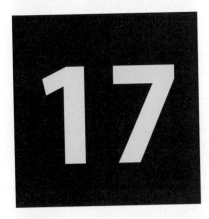

Zollinger-Ellison Syndrome (Gastrinoma)

Edward Lew, MD, MPH

ESSENTIALS OF DIAGNOSIS

▶ Peptic ulcer disease, abdominal pain, and diarrhea are common presentations.

▶ Patients have marked gastric acid secretion arising from a gastrin-secreting non–β islet cell tumor.

▶ Multiple endocrine neoplasia syndrome type 1 (MEN 1) is present in approximately 20–25% of patients.

▶ Serum gastrin concentration >1000 pg/mL in combination with acidic stomach pH <2.0 is diagnostic.

▶ Up to 40% of patients have elevated serum gastrin levels that are <500 pg/mL and warrant a secretin test.

▶ Significant hypergastrinemia can occur with proton pump inhibitor (PPI) use, *Helicobacter pylori* infection, or chronic atrophic gastritis and hypochlorhydria.

General Considerations

Zollinger-Ellison syndrome (ZES) is characterized by peptic ulcers, diarrhea, and marked gastric acid hypersecretion in association with a gastrin-secreting non–β islet cell neuroendocrine tumor (NETs) (gastrinoma). Although the true incidence of gastrinoma is unknown, estimates range from 0.1 to 3 persons per million of the population per year. ZES is a rare cause of peptic ulcer disease and accounts for about 0.1–1% of ulcers. The mean age of onset of symptoms is 41 years, and slightly more males than females are affected, with a ratio of about 3:2. The diagnosis of ZES from onset of symptom is typically delayed by at least 4–7 years. Although the majority of gastrinomas develop as a sporadic tumor, approximately 20–25% of ZES patients have this tumor as part of the inherited MEN 1. MEN 1 is an autosomal-dominant inherited syndrome characterized by pancreatic NETs, pituitary tumors, and hyperparathyroidism, and is caused by mutations of the MEN 1 tumor suppressor gene on chromosome 11q13. Treatment of ZES involves control of the profound gastric acid

hypersecretion as well as control of the gastrinoma which is malignant in 60–90% of cases. Most patients with ZES as part of the MEN 1 syndrome will only require medical therapy. In contrast, patients with sporadic ZES without metastatic spread should not only receive medical therapy but also undergo exploratory laparotomy and resection with curative intent.

Pathogenesis

Patients with ZES most often present with symptoms arising from excessive gastric acid secretion. The unregulated gastrin production from the gastrinoma binds to CCK-2 receptors located on enterochromaffin-like (ECL) cells causing the release of histamine. Histamine then binds to H_2 receptors on parietal cells to stimulate the release of acid. In addition, gastrin also has trophic effects on gastric epithelial and ECL cells. Chronic hypergastrinemia increases parietal cell mass, which further augments acid hypersecretion, causing stomach and duodenal ulceration and deactivates pancreatic enzymes, resulting in fat malabsorption and diarrhea.

Classification

Gastrinomas are derived from the enteroendocrine cells that arise from the embryologic endoderm and primarily form tumors in the duodenum and pancreas, but can also form tumors in the jejunum, lymph nodes, mesentery, hepatobiliary tract, and ovary. Histologically, the enteroendocrine cells that make up the gastrinoma are well differentiated and round, with small nuclei and prominent nucleolus. The cells produce abundant neurosecretory granules and have immunohistochemical expression of neuroendocrine markers such as synaptophysin and chromogranin. Although gastrin is typically the predominant peptide within the secretory granules of gastrinoma cells, other neuroendocrine peptides such as vasoactive intestinal peptide and glucagon can also be present.

Gastrinomas are neuroendocrine neoplasms (NENs) which are further classified by the World Health Organization based on morphology (histological differentiation) and proliferation (grade). The main groups of NENs include well differentiated NET, poorly differentiated, neuroendocrine carcinoma (NEC), and mixed neuroendocrine/non-neuroendocrine neoplasm (MiNEN). NETs are distinguished from NECs using morphology and specific cellular and architectural criteria. NETs are then graded based on the proliferation index (mitotic count and Ki67-related proliferation index).

Functional tumors overproduce hormones that cause distinct clinical syndromes. In contrast, tumors that either do not secrete hormones, secrete them in minimal amounts, or secrete peptides that do not result in any obvious syndrome are termed nonfunctional tumors. NENs that produce multiple hormones are referred by the name of the hormone whose effects dominate the clinical picture such as gastrinoma or insulinoma. Accurate classification not only provides prognostic implications but also affects treatment. Most gastrinomas are well-differentiated NETs grade 1. The incidence of NETs has reportedly been steadily rising. Survival for all NETs has also improved over time, especially for distant-stage gastrointestinal NETs and pancreatic NETs which may be related to improvement in therapies.

Dasari A, Shen C, Halperin D, et al. Trends in the incidence, prevalence, and survival outcomes in patients with neuroendocrine tumors in the United States. *JAMA Oncol.* 2017;3(10):1335–1342. [PMID: 28448665]

Niederle B, Selberherr A, Bartsch D, et al. Multiple Endocrine Neoplasia Type 1 (MEN1) and the pancreas - diagnosis and treatment of functioning and non-functioning pancreatic and duodenal neuroendocrine neoplasia within the MEN1 syndrome - An International Consensus Statement. *Neuroendocrinology.* 2021;111(7):609-630. [PMID: 32971521]

Pobłocki J, Jasińska A, Syrenicz A, et al. The neuroendocrine neoplasms of the digestive tract: diagnosis, treatment and nutrition. *Nutrients.* 2020;12(5):1437–1458. [PMID: 32429294]

▶ Clinical Findings

A. Symptoms & Signs

Abdominal pain and diarrhea are the most common symptoms experienced by ZES patients. Gastroesophageal reflux, nausea, weight loss, and bleeding are other typical symptoms. The widespread use of acid-suppressive medications such as PPIs may mask symptoms and delay diagnosis. Table 17–1 shows the frequency of these presenting symptoms in ZES patients. Diarrhea arises from the hypersecretion of acid which exceeds the neutralizing capacity of pancreatic bicarbonate secretion and damages enterocytes, inactivates pancreatic digestive enzymes (leading to malabsorption and steatorrhea), and causes primary bile acids to become insoluble. Over 70% of ZES patients suffer from diarrhea which may be the only presenting symptom in 3–10% of cases.

Table 17–1. Clinical symptoms of patients with Zollinger-Ellison syndrome.

Clinical Findings	Percentage Among 261 Patients at NIH	Range of Percentages of Patients in Literature
Abdominal pain	75	26–98
Diarrhea	73	17–73
Gastroesophageal reflux symptoms	44	0–56
Nausea	30	0–37
Vomiting	25	0–51
Bleeding	24	8–75
MEN 1 present	22	10–48
History of peptic ulcer	71	71–93
History of esophageal stricture	4	41–53
History of abdominal perforation	5	4–6
Mean age of onset (years)	41	41–53
MEN1 present	22	10–48

MEN, multiple endocrine neoplasia; NIH, National Institutes of Health. Data from Feingold KR, Anawalt B, Boyce A, et al., Endotext [Internet]. South Dartmouth (MA): MDText.com, Inc; 2000.

Nasogastric suctioning can alleviate the diarrhea. In advanced cases, patients experience symptoms directly from the growth of the gastrinoma. Patients with ZES and MEN 1 syndrome may also present with primary hyperparathyroidism as well as anterior pituitary tumors, and up to 37% develop gastric carcinoids.

The majority of ZES patients develop peptic ulcers, which can appear similar to ulcers associated with *H pylori* and nonsteroidal anti-inflammatory drug (NSAID) use. ZES patients often also have prominent gastric folds that can be seen on upper endoscopy. Only a small fraction present with a perforated ulcer or esophageal stricture. ZES should be suspected in patients who have had peptic ulcers in unusual locations (eg, second part of the duodenum and jejunum), patients with severe ulcers refractory to acid-suppressive medications, ulcer patients with hypercalcemia, and those with a personal history or family history of MEN 1 syndrome. Clinicians should also consider ZES among patients who present with the triad of abdominal pain, diarrhea, and weight loss as well as patients with prominent gastric folds on endoscopy. ZES may also be considered as a rare cause of ulcers in patients without *H pylori* infection who have not taken any aspirin or NSAIDs.

Beek DJV, Nell S, Pieterman CRC, et al. Prognostic factors and survival in MEN1 patients with gastrinomas: results from the Dutch-MEN study group (DMSG). *J Surg Oncol.* 2019;120(6):966–975. [PMID: 31401809]

Jensen RT, Ito T. Gastrinoma. 2020. In: Feingold KR, Anawalt B, Boyce A, Chrousos G, et al. editors. Endotext. South Dartmouth (MA): MDText.com, Inc. [PMID: 25905301]

B. Laboratory Findings

The diagnosis of ZES is based on finding an elevated fasting serum gastrin level associated with gastric acid hypersecretion. Unfortunately, the diagnosis is often missed or delayed because the manifestations of patients with ZES as compared to patients with peptic ulcers due to other causes closely resemble each other. Figure 17–1 is an algorithm outlining an approach to the evaluation of ZES. Patients suspected of having ZES should have a measurement of a fasting serum gastrin level, ideally while they are off all acid-suppressive medications. A known reliable and accurate gastrin assay should be used, and all PPIs should be stopped at least 1 week before testing. Patients who develop significant gastrointestinal symptoms after temporarily stopping their PPIs may require high-dose histamine-2 (H_2)-receptor blockers and frequent antacids. The H_2-receptor blockers should be stopped at least 2 days before testing while the patient continues to frequently take high doses of antacids.

A serum gastrin concentration above 1000 pg/mL in a patient with an acidic stomach pH below 2.0 is considered diagnostic of ZES (in patients who do not have a retained gastric antrum), and no other diagnostic studies are necessary. Unfortunately, this occurs in only 5–9% of ZES patients. Patients with more moderate degrees of hypergastrinemia may require more detailed investigations. Up to 40% of ZES patients have elevated serum gastrin levels of <500 pg/mL. This range of hypergastrinemia can overlap with non-ZES patients having low acid secretion. Many of these patients without ZES develop a secondary or appropriate hypergastrinemia in response to high gastric pH and decreased acid feedback inhibition of gastrin release. Patients taking PPIs as well as those with *H pylori* infection or chronic atrophic gastritis/pernicious anemia and hypochlorhydria can develop significant hypergastrinemia. The widespread use of PPIs has increased the difficulty in diagnosing ZES. In some patients with ZES, PPIs may adequately control the acid secretion and symptoms, while in other patients without ZES, PPIs may also lead to more false positive diagnoses due to the secondary hypergastrinemia. Other causes of hypergastrinemia that are not associated with excessive acid secretion include renal failure or uremia, short gut syndrome, or status post vagotomy. Disorders causing hypergastrinemia with excessive acid secretion include G-cell hyperplasia or hyperfunction, retained gastric antrum (eg, intact antrum after Billroth type II partial gastrectomy), and gastric outlet obstruction. Conversely, there have also been rare reports of gastrinoma patients having a falsely low gastrin level. This occurs because the tumor secretes bioactive gastrin precursors while the commercially available assay only detects one subtype. If the gastrin level is low or nondiagnostic but the suspicion for a tumor is high, additional testing is recommended to diagnose and localize the lesion.

The level of fasting serum gastrin elevation alone cannot differentiate appropriate from inappropriate hypergastrinemia. Determining gastric pH and/or acid output (mEq/hr) while off antisecretory drugs will help distinguish ZES and other inappropriate causes of hypergastrinemia from physiological causes of hypergastrinemia. ZES patients will have a basal gastric pH ≤2. In order to distinguish ZES from the other causes of inappropriate hypergastrinemia such as *H. pylori* infection, additional studies such as determining basal acid output, a secretin provocative test, or advanced imaging studies for the presence of a NET should be considered. Patients suspected of having ZES should also undergo screening for MEN1 by ordering serum calcium, parathyroid hormone level, prolactin, and pancreatic polypeptide.

Scott AT, Howe JR. Evaluation and management of neuroendocrine tumors of the pancreas. *Surg Clin North Am.* 2019;99(4):793–814. [PMID: 31255207]

Stawarski A, Maleika P. Neuroendocrine tumors of the gastrointestinal tract and pancreas: is it also a challenge for pediatricians? *Adv Clin Exp Med.* 2020;29(2):265–270. [PMID: 32091671]

C. Special Tests

The secretin stimulation test can establish the diagnosis of ZES and is the provocative test of choice because of its high sensitivity, ease of administration, and minimal side effects. Some studies suggest that secretin can stimulate gastrin release by directly interacting with receptors on gastrinoma cells. Intravenous administration of secretin stimulates an exaggerated serum gastrin increase in ZES patients, while the serum gastrin level falls or remains unchanged in other disorders. In previous years, secretin had been difficult to obtain but there is now a fully biologically active synthetic human secretin which can be used to diagnose ZES.

During secretin stimulation testing, a baseline serum gastrin is measured and then 2 μg/kg of secretin is administered intravenously over 1 minute. Repeated measurements of serum gastrin are subsequently made 2, 5, 10, 15, and 20 minutes later. An increase of greater than 100 pg/mL in serum gastrin levels is considered positive, whereas a rise of 200 pmg/mL above baseline is virtually diagnostic for detecting gastrinomas. Alternatively, Jensen and colleagues examined this criterion for the diagnosis of ZES as part of a large study involving 293 ZES patients from the National Institutes of Health who were compared with 537 patients in the literature. They recommend using an absolute increase in gastrin of >120 pg/mL which had a sensitivity of 94% and a specificity of 100%. The provocative secretin test is also the most sensitive indicator of recurrent or persistent disease in patients who have undergone attempted surgical resection.

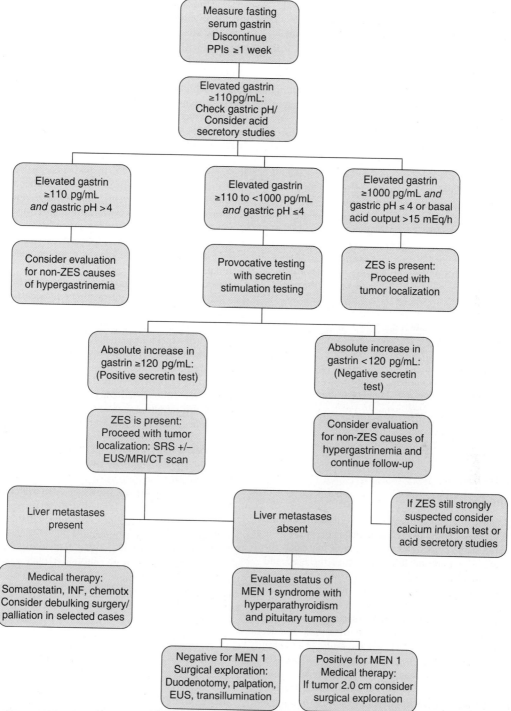

▲ **Figure 17–1.** Algorithm for evaluation of suspected Zollinger-Ellison syndrome (ZES). chemotx, chemotherapy; CT, computed tomography; EUS, endoscopic ultrasound; INF, alfa-interferon; MEN 1, multiple endocrine neoplasia syndrome type 1; MRI, magnetic resonance imaging; PPIs, proton pump inhibitors; somatostatin, somatostatin analog therapy; SRS, somatostatin receptor scintigraphy.

In such cases, another positive test necessitates further evaluation for the persistence of another lesion.

The calcium infusion study has less diagnostic accuracy (with a sensitivity of 62%) and is difficult to perform. It is also associated with adverse side effects but may be positive in the rare gastrinoma patient with a negative or equivocal secretion stimulation result. During meal provocative testing, the gastrin response unfortunately overlaps with those seen in patients with antral syndromes and is thus generally not useful. Gastric acid secretion studies have previously aided in the diagnosis of ZES through a determination of the basal acid output (BAO) and pentagastrin-stimulated acid output (MAO) but are not widely available. Hypergastrinemia with a BAO >15 mEq/h or >5 mEq/h in patients with a prior vagotomy and partial gastrectomy is suggestive of ZES. These acid output studies are mainly reserved to monitor response and determine an adequate dose of acid-suppressive medications with the goal of reducing gastric acid secretion to below 10 mEq/hr. Some reports suggest that serum levels of chromogranin A may also be helpful, because this value is frequently elevated in patients with NETs including those with gastrinomas.

Berna MJ, Hoffman KM, Long SH, et al. Serum gastrin in Zollinger-Ellison syndrome: II. Prospective study of gastrin provocative testing in 293 patients from the National Institutes of Health and comparison with 537 cases from the literature. Evaluation of diagnostic criteria, proposal of new criteria, and correlations with clinical and tumoral features. *Medicine (Baltimore)*. 2006;85(6):331–364. [PMID: 17108779]

Metz DC, Cadiot G, Poitras P, et al. Diagnosis of Zollinger-Ellison syndrome in the era of PPIs, faulty gastrin assays, sensitive imaging and limited access to acid secretory testing. *Int J Endocr Oncol*. 2017;4(4):167–185. [PMID: 29326808]

D. Imaging Studies

It is estimated that approximately 80% of gastrinomas are localized in a gastrinoma triangle area that is defined by the convergence of the cystic duct and common bile duct, the junction of the second and third portion of the head and body of the duodenum, and the junction of the head and body of the pancreas. In contrast to past reports, most gastrinomas are localized in the duodenum (70–90%) or in the pancreas (2–30%). Among these duodenal gastrinomas, over 80% are located in the first and second portion of the duodenum, which tend to be small (<1 cm) and multiple and have a relatively low rate of liver metastasis at diagnosis (in 0–10% of cases). In contrast, pancreatic gastrinomas are larger and tend to metastasize to the liver in 22 to 35% of cases. The gastrinomas associated with MEN 1 syndrome are also multiple and localized in the duodenum. A common site for metastases is the liver followed by bone, such as the spine or sacrum. Other rare extra-pancreatic sites include the gastric antrum-pyloric area, ovaries, mesentery, hepatobiliary tract, heart, and lymph nodes. In general, most patients undergo multiple imaging modalities and other investigations to try to localize the tumor and evaluate for metastases. This includes cross-sectional imaging with CT scanning, magnetic-resonance imaging (MRI), and transabdominal ultrasound. The sensitivities and specificities vary and are affected by the size of the gastrinoma. For example, some studies suggest that cross-sectional imaging only detects about 30–50% of primary gastrinomas that are <1 cm in size and detects 70–80% of hepatic metastases in affected patients. Endoscopic ultrasound (EUS) is useful for localizing pancreatic gastrinomas (with a sensitivity of about 67%), especially for tumors in the head and body of the pancreas. Other methods used include the assessment of serum gastrin gradients either determined in the portal venous drainage through transhepatic venous sampling or in hepatic veins after selective, intra-arterial secretin injections but these evaluations are costly, time consuming, and highly operator dependent. While these invasive techniques are also very accurate, they are performed less often because of the development of novel imaging techniques.

The fact that gastrinomas express somatostatin receptors has led to the development of tumor localization through somatostatin receptor scintigraphy (SRS). Conventional SRS initially used 111-Indium-labeled somatostatin analogues, such as 111-In pentetreotide with SPECT imaging. One study reported a sensitivity of 71% and specificity of 86%, and a positive predictive value of 85% which are higher than the other noninvasive modalities. SRS has now evolved using newer radiolabeled tracers with a higher affinity to somatostatin receptors such as 68-Gallium DOTA (9,4,7,10-tetraazacyclododecane-1,4,7,10-tetracetic acid). Integrated positron-emission tomography detection (PET)/CT using 68-Ga-DOTATOC or 68-Ga-DOTATATE has much greater sensitivity and is preferred over conventional SRS using 111-In pentetreotide.

In order to localize the gastrinoma and evaluate for liver metastases, most patients initially undergo an upper endoscopy and a combination of cross-sectional imaging with a CT scan or MRI and integrated PET/CT using 68-Ga-DOTATOC/or 68-Ga-DOTATATE. If these studies are unrevealing and surgery is being considered, then some patients undergo EUS with possible fine needle aspiration, and even angiography or selective arterial stimulation and venous sampling with secretin injection.

Jensen RT, Ito T. Gastrinoma. 2020. In: Feingold KR, Anawalt B, Boyce A, Chrousos G, et al., editors. Endotext. South Dartmouth (MA): MDText.com, Inc. [PMID: 25905301]

Lee L, Ito T, Jensen RT. Imaging of pancreatic neuroendocrine tumors: recent advances, current status, and controversies. *Expert Rev Anticancer Ther*. 2018;18(9):837–860. [PMID: 29973077]

Norton JA, Foster DS, Blumgart LH, et al. Incidence and prognosis of primary gastrinomas in the hepatobiliary tract. *JAMA Surg*. 2018;153(3):e175083. [PMID: 29365025]

E. Special Examinations

The more invasive localization methods such as portal venous sampling and selective intra-arterial injection of secretin combined with venous sampling have high sensitivity but only provide for a regionalization and not an exact localization of the tumor. Among select patients who do undergo surgical exploration, it is recommended to perform intraoperative ultrasound, transillumination of the duodenum, and a duodenotomy to localize small duodenal tumors. The use of intraoperative ultrasonography and endoscopic transillumination of the duodenal wall increases detection of small duodenal tumors not seen on other imaging studies. However, even after extensive imaging and detail surgical exploration, up to 10–30% of patients will not have any primary tumor found in the duodenum or pancreas.

▶ Treatment

The principal goals of treating ZES patients are to medically control gastric acid hypersecretion (which reduces symptoms and complications) and control of the tumor itself, ideally through attempted surgical cure in selected patients (which is only successful in less than 30% of patients). Prior to the 1970's, the only effective control of acid hypersecretion had been total gastrectomy. The acid hypersecretion can now be effectively treated acutely and long term using high doses of oral PPIs such as omeprazole, 40 mg twice daily, or pantoprazole, 80 mg twice daily. Some patients require an increased titration of these doses, whereas other patients may undergo a gradual dose reduction after successful control of their acid secretion and symptoms. Due to these powerful acid-suppressive medications, the survival of patients with gastrinomas now mainly depends on tumor growth and the extent of disease involvement. Patients with potentially resectable localized sporadic gastrinoma (ie, without MEN 1 syndrome) should undergo surgical exploration as the cure rate by experienced surgeons is as high as 50%. The tumor is most commonly found in the duodenum. In patients with liver metastases, surgery may be considered if all identifiable tumors can be safely removed. A multidisciplinary approach including surgical and nonsurgical therapies should be taken in patients with advanced disease.

Surgical exploration with possible curative resection is recommended for all sporadic ZES patients. This not only includes patients free of liver and distant metastases, but also those with localized resectable tumors, or patients with no identified tumor on imaging studies. Intraoperative methods, such as duodenotomy, palpation, transillumination of the duodenal wall, ultrasonography, or a combination of these techniques, greatly help to localize the gastrinoma. The goal of surgery in sporadic ZES is to cure the disease. Experienced surgeons have recommended an exploratory laparotomy with extended Kocher maneuver and careful palpation of the pancreas and duodenum for nodules. Reports suggest that duodenotomy is very effective in identifying duodenal gastrinomas, which account for 60% of gastrinomas. If possible, appropriate patients should undergo enucleation of pancreatic head tumors, or distal pancreatectomy for tail lesions, and duodenotomy and regional lymphadenopathy. Lymphadenectomy of more than 10 lymph nodes results in a higher biochemical cure as compared to selective or no lymphadenectomy. Whipple resection is not routinely performed and mainly reserved for duodenal or pancreatic head tumors that cannot be removed by enucleation. One study reported an immediate postsurgical cure rate of 51% with a subsequent 10-year cure rate of 34%. Another large study of 195 ZES patients followed for 12 years after diagnosis demonstrated that surgical exploration for gastrinoma removal or cure significantly increased patient survival. Patients undergoing surgery had greater disease-related survival than nonoperated patients, which was attributed to significant reductions in (the remaining) tumor growth and progression as well as liver metastases.

The role of surgery in patients with ZES as part of the MEN 1 syndrome remains controversial because these gastrinomas tend to be multifocal and surgery is rarely curative. As a result, an individualized approach to these patients should be considered. Several studies have shown that MEN 1 patients with small gastrinomas (<1.5–2 cm in diameter) usually have an indolent clinical course and excellent long-term prognosis. Current guidelines thus suggest that these patients should not undergo routine surgical exploration or routine Whipple resections. However, because the primary tumor size affects the subsequent development of liver metastases and a minority of these ZES patients with MEN 1 can have aggressive growth, surgical exploration should be considered for tumors greater than 2–2.5 cm to decrease the risk of malignant spread. In patients with MEN 1/ZES with hyperparathyroidism, surgical resection is recommended after surgery for the primary hyperparathyroidism and only if there is an identifiable tumor larger than 2 cm. Successful parathyroidectomy can markedly reduce fasting gastrin levels and the BAO, while increasing the sensitivity to gastric antisecretory drugs.

As previously indicated, the presence of liver metastases is an important prognostic marker of outcomes in these patients. ZES patients with diffuse liver metastases, especially those that are rapidly increasing in size, have substantially reduced survival. Aggressive surgical resection or cytoreductive surgery in patients with advanced disease may be considered to improve outcomes. Multiple other therapies have been developed for unresectable gastrinomas with liver metastases including radio-frequency ablation (RFA), cryoablation, trans-arterial embolization (TAE) or chemoembolization (TACE), radio-embolization or selective internal radiation therapy (SIRT). In addition, patients may also be treated with chemotherapy, biotherapy with somatostatin analogues or interferon-Alfa, molecular targeted therapy with mTOR (everolimus), tyrosine kinase inhibitors, peptide radio-receptor therapy (PRRT), liver transplantation, and immunotherapy.

Somatostatin analogs such as octreotide and lanreotide are effective in controlling the symptoms associated with hormone hypersecretion in pancreatic islet cell tumors that express somatostatin receptors. Lanreotide is available in a long-acting depot form (Lanreotide-SR). The somatostatin analogues may also potentially slow tumor growth with disease stabilization and prolongation of progressive free survival. However, the anti-tumor effect appears modest as some studies suggest that less than 10–15% of treated tumors decrease in size. In comparison, systemic chemotherapy using streptozotocin and doxorubicin has radiologic response rates ranging from 10% to 40% but these drugs also have substantial toxicity such as myelosuppression and renal failure. The use of the orally active alkylating agent temozolomide with capecitabine has been reported to have a 54% radiographic response to therapy. Further studies are also being conducted on the use of novel targeted-molecular therapies such as mammalian target of rapamycin (mTor) inhibitors (everolimus and Afinitor), tyrosine-kinase inhibitors (sunitinib and Sutent), small molecule vascular endothelial growth factor (VEGF), and lutetium Lu177 dotatate peptide receptor radioligand therapy. For example, the activation of the mTOR cascade plays an important role in the proliferation, growth, and apoptosis of pancreatic NENs. Everolimus was significantly associated with a nearly 3 fold increase in progression-free survival in clinical trials and has been approved by the FDA for patients with these advanced tumors. The role of liver transplantation is still under investigation but may be considered for younger patients with metastases limited to the liver.

Albers MB, Manoharan J, Detlef K Bartsch DK. Contemporary surgical management of the Zollinger-Ellison syndrome in multiple endocrine neoplasia type 1. *Best Pract Res Clin Endocrinol Metab.* 2019;33(5):101318. [PMID: 31521501]

Cives M, Ghayouri M, Morse B, et al. Analysis of potential response predictors to capecitabine/temozolomide in metastatic pancreatic neuroendocrine tumors. *Endocr Relat Cancer.* 2016;23(9):759.

Jensen RT, Norton JA. Treatment of pancreatic neuroendocrine tumors in multiple endocrine neoplasia type 1: some clarity but continued controversy. *Pancreas.* 2017;46:589–594.

Norton JA, Krampitz G, Jensen RT. Multiple endocrine neoplasia: genetics and clinical management. *Surg Oncol Clin N Am.* 2015;24:795–832.

Qu Y, Li H, Wang X, et al. Clinical characteristics and management of functional pancreatic neuroendocrine neoplasms: a single institution 20-year experience with 286 patients. *Int J Endocrinol.* 2020;1030518. [PMID: 33204258]

Prognosis

Several reports suggest that 60–90% of gastrinomas are malignant and most are not cured by surgery. Tumor progression and the presence of metastases are the main determinants of survival. Patients with a gastrinoma and diffuse liver metastases have a 10-year survival rate of 15–30%, whereas gastrinoma patients without liver metastases have a much better prognosis with a 20-year survival of over 95%. In part due to a larger tumor size and hence a greater propensity for liver metastases, the survival rate of patients with pancreatic gastrinomas tends to be lower than that of patients with duodenal gastrinomas. The 10-year survival rate was 57% in patients with sporadic pancreatic gastrinomas and 84% in patients with duodenal gastrinomas. An aggressive form of gastrinoma develops more commonly among female ZES patients without the MEN 1 syndrome who have shorter disease duration but large pancreatic tumors with liver metastases.

Ito T, Lee L, Jensen RT. Treatment of symptomatic neuroendocrine tumor syndromes: recent advances and controversies. *Expert Opin Pharmacother.* 2016;17(16):2191–2205. [PMID: 27635672]

Lee L, Ito T, Jensen RT. Prognostic and predictive factors on overall survival and surgical outcomes in pancreatic neuroendocrine tumors: recent advances and controversies. *Expert Rev Anticancer Ther.* 2019;19(12):1029–1050. [PMID: 31738624]

Norton JA, Foster DS, Ito T, Jensen RT. Gastrinomas: medical or surgical treatment. *Endocrinol Metab Clin North Am.* 2018;47(3):577–601. [PMID: 30098717]

Functional Dyspepsia

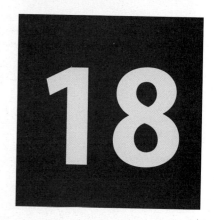

Molly L. Perencevich, MD

▶ Dyspepsia is a common symptom having either an organic or a functional cause.

▶ Clinical features of functional dyspepsia, gastroesophageal reflux disease (GERD), and gastrointestinal motility disorders overlap, making diagnosis difficult.

▶ Endoscopy is indicated for patients with new-onset symptoms who are ≥60 years of age, or have significant or more than one alarm feature.

▶ Most patients with functional dyspepsia have normal esophagogastroduodenoscopy (EGD) findings.

▶ Functional dyspepsia is a clinical diagnosis established after appropriate testing.

General Considerations

This chapter outlines the evaluation and management of dyspepsia, with a primary focus on functional dyspepsia. The term *dyspepsia* derives from the Greek "dys," meaning bad, and "pepsis," meaning digestion. The term dyspepsia encompasses a broad spectrum of symptoms that include upper abdominal pain or discomfort, postprandial fullness, early satiety, epigastric bloating, nausea, and belching. Dyspepsia is differentiated from GERD, characterized by retrosternal burning and regurgitation, but both can occur in patients.

A. Classification

The multiple causes of dyspepsia can be classified as organic or functional. Among the organic causes are peptic ulcer disease, gastritis, hepatobiliary diseases, chronic pancreatitis, upper gastrointestinal malignancies, Crohn's disease, chronic intestinal ischemia, small intestinal bacterial overgrowth or dysbiosis, infections, infiltrative diseases. In addition, several medications can cause dyspeptic symptoms (Table 18–1),

most common are nonsteroidal anti-inflammatory drugs (NSAIDs). Functional disorders such as GERD, gastroparesis, and irritable bowel syndrome (IBS) can also have overlapping symptoms with functional dyspepsia.

Functional dyspepsia, sometimes also referred to as nonulcer dyspepsia, is dyspepsia that is not due to organic causes after an appropriate evaluation. Notably, functional dyspepsia is more common (approximately 75%) than organic causes of dyspepsia. Other functional disorders can overlap with functional dyspepsia. Some patients with dyspepsia also have evidence of gastroparesis. IBS is characterized by lower abdominal discomfort and a chance in stool form or frequency.

The Rome IV criteria defines functional dyspepsia as one or more of the following symptoms: postprandial fullness, early satiation, and/or epigastric pain or burning (Table 18–2). In addition, functional dyspepsia can be further defined as two subtypes: postprandial distress syndrome and epigastric pain syndrome. Postprandial distress syndrome is characterized by bloating, fullness, and/or early satiety with meals. Epigastric pain syndrome is characterized by epigastric burning or pain that may not be related to meals. These two subtypes often coexist in patients with functional dyspepsia. Epigastric bloating, belching, and nausea can also be present, but frequent vomiting is not common in functional dyspepsia.

Ford AC, Mahadeva S, Carbone MF, et al. Functional dyspepsia. *Lancet.* 2020;396:1689–1702. [PMID: 33049222]

Stanghellini V, Talley NJ, Chan F, et al. Gastroduodenal disorders. *Gastroenterology.* 2016;150:1380–1392. [PMID: 27147122]

Talley NJ, Ford AC. Functional dyspepsia. *N Engl J Med.* 2015;373:1853–1863. [PMID: 26535514]

B. Epidemiology

The prevalence of dyspepsia is approximately 20%, the majority of which is functional dyspepsia, although this varies

Table 18–1. Medications that can cause dyspepsia.

Acarbose
Aspirin, nonsteroidal anti-inflammatory drugs
Colchicine
Digitalis preparations
Estrogens
Gemfibrozil
Glucocorticoids
Iron
Levodopa
Narcotics
Niacin
Nitrates
Orlistat
Potassium chloride
Quinidine
Sildenafil
Theophylline

somewhat based on country and how dyspepsia is defined. Dyspepsia is not associated with increased mortality but can have a significant impact on quality of life and health care expenditure.

A population-based survey study of 6000 adults in the US, Canada, and UK found that 10% fulfilled symptom-based criteria for Rome IV functional dyspepsia. The subtype distribution was 61% postprandial distress syndrome, 18% epigastric pain syndrome, and 21% overlapping variant with both syndromes. In addition, participants with functional dyspepsia had significantly greater health impairment and health care usage than those without dyspepsia.

Table 18–2. Rome IV criteria for functional dyspepsia.

Functional Dyspepsia[a] — one or more of the following:
- Bothersome postprandial fullness
- Bothersome early satiation
- Bothersome epigastric pain
- Bothersome epigastric burning

And
- No evidence of structural disease (including at upper endoscopy) that is likely to explain the symptoms

Subtypes
a. Postprandial Distress Syndrome[a] — one or both of the following at least 3 days per week:
   - Bothersome postprandial fullness (occurs after ordinary-sized meals, impacts usual activities)
   - Bothersome early satiation (prevents finishing a regular meal)
b. Epigastric Pain Syndrome[a] — one of the following at least 1 day per week:
   - Bothersome epigastric pain (impacts usual activities)
   - Bothersome epigastric burning (impacts usual activities)

[a]Criteria are met for the last 3 months, with onset at least 6 months previously.

Aziz I, Palsson OS, Törnblom H, et al. Epidemiology, clinical characteristics, and associations for symptom-based Rome IV functional dyspepsia in adults in the USA, Canada, and the UK: a cross-sectional population-based study. *Lancet Gastroenterol Hepatol*. 2018;3:252–262. [PMID: 29396034]

Ford AC, Forman D, Bailey AG, et al. Effect of dyspepsia on survival: a longitudinal 10-year follow-up study. *Am J Gastroenterol*. 2012;107:912–921. [PMID: 22472745]

Ford AC, Marwaha A, Sood R, et al. Global prevalence of, and risk factors for, uninvestigated dyspepsia: a meta-analysis. *Gut*. 2015;64:1049–1057. [PMID: 25147201]

► Pathogenesis

Organic dyspepsia can develop in the setting of the varied disease processes mentioned in this chapter and described elsewhere in this text. The pathogenesis of functional dyspepsia is unclear. Factors that play a role in causation include disturbances in motility, altered visceral sensitivity, dietary factors, and psychosomatic factors. The role of *Helicobacter pylori* in the genesis of symptoms is controversial.

A. Altered Gastrointestinal Motility

Disturbances in gastrointestinal motility may be associated with functional dyspepsia. including delayed gastric emptying, rapid gastric emptying, and gastric accommodation. There is an overlap of symptoms and pathophysiology between gastroparesis and some patients with functional dyspepsia, and approximately one quarter of patients with functional dyspepsia have evidence of delayed gastric emptying.

Gastric accommodation may also play a role in functional dyspepsia. During normal ingestion of food, the gastric fundus relaxes to "accommodate" the food particles. This accommodation is mediated by serotonin ($5\text{-}HT_{1p}$) and nitric oxide via vagal inhibitory neurons of the enteric nervous system.

The prevalence of motility disorders has varied markedly between studies, likely due to subject selection criteria and study methodology. In one study of 1287 patients with functional gastroduodenal symptoms, 29.8% had normal gastric emptying and accommodation, 21.9% had abnormal gastric accommodation only, 27.1% had abnormal gastric emptying only, and 21.1% had abnormal gastric emptying and accommodation. Increased gastric accommodation was more prevalent in patients with delayed gastric emptying compared to accelerated gastric emptying, and decreased gastric accommodation was associated with accelerated gastric emptying compared to normal emptying. Vomiting was more prevalent, and bloating less prevalent, in patients with delayed compared to accelerated or normal gastric emptying.

Other motor disorders, such as gastroesophageal reflux, small bowel dysmotility, and biliary dyskinesia, may also cause dyspeptic symptoms. As mentioned, symptoms of GERD often overlap with dyspepsia symptoms. Poor visceral localization of symptoms can often cause a reflux event to be confused with other upper gastrointestinal sources of discomfort. A study of patients with functional dyspepsia revealed that almost one-third had pathologic signs of acid reflux. In addition, both acid and nonacid reflux can cause symptoms.

Park SY, Acosta A, Camilleri M, et al. Gastric motor dysfunction in patients with functional gastroduodenal symptoms. *Am J Gastroenterol*. 2017;112:1689–1699. [PMID 28895582]

Sarnelli G, Caenepeel P, Geypens B, et al. Symptoms associated with impaired gastric emptying of solids and liquids in functional dyspepsia. *Am J Gastroenterol*. 2003;98:783–788. [PMID: 12738456]

Stanghellini V, Tack J. Gastroparesis: separate entity of just part of dyspepsia? *Gut*. 2014;63:1972–1978. [PMID: 25260920]

Xiao YL, Peng S, Tao J, et al. Prevalence and symptom pattern of pathologic esophageal acid reflux in patients with functional dyspepsia based on the Rome III criteria. *Am J Gastroenterol*. 2010;105:2626–2631. [PMID: 20823838]

B. Visceral Hypersensitivity

Some patients with functional dyspepsia may instead have normal gastric motility, but a lowered pain threshold. With visceral hypersensitivity or hyperalgesia, patients begin to experience pain or discomfort at a level of gastric distention normally not associated with symptoms in healthy individuals, resulting from increased sensory input to and from the stomach. Such enhanced perception is not limited to mechanical distention, but may also occur in response to temperature stress, acid exposure, chemical or nutrient stimuli, or hormones, such as cholecystokinin and glucagon-like peptide 1.

In patients with visceral hypersensitivity, there may be altered central nervous system processing of these stimuli. Studies have demonstrated hypersensitivity to balloon distention in the stomach in as many as 50% of patients with functional dyspepsia. Compared with controls, patients with functional dyspepsia had a significantly lower threshold to both initial sensation of balloon distention and to sensation of pain. Studies also suggest that lower postprandial gastric distention thresholds significantly correlate with severity of meal-related symptoms, including fullness, bloating, nausea, discomfort, and impaired accommodation to a meal. Visceral hypersensitivity is also thought to play a role in the pathogenesis of IBS.

Farré R, Vanheel H, Vanuytsel T, et al. In functional dyspepsia, hypersensitivity to postprandial distention correlates with meal-related symptom severity. *Gastroenterology*. 2013;145:566–573. [PMID: 23702005]

Mertz H, Fullerton S, Naliboff B, et al. Symptoms and visceral perception in severe functional and organic dyspepsia. *Gut*. 1998;42:814–822. [PMID: 9691920]

C. Dietary Factors

Dietary factors may be a potential cause of symptoms in functional dyspepsia. Patients with functional dyspepsia appear to have altered eating patterns as well as food intolerances. They frequently report being able to tolerate only small quantities of food, more commonly snacking and less likely to eat large meals. Food intolerances are also common among patients with functional dyspepsia. Enteral hormones may mediate increased intestinal sensitivity to nutrients in functional dyspepsia. Fatty foods, in particular, have been linked to dyspepsia. Other possible dietary factors include wheat, gluten, FODMAPs (fermentable oligosaccharide, disaccharide, monosaccharide and polyols), spicy foods, and caffeine. The effect of alcohol related to functional dyspepsia is not clear.

Bharucha AE, Camilleri M, Burton DD, et al. Increased nutrient sensitivity and plasma concentrations of enteral hormones during duodenal nutrient infusion in functional dyspepsia. *Am J Gastroenterol*. 2014;109:1910–1920. [PMID: 25403365]

Duncanson KR, Talley NJ, Walker MM, et al. Food and functional dyspepsia: a systemic review. *J Hum Nutr Diet*. 2018;31:390–407. [PMID: 28913843]

D. *Helicobacter pylori* Infection

The role of *H pylori* in functional dyspepsia is controversial, and no clear association has been established. Although no clear pathophysiologic mechanisms have been delineated, hypotheses include chronic mucosal inflammation causing alterations in gastroduodenal motility or sensitivity, as well as potentially affecting gastrointestinal hormones and neurotransmitters.

Although there has been some debate about whether *H pylori* eradication is beneficial in functional dyspepsia, there seems to be a small but statistically significant improvement in symptoms. It is also possible that treatment could improve symptoms by treating undiagnosed peptic ulcer disease or impacting the microbiome.

Kim YJ, Chung WC, Wook B, et al. Is *Helicobacter pylori* associated functional dyspepsia correlated with dysbiosis? *J Neurogastroenterol Motil*. 2017;23:504–516. [PMID: 28992674]

Mazzoleni LE, Sander GB, de Magalhães Francesconi CF, et al. *Helicobacter pylori* eradication in functional dyspepsia: HEROES trial. *Arch Intern Med*. 2011;171:1929–1936. [PMID: 22123802]

Suzuki H, Moayyedi P. *Helicobacter pylori* infection in functional dyspepsia. *Nat Rev Gastroenterol Hepatol*. 2013;10:168–174. [PMID: 23358394]

E. Altered Microbiome

Alterations in the microbiome of the upper small bowel may be associated with functional dyspepsia. Similar to IBS, an episode of infectious gastroenteritis is considered a risk factor for functional dyspepsia. As above, treatment of *H pylori* may be improving functional dyspepsia symptoms by altering the microbiome.

Pike BL, Porter CK, Sorrell TJ, et al. Acute gastroenteritis and the risk of functional dyspepsia: a systematic review and meta-analysis. *Am J Gastroenterol*. 2013;108:1558–1563. [PMID: 23711623]

F. Duodenal Eosinophilia

Some have hypothesized that duodenal eosinophilia may play a role in a subset of patients with functional dyspepsia. Several studies have shown significantly greater eosinophil counts in duodenal biopsies from patients with functional dyspepsia compared to those from healthy controls. However, eosinophilic infiltration has also been described in many different clinical scenarios, including healthy individuals. Therefore, the role of duodenal eosinophils in functional dyspepsia remains to be elucidated.

Talley NJ, Walker MM, Aro P, et al. Non-ulcer dyspepsia and duodenal eosinophilia: an adult endoscopic population-based case-control study. *Clin Gastroenterol Hepatol.* 2007;5:1175–1183. [PMID: 17686660]

G. Psychological Factors

Psychosocial factors may play a role in functional dyspepsia. Dyspepsia has been associated with depression, anxiety, and somatization disorders. In addition, studies have demonstrated significant associations between dyspepsia symptoms and a history of abuse in childhood or adulthood. There may be multiple mechanisms related to the brain-gut axis. One study found acute anxiety and anxiety disorders to be associated with impacted gastric accommodation.

Castillo EJ, Camilleri M, Locke GR, et al. A community-based, controlled study of the epidemiology and pathophysiology of dyspepsia. *Clin Gastroenterol Hepatol.* 2004;2:985–996. [PMID: 15551251]

Ly HG, Weltens N, Tack J, et al. Acute anxiety and anxiety disorders are associated with impaired gastric accommodation in patients with functional dyspepsia. *Clin Gastroenterol Hepatol.* 2015;13:1584–1591. [PMID: 25869636]

Talley NJ, Fett SL, Zinsmeister R, et al. Gastrointestinal tract symptoms and self-reported abuse: a population-based study. *Gastroenterology.* 1994;107:1040–1049. [PMID: 7926457]

▶ Clinical Findings

A. Symptoms & Signs

The initial clinical evaluation should focus on symptom characteristics, onset, and chronicity. Other important history to obtain includes comorbidities, surgical history, family history of upper gastrointestinal malignancy, alcohol and tobacco use, dietary factors, stressful life events, and psychological factors. Symptoms of functional dyspepsia include upper abdominal pain or discomfort, postprandial fullness, and/or early satiety. Epigastric bloating, nausea, and belching can occur, but vomiting is less common. GERD symptoms can overlap with dyspepsia. The clinician should consider a broad differential diagnosis for upper abdominal pain including

Table 18–3. "Alarm" features suggestive of the presence of upper gastrointestinal malignancy.

Unintentional weight loss
Dysphagia
Odynophagia
Persistent vomiting
Unexplained iron deficiency anemia
Jaundice
Abdominal mass
Lymphadenopathy
History of previous GI malignancy
Family history of upper GI malignancy

GERD, gallstones, medications (particularly NSAIDs), gastroparesis, chronic pancreatitis, IBS, and malignancy.

In most cases, however, the clinical history is of limited use in distinguishing organic causes from functional dyspepsia. A large systematic review of the literature showed that neither clinical impression nor computer models were able to adequately distinguish organic from functional disease.

Alarm features should be elicited as the presence of one or more of these may indicate that a patient needs earlier and more aggressive testing (Table 18–3). However, research has suggested that alarm features in the setting of dyspepsia symptoms have a low positive predictive value and are of limited value in stratifying patients for endoscopy.

The physical examination may elicit abdominal tenderness, usually in the epigastrium. Although this finding is nonspecific, several features may aid in identifying possible underlying etiologies. More focal right upper quadrant tenderness may suggest a biliary etiology such as chronic cholecystitis. A positive Carnett's sign, or focal tenderness that increases with abdominal wall contraction and palpation, suggests an etiology involving the abdominal wall musculature. Cutaneous dermatomal distribution of pain may suggest a thoracic polyradiculopathy. Most commonly, however, the physical examination is normal. Exam features of jaundice, abdominal mass, and lymphadenopathy are considered alarm features.

Moayyedi P, Lacy BE, Andrews CN, et al. ACG and CAG clinical guideline: management of dyspepsia. *Am J Gastroenterol.* 2017;112:988–1013. [PMID: 28631728]

Moayyedi P, Talley NJ, Fennerty MB, et al. Can the clinical history distinguish between organic and functional dyspepsia? *JAMA.* 2006;295:1566–1576. [PMID: 1659759]

B. Diagnostic Evaluation

Laboratory testing should include a complete blood count, liver enzymes, lipase, and amylase. Additional evaluation is based on the history, physical examination, and results of the laboratory tests.

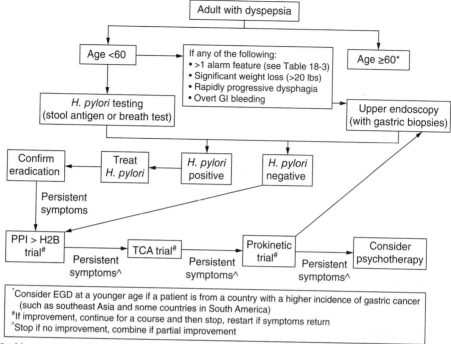

▲ **Figure 18–1.** Management of dyspepsia, including functional dyspepsia. EGD, esophagogastroduodenoscopy; H2B, H_2-receptor blocker; PPI, proton pump inhibitor; TCA, tricyclic antidepressant.

Several studies can be considered in the evaluation of dyspepsia. These were reviewed by the American College of Gastroenterology (ACG) and Canadian Association of Gastroenterology (CAG) 2017 guideline for the management of dyspepsia (Figure 18–1).

1. Esophagogastroduodenoscopy—Patients with new-onset dyspepsia at age ≥60 should undergo an EGD to exclude organic pathology. Patients with dyspepsia at age <60 are generally at very low risk (<1%) of having malignancy, even with an alarm feature. Therefore, EGD is not generally recommended as an initial test in this group. However, EGD should be recommended if they have clinically significant weight loss (>20 lbs. or >5% usual body weight over 6–12 months), overt gastrointestinal bleeding, >1 alarm feature, or rapidly progressive alarm features. In addition, patients at higher risk of malignancy, such as spending their childhood in a country with a higher incidence of gastric cancer (eg, Southeast Asia and some countries in South America) or having a family history of upper gastrointestinal cancer, should be offered EGD at a younger age. The ACG/CAG guidelines are conditional based on the available data, and the need for endoscopy should be evaluated on an individual basis using clinical judgment.

During EGD, biopsies of the stomach should be obtained to evaluate for *H pylori* even if the mucosa appears normal. Biopsies should also be obtained of any abnormal-appearing mucosa. It is not generally recommended to biopsy normal-appearing esophagus or duodenum for the indication of dyspepsia.

In younger patients without alarm features who do not have an endoscopy as part of their initial evaluation, the ACG/CAG guidelines recommend an EGD be performed after a patient has failed trials of acid suppression, antidepressants, and promotility agents (see Treatment below).

Moayyedi P, Lacy BE, Andrews CN, et al. ACG and CAG clinical guideline: management of dyspepsia. *Am J Gastroenterol.* 2017;112:988–1013. [PMID: 28631728]

Yang YX, Brill J, Krishnan P, et al. American Gastroenterological Association Institute Guideline on the role of upper gastrointestinal biopsy to evaluate dyspepsia in the adult patient in the absence of visible mucosal lesions. *Gastroenterology.* 2015;149:1082–1087. [PMID: 26283143]

2. *Helicobacter pylori* testing—For patients younger than 60 years and without significant or multiple alarm features, noninvasive *H pylori* testing should be performed prior to a trial of proton pump inhibitors (PPIs). The optimal test for *H pylori* is either a ^{13}C-urea breath test or stool antigen test, which test for the presence of active infection. It is important that patients are not taking antibiotics/bismuth for 4 weeks or PPIs for 2 weeks to prevent false negative tests. *H pylori* serology can also be used, but it can be positive in patients who had a prior infection, potentially leading to treating people who do not have current infection. For patients who undergo EGD, biopsies of the stomach should be obtained to evaluate for *H pylori* infection.

Patients with *H pylori* infection should be treated with regimens consisting of antibiotics and PPI, which is reviewed in Chapter 17.

Moayyedi P, Lacy BE, Andrews CN, et al. ACG and CAG clinical guideline: management of dyspepsia. *Am J Gastroenterol.* 2017;112:988–1013. [PMID: 28631728]

3. Other studies—Gastric scintigraphy can be considered in patients with persistent nausea and vomiting who fail initial therapy or have risk factors for gastroparesis. A 4-hour solid phase study is generally recommended. There is significant overlap of symptoms and potential pathophysiology between functional dyspepsia and gastroparesis. Upper gastrointestinal series and tests of small bowel motility may also be considered in selected patients with persistent dyspeptic symptoms despite routine evaluation and treatment.

▶ Differential Diagnosis

The differential diagnosis of dyspepsia is broad. The findings from history and physical examination and judicious use of the diagnostic studies outlined in the preceding section can aid in distinguishing the various organic causes of dyspepsia from functional dyspepsia.

A. GERD

GERD and dyspepsia overlap frequently, often coexisting in the same patient. Thus, GERD should always be considered in the dyspeptic patient. Symptoms such as regurgitation and substernal burning are more likely to be related to GERD. Erosive esophagitis on EGD may suggest acid reflux, but a normal appearing esophagus does not exclude GERD. Formal reflux testing with a 24-hour pH study with esophageal impendence off antisecretory medications (eg, PPI) can help identify the role of acid reflux, nonacid reflux, esophageal hypersensitivity, and functional heartburn as a potential cause of symptoms.

Quigley EM, Lacy BE. Overlap of functional dyspepsia and GERD—diagnostic and treatment implications. *Nat Rev Gastroenterol Hepatol.* 2013;10:175–186. [PMID: 23296247]

B. Peptic Ulcer Disease

About 15% of patients with dyspeptic symptoms have gastric or duodenal ulcers. Once diagnosed, the underlying cause of the ulcer(s) should be investigated, as many risk factors for peptic ulcers may also lead to dyspepsia symptoms, including the use of NSAIDs and the presence of *H pylori* infection.

C. Upper Gastrointestinal Malignancy

Upper gastrointestinal malignancy is an uncommon cause of dyspepsia in westernized countries. However, older patients have a higher risk. Therefore, patients with new-onset symptoms at age ≥60 should undergo early endoscopic evaluation. Other risk factors for gastric cancer include spending childhood in a country with a higher risk of gastric cancer (eg, Southeast Asia and some countries in South America) or having a family history of upper gastrointestinal cancer. These patients should be offered EGD at a younger age. CT may also be recommended in patients with unexplained epigastric pain and age ≥60 to evaluate for malignancy.

D. Chronic Intestinal Ischemia

Chronic intestinal ischemia is characterized by chronic postprandial pain with marked weight loss due to mesenteric blood flow that is inadequate to the demands required by digestion. Typically, the patient has a history of tobacco use or underlying atherosclerotic disease. A diagnosis may be made by magnetic resonance angiography (MRA) or CT angiography (CTA).

E. Pancreaticobiliary Disease

Classic biliary colic is characterized by sudden onset of right upper quadrant pain that is constant, lasting 2–6 hours, associated with nausea, and worsened postprandially. Because of the visceral nature of the pain, it is poorly localizable, and some patients may have epigastric rather than clear right upper quadrant pain. If a patient's symptoms are suggestive of biliary pain, an ultrasound of the abdomen should be obtained to evaluate the gallbladder for cholelithiasis or cholecystitis. A quantitative cholescintigraphy scan with cholecystokinin challenge may suggest chronic cholecystitis or functional gallbladder disorder as the diagnosis if the ejection fraction is less than 35–40%.

The pain associated with chronic pancreatitis and pancreatic cancer may be epigastric or localized to the central abdomen, classically with radiation to the mid back. Weight loss may occur. Pancreatic endocrine or exocrine insufficiency (eg, diabetes, steatorrhea) may or may not be present. Jaundice can also occur with pancreatic cancer. Abdominal computed tomography (CT) should be considered in patients with symptoms suggestive of pancreatic pathology, prior acute pancreatitis, and/or a family history of pancreatic disease.

F. Motility Disorders

Upper gastrointestinal motility disorders such as gastroparesis may overlap with dyspepsia. Both disorders can cause symptoms of epigastric discomfort, bloating, fullness, early satiety, and nausea. However, persistent nausea and vomiting are more common with gastroparesis. Causes of motility disturbance may include diabetic gastroparesis, chronic intestinal pseudo-obstruction, scleroderma, or postvagotomy syndromes. Gastric scintigraphy (4-hour solid phase study), upper gastrointestinal series, and tests of small bowel motility may also be considered.

Kim BJ, Kuo B. Gastroparesis and functional dyspepsia: a blurring distinction of pathophysiology and treatment. *J Neurogastroenterol Motil.* 2019;25:27–35. [PMID: 30509017]

G. Infections

Gastric infections other than *H pylori* can cause dyspepsia. These include cytomegalovirus, tuberculosis, fungal infections, *Giardia lamblia*, and *Strongyloides stercoralis*.

H. Irritable Bowel Syndrome

IBS is another functional gastrointestinal disorder which can have overlapping symptoms with dyspepsia. However, unlikely dyspepsia, IBS is more likely to have lower abdominal discomfort and is defined by a change in stool form or frequency. It is also common to have an overlap of functional dyspepsia and IBS.

von Wulffen M, Talley NJ, Hammer J, et al. Overlap of irritable bowel syndrome and functional dyspepsia in the clinical setting: prevalence and risk factors. *Dig Dis Sci.* 2019;64:480–486. [PMID: 30368683]

I. Small Intestinal Bacterial Overgrowth

Small intestinal bacterial overgrowth is associated with nonspecific symptoms such as bloating, gas, and general abdominal discomfort. It is often associated with diarrhea which may distinguish it from dyspepsia. If suspected, diagnosis can be established by breath testing or a trial of antibiotics.

J. Other Considerations

Other conditions to consider in the differential diagnosis include chronic gastric volvulus, infiltrative diseases (sarcoidosis, amyloidosis, eosinophilic gastroenteritis, Ménétrier disease, lymphoma), inflammatory bowel disease (in particular Crohn's disease), celiac disease, food allergy or intolerances, celiac artery compression syndrome, mesenteric artery syndrome, and abdominal wall pain. Endoscopy and abdominal CT or MRI may be helpful in evaluating for some of these etiologies. Abdominal wall pain is best diagnosed by history and physical exam maneuvers such as Carnett's sign.

▶ Treatment

The treatment of organic dyspepsia is targeted to the cause. Specific treatment regimens for GERD, peptic ulcer disease, and other disorders that may cause dyspepsia can be found in their respective chapters in this book.

The treatment of functional dyspepsia primarily targets symptom relief. Studies have shown moderate success in response to PPIs, antidepressants, and motility agents. An effective physician-patient relationship is important to treatment success.

Masuy I, van Oudenhove, Tack J. Review article: treatment options for functional dyspepsia. *Aliment Pharmacol Ther.* 2019;49:1134–1172. [PMID: 30924176]
Moayyedi P, Lacy BE, Andrews CN, et al. ACG and CAG clinical guideline: management of dyspepsia. *Am J Gastroenterol.* 2017;112:988–1013. [PMID: 28631728]

A. General Measures

The physician-patient relationship is crucial to the treatment of functional dyspepsia. Fears of having cancer or a life-threatening condition, anxiety levels, and stressful factors in the patient's life should be assessed and addressed early in the evaluation. After an appropriate evaluation has been conducted, the diagnosis of functional dyspepsia should also be explained as a recognized clinical entity with the emphasis on the understood pathophysiology of the problem.

B. Dietary Modification

The efficacy of dietary or lifestyle modifications in functional dyspepsia has not been well studied. Possible dietary factors include fat content, wheat, gluten, FODMAPs (fermentable oligosaccharide, disaccharide, monosaccharide and polyols), spicy foods, and caffeine. The effect of alcohol related to functional dyspepsia is not clear. More research is needed in this area before formal recommendations can be made. A food diary may help identify triggers, and trials of limiting possible dietary triggers can be considered. In addition, smaller and more frequent meals may be beneficial in patients with impaired gastric accommodation and delayed gastric emptying.

Duncanson KR, Talley NJ, Walker MM, et al. Food and functional dyspepsia: a systemic review. *J Hum Nutr Diet.* 2018;31:390–407. [PMID: 28913843]

C. Pharmacotherapy

Studies on treatment of functional dyspepsia have often been limited by insufficient sample size, single-center trials, variability in the definition of functional dyspepsia, and high placebo response rates. Given the multifactorial nature and variability in clinical symptoms associated with dyspepsia, each pharmacologic agent may be effective only in a subset of patients with dyspepsia symptoms, and drug selection may need to be targeted based on patient factors, clinical history, or symptom characteristics. The pharmacologic therapy for functional dyspepsia includes *H pylori* eradication, antisecretory agents, antidepressants, promotility agents, and other classes of drugs.

1. *H pylori* eradication—*H pylori* eradication appears to provide a small but significant benefit to patients with functional dyspepsia. However, some patients continue to have functional dyspepsia symptoms after *H. pylori* eradication.

Treatment recommendations for *H pylori* can be found in Chapter 17. After treatment for *H. pylori*, eradication testing should be performed to ensure that the infection has been cleared. If it has not, additional treatment can be provided for persistent *H pylori* infection.

After confirmation of *H pylori* eradication, or if the patient does not have *H pylori* infection, a trial of acid suppression is suggested.

Mazzoleni LE, Sander GB, de Magalhães Francesconi CF, et al. *Helicobacter pylori* eradication in functional dyspepsia: HEROES trial. *Arch Intern Med.* 2011;171:1929–1936. [PMID: 22123802]

2. Antisecretory agents—PPIs have been extensively studied in several large randomized controlled trials. A 2017 Cochrane systematic review of 18 studies with a total of 6172 patients found that PPIs were effective compared to placebo (RR = 0.88; 95% CI, 0.82–0.94; NNT = 11). It was noted that low-dose PPI had similar efficacy as standard-dose PPI. The evidence for H_2-receptor blockers is less clear. A 2006 Cochrane systematic review suggests a small benefit of H_2-receptor blockers compared to placebo for functional dyspepsia. The 2017 Cochrane review included 2 studies with a total of 740 patients that compared PPI and H_2-receptor blockers and found there was little to no effect (RR 0.88, 95% CI, 0.74–1.04).

Some data has suggested that acid suppression may be more likely to improve symptoms in EPS than PDS. However, the 2017 Cochrane systemic review reported no differences in response based on functional dyspepsia subtype.

Based on the available data, the ACG/CAG 2017 guidelines for dyspepsia recommend empirical PPI over H_2-receptor blockers after *H pylori* testing is negative or it has been eradicated. Standard-dose PPI is recommended for 8 weeks. If the patient improves on this, the PPI can be tapered down to the lowest dose needed to control symptoms. In addition, intermittent trials of stopping PPI or switching to an H_2-receptor blocker should be considered to avoid chronic PPI use if not needed.

Moayyedi P, Soo S, Deeks J, et al. Pharmacological interventions for non-ulcer dyspepsia. *Cochrane Database Syst Review.* 2006;CD001960. [PMID: 17054151]

Pinto-Sanchez MI, Yuan Y, Hassan A, et al. Proton pump inhibitors for functional dyspepsia. *Cochrane Database Syst Review.* 2017;11:CD011194. [PMID: 29161458]

3. Antidepressants—Antidepressants may improve visceral hypersensitivity or other mechanisms. Low-dose tricyclic antidepressants (TCAs), such as amitriptyline or desipramine, have been used in patients with various functional disorders, including functional dyspepsia and IBS. A systemic review and meta-analysis of three randomized controlled trials showed that TCAs were more effective than placebo for functional dyspepsia (RR 0.76; 95% CI, 0.62–0.94; NNT 6). In this review of two trials, selective serotonin reuptake inhibitors (SSRIs) were not effective (RR 1.00; 95% CI, 0.86–1.17). Mirtazapine is another antidepressant that may have benefit in patients with functional dyspepsia, in particular those with early satiety and weight loss.

Antidepressants are generally considered after a patient has not had adequate symptom improvement after a trial of acid suppression. As TCAs can slow gastric emptying due to their anticholinergic effect, they should generally be avoided in patients with gastroparesis. A trial of 8–12 weeks is generally done with slow up-titration in dose while monitoring for side effects. Lower doses (10–75 mg/day) of TCAs are typically needed for functional dyspepsia than for depression. Patients should be warned about possible side effects prior to use. TCAs can cause anticholinergic symptoms such as dry mouth, drowsiness, urinary retention, and constipation. Mirtazapine commonly causes drowsiness.

Lacy BE, Saito YA, Camilleri M, et al. Effects of antidepressants on gastric function in patients with functional dyspepsia. *Am J Gastroenterol.* 2018;113:216–224. [PMID: 29257140]

Lu Y, Chen M, Huang Z, et al. Antidepressants in the treatment of functional dyspepsia: a systematic review and meta-analysis. *PLoS One.* 2016;11:e0157798. [PMID: 27310135]

Tack J, Ly HG, Carbone F, et al. Efficacy of mirtazapine in patients with functional dyspepsia and weight loss. *Clin Gastroenterol Hepatol.* 2016;14:385–392. [PMID: 26538208]

4. Promotility agents—Promotility agents are drugs that accelerate peristalsis by interacting with receptors for serotonin, acetylcholine, dopamine, and motilin (Table 18–4). Use of these drugs has shown no clear relationship between pharmacologic enhancement of motility and improvement in symptoms of functional dyspepsia, so there may be other mechanisms by which they improve symptoms. Of note, some drugs may worsen symptoms. For example, some promotility drugs (eg, erythromycin and metoclopramide) can have a negative impact on postprandial fundic relaxation/accommodation. Higher doses of these medications often cause more side effects than additional benefit.

There is overall low-quality evidence for the benefit of promotility agents in the treatment of functional dyspepsia. A systematic review of 29 randomized controlled trials reported prokinetics to be more effective than placebo in functional dyspepsia (RR 0.81; 95% CI, 0.74–0.89; NNT 7), and there was no difference in subtypes. However, the drugs in these studies (including cisapride, mosapride, tegaserod, acotiamide, and itopride) are not available for use in the United States (US) or Canada, although some are available in other countries.

Table 18–4. Mechanism of action of promotility agents.

	Serotonin (5-HT$_4$) Agonist	5-HT$_3$ Antagonist	Dopamine (D$_2$) Antagonist	Motilin Receptor Agonist	Muscarinic receptor antagonist
Cisapride	√	√			
Mosapride	√	√			
Tegaserod[a]	√				
Metoclopramide[b]	√	√	√		
Domperidone[c]			√		
Itopride			√		
Erythromycin[a]				√	
Acotiamide					√

[a]Withdrawn from the US market in 2007 due to a concern for cardiovascular side effects, but in 2019 the FDA approved its use for women age <65 with constipation-predominant irritable bowel syndrome (with additional contraindications).
[b]Available in the US.
[c]Available in the US through a FDA Investigational New Drug application.

There are limited studies of the effect of metoclopramide and domperidone in functional dyspepsia. The ACG/CAG 2017 guidelines suggest that patients with functional dyspepsia who do not respond to PPI and TCA therapy should be offered prokinetic therapy. In the US this is generally metoclopramide (5–10 mg before meals and at night) for a 4-week trial. Potential side effects of metoclopramide should be discussed with patients, especially related to long-term use, particularly movement disorders such as extrapyramidal reactions and tardive dyskinesia. Domperidone can be considered if available. It is not Food and Drug Administration (FDA) approved in the US due to concern for risk of cardiac arrhythmia but does not have the risk of extrapyramidal reactions and tardive dyskinesia.

Pittayanon R, Yuan Y, Bollegala, et al. Prokinetics for functional dyspepsia: a systemic review and meta-analysis of randomized controlled trials. *Am J Gastroenterol.* 2019;114:233–243. [PMID: 30337705]

5. Other drugs—Antacids, bismuth, and sucralfate has been studied in several limited trials and found to be no more effective than placebo. There are not recommended for the treatment of functional dyspepsia.

Buspirone, a 5-hydroxytryptamine 1A receptor agonist, has been demonstrated to relax the proximal stomach in healthy individuals. A randomized controlled trial buspirone for 4 weeks in patients with functional dyspepsia showed a significant improvement in gastric accommodation and reduction in symptoms compared to placebo. It represents another potential treatment option for functional dyspepsia, especially in patients with symptoms suggestive of altered gastric accommodation, including early satiety and postprandial fullness.

Antinociceptive agents such as gabapentin or pregabalin have been suggested as potential agents for management of discomfort or distress related to functional gastrointestinal disorder. These drugs have been found to modulate the central processing of pain and may impact autonomic functions. In a post hoc analysis of six randomized controlled trial of patients with general anxiety disorder and gastrointestinal symptoms, pregabalin led to significant improvement in the anxiety and gastrointestinal symptoms over placebo. Studies of these medications in the treatment of functional dyspepsia are needed.

Stein DJ, Bruce Lydiard R, Herman BK, et al. Impact of gastrointestinal symptoms on response to pregabalin in generalized anxiety disorder: results of a six-study combined analysis. *Int Clin Psychopharmacol.* 2009;24:126–132. [PMID: 19352198]

Tack J, Janssen P, Masaoka T, et al. Efficacy of buspirone, a fundus-relaxing drug, in patients with functional dyspepsia. *Clin Gastroenterol Hepatol.* 2012;10:1239–1245. [PMID: 22813445]

6. Recommendations for pharmacotherapy—A stepwise approach to the pharmacologic treatment of functional dyspepsia can be used (Figure 18–1). If *H pylori* testing yields a positive result, treatment is recommended with the understanding that eradication may or may not improve symptoms. If *H pylori* testing is negative or after eradication of *H pylori*, antisecretory medications can then be tried with PPIs (standard-dose) or H$_2$-blockers (may not be as effective as PPIs) for 4–8 weeks. If a patient has no or partial response to PPI, an antidepressant, most commonly a low-dose TCA can be tried for 8–12 weeks. If it is effective, it can be continued. If the TCA is not effective, a trial of a prokinetic, most commonly metoclopramide, can be considered for 4 weeks. Buspirone and antinociceptive agents can also be considered in the treatment of functional dyspepsia in patients with refractory symptoms.

Moayyedi P, Lacy BE, Andrews CN, et al. ACG and CAG clinical guideline: management of dyspepsia. *Am J Gastroenterol.* 2017;112:988–1013. [PMID: 28631728]

D. Psychological Therapy

Psychological therapy addresses the cognitive aspects of the pathophysiology of functional dyspepsia. Several modalities have been used, including cognitive-behavioral therapy and different forms of psychotherapy. There overall is overall limited data for the use of psychological therapy in the treatment of functional dyspepsia. A systemic review in 2005 of only 4 trials randomized controlled trials suggested that there was insufficient evidence. As a part of the ACG/CAG 2017 guidelines, the authors updated this review to a total of 12 trials and found a benefit of psychological therapies. Additional research is needed in this area, but psychological therapy can be considered in patients with refractory functional dyspepsia and those whose symptoms seem triggered by psychological stress.

Moayyedi P, Lacy BE, Andrews CN, et al. ACG and CAG clinical guideline: management of dyspepsia. *Am J Gastroenterol.* 2017;112:988–1013. [PMID: 28631728]

Soo S, Moayyedi P, Deeks J, et al. Psychological interventions for non-ulcer dyspepsia. *Cochrane Database Syst Rev.* 2005;CD002301. [PMID: 21328255]

E. Complementary & Alternative Medical Therapy

Nonprescription therapies have been tried in functional dyspepsia. These therapies are not regulated by the US FDA. Therefore, standardization of purity and potency is not enforced, and safety and efficacy are not regulated. Nevertheless, limited studies have been conducted with several of these therapies. Products containing peppermint (or L-menthol) and caraway may have some benefit in functional dyspepsia. Acupuncture has also been evaluated by a Cochrane review but the data was felt to be too limited to provide a clear conclusion. These therapies can be considered, but patients should be informed of the limited data related to benefits and risks.

Chey WD, Lacy BE, Cash BD, et al. A novel, duodenal-release formulation of a combination of caraway oil and L-menthol for the treatment of functional dyspepsia: a randomized controlled trial. *Clin Transl Gastroenterol.* 2019;10:e00021. [PMID: 30939487]

Deutsch JK, Levitt J, Hass DJ. Complementary and alternative medicine for functional gastrointestinal disorders. *Am J Gastroenterol.* 2020;115:350–364. [PMID: 32079860]

Lan L, Zeng F, Liu GJ, et al. Acupuncture for functional dyspepsia. *Cochrane Database Syst Rev.* 2014;CD008487. [PMID: 25306866]

von Arnim U, Peitz U, Vinson B, et al. STW 5, a phytopharmacon for patients with functional dyspepsia: results of a multicenter, placebo-controlled double-blind study. *Am J Gastroenterol.* 2007;102:1268–1275. [PMID: 17531013]

▶ Course & Prognosis

Similar to other functional gastrointestinal disorders, functional dyspepsia can cause chronic symptoms which can be variable in intensity and change over time. Population-based studies in the US and Iceland suggest that during 10–12 years of follow-up, approximately 15–20% of people have persistent symptoms, 40–52% of patients have resolution of symptoms, and 30–35% of patients symptoms change and meet criteria for another functional gastrointestinal disorder.

Halder SLS, Locke GB, Schleck CD, et al. Natural history of functional gastrointestinal disorders: a 12-year longitudinal population-based study. *Gastroenterology.* 2007;133:799–807. [PMID: 17678917]

Olafsdottir LB, Gudjonsson H, Jonsdottir HH, et al. Natural history of functional gastrointestinal disorders: comparison of two longitudinal population-based studies. *Dig Liver Dis.* 2012;44:211–217. [PMID: 22137573]

Disorders of Gastric & Small Bowel Motility

19

Jennifer X. Cai, MD, MPH

Walter W. Chan, MD, MPH

ESSENTIALS OF DIAGNOSIS

▶ The three most common causes of gastroparesis are idiopathic, diabetic, and postsurgical.

▶ Chronic intestinal pseudo-obstruction (CIPO) involves intermittent failure of intestinal peristalsis in the small or large intestine, or both.

▶ Noninvasive imaging or endoscopy, or both, should be used to rule out mechanical obstruction in patients being worked up for gastroparesis or CIPO.

▶ The standardized 4-hour gastric emptying scintigraphy scan using a low-fat, egg-white meal is the recommended test for gastroparesis.

▶ Accelerated gastric emptying and dumping syndrome are often related to postgastric surgery and may have symptoms that mimic delayed emptying.

General Considerations

Altered gastric and small bowel motility result in either delayed gastric emptying or rapid transit. Among the disorders of gastric and small bowel motility discussed in this chapter are gastroparesis, CIPO, dumping syndrome, and rapid transit dysmotility of the small bowel.

Gastroparesis and CIPO are chronic long-term problems that have a variety of causes and can be neuropathic or myopathic. Treatment of these conditions includes dietary, medical, and, rarely, surgical therapies. Research in gastroparesis is ongoing with a focus on improving diagnostics and newer therapeutic agents. Dumping syndrome is a postsurgical iatrogenic problem that is occurring less often in relation to gastric ulcer surgery, but may be increasing among bariatric surgery patients in tandem with the increase in surgical treatment of obesity. Patient education, dietary change, and treatment of underlying medical problems are important factors in the overall management of these motility disorders.

Pathogenesis

Normal gastric emptying requires coordinated efforts by the muscles that control the four regions of the stomach, nerves that modulate the actions of these muscles, and chemical mediators. Important events that occur during gastric filling and emptying include fundic relaxation (accommodation) in response to food ingestion, antral contractions and churning (trituration) of large food particles, and finally pyloric relaxation.

The neurogenic network of the stomach includes elements of both the central nervous system (CNS) and the enteric nervous system (ENS). The CNS elements involve both sympathetic and parasympathetic fibers. Sympathetic fibers arise from the thoracic spinal nerves, extending to postganglionic nerves that run along the celiac plexus and the vascular supply to the stomach. The sympathetic innervation includes afferent pain fibers that arise from the stomach, as well as motor fibers that innervate the pyloric sphincter. The parasympathetic innervation stems from the right and left vagal trunks, which eventually divide into multiple branches that course throughout the stomach wall and synapse with the ENS.

The ENS is an independent branch of the peripheral nervous system that is divided into two plexuses: the submucosal (Meissner) and the myenteric (Auerbach) plexuses. The submucosal plexus receives only parasympathetic input and innervates the cells of epithelial layer and muscular externa. The myenteric plexus, on the other hand, is situated between the middle circular and the outer longitudinal muscle layers, receiving both sympathetic and parasympathetic input. It mediates the motor function of both muscle layers and the secretory functions of the mucosa.

The interstitial cells of Cajal (ICCs) are the "pacemaker" cells of the stomach. They are located in the myenteric plexus and are responsible for basal slow-wave activity, which occurs at 3 cycles per minute. This slow-wave activity is also called the electronic control activity or the pacesetter potential. The ICCs are also responsible for bridging the myogenic and neurogenic control mechanisms.

The migrating motor complex (MMC) is the pattern of motility activity that occurs in the fasted state. It is a 1–2 hour cycle beginning in the stomach or small intestine and divided into three phases. Phase I (45–60 minutes) is a quiescent period. Phase II (30 minutes) is a period of random intermittent contractions. Lastly, phase III (5–15 minutes), also called the activity front, is a period in which bursts of rapid, even-paced uninterrupted peristaltic contractions occur.

Upon ingesting a meal, the MMC is abolished. Gastric accommodation occurs with distention of the fundus to make room for the incoming ingested contents. This response is mediated by the parasympathetic activity from the vagal nerve through cholinergic neurotransmitters, and inhibitory input by neurotransmitters such as nitric oxide, vasointestinal peptide, and serotonin.

The ingested contents upon entering the stomach are distributed, triturated, and then emptied into the duodenum. Liquids are usually dispersed and emptied immediately. The rate of liquid emptying is slowed by increased osmolarity, nutrient content, and carbonation. Solids, on the other hand, are stored in the fundus, churned in the antrum, and emptied in two phases: a lag period and a linear emptying period. The two periods occur over 3–4 hours, with the lag period lasting 1–3 hours. During the lag period, food particles move proximally to distally and undergo trituration and redistribution. Trituration occurs in the antrum with high-amplitude contraction waves that propagate proximally to distally. The food particles are reduced to a size of approximately 1–2 mm in diameter prior to emptying. The pylorus ultimately regulates how much content is emptied into the duodenal bulb by coordinated contractions and maintenance of the lumen with fixed tone.

Besides mechanical factors, neurohormonal factors also control the rate of emptying. Glucagon and incretins (eg, amylin and glucagon-like peptide 1) slow gastric emptying. The vagus provides both excitatory and inhibitory innervation. The presence of chyme in the duodenum provides negative feedback on the rate of emptying as mediated by duodenal distention, acidification, or perfusion with fats and protein. The regulation of duodenal intake controls the level of postprandial hyperglycemia from nutrient absorption.

Camilleri M. Integrated upper gastrointestinal response to food intake. *Gastroenterology*. 2006;131:640–658. [PMID: 16890616]

Kindt S, Tack J. Impaired gastric accommodation and its role in dyspepsia. *Gut*. 2006;55:1685–1691. [PMID: 16854999]

GASTROPARESIS & CHRONIC INTESTINAL PSEUDO-OBSTRUCTION

▶ General Considerations

Gastroparesis is characterized by delayed gastric emptying that is not associated with the presence of an obstructing structural lesion in the stomach or distally in the gastrointestinal tract. Many disorders that interfere with the normal neuromuscular coordination of the stomach can lead to gastroparesis (Table 19–1). The three most common causes are idiopathic, diabetic, and postsurgical. A tertiary referral series of 146 patients showed the causes of gastroparesis to be 36% idiopathic, 29% diabetic, 14% postgastric surgery, 7.5% Parkinson disease, 4.8% collagen vascular disorders, 4.1% intestinal pseudo-obstruction, and 6% miscellaneous causes (eg, paraneoplastic syndrome, superior mesenteric artery syndrome, and median arcuate ligament syndrome). The idiopathic causes included acute viral-like gastroenteritis (23%), gastroesophageal reflux disease (GERD) and nonulcer dyspepsia (19%), and cholecystectomy.

CIPO is characterized by obstructive symptoms generated from the small or large bowel occurring in the absence of anatomic obstruction. It is a severe form of dysmotility that is considered a failure or insufficiency of the "intestinal pump." Like gastroparesis, CIPO has a wide variety of causes (Table 19–2). These can generally be separated into congenital

Table 19–1. Causes of gastroparesis.

Gastroesophageal diseases
 Gastroesophageal reflux
 Gastritis (chronic or acute)
 Acute gastroenteritis (cytomegalovirus)
 Atrophic gastritis
 Peptic ulcer disease

Neuromuscular disorders
 Muscular dystrophy
 Parkinson disease

Systemic disorders
 Diabetes mellitus
 Hypothyroidism
 Uremia
 Chronic liver disease
 Anorexia nervosa

Rheumatologic disorders
 Scleroderma

Surgical procedures
 Gastrectomy
 Roux-en-Y syndrome
 Vagotomy
 Pyloromyotomy
 Pancreatectomy
 Antireflux operations
 Combined heart-lung transplantation

Trauma
 Head injuries
 Spinal cord injuries

Other etiologies
 Idiopathic
 Medications
 Idiopathic pseudo-obstruction
 Amyloidosis

Table 19–2. Causes of chronic intestinal pseudo-obstruction.

Myopathic processes
  Myotonic dystrophy
  Duchenne muscular dystrophy

Postoperative states
  Ileus
  Ogilvie syndrome (colonic pseudo-obstruction)

Autoimmune disorders
  Systemic lupus erythematosus
  Scleroderma
  Dermatomyositis
  Polymyositis
  Celiac disease
  Autoimmune myositis or ganglionitis

Oncologic disorders
  Pheochromocytoma
  Paraneoplastic syndrome (small cell cancer,
    ganglioneuroblastoma)
  Multiple myeloma

Hematologic disorders
  Sickle cell disease

Infectious/postinfectious disorders
  Chagas disease
  Cytomegalovirus
  Varicella-zoster virus
  Epstein-Barr virus
  Kawasaki disease

Endocrine disorders
  Diabetes mellitus
  Hypoparathyroidism
  Hypothyroidism

Metabolic disorders
  Mitochondrial cytopathies

Toxins
  Fetal alcohol syndrome
  Jellyfish envenomation

Drugs
  Chemotherapy
  Diltiazem and nifedipine

Developmental disorders
  Delayed maturation of interstitial cells of Cajal

Other etiologies
  Ehlers-Danlos syndrome
  Eosinophilic gastroenteritis
  Angioedema
  Crohn's disease
  Radiation enteritis

The true prevalence of gastroparesis has been difficult to study due to underdiagnosis and the lack of inexpensive diagnostic testing that is also widely available. A large population-based study in Olmsted County, Minnesota, estimated the age-adjusted prevalence of definite gastroparesis, defined as delayed gastric emptying on scintigraphy and typical symptoms for more than 3 months, to be 24.4 per 100,000 persons (95% confidence interval [CI], 15.7–32.6). Other population studies have shown upper gastrointestinal symptoms to be present in 11–18% of diabetic patients, with 50–65% of them having delayed gastric emptying. The mean age of gastroparetic patients in one study was 45 years, with a mean age of onset of 33.7 years. The prevalence of gastroparesis per 100,000 persons was 9.6 among men versus 37.8 among women. It is unclear whether gender influences the pathophysiology of gastroparesis or if this represents a difference in health care–seeking behavior between men and women. A recent study found a higher proportion of women had gastroparesis of idiopathic etiology compared to men (69% vs 46%) as well as more severe symptoms including stomach and postprandial fullness, early satiety, bloating, and upper abdominal pain. An overlap syndrome of gastroparesis and functional dyspepsia has been noted, and 25–42% of patients with functional dyspepsia have concomitant gastroparesis.

Bytzer P, Talley NJ, Leemon M, et al. Prevalence of gastrointestinal symptoms associated with diabetes mellitus: a population-based survey of 15000 adults. *Arch Intern Med.* 2001;10:1989–1096. [PMID: 11525701]

Jung HK, Choung RS, Locke GR 3rd, et al. The incidence, prevalence, and outcomes of patients with gastroparesis in Olmsted County, Minnesota, from 1996 to 2006. *Gastroenterology.* 2009;136:1225–1233. [PMID: 19249393]

Maleki D, Locke GR 3rd, Camilleri M, et al. Gastrointestinal tract symptoms among persons with diabetes mellitus in the community. *Arch Intern Med.* 2000;9:2808–2816. [PMID: 11025791]

Parkman HP, Yamada G, Van Natta ML, et al. Ethinic, racial, and sex differences in etiology, symptoms, treatment, and symptom outcomes of patients with gastroparesis. *Clin Gastroenterol Hepatol.* 2019;17(8):1489–1499. [PMID: 30404035]

▶ **Clinical Findings**

A. Symptoms & Signs

Typical complaints of gastroparesis include postprandial nausea, vomiting, belching, early satiety, bloating, discomfort, or pain. Reflux symptoms are also common. Chronic symptoms include weight loss or electrolyte disturbances, or both. Signs and symptoms of nutritional and vitamin deficiencies that may be noted include temporal wasting and loss of subcutaneous fat (malnutrition), gum bleeding (vitamin C), visual changes with night blindness (vitamin A), neuropathy, or impaired memory and confusion (folate, vitamin B_{12}). Dysphagia or odynophagia may occur as a result of reflux esophagitis. Diarrhea and malabsorption may be a consequence of bacterial overgrowth caused by altered peristalsis.

versus acquired causes, and myopathic versus neuropathic processes. Because gastroparesis and CIPO have very similar clinical approaches, this section discusses the assessment and treatment of these conditions together.

Table 19–3. Common medications that may affect gastric emptying.

Delay Gastric Emptying	Accelerate Gastric Emptying
Calcium channel blockers (nifedipine diltiazem, verapamil, others) Potassium Dopamine Sucralfate Aluminum hydroxide Opiates Tricyclic antidepressants (imipramine, amitriptyline, desipramine) L-Dopa	Bulk laxatives Diazepam Macrolide antibiotics (erythromycin, clarithromycin, azithromycin) Antiemetics (metoclopramide)

Symptoms to look for include dry mouth, eyes, or vagina; difficulties with visual accommodation in bright light; anhidrosis (absence of sweating); impotence; dizziness on standing; scleroderma symptoms such as Raynaud phenomenon, skin tightening, and peripheral paresthesia; and numbness or focal weaknesses. A medication history can elicit drugs that may contribute to altered gastric motility (Table 19–3).

The examination should include assessment of volume status for dehydration (eg, orthostasis, pallor, and poor skin turgor) and signs of metabolic alkalosis, such as decreased respirations. Abdominal examination may reveal distention or surgical scars. The examiner should auscultate for obstructive high-pitched or absent bowel sounds, and palpate for focal tenderness or mass. A succussion splash may be heard when auscultating over the stomach while shaking the abdomen from side to side for 1 hour or more postprandially. The examiner should also test for abdominal wall-related pain by observing for Carnett sign (positive when tenderness is increased upon tensing of the abdominal muscles). Findings suggesting diabetic microvascular complications should be noted (eg, retinopathy and sensory or autonomic neuropathy). Signs of recurrent vomiting may include worn tooth enamel. Nutritional deficiencies may manifest as brittle hair and nails, cheilosis, glossitis, and tetany.

Symptoms can also be assessed by a validated instrument, the Gastroparesis Cardinal Symptom Index (GCSI), which was developed for measurement of three subsets of symptoms, including postprandial fullness/early satiety, nausea/vomiting, and bloating. The GCSI, which utilizes a two-week recall period, as well as a daily diary version, GCSI-DD, have been validated for measuring symptom severity, however, their use have been mostly limited to clinical trials.

B. Imaging & Endoscopic Studies

Radiologic studies include plain film abdominal radiographs, computed tomography of the abdomen, small bowel follow-through examination, and magnetic resonance imaging (MRI). Oral contrast should be water soluble to prevent

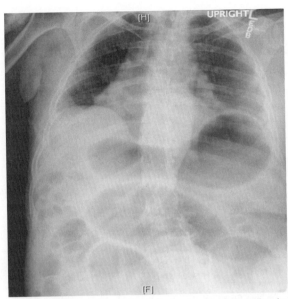

▲ **Figure 19–1.** Chronic intestinal pseudo-obstruction is seen on plain upright abdominal film. The stomach and small bowel are distended with intestinal gas.

formation of barium concretions in the gastrointestinal tract with dysmotility. Gastroparesis may be demonstrated by retained contrast in the stomach or its slow gastric transit into the small bowel. In CIPO, abdominal films may show dilated loops of small bowel and air-fluid levels (Figure 19–1), and small bowel follow-through studies may help rule out obstructive lesions and estimate small bowel transit time. MRI can measure gastric emptying and accommodation, and may provide additional information including gastroduodenal motility. However, its use in the evaluation for gastroparesis is still limited to the research setting.

Upper endoscopy is useful for ruling out a mechanical obstruction of the upper gastrointestinal tract (eg, masses, peptic ulcer disease [PUD], complications of pyloric stenosis, or acute PUD with antral edema). Retained food despite overnight fast may also be seen in the stomach during upper endoscopy in patients with gastroparesis.

C. Scintigraphy

The best current clinical test for delayed gastric emptying is gastric emptying scintigraphy using radionuclide technetium 99–labeled food. The test involves ingestion of a radiolabeled meal prepared by cooking radioisotope into the solid portion, which is usually a soft-textured food such as eggs. Scintigraphy is then performed 1–4 hours after ingestion (Figures 19–2A and B). Retention is abnormal when more than 90% of the tracer remains in the stomach at 1 hour, more than 60% at 2 hours, or more than 10% at 4 hours.

Tests shorter than 4 hours are less accurate for several reasons, including reduced sensitivity. Furthermore, the lag

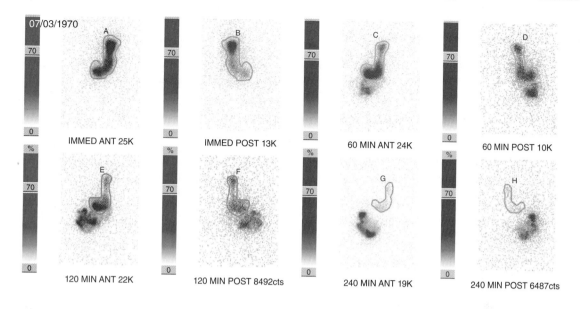

07/03/1970

IMMED ANT 25K   IMMED POST 13K   60 MIN ANT 24K   60 MIN POST 10K

120 MIN ANT 22K   120 MIN POST 8492cts   240 MIN ANT 19K   240 MIN POST 6487cts

500μCi 99m TCSC EGG sandwich (120 ml H$_2$O)
GASTRIC EMPTYING at 60 MIN is 32%
120 MIN is 60%
240 MIN is 96%

▲ **Figure 19–2A.** A normal ^{99m}Tc-labeled 4-hour gastric emptying scintigraphy showing normal volume of gastric residuals at baseline, 1, 2, and 4 hours after ingestion of test meal. (Reproduced with permission from Dr. Carlos A. Rabito, Massachusetts General Hospital.)

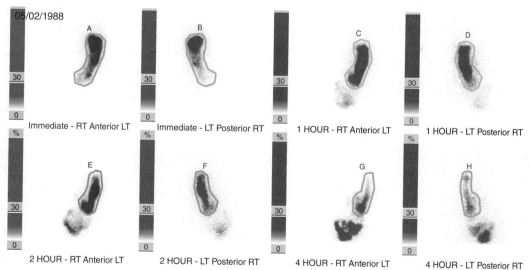

05/02/1988

Immediate - RT Anterior LT   Immediate - LT Posterior RT   1 HOUR - RT Anterior LT   1 HOUR - LT Posterior RT

2 HOUR - RT Anterior LT   2 HOUR - LT Posterior RT   4 HOUR - RT Anterior LT   4 HOUR - LT Posterior RT

99mTc Sulfur Colloid 0.53 mCi
EGG SANDWICH + 120 mL WATER
Gastric Emptying @ 1 HOUR is 12%
2 HOUR is 26%
4 HOUR is 76%

▲ **Figure 19–2B.** An abnormal ^{99m}Tc-labeled 4-hour gastric emptying scintigraphy showing decreased clearance (or increased retention) at 1, 2, and 4 hours after ingestion. (Reproduced with permission from Dr. Carlos A. Rabito, Massachusetts General Hospital.)

period is variable; some patients with prolonged lag phases have apparently normal 4-hour tests due to a "catch-up" in gastric emptying. Gastric residual measured at 4 hours after ingestion has a 100% sensitivity and 70% specificity for gastroparesis.

There had been some concerns about the lack of standardization of the procedure, and several proposed protocols have been suggested. A consensus statement from experts of the American Neurogastroenterology and Motility Society and the Society of Nuclear Medicine recommends a standardized protocol with a 4-hour test using low-fat, egg-white meal. Scintigraphy measurements are then taken at 0, 1, 2, and 4 hours after ingestion.

Another use of scintigraphy is the assessment of gastric accommodation. By dividing the area of interest into a distal and proximal segment and radiographically measuring the gastric volume in each segment, the regional changes over time can be assessed. A normal stomach with appropriate accommodation usually shows redistribution of the meal to the distal segment after accumulation in the proximal segment. Impaired gastric accommodation can be seen in diabetic vagal neuropathy, postvagotomy surgery, postfundoplication dyspepsia, and functional dyspepsia.

Abell TL, Camilleri M, Donohoe K, et al. Consensus recommendations for gastric emptying scintigraphy: a joint report of the American Neurogastroenterology and Motility Society and the Society of Nuclear Medicine. *Am J Gastroenterol.* 2008;103: 753–763. [PMID: 18028513]

Guo JP, Maurer AH, Fisher RS, et al. Extending gastric emptying scintigraphy from 2 to 4 hours detects more patients with gastroparesis. *Dig Dis Sci.* 2001;46:24–29. [PMID: 11270790]

Revicki DA, Camilleri M, Kuo B, et al. Evaluating symptom outcomes in gastroparesis clinical trials: validity and responsiveness of the Gastroparesis Cardinal Symptom Index-Daily Diary (GCSI-DD). *Neurogastroenterol Motil.* 2012;24(5):456–463. [PMID: 22284754]

Tougas G, Eaker EY, Abell TL, et al. Assessment of gastric emptying using a low fat meal: establishment of international control values. *Am J Gastroenterol.* 2000;95:1456–1462. [PMID: 10894578]

Ziessman HA, Bonta DV, Goetze S, et al. Experience with a simplified, standardized 4-hour gastric-emptying protocol. *J Nucl Med.* 2007;48:568–572. [PMID: 17401093]

D. Breath Testing

Another tool to measure gastric emptying is breath testing using a solid meal with nonradioactive isotope ^{13}C-labeled medium-chain triglycerides, octanoate, or spirulina. When ingested, the ^{13}C-labeled octanoate or spirulina is rapidly absorbed in the small intestine and metabolized by the liver into $^{13}CO_2$, which is excreted in the lungs and can then be measured in breath samples to indirectly estimate the rate of gastric emptying. This test has been shown to correlate strongly with scintigraphy by some clinical studies, and the ^{13}C spirulina technique has been approved by the US Food and Drug Administration (FDA). Further research in this

method of measuring gastric emptying is ongoing with the goal of using breath testing possibly as an office-based test in the future.

E. Special Tests of Motility

Ingestion and counting of radiopaque markers at 6 hours has been used to help identify the location of functional dysmotility. However, the clinical utility of this test is limited due to lack of standardization and possible uncertainty about whether markers are located in the stomach or within a segment of small bowel that overlaps the stomach.

For evaluation of small bowel motility, upper gastrointestinal and small bowel film series provide rough assessments at best. Quantification can be done by scintigraphy.

Antroduodenal manometry, which is not widely available, can provide information about the coordination of gastric and duodenal motility and can help differentiate between a neuropathic and a myopathic motility problem. It involves inserting a large catheter with multiple manometric sensors down to the antrum and the proximal small bowel, usually with the aid of fluoroscopy. The test is then performed over several hours in the fasting state, with a test meal, and sometimes with motility agents such as erythromycin. A neuropathic process that is intrinsic or visceral is usually characterized by uncoordinated contractions of normal amplitude, and abnormal or even absent phase III contractions of the MMC. The presence of phase III of the MMC is associated with a favorable prognosis, with better tolerance of enteral feedings and response to prokinetic drugs. In contrast, contraction amplitudes are reduced with myopathic processes, while spatial and temporal organization is preserved. Other antroduodenal manometric findings in CIPO may include simultaneous waveforms, retrograde propagation of phase III of the MMC, high-amplitude and high-frequency bursts during both fasting and fed periods, and sustained high-pressure zones in limited small bowel segments, or inability of a meal to initiate the fed period activity pattern.

F. Electrogastrography

Electrogastrography can record gastric muscular activity waveforms via cutaneously placed pads, similar to an electrocardiogram for the myocardium. Abnormal electrogastrograms are defined as observed dysrhythmia for more than 30% of the recording time or failure of an ingested meal to elicit increased amplitude in gastric signals. However, the electrogastrogram has not been widely used clinically. Furthermore, there has been little evidence that electrogastrography aids in the management of patients with gastroparesis.

G. Wireless Motility Capsule

The wireless motility capsule (SmartPill GI Monitoring System) is an ingested capsule that can deliver information on pressure, pH, and temperature wirelessly to a data recorder

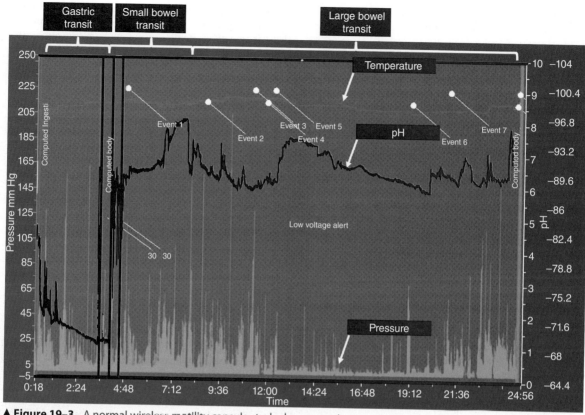

▲ **Figure 19–3.** A normal wireless motility capsule study demonstrating gastric transit, small bowel transit, and large bowel transit times as estimated by changes in pH, temperature, and pressure measurements.

worn by the patient (Figure 19–3). The pill is swallowed after ingesting a standard 220-kcal meal. The data permit estimates of gastric emptying time, combined small and large bowel transit time, colonic transit time, and total transit time, as well as study of pressure patterns from the gastrointestinal tract in the stomach, small bowel, and colon. The capsule has been approved by the FDA for use in studying gastroparesis. The device has been compared with gastric scintigraphy at a 2-hour emptying time (r = 0.63) and at a 4-hour emptying time (r = 0.73). The better correlation with 4-hour emptying time is likely due to the capsule, a nondigestible solid, being emptied from the stomach after the emptying of most of the test meal in the subject. The device is a reasonable alternative to conventional scintigraphy for gastroparesis. It has also been demonstrated to be useful in the study of small and large intestinal dysmotility. In the evaluation of constipation, the colonic transit time measured on the wireless motility capsule correlates with results from the conventional radiopaque markers study (r = 0.69) and demonstrates comparable diagnostic accuracy. This diagnostic modality may be particularly advantageous in patients with suspected multiregional dysmotility.

Kuo B, McCallum RW, Koch KL, et al. Comparison of gastric emptying of a nondigestible capsule to a radio-labelled meal in healthy and gastroparetic subjects. *Aliment Pharmacol Ther.* 2008;27:186–196. [PMID: 17973643]

Rao SS, Kuo B, McCallum RW, et al. Investigation of colonic and whole-gut transit with wireless motility capsule and radiopaque markers in constipation. *Clin Gastroenterol Hepatol.* 2009;7:537–544. [PMID: 19418602]

▶ **Differential Diagnosis**

Once mechanical obstruction is ruled out, vomiting related to gastroparesis must be distinguished from regurgitation, rumination syndrome, and the eating disorders of anorexia nervosa and bulimia. Rumination syndrome is characterized by daily, early postprandial regurgitation of food that occurs effortlessly without nausea, likely as a learned behavior. Daily vomiting is seen only in severe gastroparesis. In addition, associated symptoms of abdominal pain, discomfort, and bloating are more suggestive of gastroparesis. Other nonobstructive disorders with symptoms that may mimic gastroparesis include functional dyspepsia (postprandial distress syndrome subtype), accelerated gastric emptying, and esophageal dysmotility.

Treatment

Treatment should be tailored for each individual. The general approach to management involves correction of dehydration, malnutrition, and nutritional deficiencies; dietary modifications; use of pharmacologic motility agents, including prokinetics and antiemetics; and normalization of hyperglycemia in diabetic gastroparesis. For patients with refractory gastroparesis, more aggressive therapies include decompression by gastrostomy tubes, consideration of gastric electrical stimulation (GES), pyloric injection with botulinum toxin, and surgical treatment.

Camilleri M. Clinical practice. Diabetic gastroparesis. *N Engl J Med.* 2007;356:820–829. [PMID: 17314341]

Camilleri M, Bharucha AE, Farrugia G. Epidemiology, mechanisms, and management of diabetic gastroparesis. *Clin Gastroenterol Hepatol.* 2011;9:5–12. [PMID: 20951838]

Connor FL, Di Lorenzo C. Chronic intestinal pseudo-obstruction: assessment and management. *Gastroenterology.* 2006;130: S29–S36. [PMID: 16473068]

Park MI, Camilleri M. Gastroparesis: clinical update. *Am J Gastroenterol.* 2006;101:1129–1139. [PMID: 16696789]

Parkman HP, Hasler WL, Fisher RS; American Gastroenterological Association. American Gastroenterological Association medical position statement: diagnosis and treatment of gastroparesis. *Gastroenterology.* 2004;127:1589–1591. [PMID: 15521025]

A. Correction of Dehydration & Nutritional Deficiencies

During acute exacerbation of gastroparesis, dehydration and electrolyte imbalances should be corrected promptly. Hypokalemia and metabolic alkalosis are common in patients with persistent vomiting. Repletion can be instituted orally, enterally through feeding tubes, or parenterally. If the gastrointestinal tract is severely impaired, parenteral nutrition should be considered. Prolonged enteral feeding may require a jejunostomy tube to bypass the pylorus.

B. Dietary Modifications

Dietary recommendations include eating frequent, smaller sized meals. Solid foods can also be substituted for those that are pureed or liquid, such as soups. High-fat foods delay gastric emptying, as do high-fiber foods. In a randomized controlled study of patients with diabetic gastroparesis, small particle size reduced nausea, vomiting, postprandial fullness, bloating, regurgitation/heartburn, but not abdominal pain, compared to a control diet of large particle size and low glycemic index.

C. Pharmacotherapy

1. Prokinetics—Prokinetics available in the United States include metoclopramide and erythromycin, both of which can be administered orally and intravenously. Erythromycin (40–250 mg three times daily) is a macrolide antibiotic that has activity on motilin receptors on both neurons and smooth muscles. Metoclopramide (starting with 5 mg twice daily to 10–20 mg two to three times daily) is a $5\text{-}HT_4$ agonist and dopamine antagonist, and, therefore, contains both antiemetic and prokinetic activity. Both of these drugs have been shown in randomized controlled trials to improve symptoms by 25–68% and to increase gastric emptying in objective tests by 25–72%. Elixir forms of both drugs may have better absorption and subsequent bioavailability than pill forms. Intravenous erythromycin at 3 mg/kg (given at 125–250 mg three to four times daily) is more effective than placebo in hospitalized patients with gastroparesis and has been demonstrated to decrease symptoms, with positive objective measures of improved emptying. Unfortunately, the beneficial effect of erythromycin is often short lived due to tachyphylaxis, or tolerance to the medication. Rapid development of tolerance to the medication may be due to saturation of motilin receptors and their subsequent downregulation. The treatment effect of erythromycin significantly drops after 4 weeks, although some patients may continue to experience benefit. Therefore, erythromycin may be best used during exacerbations of symptoms or on an intermittent basis in those unable to tolerate, those who need a holiday from, or those unresponsive to metoclopramide.

Several other prokinetics have been used clinically for gastroparesis but are not widely available in the United States. Other agents include cisapride, a parasympathomimetic that acts as a serotonin $5\text{-}HT_4$ agonist, and domperidone, a dopamine (D_2) receptor antagonist. Both drugs are available in Canada, Mexico, and Europe. Domperidone is available in the United States through an FDA investigational new drug (IND) program. Cisapride has been associated with long QT syndrome, which can predispose to torsades de pointes, causing the drug to be taken off the US market in March 2000. Likewise, domperidone has not been approved by the FDA due to risk of cardiac arrhythmia and its bioavailability in breast milk. However, both drugs have been found to be efficacious in treating gastroparesis. Additional concerns with metoclopramide and domperidone relate to CNS side effects, which include somnolence, mental function, anxiety, and depression. There are also medicolegal concerns about the chronic use of metoclopramide owing to adverse reactions (ie, neurologic effects and movement disorders). Early effects include akathisia (a sensation of "inner restlessness") and dystonia, and later effects may include tardive dyskinesia and parkinsonism. Because domperidone does not cross the blood-brain barrier, its CNS effects are notably less compared to metoclopramide. On the other hand, both domperidone and metoclopramide are equally effective in controlling symptoms of diabetic gastroparesis in comparative trials.

Another prokinetic agent, prucalopride, recently approved for chronic idiopathic constipation, is a highly selective 5-hydroxytryptamine 4 ($5\text{-}HT_4$) receptor agonist that was shown to significantly improve symptoms, quality of life, as well as gastric half emptying time in a randomized controlled trial of 34 patients with predominantly idiopathic gastroparesis.

2. Antiemetics—Antiemetics such as diphenhydramine, phenothiazine compounds, and even metoclopramide can help control symptoms of nausea. The more commonly used agents include prochlorperazine, trimethobenzamide, and promethazine. Serotonin (5-HT$_3$) antagonists, such as granisetron and ondansetron, are frequently used in chemotherapy patients but are also useful in gastroparesis. They act on the area postrema and peripheral afferent nerves. A neurokinin-1 receptor antagonist, aprepitant, failed to significantly improve nausea among gastroparesis patients in a randomized controlled trial (APRON) using a visual analogue scale as the primary outcome, however, the drug did result in improvement of several secondary outcome measures for nausea, vomiting, and overall symptoms using the GCSI score. Other agents used in clinical practice, albeit without strong supportive data, include benzodiazepines, synthetic cannabinoids, and transdermal scopolamine.

3. Alternative agents—Multiple other agents with different mechanisms have also been tried. Tegaserod (Zelnorm; 2–6 mg twice daily) is a partial 5-HT$_4$ receptor agonist that enhances gastric emptying, but no clinical trials have been undertaken specifically in patients with gastroparesis. It had been used with anecdotal success, but was removed from the market in early 2007 due to concerns about increased risk of myocardial infarction and stroke. More recently, the FDA approved the reintroduction of tegaserod in 2019 for irritable bowel syndrome with constipation in women under the age of 65 years. Agents with limited success and also with notable adverse cholinergic side effects include bethanechol (10–20 mg two to three times daily), a muscarinic cholinergic agent, and pyridostigmine (30 mg four times daily), an anticholinesterase.

4. Pain management—The management of pain in gastroparesis has not been specifically addressed in clinical studies. Currently, the most commonly used agents are tricyclic antidepressants (nortriptyline, amitriptyline), which have been shown to be effective in treating functional bowel disorders. Gabapentin, a γ-aminobutyric acid analog, has also been used as a motility-neutral pain modulator in patients with functional or dysmotility-related abdominal pain. Opioids commonly prescribed for chronic pain syndromes should be avoided given their adverse effects on gastrointestinal motility.

5. Other drugs—Pharmacologic treatment for disorders associated with CIPO include antibiotic regimens for bacterial overgrowth, which is usually treated with common antibiotics such as doxycycline, ciprofloxacin, metronidazole, or double-strength trimethoprim–sulfamethoxazole for 7–10 days. Rifaximin (400–1200 mg/day), a nonabsorbable antibiotic approved for use in traveler's diarrhea and irritable bowel syndrome, has also been shown to be effective for small bowel bacterial overgrowth and normalizing hydrogen breath tests.

Short-acting subcutaneous octreotide (50 μg subcutaneously at night) has been tried in patients with CIPO, and studies have shown that it increases MMCs in the small bowel. This therapy should be avoided in patients with concomitant bacterial overgrowth.

6. Investigational drugs—Some of the drugs currently under investigation include other prokinetics such as itopride, a dopamine receptor antagonist, and mosapride, a 5-HT$_4$ receptor agonist. Ghrelin agonists such as relamorelin are also under investigation. Several motilitides, which are motilin receptor agonists without some of the undesirable features of erythromycin, are also being studied. Azithromycin given intravenously has been compared with erythromycin and was found to result in higher antral contraction amplitude and motility index. Further study of its effects on symptom improvement is needed.

D. Normalization of Hyperglycemia

There is little evidence that controlling hyperglycemia has a direct relationship to symptom improvement. However, there is a well-established inverse relationship between blood glucose levels and rate of gastric emptying. Hyperglycemia is associated with delayed gastric emptying, as are euglycemia with normal gastric emptying and hypoglycemia with accelerated gastric emptying. Moreover, acute changes in blood glucose concentration have an effect on both gastric motor function and upper gastrointestinal symptoms. Evidence also suggests that response to prokinetics is partially determined by hyperglycemia. With regard to practical care of diabetic patients with gastroparesis, short-acting insulin should be dosed after, rather than prior, to eating to ensure that the patient tolerates the entire meal and to avoid hypoglycemia.

E. Decompression Gastrostomy Tubes & Jejunal Feeding Tubes

Advanced gastroparesis or CIPO may require decompression. Venting can be accomplished by a nasogastric tube or by a percutaneous endoscopic gastrostomy (PEG) or jejunostomy tube. Several feeding tubes have both a venting port upstream and a feeding port downstream. However, before placing the tube in a patient with severe symptoms, it is prudent to try nasal jejunal tube feeding first to test whether the patient can tolerate enteral feeding. Criteria for tube feeding include severe weight loss, multiple hospitalizations, and malnutrition.

F. Gastric Electrical Stimulation

Electrical stimulation of the stomach for treatment of gastroparesis is done laparoscopically by implanting a device into the antral muscular wall, with electrodes that connect to a pacemaker pocketed into the abdominal wall. The stimulation is classified based on the frequency of the electrical stimulus (high or low frequency). A high-frequency electrical stimulation device (Enterra, Medtronic) has been approved by the FDA through a humanitarian device exemption. An early crossover controlled trial of 33 patients with idiopathic or diabetic gastroparesis showed that the frequency of vomiting was decreased significantly, but overall effect on symptoms was not significant. Open-label long-term studies with follow-up of 3.4–3.7 years have shown relief of symptoms and decreased need for nutritional supplementation. More recent studies have demonstrated the efficacy of GES in decreasing vomiting symptoms associated with diabetic gastroparesis and idiopathic gastroparesis. However, gastric retention has only been shown to be decreased among diabetic, but not idiopathic, gastroparesis. This suggests that the effect of GES in decreasing gastroparesis symptoms may involve sensory modulation, rather than motility stimulation. Predictors of treatment success in patients receiving GES include diabetic gastroparesis, symptoms that are predominantly nausea and vomiting, and symptoms that do not require narcotic therapy. Although GES is a promising therapy, further studies are needed in this area.

Abell T, McCallum R, Hocking M, et al. Gastric electrical stimulation for medically refractory gastroparesis. *Gastroenterology*. 2003;125:421–428. [PMID: 12891544]

Abidi N, Starkebaum WL, Abell TL. An energy algorithm improves symptoms in some patients with gastroparesis and treated with gastric electrical stimulation. *Neurogastroenterol Motil*. 2006;18:334–338. [PMID: 16553589]

Carbone F, Van den Hooute K, Clevers E, et al. Prucalopride in gastroparesis: a randomized placebo-controlled crossover study. *Am J Gastroenterol*. 2019;114(8):1265–1274. [PMID: 31295161]

Hou Q, Lin Z, Mayo MS, et al. Is symptom relief associated with reduction in gastric retention after gastric electrical stimulation treatment in patients with gastroparesis? A sensitivity analysis with logistic regression models. *Neurogastroenterol Motil*. 2012;24:639–645. [PMID: 2249777]

McCallum RW, Sarosiek I, Parkman HP, et al. Gastric electrical stimulation with Enterra therapy improves symptoms of idiopathic gastroparesis. *Neurogastroenterol Motil*. 2013;25:815–e636. [PMID: 23895180]

Olausson EA, Störsrud S, Grundin H, et al. A small particle size diet reduces upper gastrointestinal symptoms in patients with diabetic gastroparesis: a randomized controlled trial. *Am J Gastroenterol*. 2014;109(3):375–385. [PMID: 24419482]

Pasricha PJ, Yates KP, Sarosiek I, et al. Aprepitant has mixed effects on nausea and reduces other symptoms in patients with pastroparesis and related disorders. *Gastroenterology*. 2018;154(1):65–76. [PMID: 29111115]

G. Pyloric Injection with Botulinum Toxin

Gastric emptying may be facilitated by keeping the pylorus relaxed. Injection of botulinum A toxin into the pyloric sphincter has been thought to paralyze the smooth muscle of the pylorus and antrum by inhibiting acetylcholine release. Several uncontrolled open-label trials have previously reported its efficacy in gastroparesis. However, two randomized, controlled trials have shown no treatment benefit in both subjective (symptoms) and objective (gastric emptying)

end points. These results suggest no role for pyloric sphincter botulinum toxin injection in the widespread treatment of gastroparesis.

H. Endoscopic Pyloromyotomy

Gastric peroral endoscopic myotomy (G-POEM) has recently emerged as a treatment for severe refractory gastroparesis. Initially described in 2013, G-POEM is a minimally invasive technique that consists of creating a submucosal tunnel extending to the pylorus, dissecting circular and oblique muscle layers, and closing the tunnel with endoscopic clips. The first systematic review of early outcomes of G-POEM across 10 studies and 292 patients revealed 100% technical success, symptomatic improvement in 84%, and an adverse event rate of 6.8%, however, controlled trials are still needed to assess longterm efficacy and identify predictors for treatment response.

Arts J, Holvoet L, Caenepeel P, et al. Clinical trial: a randomized-controlled crossover study of intrapyloric injection of botulinum toxin in gastroparesis. *Aliment Pharmacol Ther*. 2007;26:1251–1258. [PMID: 17944739]

Friedenberg FK, Palit A, Parkman HP, et al. Botulinum toxin A for the treatment of delayed gastric emptying. *Am J Gastroenterol*. 2008;103:416–423. [PMID: 18070232]

Spadaccini M, Maselli R, Chandrasekar VT, et al. Gastric peroral endoscopic pyloromyotomy for refractory gastroparesis: a systematic review of early outcomes with pooled analysis. *Gastrointest Endosc*. 2019;91(4):746–752. [PMID: 31809720]

I. Surgical Treatment

Surgical treatment is the last resort for both gastroparesis and CIPO and is rarely indicated. For gastroparesis, surgical placement of gastrostomy and jejunostomy tubes may be done for feeding and decompression. Definitive surgical treatment for gastroparesis includes a subtotal or complete gastrectomy. A systematic review of surgical therapy for gastroparesis found that gastrectomy may help postsurgical gastroparesis, but issued caution on surgical therapy for diabetic or idiopathic gastroparesis.

For CIPO, the surgical therapy aims to bypass areas of localized disease in the small intestine, or resect the colon for severe constipation. Again, caution is warranted when considering surgery in this condition as the original problem may manifest itself in unresected portions of the gut. If the disease is within both the upper and lower intestinal tract, colectomy is less likely to be beneficial. Gastrostomy, jejunostomy, or loop enterostomy may be done to shorten the gut, facilitate transit, and vent the bowel. Percutaneous colonoscopy in adult CIPO patients has shown success in reducing distention.

Small bowel transplantation is indicated for patients with end-stage parenteral nutrition–dependent pseudo-obstruction and complications of prolonged parenteral nutrition or line access.

Prognosis

Little is known about either the overall prognosis or the quality of life of patients with gastroparesis and CIPO. The disease can be long-standing and have a substantial impact on well-being. Symptom severity scales have been developed and validated and may be useful in clinical and research settings. The overall long-term prognosis is determined by the underlying disease process, if known. In general, postinfectious or postsurgical gastroparesis or CIPO are more likely to improve or resolve over time, while diabetic or idiopathic dysmotility tend to be chronic and require long-term therapy.

DUMPING SYNDROME & ACCELERATED GASTRIC EMPTYING

General Considerations

Dumping syndrome and accelerated gastric emptying are diseases that can occur after gastric surgery when a truncal vagotomy or gastrectomy has been performed. With the onset of medical treatment for PUD and *Helicobacter pylori* eradication, gastric ulcer surgery has significantly decreased, and expectedly, these postoperative accelerated gastric states have also decreased. Presently, bariatric surgery with Roux-en-Y gastric bypass causes dumping syndrome in as many as 50% of patients. Aside from the iatrogenic causes, diabetes with vagal dysfunction and Zollinger-Ellison syndrome can also be associated with rapid gastric emptying. Rapid gastric emptying is caused by high gastric pressures, impaired gastric accommodation, and the lack of a regulating pyloric sphincter.

Clinical Findings

A. Symptoms & Signs

Dumping syndrome can be characterized as early or late, each with different symptoms. Both types of dumping syndrome can occur in the same patient. Early dumping syndrome occurs during or immediately after a meal and is characterized by nausea, vomiting, bloating, cramping, diarrhea, dizziness, and fatigue. These early symptoms are hypothesized to be a result of neuroendocrine changes associated with a hyperosmolar load in the small bowel. Some of the postprandial upper abdominal symptoms associated with early dumping syndrome can be indistinguishable from those of delayed gastric emptying. Late dumping happens 1–3 hours after a meal and is characterized by hypoglycemia, weakness, sweating, and dizziness. Hypoglycemia occurs because a high carbohydrate content absorption into the small bowel evokes a strong insulin response with secondary hypoglycemia.

B. Diagnostic Tests

Dual-phase gastric scintigraphy using radiolabeled solids and liquids is the best diagnostic test. Hydrogen breath tests can be diagnostic in the appropriate clinical scenario. If early dumping is suspected, an early peak will be noted, usually within 1 hour of ingestion.

Treatment

The treatment of dumping syndrome involves mainly dietary modifications. These include switching to smaller, more frequent meals; minimizing ingestion of simple carbohydrates; avoiding simultaneous fluid intake with solids; and adding supplemental fiber (pectin, guar gum) to increase the viscosity of the ingested food and delay gastric emptying. Medical therapy includes acarbose (50–100 mg three times daily), an α-glucosidase inhibitor that blunts the rapid absorption of glucose. Short-acting (50 μg subcutaneously three times daily) or long-acting (10 mg intramuscularly every 4 weeks) octreotide acts by inhibiting effects on insulin and gut hormone release, as well as decreasing intestinal transit time. Short-term use is initially effective, but response is less optimal with longer use.

Didden P, Penning C, Masclee AA. Octreotide therapy in dumping syndrome: analysis of long-term results. *Aliment Pharmacol Ther.* 2006;24:1367–1375. [PMID: 17059518]

Hasler WL. Dumping syndrome. *Curr Treat Options Gastroenterol.* 2002;5:139–145. [PMID: 11879594]

RAPID TRANSIT DYSMOTILITY OF THE SMALL BOWEL

Rapid transit of small bowel contents occurs in postvagotomy diarrhea, short bowel syndrome, irritable bowel, diabetic enteropathy, or carcinoid syndrome. These syndromes, except for irritable bowel syndrome, can cause severe dehydration and electrolyte disturbances.

Scintigraphy or the lactulose hydrogen breath test can be diagnostic. Small bowel manometry is not widely available but may show high-amplitude contractions, rapid peristalsis, and prolonged duration.

Treatment

The initial focus of treatment is on correction of dehydration and electrolyte imbalance. Patients, once stabilized, should avoid hyperosmolar drinks and receive rehydration with iso-osmolar fluids. Parenteral support with intravenous fluids or even parenteral nutrition may be necessary for patients with <1 m of small bowel.

Loperamide (4 mg, 30 minutes prior to meals and bedtime) can decrease the gastrocolic reflex and slow motility. Verapamil (40 mg twice daily) or clonidine (0.1 mg twice daily), or both, may be used in conjunction with loperamide. Subcutaneous octreotide (50 μg twice daily) can be considered if other drugs fail.

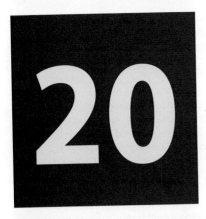

20

Acute Upper Gastrointestinal Bleeding

John R. Saltzman, MD

ESSENTIALS OF DIAGNOSIS

▶ Patients with acute upper gastrointestinal (GI) bleeding can present with hematemesis, melena, or hematochezia.

▶ Prognostic risk scores help predict low-risk and high-risk clinical outcomes.

▶ Stigmata of recent hemorrhage are endoscopic findings that predict further bleeding.

▶ Endoscopy provides diagnosis, prognosis, and therapy.

General Considerations

Nonvariceal upper GI bleeding is a common reason for emergency department visits and admissions to the hospital. It has been estimated that upper GI bleeding is responsible for over 230,000 Emergency Department visits per year and about 200,000 hospitalizations per year in the United States. In addition, about 100,000 patients per year develop upper GI bleeding during hospitalizations for other reasons.

Upper GI bleeding is by defined by a source of bleeding proximal to the ligament of Treitz. The natural history of nonvariceal upper GI bleeding is that approximately 80% of patients will stop bleeding spontaneously and in this group, no further urgent intervention will be needed. Thus about 20% of patients will undergo an endoscopic intervention to stop or prevent further bleeding. In patients treated endoscopically 10–20% will experience rebleeding, and if a patient rebleeds, there is a 10-fold increased mortality rate.

The overall in hospital mortality rate is 2–3% for patients with nonvariceal upper GI bleeding. Mortality is typically due to factors other than GI bleeding and occurs primarily in patients who are older and due to cardiovascular complications and comorbidities, and not from uncontrollable GI hemorrhage.

Abougergi MS, Travis AC, Saltzman JR. The in-hospital mortality rate for upper gastrointestinal hemorrhage is decreasing over two decades in the United States: a nationwide analysis. *Gastrointest Endosc.* 2015;81:882–888. [PMID: 25484324]

Laine L, Barkun AN, Saltzman JR, Martel M, Leontiadis GI. ACG Clinical Guideline: Upper Gastrointestinal and Ulcer Bleeding. *Am J Gastroenterol.* 2021;116(5):899–917. [PMID: 33929377]

Peery AF, Crockett SD, Murphy CC, et al. Burden and cost of gastrointestinal, liver, and pancreatic diseases in the United States: update 2018. *Gastroenterology.* 2019;156(1):254–272. [PMID: 30315778]

▶ Clinical Findings

A. Symptoms & Signs

The clinical characteristics of bleeding should be accurately described at the time of presentation. Hematemesis is overt bleeding with vomiting of fresh blood or clots. Melena refers to dark black and tarry-appearing stool, with a distinctive smell. The term "coffee grounds" describes gastric aspirates or vomitus that contains dark specks of old blood. Hematochezia is the passage of fresh blood or clots per rectum. Although bright red blood per rectum is usually indicative of a lower GI source, it may be seen in patients with brisk upper GI bleeding.

Concurrent with the initial evaluation of patients with suspected upper GI bleeding, resuscitation must be promptly instituted, with the goal of achieving hemodynamic stability. The evaluation must assess vital signs, the presence or absence of shock and hypovolemia, and medical comorbidities (malignancy, chronic obstructive pulmonary disease, coronary artery disease, etc.). Patients with postural hypotension have a significant blood volume loss of at least 10% and those with shock have a blood volume loss of at least 20%, a predictor of poor outcome. Medications used by the patient need to be reviewed with special attention given to antithrombotics, including the anticoagulant and antiplatelet agents.

Table 20–1. Risk factors for poor outcome in upper gastrointestinal bleeding.

Age >60
Shock (systolic blood pressure <100 mm Hg); pulse >100 beats/min
Malignancy or varices as bleeding source
Onset in hospital
Comorbid illness
Active bleeding (hematemesis, bright red blood in nasogastric tube, or hematochezia)
Recurrent bleeding
Severe coagulopathy

B. Risk Assessment

1. Clinical predictors—Factors that predict a good or a poor prognosis in patients with nonvariceal upper GI bleeding can be used to appropriately triage and manage patients. In patients presenting with upper GI bleeding, several clinical prognostic factors have been shown to be helpful in predicting a poor outcome (Table 20–1). Patients who experience onset of GI bleeding as inpatients hospitalized for other reasons have a higher rate of mortality compared with those who are outpatients. Age greater than 60 years is associated with an increased mortality. The mortality rate increases with the number of patient comorbidities.

Bethea ED, Travis AC, Saltzman JR. Initial assessment and management of patients with nonvariceal upper gastrointestinal bleeding. *J Clin Gastroenterol.* 2014;48:823–829. [PMID: 25090451]

2. Risk stratification scores—Clinical risk stratification scores have been developed to help optimize the management of patients with nonvariceal upper GI bleeding. The aims of these scores are to identify low-risk patients who can be discharged either directly from the emergency department or at an early stage of hospitalization, and to identify high-risk patients who are at risk for bad outcomes and need the most resources. These prognostic risk scores should be incorporated as part of routine clinical care to help direct triage decisions. Both the International Consensus Guidelines and the ACG guidelines on the management of patients with nonvariceal upper GI bleeding recommend the use of prognostic scales for the early risk stratification of patients into low- and high-risk categories for rebleeding and mortality.

A widely used prognostic risk score that only uses clinical information obtained at the time of presentation is the Glasgow-Blatchford score (GBS). The clinical information incorporated in this scoring system includes hemoglobin, blood urea nitrogen, pulse, systolic blood pressure, presence of syncope, melena, liver disease, and heart failure (Table 20–2). This scoring system for upper GI bleeding is valuable because all the information is available at initial presentation, and it does not require endoscopic performance to calculate. The GBS can be used to predict low-risk bleeders who may be able to be managed as an outpatient as well

Table 20–2. Glasgow-Blatchford score.

Variable	Points
Systolic Blood Pressure (mm Hg)	
100–109	1
90–99	2
<90	3
Blood Urea Nitrogen (mg/dL)	
>18 and <22	2
>22 and <28	3
>28 and <70	4
>70	6
Hemoglobin for Men (g/dL)	
12.0–12.9	1
10.0–11.9	3
<10.0	6
Hemoglobin for Women (g/dL)	
10.0–11.9	1
<10.0	6
Other Markers at Presentation	
Heart rate >100 beats/min	1
Melena	1
Syncope	2
Liver disease	2
Cardiac disease/failure	2

Data from Blatchford O, Murray WR, Blatchford M. A risk score to predict need for treatment for upper-gastrointestinal haemorrhage. *Lancet.* 2000;356(9238):1318–21. [PMID: 11073021].

as high-risk bleeders who may need blood transfusions and endoscopic interventions. The GBS has been best validated to predict low risk patients and a GBS score of 0–1 has been recommended by the European Society of Gastrointestinal Endoscopy, as it is 98% sensitive at predicting low-risk (although specificity is 27%). Patients triaged to outpatient management should be informed of the risk of further bleeding and be scheduled for prompt evaluation by a gastroenterologist and endoscopy.

A high-risk stratification score for upper GI bleeding derived in the United States that also only uses information at the time of the initial presentation is called the AIMS65 score. This score is highly predictive of mortality and is easy to calculate as it uses an equal weighting of its five components: Albumin <3.0 g/dL, INR >1.5, Mental status changes, Systolic blood pressure less than 90 mm Hg, and age greater than 65 years. Patients at high risk have two or more of these risk factors present. The AIMS65 score has been directly compared to the GBS in several studies and may be superior to the GBS for predicting mortality.

Although the International Consensus and ACG guidelines recommend incorporation of risk stratification scores in the care of patients with upper GI bleeding, there has not been widespread adoption of these scores in clinical practice. Barriers to implementation of risk scores vary by physician's specialty and training status; and include a lack in knowledge of GI bleeding risk scores, and perceived lack of utility. Risk scores in GI bleeding should be used in conjunction with clinical judgment and should be understood to be a useful evidence-based adjunct to help with patient triage and to determine the severity of bleeding (Figure 20–1).

Banister T, Spiking J, Ayaru L. Discharge of patients with an acute upper gastrointestinal bleed from the emergency department using an extended Glasgow-Blatchford Score. *BMJ Open Gastroenterol.* 2018;5:e000225. [PMID: 30233807]

Barkun A, Almadi M, Kuipers EJ, et al. Management of nonvariceal upper gastrointestinal bleeding: guideline recommendations from the International Consensus Group. *Ann Intern Med.* 2019;171(11):805–822. [PMID: 31634917]

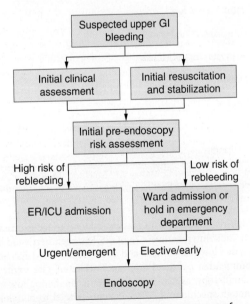

▲ **Figure 20–1.** Algorithm for the management of acute upper gastrointestinal bleeding. ER, emergency room; ICU, intensive care unit. (Adapted with permission from Eisen GM, Dominitz JA, Faigel DO, et al. Standards of Practice Committee. An annotated algorithmic approach to upper gastrointestinal bleeding. *Gastrointest Endosc.* 2001;53(7):853–858.)

Barkun A, Bardou M, Kuipers EJ, et al, International Consensus Upper Gastrointestinal Bleeding Conference Group. International consensus recommendations on the management of patients with nonvariceal upper gastrointestinal bleeding. *Ann Intern Med.* 2010;152:101–113. [PMID: 20083829]

Gralnek IM, Dumonceau JM, Kuipers EJ, et al. Diagnosis and management of nonvariceal upper gastrointestinal hemorrhage: European Society of Gastrointestinal Endoscopy (ESGE) Guideline. *Endoscopy.* 2015;47(10):a1–a46.

Kumar NL, Travis AC, Saltzman JR. Initial management and timing of endoscopy in nonvariceal upper GI bleeding. *Gastrointest Endosc.* 2016;84(1):10–17.

Laine L. Clinical Practice. Upper gastrointestinal bleeding due to a peptic ulcer. *N Engl J Med.* 2016;374(24):2367–2376. [PMID: 27305194]

Robertson M, Majumdar A, Boyapati R, et al. Risk stratification in acute upper GI bleeding: comparison of the AIMS65 score with the Glasgow-Blatchford and Rockall scoring systems. *Gastrointest Endosc.* 2016;83(6):1151–1160. [PMID: 26515955]

Saltzman JR, Tabak YP, Hyett BH, et al. A simple risk score accurately predicts in-hospital mortality, length of stay, and cost in acute upper GI bleeding. *Gastrointest Endosc.* 2011;74:1215–1224.

▶ **Treatment of Upper Gastrointestinal Bleeding**

A. Medical Therapy

1. Initial therapy—Patients need to have at minimum two large-bore peripheral intravenous access catheters (18 gauge or larger). Crystalloid fluids (normal saline or lactated Ringers solution) should be initially administered to maintain an adequate blood pressure. Supplemental oxygen should be administered routinely. Patients who are not able to adequately protect their airways or patients with ongoing severe hematemesis and at increased risk for aspiration should be considered for elective endotracheal intubation.

Concurrent with the initial evaluation of patients with suspected upper GI bleeding is resuscitation, with the goal of achieving hemodynamic stability. Red blood cell transfusions should target a hemoglobin >7 g/dL. The most direct evidence favoring a restrictive transfusion strategy comes from a randomized trial that included over 900 adults with acute upper GI bleeding. The patients were randomly assigned to receive transfusions if the hemoglobin was <9 g/dL or to receive transfusions if the hemoglobin was <7 g/dL. Patients in the <7 g/dL transfusion arm had lower mortality rates than those in the <9 g/dL transfusion arm (5% vs 9%; adjusted hazard ratio 0.55), supporting the use of a more restrictive approach to transfusion. However, in patients with clinical evidence of intravascular volume depletion, hemodynamic instability or comorbidities such as acute coronary syndrome or active neurologic disease, a higher hemoglobin level of 9–10 g/dL may need to be targeted.

In patients with a coagulopathy, if needed to help with hemostasis the coagulopathy should be corrected to an INR <2.5, preferably with transfusion of prothrombin complex concentrate as it allows for rapid reversal. Alternatively reversal can be accomplished with fresh frozen plasma (slower and higher volume) or administration of vitamin K (although may cause a hypercoagulable state). In patients with a low platelet count (<50,000), platelet transfusion should be considered.

2. Medications—Various medications have been used to treat patients with nonvariceal upper GI bleeding, including antacids, histamine-2 (H_2)-receptor antagonists, proton pump inhibitors (PPIs), and octreotide. The use of antacids and H_2-receptor antagonists has not been shown to alter the natural history of patients with acute upper GI bleeding and is not recommended.

A. Proton pump inhibitors—In studies of PPIs in select patients with nonvariceal upper GI bleeding, a benefit of medical treatment has been demonstrated. PPIs are the only drugs that can maintain a gastric pH of greater than 6.0 and can prevent fibrinolysis of an ulcer clot. The use of PPIs in the treatment of patients with upper GI bleeding has been widely adopted.

There have now been multiple studies showing the benefits of the use of PPIs in patients with high-risk stigmata of hemorrhage who undergo endoscopic therapy. This was initially shown in a study of patients who had successful hemostasis using combination therapy. Patients were then randomized to a bolus infusion of omeprazole, 80 mg, followed by a continuous infusion of 8 mg/h, versus a placebo infusion. This study showed that bleeding is reduced in patients who undergo endoscopic therapy and receive high-dose PPIs relative to those who undergo endoscopic therapy alone.

In patients initially treated in the emergency department with a bolus infusion of omeprazole followed by a continuous infusion, the need for endoscopic therapy is reduced, however patient clinical outcomes are not changed. The natural history of peptic ulcers treated with endoscopic therapies shows that it typically takes about 3 days for most high-risk lesions for further bleeding to become low-risk lesions.

The benefit of PPIs in the management of acute upper GI bleeding appears to be a class effect and PPI dosing should be similar. Guidelines recommend high dose PPIs such as an 80-mg bolus followed by an 8 mg/h infusion for 72 hours in patients who have received successful endoscopic therapy. An alternative option is a twice daily dosing of a PPI (after an 80 mg intravenous bolus) such as omeprazole 40 mg intravenously twice daily. Patients who remain stable for 72 hours after endoscopic treatment should be switched to a twice-daily standard dose of an oral PPI for 14 days before being changed to a once daily PPI.

B. Octreotide—Octreotide can be used to treat patients with nonvariceal upper GI bleeding. Although this medication is widely used in patients with variceal bleeding, it is also helpful as an adjunctive treatment in some patients with nonvariceal bleeding. However, octreotide should not be given as the primary treatment in patients with nonvariceal upper GI bleeding. The use of octreotide can be considered in patients who have persistent bleeding on optimal medical management, including PPIs, and are poor surgical risks (eg, those with multiple comorbidities already in the hospital).

Cheng HC, Wu CT, Chang WL, Cheng WC, Chen WY, Sheu BS. Double oral esomeprazole after a 3-day intravenous esomeprazole infusion reduces recurrent peptic ulcer bleeding in high-risk patients: a randomised controlled study. *Gut.* 2014;63:1864–1872. [PMID: 24658598]

Jairath V, Kahan BC, Gray A, et al. Restrictive versus liberal blood transfusion for acute upper gastrointestinal bleeding (TRIGGER): a pragmatic, open-label, cluster randomised feasibility trial. *Lancet.* 2015;386:137–144. [PMID: 25956718]

Lau JY, Leung WK, Wu JC, et al. Omeprazole before endoscopy in patients with gastrointestinal bleeding. *N Engl J Med.* 2007;356:1631–1640. [PMID: 17442905]

Lau JY, Sung JJ, Lee KK, et al. Effect of intravenous omeprazole on recurrent bleeding after endoscopic treatment of bleeding peptic ulcers. *N Engl J Med.* 2000;343:310–316. [PMID: 10922420]

Sung JJ, Chan FK, Lau JY, et al. The effect of endoscopic therapy in patients receiving omeprazole for bleeding ulcers with non-bleeding visible vessels or adherent clots: a randomized comparison. *Ann Intern Med.* 2003;139:237–243. [PMID: 12965978]

Villanueva C, Colomo A, Bosch A, et al. Transfusion strategies for acute upper gastrointestinal bleeding. *N Engl J Med.* 2013;368:11–21. [PMID: 23281973]

B. Endoscopic Therapy

The goal of endoscopic therapy is to control active bleeding and prevent rebleeding. Further bleeding is the greatest contributor to both morbidity and mortality. The ability to endoscopically achieve sustained hemostasis is dependent on controlled access to the bleeding vessel, a relatively small vessel size that is amenable to endoscopic therapy, and the absence of significant coagulation defects.

Upper endoscopy provides diagnosis, prognosis, and therapy in patients with acute upper GI bleeding and is reasonably safe to perform (50% of complications are cardiopulmonary). Upper endoscopy is 90–95% sensitive at locating the bleeding site. Sensitivity increases when the procedure is done closer to the onset of the bleeding and decreases with increasing duration of time. Most patients with upper GI bleeding should undergo an upper endoscopy within 24 hours of presentation as is currently recommended by guidelines. Studies in patients with nonvariceal upper GI bleeding have not found an overall advantage of emergent endoscopy (within 12 hours) in terms of rebleeding rate, need for surgery, or mortality. Furthermore, there may be an increase in mortality with emergent endoscopy, especially in patients with multiple comorbidities (ASA score of III–V).

Endoscopy can offer therapeutic options including injection, cautery, placement of clips, use of a hemostatic spray, or a combination of therapies. Endoscopy can also predict the likelihood of persistent or recurrent bleeding based on recognition of the endoscopic stigmata of recent hemorrhage.

Table 20–3. Stigmata of recent hemorrhage: risk of rebleeding, mortality, and prevalence.

Stigmata	Risk of Rebleeding[a] (%)	Mortality (%)	Prevalence (%)
Active arterial bleeding	55–90	11	10
Nonbleeding visible vessel	40–50	11	25
Adherent clot	20–35	7	10
Oozing (without visible vessel)	10–25	NA	10
Flat spot	<10	3	10
Clean ulcer base	<5	2	35

[a]With medical management alone.
NA, not applicable.

1. Stigmata of recent hemorrhage—It is important to recognize the stigmata of recent hemorrhage, which are endoscopic findings in patients with bleeding peptic ulcers (Table 20–3). Patients with active bleeding seen at the time of upper endoscopy have a very high rate of ongoing bleeding, with rates as high as 90% with spurting bleeding if no intervention is performed (Plate 21). Patients who have nonbleeding visible vessels are also at high risk of further bleeding, as despite not having active bleeding at the time of endoscopy, rebleeding occurs in approximately 45% (Plates 22 and 23). Patients who have adherent clots that do not easily wash off have an intermediate probability of further bleeding (Plate 24). Approximately 20–35% of patients with adherent clots will have further bleeding, depending on what is underneath the clot. The risk is 40–50% if there is an underlying nonbleeding visible vessel, and <5% if the clot base is clean. Patients who are considered to be at low risk based on endoscopic stigmata of recent hemorrhage include those with flat spots, which have a <10% risk of further bleeding (Plate 25). Patients who have clean ulcer bases (Plate 26) or Mallory-Weiss tears, who do not have concomitant coagulopathies or use of medications that alter clotting, have a very low rate of further bleeding (<5%).

The endoscopic stigmata of hemorrhage can be difficult to interpret. Nonbleeding visible vessels cause the most difficulty and may be missed or misinterpreted. Nonbleeding visible vessels are raised protuberances from an ulcer bed that can be of any color, but they can be confused with flat spots. These may represent vessels, pseudoaneurysms, or clots and have a variable appearance.

2. Utility of endoscopic therapy—Endoscopic therapy for patients with bleeding peptic ulcers is the standard of care for patients with high-risk stigmata of recent hemorrhage. Patients who have active bleeding or are found to have nonbleeding visible vessels should undergo endoscopic hemostasis to improve outcomes.

The optimal management of adherent clots is controversial. Although some physicians recommended against endoscopic treatment of adherent clots, this practice has been challenged by several studies showing a possible benefit of endoscopic treatment. The technique to treat an adherent clot starts with the use of epinephrine injection in four quadrants at the pedicle of the clot. A snare is used to cold guillotine the clot 3–4 mm above its base. Care is taken not to shear off the clot, which can irritate the area and provoke bleeding. The base of the ulcer is then vigorously irrigated with fluid to expose any underlying stigmata. Any visible vessel exposed or active bleeding provoked is treated with cautery therapy or hemostatic clips. This technique in areas assessable for endoscopic treatment appears safe and facilitates endoscopic therapy.

3. Optimizing endoscopic visualization—One of the challenges of managing patients with GI bleeding is visualization due to blood within the GI tract. This problem can be overcome by the use of a variety of techniques, individually or in combination. It is helpful for endoscopists to use double-channel or large-channel endoscopes, which allow for vigorous aspiration (Figure 20–2). Gastric lavage with large volumes of fluid is no longer recommended, even in those

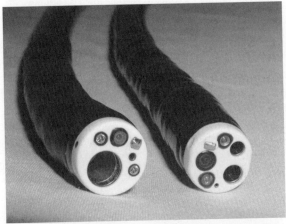

▲ **Figure 20–2.** Large channel therapeutic endoscope (*left*) and double-channel therapeutic endoscope (*right*).

with large upper GI bleeds. Additional suction devices can be placed over the biopsy channel of the endoscope to facilitate removal of large amounts of blood and clots efficiently during endoscopy.

Intravenous erythromycin (250 mg bolus or 3 mg/kg over 30 minutes) is a prokinetic drug that can be used to increase gastric emptying and clear the stomach of blood. Erythromycin is given intravenously 30–120 minutes prior to endoscopy. The use of erythromycin significantly improves the quality of the gastric examination. This is a useful adjunctive treatment in patients with large GI bleeds with retained blood in the stomach. It is usually used before the initial endoscopy but can be given after endoscopy if there is a large amount of blood in the stomach that prohibits the identification or treatment of the bleeding source, with withdrawal of the endoscope and erythromycin infusion before proceeding with repeat endoscopy. The data on other possible prokinetics including metoclopramide and azithromycin is not as robust as that for erythromycin and thus these should not be used unless erythromycin is not readily available. In general, promotility agents should be considered in patients suspected or found to have large amounts of blood or clot in their stomachs.

Kumar NL, Cohen AJ, Nayor J, Claggett BL, Saltzman JR. Timing of upper endoscopy influences outcomes in patients with acute nonvariceal upper GI bleeding. *Gastrointest Endosc.* 2017;85(5):945–952. [PMID: 27693643]

Laursen SB, Leontiadis GI, Stanley AJ, Møller MH, Hansen JM, Schaffalitzky de Muckadell OB. Relationship between timing of endoscopy and mortality in patients with peptic ulcer bleeding: a nationwide cohort study. *Gastrointest Endosc.* 2017;85(5): 936–944. [PMID: 27623102]

Lau JYW, Yu Y, Tang RSY, et al. Timing of endoscopy for acute upper gastrointestinal bleeding. *N Engl J Med.* 2020;382(14): 1299–1308. [PMID: 32242355]

Rahman R, Nguyen DL, Sohail U, et al. Pre-endoscopic erythromycin administration in upper gastrointestinal bleeding: an updated meta-analysis and systematic review. *Ann Gastroenterol.* 2016;29(3):312–317. [PMID: 27366031]

4. Methods to control bleeding—The current endoscopic modalities to treat nonvariceal GI bleeding include the use of injection therapies (primarily dilute epinephrine), contact thermal therapies including heater probes, monopolar probes and bipolar probes, the use of noncontact thermal methods (argon plasma coagulation), mechanical treatments including a variety of hemostatic clips and band ligation techniques, and a combination of the preceding treatment modalities (typically injection therapy combined with one of the other modalities).

Injection therapies reduce blood flow primarily by local tamponade. The use of vasoconstricting agents, such as epinephrine (diluted 1:10,000 to 1:100,000), reduces blood flow. This type of therapy may not be beneficial in the setting of active bleeding within fibrotic or penetrating ulcers. Injection therapy as monotherapy is not felt to be as efficacious as other monotherapies as there is a higher rate of further bleeding, and thus should not be used as the only modality of treatment. Higher doses of injected epinephrine are more likely to cause cardiovascular side effects (especially when injected in the region of the distal esophagus in patients with cardiovascular disease). Injection of absolute alcohol in very small volumes has been shown to be effective at treating bleeding ulcers, however this is not routinely used in practice possibly due to the potential of injected alcohol to cause significant tissue injury.

Use of thermal methods to control nonvariceal upper GI bleeding is quite widespread. Bipolar cautery is the thermal modality used most extensively, as it has the advantage over heater probes of being able to be used perpendicularly or tangentially. The bleeding vessel is compressed and then coagulated to provide "coaptive coagulation." The larger 10 French probes are generally more effective than the smaller 7 French probes, but need to be placed via a therapeutic scope with a large channel. It is optimal to use a relatively low wattage (eg, 10–15 watts in the duodenum; 15–20 watts in the stomach) for a prolonged contact time (8–12-second pulses) for each treatment pulse. With each treatment pulse, the technique includes using the water jet after each pulse to separate the probe from the underlying coagulum in order to avoid the probe sticking and provoking further bleeding when repositioned. Four to six pulses are typically used to provide effective treatment using moderate pressure in the stomach and lighter pressure in the duodenum. The end point of treatment is reached when the involved vessel completely flattens out and there is no further bleeding.

Monopolar cautery with soft coagulation current has recently been recognized to be effective for the treatment of upper GI bleeding. There is a rotating grasping monopolar forceps available that is widely used in the performance of endoscopic submucosal dissection (ESD). Monopolar cautery is applied by grasping the vessel and tenting the mucosa toward the endoscope or by placing the closed forceps next to the vessel and then applying cautery. Cautery is given in short 1–2 second bursts and repeated as needed. Several small trials have shown this technique to be similar in efficacy as the other standard endoscopic therapies. Although monopolar cautery with soft coagulation can be used as first line treatment to control bleeding, in practice it is often used as a rescue treatment for persistent bleeding after other standard therapies have failed.

Combination therapies are a safe and effective method and typically involve injection therapy with dilute (eg, 1:10,000) epinephrine, combined with a thermocoagulation technique or hemostatic clip placement. Combination therapy appears to provide a more durable control of bleeding than monotherapies.

Endoscopic hemostatic clips are a method of hemostatic control that is widely used and has the theoretical advantage over cautery therapies of not causing further tissue damage or injury (Plates 27 and 28). Hemostatic clips have a similar primary efficacy at providing hemostasis compared with other endoscopic cautery techniques. The combination of dilute epinephrine injection along with hemostatic clips is an effective endoscopic treatment option. Combination treatment that includes hemostatic clips is effective in patients with major upper GI bleeding or large blood vessels with injection of dilute epinephrine before the application of hemostatic clips. Epinephrine can also be injected for treatment of persistent bleeding or oozing after the application of hemostatic clips.

Large over-the-scope clips (much larger than standard hemostatic clips) are now available for endoscopic therapy of upper GI bleeding. These clips are placed over the tip of the endoscope and deployed with a technique similar to band ligation. Over-the-scope clips may successfully control bleeding of large arteries such as the gastroduodenal artery or left gastric artery whereas other therapies are not as effective in such large blood vessels. In addition these over-the-scope clips potentially provide more durable bleeding control with less rebleeding, which may be especially beneficial in patients who need to resume anti-thrombotic medications. In addition, the use of these large clips has shown to be effective in patients with rebleeding after initial endoscopic hemostasis.

A novel therapy for hemostasis is the use of a hemostatic nanopowder spray, (approved by the FDA as Hemospray for both nonvariceal upper and lower GI bleeding). This spray acts like a procoagulant and stops bleeding by tamponade, dehydration of blood, and activation of the clotting cascade and platelets. Many cohort studies have demonstrated the effectiveness of this new treatment modality at stopping active bleeding (>90% effective at stopping active bleeding). A recent randomized controlled trial of hemostatic spray versus standard of care endoscopic therapies for initial treatment of upper GI bleeding showed similar efficacy at controlling bleeding. However, there is a risk of rebleeding after initial control, especially in patients with large vessels and spurting bleeding such that a second treatment modality may be needed to prevent further bleeding, which is typically provided at a repeat upper endoscopy (due to difficulties in visualization due to the adherent powder). This hemostatic spray also appears to be effective in the difficult to control situation of active bleeding from an upper GI malignancy. Hemostatic sprays are only effective at treating actively bleeding lesions and have no role in the management of nonbleeding high risk stigmata such as nonbleeding visible vessels.

Patients requiring endoscopic therapy for nonvariceal bleeding should typically be treated with combination therapy using an injection of dilute epinephrine combined with a thermocoagulation method or with hemostatic clip application. Because some lesions or locations are better suited to one type of therapy, ideally an endoscopist should be familiar with both treatment options. Treatment with an over-the-scope clip is an option for initial control in patients with severe bleeding and/or from large vessels or with rebleeding. Hemostatic spray can be used as a rescue therapy after other endoscopic treatments have failed to control active bleeding or can be used as an initial therapy to treat active bleeding.

ASGE Standards of Practice Committee, Hwang JH, Fisher DA, Ben-Menachem T, et al. The role of endoscopy in the management of acute non-variceal upper GI bleeding. *Gastrointest Endosc.* 2012;75:1132–1138. [PMID: 22624808]

Aziz M, Weissman S, Mehta TI, et al. Efficacy of Hemospray in non-variceal upper gastrointestinal bleeding: a systematic review with meta-analysis. *Ann Gastroenterol* 2020;33:145–154. [PMID: 32127735]

Baracat FI, de Moura DTH, Brunaldi VO, et al. Randomized controlled trial of hemostatic powder versus endoscopic clipping for non-variceal upper gastrointestinal bleeding. *Surg Endosc* 2020;34:317–324. [PMID: 30927124]

Chen YI, Wyse J, Lu Y, Martel M, Barkun AN. TC-325 hemostatic powder versus current standard of care in managing malignant GI bleeding: a pilot randomized clinical trial. *Gastrointest Endosc.* 2020;91(2):321–328. [PMID: 31437456]

Hussein M, Alzoubaidi D, Fraile-López M, et al. Hemostatic spray powder TC-325 in the primary endoscopic treatment of peptic ulcer related bleeding: multicentre international registry. *Endoscopy.* 2021;53(1):36–43.

Jensen DM, Kovacs T, Ghassemi KA, Kaneshiro M, Gornbein J. Randomized controlled trial of over-the-scope clip as initial treatment of severe non-variceal upper gastrointestinal bleeding. *Clin Gastroenterol Hepatol.* 2021;19(11):2315–2323. [PMID: 32828873]

Lau JY, Pittayanon R, Kwek A, et al. A non-inferiority randomized controlled trial to compare hemostatic powder TC325 and standard therapy in bleeding from non-variceal upper gastrointestinal causes (abstract). *Ann Intern Med.* 2021 Dec 7. [PMID: 34871051]

Saltzman J, Strate L, Di Sena V, et al. Prospective trial of endoscopic clips versus combination therapy in upper GI bleeding (PROTECCT—UGI Bleeding). *Am J Gastroenterol.* 2005;100:1503–1508. [PMID: 15984972]

Schmidt A, Gölder S, Goetz M, et al. Over-the-scope clips are more effective than standard endoscopic therapy for patients with recurrent bleeding of peptic ulcers. *Gastroenterology.* 2018;155(3):674–686. [PMID: 29803838]

Sung JJ, Chiu PW, Chan FKL, et al. Asia-Pacific working group consensus on non-variceal upper gastrointestinal bleeding: an update 2018. *Gut.* 2018;67:1757–1768. [PMID: 29691276]

Toka B, Eminler AT, Karacaer C, Uslan MI, Koksal AS, Parlak E. Comparison of monopolar hemostatic forceps with soft coagulation versus hemoclip for peptic ulcer bleeding: a randomized trial (with video). *Gastrointest Endosc.* 2019;89(4):792–802. [PMID: 30342026]

C. Treatment of Patients with Recurrent Gastrointestinal Bleeding

The natural history of patients who are treated with endoscopic therapy is that 80–90% of patients will have permanent control of their bleeding (Figure 20–3). However, 10–20% of patients will have recurrent bleeding despite initially successful endoscopic therapy. In these patients, further attempts

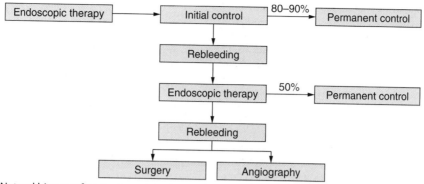

▲ **Figure 20–3.** Natural history of patients undergoing endoscopic therapy.

at endoscopic therapy are less effective at achieving permanent control, as 50–75% of those patients will ultimately be controlled by a second endoscopic therapy. In patients with rebleeding, over-the-scope clips are a possible option to improve efficacy. In addition, there is Doppler probe that can be utilized to interrogate the region of the bleeding vessel after endoscopic therapy such that additional therapy should be applied until flow has stopped. This approach has also been shown effective at decreasing rates of further bleeding. In patients who fail a second therapeutic endoscopy, other modalities or treatments should be offered, including angiography and surgery.

Some patients with rebleeding after an initially successful therapeutic endoscopy including those with very large vessels and those with massive bleeding, should be considered to directly proceed with a more definitive treatment such as angiography or surgery. It is important to identify patients who will ultimately need angiography or surgery and to proceed to further therapeutic interventions as appropriate. It is critical to consult and communicate with invasive radiologists and surgeons early in the care of patients who may need these treatments, such as those with massive bleeding or who are at high risk for poor outcomes.

Lau JY, Sung JJ, Lam YH, et al. Endoscopic retreatment compared with surgery in patients with recurrent bleeding after initial endoscopic control of bleeding ulcers. *N Engl J Med.* 1999;340:751–756. [PMID: 10072409]

D. Impact of Antithrombotics on Rebleeding

A major factor that has made the management of patients with GI bleeding more difficult in recent years is the increased use of antithrombotic medications. These medications are now a major etiologic contributor to upper GI bleeding. Antithrombotics consist of the antiplatelet and anticoagulant classes of medications.

The antiplatelet agents include aspirin, nonsteroidal anti-inflammatory drugs (NSAIDs) and the P2Y$_{12}$ inhibitors

(clopidogrel, prasugrel, and ticagrelor). Among patients on long-term, low-dose aspirin, the risk of overt GI bleeding is increased twofold compared to placebo. There is an additional increased risk of GI bleeding with certain combinations of drugs. Dual antiplatelet therapy is the combination of aspirin and a P12Y$_{12}$ inhibitor, and is widely used in patients with cardiovascular diseases, especially after coronary stent placement. Compared with aspirin alone, the dual antiplatelet therapy causes a two- to threefold increase in patients with major GI bleeding. Risk factors for bleeding in patients taking dual antiplatelet therapy are a history of peptic ulcers and prior GI bleeding, and possibly male gender, age more than 70, and *Helicobacter pylori* (*H pylori*) infection.

Concomitant use of NSAIDs, COX-2 inhibitors, or low-dose aspirin, and corticosteroid therapies increased the risk for upper GI bleeding. Concomitant use of NSAIDs and low-dose aspirin with aldosterone antagonists (eg, spironolactone) has been associated with an increased risk for upper GI bleeding. The serotonin reuptake inhibitors (SSRIs) have also been implicated as a possible cause of GI bleeding, possibly due to SSRIs blocking serotonin reuptake in platelets and thus inhibiting platelet aggregation. The combination of NSAIDs and SSRIs increases bleeding risk by 1.6 fold.

There are no reversal drugs available for the antiplatelet agents and transfusion of platelets in active bleeding has not been shown to be beneficial if the platelet count is above 50,000 mm^3. It is important to resume these medications if given for secondary prophylaxis, such as postacute coronary syndrome. In a trial of patients who were on aspirin for secondary prophylaxis with bleeding peptic ulcers that were successfully treated endoscopically, patients were randomized to prompt resumption of aspirin or withholding of aspirin for 30 days. Patients who resumed aspirin had twice the rebleeding rate of those who withheld aspirin, however they also had a nine fold increased mortality rate. We need to balance the risk of bleeding versus the risks of thromboembolism in patients restarted on anti-thrombotics. Communication with the prescribing physician is a key aspect of management. These medications should generally be restarted as soon as the bleeding is stabilized, usually after 72 hours of endoscopic therapy and almost always within 7 days.

The anticoagulants include heparin, warfarin and the direct oral anticoagulants (DOACs). In general with acute GI bleeding, anticoagulation is withheld if possible and the INR is reduced or normalized with reversal agents includes prothrombin complex concentrate or fresh frozen plasma in these patients. In a retrospective study of 233 patients with nonvariceal upper GI bleeding receiving endoscopic therapy, the presence of mild to moderate anticoagulation (INR 1.3–2.7) did not appear to alter the outcomes of endoscopic therapy. Upper endoscopy with endoscopic therapy appears appropriate to perform in patients with upper GI bleeding who are mildly to moderately anticoagulated. International Consensus and ACG guidelines recommend that a moderate coagulopathy (INR up to 2.5) should not delay therapeutic endoscopy.

The DOACS are comprised of the Xa inhibitors (apixaban, rivaroxaban, and edoxaban) and the IIa/thrombin inhibitors (eg, dabigatran). These oral drugs are convenient for patients as they are given as a fixed dose that does not require coagulation management and are highly effective anticoagulants. Although they generally are considered safer than warfarin, especially in terms of risk for intracranial hemorrhage, the risk of GI bleeding is increased with this class of drugs. However, this risk of GI bleeding seems to vary by drug, as dabigatran and rivaroxaban clearly are associated with an increased bleeding risk whereas apixaban has a similar rate of bleeding as compared with warfarin.

In managing patients with upper GI bleeding on DOACs, it is important to understand a few principles. The pharmacodynamics of these drugs show a rapid onset and offset of anticoagulation such that after ingestion of an oral dose, full therapeutic anticoagulation is achieved within a few hours. In addition, the percent anticoagulation declines to about 20% in 24 hours and <5% in 48% in patients with normal renal function. As the DOACs are renally cleared, impaired renal function prolongs the duration of anticoagulation. Thus withholding the DOAC and providing IV fluid hydration is sufficient management in most patients. There are specific reversal agents for the DOACS now available in the event that rapid reversal is needed such as massive GI bleeding. Idarucizumab is a monoclonal antibody that is given in two doses to reverse dabigatran and andexanet alpha is a decoy protein that is administered as a continuous infusion to reverse the Xa inhibitors.

ASGE Standards of Practice Committee, Acosta RD, Abraham NS, et al. The management of antithrombotic agents for patients undergoing GI endoscopy [published correction appears in Gastrointest Endosc. 2016 Mar;83(3):678]. *Gastrointest Endosc.* 2016;83(1):3–16. [PMID: 26621548]

Guo CG, Chen L, Chan EW, et al. Systematic review with meta-analysis: the risk of gastrointestinal bleeding in patients taking third-generation P2Y$_{12}$ inhibitors compared with clopidogrel. *Aliment Pharmacol Ther.* 2019;49(1):7–19. [PMID: 30506985]

Masclee GM, Valkhoff VE, Coloma PM, et al. Risk of upper gastrointestinal bleeding from different drug combinations. *Gastroenterology.* 2014;147:784–792. [PMID: 24937265]

Ray WA, Chung CP, Murray KT, et al. Association of oral anticoagulants and proton pump inhibitor cotherapy with hospitalization for upper gastrointestinal tract bleeding. *JAMA.* 2018;320(21):2221–2230. [PMID: 30512099]

Saltzman JR. The challenge of nonvariceal upper GI bleeding management in patients with acute coronary syndrome receiving dual-antiplatelet therapy. *Gastrointest Endosc.* 2020;92:75–77. [PMID: 32586567]

Sung JJ, Lau JY, Ching JY, et al. Continuation of low-dose aspirin therapy in peptic ulcer bleeding: a randomized trial. *Ann Intern Med.* 2010;152:1–9. [PMID: 19949136]

Wolf AT, Wasan SK, Saltzman JR. Impact of anticoagulation on rebleeding following endoscopic therapy for non-variceal upper gastrointestinal hemorrhage. *Am J Gastroenterol.* 2007;102: 290–296. [PMID: 17100959]

Zakko L, Rustagi T, Douglas M, Laine L. No benefit from platelet transfusion for gastrointestinal bleeding in patients taking antiplatelet agents. *Clin Gastroenterol Hepatol.* 2017;15(1):46–52.

E. *Helicobacter pylori* Infection

Patients with acute nonvariceal upper GI bleeding should be tested for the presence of *H pylori* infection. Diagnostic tests for *H pylori* include biopsy for histology or rapid urease testing, serology, stool antigen, and urea breath testing. In the setting of acute upper GI bleeding, these tests have a high positive predictive value but a low negative predictive value. Thus initially negative results may need to be repeated at follow-up. Patients who have a positive *H pylori* test must be treated with antibiotics. In addition, they should have a repeat evaluation for *H. pylori* infection, such as with a breath test, at least 4 weeks after completion of the antibiotic therapy to document eradication. If *H pylori* infection is persistent, a different treatment regimen should be chosen that includes different antibiotics and again a test for *H pylori* should be performed after completion of the antibiotic therapy to document eradication.

Chey WD, Leontiadis GI, Howden CW, Moss SF. ACG Clinical Guideline: treatment of *Helicobacter pylori* infection [published correction appears in Am J Gastroenterol. 2018 Jul;113(7):1102]. *Am J Gastroenterol.* 2017;112(2):212–239. [PMID: 28071659]

Lanas A, Chan FKL. Peptic ulcer disease. *Lancet.* 2017;390(10094): 613–624. [PMID: 28242110]

▼ SPECIFIC CAUSES OF ACUTE UPPER GI BLEEDING

This section discusses the diagnosis and treatment of common (Table 20–4) and uncommon (Table 20–5) sources of upper GI bleeding, including several specific causes of upper GI bleeding, both nonvariceal and variceal in origin.

Table 20–4. Common sources and prevalence of upper gastrointestinal bleeding.[a]

Source	Prevalence (%)
Duodenal ulcer	24.3
Gastric erosions	23.4
Gastric ulcer	21.3
Esophagogastric varices	10.3
Mallory-Weiss tear	7.2
Esophagitis	6.3
Erosive duodenitis	5.8

[a]Frequency >5% in American Society for Gastrointestinal Endoscopy bleeding survey of 2225 patients.

Table 20–5. Uncommon causes of upper gastrointestinal bleeding.[a]

Gastroesophageal reflux disease
Trauma from foreign bodies
Esophageal ulcer
Cameron lesion
Dieulafoy syndrome
Stress ulcer
Drug-induced erosions
Angioma
Watermelon stomach
Portal hypertensive gastropathy
Aortoenteric fistula
Radiation-induced telangiectasia
Benign tumors
Malignant tumors
Blue rubber bleb nevus syndrome
Osler-Weber-Rendu syndrome (hereditary hemorrhagic telangiectasias)
Hemobilia
Hemosuccus pancreatitis
Infections (cytomegalovirus, herpes simplex virus)
Stomal ulcer
Zollinger-Ellison syndrome

[a]Frequency <5%.

NONVARICEAL BLEEDING

1. Peptic Ulcer Disease

 ESSENTIALS OF DIAGNOSIS

▶ Peptic ulcers are the most common cause of upper GI bleeding.

▶ Most ulcers are caused by *H pylori* infection or medication use.

▶ Peptic ulcer may not cause symptoms before bleeding.

▶ Upper endoscopy is the best test for diagnosis.

General Considerations

The most common cause of acute upper GI bleeding is peptic ulcer disease, which accounts for over 50% of cases admitted to the hospital in the United States. The annual incidence of peptic ulcer disease in patients infected with *H pylori* is about 1% per year, which is 6–10 times higher than in patients who are uninfected.

Pathogenesis

A variety of conditions can lead to development of erosive or ulcerative diseases of the upper GI tract. In addition to peptic ulcer disease, which develops from an imbalance of protective and disruptive factors of the GI mucosa, medications including NSAIDs and aspirin, Zollinger-Ellison syndrome, esophagitis, stress-induced gastric injury, and infections can cause erosions or ulcers. Disruptive factors that can damage the mucosa of the GI tract include acid, pepsin, bile salts, ischemia, and *H pylori*. Exogenous causes are predominately medications. Stress-induced ulcers are a common cause of bleeding in patients hospitalized for other severe illnesses. Risk factors for stress-induced ulcers include respiratory failure and coagulopathy. The defensive forces of the upper GI tract include esophageal motility with clearance of refluxed materials, the lower esophageal sphincter to prevent reflux, and salivary secretions that contain bicarbonate. The gastric protective factors include the mucous layer as well as tissue mediators.

Clinical Findings

A. Symptoms & Signs

Clinical manifestations of peptic ulcer disease range from silent, asymptomatic disease to severe abdominal pain with bleeding. Peptic ulcers classically cause dyspepsia with epigastric burning pain, and are relieved with anti-acid therapies. Classic duodenal ulcer symptoms occur when acid is secreted without a food buffer, 2–5 hours after meals or on an empty stomach (such as nocturnally). Although symptoms are typically in the epigastric area, they may localize to either the left or right upper quadrants or the hypochondrium. In patients with ulcer symptoms, symptomatic periods may be followed by symptom-free periods of weeks or months. Other symptoms that have been associated with ulcers include anorexia, early satiety, nausea, belching, vomiting, and weight loss. It is important to note that only 30–40% of patients with severe bleeding from peptic ulcer disease have ulcer symptoms prior to the GI bleeding.

B. Laboratory Findings

The laboratory findings for bleeding peptic ulcer disease are nonspecific and include anemia with a decrease in hemoglobin and an elevated ratio of blood urea nitrogen to creatinine of greater than 30:1 in some patients. *H pylori* serology may be indicative of current or prior infection and thus tests for active infections are best including breath tests, stool antigen, and endoscopic biopsies. In the rare patient with Zollinger-Ellison syndrome, the serum gastrin level will be elevated, although a mildly to moderately elevated gastrin level (typically less than 400 pg/mL) is seen in > 80% with PPI use.

C. Imaging Studies

Upper endoscopy is the primary modality to detect peptic ulcers, due to its combination of both high sensitivity and specificity, as well as its capability of providing endoscopic therapy. Barium studies, although capable of detecting peptic ulcers, should be avoided in the acute setting, as barium interferes with further endoscopic treatments and other imaging modalities. An abdominal CT exam should be performed in patients with suspected perforation. In patients with ongoing upper GI bleeding without an identifiable cause on upper endoscopy, or who have recurrent bleeding uncontrolled by upper endoscopy, CT angiography with intravenous contrast may be useful to define the source of the bleeding as it is readily obtained and accurate at localizing active bleeding. Although upper endoscopy is the standard therapy of bleeding ulcers, in patients with massive bleeding or who are unable to be controlled endoscopically, angiography can provide treatment either with placement of a coil or embolization of the involved artery.

▶ Differential Diagnosis

As the symptoms of peptic ulcer disease are nonspecific, other causes of upper abdominal pain should be considered, including gastroesophageal reflux disease, nonulcer dyspepsia, cholelithiasis, choledocholithiasis, pancreatic disease, and malignancy. These conditions, however, are not typically associated with GI bleeding. Patients who appear to have an upper GI bleed may actually have a bleeding source in their small bowel or colon. Thus if no source of bleeding is found on upper endoscopy, a source distal to the ligament of Treitz needs to be considered. The differential diagnosis of lesions seen at endoscopy that appear as peptic ulcers includes NSAID-induced damage, infectious etiologies, and malignant disease, including adenocarcinoma and lymphoma. Ischemic disease as a cause of bleeding in the upper GI tract is unusual.

▶ Complications

Complications of peptic ulcer disease include bleeding, perforation, and obstruction. However, most patients with peptic ulcers do not develop these complications. Patients with bleeding peptic ulcers may develop aspiration pneumonia or complications of endoscopic therapy, such as respiratory depression and perforation. The tissue damage associated with ulcers may worsen with endoscopic treatment, particularly with cautery methods. This is a potential advantage of hemostatic clip use, which should not further damage an already compromised mucosa.

▶ Treatment

The principles of treatment of peptic ulcer disease are those outlined previously for treatment of upper GI bleeding and are detailed in Figure 20–4. Initial management must be centered on adequate resuscitation and stabilization. Decisions on whether to admit patients and how to optimally manage them depend on the clinical presentation and initial bleeding severity. Patients admitted should be kept NPO and evaluated with upper endoscopy within 24 hours.

In patients requiring endoscopic therapy, use of adjuvant medical therapy with high-dose PPIs should be administered. In patients who do not have high-risk endoscopic stigmata of hemorrhage and who do not require endoscopic therapy, medical treatment should be initiated with low-dose PPIs to begin the healing process. The presence of *H pylori* should be sought by endoscopic biopsy, stool antigen testing, or breath testing, and patients who have *H pylori* should undergo eradication therapy to decrease the risk of recurrent bleeding and peptic ulcer disease. If other identifiable modifiable factors are present such as medications associated with ulcers and GI bleeding, these should be discontinued if possible. However, patients on antithrombotic medications for secondary prevention should be restarted as soon as the GI bleeding has been stabilized.

Endoscopic therapy should be performed in patients with high-risk endoscopic stigmata of recent hemorrhage, as detailed previously.

▶ Course & Prognosis

The natural history of patients with bleeding peptic ulcers is that the majority will spontaneously stop bleeding and will not require interventional therapies. In patients who have bleeding requiring endoscopic treatment, the majority will be controlled with endoscopic measures. An angiographic intervention or surgery is needed only in a small minority of patients who have severe ongoing or upper GI bleeding, not controllable by endoscopic and medical therapies. Mortality, typically from comorbid illnesses including underlying malignancy, liver and cardiac disease and in patients who were already hospitalized, remains significant in patients who have upper GI bleeding due to peptic ulcer disease. After discharge from the hospital, it is unusual for patients to require readmission for recurrent bleeding if the previously described management measures have been instituted and if the patient does not have further need for antithrombotics.

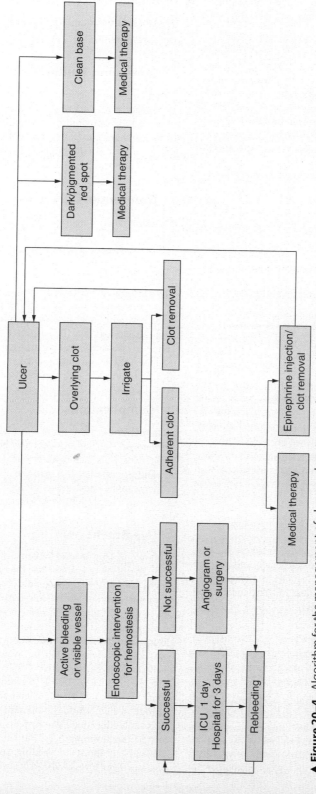

▲ **Figure 20–4.** Algorithm for the management of ulcers and acute gastrointestinal bleeding. ICU, intensive care unit. (Adapted with permission from Eisen GM, Dominitz JA, Faigel DO, et al. Standards of Practice Committee. An annotated algorithmic approach to upper gastrointestinal bleeding. *Gastrointest Endosc.* 2001;53(7):853–858.)

An evidence-based, comprehensive, and multidisciplinary approach to the management of patients with bleeding peptic ulcers results in optimal outcomes.

Lau JYW, Pittayanon R, Wong KT, et al. Prophylactic angiographic embolisation after endoscopic control of bleeding to high-risk peptic ulcers: a randomised controlled trial. *Gut* 2019;68: 796–803. [PMID: 29802172]

Stanley AJ, Laine L. Management of acute upper gastrointestinal bleeding. *BMJ.* 2019;364:l536. [PMID: 30910853]

Tarasconi A, Baiocchi GL, Pattonieri V, et al. Transcatheter arterial embolization versus surgery for refractory non-variceal upper gastrointestinal bleeding: a meta-analysis. *World J Emerg Surg* 2019;14:1–13. [PMID: 30733822]

2. Mallory-Weiss Tears

 ESSENTIALS OF DIAGNOSIS

▶ Associated with repeated vomiting and retching.
▶ Endoscopy is the best test for diagnosis.

General Considerations

A Mallory-Weiss tear is a common cause of upper GI bleeding, accounting for approximately 5% of all cases. As the tears are relatively superficial, most heal within 24–48 hours. Mallory-Weiss tears may be difficult to visualize on upper endoscopy as they be subtle in appearance (like a papercut), especially if endoscopy is not performed promptly. Although in most patients the tears resolve spontaneously, massive bleeding can occur from Mallory-Weiss tears in patients who have portal hypertension, especially if esophageal varices are present.

Pathogenesis

Mallory-Weiss tears occur at the gastroesophageal junction in the distal esophagus or proximal stomach and may be single or multiple. Typically these tears form after repeated or severe vomiting or retching. The tears may extend into the underlying venous or arterial plexuses.

Clinical Findings

A. Symptoms & Signs

The typical presentation of a Mallory-Weiss tear is acute upper GI bleeding in a young to middle-aged man, following repeated vomiting or retching after drinking alcohol. The history of antecedent retching and vomiting may not always be obtained. If there are additional systemic signs, such as fever, chest pain, and shortness of breath, the Boerhaave syndrome with esophageal perforation should be considered.

B. Laboratory Findings

The laboratory findings for a Mallory-Weiss tear are nonspecific and are similar to those for peptic ulcer disease.

C. Imaging Studies

Upper endoscopy, performed promptly, is the diagnostic and therapeutic procedure of choice. The tears can be seen as single or multiple longitudinal disruptions of the mucosa of the distal esophagus, at the gastroesophageal junction, within a hiatal hernia, or in the stomach just below the gastroesophageal junction with associated bleeding (Plate 29).

Differential Diagnosis

The differential diagnosis of Mallory-Weiss tears includes other lesions of the gastroesophageal junction, including reflux esophagitis, infectious esophagitis, pill-induced esophagitis, Cameron lesion, and Dieulafoy lesion. Mallory-Weiss tears are focal lesions within an otherwise normal-appearing region of mucosa, which distinguishes them from reflux or infectious esophagitis. Patients with pill-induced esophagitis often have additional areas of injury higher up the esophagus, and this etiology may be suspected by history. A Dieulafoy lesion is associated with normal-appearing adjacent mucosa and the presence of a protuberant artery typically several centimeters below the gastro-esophageal junction.

Complications

Although the natural history of Mallory-Weiss tears is that they are self-healing, patients may have ongoing bleeding or rebleeding. This is more likely with deeper tears or in patients on antithrombotics. It is also possible to have a perforation either spontaneously, due to repeated vomiting, or after endoscopic therapy leading to mediastinitis.

Treatment

Endoscopic treatment of patients with Mallory-Weiss tears is indicated if there is active bleeding or a nonbleeding visible vessel seen at the time of endoscopy. Combination therapy with injection initially to slow or stop the bleeding followed by cautery or application of hemostatic clips is effective in most patients. However, because the injury is a tear of the lining (and the esophagus lacks a serosa), over injection and over cauterization should be avoided. In cases of associated portal hypertension or esophageal varices, endoscopic therapy must be cautiously performed and cautery therapy should be avoided. These patients are best treated with band ligation or hemostatic clip placement. Medical therapy with PPIs should be initiated in patients with Mallory-Weiss tears to start the healing process but has not been shown to alter the course of the acute bleeding. Surgical intervention, with over sewing of a vessel, is rarely needed.

Course & Prognosis

The natural history of Mallory-Weiss tears is that most bleeding will stop spontaneously and healing will start to occur within 24–48 hours in the majority of patients. Further bleeding is unusual once bleeding has ceased.

Chang MA, Savides TJ. Endoscopic management of nonvariceal, nonulcer upper gastrointestinal bleeding. *Gastrointest Endosc Clin N Am.* 2018;28(3):291–306. [PMID: 29933776]

3. Dieulafoy Lesion

ESSENTIALS OF DIAGNOSIS

▶ Massive bleeding.

▶ Most often located below the gastroesophageal junction in cardia.

▶ Difficult to diagnose.

Pathogenesis

A Dieulafoy lesion is a dilated, aberrant submucosal vessel that erodes through otherwise normal surrounding epithelium not associated with an ulcer. Although originally described in 1884 by Gallard, the lesion is named after the French surgeon Georges Dieulafoy, who 14 years later described the lesion as "exulceratio simplex." The arteries are usually 1–2 mm in size, which is approximately 10 times the caliber of mucosal capillaries, but can be larger. The typical location is in the upper stomach along the high lesser curvature, within 6 cm of the gastroesophageal junction and often within 2 cm. Dieulafoy lesions have been reported in other areas throughout the GI tract, including the esophagus, duodenum, and colon. The cause of a Dieulafoy lesion is unknown, although the lesion may be congenital. When a Dieulafoy lesion bleeds, massive arterial bleeding will occur. The typical patient with a Dieulafoy lesion is a man, with multiple comorbidities, already hospitalized for other problems who abruptly has a major upper GI bleed.

Clinical Findings

A. Symptoms & Signs

A patient with a Dieulafoy lesion often presents with a massive acute upper GI bleed. However, the bleeding may be self-limited in nature or follow a stuttering course. In active bleeding, the diagnosis is confirmed by finding a visible vessel with active arterial pumping, without an associated ulcer or mass. The diagnosis can be difficult or missed, as the lesion does not have a surrounding ulcer, the location may be dependent within the stomach during endoscopy and as bleeding is often massive that the area may be covered with blood. In the absence of active bleeding, the lesion is difficult to visualize, as it may appear as a small and subtle raised area, such as a nipple or visible vessel without an associated ulcer. In patients with massive bleeding and no obvious cause, the lesser curvature within 6 cm of the gastroesophageal junction should always be carefully inspected for a Dieulafoy lesion.

B. Imaging Studies

Upper endoscopy is the primary modality to detect a Dieulafoy lesion. If bleeding has stopped and there is doubt about the nature of the lesion, the use of a Doppler probe if available or endoscopic ultrasound with Doppler flow may be helpful to confirm the diagnosis.

Treatment

Endoscopic treatment is the primary modality for bleeding control of a Dieulafoy lesion. Combination therapy with injections of epinephrine followed by cautery may be used, or hemostatic clips may be placed. Band ligation or over-the-scope clips may also be placed over a Dieulafoy lesion. The risk of recurrent bleeding following endoscopic treatment is relatively high due to the large size of the underlying artery. It may be helpful to tattoo the area with ink or place a hemostatic clip at or near the site (if not already utilized) to help localize the area for subsequent endoscopic therapy or future operative treatment. In patients with recurrent bleeding, an attempt to repeat endoscopic therapy is reasonable; however, surgical therapy may be necessary. Surgical treatment of a Dieulafoy lesion is typically a wedge resection, as simple over sewing has a high rebleeding rate.

Awadalla M, Mahmoud M, McNamara P, Wassef W. Gastric vascular abnormalities: diagnosis and management. *Curr Opin Gastroenterol.* 2020;36(6):538–546. [PMID: 32925176]

Lai Y, Rong J, Zhu Z, et al. Risk factors for rebleeding after emergency endoscopic treatment of Dieulafoy lesion. *Can J Gastroenterol Hepatol.* 2020;2020:2385214. Published 2020 Aug 24. [PMID: 32908851]

Lara LF, Sreenarasimhaiah J, Tang SJ, Afonso BB, Rockey DC. Dieulafoy lesions of the GI tract: localization and therapeutic outcomes. *Dig Dis Sci.* 2010;55:3436–3441. [PMID: 20848205]

4. Vascular Malformations

ESSENTIALS OF DIAGNOSIS

▶ Wide spectrum of disorders.

▶ Can cause acute or chronic bleeding.

▶ Variable bleeding rates.

General Considerations

Various terms are used to describe vascular malformations of the upper GI tract, including arteriovenous malformations, vascular ectasia, angiodysplasia, and telangiectasia. Although these lesions can present as acute, overt upper GI bleeding, they are frequently a source of chronic occult GI bleeding and iron deficiency anemia. Vascular malformations of the upper GI tract may be associated with small bowel angioectasias (also of obscure origin).

Pathogenesis

Vascular malformations of the upper GI tract may be arterial or venous in origin. The majority are idiopathic with unknown causes. The spectrum of vascular malformations includes Dieulafoy lesions, as previously discussed, watermelon stomach (gastric antral vascular ectasia [GAVE]), Osler-Weber-Rendu syndrome (hereditary hemorrhagic telangiectasia), blue rubber bleb nevus syndrome, and radiation-induced telangiectasias.

Clinical Findings

Bleeding from upper GI vascular malformations is typically intermittent and low-grade in nature, although it can be acute and overt. The endoscopic appearance can be variable, but includes a superficial collection or tuft of blood vessels (Plate 30). These also can be detected by angiography, with findings including an early filling vein, a vascular tuft, and a late draining vein.

Treatment

The primary treatment of vascular malformations is with endoscopic therapy. Endoscopic therapy with thermal coagulation is the treatment of choice, with cautery applied initially to the periphery and then at the center of the lesion. There should be whitening of the mucosa and ablation of all visible vascular tissue. Argon plasma coagulation is an effective noncontact cautery treatment of vascular malformations. It is important to avoid overdistention (by the argon gas) of the stomach or small intestine during therapy, as well as to avoid contact with tissue when using argon plasma coagulation therapy. Repeated therapy should not be applied to the same location due to the risk of transmural injury and perforation, especially in the small bowel.

Various medications have been used in an attempt to treat vascular malformations in the upper GI tract. Combination estrogen–progesterone therapy has been widely used, but overall has yielded inconsistent results. There has been some success with the use of thalidomide, however this cannot be used in women of childbearing potential due to the well-known fetal risks. Angiography and surgery can be offered for failures of endoscopic and medical therapy but are rarely necessary.

Bayudan AM, Chen CH. Thalidomide for refractory gastrointestinal bleeding from vascular malformations in patients with significant comorbidities. *World J Clin Cases.* 2020;8(15):3218–3229. [PMID: 32874976]

Nardone G, Compare D, Martino A, Rocco A. Pharmacological treatment of gastrointestinal bleeding due to angiodysplasias: a position paper of the Italian Society of Gastroenterology (SIGE). *Dig Liver Dis.* 2018;50(6):542–548. [PMID: 29610020]

5. Watermelon Stomach (Gastric Antral Vascular Ectasia)

 ESSENTIALS OF DIAGNOSIS

▶ Idiopathic or associated with portal hypertension or systemic sclerosis.
▶ Characteristic endoscopic appearance of radiating rows of vascular malformations extending outward from the pylorus.

Pathogenesis

Watermelon stomach or GAVE is a relatively unusual cause of upper GI bleeding. This condition can occur along with, or be confused with, portal hypertensive gastropathy. In this condition vascular malformations typically occur in rows of reddish stripes that radiate outward from the pylorus, in a pattern that can resemble the stripes on a watermelon. These stripes represent rows of vascular malformations and watermelon stomach is easy to recognize in the classic form. However, watermelon stomach may have a less organized appearance, with more scattered erythema and vascular malformations, making it more difficult to diagnose.

The cause of watermelon stomach is idiopathic; however, it may be due to gastroduodenal prolapse and has been noted to occur more commonly in patients with cirrhosis, portal hypertension, and systemic sclerosis. Patients with concomitant portal hypertension have bleeding that is more difficult to control, requiring treatment of the underlying portal hypertension.

Clinical Findings

The diagnosis of watermelon stomach is based on the classic endoscopic appearance of radiating rows of vascular malformations originating from the pyloric area (Plate 31). Although the diagnosis is made by the characteristic endoscopic appearance, it can be confirmed by histology from endoscopic biopsy. Biopsies of watermelon stomach show areas of vascular ectasia associated with spindle cell proliferation and fibrohyalinosis. The bleeding that occurs is typically chronic and low grade, often associated with iron deficiency anemia and occult bleeding. It is unusual to have acute or massive upper GI bleeding from watermelon stomach.

Treatment

Endoscopic therapy is effective at treating watermelon stomach, especially in the absence of concomitant portal hypertension. This may be done with multipolar electrocoagulation or argon plasma coagulation. Several courses of treatment are required to obliterate the vascular ectasias and decrease or stop bleeding. In refractory patients with watermelon stomach, radiofrequency ablation, band ligation, and cryotherapy have been used with success. Although most patients respond to endoscopic therapy, surgery may be needed for patients who have persistent bleeding despite endoscopic management. Surgical management with antrectomy prevents further bleeding.

Hsu WH, Wang YK, Hsieh MS, et al. Insights into the management of gastric antral vascular ectasia (watermelon stomach). *Therap Adv Gastroenterol.* 2018;11:1756283X17747471. Published 2018 Jan 14. [PMID: 29399041]

McGorisk T, Krishnan K, Keefer L, Komanduri S. Radiofrequency ablation for refractory gastric antral vascular ectasia (with video). *Gastrointest Endosc.* 2013;78:584–588. [PMID: 23660565]

LESS COMMON CAUSES OF NONVARICEAL BLEEDING

1. Aortoenteric Fistula

ESSENTIALS OF DIAGNOSIS

► High index of suspicion is needed for diagnosis.

► Massive bleeding may cause exsanguination.

► Rapid diagnosis and progression to surgery are required.

Aortoenteric fistulas occur when there is a direct communication between the aorta and the GI tract. These typically occur in patients who have had a prosthetic aortic graft that erodes into the intestine. They also can occur from aortic aneurysms, after radiation therapy, or from postinfectious aortitis (eg, from syphilis or tuberculosis), trauma, or tumor invasion.

The third and fourth portions of the duodenum are the most common sites of aortoenteric fistulas, followed by the jejunum and the ileum. Patients may have a "herald" bleed with initial hematemesis or hematochezia, which may spontaneously remit. This may then be followed by massive bleeding, including exsanguination, making it important to diagnose this condition as early as possible. Intermittent bleeding can occur if a blood clot temporarily seals a fistulous connection. Abdominal or back pain occurs in about half of patients. Signs of fever or infection may be present.

On physical examination, a bruit may be heard or a pulsatile mass may be palpable.

A high index of suspicion is needed to properly diagnose a patient with an aortoenteric fistula while there is still time for successful management. In a patient who has a known risk factor, such as previous aortic grafting, this diagnosis should be considered. It should also be suspected in patients with bleeding from the third or fourth portion of the duodenum, particularly with massive bleeding. Aortic graft material may occasionally be seen at endoscopy protruding into the bowel lumen. The diagnosis can be confirmed by CT with angiography or angiography directly. Diagnostic tests need to be done in an expeditious manner along with surgical evaluation.

The management of an aortoenteric fistula is surgical. The mortality rate of an unrecognized fistula is 100%, whereas the mortality for a recognized fistula is 30%. Treatment consists of surgical repair of the aortoenteric fistula.

Perencevich M, Saltzman JR, Levy BD, Loscalzo J. Clinical problem-solving. The search is on. *N Engl J Med.* 2013;368:562–567. [PMID: 23388008]

2. Hemobilia

ESSENTIALS OF DIAGNOSIS

► Triad of jaundice, biliary colic, and GI bleeding.

► Consider in patients after trauma or hepatic intervention.

Hemobilia, bleeding that occurs from the hepatobiliary tract, is a rare cause of acute upper GI bleeding. Hemobilia should be considered in patients who have had a recent history of hepatic or biliary tract injury. This includes trauma to the area and percutaneous (or transjugular) liver biopsies, and percutaneous transhepatic cholangiograms. Hemobilia can also occur from gallstones, cholecystitis, hepatobiliary tumors, hepatic abscesses, and aneurysms.

The classic Quincke's triad of hemobilia is biliary colic, obstructive jaundice, and GI bleeding. Obstructive jaundice may be associated with biliary sepsis. Patients with this triad should be considered as potentially having hemobilia.

The diagnosis of hemobilia can be difficult by upper endoscopy. A side-viewing duodenoscope is usually needed to look at the ampulla directly or to perform endoscopic retrograde cholangiopancreatography to remove blood in the biliary tract causing obstruction (ERCP) (Plate 32). A CT angiogram or angiography can be done to localize the source of bleeding.

Treatment is directed at the primary cause of bleeding. Although occasionally treatment can be done endoscopically, it usually needs to be performed angiographically (such as by arterial embolization) or surgically.

Zhornitskiy A, Berry R, Han JY, Tabibian JH. Hemobilia: historical overview, clinical update, and current practices. *Liver Int.* 2019;39(8):1378–1388.

3. Hemosuccus Pancreaticus

ESSENTIALS OF DIAGNOSIS

▶ Suspect when bleeding is associated with pancreatic disease.

▶ Best detected with a side-viewing duodenoscope.

Hemosuccus pancreaticus occurs when there is bleeding from the pancreatic duct. This is a rare cause of upper GI bleeding that can be due to chronic pancreatitis, pancreatic pseudocysts, or pancreatic tumors. Bleeding occurs when there is erosion into a vessel, forming a direct communication with the pancreatic duct. It can also occur after a therapeutic endoscopy of the pancreas, including pancreatic sphincterotomy or stone removal.

The diagnosis of hemosuccus pancreaticus should be suspected when upper GI bleeding occurs in the setting of pancreatic disease. Although it can be difficult to detect by routine endoscopy, a side-viewing duodenoscope and ERCP may reveal the pancreatic duct as the source of the bleeding. The diagnosis can be confirmed by abdominal CT angiography or angiography. Mesenteric angiography is an important treatment modality, often with therapy using coil embolization to control the acute bleeding. For persistent or massive bleeding, surgery with resection of the bleeding area or ligation of the bleeding vessel may be required.

Shetty S, Shenoy S, Costello R, Adeel MY, Arora A. Hemosuccus Pancreaticus. *J Ayub Med Coll Abbottabad.* 2019;31(4):622–626. [PMID: 31933323]

Yu P, Gong J. Hemosuccus pancreaticus: a mini-review. *Ann Med Surg (Lond).* 2018;28:45–48. [PMID: 29744052]

4. Cameron Lesion

ESSENTIALS OF DIAGNOSIS

▶ Close inspection of hiatal hernia during endoscopy is needed.

▶ Acute or chronic GI bleeding.

Cameron lesions are erosions or ulcers that occur in the distal aspect of a hiatal hernia. Although this may be an incidental finding, a Cameron lesion can be responsible for acute or chronic upper GI bleeding and iron deficiency anemia.

The mechanism of formation of a Cameron lesion is incompletely understood, although potential causative factors include gastroesophageal reflux and mechanical trauma of the area. The diagnosis requires an upper endoscopy and if not actively bleeding the lesion can be easily missed or mistaken as an incidental finding.

Management of a Cameron lesion depends on the clinical situation. Patients with acute bleeding can be effectively treated by standard endoscopic methods. Patients who do not have acute bleeding, but have chronic blood loss may be treated with medical therapy, such as PPI therapy and iron repletion. Surgical repair of the hiatal hernia is curative, but rarely needed.

Parikh K, Ali MA, Wong RC. Unusual causes of upper gastrointestinal bleeding. *Gastrointest Endosc Clin N Am.* 2015;25(3): 583–605. [PMID: 26142040]

5. Upper Gastrointestinal Tumors

ESSENTIALS OF DIAGNOSIS

▶ Benign and malignant tumors can bleed.

▶ Bleeding may be slow or massive.

Neoplasms of the upper GI tract account for less than 3% of upper GI bleeding. These tumors may be malignant tumors (primary or metastatic) such as adenocarcinomas, lymphomas, and melanomas, or can be benign, such as leiomyomas, GI stromal tumors, or lipomas.

The symptoms that suggest bleeding may be from a GI tumor include those that may be attributable to the primary tumor, such as dysphagia from esophageal cancer or gastric outlet obstruction due to carcinoma of the stomach. Other symptoms are nonspecific, including cachexia, weight loss, and early satiety.

Bleeding from an upper GI tumor can be from diffuse mucosal erosions or ulcerations, or from erosion of the tumor into an underlying vessel (Plates 33 and 34). The bleeding may be slow or may be massive. If the diagnosis of a tumor is not previously known, it may be detected at the time of endoscopy and confirmed by biopsies. Endoscopic ultrasound may be needed to evaluate submucosal masses to fully characterize or biopsy.

Endoscopic treatment of patients with upper GI bleeding can be performed, but is less effective in the setting of tumors. Typically the standard endoscopic treatments, although they may be effective, often are used as a temporizing measure prior to more definitive measures such as angiography surgery, because rebleeding will frequently occur after endoscopic control of bleeding, thus requiring a more durable approach. Hemostatic spray has been found to control active malignant bleeding and can treat be successful at treating multiple oozing sites and can result in long-term hemostasis.

However when spurting bleeding occurs from a erosion of the tumor into a large underlying artery, hemostatic spray will likely only provide temporizing therapy. Medical therapy is ineffective in this setting, although palliative measures may be provided, including chemotherapy and radiation of the primary tumor.

Patients who have bleeding due to an upper GI malignancy have a very poor prognosis. The majority of patients will die within 3 months. However, patients who have a benign upper GI tumor that bleeds should be cured by surgical resection.

Meng ZW, Marr KJ, Mohamed R, James PD. Long-term effectiveness, safety and mortality associated with the use of TC-325 for malignancy-related upper gastrointestinal bleeds: a multicentre retrospective study. *J Can Assoc Gastroenterol.* 2019;2(2):91–97. [PMID: 31294371]

Ofosu A, Ramai D, Latson W, Adler DG. Endoscopic management of bleeding gastrointestinal tumors. *Ann Gastroenterol.* 2019;32(4):346–351. [PMID: 31263356]

VARICEAL BLEEDING

1. Gastroesophageal Varices

ESSENTIALS OF DIAGNOSIS

▶ Sign of advanced liver disease.

▶ Larger varices bleed more often.

▶ Associated with a high rate of bacterial infections.

▶ May involve the esophagus, stomach, or both.

General Considerations

Esophageal and gastric varices may occur without any clinical symptoms. In patients with cirrhosis, particularly in more advanced stages, screening measures are performed to detect varices in an attempt to decrease the risk of initial bleeding. Acute variceal bleeding is different from nonvariceal bleeding in many respects. Only 50% of patients with a variceal hemorrhage stop bleeding spontaneously (compared with approximately 80–90% of patients with nonvariceal upper GI bleeding). Following cessation of active variceal bleeding, there is a high risk of recurrent bleeding within 6 weeks. The time of greatest risk is within the first 48–72 hours, and over 50% of all rebleeding episodes occur within the first 10 days. Mortality during the 6 weeks following the index bleed is directly related to rebleeding. Risk factors for rebleeding include age greater than 60 years, large varices, severe initial bleed (hemoglobin <8 g/dL on admission), and renal failure. Mortality is between 5% and 50% for each bleeding episode, and 70–80% in those with continuous bleeding.

In recent years there has been a decrease in the mortality due to the prevention of rebleeding by the use of earlier, more effective endoscopic therapy along with effective vasoactive medications as well as the prevention of infection due to the use of prophylactic antibiotics. Variceal hemorrhage is responsible for one-third of all deaths due to cirrhosis.

Pathogenesis

Esophageal and gastric varices develop as a result of portal hypertension. Portal hypertension can be from prehepatic causes (eg, portal vein thrombosis and schistosomiasis), hepatic disease (cirrhosis most commonly), and post hepatic disease (eg, hepatic vein thrombosis, cardiac failure, and constrictive pericarditis). Varices are dilated venous collaterals that have a relatively weak wall that has a tendency to rupture and can bleed massively. Varices may be isolated to the stomach if they are due to splenic vein thrombosis, acute pancreatitis, or a pancreatic tumor.

Clinical Findings

A. Symptoms & Signs

The symptoms of variceal bleeding are nonspecific and include hematemesis, melena, and hematochezia. Patients may feel light-headed and dizzy, and those with severe liver disease may have hepatic encephalopathy. Other associated signs and symptoms are manifestations of cirrhosis, including jaundice, spider telangiectasia, palmar erythema, ascites, and Dupuytren contractures.

B. Laboratory Findings

Abnormalities of the liver enzymes (alanine aminotransferase and aspartate aminotransferase) are seen in patients with active hepatocellular damage. Patients may have hyperbilirubinemia and poor synthetic function, with hypoalbuminemia and an elevated INR. Patients with bone marrow suppression from alcohol may have pancytopenia; those with hypersplenism may have low platelets. In patients with liver failure, hypoglycemia may occur, and in those with hepatorenal syndrome, blood urea nitrogen and creatinine are elevated.

C. Imaging Studies

Upper endoscopy is the primary diagnostic modality and allows for endoscopic therapy. The Japanese Research Society for Portal Hypertension criteria includes a size (or form) classification. Small straight varices are classified as F1, enlarged tortuous varices occupying less than one-third of the esophageal lumen are F2, and large coil-shaped varices that occupy more than one-third of the esophageal lumen are F3. Abdominal CT or abdominal ultrasound may show the presence of collateral vessels or recanalization of the umbilical vein. Hepatic venous pressure gradients of more than 12 mm Hg are a predictor of bleeding.

Differential Diagnosis

The differential diagnosis includes the nonvariceal causes of upper GI bleeding. Patients with cirrhosis and upper GI bleeding are found to have a variceal source of bleeding in 50–90% of cases. However, patients with cirrhosis can also bleed from esophagitis, peptic ulcer disease, Mallory-Weiss tears, and other nonvariceal sources.

Complications

Bleeding from esophageal or gastric varices may be massive and uncontrollable, resulting in severe hemorrhage and death. Acute variceal bleeding in a patient with cirrhosis may precipitate further worsening of liver disease, with increasing hepatic encephalopathy and development of the hepatorenal syndrome. Bacterial infections are present in up to 20% of cirrhotic patients with GI bleeding, and subsequently develop in an additional 50% of patients during hospitalization for variceal bleeds. The use of prophylactic antibiotics in patients with acute variceal bleeding has been shown to decrease the rates of subsequent infection, spontaneous bacterial peritonitis, bacteremia, and death.

Treatment

Patients with acute variceal bleeding are typically treated with multiple modalities simultaneously, including medical therapies and endoscopic management. Over-resuscitation should be avoided, as over vigorous volume repletion has been associated with precipitation of further bleeding. Due to the acuity and severity of bleeding, radiologic and surgical treatments may be needed. Similar to nonvariceal upper GI bleeding, blood transfusions in general should target hemoglobin >7 g/dL. Patients with variceal bleeding treated with a restrictive transfusion strategy have lower mortality rates than those treated with a liberal transfusion strategy.

A. Medical Therapy

In patients with suspected variceal bleeding, medical therapy to reduce bleeding should be initiated prior to endoscopic evaluation. The use of prophylactic antibiotics (typically a quinolone or ceftriaxone) given before endoscopy in cirrhotic patients reduces infectious complications and decreases mortality.

Medications have been shown to decrease active variceal bleeding. Terlipressin is a synthetic analog of vasopressin that is released in a sustained and slow manner. It is effective at controlling bleeding reducing mortality as vasopressin. Unfortunately, terlipressin is not currently available in the United States, but is widely used in other countries.

Octreotide, an analog of somatostatin, has been extensively studied in patients with bleeding esophageal and gastric varices. It indirectly causes vasoconstriction and decreases portal blood flow. Octreotide is typically given as a bolus injection of 50 µg followed by a continuous infusion of 50 µg/h intravenously. Octreotide is useful in achieving hemostasis and preventing early rebleeding. Once patients are stabilized from the acute variceal bleeding episode, β-blockers are given to prevent rebleeding. (See Chapter 49 for additional discussion of portal hypertension.)

B. Endoscopic Therapy

The treatment of choice for bleeding esophageal varices is endoscopic hemostasis (Plates 35 and 36). The objective of endoscopic therapy is to find the source of the bleeding and to effectively treat it. Varices are evaluated for signs of either active bleeding or markers of recent bleeding. These markers include large tortuous varices with red wale marks (longitudinal red streaks on varices that resemble red, corduroy wales), cherry red spots (discrete cherry red spots that are flat on a varix), and hemocystic spots (raised discrete red spots that overlie varices that appear as "blood blisters"). Platelet or fibrin plugs are white nipple-like projections that project from a varix indicative of a site with recent bleeding and with a very high risk of bleeding.

Endoscopic therapies for esophageal varices are initially applied to the distal esophagus at the gastroesophageal junction and then extended proximally. Most variceal bleeding is from the distal 5–10 cm of the esophagus. Gastric varices are poorly responsive to traditional endoscopic therapies and do not respond to typical endoscopic banding and injection treatments (Plate 37). The use of cyanoacrylate injections for bleeding gastric varices are effective, although occasionally associated with severe complications including pulmonary embolism not approved for use in the United States. Recently the combination of endoscopic ultrasound placed vascular coils into the varices along with injection of glue or gel foam has been shown to be effective and may reduce the possibility of embolism.

Endoscopic injection sclerotherapy is an older method of injecting esophageal varices directly using a freehand technique with 1–3 mL of a sclerosing agent (sodium morrhuate or ethanolamine) at each site. Numerous techniques and agents have been used to sclerose varices. Although this technique is effective, esophageal variceal band ligation is more effective, associated with less rebleeding, fewer complications, and a lower mortality rate, and requiring fewer treatment sessions to obliterate the varices. Thus this technique is generally not used as primary therapy, although there may still be a role for injection of residual varices after band ligation therapy that are not amenable to further banding.

Endoscopic variceal ligation is the treatment of choice for controlling acute esophageal variceal hemorrhage. Endoscopic esophageal variceal band ligation therapy is a method of placing elastic bands over varices. This is typically initially performed within the distal 5 cm of the esophagus and extended proximally depending on the length of the variceal chain. Varices are suctioned into a banding device, and the bands are released around the base of the varices. Esophageal variceal band ligation controls acute bleeding in >90% of patients, but with a rebleeding rate of up to 30%. A drawback of the banding technique is that it can be difficult to perform in the setting of active bleeding; it may be hard to localize the exact source of bleeding with the restricted endoscopic view afforded by the banding device, and blood may pool within the banding mechanism.

There are several new methods reported to endoscopically control bleeding if standard methods are not effective. Similar to nonvariceal bleeding, hemostatic spray has been successfully utilized to control active variceal bleeding, although not approved by the FDA for this indication in the United States. In addition, specially designed self-expanding covered metal stents may be deployed for control of refractory esophageal variceal bleeding with good success rates.

C. Balloon Tamponade

Balloon tamponade is an effective way to achieve short-term hemostasis but should be reserved for patients whose variceal bleeding cannot be controlled by endoscopic therapy or who are having massive bleeding that prohibits an endoscopic attempt. A commonly used device is the Sengstaken-Blakemore tube, which has a large 250-mL gastric balloon and an esophageal balloon, as well as a gastric suctioning port. In patients with massive bleeding uncontrollable by other measures, this tube can be placed with the gastric balloon first inflated after radiographic confirmation of proper position. A nasogastric tube is also usually placed into the esophagus above the level of the balloon for suction. If necessary, the esophageal balloon can be carefully inflated. However, the use of the esophageal balloon is associated with esophageal wall necrosis and rupture, a lethal complication. If definitive therapy is not performed, recurrent bleeding likely will occur when the balloon is deflated. In general, balloon tamponade should be used in an effort to temporarily stabilize a patient prior to the performance of a more definitive radiologic treatment.

D. Radiologic Therapy

The main radiologic therapy is transjugular intrahepatic portosystemic shunt (TIPS). TIPS is a radiologic procedure that creates a portosystemic shunt via a transjugular approach. In this procedure, a connection is made between the portal and hepatic veins and a stent is placed between the two veins. Complications include encephalopathy due to the shunting, shunt occlusion with rebleeding, and shunt migration. Although TIPS is very effective at controlling bleeding (immediate hemostasis in >90% and rebleeding in about 10% of patients), in general TIPS is performed for patients who have persistent variceal bleeding despite endoscopic and medical attempts to control. However, a randomized multicenter trial that compared TIPS with optimal medical and endoscopic therapies in patients at a high risk of rebleeding found improved rates of rebleeding and mortality with TIPS treatment. In consideration of these results, Child-Pugh B or C disease patients who are at very high risk of rebleeding should be considered for TIPS treatment early in their hospital course.

For patients with bleeding gastric varices, another angiographic option is balloon-occluded retrograde transvenous obliteration (BRTO). In the BRTO procedure, a catheter is directed to the gastrorenal or gastrocaval shunt and a balloon is expanded to block the shunt. Sclerosant is then directly injected into the gastric varices until flow is obliterated. BRTO has similar efficacy as a TIPS procedure, but has fewer side effects including postoperative bleeding, encephalopathy, and mortality.

E. Surgical Therapy

Various surgical therapies can be performed to control esophageal and gastric variceal bleeding. These include creation of a portosystemic shunt, which may be a portacaval shunt (nonselective) or a distal splenorenal shunt (selective). Alternately, esophageal transection can be performed, in which the distal esophagus is transected and then stapled back together after ligation of varices, with devascularization of the gastroesophageal junction (Sugiura procedure). In general, the patients who have the best outcomes with surgical shunt therapy have relatively well-preserved liver function (Child-Turcotte-Pugh class A), but have failed endoscopic treatment. The definitive operation to control variceal bleeding is liver transplantation. This is an option only in patients who already listed for liver transplantation due to poor liver function.

▶ Course & Prognosis

Variceal bleeding is a significant cause of rebleeding and mortality. Patients have a high risk of rebleeding until the gastroesophageal varices are obliterated. If a patient survives the initial bleeding episode, repeated courses of band ligation are performed approximately every 2–4 weeks until the varices are obliterated. This technique is often combined with medical therapy using β-blockade. The prognosis for patients with bleeding gastroesophageal varices is poor, even with control of bleeding varices, as this is indicative of progressive liver disease. Patients die from hepatic decompensation, rebleeding, infections, renal failure, and other complications.

2. Portal Hypertensive Gastropathy

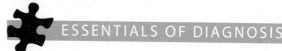

ESSENTIALS OF DIAGNOSIS

▶ Characteristic "snakeskin" endoscopic appearance.
▶ Rare cause of acute bleeding.

▶ Clinical Findings

Portal hypertensive gastropathy, also called congestive gastropathy, occurs with edema and capillary venous dilation in the submucosa and mucosa of the stomach. This causes friability and can result in bleeding with rupture of the ectatic vessels. Endoscopically, the appearance is a reticular, mosaic-like pattern of pink mucosa, with a characteristic "snakeskin" appearance. In patients with cirrhosis and portal hypertension, gastric mucosal blood flow is increased, leading to congestion and hyperemia of the stomach.

Portal hypertensive gastropathy may develop after the endoscopic treatment of esophageal varices. It is postulated that treatment of the esophageal varices increases backpressure into the stomach, leading to the development of gastric congestion. Overall this is a relatively rare cause of acute upper GI bleeding, although it may be a source of chronic blood loss in cirrhotic patients.

▶ Treatment

The goal of treatment of portal hypertensive gastropathy is to decrease portal pressures and therefore stop bleeding. Endoscopic treatments are generally not effective in this disorder, although hemostatic spray may be used as temporizing therapy. The affected area is diffuse, and pharmacologic agents that decrease blood flow, such as octreotide, can be used acutely. Low-dose β-blockers such as propranolol (20–40 mg/day) are often given initially, with the dose increased and adjusted until bleeding stops or side effects occur. Patients with uncontrolled bleeding may need TIPS therapy or shunt surgery. In patients with decompensated liver disease, liver transplantation is indicated.

Abid S, Jafri W, Hamid S, et al. Terlipressin vs octreotide in bleeding esophageal varices as an adjuvant therapy with endoscopic band ligation: a randomized double-blind placebo-controlled trial. Am J Gastroenterol. 2009;104:617–623. [PMID: 19223890]

ASGE Standards of Practice Committee, Hwang JH, Shergill AK, Acosta RD, et al. The role of endoscopy in the management of variceal hemorrhage. Gastrointest Endosc. 2014;80:221–227. [PMID: 25034836]

Bazarbashi AN, Wang TJ, Jirapinyo P, Thompson CC, Ryou M. Endoscopic ultrasound-guided coil embolization with absorbable gelatin sponge appears superior to traditional cyanoacrylate injection for the treatment of gastric varices. Clin Transl Gastroenterol. 2020;11(5):e00175. [PMID: 32677809]

Chavez-Tapia NC, Barrientos-Gutierrez T, Tellez-Avila F, et al. Meta-analysis: antibiotic prophylaxis for cirrhotic patients with upper gastrointestinal bleeding—an updated Cochrane review. Aliment Pharmacol Ther. 2011;34:509.

Garcia-Tsao G, Abraldes JG, Berzigotti A, et al. Portal hypertensive bleeding in cirrhosis: Risk stratification, diagnosis, and management: 2016 practice guidance by the American Association for the study of liver diseases. Hepatology 2017; 65:310–335. [PMID: 27786365]

García-Pagán JC, Caca K, Bureau C, et al. Early TIPS (Transjugular Intrahepatic Portosystemic Shunt) Cooperative Study Group. Early use of TIPS in patients with cirrhosis and variceal bleeding. N Engl J Med. 2010;362:2370–2379. [PMID: 20573925]

García-Pagán JC, Saffo S, Mandorfer M, Garcia-Tsao G. Where does TIPS fit in the management of patients with cirrhosis? JHEP Rep. 2020;2(4):100122. Published 2020 May 23. [PMID: 32671331]

Ibrahim M, El-Mikkawy A, Mostafa I, Devière J. Endoscopic treatment of acute variceal hemorrhage by using hemostatic powder TC-325: a prospective pilot study. Gastrointest Endosc. 2013;78:769–773. [PMID: 24120338]

Jakab SS, Garcia-Tsao G. Evaluation and management of esophageal and gastric varices in patients with cirrhosis. Clin Liver Dis. 2020;24(3):335–350. [PMID: 32620275]

Li L, Yu C, Li Y. Endoscopic band ligation versus pharmacological therapy for variceal bleeding in cirrhosis: a meta-analysis. Can J Gastroenterol. 2011;25:147–155. [PMID: 21499579]

Maufa F, Al-Kawas FH. Role of self-expandable metal stents in acute variceal bleeding. Int J Hepatol. 2012;2012:418369. [PMID: 22928113]

Mishra SR, Chander Sharma B, Kumar A, Sarin SK. Endoscopic cyanoacrylate injection versus beta-blocker for secondary prophylaxis of gastric variceal bleed: a randomized controlled trial. Gut. 2010;59:729–735. [PMID: 20551457]

Tripathi D, Stanley AJ, Hayes PC, et al. U.K. guidelines on the management of variceal haemorrhage in cirrhotic patients. Gut. 2015; 64:1680. [PMID: 25887380]

Wang ZW, Liu JC, Zhao F, et al. Comparison of the effects of TIPS versus BRTO on bleeding gastric varices: a meta-analysis. Can J Gastroenterol Hepatol. 2020 Feb 11;2020:5143013. [PMID: 32104670]

Wells M, Chande N, Adams P, et al. Meta-analysis: vasoactive medications for the management of acute variceal bleeds. Aliment Pharmacol Ther. 2012;35:1267. [PMID: 22486630]

Intestinal Malabsorption & Nutrition

Walter M. Kim, MD PhD

Joshua R. Korzenik, MD

21

ESSENTIALS OF DIAGNOSIS

- ▶ Celiac disease—characteristic though not specific small bowel mucosal lesion, positive antitissue transglutaminase (anti-tTG) or antiendomysium (anti-EmA) serology, and clinical response to gluten withdrawal. HLA-DQ2 and/or HLA-DQ8 present in >99%.

- ▶ Tropical sprue—appropriate geographic exposure; exclude other mucosal diseases (eg, celiac disease and protozoal infestation), exclude small intestinal bacterial overgrowth (SIBO), and assess response to antibiotics and folate.

- ▶ Eosinophilic gastroenteritis—histologic demonstration of increased gastric, intestinal, or colonic mucosal or mural eosinophilic infiltration or eosinophilic ascites.

- ▶ Systemic mastocytosis—demonstration of increased mucosal mast cells (>20 per high-power field) in stomach, small bowel, colon; elevated serum tryptase.

- ▶ Radiation enteritis—history of radiation with mucosal telangiectasias, obliterative endarteriolitis, fibrosis, and strictures; SIBO may develop.

- ▶ Whipple disease—demonstrates *Tropheryma whipplei* and characteristic periodic acid–Schiff-positive macrophages in the intestinal mucosa or other tissue.

- ▶ SIBO—documented evidence of malabsorption, positive breath test (lactulose, glucose) or culture of jejunal aspirate (>10^5 CFU/mL) if available and response to antibiotics.

- ▶ Short bowel syndrome—history of small bowel resection.

- ▶ Intestinal lymphangiectasia—hypoproteinemia, lymphocytopenia, evidence of protein-losing enteropathy, increased fecal loss of α_1-antitrypsin.

General Considerations

Normally the human gastrointestinal tract digests and absorbs dietary nutrients with remarkable efficiency. A typical Western diet ingested by an adult includes approximately 100 g of fat, 400 g of carbohydrate, 100 g of protein, 2 L of fluid, and the required vitamins and electrolytes including sodium, potassium, chloride, calcium, and magnesium. Salivary, gastric, intestinal, hepatic, and pancreatic secretions add an additional 7–8 L of protein-, lipid-, and electrolyte-containing fluid to intestinal contents. This massive load is reduced by the small and large intestines to less than 200 g of stool that contains less than 8 g of fat, 1–2 g of elemental nitrogen, and less than 20 mM each of Na^+, K^+, Cl^-, HCO_3^-, Ca^{2+}, or Mg^{2+} ions.

If there is impairment of any of the many steps involved in the complex process of nutrient digestion and absorption, intestinal malabsorption may ensue. If the abnormality involves a single step in the absorptive process, as in primary lactase deficiency, or if the disease process is limited to the very proximal small intestine, *selective malabsorption* of only a single nutrient (iron or folate) may occur. However, *generalized malabsorption* of multiple dietary nutrients develops when the disease process is extensive, thus disturbing several digestive and absorptive processes, as occurs in celiac disease with extensive involvement of the small intestine.

Pathogenesis

Diseases associated with malabsorption can be segregated into three major categories: those associated with (1) impaired intraluminal digestion, (2) impaired mucosal digestion and absorption, and (3) impaired postmucosal nutrient transport (Table 21–1). Indeed, these are the major mechanisms of intestinal absorption and some disease entities fit neatly into these specific categories. As an example of intraluminal digestive disease, impaired delivery of pancreatic lipase, proteases, and bicarbonate in exocrine pancreatic insufficiency

Table 21–1. Classification of causes of intestinal malabsorption.

1. **Diseases in which impaired intraluminal digestion is dominant**
   - Pancreatic diseases (see Chapter 29)
   - Hepatobiliary disease
   - Postgastrectomy malabsorption
2. **Diseases in which impaired mucosal digestion, uptake, and transport are dominant**
   - Celiac disease
   - Refractory sprue
   - Immunoproliferative small intestinal disease (IPSID) and lymphoma
   - Tropical sprue
   - Eosinophilic gastroenteritis (EGE)
   - Systemic mastocytosis
   - Radiation enteritis
   - Amyloidosis
   - Whipple disease
   - Crohn's disease (see Chapter 3)
   - Abetalipoproteinemia
   - Parasitic infestations
   - Carbohydrate intolerance
3. **Diseases and syndromes in which both impaired intraluminal digestion and mucosal function are often operative**
   - Small intestinal bacterial overgrowth (SIBO)
   - Short bowel syndrome
   - Gastrinoma (Zollinger-Ellison syndrome)
4. **Diseases or syndromes in which impaired postmucosal transport is dominant**
   - Primary intestinal lymphangiectasia
   - Secondary intestinal lymphangiectasia

(EPI) and reduced delivery of hepatobiliary secretions, notably bile salts in biliary obstruction, into the intestinal lumen may result in profound intraluminal maldigestion and may induce malabsorption, especially steatorrhea. As an example of a disease in which the evident pathology is confined to the intestinal mucosa, such as abetalipoproteinemia or lactase deficiency impaired mucosal digestion or absorption, or both, produce nutrient malabsorption. Reduced intestinal lymphatic drainage, an example of impaired postmucosal nutrient transport, whether due to primary or secondary postmucosal obstruction of intestinal lymphatics, results in diminished fat absorption and fecal protein loss.

However, such a classification of malabsorption diseases has its limitations; although one mechanism may dominate in any given disease, in many instances, others contribute. For example, in short bowel syndrome, the marked reduction in mucosal surface and brush border hydrolases results in reduced mucosal absorption and digestion, but if the ileum is absent, bile salt deficiency results in impaired intraluminal digestion; in SIBO, bacteria impair intraluminal lipid digestion but also damage brush border hydrolases and may induce significant mucosal inflammation impairing mucosal digestion and absorption as well; in Whipple disease, the mucosal

infiltration by macrophages and *T whipplei* impair mucosal absorption, but mesenteric and retroperitoneal lymph node involvement may produce lymphatic obstruction, impairing postmucosal delivery and systemic distribution of absorbed dietary lipids.

► Clinical Findings

See Table 21–2.

A. Signs & Symptoms

1. Gastrointestinal manifestations—Depending on the nature of the disease process causing malabsorption and its extent, gastrointestinal symptoms may range from severe to subtle or may even be totally absent. Diarrhea, flatulence, abdominal bloating, abdominal cramping, weight loss, and pain may be present. Although diarrhea is a common complaint, the character and frequency of stools may vary considerably, ranging from over 10 watery stools per day to less than one voluminous putty-like stool, the latter causing some patients to complain of constipation. Small bowel diarrhea tends to have fewer stools compared to the urgency and frequency that is more characteristic of rectal inflammation. On the other hand, stool mass is invariably increased above the normal of 150–200 g/day in patients with generalized malabsorption and significant steatorrhea. Not only do unabsorbed nutrients contribute to stool mass, but secretion of mucosal fluid and electrolyte is also increased in diseases associated with mucosal inflammation such as celiac disease. In addition, unabsorbed fatty acids, converted to hydroxy-fatty acids by colonic flora, as well as unabsorbed bile acids impair absorption and induce secretion of water and electrolytes by the colon adding to stool mass.

Weight loss is common among patients with significant intestinal malabsorption but must be evaluated in the context of caloric intake. Some patients compensate for fecal wastage of unabsorbed nutrients by significantly increasing their oral intake. Others reduce caloric intake as a means of trying to minimize diarrhea. Eliciting a careful dietary history from patients with suspected malabsorption is therefore crucial.

Excessive flatus and abdominal bloating may reflect excessive gas production due to fermentation of unabsorbed carbohydrate, especially among patients with primary or secondary disaccharidase deficiency. Malabsorption of dietary nutrients and excessive fluid secretion by inflamed small intestine also contribute to abdominal distention and bloating.

Prevalence, severity, and character of abdominal pain vary considerably among the various disease processes associated with intestinal malabsorption. For example, pain is common in patients with chronic pancreatitis, pancreatic cancer or Crohn's disease, but it is absent in most patients with celiac disease or postgastrectomy malabsorption.

2. Extraintestinal manifestations—A substantial number of patients with intestinal malabsorption present initially with symptoms or laboratory abnormalities that point to other

Table 21–2. Clinical findings in intestinal malabsorption.

Organ System	Clinical Feature	Cause
Gastrointestinal tract	Diarrhea	Nutrient malabsorption; small intestinal secretion of fluid and electrolytes; action of unabsorbed bile acids and hydroxy-fatty acids on colonic mucosa
	Weight loss	Nutrient malabsorption; decreased dietary intake
	Flatus	Bacterial fermentation of unabsorbed dietary carbohydrates
	Abdominal pain	Distention of bowel, muscle spasm, serosal and peritoneal involvement by disease process
Hematopoietic system	Glossitis, stomatitis, cheilosis	Iron, riboflavin, niacin deficiency
	Anemia, microcytic	Iron, pyridoxine deficiency
	Anemia, macrocytic	Folate, vitamin B_{12} deficiency
	Bleeding	Vitamin K deficiency
Musculoskeletal system	Osteopenic bone disease	Calcium, vitamin D malabsorption
	Osteoarthropathy	Not known
	Tetany	Calcium, magnesium, and vitamin D deficiency
Endocrine system	Amenorrhea, impotence, infertility	Generalized malabsorption and malnutrition
	Secondary hyperparathyroidism	Protracted calcium and vitamin D deficiency
Skin	Purpura	Vitamin K deficiency
	Follicular hyperkeratosis and dermatitis	Vitamin A, zinc, essential fatty acids, niacin deficiency
	Edema	Protein-losing enteropathy, malabsorption of dietary protein
	Hyperpigmentation	Secondary hypopituitarism and adrenal insufficiency
	Vesicular eruption	Dermatitis herpetiformis
Nervous system	Xerophthalmia, night blindness	Vitamin A deficiency
	Peripheral neuropathy	Vitamin B_{12}, thiamine deficiency

organ systems in the absence of or overshadowing symptoms referable to the gastrointestinal tract (see Table 21–2). For example, there is increasing epidemiologic evidence that more patients with celiac disease present with anemia and osteopenic bone disease in the absence of significant gastrointestinal symptoms than present with classic gastrointestinal symptomatology. Microcytic or macrocytic anemia may reflect impaired iron or folate/vitamin B_{12} malabsorption, respectively. Purpura, subconjunctival hemorrhage, or even frank bleeding may reflect hypoprothrombinemia secondary to vitamin K malabsorption. Osteopenic bone disease is common, especially in the presence of steatorrhea. Impaired calcium and vitamin D absorption and chelation of calcium by unabsorbed fatty acids resulting in fecal loss of calcium may all contribute. If calcium deficiency is prolonged, secondary hyperparathyroidism may develop. Prolonged malnutrition may induce amenorrhea, infertility, and impotence. Edema and even ascites may reflect hypoproteinemia associated with

protein-losing enteropathy caused by lymphatic obstruction or extensive mucosal inflammation. Dermatitis and peripheral neuropathy may be caused by malabsorption of specific vitamins or micronutrients and essential fatty acids. These findings may occur in the absence of specific gastrointestinal symptoms.

Bernstein CN, Leslie WD, Leboff MS. AGA technical review on osteoporosis in gastrointestinal disease. *Gastroenterology*. 2003;124:795–841. [PMID: 12612917]

Fine KD, Schiller LR. AGA technical review on the evaluation and management of chronic diarrhea. *Gastroenterology*. 1999;116:1464–1486. [PMID: 10348832]

B. Laboratory & Imaging Studies

1. Stool studies—Descriptions of bowel movements by patients are subjective and often inaccurate. Therefore, careful inspection of the stool by the physician is an important component of the malabsorption evaluation. Although some fat is present in normal stool, the number and size of fat droplets are markedly increased if there is substantial steatorrhea. Steatorrheic stool may be loose or formed but is usually pale, greasy, often bulky with low density and has a characteristic rancid odor. Sudan stain of a spot stool sample for fat is a simple and useful screening test for steatorrhea. Alternatively, stool microscopy using Oil Red O dye to stain lipids and triglycerides offers a moderately sensitive (72%) and highly specific (95%) assessment of fat malabsorption. Quantitative determination of fat in a pooled 48- or 72-hour stool collection, although cumbersome, remains the definitive test for steatorrhea. Ideally, the patient should be placed on an 80–100-g fat diet for 1–2 days before the stool collection is begun and maintain that intake throughout the collection period. Unabsorbable fat, such as mineral oil, olestra (Olean), and fat-based suppositories, must be avoided. The collection should be refrigerated to minimize bacterial metabolism of long-chain fatty acids. Excretion of more than 7–8% of fat intake connotes steatorrhea. The collection should be weighed so that stool fat concentration can be calculated; a stool fat concentration over 9.5% suggests intraluminal maldigestion, whereas a stool fat concentration less than 9.5% suggests mucosal disease as intestinal fluid secretion and malabsorption of other nutrients dilute stool fat in the latter situation (Table 21–3).

Measurements of the pancreatic enzyme, elastase, in the stool assayed using a monoclonal or polyclonal enzyme-linked immunosorbent assay (ELISA) is useful for detecting severe pancreatic exocrine deficiency, but its role in detecting milder disease is limited due to its lack of sensitivity (50–93%)

Table 21–3. Useful laboratory tests in evaluation of intestinal malabsorption.

Test	Impaired Intraluminal Digestion	Mucosal Disease	Lymphatic Obstruction	Limitations
Stool fat (qualitative, quantitative)	Increased (concentration usually >9.5%)	Increased (concentration usually <9.5%)	Increased	False-negative result if inadequate ingestion of dietary fat or recent barium ingestion; false-positive result with castor oil or mineral oil ingestion
Stool elastase	Low in moderate and severe pancreatic exocrine insufficiency	May be low due to dilution	Usually normal	Low specificity for pancreatic disease if small intestinal disease is present
Stool ova and parasites and specific parasitic antigens	May be positive in parasitic biliary cholangiopathy	May diagnose *Giardia*, *Cystoisospora*, cryptosporidia, microsporidia, tapeworms	Negative	False-negative result may occur if recent barium ingestion
Serum carotene	Decreased	Decreased	Decreased	Low values may occur in normal subjects who ingest little dietary carotene
Serum cholesterol	Decreased	Decreased	Decreased	May be normal or increased in patients with untreated lipoprotein abnormality
Serum albumin	Usually normal, except with bacterial overgrowth	Often decreased	Often decreased	Hypoalbuminemia may reflect impaired synthesis in liver disease
Prothrombin activity	Decreased if severe	Decreased if severe	Decreased if severe	May also be decreased in liver disease but parenterally administered vitamin K should induce normalization if caused by malabsorption
Serum calcium	Usually normal if pancreas is the cause	Decreased	Decreased	May reflect hypoalbuminemia
Serum 25-OH vitamin D	Decreased	Decreased	Decreased	
Serum iron	Normal	Often decreased	Normal	

(Continued)

Table 21–3. Useful laboratory tests in evaluation of intestinal malabsorption. (Continued)

Test	Impaired Intraluminal Digestion	Mucosal Disease	Lymphatic Obstruction	Limitations
Serum folate	Normal, may be increased with bacterial overgrowth	Often decreased	Normal	
Xylose absorption	Normal, except with bacterial overgrowth	Abnormal, unless disease confined to distal small intestine	Normal	Requires normal gastric emptying and renal function
Lactose absorption (lactose tolerance test or breath hydrogen after lactose load)	Normal, except in some instances of bacterial overgrowth	Increase in plasma glucose <20 mg/dL; increase in breath H_2 >20 ppm above fasting baseline	Normal	May be abnormal in all categories if patient has primary intestinal lactase deficiency; requires normal gastric emptying
Vitamin B_{12} absorption (Schilling test)	Decreased in bacterial overgrowth and exocrine pancreatic insufficiency	Decreased in extensive ileal disease	Normal	Requires good renal function
Lactulose and glucose breath hydrogen test	Early appearance of H_2 in breath in bacterial overgrowth	Normal	Normal	Requires normal gastric emptying; false-positive results may occur in patients with rapid small intestinal transit
Secretin/cholecystokinin stimulation tests	Abnormal in chronic pancreatic exocrine insufficiency	Normal	Normal	Relatively low sensitivity, cumbersome, and labor intensive
Anti–tissue transglutaminase IgA and antiendomysial IgA antibodies	Absent	Present in celiac disease	Absent	Lower sensitivity in infants and all ages in mild disease, false-negative results in IgA deficiency
Endoscopic intestinal biopsy	Normal except in severe bacterial overgrowth	Often abnormal	Often abnormal	May miss patchy mucosal disease
Video capsule endoscopy	Usually normal	Often abnormal	Often abnormal	Labor intensive, cannot biopsy lesions, may obstruct strictured intestine

and specificity (62–93%). The secretin/cholecystokinin stimulation test, although cumbersome and rarely performed, remains the gold standard for detecting pancreatic insufficiency (see Chapter 29).

Stool samples should be evaluated for ova and parasites and for specific parasitic antigens in patients with suspected malabsorption, especially if diarrhea is present. Several protozoal diseases, including giardiasis, cryptosporidiosis, microsporidiosis, and *Cystoisospora belli* infection, can produce significant malabsorption.

Assessment of fecal calprotectin can be an effective screening test for inflammation and Crohn's disease of the small bowel for purposes of this discussion, though the test is less reliable with more proximal small bowel involvement. As a product associated with neutrophil-mediated inflammation, it also does not serve as a useful marker of eosinophilic or lymphocytic disease as it would reflect neutrophilic infiltration of the mucosa.

Bo-Linn GW, Fordtran JS. Fecal fat concentration in patients with steatorrhea. *Gastroenterology*. 1984;87:318–322. [PMID: 6735076]

Leeds JS, Oppong K, Sanders DS. The role of fecal elastase-1 in detecting exocrine pancreatic disease. *Nat Rev Gastroenterol Hepatol*. 2011;8:405–415. [PMID: 21629239]

Nikaki K, Gupte GL. Assessment of intestinal malabsorption. *Best Pract Res Clin Gastroenterol*. 2016;30(2):225–235. [PMID: 27086887]

Stein J, Jung M, Sziegoleit A, Zeuzem S, Caspary WF, Lembcke B. Immunoreactive elastase I: clinical evaluation of a new noninvasive test of pancreatic function. *Clin Chem*. 1996;42(2):222–226. [PMID: 8595714]

2. Blood studies—Abnormalities in the formed elements of the peripheral blood are quite common in patients with diseases that produce malabsorption. Anemia is common. Diffuse lesions of the proximal intestine as occur in celiac disease or Whipple disease interfere with iron absorption and folate absorption resulting in microcytic (iron deficiency or blood loss), macrocytic (folate or vitamin B_{12} deficiency), or dimorphic anemia (combined iron and folate or vitamin B_{12} deficiency). Ileal resection or severe ileal disease as well as intraluminal bacterial overgrowth and, rarely, severe EPI interfere with vitamin B_{12} absorption and may produce macrocytic anemia. Concomitantly, serum iron saturation, ferritin, iron, folate, and vitamin B_{12} levels are decreased. Normocytic anemia may reflect acute or subacute blood loss as may occur in Crohn's disease, intestinal lymphoma, or Whipple disease. Peripheral leukocytosis is unusual, but the differential count may reveal eosinophilia in eosinophilic enteritis or some parasitic diseases or profound lymphopenia in patients with intestinal lymphangiectasia. Thrombocytosis, if present, may reflect hyposplenism, which occurs in some adults with celiac disease.

A number of other blood chemistries and serologies may be abnormal and may provide clues that malabsorption is present, and, in some instances, help define a specific diagnosis. Low serum carotene and cholesterol are nonspecific indicators of fat malabsorption, but the serum carotene also largely reflects recent dietary carotene intake. Low serum calcium in patients with malabsorption may reflect poor absorption in mucosal disease, intraluminal formation of insoluble calcium soaps by interaction with unabsorbed fatty acids, as well as coexistent vitamin D deficiency, all resulting in fecal wastage of calcium. Low serum calcium may also accompany hypoalbuminemia, especially in patients with mucosal disease or lymphangiectasia, causing exudative enteric protein loss. The prothrombin time may be prolonged as vitamin K is fat soluble, but in the absence of liver disease, the international normalized ratio (INR) should normalize following intravenous vitamin K replacement. Levels of anti–tissue trans-glutaminase immunoglobulin A antibody (anti-tTG IgA), which is positive in 98% of individuals with celiac assuming they do not have an IgA deficiency should be obtained if celiac disease is suspected with subsequent antiendomysial IgA antibody evaluation, which is positive in 90–95% of individuals with celiac and essentially 100% specific, or endoscopy with duodenal biopsy sampling if diagnosis of celiac disease is uncertain.

3. Specific oral absorption tests and breath tests—
Where available, the D-xylose absorption test may help to differentiate malabsorption caused by small intestinal mucosal disease from malabsorption due to impaired intraluminal digestion or lymphatic obstruction. This pentose sugar requires no intraluminal processing and is absorbed by facilitated diffusion. After administration of an oral 25 g dose to a well-hydrated patient, 5 g or more are normally excreted in the urine over 5 hours, and blood levels should reach 25 mg/dL 2 hours after the test dose. Reduced urine excretion and blood levels suggest disease of the mucosa of the proximal small intestine such as celiac disease. However, the test has significant limitations. It is dependent on normal gastric emptying and normal renal function; delayed gastric emptying will lower both urine xylose excretion and blood xylose levels giving a potentially false-positive result and impaired renal function will reduce urine xylose excretion but not blood xylose levels in the face of normal gastric emptying. Ascites and edema may result in sequestration of absorbed xylose and produce a false-positive test result. Additionally, in patients with bacterial overgrowth in the proximal small intestine, the xylose absorption test may be positive as some bacterial species metabolize xylose, reducing its availability for absorption.

To screen for intestinal lactase or, less commonly, sucrase deficiency, either breath hydrogen excretion or blood glucose can be measured following an orally administered test dose of lactose or sucrose. Determination of breath hydrogen excretion has virtually supplanted measurement of blood glucose when testing for lactase deficiency because of its simplicity and because no venipuncture is needed. If lactose is malabsorbed, it travels to the distal small intestine where the bacterial flora metabolizes the sugar releasing hydrogen, which is excreted by the lungs and can be readily measured in the breath. After a test lactose dose of 2 g/kg (25 g maximum), a rise of less than 10 parts per million (ppm) is normal, whereas a rise to 20 ppm suggests lactase deficiency. Limitations include impaired gastric emptying, chronic pulmonary disease, recent antibiotic usage, or absence of hydrogen-producing bacteria, all of which reduce breath hydrogen excretion, potentially giving rise to falsely negative results. On the other hand, proximal SIBO may result in a false-positive result, causing hydrogen release before the sugar can be normally absorbed. Disaccharidase enzyme levels can also be directly measured biochemically if fresh mucosal biopsy tissue is available for this purpose; however, this is rarely performed in the clinical setting. It is important to emphasize that neither oral absorption tests, hydrogen breath tests nor direct measurements of disaccharidase enzymes in mucosal tissues, distinguish primary enzyme deficiency from secondary enzyme deficiency caused by other disease processes that damage the epithelium mucosa of the small intestine.

Several substrates have been used in breath tests to screen for small intestinal intraluminal bacterial overgrowth. These include glucose, lactulose, and radio-isotope labeled ^{14}C-xylose. In all instances, the presence of bacteria in the proximal small intestine should result in rapid bacterial metabolism of the sugars and hence appearance in the breath of $^{14}CO_2$ after ^{14}C-xylose and of hydrogen after glucose as well as early peak breath hydrogen levels after lactulose administration. Under normal circumstances, lactulose is not metabolized until it reaches the distal ileal and colonic flora, resulting in later peak hydrogen levels, whereas glucose and xylose are fully absorbed in the proximal intestine before there is opportunity for bacterial metabolism. All three tests have significant limitations. Delayed gastric emptying, rapid small intestinal transit, absence of hydrogen-producing colonic flora in those whose microbiota instead produce methane (CH_4), and significant pulmonary disease all reduce sensitivity or specificity when compared with the gold standard for diagnosing intraluminal bacterial overgrowth, namely, quantitative culture analysis of an aspirate of proximal jejunal intraluminal contents. These tests are at best 70–80% sensitive in confirming a diagnosis of SIBO.

Abdelshaheed NN, Goldberg DM. Biochemical tests in diseases of the intestinal tract: their contribution to diagnosis, management, and understanding the pathophysiology of specific disease states. *Crit Rev Clin Lab Sci.* 1997;34:141–223. [PMID: 9143817]

Craig RM, Ehrenpreis ED. D-xylose testing. *J Clin Gastroenterol.* 1999;29:143–150. [PMID: 10478874]

Gasbarrini AA, Corazza GRG, Gasbarrini GG, et al. Methodology and indications of H2-breath testing in gastrointestinal diseases: the Rome Consensus Conference. *Aliment Pharmacol Ther.* 2009;29(suppl 1):1–49. [PMID: 19344474]

Losurdo G, Leandro G, Ierardi E, et al. Breath tests for the noninvasive diagnosis of small intestinal bacterial overgrowth: a systematic review with meta-analysis. *J Neurogastroenterol Motil.* 2020;26(1):16–28. [PMID: 31743632]

Thomas PD, Forbes A, Green J, et al. Guidelines for the investigation of chronic diarrhoea, 2nd edition. *Gut.* 2003;52(suppl 5):1–15. [PMID: 12801941]

4. Imaging studies—Various imaging studies are available to help clarify the nature of pancreatic and hepatobiliary disease that may cause or contribute to intestinal malabsorption. These include endoscopic retrograde cholangiopancreatography (ERCP), magnetic resonance cholangiopancreatography (MRCP), abdominal computed tomography (CT), abdominal magnetic resonance imaging (MRI), and abdominal and endoscopic ultrasonography. They are discussed in some detail in Chapter 9 of this text.

For many years, conventional barium contrast studies of the small intestine (small bowel follow through x-ray series) were the standard for evaluating the gross structure of the small intestine in suspected or proven malabsorption. However, both sensitivity and specificity of the conventional small intestinal contrast series are low. Sensitivity, especially for detection of focal lesions, can be improved by utilizing double-contrast enteroclysis performed by instilling both barium and carboxymethyl cellulose into the duodenal lumen and fluoroscopically following the contrast material as it transits the small intestine. However, enteroclysis is labor intensive, limited by body habitus and results in substantial exposure of the patient to radiation. More recently, computed tomographic enterography (CTE), has become widely used for detecting small intestinal abnormalities. CTE is performed with administration of oral and intravenous contrast material. Both sagittal and cross-sectional images are obtained. MRI enterography provides similar information as CTE. Both techniques are useful, for example, in the detection of diffuse mucosal disease as well as focal abnormalities such as strictures and neoplasms, evaluation of bowel wall thickness, evaluation of visceral as well as mucosal blood flow, and assessing the length of remaining small intestine after major intestinal resections. MRI enterography has the distinct benefit of avoiding exposure to ionizing radiation, especially important in the evaluation of pregnant patients, pediatric patients and patients such as those with Crohn's disease likely to require multiple studies over time.

Masselli G, Gualdi G. CT and MR enterography in evaluating small bowel diseases: when to use which modality?. *Abdom Imaging.* 2013;38:249–259. [PMID: 23011551]

Park SH, Ye BD, Lee TY, Fletcher JG. Computed tomography and magnetic resonance small bowel enterography: current status and future trends focusing on Crohn's disease. *Gastroenterol Clin North Am.* 2018;47(3):475–499. [PMID: 30115433]

5. Endoscopic and biopsy studies—Visualization of the mucosal surface of the small intestine within the reach of the endoscope allows the macroscopic detection of abnormal gross mucosal surface features. These include the diminution and scalloping of mucosal folds, absence or apparent blunting of villi (common in celiac disease), and whitish-appearing dilated lymphatic lacteals within villi commonly found in Whipple disease and intestinal lymphangiectasia. However, both the sensitivity and specificity of such endoscopic findings are low. Rather, the greatest contribution of direct endoscopy to the evaluation of patients with malabsorption is its facilitation of mucosal biopsy under direct visualization. As indicated in Table 21–4, some diseases, such as Whipple disease, amyloidosis, and giardiasis, are associated with a specific lesion, and biopsy is often diagnostic. Other diseases are characterized by histologic features that, although abnormal, lack specificity and require additional clinical information for a definitive diagnosis. However, even when the biopsy specimen is not in and of itself diagnostic, it is often of great value as it establishes unequivocally the presence of mucosal disease. The definitive diagnosis is then established by additional diagnostic studies or by response to specific therapy.

Because intestinal malabsorption may occur in a number of diseases in which mucosal involvement may be patchy (see Table 21–4), multiple biopsy specimens (at least four, preferably six to eight) should be obtained from several sites in the duodenum or proximal jejunum. A biopsy or two should be obtained from the duodenal bulb as lesions consistent with celiac disease were observed only in the bulb in about 10% of patients in several recent studies. Samples of luminal fluid can also be obtained at the time of endoscopy, facilitating the diagnosis of parasitic infestation such as giardiasis and coccidioses and, if sophisticated culture facilities are available, intestinal intraluminal bacterial overgrowth.

Wireless video capsule endoscopy (VCE) using a swallowed camera that transmits high resolution color images of the mucosal surface as it tumbles through the gastrointestinal tract is an established imaging modality of the intestinal mucosa, including that of the mid and distal small intestine (see Chapter 34). It has been particularly useful in detecting

Table 21–4. Information provided by mucosal biopsy of the small intestine.

1. **Disorders in which biopsy result is diagnostic: diffuse lesions**
   a. Whipple disease
      - Lamina propria infiltrated with periodic acid–Schiff-positive macrophages
      - Characteristic bacilli in mucosa
   b. *Mycobacterium avium–intracellulare* enteritis: similar to Whipple disease but bacilli are acid fast
   c. Severe immunoglobulin deficiency
      - Mucosal architecture from normal to flat
      - Plasma cells absent or markedly diminished in lamina propria
      - Giardia trophozoites may be present
   d. Abetalipoproteinemia
      - Mucosal architecture normal
      - Lipid-laden absorptive cells appear vacuolated
2. **Disorders in which biopsy result may be diagnostic: patchy lesions**
   a. Intestinal lymphoma
      - Villi widened, shortened, or absent
      - Malignant lymphoma cells infiltrate epithelium lamina propria and submucosa
   b. Intestinal lymphangiectasia
      - Mucosal architecture normal
      - Dilated lymphatics in lamina propria and submucosa
   c. Eosinophilic gastroenteritis
      - Mucosal architecture from normal to flat
      - Patchy infiltration of lamina propria with aggregates of eosinophils
   d. Mastocytosis
      - Mucosal architecture from normal to flat
      - Patchy infiltration of lamina propria with mast cells, eosinophils, and neutrophils
   e. Amyloidosis
      - Mucosal architecture normal
      - Amyloid in lamina propria and submucosa, often in blood vessel walls, shown with Congo red stain and polarized light
   f. Crohn's disease
      - Mucosal architecture variable
      - Noncaseating granulomata and inflammation in lamina propria and submucosa
   g. Giardiasis
      - Mucosal architecture from normal to flat
      - Trophozoites in lumen and on surface of absorptive cells
      - Minimal to severe inflammation in lamina propria
   h. Coccidiosis
      - Villi shortened
      - Crypts hyperplastic
      - Coccidial forms in apical cytoplasm of (cryptosporidiosis) or anywhere within (Cystoisospora) absorptive cells
      - Inflammation of lamina propria
3. **Disorders in which biopsy result is abnormal but not diagnostic**
   a. Celiac disease
      - Villi shortened or absent
      - Crypts hyperplastic
      - Damaged absorptive cells
      - Increased intraepithelial lymphocytes (IELs)
      - Inflammation of lamina propria
   b. Refractory sprue: histology indistinguishable from celiac disease; immunocytochemistry may show phenotypically abnormal IELs
   c. Tropical sprue
      - Mucosal architecture from nearly normal to flat mucosa (as in celiac sprue)
      - Absorptive cell damage mild
      - Inflammation of lamina propria
   d. Viral gastroenteritis: indistinguishable from mild to moderate tropical sprue or celiac disease lesion
   e. Intraluminal bacterial overgrowth: may be normal or indistinguishable from mild to moderate tropical sprue or celiac disease lesion
   f. Folate or vitamin B_{12} deficiency, acute radiation enteritis
      - Villi shortened
      - Crypts hypoplastic
      - Megalocytic epithelium
      - Diminished mitoses
      - Inflammation of lamina propria

focal lesions beyond the reach of the endoscope, especially among patients with occult gastrointestinal bleeding. Like direct endoscopy, it also provides useful views of the gross structure of the mucosa and detects the fold scalloping, flat mucosa, and distended lymphatic lacteals when these lesions are well developed. A limitation of capsule endoscopy is that it provides no tissue for pathologic evaluation. Hence, its role in the diagnosis of intestinal malabsorption is complementary to endoscopy and biopsy. However, the capsule camera may cause intestinal obstruction if tight strictures are present; hence, it must be used with caution in patients with suspected malignancy or suspected stricturing Crohn's disease and should be preceded by patency capsule evaluation in those types of cases.

Babbin BA, Crawford K, Sitaraman SV. Malabsorption work-up: utility of small bowel biopsy. *Clin Gastroenterol Hepatol.* 2006;4:1193–1198. [PMID: 16979950]

Eliakim R. Video capsule endoscopy of the small bowel. *Curr Opin Gastroenterol.* 2013;29:133–139. [PMID: 23221650]

SPECIFIC CONDITIONS RESULTING IN INTESTINAL MALABSORPTION

DISEASES ASSOCIATED WITH INTRALUMINAL MALDIGESTION

1. Pancreatic & Hepatobiliary Diseases

Delivery of adequate amounts of pancreatic lipase, colipase, proteases, and amylases as well as bicarbonate into the proximal intestine is essential for normal intraluminal digestion of dietary lipids, proteins, and complex carbohydrates. Pancreatic reserve is substantial, and significant malabsorption generally does not occur unless there is 85–90% reduction in pancreatic enzyme secretion. The diagnostic and clinical ramifications of chronic pancreatic insufficiency are discussed in detail in the chapters that deal with pancreatitis (see Chapter 28) and pancreatic neoplasms (see Chapter 31). As described earlier, determination of stool fat concentration

(see Table 21–3) is useful in distinguishing malabsorption caused by EPI resulting in impaired intraluminal digestion from malabsorption caused by mucosal disease. In malabsorption caused by pancreatic disease, tests of mucosal absorption, such as oral tolerance tests and intestinal mucosal structure as assessed by biopsy and imaging studies, are usually normal unless there is coexisting mucosal disease.

Delivery of bile salts into the proximal intestinal lumen is essential for normal dispersion and intraluminal digestion of dietary lipids prior to their absorption by the intestinal mucosa. Hence, hepatobiliary disease that significantly reduces bile salt synthesis and delivery of bile salts into the proximal intestinal lumen causes significant malabsorption as does fecal bile salt loss caused by ileal disease or resection sufficient to deplete the circulating bile salt pool. (See the discussion of "short bowel syndrome.")

2. Postgastrectomy Malabsorption

With the recognition of gastric *Helicobacter pylori* colonization as a cause of peptic ulcer disease, the development of histamine-2 (H_2) receptor antagonists and proton pump inhibitors for therapy of peptic ulcer disease as well as endoscopic interventional techniques to control ulcer bleeding, the need for surgical intervention to treat peptic ulcer disease has diminished strikingly in recent decades. However, occasionally patients still require surgery to control ulcer bleeding and others require partial or total gastric resection for malignancy, vascular compromise, or gastric infections. Hence, a pool of individuals at risk for malabsorption after gastric surgery persists. The risk of significant malabsorption correlates with the extent of alteration of normal anatomy. Thus, the risk is greatest after total gastrectomy and progressively decreases after partial gastrectomy and gastrojejunal anastomoses (Billroth II), antrectomy and gastric duodenal anastomoses (Billroth I), and vagotomy and pyloroplasty and is virtually nonexistent after selective proximal vagotomy.

Several mechanisms may cause malabsorption after gastric surgery, and treatment varies depending on the causes (Table 21–5). The most common has been termed "poor

Table 21–5. Malabsorption associated with gastric surgery.

Cause	Onset	Diagnosis	Treatment
"Poor mixing, poor timing"	Immediate	Exclusion of other causes	Antimotility agents, supplemental pancreatic enzymes
Intraluminal bacterial overgrowth	Delayed	Vitamin B_{12} absorption tests, breath tests, cultures of luminal contents	Antibiotics, surgical revision if refractory to antibiotics
Unmasked latent celiac disease	Immediate	Antitissue transglutaminase or antiendomysial antibodies, intestinal mucosal biopsy	Dietary gluten withdrawal
Gastrocolic or jejunocolic fistula	Delayed	Barium enema, endoscopy	Antibiotics and surgery
Inadvertent gastroileostomy	Immediate	Upper gastrointestinal series	Surgery

mixing and poor timing." Rapid gastric emptying coupled with decreased release of secretin and cholecystokinin results in suboptimal exposure of the nutrient bolus to both bile salts and pancreatic enzyme as it traverses the small intestine. This diagnosis is made after excluding more treatable causes of postgastrectomy malabsorption.

Intraluminal bacterial overgrowth should be excluded as a cause of postgastrectomy malabsorption. Reduced acid secretion and intraluminal stasis, especially in patients with an afferent loop following total gastrectomy or a Billroth II operation, are predisposing causes.

Patients with silent or latent celiac disease may develop symptomatic celiac disease after gastrectomy most likely caused by the rapid delivery of gluten to the small intestine and its impaired digestion in the remaining gastric remnant and proximal intestine.

Recurrent ulcer disease, especially in patients who have undergone a gastrojejunostomy, may cause a gastrocolic or jejunocolic fistula. Reflux of colonic contents into the gastric remnant and proximal intestine through the fistula results in massive bacterial overgrowth. As intracolonic pressure exceeds intrajejunal pressure, a barium enema is the diagnostic procedure of choice as infused barium will flow through the fistula into the stomach or proximal bowel, bypassing the distal small intestine. Control with antibiotics is usually unsuccessful, and further surgery is indicated to correct the cause of the recurrent ulcer and to remove or repair the fistula.

Severe malabsorption immediately after surgery has been reported if a surgeon inadvertently creates a gastroileostomy rather than a gastrojejunostomy. Fortunately, such surgical misadventure is very rare, and treatment is surgical revision of the anastomoses.

Malabsorption of specific vitamins and minerals may occur. For example, calcium and vitamin D malabsorption may result in osteopenia and iron malabsorption may result in anemia, especially among those in whom the duodenum and proximal jejunum have been bypassed. Vitamin B_{12} malabsorption may result from major gastric resections or atrophy of the remaining gastric mucosa. Specific therapy for these deficiencies should be provided as indicated.

Lactose intolerance may be aggravated or first become evident after gastric surgery due to rapid delivery of lactase-containing nutrients into the small intestine. Treatment with supplemental lactase or low-lactose dairy products is usually effective.

DISEASES ASSOCIATED WITH IMPAIRED MUCOSAL DIGESTION & ABSORPTION

1. Celiac Disease (Celiac Sprue)

Celiac disease is an immune-mediated gluten intolerance in genetically predisposed individuals in whom exposure to wheat, barley, rye, or triticale induces a characteristic though not specific mucosal pathology that responds to withdrawal

of dietary gluten. With the increase in availability during the past 20 years of reliable serologic screening tests, it has become evident that the disease is far more common than was previously appreciated. It occurs in 0.5–1% of the general population and is rarest among those of Chinese, Japanese, Korean, and African heritage where gluten consumption is low. Females are at higher risk of developing celiac disease where there is a 1.5:1 female-to-male ratio of positive serological testing. Symptoms may initially present at virtually any age, ranging from infancy (upon addition of gluten-containing cereal to feedings) to late adulthood. There is accumulating evidence that the true incidence of celiac disease is increasing. Its prevalence is increased among those with a number of autoimmune diseases which include, for example, dermatitis herpetiformis (>90%), type 1 diabetes (3–16%), Sjögren syndrome, Inflammatory Bowel Disease, microscopic colitis, and autoimmune liver and thyroid diseases. The minority of individuals with celiac disease have classical symptoms of malabsorption whereas the majority have either nonclassical symptoms or only mild or no gastrointestinal symptoms.

Caio G, Volta U, Sapone A, Leffler DA, De Giorgio R, Catassi C, Fasano A. Celiac disease: a comprehensive current review. *BMC Med.* 2019;17(1):142. [PMID: 31331324]

Ludvigsson JF, Leffler DA, Bai JC, et al. The Oslo definitions for coeliac disease and related terms. *Gut.* 2013;62:43–52. [PMID: 22345659]

Ludvigsson JF, Rubio-Tapia A, van Dyke CT, et al. Increasing incidence of celiac disease in a North American population. *Gastroenterol.* 2013;108:818–824. [PMID: 23511460]

Pathogenesis

Genetic factors and altered immune function both play a major role in the pathogenesis of celiac disease. The disease has a prevalence of 10–15% in first-order relatives (parents, children, and siblings) of affected individuals. Concordance is approximately 75–80% among identical twins, and approximately 25–30% among HLA-identical siblings; 90–95% of affected individuals carry the HLA-DQ2 heterodimer; over 90% of the remaining 5–10% carry the HLA-DQ8 heterodimer. Thus HLA-DQ2 and/or HLA-DQ8 is present in >99% of celiac patients; however, it is worth noting that only 3% of HLA-DQ2 or HLA-DQ8-containing individuals develop celiac disease. Those who are homozygous for HLA-DQ2 and/or HLA-DQ8 are at greater risk of developing celiac disease than those who are heterozygous.

Because of their high proline content, the gluten proteins in wheat, barley, and rye resist intraluminal proteolytic digestive processes. This results in the accumulation of large peptide fragments, some of which result in damage of the mucosa of individuals with celiac disease both *in vivo* and *in vitro*. Mucosal tissue transglutaminase (tTG) deamidates glutamine residues in the immunogenic peptide fragments.

These now negatively charged fragments bind to the antigen-binding grooves of intestinal antigen-presenting cells from individuals with celiac disease which, in turn, present these dietary gluten peptides in the context of HLA-DQ2 and/or HLA-DQ8 and thus activate DQ2-restricted or DQ8-restricted gluten peptide–specific mucosal T lymphocytes. Once activated, the T lymphocytes release inflammatory mediators that contribute to the development of mucosal damage.

Recent studies suggest that activation of the innate immune system may participate in the pathogenesis of celiac disease in concert with the adaptive immune system. Upregulation of mucosal interleukin-15 expression during gluten exposure ultimately imparts natural killer cell–like properties to the lymphocytes residing among the mucosal epithelial cells (intraepithelial lymphocytes [IELs]), resulting in epithelial cell damage and increased mucosal permeability. This, in turn, likely facilitates the exposure of mucosal antigen-presenting cells to toxic gluten peptides this inducing T-cell activation of the adaptive immune response.

Dieli-Crimi R, Cénit MC, Núñez C. The genetics of celiac disease: a comprehensive review of clinical implications. *J Autoimmun.* 2015;64:26–41. [PMID: 26194613]

Jabri B, Sollid LV. Tissue-mediated control of immunopathology in celiac disease. *Nat Rev Immunol.* 2009;9:858–871. [PMID: 19935805]

Kupfer SS, Jabri B. Pathophysiology of celiac disease. *Gastrointest Endoscopy Clin N Am.* 2012;11:639–660. [PMID: 23083984]

Lundin KE, Wijmenga C. Coeliac disease and autoimmune disease-genetic overlap and screening. *Nat Rev Gastroenterol Hepatol.* 2015;12:507–515. [PMID: 26303674]

▶ Clinical Findings

A. Symptoms & Signs

The clinical spectrum of celiac disease is very broad. In those with a mild lesion involving only the proximal small intestine, the disease may be completely silent with no evident clinical manifestations. This has been termed "subclinical" or "asymptomatic" celiac disease. In others with a lesion limited to the proximal intestine, selected nutrient deficiencies, which may include iron, folate, or calcium, may be present with resultant anemia or osteopenia but with no significant gastrointestinal symptoms. This has been termed "nonclassical" or extraintestinal celiac disease. On the other hand, if a more severe lesion extends to the more distal intestine, pan malabsorption with gastrointestinal symptoms, including weight loss, diarrhea, excess flatus, and abdominal discomfort, may all be present in concert with evidence of involvement of other systems (see Table 21–2). This has been termed "classical" or intestinal celiac disease. The severity of the mucosal lesion and the extent of the intestinal involvement by the lesion are likely important factors in the clinical presentation of any given patient.

Physical findings like symptoms may vary among celiac patients and may be absent in those with subclinical and non-classical celiac disease. In those with more symptomatic disease, the physical findings described previously in the general description of intestinal malabsorption may be evident.

B. Laboratory Findings

Laboratory findings, like the clinical manifestations, may vary enormously depending on extent of disease, ranging from no abnormalities or only isolated iron or folate deficiency in nonclassical celiac disease to multiple abnormalities including steatorrhea, hypoalbuminemia, hypoprothrombinemia, hypocalcemia, and so on in classical celiac disease (see Table 21–3). Elevated serum transaminase levels may be the presenting finding in some patients with celiac disease.

To correctly diagnose celiac disease, the clinician obviously must suspect that the disease may be present. This is simple enough in those in whom gastrointestinal symptoms and malabsorption are obvious. It is more of a challenge if only subtle symptoms or a nonspecific laboratory abnormality is present. Such patients are often diagnosed as having irritable bowel syndrome (IBS), unexplained osteopenia, or unexplained iron deficiency or folate deficiency anemia. A high index of suspicion is essential for the correct diagnosis of the many patients who present with subtle findings.

Serologic tests are useful screening tests for celiac disease. Both the ELISA-based anti-tTG IgA and the immunofluorescent anti-EmA (anti-endomysium) IgA tests are useful and have reported sensitivities of 94–97% and specificities of 91–100%. Sensitivities are somewhat lower in infants, toddlers, and patients with mild or silent disease. Both tests measure the autoantibody directed against the enzyme, tissue transglutaminase. Tissue transglutaminase is found in many body tissues including the intestinal mucosa. The anti-tTG IgA test is widely used as the initial screening test owing to its higher sensitivity (97% vs 94%) with the anti-EmA IgA test, which is operator dependent and somewhat more costly, used when the anti-tTG IgA test is unexpectedly negative or to confirm a positive anti-tTG IgA test due to its higher specificity (91% vs 100%).

Both conventional anti-tTG and anti-EmA measure IgA class antibodies; therefore, some false-negative tests are inevitable as the prevalence of selective IgA deficiency among celiac disease patients is 2–4%. Thus, if an anticipated positive test is reported as negative, the serum IgA level should be quantitated. Anti-tTG IgG and anti-EmA IgG can be determined, but the sensitivity of these tests is substantially lower than that of their IgA counterparts. Recently, both anti-deamidated gliadin peptide (DGP) IgA and IgG antibody tests have become available. However, it has not been demonstrated that anti-DGP IgA provides a significant advantage over anti-tTG IgA. On the other hand, anti-DGP IgG has higher sensitivity (84.4%) and specificity (98.5%) than anti-tTG IgG and is the serological test of choice in IgA-deficient individuals.

Mucosal intestinal biopsy of the bulb, the distal duodenum or proximal jejunum, coupled with a clinical response to the dietary withdrawal of gluten, remains the gold standard for the diagnosis of celiac disease. Because dietary gluten withdrawal is a lifetime commitment with substantial cost and social liability, a diagnostic trial of a gluten-free diet (GFD) should not be undertaken without first obtaining biopsy evidence consistent with celiac sprue. The one exception to this rule is recommended in recently published pediatric association guidelines for children and adolescents whose anti-tTG IgA levels exceed 10 times the upper limit of normal, who are also anti-EmA positive using a separate blood sample and who are HLA-DQ2 and/or HLA-DQ8 positive. If these criteria are met in the pediatric population, biopsy prior to institution of a GFD may be omitted.

In biopsies from untreated celiac patients, villi may be blunted or the mucosal surface may appear to be flat with complete absence of villi. Crypts are hyperplastic, with increased numbers of mitotic figures. Surface absorptive cells are damaged and infiltrated by increased numbers of IELs. There is also extensive infiltration of the lamina propria by a lymphoplasmacytic infiltrate. The mucosal lesion, although characteristic, is not specific (Plate 38, 39). Other diseases that may have similar clinical manifestations and may have similar mucosal histology include refractory sprue, tropical sprue, viral gastroenteritis (especially when caused by rotavirus in children), intraluminal bacterial overgrowth, olmesartan-induced enteropathy, and eosinophilic gastroenteritis. Hence, a clinical response to gluten withdrawal is a crucial step in establishing the diagnosis.

Human leukocyte antigen (HLA) testing is of value in patients with atypical features or incongruent serologic and biopsy results for excluding celiac disease. It is also of value in patients who have begun a GFD in the absence of definitive studies establishing a diagnosis of celiac disease. The absence of both HLA-DQ2 and HLA-DQ8 effectively excludes the diagnosis of celiac disease. On the other hand, the detection of either of these haplotypes is of no direct diagnostic value in establishing the diagnosis of celiac disease as they are present in approximately 25–35% of Caucasians of European heritage.

Lebwohl B, Sanders DS, Green PHR. Coeliac disease. *Lancet.* 2018;391(10115):70–81. [PMID: 28760445]

Leffler DA, Schuppan D. Update on serological testing in celiac disease. *Am J Gastroenterol.* 2010;105:2520–2524. [PMID: 21131921]

Zucchini L, Giusti D, Gatouillat G, Servettaz A, Tabary T, Barbe C, Pham BN. Interpretation of serological tests in the diagnosis of celiac disease: anti-deamidated gliadin peptide antibodies revisited. *Autoimmunity.* 2016;49(6):414–420. [PMID: 27452003]

▶ Treatment

The cornerstone of treatment of celiac disease is adherence to a GFD through the elimination of products containing wheat, barley, rye, and triticale (Table 21–6). There is convincing

Table 21–6. Initial treatment of celiac disease.

- Avoid all wheat, barley, rye, and oat gluten
- Rice, corn, millet, potato, buckwheat, and soybeans are safe
- Read all labels of processed foods; be suspicious of all additives such as hydrolyzed vegetable protein
- Limit intake of dairy products until diarrhea disappears
- Replace all deficient micronutrients with specific supplements as needed (calcium, iron, folate, vitamins)
- Pneumococcal vaccination if hyposplenism is present
- Join a local celiac disease support group

evidence that at least moderate quantities of oats (50 g/day) are well tolerated by celiac patients, but some brands of commercially available oats may be contaminated with wheat and other cereal grains during processing and shipping. Hence, it is wise, at least initially, to avoid oats unless obtained from a reliable source that is known to supply oats free of other contaminating cereal grains. Many other dietary carbohydrate staples including rice, corn, potatoes, millet, and soybeans are well tolerated by celiac patients. Micronutrient deficiencies including iron and folate deficiencies should be treated. If osteopenia is present (bone density should be determined), calcium and vitamin D should be prescribed. Pneumococcal vaccine should be administered to those with evidence of hyposplenism.

Although implementation of GFD sounds simple, it is not. Wheat is ubiquitous in the Western diet and is particularly hard to spot in processed foods such as ice cream, sauces, and candies. For example, an additive as benign sounding as "hydrolyzed vegetable protein" is often derived from wheat and therefore may be rich in gluten. Hence, counseling by a knowledgeable dietician and physician as well as participation in local celiac disease lay support groups are important facets in the education of celiac patients and facilitation of long-term dietary compliance.

If diarrhea and steatorrhea are present, lactose restriction may be needed initially as clinically significant secondary lactase deficiency is often present. However, dairy products are a good source of many nutrients, including calcium and protein, and should be encouraged as symptoms disappear unless primary lactase deficiency is also present. Pure oats from a reliable source can be added if desired by the patients once symptoms have cleared with gluten withdrawal. Dietary compliance should be monitored on follow-up visits every 6–12 months. A repeat serologic test (anti-tTG or anti-EmA IgA) is helpful 6–12 months after initiation of gluten withdrawal as the antibodies disappear in fully compliant celiac patients. With those exceptions and perhaps an annual hemoglobin or hematocrit and monitoring of bone density, no other specific follow-up beyond routine medical care is needed in the absence of symptoms and signs.

▶ Course & Prognosis

By and large, the prognosis of patients with celiac disease is excellent. There is a higher incidence of lymphoma, especially of the T-cell type derived from IELs (see next section), among celiac patients (see Figure 9–14). But the risk is greatest among symptomatic patients who have had many years of gluten exposure. In contrast, the risk is low among those with latent or silent disease. Most of the celiac disease-associated lymphomas that do develop occur in the intestine, but lymphoma at distant sites may also develop, including B-cell lymphomas. There is increasing evidence that strict adherence to a GFD substantially reduces the risk of subsequent lymphoma development; screening for lymphoma is not recommended unless suggestive symptoms develop. The incidence of small intestinal, esophageal, and pharyngeal carcinomas may also be increased in celiac disease, but available evidence is less convincing than for lymphomas.

Some patients may fail to respond to gluten withdrawal, whereas others may respond initially but then develop recurrent symptoms while claiming to adhere to a GFD. In these instances, advertent or inadvertent gluten ingestion is the most common cause of continuing symptoms. Dietary compliance should be carefully evaluated by a dietician expert in the celiac diet. Celiac serologies can be helpful if sufficient time on the diet has elapsed (at least 6 months). If positive, they suggest continued gluten ingestion. If negative, they are not sufficiently sensitive to exclude some continued gluten intake. If continued gluten intake appears unlikely, thorough evaluation is needed to exclude other gastrointestinal diseases with symptoms that may mimic those of celiac disease such as lymphoma, refractory sprue (see next section), microscopic colitis, and IBS (Table 21–7).

Given the known high prevalence of celiac disease in first-order relatives or patients with the disease, all immediate family members should be screened for celiac disease; young individuals should be screened after 24 months of age when they have developed their own antibodies. The prevalence of celiac disease also is high in several other diseases, many of which are associated with autoimmunity (Table 21–8). Although studies of the cost-effectiveness of screening for celiac disease in these conditions are limited, evidence that persistent gluten ingestion increases the risk of malignancy and that clinical manifestations of celiac disease are often subtle yet damaging (eg, osteopenia) provides a strong argument for increased serologic screening.

Table 21–7. Considerations in patients unresponsive to a gluten-free diet.

Poor dietary compliance or inadvertent gluten consumption
Coexistent irritable bowel syndrome
Microscopic colitis
Primary lactase deficiency
Small intestinal bacterial overgrowth (SIBO)
Drug-induced (olmesartan) enteropathy
Autoimmune enteropathy
Lymphoma
Refractory celiac disease

Table 21–8. Prevalence of celiac sprue in selected diseases.

Disease or Finding	Prevalence of Celiac Sprue
Dermatitis herpetiformis	>90%
Diabetes mellitus type 1	2–8%
Autoimmune thyroid disease	~3%
Down syndrome	3–12%
Turner syndrome	2–10%
Unexplained infertility	2–4%
Unexplained osteopenia	2–3%
Unexplained anemia	2–8%
Irritable bowel syndrome	Up to 10%
Liver function tests	1.5–9.0%
Selective IgA deficiency	2–4%

Elfström P, Granath F, Smedby KE, et al. Risk of lymphoproliferative malignancy in relation to small intestinal histopathology among patients with celiac disease. *J Natl Cancer Inst.* 2011;103:436–444. [PMID: 21289299]

Green PHR, Cellier C. Celiac disease. *N Engl J Med.* 2007;357: 1731–1743. [PMID: 17960014]

Husby S, Murray JA, Katzka DA. AGA clinical practice update on diagnosis and monitoring of celiac disease-changing utility of serology and histologic measures: expert review. *Gastroenterology.* 2019;156(4):885–889. [PMID: 30578783]

Ludvigsson JF, Bai JC, Biagi F, et al. Diagnosis and management of adult cœliac disease: guidelines from British Society of Gastroenterology. *Gut.* 2014;63:1210–1228. [PMID: 24917550]

Rubio-Tapia A, Hill ID, Kelly CP, et al. ACG clinical guidelines: diagnosis and management of celiac disease. *Am J Gastroenterol.* 2013;108:656–676. [PMID: 23609613]

Tack GJ, Verbeek WHM, Schruers MWJ, et al. The spectrum of celiac disease: epidemiology, clinical aspects and treatment. *Nat Rev Gastroenterol Hepatol.* 2010;7:204–213. [PMID: 20212505]

2. Refractory Celiac Disease (RCD, Refractory Sprue)

The clinical presentation and small intestinal mucosal histology of refractory celiac disease (RCD) mimic those of severe untreated celiac disease; generalized malabsorption, its associated complications and blunted/absent villi, crypt hyperplasia, mucosal inflammation, and increased IELs on histology are all present. However, unlike celiac disease, there is no or, at best, an incomplete response to dietary gluten withdrawal. Some patients initially respond to gluten withdrawal and exhibit serologic tests consistent with celiac disease but then, after months or years, become refractory to gluten withdrawal. Others are refractory to gluten elimination at presentation and may lack the serologic celiac markers even before a trial of gluten withdrawal. In all, other potential causes for the symptoms, including poor dietary compliance or other diseases such as lymphoma, lymphocytic colitis, tropical sprue, SIBO, drug-induced enteropathy, and eosinophilic enteritis, must be excluded as RCD is largely a diagnosis of exclusion.

There are two major categories of RCD. In the first (type 1), the expanded population of IELs consists of phenotypically normal polyclonal T cells. Many patients in this category improve with corticosteroids or other immunosuppressive treatments; gluten withdrawal should also be maintained. Oral budesonide should be tried first, and systemic corticosteroids or other immunosuppressant agents such as azathioprine should be reserved for those who fail budesonide, given the need for long-term treatment and potential side effects. Once patients respond, they should be tapered to the lowest dose of corticosteroid that controls symptoms. In the second category (type 2), epithelial cell interleukin-15 (IL-15) overexpression promotes the emergence of clonal populations of phenotypically aberrant IELs, which may represent a low-grade intraepithelial lymphoma. These abnormal T cells fail to express surface CD3, CD8, or the T-cell receptor for β-chain while retaining CD3 in the intracellular compartment. Patients with type 1 RCD may, with time, progress to type 2.

The prognosis is guarded for patients with RCD, especially those with type 2 disease. Many develop intractable nutritional deficiencies requiring long-term parenteral alimentation that may lead to complicating infections. Some ultimately progress to T-cell lymphoma. Attempts at treatment when conventional immunosuppression fails have included infliximab, cladribine, and autologous stem cell transplantation resulting in anecdotal reports of responses in some but not all patients, but there is concern that these treatments may hasten progression to lymphoma.

Lui H, Brais R, Lavergne-Slove A, et al. Continual monitoring of intraepithelial lymphocyte immunophenotype and clonality is more important than snapshot analysis in the surveillance of refractory celiac disease. *Gut*. 2010;59:452–460. [PMID: 19996326]

Malamut G, Afchain P, Verkarre V, et al. Presentation and long-term follow-up of refractory celiac disease: comparison of type I with type II. *Gastroenterology*. 2009;136:81–90. [PMID: 19014942]

Malamut G, Cellier C. Refractory celiac disease. *Gastroenterol Clin North Am*. 2019;48(1):137–144. [PMID: 30711206]

3. Immunoproliferative Small Intestinal Disease & Intestinal Lymphoma

Primary small intestinal lymphoma is uncommon in developed countries, occurring most often in middle-aged men with focal involvement and with a predilection for the ileum. As primary focal intestinal lymphomas are not usually associated with diarrhea and malabsorption but usually present as bleeding or mass-related abdominal pain and obstruction,

they will not be considered further in this chapter. In contrast, two variants of small intestinal lymphoma regularly cause malabsorption and downstream nutritional deficiencies: immunoproliferative small intestinal disease (IPSID)-associated lymphoma and enteropathy-associated T-cell lymphoma (EATL).

IPSID occurs primarily in young adults among native Middle Eastern populations as well as in South Africa and Pakistan. It is exceedingly rare in more industrialized nations. Its cause is largely unknown, but because IPSID occurs where hygiene is poor, it has been suggested that bacteria or other antigens cause excessive proliferation of immunocompetent cells in the lamina propria and that poor nutrition in the at-risk population plays a permissive role. However no specific causative pathogen has been identified, although an association of IPSID with *Campylobacter jejuni* has been suggested. In the early stages of the disease, there is diffuse infiltration of the mucosa and submucosa with B lymphocytes and plasma cells. As the disease progresses, the infiltrating cells develop histologically malignant characteristics with mesenteric lymph nodes involvement. Early clinical features include anorexia, weight loss, diarrhea, steatorrhea, and abdominal pain whereas edema, ascites, and hepatic splenomegaly and palpable abdominal masses may become evident in later stages of disease.

A distinctive laboratory feature found in the majority of patients with IPSID and IPSID-associated lymphoma is the presence of a paraprotein consisting of the Fc portion of IgA that migrates as a broad band on protein electrophoresis in the α2 and β regions.

Early in the disease before malignant cells are observed, prolonged treatment (6 months or more) with antibiotics such as tetracycline, ampicillin, and metronidazole has induced prolonged remission and even cures. Hence, this stage of the disease has been likened to *H. pylori*–associated gastric early mucosa-associated lymphoid tissue (MALT) lymphomas. If the process fails to respond to antibiotics, or once lymphoma has been established, either by endoscopic biopsy or staging laparotomy, combination chemotherapy with or without radiotherapy and nutritional support are the only therapeutic options as the extent of intestinal involvement usually precludes surgical resection.

EATL is a complication of both celiac disease and RCD. It occurs primarily in patients over the age of 50 who have had prolonged gluten exposure and symptomatic celiac disease, although occasionally celiac disease may be undiagnosed until the initial presentation of EATL. Clinical deterioration in a patient with established celiac disease despite strict compliance with a GFD or failure of a patient recently diagnosed with celiac disease to respond to a strict GFD should raise suspicion and trigger further diagnostic evaluation (see Table 21–7). Signs and symptoms are similar to those seen in IPSID including anorexia, weight loss, diarrhea, steatorrhea, bleeding, and abdominal pain. Rarely, perforation with resultant peritonitis may occur. Useful studies include push enteroscopy with mucosal biopsies from multiple levels of the small intestine, VCE, conventional abdominal CT, and CT or MRI enterography; the value of positron emission tomography (PET) imaging is controversial. If suspicious lesions are detected but are not accessible by endoscopy or if results of studies are negative but the suspicion of EATL is high, laparoscopy or laparotomy with full-thickness small intestine biopsies and mesenteric lymph node biopsies must be considered.

The prognosis of EATL once diagnosed is dismal. With few exceptions, responses to intensive chemotherapy have been transient. More recently, autologous stem cell transplantation following intensive chemotherapy has shown some promise, but further studies are needed.

Catassi C, Bearzi I, Holmes GK. Association of celiac disease and intestinal lymphomas and other cancers. *Gastroenterology*. 2005;128:S79–S86. [PMID: 15825131]

Salem PA, Estephan FF. Immunoproliferative small intestinal disease: current concepts. *Cancer J*. 2005;11:374–382. [PMID: 16259867]

4. Tropical Sprue

Tropical sprue occurs among natives of, visitors to, and expatriates from selected countries located primarily between the Tropic of Cancer and the Tropic of Capricorn. Major epidemics have been described historically in south Indian villages. Tropical sprue remains a major endemic cause of malabsorption in parts of India, responsible for 22–37% of patients presenting with intestinal malabsorption in two recent studies. Sporadic cases seen in the United States are largely among immigrants and visitors from the Caribbean or tropical Asia as well as returning tourists who have spent at least a month or more in endemic areas. The cause of tropical sprue remains obscure, but its epidemiology and its response to antibiotic therapy strongly suggest that colonization of the intestine by an infectious agent or alteration in the intestinal bacterial flora induced by the exposure to another environmental agent underlies its pathogenesis. However, to date no single causative infectious agent has been identified.

Clinical signs and symptoms are nonspecific and include diarrhea, steatorrhea, weight loss, nausea, and anorexia. Anemia is common and more often observed in tropical sprue than celiac disease. Tropical sprue-associated anemia is most often megaloblastic, reflecting vitamin B_{12} or folate deficiency, or both, although coexistent iron deficiency may result in a dimorphic anemia. Mucosal biopsy of the small intestine reveals a nonspecific lesion of variable severity, which may involve the length of the small intestine in patchy fashion. Architectural changes range from minimal villous blunting to complete absence of villi with underlying infiltration of the lamina propria with mononuclear cells and IELs. Thus, the histologic lesion cannot be distinguished with certainty from that observed in celiac disease, viral gastroenteritis, or intraluminal bacterial overgrowth. As there is no specific diagnostic test for tropical sprue, the diagnosis relies

Table 21–9. Features that distinguish tropical sprue from celiac disease.

History of exposure to an endemic region
Antitissue transglutaminase and antiendomysial antibodies are absent
Vitamin B_{12} deficiency more common
No response to gluten-free diet
Response to treatment with folic acid and antibiotics in most cases
Biopsy histology does not distinguish between tropical sprue and celiac disease

on excluding celiac disease (Table 21–9) and other diseases that cause malabsorption including protozoal infestations that can cause similar symptoms and are also endemic to the tropics where sanitation may be suboptimal.

Recommended treatment is based on observational studies and includes an antibiotic such as tetracycline and high-dose folic acid. The optimal duration of treatment is unclear, although treatment for 1–2 months appears to be sufficient for most travelers and expatriates. Treatment lasting 6 months to 1 year is recommended for chronically ill residents in the tropics. Poorly absorbed sulfonamides are suggested for those in whom tetracycline is contraindicated such as young children and pregnant women. Specific nutritional deficiencies such as vitamin B_{12}, vitamin D, and calcium deficiencies should also be corrected. The response to treatment is usually prompt; hence, the prognosis with proper treatment is excellent, although relapses occurring months to years after treatment have been noted. It has been suggested that the response among those with tropical sprue acquired in the Caribbean is more predictable than that observed among those with tropical sprue acquired in Asia, but rigorous comparative studies are not available, and this perception may be confounded by the presence of other causes of gastrointestinal symptoms among Asian population.

Brown IS, Bettington A, Bettington M, et al. Tropical sprue: revisiting an underrecognized disease. *Am J Surg Pathol*. 2014;38: 666–672. [PMID: 24441659]

Nath SK. Tropical sprue. *Curr Gastroenterol Rep*. 2005;7:343–349. [PMID: 16168231]

Sharma P, Baloda V, Gahlot GP, et al. Clinical, endoscopic, and histological differentiation between celiac disease and tropical sprue: a systematic review. *J Gastroenterol Hepatol*. 2019;34(1):74–83. [PMID: 30069926]

5. Eosinophilic Gastroenteritis

Eosinophilic gastroenteritis is an uncommon, poorly understood disease characterized by infiltration of the stomach, small intestine, or colon with mature eosinophils, and, in about 80% of those affected, pronounced peripheral eosinophilia. More than 50% of patients have a history of significant atopy or specific food intolerance however the underlying pathogenesis is poorly understood. Presumably, chemokines such as eotaxin-1 and eotaxin-2 recruit eosinophils to the gut where they are activated to release proinflammatory mediators, including major basic protein, eosinophilic peroxidase, eosinophilic cationic protein, and leukotrienes, but the initiating trigger is unknown.

Clinical Findings

Three major patterns of eosinophilic infiltration induce distinctive clinical features, although the features are not necessarily syndromic and there may be substantial overlap. The most common is associated with mucosal and submucosal eosinophilic infiltration most pronounced in the small intestine. Characteristic clinical features of this subset include diarrhea, steatorrhea (usually mild), abdominal pain, nausea, and, in some cases, vomiting. Iron deficiency and hypoalbuminemia associated with protein-losing enteropathy may be present. Imaging of the small intestine may reveal small bowel wall thickening and mucosal nodularity.

The second pattern is associated primarily with submucosal and visceral muscle wall eosinophil infiltration sometimes sufficient to produce mass lesions evident on imaging studies of the stomach, small intestine, and, rarely, colon. Obstructive symptoms including nausea and vomiting are often accompanied by abdominal pain. These findings may mimic those of malignancy. Weight loss is common, and diarrhea may be present.

The third and, in most series, the least common pattern is characterized primarily by serosal and subserosal eosinophilic infiltration. It is associated with ascites containing large numbers of eosinophils as well as with abdominal discomfort, nausea, and diarrhea.

The diagnosis rests on the presence of gastrointestinal symptoms, the histologic demonstration of visceral eosinophil infiltration or eosinophilic ascites, and the exclusion of other entities that produce eosinophilia and gastrointestinal symptoms. These include parasitic disease, specific food or drug hypersensitivities, mastocytosis, polyarteritis nodosa, eosinophilic granulomatosis with polyangiitis (EGPA or Churg-Strauss syndrome), lymphoma, inflammatory bowel disease, and the hypereosinophilic syndrome. In patients with mucosal involvement of the small intestine, eosinophilic infiltration is often patchy, and the mucosa from adjacent areas can be normal or have the features of a nonspecific enteritis. Hence, multiple biopsies should be obtained at endoscopy from several intestinal levels for diagnosis. Even then, while the observation of extensive eosinophilic infiltration helps to establish the diagnosis, its absence does not exclude it given the patchy nature of mucosal involvement. Serum IgE levels are elevated in most but not all patients thereby limiting its diagnostic capacity. Correct diagnosis is especially important in patients with muscle wall eosinophilic infiltration mimicking malignancy and may require full-thickness biopsy at laparoscopy or laparotomy to avoid unnecessary radical resective surgery.

Treatment

Spontaneous remission is reported in 30–40% of cases of eosinophilic gastroenteritis. In patients with persistent disease activity, corticosteroids are the mainstay of treatment regardless of the pattern of clinical presentation and provide a good overall prognosis. In most patients, sustained symptomatic remission is induced with a 2–4 week course at moderate corticosteroid dosages (prednisone 20–40 mg/day) followed by a gradual taper. Recently, non–enteric-coated budesonide has been used successfully. A minority of patients may relapse and require repeated courses of corticosteroids. A few unfortunate patients require continuous steroid maintenance or fail to respond to corticosteroids. Elimination diets based on skin sensitivity and radioallergosorbent testing have been disappointing in that sustained responses are uncommon. Responses in some patients to six food elimination and elemental diets have been reported but compliance and quality of life issues are limitations. There are anecdotal reports of responses to oral cromolyn, ketotifen, and montelukast in some but not all refractory patients. With the identification of the role of Il-4 and Il-5 in eosinophilic disorders, monoclonal antibodies targeting Il-4 such as dupilumab, a receptor alpha antagonist or mepolizumab an Il-5 antagonist are changing the landscape and options considerably with more effective approaches.

Walker MM, Potter M, Talley NJ. Eosinophilic gastroenteritis and other eosinophilic gut diseases distal to the oesophagus. *Lancet Gastroenterol Hepatol.* 2018;3(4):271–280. [PMID: 29533199]

Zhang M, Li Y. Eosinophilic gastroenteritis: a state-of-the-art review. *J Gastroenterol Hepatol.* 2017;32(1):64–72. [PMID: 27253425]

6. Systemic Mastocytosis

Given the multiple forms of systemic mastocytosis and its diverse clinical features, comprehensive discussion of the disease is beyond the scope of this chapter and the focus will be on the small intestinal involvement that may produce malabsorption. Similarly, other mast cell–mediated disease, such as the recently characterized mast cell activation syndrome which causes gastrointestinal symptoms but not associated with malabsorption, is not discussed here.

Although many patients with systemic mastocytosis have gastrointestinal symptoms, in selected patients with systemic mastocytosis, there is extensive infiltration of the intestinal mucosa and submucosa with mast cells, and especially CD25- or CD117-positive mast cells, occasionally in the absence of the obvious skin lesions usually associated with this disease entity. The observed mast cell infiltration can be focal or quite diffuse. In and of itself, it may produce malabsorption and can contribute to the gastrointestinal symptoms associated with mediator release, which may include weight loss, diarrhea, steatorrhea, nausea, vomiting, and abdominal pain. In addition, excessive gastric acid secretion related to mast cell histamine release may inactivate pancreatic lipase and cause intestinal mucosal damage, predisposing to malabsorption. Release of mediators such as prostaglandin D_2 from local or distant mast cells may increase motility, contributing to diarrhea, malabsorption, and abdominal discomfort.

The presence of classic skin manifestations of mastocytosis, including dermatographia and urticaria pigmentosa, coexistent splenomegaly, or peptic ulcer disease, the latter caused by mast cell histamine release, should arouse suspicion and facilitate the diagnosis of symptomatic intestinal mast cell disease. Serum tryptase concentration and serum and urinary histamine levels are usually elevated. Small bowel imaging studies reveal an infiltrative pattern with thickened or nodular folds. Increased mast cells and eosinophil infiltration of the mucosa and submucosa in biopsy specimens are diagnostic if present in the appropriate clinical setting.

Sodium cromoglycate, ketotifen, antileukotrienes, oral prednisone, H_2-receptor antagonists, proton pump inhibitors, and low-dose aspirin have been reported as being beneficial in relieving diarrhea, abdominal pain, and other symptoms, but treatment is empiric as controlled therapeutic trials are lacking. Direct treatment of mast cell proliferation with tyrosine kinase inhibitors such as imatinib mesylate has been disappointing as resistance is conferred by the D816V mutation in the tyrosine kinase domain of c-KIT (CD117; this mutation is present in 90% or more of systemic mastocytosis patients). Recently, omalizumab, an anti-IgE monoclonal antibody, has been demonstrated to reduce and resolve systemic mastocytosis-associated gastrointestinal symptoms in 90% and 30% of patients, respectively, but in only limited studies that require more extensive controlled trials.

Shih AR, Deshpande V, Ferry JA, Zukerberg L. Clinicopathological characteristics of systemic mastocytosis in the intestine. *Histopathology*. 2016;69(6):1021-1027. [PMID: 27391777]

Sokol H, Georgin-Lavialle S, Grandpeix-Guyodo C, et al. Gastrointestinal involvement and manifestations in systemic mastocytosis. *Inflamm Bowel Dis*. 2010;16:1247–1253. [PMID: 20162539]

7. Radiation Enteritis & Colitis

The small intestine and colon are especially susceptible to the acute inhibitory and destructive effects of ionizing radiation given the rapid renewal rate of their epithelia. Radiation exposure of the intestine results in iatrogenic mucosal atrophy with decreased villus and crypt height in the small intestine and decreased crypt height in the colon and the rectum. In addition, substantial mucosal inflammation occurs in the mucosa of both organs that lie within the field of radiation. Although the damaged segment of the small intestine is functionally impaired, clinically evident malabsorption is unusual as there is sufficient unexposed small intestine to compensate and the mucosal lesion heals rapidly once radiation exposure ceases. On the other hand, diarrhea and hematochezia are common features of colitis and proctitis that can accompany radiation therapy. These symptoms also remit promptly in the majority of cases after radiation therapy has been completed.

In contrast, the delayed effect of radiation therapy to the intestine can cause serious debilitating disease and may manifest months to years after radiation exposure. The threshold dose is in the range of 4000–5000 cGy and is influenced by associated risk factors, including concomitant chemotherapy and prior surgery causing fixation of the intestine in the radiation field through adhesions and by radiation technique. An obliterative endarteriolitis of submucosal arterioles develops resulting in fibrosis, strictures, fistula formation, telangiectasias, and ischemic ulceration of the overlying mucosa. Malabsorption develops in some patients due to (1) bacterial overgrowth caused by stricture-induced stasis and impaired motility if there is neuromuscular involvement, (2) bile salt deficiency if ileal involvement is severe, (3) lymphatic obstruction, or (4) enterocolic fistula formation.

Clinical Findings

Acute symptoms include diarrhea, abdominal pain, and anorexia and can develop within hours to days after radiation exposure. Chronic radiation enteritis or colitis leads to a chronic malabsorption syndrome and/or obstructive pathology that occurs at least two months after the completion of radiation therapy. Strictures may produce partial or even complete intestinal obstruction with nausea, vomiting, and painful abdominal distention. Imaging studies such as CT or MRI enterography, barium enema, and small intestinal series help to characterize the extent of disease and localize the site of stricture, but the images may resemble closely the features of other ischemic or inflammatory lesions. If the involved intestine is within the reach of an endoscope, biopsy is usually diagnostic with demonstration of the endarteriolaritis, fibrosis, and the presence of bizarre-appearing submucosal fibroblasts.

Treatment

Overall, treatment is disappointing. If there is associated bacterial overgrowth caused by stasis and strictures, treatment with antibiotics as detailed in the later section dealing with that entity is often beneficial. If ileal disease is present, bile salt–binding resins may reduce the bile salt–induced diarrhea but may also aggravate steatorrhea by further reducing the bile salt pool. Supportive measures such as polymeric dietary supplements containing medium-chain triglycerides or even parenteral nutrition may be needed. Dilation of strictures within endoscopic reach may be helpful. There are a few anecdotal reports of benefit from hyperbaric oxygen treatments but lack of general availability and cost are limitations.

Surgery should be reserved for severe intestinal or colonic strictures and enterocolic, enterovesical, or rectovesical fistulas. Surgery is associated with substantial morbidity because the compromised circulation of the affected bowel interferes with normal healing. For bleeding rectal and colonic telangiectatic lesions, laser or argon plasma coagulation is often helpful, but treatments used for idiopathic inflammatory bowel disease including local or oral corticosteroids or 5-aminosalicylate have not shown consistent benefit. Radiation enteritis and colitis are often progressive and therefore the prognosis is guarded.

Chater C, Saudemont A, Zerbib P. Chronic radiation enteritis. *J Visc Surg.* 2019;156(2):175–176. [PMID: 30249429]

Theis VS, Sripadam R, Ramani V, et al. Chronic radiation enteritis. *Clin Oncol.* 2010;22:70–83. [PMID: 19897345]

8. Intestinal Amyloidosis

Intestinal amyloid deposits are most often seen among patients with secondary amyloidosis (acute phase serum amyloid A [AA type] that deposits superficially) but have also been noted among patients with primary amyloidosis (monoclonal immunoglobulin light chains [AL type]) and dialysis-associated amyloidosis (β_2-microglobulin retention) that are more likely to deposit in the submucosa. Several mechanisms may contribute to the malabsorption that may accompany intestinal amyloid deposition. Neuromuscular infiltration results in impaired motility predisposing to stasis, resulting in intestinal pseudo-obstruction often with associated intraluminal bacterial overgrowth. On the other hand, autonomic dysfunction may be associated with rapid intestinal transit resulting in diarrhea. Vascular infiltration may induce small vessel ischemia. In advanced disease, mucosal amyloid deposits may impair enterocyte function and diffusion of absorbed nutrients from the lumen to the mucosal vasculature and lymphatics.

▶ Clinical Findings

Symptoms and signs vary significantly from patient to patient. In some patients, a pseudo-obstruction-like picture may exist with abdominal distension, nausea, anorexia, constipation, or diarrhea dominating the clinical presentation. Weight loss may be severe, resulting from impaired oral intake and malabsorption. Orthostasis may be prominent. In other patients, gastrointestinal bleeding from ulcerated mucosa usually related to vascular amyloid deposition may be the presenting feature. Protein-losing enteropathy may produce edema and ascites. The diagnosis should be suggested by the presence of conditions known to be associated with secondary amyloidosis. Examples include rheumatoid or psoriatic arthritis, inflammatory bowel disease, tuberculosis or other chronic infections, amyloid deposition in other organs such as the kidney or liver, or a history of chronic dialysis. Imaging studies suggesting intestinal stasis and pseudo-obstruction or mucosal infiltrative disease are helpful but not specific. Demonstration of amyloid deposition by biopsy of the rectum, stomach or small intestine is definitive; congo red stains should be obtained and examined with polarized light as the vascular amyloid infiltration can be subtle.

▶ Treatment

Treatment of primary amyloidosis is based on oncologic chemotherapy. Treatment of secondary amyloidosis should be directed at the underlying cause to minimize progression or even induce improvement. Bacterial overgrowth, if present, should be treated with antibiotics. Prokinetic agents may be useful if pseudo-obstruction is present whereas antimotility agents may benefit those with diarrhea associated with rapid transit. Other treatment of malabsorption is generally supportive, with dietary counseling and, if needed, parenteral nutrition.

Bansal R, Syed U, Walfish J, Aron J, Walfish A. Small bowel amyloidosis. *Curr Gastroenterol Rep.* 201826;20(3):11. [PMID: 29582184]

Iida T, Yamano H, Nakase H. Systemic amyloidosis with gastrointestinal involvement: diagnosis from endoscopic and histological views. *J Gastroenterol Hepatol.* 2018;33(3):583–590. [PMID: 28940821]

Petre S, Shah IA, Gilani N. Review article: gastrointestinal amyloidosis-clinical features, diagnosis and therapy. *Aliment Pharmacol Ther.* 2008;27:1006–1016. [PMID: 18363891]

9. Whipple Disease

Whipple disease is an unusual and uncommon systemic infectious disease with protean clinical manifestations that occurs primarily in Caucasian middle-aged men. The small intestine is often involved, producing malabsorption in the majority of patients. Although the disease was described in 1907, the role of bacterial infection in its pathogenesis was not recognized until more than 50 years later. Identification, culture, and molecular characterization of the organism, the actinobacteria *T whipplei*, was finally achieved in the early 1990s.

Despite characterization of *T. whipplei*, many aspects of the pathogenesis of Whipple disease remain enigmatic. There is evidence that *T. whipplei* is a widely present commensal in the environment and *T. whipplei* DNA has been found in the saliva and feces of up to 30% of the general population with an especially high prevalence among sewage treatment workers. Over 70% of people have been reported to have serum IgG antibodies directed against *T. whipplei* suggestive of widespread exposure. *T. whipplei* has also recently been suggested as a cause of acute gastroenteritis in young children. However, the scarcity of the classical disease and the lack of documented human-to-human transmission are most unusual for a disease that is caused by an infectious agent. Although the pathogenesis is not well understood, there is some evidence of altered macrophage function and activation and an impaired type 1 T-cell response in predisposed individuals but, interestingly, little to suggest chronic immunodeficiency or increased susceptibility to other infections.

Clinical Findings

The clinical features of disease activity may include virtually any of the body's organ systems. In the classic presentation, gastrointestinal symptoms are usually striking and resemble those seen in other diseases with generalized malabsorption. Weight loss, diarrhea, steatorrhea, and abdominal distention are present in 80–90% of patients, and both peripheral edema reflecting hypoproteinemia from protein-losing enteropathy and poor nutrition are common. Fever is present in 30–50% of patients and occasionally is the sole presenting symptom. Arthralgia and arthritis occur in 60–75%, often involving multiple joints and preceding the onset of gastrointestinal symptoms by months to even years. Patients with Whipple disease may present with extraintestinal symptoms in the absence of or overshadowing gastrointestinal manifestations. In addition to the joint symptoms, diverse central nervous system (CNS) symptoms such as cognitive deterioration, ophthalmoplegia, hypothalamic dysfunction, oculomasticatory or oculofacial myorhythmia, seizures, or ataxia may be among the presenting complaints. In other patients, cardiac manifestations, including pericarditis and culture-negative endocarditis, or pleuropulmonary involvement, including pleural effusions, cough, and sarcoid-like pulmonary infiltrates, may be the initial manifestations. Occasional patients have presented just with fever of unknown origin.

In addition to the physical findings characteristic of malabsorption, skin hyperpigmentation, peripheral lymphadenopathy, cardiac murmurs, signs of arthritis, and neurologic abnormalities may be present. Anemia with or without occult gastrointestinal bleeding, hypoalbuminemia, and hypocalcemia are relatively common.

The diagnosis is established by demonstration of *T. whipplei* in involved tissues by microscopy together with the characteristic infiltration of periodic acid–Schiff (PAS)-positive macrophages (Plate 40). In the small intestine, mucosal architecture is distorted by the macrophage infiltrate, and mucosal and submucosal lymphatics are dilated. Electron microscopy reveals the characteristic bacteria in the mucosa. Biopsy of the mucosa of the proximal intestine is the diagnostic procedure of choice due to the high prevalence of small intestinal mucosal involvement. Care must be taken to exclude *Mycobacterium avium* infection in immunocompromised patients that can mimic the intestinal histologic features of Whipple disease but can easily be distinguished with Ziehl-Neelsen staining, as *M. avium* is acid fast whereas *T. whipplei* is not. Alternatively, polymerase chain reaction (PCR) amplification against *T. whipplei* of involved tissues and tissue fluids can be used for diagnosis. In suspected CNS involvement, *T. whipplei*-directed PCR and cytology of cerebral spinal fluid sediment are of major diagnostic value.

Treatment

Empiric treatment with antibiotics results in prompt improvement in most patients and in permanent cure in many. Because of the danger of CNS involvement even in the absence of symptoms, use of antibiotics that penetrate the blood-brain barrier is desirable. One recommended regimen is ceftriaxone 2 g IV daily for 2 weeks followed by trimethoprim/ sulfamethoxazole 160 mg/800 mg orally twice daily for 1–3 years; trimethoprim–sulfamethoxazole alone has also been successful in many patients. There are no evidence-based studies that establish the optimal duration of antibiotic treatment to prevent relapses. Replacement therapy to correct specific nutritional deficiencies is important for supportive management. Immunosuppressants and anti-TNF agents, often used for non-Whipple disease arthritis, should be avoided as they may aggravate Whipple disease; following the start of antibiotic treatment, immunosuppressants may precipitate an immune reconstitution syndrome.

The overall prognosis in the absence of CNS involvement is excellent, although patients should be carefully monitored indefinitely for signs of relapse that may occur even years after apparently successful treatment. CNS symptoms may be the first sign of relapse.

Dolmans RA, Boel CH, Lacle MM, Kusters JG. Clinical manifestations, treatment, and diagnosis of *Tropheryma whipplei* infections. *Clin Microbiol Rev.* 2017;30(2):529–555. [PMID: 28298472]

Fenollar F, Puéchal X, Raoult D. Whipple's disease. *N Engl J Med.* 2007;356:55–66. [PMID: 17202456]

Fuerle GE, Junga NS, Marth T. Efficacy of ceftriaxone or meropenem as initial therapies in Whipple's disease. *Gastroenterology.* 2010;138:478–486. [PMID: 19879276]

Marth T, Moos V, Müller C, Biagi F, Schneider T. *Tropheryma whipplei* infection and Whipple's disease. *Lancet Infect Dis.* 2016;16(3):e13–22. [PMID: 26856775]

10. Crohn's Disease

Crohn's disease patients with extensive ileal involvement, extensive intestinal resections, enterocolic fistulas, and strictures leading to SIBO may develop significant and occasionally devastating malabsorption (see Chapter 3).

11. Abetalipoproteinemia

In this rare autosomal-recessive disease, mutations in the gene encoding microsomal triglyceride transfer protein interfere with posttranslational processing of apoprotein B, resulting ultimately in the absence of apoprotein B–containing lipoproteins in the circulating blood. Absorptive cells of the small intestine are packed with massive lipid droplets reflecting the impaired export of lipid from the epithelium following its uptake from the gut lumen.

The disease is usually evident in infancy or childhood when diarrhea and steatorrhea are noted. Acanthocytic red blood cells, reflecting their altered membrane lipid content, appear early, whereas the onset of retinitis pigmentosa and neurologic manifestations, including ataxia, tremors, peripheral neuropathy, and nystagmus, appear later in childhood or adolescence in untreated patients. Progression to hepatic steatosis and more rarely cirrhosis has been described. Laboratory features in addition to acanthocytosis and steatorrhea include absent serum β-lipoproteins and very low serum cholesterol and triglycerides, abnormal liver chemistries, and specifically low levels of vitamin E and other fat-soluble vitamins in untreated patients.

Although targeted treatment of the genetic defect is not available, prompt institution of high-dose oral vitamin E and A replacement at an early age markedly attenuates and sometimes prevents the development of the retinal lesions and the neurologic complications. Other fat-soluble vitamins should also be replaced. Cautious substitution of long-chain dietary fats with medium-chain triglycerides can be tried to improve nutrition, but in a few individuals, cirrhosis has been attributed to medium-chain triglyceride use.

Gregg RE, Wetterau JR. The molecular basis of abetalipoproteinemia. *Curr Opin Lipidol.* 1994;5:81–86. [PMID: 8044420]

Zamel R, Khan R, Pollex, RL, et al. Abetalipoproteinemia: two case reports and literature review. *Orphanet J Rare Dis.* 2008;3:19. [PMID: 18611256]

12. Parasitic Infestations

Whereas mild infestation of the intestine with *Strongyloides stercoralis* usually causes no symptoms, heavy infestation may induce fever, nausea, vomiting, weight loss, abdominal pain, and steatorrhea. The clinical picture may resemble tropical sprue, but eosinophilia is usually evident in severe infestations. If stool studies are negative, duodenal aspiration is indicated. A highly specific ELISA serology test is available but has limited clinical value as it but may remain positive for several years after parasitic eradication and may be negative in immunocompromised hosts. Ivermectin is the most effective therapy; in severe infestations, it can be combined with albendazole for greatest efficacy.

Giardia, coccidial, and microsporidial infestations can also produce malabsorption. These protozoal infestations are discussed in Chapter 5.

13. Carbohydrate Intolerance

The terminal phase of digestion of ingested complex carbohydrates such as starch as well as disaccharides including lactose, sucrose, maltose, and trehalose, occurs at the brush border membrane of intestinal absorptive cells where glycoprotein enzymes including lactase, sucrase-isomaltase, maltase-glucoamylase, and trehalase are located. Deficiency of any of these enzymes or defects in the monosaccharide transport process produces retention of unabsorbed sugars in the gut lumen. These, if present in sufficient quantity,

produce osmotic diarrhea and flatulence, the latter caused by intraluminal bacterial fermentation of the unabsorbed sugars. In addition, approximately 50% of healthy individuals are unable to fully absorb 25 g of free fructose. Ingestion of glucose or galactose in concert with fructose has been shown to enhance fructose absorption. Additionally, the fructose from the fructose-glucose combination of sucrose is more readily absorbed than the free monosaccharide. Ingestion of nonabsorbable sugars such as sorbitol, used to sweeten dietary foods, or of excessive amounts of fruit juices or of high-fructose corn syrup–containing carbonated beverages may cause gastrointestinal symptoms in some individuals.

Congenital disaccharidase deficiencies and monosaccharide transport defects are uncommon and produce symptoms in infancy upon introduction of the offending carbohydrate into the diet. Isolated lactase deficiency is the most common cause of carbohydrate intolerance and may become symptomatic after the age of 5. Low mucosal lactase levels are observed in 5–20% of adult North American and Western European Caucasians, 50–95% of African Americans and Africans, 50% of Hispanics, and over 90% of Asians; decrease or loss of lactase expression correlates with age progression. The diagnosis of lactase deficiency is suggested by a history of the induction of diarrhea, abdominal discomfort, bloating, and flatulence following the ingestion of dairy products or other foods rich in lactose. However, as these symptoms lack specificity, it is not uncommon to ascribe the symptoms of another clinical entity, such as IBS, to lactase deficiency or vice versa. The diagnosis is confirmed by the lactose breath hydrogen test that measures the level of expired hydrogen gas as a marker of bacterial breakdown of undigested lactose. Alternatively, a lactose tolerance test can be performed that measures a patient's blood glucose levels after they are given a dose of lactose.

Diseases that are associated with substantial mucosal damage such as celiac disease may produce clinically significant carbohydrate intolerance caused by impaired mucosal digestion and absorption of carbohydrates. Unless the individual also has isolated lactase deficiency, carbohydrate digestion and absorption should normalize as the mucosa heals with effective therapy of the underlying disorder.

Treatment of carbohydrate intolerance consists of decreasing or removing the offending carbohydrate from the diet. For lactase deficiency, reduction of dietary lactose by limiting dairy products and lactose-rich baked or processed foods is usually sufficient. A completely lactose-free diet is rarely necessary. Indeed, elegant studies have demonstrated unequivocally that most individuals with isolated acquired lactase deficiency can tolerate moderate amounts of lactose (12–15 g, the equivalent of 8 oz of milk twice daily) in their diet. Alternatively, commercially available lactase preparations can be ingested in concert with lactose-containing foods or foods pretreated with lactase can be utilized. Supplemental calcium and vitamin D should be recommended if there is significant dietary restriction of dairy products.

Gibson PR, Newnham E, Barrett JS, et al. Fructose malabsorption and the bigger picture. *Aliment Pharmacol Ther.* 2007;25:349–363. [PMID: 17217453]

Misselwitz B, Butter M, Verbeke K, Fox MR. Update on lactose malabsorption and intolerance: pathogenesis, diagnosis and clinical management. *Gut.* 2019;68(11):2080–2091. [PMID: 31427404]

Suchy FJ, Brannon PM, Carpenter TO, et al. National Institutes of Health Consensus Development Conference: lactose intolerance and health. *Ann Intern Med.* 2010;152:792–796. [PMID: 20404261]

DISEASES CAUSED BY IMPAIRMENT OF BOTH INTRALUMINAL DIGESTION & MUCOSAL DIGESTION/ABSORPTION

1. Small Intestinal Bacterial Overgrowth

Under normal circumstances, the proximal small intestinal lumen harbors less than 10^5 bacteria per milliliter of intestinal contents, most of which are gram-positive organisms derived from the oropharyngeal flora. The major mechanisms limiting excessive bacterial growth in the proximal intestine are normal intestinal motor function and normal gastric acid secretion. Secretion of immunoglobulins into the gut lumen also inhibits proximal bacterial proliferation. The presence of any condition that interferes with these protective mechanisms, notably impaired intestinal motility, structural lesions predisposing to intestinal stasis, profound reduction or absence of gastric acid secretion, and immunodeficiency syndromes, may precipitate SIBO (Table 21–10).

▶ Pathogenesis

Several mechanisms contribute to the malabsorption that develops in SIBO. Normally, bile salts secreted by the liver are conjugated to glycine or taurine and are absorbed by a specific active transport process in the distal ileum. In SIBO, the bacteria produce enzymes that deconjugate the bile salts. The more lipid-soluble deconjugated bile salts are absorbed prematurely in the proximal gut by passive nonionic diffusion resulting in their decreased availability intraluminally. Moreover, the deconjugated bile salts are weakly soluble at the normal intraluminal pH and are less effective detergents, resulting in less effective intraluminal dispersion of dietary lipids for absorption. Additionally, the bacteria produce proteases and glycosidases and, in some instances, toxins that damage the epithelium, especially brush border hydrolases, thus interfering with the terminal phase of carbohydrate and protein digestion. The interaction of the bacteria with the mucosa may also produce an inflammatory mucosal lesion further contributing to impaired absorption. Finally, within the gut lumen, the bacteria bind and metabolize vitamin B_{12}, preventing its absorption in the distal ileum.

Table 21–10. Causes of bacterial overgrowth in the proximal intestine.

1. **Motility disorders**
   a. Scleroderma
   b. Amyloidosis
   c. Pseudo-obstruction
   d. Vagotomy
   e. Diabetes with visceral neuropathy
   f. Irritable bowel syndrome
2. **Structural abnormalities**
   a. Diverticula
   b. Strictures
      • Crohn's disease
      • Vascular disease
      • Radiation enteritis
   c. Adhesions causing partial obstruction
   d. Afferent loop stasis after Billroth II gastrectomy
   e. Fistulas
      • Gastrocolic
      • Jejunocolic
      • Jejunoileal
3. **Hypochlorhydria or achlorhydria**
   a. Gastric atrophy with or without pernicious anemia
   b. Vagotomy or gastric resection
   c. Prolonged use of high-dose proton pump inhibitors
4. **Hypogammaglobulinemia or agammaglobulinemia**

▶ Clinical Findings

The clinical features of SIBO that are caused by bacterial overgrowth are typical of those seen in other malabsorptive states, with weight loss, diarrhea, steatorrhea, flatulence, and abdominal pain and distention being common. Extraintestinal manifestations especially those due to deficiencies in specific vitamins (A, B_{12}, D, E) and minerals (iron, calcium) may be prominent. In the elderly, SIBO is probably an under-recognized cause of poor nutrition; weight loss and mild diarrhea may be the major features. If the condition has persisted long enough to deplete vitamin B_{12} stores, megaloblastic anemia and neurologic manifestations identical to those observed in pernicious anemia may develop. In addition, a spectrum of additional symptoms, such as abdominal pain, nausea, and vomiting, may reflect the primary disease process predisposing to SIBO.

Quantitative culture of the duodenal or proximal jejunal fluid ($>10^5$ CFU/mL) is widely considered the diagnostic gold standard for documenting SIBO but is not generally available, as it is invasive, costly, and the fastidious growth requirements of the gut flora require the use of multiple media and growth conditions not available in most clinical microbiology laboratories. Moreover, collection and culture techniques lack standardization making interpretation and comparison of available studies difficult. Breath tests utilizing lactulose, xylose, and glucose are reasonable surrogates but are subject to major limitations of sensitivity and specificity.

If there is no ileal disease, the two-stage radiolabeled vitamin B_{12} absorption test (Schilling test) is helpful if available; the bacteria impair absorption both of free vitamin B_{12} and intrinsic factor-bound vitamin B_{12} and thus urinary excretion is low. Tissue retrieved by small intestinal mucosal biopsy may range from normal histology to a severe but nonspecific lesion with villus blunting, crypt hyperplasia, damaged absorptive cells, and substantial mucosal inflammation. Often a clinical response to empiric antibiotic treatment is used diagnostically.

▶ Treatment

If a correctable lesion such as a gastrocolic fistula or a discrete intestinal stricture is the cause of SIBO, surgical repair is the treatment of choice. If SIBO is associated with chronic motor abnormalities, achlorhydria, or noncorrectable anatomic abnormalities such as multiple jejunal diverticula, antibiotics are the treatments of choice. Some patients respond to amoxicillin/clavulanate alone; others require broader coverage with the addition of metronidazole. Promising responses have been obtained with rifaximin, a poorly absorbed although costly antibiotic. A single 2-week course of therapy may effect a prolonged remission in up to 70% of patients; others require frequent intermittent courses of antibiotics when symptomatic or even continuous treatment for maximum benefit. Use of prokinetic agents has shown little or no benefit. As with all diseases associated with malabsorption, nutritional deficiencies, including vitamin B_{12} deficiency, should be corrected. Modified diets such as the low fermentable oligo-, di-, and monosaccharides and polyols (FODMAP) diet diminish the load of fermentable substrates metabolized by the small intestinal microbiota and show efficacy in reducing symptoms of bloating and flatulence in IBS however their role in treatment of SIBO at present is not well defined.

Recently, SIBO has been incriminated in some patients with IBS, especially in the subset with diarrhea. However, the reported prevalence of SIBO in IBS ranges from 4% to 64%, highlighting the controversy and lack of standardized diagnostic criteria in this area. Clinical improvement with antibiotic treatment in this group of patients has been reported in some series.

Gatta L, Scarpignato C. Systematic review with meta-analysis: Rifaximin is effective and safe for the treatment of small intestine bacterial overgrowth. *Aliment Pharmacol Ther.* 2017;45: 604–616. [PMID: 28078798]

Grace E, Shaw C, Whelan H, et al. Review article: small intestinal bacterial overgrowth-prevalence, clinical features, current and developing diagnostic tests, and treatment. *Aliment Pharmacol Ther.* 2013;38:674–688. [PMID: 23957651]

Quigley EM. Small intestinal bacterial overgrowth: what it is and what it is not. *Curr Opin Gastroenterol.* 2014;30:1141–1146. [PMID: 24406476]

Rao SSC, Bhagatwala J. Small intestinal bacterial overgrowth: clinical features and therapeutic management. *Clin Transl Gastroenterol.* 2019;10(10):e00078. [PMID: 31584459]

Rezaie A, Pimentel M, Rao SS. How to test and treat small intestinal bacterial overgrowth: an evidence-based approach. *Curr Gastroenterol Rep.* 2016;18(2):8. [PMID: 26780631]

2. Short Bowel Syndrome (Intestinal Failure)

The small intestine has sufficient reserve so that resection of 50% is well tolerated provided that the duodenum and proximal jejunum and the distal 100 cm of the ileum are not removed and are devoid of any disease. Resection of smaller lengths that include the proximal or distal segments often produce symptoms and signs related to their selective absorptive functions (iron, folate, and calcium malabsorption for the proximal intestine and bile salt and vitamin B_{12} malabsorption for the distal ileum). On the other hand, resection of 70–80% of the small intestine often produces catastrophic malabsorption with massive diarrhea, severe electrolyte imbalances and steatorrhea, especially if the distal ileum, ileocecal valve, and colon have been lost. Factors contributing to malabsorption include the reduction of the available absorptive surface, depletion of the bile salt pool, SIBO and acid hypersecretion that can induce intestinal mucosal damage and inactive pancreatic lipase. Conditions that may require small bowel resection of such magnitude to result in short bowel syndrome in adults include vascular catastrophes involving the mesenteric circulation, refractory long-standing Crohn's disease, radiation enterocolitis, severe trauma, and malignant disease. Historically, bariatric jejunoileal bypass and inadvertent gastroileal anastomosis at the time of partial gastrectomy were additional but uncommon causes.

Prompt and vigorous fluid and electrolyte replacement based on careful monitoring of losses is essential, as is early implementation of parenteral alimentation with meticulous vitamin and mineral supplementation. Early initiation of continuous enteral feedings is desirable to minimize intestinal mucosal atrophy and maximize adaptive mucosal hyperplasia. Protein hydrolysate–based polymeric supplements, which contain more fat and less carbohydrates and less of an osmotic load, are usually better tolerated than elemental supplements after the first few weeks. Acid hypersecretion during the early period following massive resection should be controlled with liberal proton pump inhibitor administration. Although growth hormone and glutamine have been advocated to facilitate adaptive changes in the residual small intestine, their use is controversial due to conflicting evidence as to their efficacy. The supplementation of TPN with glutamine has been suggested to assist some who are TPN dependent to be less dependent or freed from TPN perhaps through hypertrophying of the mucosa. Liberal use of agents such as loperamide or codeine to decrease intestinal transit time and increase contact of nutrients with the intestinal mucosa is desirable. Octreotide has been used to reduce secretion of pancreatic enzymes but there is concern that octreotide may interfere with intestinal protein synthesis and subsequent adaptation. Suspected SIBO should be treated as described previously with antibiotics including rifaximin or amoxicillin/clavulanate. Transition to oral feedings, starting with multiple small meals while tapering parenteral nutrition, is a major goal and often feasible as intestinal adaptation progresses over time. The supplementation of TPN with glutamine has been suggested to assist some who are TPN dependent to be less dependent or freed from TPN perhaps through hypertrophy of the mucosa and augmenting absorption. Teduglutide, a Food and Drug Administration (FDA)-approved glucagon-like peptide 2 analog, has been shown in one study to significantly reduce parenteral nutrition requirements in some patients over a 52-week period. Indeed, in 4 of 52 patients, parenteral nutrition could be stopped completely. Bowel lengthening procedures such as serial transverse enteroplasty may be beneficial in selected patients, especially young children. In patients in whom adaptation is not adequate and long-term parenteral nutrition is not feasible due to loss of venous access, recurrent line sepsis, or progressive liver disease, small intestinal transplantation is an alternative. Three to five year survival exceeds 50% in expert hands, but the shortage of organ donors and the relatively few tertiary care centers equipped with the requisite surgical skills and experience limit this option to a selected few.

There are a number of complications that may develop with time in patients with short bowel syndrome. Cholelithiasis may form, especially if long-term parenteral alimentation is required and the enterohepatic bile salt circulation is interrupted. Prophylactic ursodeoxycholate may be useful in certain settings. If feasible, a surgeon may perform prophylactic cholecystectomy at the time of bowel resection to reduce the risk of downstream gallstone complications. Renal calculi, often composed of calcium oxalate, may develop if the colon is retained. Unabsorbed fatty acids bind calcium, reducing its availability to form calcium oxalate in the gut lumen. Free oxalate is then absorbed in the colon, especially if bile acids also spill, increasing colonic permeability to oxalate. Supplemental calcium, low-oxalate diet, and high fluid intake are therapeutic approaches. Steatotic and cholestatic liver disease may develop and progress to cirrhosis and its complications, especially if long-term parenteral nutrition is required and the distal ileum is absent. D-Lactic acidosis, likely reflecting bacterial metabolism of unabsorbed carbohydrates to D-lactic acid, may develop, especially in children.

Buchman AL. Etiology and initial management of short bowel syndrome. Gastroenterology. 2006;130:S5–S15. [PMID: 16473072]

Carroll RE, Benedetti E, Schowalter JP, Buchman AL. Management and complications of short bowel syndrome: an updated review. Curr Gastroenterol Rep. 2016;18(7):40. [PMID: 27324885]

Fishbein TM. Intestinal transplantation. N Engl J Med. 2009;361:998–1008. [PMID: 19726774]

Kochar B, Herfarth HH. Teduglutide for the treatment of short bowel syndrome - a safety evaluation. Expert Opin Drug Saf. 2018;17(7):733–739. [PMID: 29848084]

3. Gastrinoma & Zollinger-Ellison Syndrome

Patients with Zollinger-Ellison syndrome (see also Chapter 17) frequently present with symptoms and signs of malabsorption, including weight loss, diarrhea, and steatorrhea in the absence of or overshadowing acid peptic symptoms. The massive gastric acid secretion inactivates pancreatic lipase and impairs lipid emulsification by bile salts resulting in impairment of intraluminal lipid dispersion, which is required for efficient absorption. Moreover, the persistent and intense exposure to acid damages the mucosa of the proximal small intestine, impairing absorptive function. Biopsy specimens can demonstrate a striking architectural lesion with blunting or absence of villi and profound inflammation of the lamina propria. Diagnosis requires a high index of suspicion and is established by the demonstration of an elevated fasting serum gastrin, a positive secretin stimulation test, and the presence of a gastrinoma by imaging studies. Treatment includes inhibition of gastric secretion with proton pump inhibitors and surgical resection of the gastrinoma, if feasible (see Chapter 17).

Roy PK, Venzon DJ, Shojamanesh H, et al. Zollinger-Ellison syndrome. Clinical presentation in 261 patients. Medicine (Baltimore). 2000;79:379–411. [PMID: 11144036]

DISEASES CAUSED BY IMPAIRED POSTMUCOSAL TRANSPORT

Intestinal Lymphangiectasia

Intestinal lymphangiectasia may be primary or secondary. The primary form usually presents in infancy or childhood and is associated with focal or diffuse ectasia of the mucosal intestinal lymphatics, most likely reflecting impaired lymphatic formation during development. Concomitant defects in lymphatics at other body sites such as the extremities support this concept. Familial clustering of cases suggests a genetic basis in some. Secondary intestinal lymphangiectasia results from acquired obstruction of mesenteric or more proximal lymphatics. Disruption of intestinal lymphatic drainage may reflect trauma, retroperitoneal fibrosis, neoplasms, infections such as tuberculosis, congestive heart failure, or severe portal hypertension. Rupture of the lymphatics results in leakage of protein and lymphocyte-rich lymph into the gut lumen as well as impaired transport of dietary lipids to the systemic circulation by the damaged lymphatics.

Clinical features in both primary and secondary types include weight loss, growth failure in children, steatorrhea, and diarrhea if disease is extensive. Edema, chylous ascites, and chylous pleural effusions reflect associated protein-losing enteropathy and impaired transport and leakage of dietary lipids. Helpful laboratory findings include lymphocytopenia, which may be striking, and low serum albumin, immunoglobulins, transferrin, and ceruloplasmin.

Increased clearance of α_1-antitrypsin pinpoints the intestinal tract as the source of protein loss, but evaluation of the test requires adjustment in patients with diarrhea; clearance greater than 24 mL/day in the absence of diarrhea or greater than 56 mL/day in the presence of diarrhea indicates increased enteric protein loss. Imaging studies such as CT scan of the abdomen can help to localize anatomic abnormalities such as fibrosis and adenopathy and often reveal thickening and edema of the abdominal wall. Contrast or magnetic resonance lymphangiography, if available, may localize the site of lymphatic obstruction or leakage. Conventional and VCE may reveal whitish villi due to distended ectatic mucosal lymphatics. Mucosal biopsy characteristically shows tall villi, dilated lymphatics, and mucosal edema, but involvement may be patchy; hence, absence of lymphatic dilation in available biopsy specimens does not exclude the diagnosis.

Treatment includes reduction of dietary long-chain triglycerides that stimulate lymph formation, increasing intralymphatic pressure and predisposing to lymphatic rupture and lymph leakage. Addition of medium-chain triglyceride–containing supplements and use of medium-chain triglyceride oil benefit nutrition as they are transported in the portal blood, not the lymphatics. A high-protein diet utilizing supplements as needed helps counter enteric protein loss. If the responsible disease process involves a limited segment of the intestine, resection can sometimes be beneficial. Likewise, if a surgically correctable focal obstruction of a major lymphatic is found, surgery should be considered. Treatment of underlying specific diseases such as retroperitoneal neoplasm or infection is indicated.

Alshikho MJ, Talas JM, Noureldine SI, et al. Intestinal lymphangiectasia: insights on management and literature review. *Am J Case Rep.* 201621;17:512–522. [PMID: 27440277]

Freeman HJ, Nimmo M. Intestinal lymphangiectasia in adults. *World J Gastrointest Oncol.* 2011;3:19–23. [PMID: 2136484]

Chronic Constipation & Fecal Incontinence

22

Nayna A. Lodhia, MD

Walter W. Chan, MD, MPH

ESSENTIALS OF DIAGNOSIS

- A thorough digital rectal examination (DRE) is critical in the evaluation of anorectal disorders and should be performed in all patients presenting with constipation and fecal incontinence. An adequate DRE should include the assessment of anal sphincter tone, squeeze, and response to cough and bearing down or strain.

- Colonic transit can be assessed using a radio-opaque sitz marker study or wireless motility capsule. Retention of >20% of sitz marker after 5 days suggests abnormal colonic transit.

- High-resolution anorectal manometry, balloon expulsion testing, and defecography, either fluoroscopic or by magnetic resonance imaging (MRI), allow evaluation of dyssynergic defecation and pelvic floor dysfunction in patients with chronic constipation.

- Decreased resting anal sphincter pressure on anorectal manometry suggests internal anal sphincter weakness, while abnormal squeeze pressure indicates dysfunction of the external anal sphincter in patients with fecal incontinence.

- Endoscopic ultrasound may be considered in patients presenting with fecal incontinence and evidence of anal sphincters weakness or defect on anorectal manometry, particularly in those with past medical or obstetric history that may suggest anal sphincter injury or trauma.

CHRONIC CONSTIPATION

Epidemiology

Constipation is one of the most common gastrointestinal complaints in the general population, with an estimated worldwide prevalence of anywhere between 2% and 40.1%.

It accounts for nearly 1.6 million emergency and outpatient clinic visits annually in the United States of America making it the sixth most common gastrointestinal symptom prompting medical evaluation in 2014. The prevalence of constipation related complaints has increased over time with a doubling of the rates of ambulatory care diagnoses and a four-fold increase in the rates of hospital discharge diagnoses from 1992 to 2004. With the increasing prevalence, 5.4 million prescriptions were filled for constipation and approximately $821 million USD have been spent on over-the-counter laxatives. Overall, the total cost of medical therapy for constipation is estimated to be $1912-7522 USD per patient per year.

Bharucha AE, Lacy BE. Mechanisms, evaluation, and management of chronic constipation. *Gastroenterology.* 2020;158(5):1232–1249. [PMID: 31945360]

Everhart JE, Ruhl CE. Burden of digestive diseases in the United States part II: lower gastrointestinal diseases. *Gastroenterology.* 2009;136(3):741–754. [PMID: 19166855]

Higgins PD, Johanson JF. Epidemiology of constipation in North America: a systematic review. *Am J Gastroenterol.* 2004;99(4):750–759. [PMID: 15089911]

Mugie SM, Benninga MA, Di Lorenzo C. Epidemiology of constipation in children and adults: a systematic review. *Best Pract Res Clin Gastroenterol.* 2011;25(1):3–18. [PMID: 21382575]

Nellesen D, Chawla A, Oh DL, Weissman T, Lavins BJ, Murray CW. Comorbidities in patients with irritable bowel syndrome with constipation or chronic idiopathic constipation: a review of the literature from the past decade. *Postgrad Med.* 2013;125(2):40–50. [PMID: 23816770]

Peppas G, Alexiou VG, Mourtzoukou E, Falagas ME. Epidemiology of constipation in Europe and Oceania: a systematic review. *BMC Gastroenterol.* 2008;8:5. [PMID: 18269746]

Peery AF, Crockett SD, Murphy CC, et al. Burden and cost of gastrointestinal, liver, and pancreatic diseases in the United States: update 2018. *Gastroenterology.* 2019;156(1):254–272. [PMID: 30315778]

Table 22–1. Rome IV criteria for chronic constipation.

Symptom onset ≥6 months prior to diagnosis and fulfilling the following criteria for the last 3 months:

1. **Two or more of the following:**
   a. Straining during more than 25% of defecations
   b. Lumpy or hard stools more than 25% of defecations.
   c. Sensation of incomplete evacuation more than 25% of defecations
   d. Sensation of anorectal obstruction/blockage more than 25% of defecations
   e. Manual maneuvers to facilitate more than 25% of defecations (eg, digital evacuation, support of the pelvic floor).
   f. Fewer than 3 spontaneous bowel movements per week.
2. **Loose stools are rarely present without the use of laxatives**
3. **Insufficient criteria for irritable bowel syndrome.**

Rao SS. Constipation: evaluation and treatment of colonic and anorectal motility disorders. *Gastroenterol Clin North Am.* 2007;36(3):687–711.

Suares NC, Ford AC. Prevalence of, and risk factors for, chronic idiopathic constipation in the community: systematic review and meta-analysis. *Am J Gastroenterol.* 2011;106(9):1582–1591. [PMID: 21606976]

Definition

Chronic constipation is defined by multiple lower gastrointestinal symptoms such as decreased stool frequency, difficulty passing stool, or feeling incomplete evacuation that can occur alone or with another comorbid disorder such as hypothyroidism. The Rome IV consensus guidelines were developed to outline the bowel symptoms that can be used to define constipation. Per these criteria a patient must have had symptom onset at least six months prior to diagnosis and have fulfilled the criteria shown in Table 22–1 for the last three months.

In addition to the Rome criteria, the Bristol Stool Form Scale (BSFS) was developed as a simple method to assess stool type based on its visual appearance on a scale of one to seven (Table 22–2).

Types 1 and 2 on the scale indicate constipation and types 6 and 7 are suggestive of diarrhea. This scale has been shown to accurately assess colonic transit times with stools forms 1 and 2 being associated with constipation and slower transit times.

Table 22–2. Bristol stool scale.

Type 1: Separate hard lumps, nut-like
Type 2: Lumpy sausage
Type 3: Sausage with cracks on its surface
Type 4: Smooth snake
Type 5: Soft blobs with clear edges
Type 6: Fluffy pieces with ragged edges
Type 7: Watery without any solid pieces

Pathophysiology

Normal defecation includes a coordinated effort between peristalsis, water and ion absorption and excretion, and pelvic floor muscle/anorectal contraction and relaxation. Chronic constipation may be caused by anatomic changes, such as colonic elongation, altered motility, or abnormalities in normal defecation physiology. Two primary physiologic processes can contribute to chronic constipation: (1) colonic dysfunction and (2) anorectal evacuation dysfunction. Patients may have evidence of slow transit constipation and/or rectal evacuation disorders; however, a majority of patients with chronic constipation may not demonstrate evidence of either, and are thought to have normal transit constipation, also known as functional constipation. These patients often have symptoms that may overlap with constipation-predominant irritable bowel syndrome (IBS-C).

Colonic dysfunction, also known as decreased colonic inertia, can be caused by reduced coordinated peristalsis leading to a slow bowel transit time. As stools enter the cecum from the terminal ileum, water and ion absorption begins in the proximal colon. If peristalsis is affected, the resultant slow transit of stools through the proximal colon may lead to increased water absorption, thereby creating dry, lumpy stools. Alternatively, dehydration can also lead to increased colonic water absorption. Some studies have suggested that changes in the colonic bacterial content may affect motility and lead to constipation as well; however, this has not been well established.

After the stools have moved through the colon, waste and indigestible materials are stored in the rectum until they can be excreted through a coordinated contraction and relaxation of three major pelvic and anorectal muscles. First, the internal anal sphincter is made of circular smooth muscle and is innervated by the enteric nervous system. It is tonically contracted at rest to maintain the basal sphincter tone. Second, the external anal sphincter is made of striated muscle with somatic innervation through the pudendal nerve, and is responsible for voluntary squeeze. Lastly, the puborectalis muscle is striated muscle that is innervated with pelvic branches S3 and S4. At baseline, the sling-like muscle around the anorectal junction is contracted to help maintain an anorectal angle of approximately 80 degrees. During defecation, the anorectal angle increases and straightens as the puborectalis muscle relaxes to facilitate passage of stools.

During normal defecation (Figure 22–1), the presence of contents in the rectum triggers a reflexive relaxation of the internal anal sphincter, termed the rectoanal inhibitory reflex (RAIR). Relaxation of the internal anal sphincter allows sampling of the rectal content by the anal ectoderm, which distinguishes between stools and gas. The external anal sphincter also contracts to hold the content in the rectum. When the individual is ready for defecation, the rectal pressure is increased via abdominal muscle contraction, while the anal sphincters and puborectalis muscle relax to allow the stool to be expelled. Altered rectal sensation and/or impaired coordination of the pelvic floor or anal sphincter muscles would lead to defecation or outlet disorders.

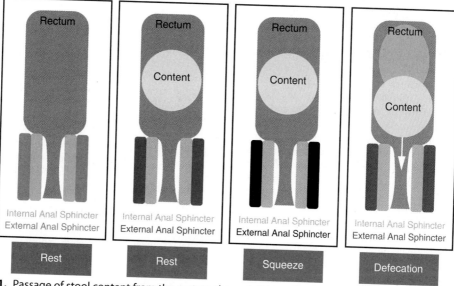

▲ **Figure 22–1.** Passage of stool content from the rectum through the anal canal. At rest the internal anal sphincter (IAS) and external anal sphincter (EAS) are inactive and the IAS is tonically contracted. As stool content enters the rectum, the IAS reflexively relaxes (rectoanal inhibitory reflex). When the individual voluntarily squeezes, the EAS contracts to prevent passage of stool. When ready to defecate, the IAS and EAS relax for passage of stool.

Ashraf W, Park F, Lof J, Quigley EM. An examination of the reliability of reported stool frequency in the diagnosis of idiopathic constipation. *Am J Gastroenterol.* 1996;91(1):26–32. [PMID: 8561138]

Chassard C, Dapoigny M, Scott KP, et al. Functional dysbiosis within the gut microbiota of patients with constipated-irritable bowel syndrome. *Aliment Pharmacol Ther.* 2012;35(7):828–838. [PMID: 22315951]

Dickson EJ, Hennig GW, Heredia DJ, et al. Polarized intrinsic neural reflexes in response to colonic elongation. *J Physiol.* 2008;586(17):4225–4240. [PMID: 18635646]

Ge X, Ding C, Zhao W, et al. Antibiotics-induced depletion of mice microbiota induces changes in host serotonin biosynthesis and intestinal motility. *J Transl Med.* 2017;15(1):13. [PMID: 28086815]

Hyland NP, Cryan JF. Microbe-host interactions: influence of the gut microbiota on the enteric nervous system. *Dev Biol.* 2016;417(2): 182–187. [PMID: 27343895]

Lewis SJ, Heaton KW. Stool form scale as a useful guide to intestinal transit time. *Scand J Gastroenterol.* 1997;32(9):920–924. [PMID: 9299672]

Manabe N, Wong BS, Camilleri M, Burton D, McKinzie S, Zinsmeister AR. Lower functional gastrointestinal disorders: evidence of abnormal colonic transit in a 287 patient cohort. *Neurogastroenterol Motil.* 2010;22(3):293-e82. [PMID: 20025692]

Mearin F, Lacy BE, Chang L, et al. Bowel disorders. *Gastroenterology.* 2016; 150(6):1393–1407. [PMID: 27144627]

Smith TK, Spencer NJ, Hennig GW, Dickson EJ. Recent advances in enteric neurobiology: mechanosensitive interneurons. *Neurogastroenterol Motil.* 2007;19(11):869–878. [PMID: 17988274]

► Diagnosis

History and physical exam are the most important part of the workup when a patient presents with chronic constipation because they inform the need for additional work up or if the patient can be treated symptomatically.

The history should assess when the patient's symptoms started and characterize the symptoms including stool frequency, consistency per the BSFS, and color (brown, red or black suggesting blood vs green suggesting bile). Prior to having a bowel movement, is there a pain or is there a sense of urgency to defecate? After bowel movement, is there rectal pain, does any preceding abdominal pain resolve, is there fecal incontinence or a sense of incomplete evacuation, and do they need to use digital maneuvers to assist stool passage? How long are they sitting on the toilet for? It is important to assess the patient's lifestyle including life stressors, dietary changes, and medication.

After the present illness is characterized, a thorough medical history should be obtained. When evaluating patients past medical history, a systems-based approach will best address other etiologies that may be contributing to constipation. Metabolic disorders such as diabetes, hypothyroidism, hyperparathyroidism, electrolyte imbalances (hypocalcemia, hypokalemia, hypomagnesemia), and obesity may all contribute to constipation. A history of neuropathies such as autonomic disease, postural orthostatic tachycardia syndrome (POTS), Hirschsprung disease, amyloidosis, central nervous system lesions, and Parkinson's disease, should be evaluated. And lastly, the past medical history should address other considerations including colonic obstruction (masses, adhesions), paraneoplastic syndromes, eating disorders, dietary changes (low fiber, high protein), and pseudo-obstruction. Inadequate caloric intake can mimic the symptoms of slow transit constipation, so this should be addressed prior to additional workup. Gastrointestinal causes including inflammatory bowel disease, anal strictures, anal fissures, and hemorrhoids can also contribute to constipation.

The past surgical history should specifically address a patient's history of abdominal and pelvic floor surgeries. Obstetric history including number of pregnancies, types of delivery (normal spontaneous vaginal delivery, cesarean section) and use of assistive devices for a vaginal delivery (vacuum extraction, forceps, episiotomy) should be obtained. History of pelvic floor surgery and anal traumas should also be discussed with the patient.

A family history suggestive of malignancy or advanced polyps should be documented. A family history of neurologic or autoimmune disorders may also affect the differential diagnosis.

Many medications can contribute to constipation and a full medication history including over-the-counter medications and recent dose changes should be carefully obtained. Pain medications including opioids, but also over the counter pain medications such as non-steroidal anti-inflammatory drugs (NSAIDs) are often the first medications that come to mind when evaluating patients with constipation. However, other medications such as antihistamines, neuropathic medications, antihypertensives, and antidepressants can all lead to decreased stool frequency.

After a thorough history has been obtained from the patient, the physical exam, specifically the DRE is the next most informative step in evaluating a patient with constipation. When done correctly, the DRE has a 75% sensitivity and an 87% specificity for dyssynergic defecation, and the positive predictive value to identify low resting and squeeze pressures of 67% and 81%, respectively. This makes it an effective, inexpensive test that can be done in the office. The DRE begins with positioning the patient in the left lateral position with their hips flexed to 90 degrees:

First, the anus and surrounding tissue, including the anal mucosa, should be inspected with a bright light. Skin excoriations, skin tags, anal fissures, scars, external hemorrhoids, prolapsed hemorrhoids, rectal prolapse, and condyloma should be noted. If a fissure is seen, consider using a lidocaine lubricant for examination, as it could be very painful for the patient otherwise.

Second, the anocutaneous reflex is elicited by stroking the perianal skin toward the anus in each quadrant with a cotton bud. A normal response is a brisk contraction of the perianal skin, the anoderm and the external anal sphincter to the cotton swab. If there is an impaired response, there is no response to the soft cotton but there is a response to the wooden end of the cotton bud. An abnormal exam suggests a neuronal injury in the sensory nerves S2, S3, and S4.

Third, advance a lubricated and gloved index finger into the rectum and feel the mucosa and surrounding muscle, bone, uterus, prostate, and pelvic structures. The presence of stool in the rectum suggests lack of stool awareness and possible rectal hyposensitivity. Hard and compact stool in the rectum indicates a fecal impaction.

Last, the anal sphincter should be assessed at rest and when contracted. At rest, the tonicity of the internal anal sphincter should be noted. Then ask the patient to squeeze to assess the strength of the external anal sphincter. Sphincter defects should be noted during the rest and squeeze maneuvers. Dyssynergic defecation is assessed with the bearing down maneuver that can be done by asking the patient to cough or have the patient bear down themselves. With either method, the clinician's hand should remain on the patient's abdomen to ensure the abdominal muscles contract and the external anal sphincter contracts in a coordinated fashion, to prevent passage of stool. If this does not occur, fecal incontinence should be suspected. There is a concern for dyssynergic defecation when the abdominal muscles cannot contract, the anal sphincter or puborectalis cannot relax, there is paradoxical contraction of the anal sphincter or puborectalis, or there is absence of the perineal descent. A rectocele is present if, when the patient bears down, the finger dips into an indentation of the rectal wall when resting anteriorly.

Forootan M, Bagheri N, Darvishi M. Chronic constipation: a review of literature. *Medicine (Baltimore)*. 2018;97(20):e10631. [PMID: 29768326]

Hadley SJ, Walsh BT. Gastrointestinal disturbances in anorexia nervosa and bulimia nervosa. *Curr Drug Targets CNS Neurol Disord*. 2003;2(1):1–9. [PMID: 12769807]

Hill J, Corson RJ, Brandon H, Redford J, Faragher EB, Kiff ES. History and examination in the assessment of patients with idiopathic fecal incontinence. *Dis Colon Rectum*. 1994;37(5):473–477. [PMID: 8181410]

Rao SSC. Rectal exam: yes, it can and should be done in a busy practice! *Am J Gastroenterol*. 2018;113(5):635–638. [PMID: 29453382]

Rao SS, American College of Gastroenterology Practice Parameters Committee. Diagnosis and management of fecal incontinence. American College of Gastroenterology Practice Parameters Committee. *Am J Gastroenterol*. 2004;99(8):1585–1604. [PMID: 15307881]

Tantiphlachiva K, Rao P, Attaluri A, Rao SS. Digital rectal examination is a useful tool for identifying patients with dyssynergia. *Clin Gastroenterol Hepatol*. 2010;8(11):955–960. [PMID: 20656061]

Diagnostic Algorithm

After a thorough history and physical exam is completed, additional workup may need to be considered. If there are any concerning signs or symptoms such as rectal bleeding, acute onset symptoms, weight loss, or family history of malignancy, a colonoscopy should be performed. However, in the absence of these red flag findings, it is extremely rare for a colonoscopy to assist in the diagnosis of constipation. In these cases, it is appropriate to begin with symptomatic management. If symptomatic management is not effective, or if there are abnormal findings on the DRE, then high resolution anorectal manometry (HRAM) can be considered.

In HRAM, catheters with closely spaced pressure sensors are inserted into the rectum and are used to assess anorectal function (Figure 22–2). Initially the resting pressure or the basal tone is measured, which represents the strength of the internal anal sphincter. Next, the patient is asked to perform a squeeze to assess their external anal sphincter strength. This measurement can be limited by patient cooperation or ability to understand the instructions, which should be kept in mind when interpreting the results.

Lastly, during HRAM, a 4 cm balloon is filled with warm water in the rectum sequentially and the individual is asked

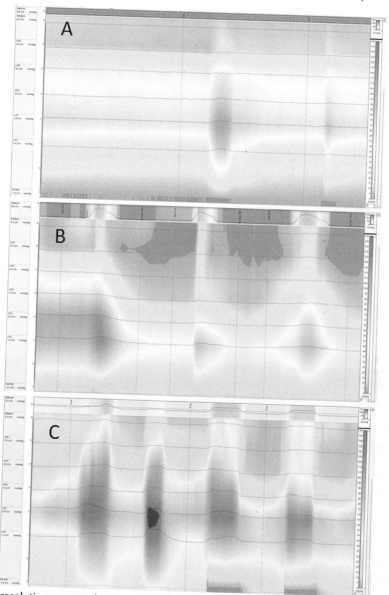

▲ **Figure 22–2.** High-resolution anorectal manometry. (A) The basal anal sphincter tone (resting pressure) and the squeeze maneuver are shown. The resting pressure estimates the internal anal sphincter tone while the squeeze pressure represents the external anal sphincter strength. (B) The recto-anal inhibitory reflux (RAIR) is estimated by inflating an intra-rectal balloon and assessing the relaxation of the internal anal sphincter. (C) An example of dyssynergic defecation during the strain or bear-down maneuver, with a paradoxical increase in anal sphincter pressure rather than relaxation during simulated defecation.

to say when they first sense something in the rectum, have an urge to have a bowel movement, or can no longer tolerate increased volume. This provides information on the sensitivity of the rectum, which is essential in bowel control and defecation. Additionally as the balloon is inflated, the rectal anal inhibitory reflex should be elicited, the absence of this reflex may be suggestive of absence of proper innervation, such as aganglionosis seen in Hirschsprung disease. Then the patient is asked to expel the balloon that is inflated to 50 mL. If the patient takes longer than two minutes to expel the balloon, the test is considered abnormal. This test has an 80–90% specificity and a 50% sensitivity.

The HRAM can also assess for dyssynergic defecation. In a normal response to increasing rectal pressures, the anal pressure should decrease to allow for passage of stools. In dyssynergia the rectal pressures or anal pressures could be abnormal. The rectal pressures can be appropriately elevated or they could be inadequate to enforce a squeeze. The anal pressures can be elevated or inappropriately normal. There are four types of dyssynergia based on the anal and rectal pressures:

1. Type I: adequate rectal push effort with paradoxical anal sphincter contraction.
2. Type II: inadequate rectal push effort with paradoxical anal sphincter contraction.
3. Type III: adequate rectal push effort but inadequate relaxation (<20%) of anal sphincter pressure.
4. Type IV: inadequate rectal push effort and also inadequate relaxation.

If the HRAM is inconclusive, additional imaging techniques such as defecography can help differentiate between a defecatory disorder and colonic transit disorders. During defecography, which can be performed under fluoroscopy or using an MRI, 150 mL of barium paste is inserted into the rectum and the patient is asked to expel the contents in a seated position on the commode. The advantage of MRI defecography is that it allows evaluation of the pelvic floor anatomy and function simultaneously; therefore, it can uniquely evaluate for rectal mucosal intussusception. It is more precise and reproducible than fluoroscopy; however, it is also four times more expensive than fluoroscopy and requires an open MRI where the patient is in the seated position passing contrast through their rectum, which can be embarrassing for the patient.

To begin analyzing an MRI defecography (Figure 22–3), the pubococcygeal line (PCL), a straight line connecting the inferior border of the pubic symphysis to the last coccygeal joint, should be identified. This line is the guiding light for the rest of the study because it has the best inter and intra observer reliability. It represents the plane of attachment of the pelvic muscles and all organs should remain above this line and go no more than 1 cm below it. If it does go more than 1 cm below this line, then it's a sign of prolapse. The anorectal angle is determined at rest, with the squeeze maneuver and while bearing down. The anorectal angle is the intersection of the posterior border of the distal part of the rectum and the central axis of the anal canal. A normal angle is between 108 and 127 degrees. As the muscles contract, the angle is decreased by about 15–20 degrees. When the muscles relax for evacuation, the angle increases about 15–20 degrees.

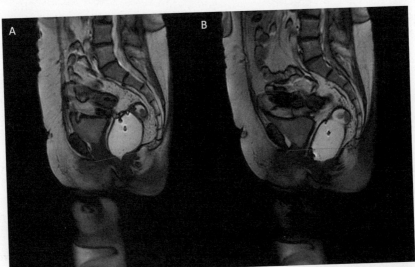

▲ **Figure 22–3.** Normal MR defecography. (A) At rest, the pelvic organs remain above or within 1 cm below the pubococcygeal line (PCL) and the anorectal angle approximates between 108 and 207 degrees. (B) During defecation, relaxation of the puborectalis and pelvic floor muscles result in descend of the anorectal junction, increase in anorectal angle, and straightening of the anorectal canal.

Slow colonic transit can be assessed using a radio-opaque marker study. In these studies, patients are asked to avoid laxatives and high fiber 2–3 days prior to the test. On the day of the test, a capsule containing 24 markers are ingested and an abdominal x-ray is obtained after 5 days. The study is considered abnormal if there are more than five markers retained in the colon. The location of the retained markers may indicate the area of slow transit. For example, if the markers are retained throughout the colon, then there is likely global decreased peristalsis; however, if they are all retained in the descending colon, the left colon is likely where peristalsis is most delayed.

A wireless motility capsule study can be used in lieu of a radio-opaque marker study. This requires a patient to ingest a wireless pH, temperature and pressure recording capsule which is used to assess regional and whole-gut transit times without any radiation exposure. Normal colonic transit time is 10–59 hours and the whole gut transit time is typically 10–73 hours.

Bond JH. Is referral for colonoscopy underutilized by primary care physicians? *Gastrointest Endosc.* 2000;52(5):693–696. [PMID: 11060206]

Chiarioni G, Kim SM, Vantini I, Whitehead WE. Validation of the balloon evacuation test: reproducibility and agreement with findings from anorectal manometry and electromyography. *Clin Gastroenterol Hepatol.* 2014;12(12):2049–2054. [PMID: 24674941]

El Sayed RF, Alt CD, Maccioni F, et al. Magnetic resonance imaging of pelvic floor dysfunction - joint recommendations of the ESUR and ESGAR Pelvic Floor Working Group. *Eur Radiol.* 2017;27(5):2067–2085. [PMID: 27488850]

Grossi U, Carrington EV, Bharucha AE, Horrocks EJ, Scott SM, Knowles CH. Diagnostic accuracy study of anorectal manometry for diagnosis of dyssynergic defecation. *Gut.* 2016;65(3):447–455. [PMID: 25765461]

Heinrich H, Misselwitz B. High-resolution anorectal manometry - new insights in the diagnostic assessment of functional anorectal disorders. *Visc Med.* 2018;34(2):134–139. [PMID: 29888243]

Hinton JM, Lennard-Jones JE, Young AC. A new method for studying gut transit times using radioopaque markers. *Gut.* 1969;10(10):842–847. [PMID: 5350110]

Lee TH, Bharucha AE. How to perform and interpret a high-resolution anorectal manometry test. *J Neurogastroenterol Motil.* 2016;22(1):46–59. [PMID: 26717931]

Lee YY, Erdogan A, Rao SS. How to assess regional and whole gut transit time with wireless motility capsule. *J Neurogastroenterol Motil.* 2014;20(2):265–270. [PMID: 24840360]

Pannu HK, Javitt MC, Glanc P, et al. ACR appropriateness criteria pelvic floor dysfunction. *J Am Coll Radiol.* 2015;12(2):134–142. [PMID: 25652300]

Rao SS, Kuo B, McCallum RW, et al. Investigation of colonic and whole-gut transit with wireless motility capsule and radio-opaque markers in constipation. *Clin Gastroenterol Hepatol.* 2009;7(5):537–544. [PMID: 19418602]

Salvador JC, Coutinho MP, Venancio JM, Viamonte B. Dynamic magnetic resonance imaging of the female pelvic floor - a pictorial review. *Insights Imaging.* 2019;10(1):4. [PMID: 30689115]

Schussele Filliettaz S, Gonvers JJ, Peytremann-Bridevaux I, et al. Appropriateness of colonoscopy in Europe (EPAGE II). Functional bowel disorders: pain, constipation and bloating. *Endoscopy.* 2009;41(3):234–239. [PMID: 19280535]

Vader JP, Pache I, Froehlich F, et al. Overuse and underuse of colonoscopy in a European primary care setting. *Gastrointest Endosc.* 2000;52(5):593–599. [PMID: 11060181]

▶ Management

The management of chronic constipation usually begins with a high fiber diet, particularly soluble fibers like psyllium or ispaghula, which are superior to insoluble dietary fibers like wheat bran. Fiber, a carbohydrate polymer, works by absorbing fluid to bulk stool and can affect the gut microbiota or epithelial permeability through fermentation. Because fiber supplements can cause bloating, fullness, and abdominal discomfort, it is important to recommend generous fluid intake along with fiber supplementation and patients should be warned that gaseous distension will typically resolve within a week. Treatment with soluble fiber has been shown to improve global symptoms, straining, the mean number of stools per week, and stool consistency. In patients where there is concern for a defecatory disorder or slow transit constipation, fiber should be used with caution as it can potentially worsen symptoms.

Surfactants, or stool softeners such as docusate, lower the surface tension of stool and allow water to enter the stool. The data for the treatment of constipation with stool softeners is inadequate to recommend its chronic use in palliative care patients with advanced disease.

Stimulant laxatives like Bisacodyl and glycerine suppositories work on the colonic mucosa to propagate colonic contractions by stimulation of the colonic myenteric plexus with independent antiabsorptive and secretory effects. Their long-term use appears to be safe; however, they are most typically used as rescue medications. It is thought that the suppository should be given 30 minutes postprandially to optimally sync the gastro-colonic response. Abdominal cramps are well known side effects as well as melanosis coli or hepatotoxicity with senna. Electrolyte imbalances can also be seen with stimulant laxatives. Contrary to conventional teachings, there is no evidence to suggest that stimulant laxatives can cause structural damage to the surface of epithelial cells.

Osmotic laxatives include PEG-based solutions, magnesium citrate–bases, sodium phosphate–bases, and non-absorbable carbohydrates (lactulose). They may be options for regular use due to the long-term efficacy data available for certain osmotic laxatives such as PEG-based solutions. Dried plums and prune juice have been traditionally used for the treatment of constipation not only for their soluble fiber but also the sorbitol and phenolic compounds that act as osmotic laxatives. As hypertonic products, they draw fluid into the lumen through osmosis. Studies show that the use of osmotic laxatives is safe up to 24 months and dosing can be titrated to symptoms. Bloating and flatulence are common side effects particularly with lactulose. There are some case reports of hypermagnesemia in patients with renal impairment so it should be used with caution in those patients. Unfortunately, 50% of chronic constipation patients report dissatisfaction with these therapies and their concerns include unpredictability (71–75%), bloating (52–67%), poor symptom relief (44–50%), or inability to improve quality of life (44–68%).

Intestinal secretagogues include lubiprostone, linaclotide, plecanatide, and tenapanor. While each medication has a slightly different mechanism of action, they all facilitate passage of chloride ions across cell membranes, which is key to maintaining fluid homeostasis for cell volume and intracellular pH. This not only accelerates transit but also facilitates the ease of defecation. None of these have been studied in pregnancy so they are all pregnancy class C; therefore, women of childbearing age should have a negative pregnancy test result before starting treatment and should remain on contraception while taking the medication.

Lubiprostone is a bicyclic fatty acid derivative that works by activating apical chloride channels. It activates prostaglandin EP receptors and the apical cystic fibrosis transmembrane regulator (CFTR), which helps mediate intestinal fluid secretion, and can stimulate small intestinal and colonic transit times. A dose of 24 micrograms is given in chronic constipation and 8 micrograms in IBS-C. Nausea is the most common side effect occurring in 31% of patients, but diarrhea (12%) and headaches (11%) are also common side effects. It is thought that the lubiprostone affects accommodation of the stomach by affecting the smooth muscles leading to nausea.

Linaclotide is a homolog of enterotoxins that can cause diarrhea. Linaclotide activates guanylyl cyclase C receptor that is expressed on the brush border of intestinal mucosa from the duodenum to the rectum. This activation converts guanosine triphosphate to cyclic guanosine monophosphate, which propagates a signal for CFTR phosphorylation, opening the CFTR chloride channel releasing ions and water into the intestinal lumen. It also has a direct neuronal effect and can affect the sensory innervation of the gut which can help with visceral hypersensitivity and pain. The effects on visceral hypersensitivity is higher at higher doses. Therefore, the dose of 290 mcg is approved for IBS-C, and chronic constipation is approved at 145 mcg. It is overall a safe medication with a dose dependent diarrhea as the main side effect; however, because it can be titrated to symptoms, it has a low rate of discontinuation due to diarrhea.

Plecanatide has the same mechanism as linaclotide; however, it is only active in the intestinal tract and is not systemically absorbed. This is only approved for use at a dose of 3 mg daily for IBS-C and chronic constipation eliminating the need for dose titration. Like the other secretagogues, diarrhea is the main adverse effect.

Serotonergic enterokinetic agents, such as prucalopride, activate the 5-HT4 receptors and stimulate peristalsis by enhancing proximal smooth muscle contractions and relaxing distal muscles. It also modulates cyclic adenosine monophosphate mediated chloride secretion and visceral sensitivity. A dose of 2 mg is recommended but it is decreased in older adults. It has a 90% bioavailability and a half-life of 24–30 hours. Side effects include headache, nausea, abdominal pain, and diarrhea.

Biofeedback therapy can be an adjunctive to the medical management of patients with chronic constipation due to defecatory disorders. Biofeedback therapy is a method of physical therapy that restores normal defecation by correcting dyssynergia of abdominal, rectal, puborectalis, and anal sphincter muscles. It facilitates normal evacuation by stimulated defecation training and enhanced rectal sensory perceptions. Biofeedback therapy can take an average of 4–6 therapy sessions and, at home, patients may be asked to do exercises with diaphragmatic breathing and attempted defecation for at least 15 minutes two to three times per a day. Studies have shown that biofeedback therapy is effective in treatment of defecatory disorders.

Botox can be used with defecatory disorders to help relax the puborectalis muscle using ultrasound guidance to inject 60–100 units of Botox. Botox injections have been found to decrease tone during straining 1–2 months post-injection ($P <0.01$) and can improve the anorectal angle from 98 to 121 degrees ($P <0.01$). Results are variable and can result in fecal incontinence, so this treatment is typically reserved for refractory cases of chronic constipation.

The role of surgical treatment, namely colectomy, should be limited to patients without rectal outlet problems who have failed to respond to aggressive medical and biofeedback treatments, and who have demonstrable colonic neuropathy only. Patients should undergo a thorough preoperative evaluation including anorectal manometry, defecography, and gastrointestinal tract motility assessment. Delayed motility elsewhere in the gastrointestinal tract is a predictor for failure of colectomy. A majority (80–93.7%) of patients have satisfactory results postoperatively; however, patients may complain of postoperative abdominal pain (41%), incontinence (21%), and diarrhea (46%) at least some of the time. Preoperatively, patients should be counseled on the risk of persistent abdominal pain and bloating, as well as the possibility of developing new gastrointestinal symptoms due to small intestinal bacterial overgrown, which occurs in 24% of patients undergoing total colectomies.

Sacral nerve stimulation is not approved for treatment in the United States of America, but has gained some traction in Europe. In patients with medically refractory chronic constipation, sacral nerve stimulation improved symptoms in

39/45 (86.7%) of patients and improved transit colonic transit times. In another study of patients with slow transit constipation and pelvic floor constipation receiving sacral nerve stimulation, only 42% of patients improved symptoms. Significantly high adverse event rates have been reported with sacral nerve stimulation treatment with 58% of patients having at least one reportable event, most commonly decreased efficacy, pain, and undesired change in sensation and 33% of patients required surgical interventions for correction or removal.

Attaluri A, Donahoe R, Valestin J, Brown K, Rao SS. Randomised clinical trial: dried plums (prunes) vs. psyllium for constipation. *Aliment Pharmacol Ther*. 2011;33(7):822–828. [PMID: 21323688]

Bharucha AE, Pemberton JH, Locke GR, 3rd. American Gastroenterological Association technical review on constipation. *Gastroenterology*. 2013;144(1):218–238. [PMID: 23261065]

Bharucha AE, Waldman SA. Taking a lesson from microbial diarrheagenesis in the management of chronic constipation. *Gastroenterology*. 2010;138(3):813–817. [PMID: 20114092]

Bijkerk CJ, de Wit NJ, Muris JW, Whorwell PJ, Knottnerus JA, Hoes AW. Soluble or insoluble fibre in irritable bowel syndrome in primary care? Randomised placebo controlled trial. *BMJ*. 2009;339:b3154. [PMID: 19713235]

Camilleri M, Bharucha AE, Ueno R, et al. Effect of a selective chloride channel activator, lubiprostone, on gastrointestinal transit, gastric sensory, and motor functions in healthy volunteers. *Am J Physiol Gastrointest Liver Physiol*. 2006;290(5):G942–G947. [PMID: 16603730]

Camilleri M, Deiteren A. Prucalopride for constipation. *Expert Opin Pharmacother*. 2010;11(3):451–461. [PMID: 20102308]

Corazziari E, Badiali D, Bazzocchi G, et al. Long term efficacy, safety, and tolerability of low daily doses of isosmotic polyethylene glycol electrolyte balanced solution (PMF-100) in the treatment of functional chronic constipation. *Gut*. 2000;46(4):522–526. [PMID: 10716682]

DiPalma JA, Cleveland MB, McGowan J, Herrera JL. A comparison of polyethylene glycol laxative and placebo for relief of constipation from constipating medications. *South Med J*. 2007;100(11):1085–1090. [PMID: 17984738]

Ford AC, Suares NC. Effect of laxatives and pharmacological therapies in chronic idiopathic constipation: systematic review and meta-analysis. *Gut*. 2011;60(2):209–218. [PMID: 21205879]

Gras-Miralles B, Cremonini F. A critical appraisal of lubiprostone in the treatment of chronic constipation in the elderly. *Clin Interv Aging*. 2013;8:191–200. [PMID: 23439964]

Holscher HD. Dietary fiber and prebiotics and the gastrointestinal microbiota. *Gut Microbes*. 2017;8(2):172–184. [PMID: 28165863]

Hurdon V, Viola R, Schroder C. How useful is docusate in patients at risk for constipation? A systematic review of the evidence in the chronically ill. *J Pain Symptom Manage*. 2000;19(2):130–136. [PMID: 10699540]

Johanson JF, Kralstein J. Chronic constipation: a survey of the patient perspective. *Aliment Pharmacol Ther*. 2007;25(5):599–608. [PMID: 17305761]

Johnston JM, Kurtz CB, Macdougall JE, et al. Linaclotide improves abdominal pain and bowel habits in a phase IIb study of patients with irritable bowel syndrome with constipation. *Gastroenterology*. 2010;139(6):1877–1886. [PMID: 20801122]

Kienzle-Horn S, Vix JM, Schuijt C, Peil H, Jordan CC, Kamm MA. Efficacy and safety of bisacodyl in the acute treatment of constipation: a double-blind, randomized, placebo-controlled study. *Aliment Pharmacol Ther*. 2006;23(10):1479–1488. [PMID: 16669963]

Lacy BE, Levy LC. Lubiprostone: a novel treatment for chronic constipation. *Clin Interv Aging*. 2008;3(2):357–364. [PMID: 18686757]

Lembo AJ, Schneier HA, Shiff SJ, et al. Two randomized trials of linaclotide for chronic constipation. *N Engl J Med*. 2011;365(6):527–536. [PMID: 21830967]

Louvel D, Delvaux M, Staumont G, et al. Intracolonic injection of glycerol: a model for abdominal pain in irritable bowel syndrome? *Gastroenterology*. 1996;110(2):351–361. [PMID: 8566580]

Manabe N, Cremonini F, Camilleri M, Sandborn WJ, Burton DD. Effects of bisacodyl on ascending colon emptying and overall colonic transit in healthy volunteers. *Aliment Pharmacol Ther*. 2009;30(9):930–936. [PMID: 19678812]

Migeon-Duballet I, Chabin M, Gautier A, et al. Long-term efficacy and cost-effectiveness of polyethylene glycol 3350 plus electrolytes in chronic constipation: a retrospective study in a disabled population. *Curr Med Res Opin*. 2006;22(6):1227–1235. [PMID: 16846556]

Mueller-Lissner S, Kamm MA, Wald A, et al. Multicenter, 4-week, double-blind, randomized, placebo-controlled trial of sodium picosulfate in patients with chronic constipation. *Am J Gastroenterol*. 2010;105(4):897–903. [PMID: 20179697]

Nyberg C, Hendel J, Nielsen OH. The safety of osmotically acting cathartics in colonic cleansing. *Nat Rev Gastroenterol Hepatol*. 2010;7(10):557–564. [PMID: 20736921]

Pare P, Fedorak RN. Systematic review of stimulant and non-stimulant laxatives for the treatment of functional constipation. *Can J Gastroenterol Hepatol*. 2014;28(10):549–557. [PMID: 25390617]

Rao SS, Rattanakovit K, Patcharatrakul T. Diagnosis and management of chronic constipation in adults. *Nat Rev Gastroenterol Hepatol*. 2016;13(5):295–305. [PMID: 27033126]

Rao SSC. Plecanatide: a new guanylate cyclase agonist for the treatment of chronic idiopathic constipation. *Therap Adv Gastroenterol*. 2018;11:1756284818777945. [PMID: 29942351]

Rao SS. Biofeedback therapy for constipation in adults. *Best Pract Res Clin Gastroenterol*. 2011;25(1):159–166. [PMID: 21382587]

Roerig JL, Steffen KJ, Mitchell JE, Zunker C. Laxative abuse: epidemiology, diagnosis and management. *Drugs*. 2010;70(12):1487–1503. [PMID: 20687617]

Schey R, Rao SS. Lubiprostone for the treatment of adults with constipation and irritable bowel syndrome. *Dig Dis Sci*. 2011;56(6):1619–1625. [PMID: 21523369]

Singh S, Rao SS. Pharmacologic management of chronic constipation. *Gastroenterol Clin North Am*. 2010;39(3):509–527. [PMID: 20951915]

Suares NC, Ford AC. Systematic review: the effects of fibre in the management of chronic idiopathic constipation. *Aliment Pharmacol Ther.* 2011;33(8):895–901. [PMID: 21332763]

Voderholzer WA, Schatke W, Muhldorfer BE, Klauser AG, Birkner B, Muller-Lissner SA. Clinical response to dietary fiber treatment of chronic constipation. *Am J Gastroenterol.* 1997;92(1):95–98. [PMID: 8995945]

Wald A. Is chronic use of stimulant laxatives harmful to the colon? *J Clin Gastroenterol.* 2003;36(5):386–389. [PMID: 12702977]

FECAL INCONTINENCE

Fecal incontinence is defined as the unintentional loss of stool or liquid stool, and anal incontinence also includes the leakage of gas. The prevalence in men and women is roughly the same and estimated to be between 7% and 15%. Risk factors include older age, poor health status, anatomical injury (obstetric trauma, hemorrhoidectomy, internal sphincterotomy, fistulotomy), vaginal delivery, radiation, neurologic disorders (stroke, multiple sclerosis, Parkinson's disease, myotonic dystrophy, spinal cord injury), endocrine (diabetes), or rheumatologic disorders (systemic sclerosis).

▶ Diagnosis

Thorough history and physical examination are the basis of diagnosis and treatment for fecal incontinence. The natural history of the symptoms should be characterized as they may inform why the patient is seeking medical attention at this time, as symptoms are often chronic. Characterization of the stool type can also narrow the etiology of the fecal incontinence. For example, solid stool incontinence is most suggestive of sphincter muscle weakness, whereas liquid stool incontinence may indicate overflow diarrhea. The urge to defecate prior to the incontinence is most consistent with external anal sphincter weakness, but passive incontinence is associated with internal anal sphincter dysfunction. Patients with diabetes or scleroderma may complain of nocturnal incontinence as well. While urinary incontinence may be a comorbid condition, it requires a separate evaluation from a urologist.

After the present illness is characterized, a thorough medical history, including obstetric, family, medication, and dietary history, should be obtained. As in chronic constipation, a systems-based approach to the past history ensures that all differential diagnoses are considered and evaluated. Surgical, obstetric, and radiation history can affect the risk of a patient developing fecal incontinence, even years after the initial surgery or delivery.

A thorough DRE as described above can help isolate the area of weakness or reason for incontinence. For example, the presence of hard, compact stool in the rectum indicates fecal impaction and suggests overflow incontinence. A poor rectal tone may suggest an internal anal sphincter defect or dysfunction, while the squeeze maneuver can assess the strength of the external anal sphincter.

Additional workup should be based on the patient's clinical history and physical exam. If there are signs of diarrhea, stool studies including inflammatory markers (fecal calprotectin) and infectious studies should be obtained. If there are any concerning systemic findings such as weight loss, night sweats, or acute onset of symptoms, consider a colonoscopy to evaluate for malignancy. The strength and function of the internal and external anal sphincters may also be quantitatively assessed using the anorectal manometry. In addition, altered rectal sensation may contribute to fecal incontinence and can be evaluated using anorectal manometry.

In patients with asymmetric weakness of the internal or external anal sphincter, endoscopic ultrasound may be used to further evaluate for sphincter defects. Internal anal sphincter tears will appear as hyperechoic breaks in the hypoechoic ring, whereas external anal sphincter tears appear as hypoechoic breaks in the hyperechoic ring. Lower endoscopic ultrasound has a sensitivity that approaches 100%; however, there is no clear correlation between symptomatic incontinence and sphincter defects.

Ditah I, Devaki P, Luma HN, et al. Prevalence, trends, and risk factors for fecal incontinence in United States adults, 2005-2010. *Clin Gastroenterol Hepatol.* 2014;12(4):636–643. [PMID: 23906873]

FitzHarris GP, Garcia-Aguilar J, Parker SC, et al. Quality of life after subtotal colectomy for slow transit constipation: both quality and quantity count. *Dis Colon Rectum.* 2003;46(4):433–440. [PMID: 12682533]

Hope C, Reilly J, Lund J, Andreyev H. Systematic review: the effect of right hemicolectomy for cancer on postoperative bowel function. *Support Care Cancer.* 2020;28(10):4549–4559. [PMID: 32430603]

Holzer B, Rosen HR, Novi G, et al. Sacral nerve stimulation in patients with severe constipation. *Dis Colon Rectum.* 2008;51(5):524–529. [PMID: 18322757]

Kamm MA, Dudding TC, Melenhorst J, et al. Sacral nerve stimulation for intractable constipation. *Gut.* 2010;59(3):333–340. [PMID: 20207638]

Maeda Y, Lundby L, Buntzen S, Laurberg S. Sacral nerve stimulation for constipation: suboptimal outcome and adverse events. *Dis Colon Rectum.* 2010;53(7):995–999. [PMID: 20551750]

Maria G, Cadeddu F, Brandara F, Marniga G, Brisinda G. Experience with type A botulinum toxin for treatment of outlet-type constipation. *Am J Gastroenterol.* 2006;101(11):2570–2575. [PMID: 17029615]

Pemberton JH, Rath DM, Ilstrup DM. Evaluation and surgical treatment of severe chronic constipation. *Ann Surg.* 1991;214(4):403–411. [PMID: 1953096]

Perry S, Shaw C, McGrother C, et al. Prevalence of faecal incontinence in adults aged 40 years or more living in the community. *Gut.* 2002;50(4):480–484. [PMID: 11889066]

Rao SS, Rattanakovit K, Patcharatrakul T. Diagnosis and management of chronic constipation in adults. *Nat Rev Gastroenterol Hepatol.* 2016;13(5):295–305. [PMID: 27033126]

Rao SSC, Tan G, Abdulla H, Yu S, Larion S, Leelasinjaroen P. Does colectomy predispose to small intestinal bacterial (SIBO) and fungal overgrowth (SIFO)? *Clin Transl Gastroenterol.* 2018;9(4):146. [PMID: 29691369]

Redmond JM, Smith GW, Barofsky I, Ratych RE, Goldsborough DC, Schuster MM. Physiological tests to predict long-term outcome of total abdominal colectomy for intractable constipation. *Am J Gastroenterol.* 1995;90(5):748–753. [PMID: 7733081]

Tian Y, Wang L, Ye JW, et al. Defecation function and quality of life in patients with slow-transit constipation after colectomy. *World J Clin Cases.* 2020;8(10):1897–1907. [PMID: 32518779]

Wald A. Update on the management of fecal incontinence for the gastroenterologist. *Gastroenterol Hepatol (N Y).* 2016;12(3):155–164. [PMID: 27231444]

Wald A, Bharucha AE, Cosman BC, Whitehead WE. ACG clinical guideline: management of benign anorectal disorders. *Am J Gastroenterol.* 2014;109(8):1141–1157. [PMID: 25022811]

Management

The management of fecal incontinence requires a multimodality approach that is tailored to each patient given the many different etiologies. Optimal management should be individualized based on the patient's underlying pathophysiology and ability to comply with the prescribed treatment. Additionally, fecal incontinence should not be attributed to age-related physiologic changes, and should always be worked up and treated regardless of the patient's age.

A. Sphincter Weakness

This is most often seen in middle-aged or older men, but may also occur in women, and patients typically complain of small amounts of fecal or mucus seepage in the absence of urge or passive incontinence.

Isolated weakness of the internal anal sphincter is typically seen in scleroderma or in patients with a history of a sphincterotomy. External anal sphincter weakness can lead to stress incontinence, which is caused by bearing down, like lifting a heavy box, and may be seen after a hemorrhoidectomy. Treatment includes an anal plug but compliance is limited as it is often poorly tolerated. Sphincter training such as Kegel exercises can also be used to help strengthen the external anal sphincter, but there is significant variation in efficacy in clinical studies.

Karoui S, Savoye-Collet C, Koning E, Leroi AM, Denis P. Prevalence of anal sphincter defects revealed by sonography in 335 incontinent patients and 115 continent patients. *AJR Am J Roentgenol.* 1999;173(2):389–392. [PMID: 10430142]

Rieger N, Tjandra J, Solomon M. Endoanal and endorectal ultrasound: applications in colorectal surgery. *ANZ J Surg.* 2004;74(8):671–675. [PMID: 15315569]

Sultan AH, Kamm MA, Talbot IC, Nicholls RJ, Bartram CI. Anal endosonography for identifying external sphincter defects confirmed histologically. *Br J Surg.* 1994;81(3):463–465. [PMID: 8173933]

Sultan AH, Nicholls RJ, Kamm MA, Hudson CN, Beynon J, Bartram CI. Anal endosonography and correlation with in vitro and in vivo anatomy. *Br J Surg.* 1993;80(4):508–511. [PMID: 8495324]

Tjandra JJ, Dykes SL, Kumar RR, et al. Practice parameters for the treatment of fecal incontinence. *Dis Colon Rectum.* 2007;50(10):1497–1507. [PMID: 17674106]

Wald A. Update on the management of fecal incontinence for the gastroenterologist. *Gastroenterol Hepatol (N Y).* 2016;12(3):155–164. [PMID: 27231444]

B. Decreased Rectal Sensation

Rectal hyposensitivity can lead to a large stool burden in the rectal vault that is not sensed by the individual. Soluble fiber supplements can bulk the stool to increase the volume of stool and increase sensation. There are inconsistent results with biofeedback therapy in these cases, but it can also be considered.

C. Overflow Incontinence

Overflow incontinence results from seepage of liquid feces around an impacted fecalith and treatment includes removal of the impacted stool for immediate relief. Abdominal radiography can be used to identify the location of the impaction if it is not within reach of a finger on the DRE. Ongoing bowel regimen is important to implement after the colon cleansing because of the high rate of recurrence in the long term.

D. Decreased Rectal Compliance

Decreased rectal compliance is typically caused by an underlying pathophysiologic process such as inflammatory bowel disease or radiation injury. If possible, the underlying cause should be addressed first. If, despite optimal management of the underlying pathophysiology, there is ongoing fecal incontinence, then modification of the stool consistency and volume can be beneficial. A combination of decreasing dietary fiber, to decrease the stool volume, with an antidiarrheal has anecdotally shown to be effective in treatment of fecal incontinence due to decreased rectal compliance. Loperamide, which does not have effects on the central nervous system and can increase internal anal sphincter tone, has been shown to be more effective in patients with fecal incontinence in randomized controlled trials when compared to diphenoxylate–atropine. Loperamide should be given in doses of 2–4 mg 45 minutes before meals or social occasions to avoid episodes of fecal incontinence. Tricyclic antidepressants (TCAs) have been shown to be effective in patients with fecal incontinence as well due to their anticholinergic effects. In some cases, when the patient has a normal storage capacity, fiber supplementation can be helpful.

If symptoms are refractory to conservative measures, more invasive treatments can be considered. In patients with mild to moderate refractory symptoms, injectable anal bulking agents can be used to augment the walls of the internal anal sphincter to close the anal canal or raise the pressure inside the anal canal. In a 2013 Cochrane review, only modest short-term improvements were found with injectable bulking agents, with better results seen with ultrasound-guided injections. In the largest prospective randomized study to date, 53% of patients treated with Dextrannomerhyaluronic acid (NASHA Dx) experienced symptom improvement, compared to only 31% who received a sham injection.

Sacral neuromodulation stimulates an afferent pathway through chemical mediating receptors to change brain activity used for continence.

In pooled analysis, sacral neuromodulation resulted in improvement in weekly fecal incontinence episodes in 79% of patients in the short term (0–12 months) and 84% in the long term (>36 months). Unfortunately, its use is limited by the high adverse event rate seen with sacral neuromodulation. Prior literatures have shown that 39.2% of patients needed a device revision, replacement or explant, 19.2% of patients experience paresthesia, 10% had an implant site infection, and 8.3% experienced urinary incontinence.

Anal sphincteroplasty is used to repair damaged or weakened anal sphincters or to create a new functional sphincter with skeletal muscle from an adjacent site. Studies have shown that the results are poor regardless of how trained the surgeon is, so its use has decrease in favor of other surgical techniques. Gracioplasty uses the gracilis muscle to form a new sphincter around the anus with or without an electoral stimulator device in the abdominal wall to sustain tone and to maintain continence. The magnetic anal sphincter consists of a magnetic anal sphincter interlinked with titanium beads and is placed to encircle the external anal sphincter and assist with continence. Gracioplasty and the magnetic anal sphincter are not FDA approved in the United States of America.

Newer devices like the artificial bowel sphincter and magnetic anal sphincter are also being studied. The artificial bowel sphincter acts as an inflatable cuff with a control pump and balloon that regulates pressure to maintain continence. While it provides a high degree of improvement in fecal incontinence symptoms, there is also a high rate of complications (infections, device erosions, anorectal ulceration, device malfunction, pain, and constipation). In a systematic review, 5 years postoperatively, 59% of devices remained functional. Given the lower safety profile, artificial bowel sphincters are typically only offered to patients who have failed other treatments or have significant sphincter injury, congenital malformations, neurogenic incontinence from spinal cord injury, or postsurgical significant bowel dysfunction with intact anal canal anatomy.

Colostomy is reserved for patients who have failed medical and behavioral therapy. Although many patients are initially resistant to the idea, it should be emphasized that this intervention is generally associated with improved quality of life and allows greater freedom of activity because of the removal of fear of incontinence episodes. Adverse events are those expected with abdominal surgery and operative anesthesia including bleeding, cardiorespiratory events related to anesthesia, and a parastomal hernia.

Chiarioni G, Bassotti G, Stanganini S, Vantini I, Whitehead WE. Sensory retraining is key to biofeedback therapy for formed stool fecal incontinence. *Am J Gastroenterol.* 2002;97(1):109–117. [PMID: 11808933]

Colquhoun P, Kaiser R, Weiss EG, et al. Correlating the Fecal Incontinence Quality-of-Life Score and the SF-36 to a proposed Ostomy Function Index in patients with a stoma. *Ostomy Wound Manage.* 2006;52(12):68–74. [PMID: 17204828]

Devesa JM, Rey A, Hervas PL, et al. Artificial anal sphincter: complications and functional results of a large personal series. *Dis Colon Rectum.* 2002;45(9):1154–1163. [PMID: 12352229]

Graf W, Mellgren A, Matzel KE, et al. Efficacy of dextranomer in stabilised hyaluronic acid for treatment of faecal incontinence: a randomised, sham-controlled trial. *Lancet.* 2011;377(9770):997–1003. [PMID: 21420555]

Hong KD, Dasilva G, Kalaskar SN, Chong Y, Wexner SD. Long-term outcomes of artificial bowel sphincter for fecal incontinence: a systematic review and meta-analysis. *J Am Coll Surg.* 2013;217(4):718–725. [PMID: 23891075]

Hull T, Giese C, Wexner SD, et al. Long-term durability of sacral nerve stimulation therapy for chronic fecal incontinence. *Dis Colon Rectum.* 2013;56(2):234–245. [PMID: 23303153]

Lacima G, Pera M, Amador A, Escaramis G, Pique JM. Long-term results of biofeedback treatment for faecal incontinence: a comparative study with untreated controls. *Colorectal Dis.* 2010;12(8):742–749. [PMID: 19486084]

Maeda Y, Laurberg S, Norton C. Perianal injectable bulking agents as treatment for faecal incontinence in adults. *Cochrane Database Syst Rev.* 2013;(2):1–35. [PMID: 23450581]

Melenhorst J, Koch SM, van Gemert WG, Baeten CG. The artificial bowel sphincter for faecal incontinence: a single centre study. *Int J Colorectal Dis.* 2008;23(1):107–111. [PMID: 17929038]

Mundy L, Merlin TL, Maddern GJ, Hiller JE. Systematic review of safety and effectiveness of an artificial bowel sphincter for faecal incontinence. *Br J Surg.* 2004;91(6):665–672. [PMID: 15164433]

Norton C, Burch J, Kamm MA. Patients' views of a colostomy for fecal incontinence. *Dis Colon Rectum.* 2005;48(5):1062–1069. [PMID: 15868244]

Norton C, Chelvanayagam S, Wilson-Barnett J, Redfern S, Kamm MA. Randomized controlled trial of biofeedback for fecal incontinence. *Gastroenterology.* 2003;125(5):1320–1329. [PMID: 14598248]

Norton C, Cody JD. Biofeedback and/or sphincter exercises for the treatment of faecal incontinence in adults. *Cochrane Database Syst Rev.* 2012;(7):1–58. [PMID: 22786479]

Pager CK, Solomon MJ, Rex J, Roberts RA. Long-term outcomes of pelvic floor exercise and biofeedback treatment for patients with fecal incontinence. *Dis Colon Rectum.* 2002;45(8):997–1003. [PMID: 12195181]

Palmer KR, Corbett CL, Holdsworth CD. Double-blind cross-over study comparing loperamide, codeine and diphenoxylate in the treatment of chronic diarrhea. *Gastroenterology.* 1980;79(6):1272–1275. [PMID: 7002706]

Paquette IM, Varma MG, Kaiser AM, Steele SR, Rafferty JF. The American Society of Colon and Rectal Surgeons' Clinical Practice Guideline for the Treatment of Fecal Incontinence. *Dis Colon Rectum.* 2015;58(7):623–636. [PMID: 26200676]

Read M, Read NW, Barber DC, Duthie HL. Effects of loperamide on anal sphincter function in patients complaining of chronic diarrhea with fecal incontinence and urgency. *Dig Dis Sci.* 1982;27(9):807–814. [PMID: 7105952]

Rao SS. Current and emerging treatment options for fecal incontinence. *J Clin Gastroenterol.* 2014;48(9):752–764. [PMID: 25014235]

Santoro GA, Eitan BZ, Pryde A, Bartolo DC. Open study of low-dose amitriptyline in the treatment of patients with idiopathic fecal incontinence. *Dis Colon Rectum.* 2000;43(12):1676–1681. [PMID: 11156450]

Solomon MJ, Pager CK, Rex J, Roberts R, Manning J. Randomized, controlled trial of biofeedback with anal manometry, transanal ultrasound, or pelvic floor retraining with digital guidance alone in the treatment of mild to moderate fecal incontinence. *Dis Colon Rectum.* 2003;46(6):703–710. [PMID: 12794569]

Sun WM, Read NW, Verlinden M. Effects of loperamide oxide on gastrointestinal transit time and anorectal function in patients with chronic diarrhoea and faecal incontinence. *Scand J Gastroenterol.* 1997;32(1):34–38. [PMID: 9018764]

Tan EK, Vaizey C, Cornish J, Darzi A, Tekkis PP. Surgical strategies for faecal incontinence--a decision analysis between dynamic graciloplasty, artificial bowel sphincter and end stoma. *Colorectal Dis.* 2008;10(6):577–586. [PMID: 18005188]

Thin NN, Horrocks EJ, Hotouras A, et al. Systematic review of the clinical effectiveness of neuromodulation in the treatment of faecal incontinence. *Br J Surg.* 2013;100(11):1430–1447. [PMID: 24037562]

Wald A. Biofeedback for fecal incontinence. *Gastroenterology.* 2003;125(5):1533–1535. [PMID: 14598270]

Wald A. Clinical practice. Fecal incontinence in adults. *N Engl J Med.* 2007;356(16):1648–1655. [PMID: 17442907]

Wexner SD, Jin HY, Weiss EG, Nogueras JJ, Li VK. Factors associated with failure of the artificial bowel sphincter: a study of over 50 cases from Cleveland Clinic Florida. *Dis Colon Rectum.* 2009;52(9):1550–1557. [PMID: 19690481]

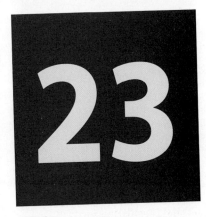

Diverticular Disease of the Colon

Navin L. Kumar, MD

Benjamin N. Smith, MD

DIVERTICULOSIS

ESSENTIALS OF DIAGNOSIS

▶ Radiographic or endoscopic demonstration of diverticula.

▶ Normal vital signs and laboratory evaluation.

▶ Absence of complications (diverticulitis, diverticular hemorrhage).

General Considerations

Diverticula are acquired herniations of the colonic mucosa and submucosa through the muscularis propria. They occur most commonly in the sigmoid colon and can vary in size and number, although typically they are between 5 and 10 mm in diameter. Diverticulosis refers to the presence of diverticula in an individual regardless of symptoms, whereas diverticular disease refers to the presence of diverticula associated with symptoms, which occurs in 20% of individuals with diverticula. This subset of patients may have symptomatic uncomplicated diverticular disease, acute diverticulitis, or diverticular bleeding, as well as the more rare segmental colitis associated with diverticula (SCAD).

Diverticulosis is the most common structural abnormality of the colon and its prevalence is age-dependent. Currently, it is estimated that diverticulosis affects less than 20% of people at age 40 and 60% by age 60. An exception to this is in vegetarians, in whom the prevalence of diverticulosis is much lower, presumably due to diets that are higher in fiber. Men and women are affected equally. The prevalence and distribution of diverticula vary throughout the world. Whereas diverticula are common and predominantly left-sided in Western countries (95% involve the sigmoid colon), in urbanized areas of Asia, such as Japan, Hong Kong, and Singapore, the prevalence is only 20% and the diverticula are predominantly right-sided, even among those who have adopted a Western-style, low-fiber diet.

▶ Pathogenesis

A. Colonic Motility

Segmentation within the colon is thought to play an important role in the development of diverticula. Segmentation refers to the process by which a short segment of the circular muscle of the colon contracts in a nonpropulsive manner. This produces a closed segment of colon with increased intraluminal pressure, and likely serves to increase water and electrolyte absorption from the colon. These elevated intraluminal pressures may ultimately result in herniation of the mucosa and submucosa at sites of weakness (namely, where the vasa recta penetrates the muscularis propria between the taeniae coli), resulting in the formation of diverticula. Diverticula are not seen in the rectum because the taeniae coalesce at the rectum to form the circumferential longitudinal muscle layer.

The *law of Laplace* (transmural pressure gradient equals the wall tension divided by the radius, $\Delta P = T/r$) may help to explain why diverticula are so common in the sigmoid colon. Compared with the remainder of the colon, the sigmoid has a smaller radius. Because the transmural pressure gradient is inversely proportional to the bowel radius, it will be highest at the level of the sigmoid, potentially favoring the formation of diverticula in this region. Additionally, myochosis (thickening of the circular muscle layer, shortening of the taeniae coli, and narrowing of the lumen, Figure 23–1) is seen in most patients with sigmoid diverticula. These changes result from increased deposition of collagen and elastin within the taeniae, and not from hypertrophy or hyperplasia of the bowel wall. In addition to increasing intraluminal pressure by narrowing the lumen, these changes may also decrease the resistance of the colon wall (see below).

B. Role of Fiber & Other Lifestyle Factors

Fiber in the diet leads to increased stool bulk and decreased colonic transit times and thus may play a role in preventing the development of diverticulosis. Individuals from countries

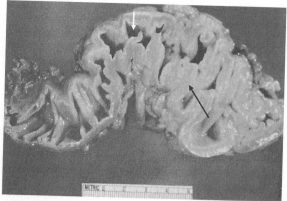

▲ **Figure 23–1.** Myochosis. Note marked thickening of muscle layer (*lower, black arrow*) and resultant lumina narrowing (*top, white arrow*) in a patient with myochosis and left lower quadrant abdominal pain.

with high-fiber diets tend to have larger diameter colons, compared with those from countries with low-fiber intake. Having a larger colonic diameter may weaken the segmental contractions of the colon that lead to higher intraluminal pressures.

The role of fiber in the development of diverticulosis was first suggested by epidemiologic evidence. Diverticula rarely develop in rural Asia or Africa (prevalence of <0.2%), where diets are high in fiber. However, in areas that have adopted Western dietary habits, diverticula become more prevalent. In addition, populations that have moved from rural to urban environments show an increased prevalence of diverticulosis. Diets higher in total fat and red meat have also shown a higher risk of diverticular disease.

In addition to a high-fiber diet, increased physical activity may also decrease the risk of diverticular disease, particularly for those who engage in more vigorous activity such as running. Similarly, obesity is associated with an increase risk of diverticular disease, with one study noting an almost two-fold increased risk of diverticular bleeding for men with the highest quintile of waist circumference compared with those in the lowest. Contrary to popular teaching, there is no strong evidence that seeds, nuts, or popcorn lead to an increase in the frequency of complications from diverticulosis.

► Clinical Findings

A. Symptoms & Signs

The majority of patients with diverticulosis are asymptomatic, with only 20% developing symptoms over their life span. For those with symptomatic uncomplicated diverticular disease, abdominal pain is the most common symptom and is usually localized in the left lower quadrant. It is important to emphasize that left lower quadrant pain may be the result of myochosis (thickening of the circular muscle layer,

shortening of the taeniae coli, and narrowing of the lumen often seen in patients with diverticular disease). In patients with right-sided diverticula, the pain can be felt in the right lower quadrant. The pain may worsen after eating and in some is relieved with the passage of stool or flatus. Patients may also complain of nausea, cramping, irregular bowel movements (intermittent diarrhea or constipation), bloating, and flatulence.

Patients do not demonstrate abnormal vital signs, such as tachycardia or fever, in uncomplicated diverticulosis. With palpation of the left lower quadrant, mild tenderness and voluntary guarding may be present.

B. Laboratory Findings

In uncomplicated diverticulosis, laboratory values, including the hematocrit, hemoglobin, and white blood cell count, are normal, and testing of the stool for occult blood is negative.

C. Imaging Studies

A double-contrast barium enema will demonstrate the presence, localization, and number of diverticula (Figure 23–2). If segmental spasm is present, a transient saw-tooth pattern may be seen. In uncomplicated diverticulosis, there should be no extravasation of contrast, nor should there be evidence of fistulae, strictures, or persistent spasm, all of which suggest diverticulitis. Diverticulosis can also be seen on abdominal computed tomography (CT) with oral or rectal contrast.

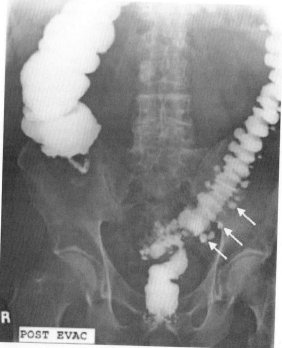

▲ **Figure 23–2.** Barium enema showing the presence of diverticula (*arrows*).

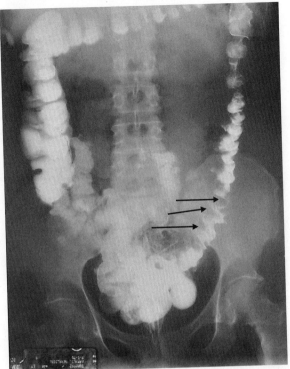

▲ **Figure 23–3.** Scalloping and luminal narrowing due to muscle enlargement (myochosis) and luminal narrowing.

In patients with myochosis, a plain abdominal x-ray may show scalloping in the left colon due to muscle hypertrophy (Figures 23–1 and 23–3).

D. Endoscopy

Diverticulosis is frequently discovered during colonoscopy as an incidental finding (Plate 41). Additionally, because disorders such as colorectal cancer, inflammatory bowel disease, and ischemic colitis are included in the differential diagnosis for patients with abdominal pain related to diverticulosis, colonoscopy is the preferred diagnostic study. Colonoscopy, however, can be difficult to perform in patients with diverticulosis due to narrowing of the colonic lumen and possible colonic fixation from prior episodes of diverticulitis resulting in inflammation and pericolic fibrosis. Colonoscopy is relatively contraindicated in patients in whom acute diverticulitis is suspected, due to an increased risk of colonic perforation.

▶ Differential Diagnosis

The nonspecific symptoms of uncomplicated diverticulosis can mimic many other conditions, and differentiation can be difficult. Many of the signs and symptoms of symptomatic diverticulosis are also seen in irritable bowel syndrome. The fact that both disorders are common, and can coexist, makes differentiation even more difficult. Irritable bowel syndrome frequently causes diffuse abdominal pain; thus, pain localized to the left lower quadrant in the setting of demonstrated diverticula supports a diagnosis of uncomplicated diverticulosis.

Mild diverticulitis can manifest similarly and is not ruled out by the absence of a fever, elevated white blood cell count, or other signs of infection. Other pelvic infections, such as appendicitis and pelvic inflammatory disease, can also mimic diverticulosis. Other causes of lower abdominal pain that need to be considered are infectious colitis, inflammatory bowel disease, ischemic colitis, colorectal cancer, and endometriosis.

▶ Complications

Diverticulosis can be complicated by acute diverticulitis, which results from the perforation of a diverticulum, as well as by hemorrhage, which occurs when the arteriole associated with the diverticulum erodes.

Of note, a subset of patients with diverticulosis (0.26–1.5%) may also develop low-grade colonic inflammation in the interdiverticular mucosa (without involvement of the diverticular orifices)—a condition known as segmental colitis with diverticula (SCAD). The inflammation is only seen in areas with diverticula and spares the rectum. Patients with SCAD typically report chronic diarrhea, crampy abdominal pain, and at times intermittent hematochezia. Treatment approaches for segmental colitis have only been studied in small groups of patients or presented as case reports. Options include oral antibiotics, mesalamine, steroids, and segmental resection for those with steroid-refractory or steroid-dependent SCAD. Whether SCAD is a distinct entity or belongs on a spectrum with inflammatory bowel disease remains uncertain. The overlap in clinical presentation and histology confounds studies of the natural history of this condition. Mild cases may go undiagnosed whereas severe cases may be misdiagnosed as diverticulitis or inflammatory bowel disease. The distinction is important as long-term treatment may not be needed in SCAD.

▶ Treatment

Most patients with diverticulosis do not require any specific treatment, and there are no medical treatments that will lead to the regression of diverticula, once present. The treatment of patients with recurrent uncomplicated diverticular disease focuses on relieving symptoms. Therapies used to treat uncomplicated diverticular disease include fiber-rich diets, probiotics, and prebiotics. Patients with myochosis may get symptom relief with the addition of a fiber supplement.

A. Fiber

Fiber is slowly fermented by gut microflora, resulting in the production of short-chain fatty acids and gas. This in turn results in shortened gut transit time, which reduces intracolonic pressure and helps with constipation.

The recommended daily fiber intake for adults is 20–35 g/day, and fiber supplements are available to help meet this requirement. Supplements contain either soluble fiber (psyllium, ispaghula, calcium polycarbophil) or insoluble fiber (corn fiber, wheat bran). Soluble fiber is more readily fermented by gut microflora, whereas insoluble fiber undergoes minimal fermentation, and likely exerts its effects by increasing stool mass and thus increasing the luminal diameter, which in turn decreases the transmural pressure gradient. (Recall that, according to the law of Laplace, $\Delta P = T/r$.) Studies looking at the effect of high-fiber diets on symptoms from uncomplicated diverticular disease, however, have not been conclusive, with some studies showing a benefit, while others do not. Despite this, increasing dietary fiber, often with fiber supplements, is currently the mainstay of treating uncomplicated diverticular disease.

B. Probiotics & Prebiotics

Probiotics contain microorganisms with beneficial properties, and the goal in using them is to alter the gut's microflora to reestablish the normal bacterial flora. *Bifidobacteria* and *Lactobacilli* are used most frequently. Some preparations also contain other bacteria and nonbacterial organisms, such as *Escherichia coli* and *Saccharomyces boulardii*. In diverticular disease, the normal bacterial flora may be altered by slowed colonic transit and stool stasis, so it is theorized that reestablishing normal gut flora may lead to symptomatic improvement. However, high-quality data is lacking to support these claims.

Prebiotics are substances that promote the growth and metabolic activity of beneficial bacteria, especially *Bifidobacteria* and *Lactobacilli*. Prebiotics are frequently indigestible complex carbohydrates. Bacteria ferment these substances, leading to a more acidic luminal environment, which suppresses the growth of harmful bacteria. Substances that have been shown to promote the growth of *Bifidobacteria* and *Lactobacilli* include psyllium fiber, lactulose, fructose, oligosaccharides, germinated barley extracts, and inulin.

Prognosis

Twenty percent of patients with diverticula will develop symptoms of uncomplicated diverticular disease, while 10–25% of patients with diverticulosis will go on to develop a complication (75% of whom will have had no preceding symptoms). Fortunately, most episodes of diverticulitis and diverticular hemorrhage are self-limited and can be managed medically. An additional small subset of patients will develop severe pain and colonic dysmotility. Although not life threatening, the symptoms can be debilitating.

Carabotti M, Annibale B. Treatment of diverticular disease: an update on latest evidence and clinical implications. *Drugs Context*. 2018;7:212526. [PMID: 29623099]

Cassieri C, Brandimarte G, Elisei W, Lecca GP, Goni E, Penna A, Picchio M, Tursi A. How to Differentiate Segmental Colitis Associated With Diverticulosis and Inflammatory Bowel Diseases. *J Clin Gastroenterol*. 2016;50(suppl 1):S36–S38. [PMID: 27622359]

DiSiena MS, Birk JW. Diverticular disease: the old, the new, and the ever-changing view. *South Med J*. 2018;111(3):144–150. [PMID: 29505648]

Freeman HJ. Segmental colitis associated diverticulosis syndrome. *World J Gastroenterol*. 2016;22(36):8067–8069. [PMID: 27688648]

Kucejko RJ, Poggio JL. Considerations and changes in the evaluation, management, and outcomes in the management of diverticular disease: the diagnosis, pathology, and treatment of diverticular colitis. *Clin Colon Rectal Surg*. 2018;31(4):221–225. [PMID: 29942211]

Peery AF, Sandler RS, Ahnen DJ, et al. Constipation and a low-fiber diet are not associated with diverticulosis. *Clin Gastroenterol Hepatol*. 2013;11:1622–1627. [PMID: 23891924]

Peery AF, Keku TO, Martin CF, et al. Distribution and characteristics of colonic diverticula in a United States screening population. *Clin Gastroenterol Hepatol*. 2016;14(7):980. [PMID: 26872402]

Petruzziello L, Iacopini F, Bulajic M, et al. Review article: uncomplicated diverticular disease of the colon. *Aliment Pharmacol Ther*. 2006;23:1379–1391. [PMID: 16669953]

Reddy VB, Longo WE. The burden of diverticular disease on patients and healthcare systems. *Gastroenterol Hepatol*. 2013;9:21–27. [PMID: 24707230]

Rezapour M, Ali S, Stollman N. Diverticular disease: an update on pathogenesis and management. *Gut Liver*. 2018;12(2):125–132. [PMID: 28494576]

Rocco A, Compare D, Caruso F, Nardone G. Treatment options for uncomplicated diverticular disease of the colon. *J Clin Gastroenterol*. 2009;43:803–808. [PMID: 19652620]

Schembri J, Bonello J, Christodoulou DK, Katsanos KH, Ellul P. Segmental colitis associated with diverticulosis: is it the coexistence of colonic diverticulosis and inflammatory bowel disease? *Ann Gastroenterol*. 2017;30(3):257–261. [PMID: 28469355]

Shaheen NJ, Hansen RA, Morgan DR, et al. The burden of gastrointestinal and liver diseases, 2006. *Am J Gastroenterol*. 2006;101:2128–2138. [PMID: 16848807]

Stollman N, Picchio M, Biondo S, et al. Critical issues on diverticular disease. *J Gastrointestin Liver Dis*. 2019;28(suppl. 4):35–38. [PMID: 31930225]

Strate LL, Liu YL, Syngal S, et al. Nut, corn, and popcorn consumption and the incidence of diverticular disease. *JAMA*. 2008;300(8):907. [PMID 18728264]

Strate LL, Liu YL, Aldoori WH, et al. Obesity increases the risks of diverticulitis and diverticular bleeding. *Gastroenterology*. 2009;136(1):115. [PMID 18996378]

Ticinesi A, Nouvenne A, Corrente V, Tana C, Di Mario F, Meschi T. Diverticular disease: a gut microbiota perspective. *J Gastrointestin Liver Dis*. 2019;28(3):327–337. [PMID: 31517330]

Tursi A. Segmental colitis associated with diverticulosis: complication of diverticular disease or autonomous entity? *Dig Dis Sci*. 2011;56:27–34. [PMID: 20411418]

Wang FW, Chuang HY, Tu MS, et al. Prevalance and risk factors of asymptomatic colorectal diverticulosis in Taiwan. *BMC Gastroenterol*. 2015;15(1):40. [PMID 25888375]

Zullo A, Gatta L, Vassallo R, et al. Paradigm shift: the Copernican revolution in diverticular disease. *Ann Gastroenterol*. 2019;32(6):541–553. [PMID: 31700230]

ACUTE DIVERTICULITIS

ESSENTIALS OF DIAGNOSIS

▶ Abdominal pain and tenderness (typically left lower quadrant).

▶ Fever or leukocytosis, or both.

▶ Characteristic radiographic findings.

General Considerations

First described in 1849, diverticulitis results from the micro- or macroperforation of a diverticulum, resulting in anything from subclinical inflammation to feculent peritonitis. It affects approximately 4% of patients with diverticulosis and can be associated with significant complications (abscess, fistula, obstruction, phlegmon, bleeding, or macroperforation). There is a male predominance in patients younger than 45 years, an equal sex distribution for patients between the ages of 45 and 54, and a female predominance after the age of 54.

Acute diverticulitis can be either complicated or uncomplicated. The severity of diverticulitis is often described using the Hinchey classification, which categorizes diverticulitis into four stages based on clinical and operative findings. Modifications of the classification have also been developed that incorporate CT findings (Table 23–1).

Pathogenesis

Previously it was thought that diverticulitis was the result of obstruction of a diverticulum by a fecalith leading to increased pressure within the diverticulum, with subsequent perforation. However, it is now understood that diverticular obstruction is a rare event and that most cases of diverticulitis are the result of erosion of the diverticular wall due to increased intraluminal pressure or inspissated food particles. This leads to inflammation and focal necrosis, with resultant perforation of the thin-walled diverticulum. Subsequent complications occur when the inflamed diverticulum is poorly contained, leading to free perforation and peritonitis in the severest of cases.

In terms of risk factors, Nonsteroidal anti-inflammatory drugs (NSAIDs) have been associated with diverticulitis and perforation. This association is postulated to be related to decreased prostaglandin synthesis and direct topical mucosal damage. By stimulating mucin and bicarbonate secretion and increasing mucosal blood flow, prostaglandins aid in maintaining the colonic mucosal barrier. In addition, NSAIDs are weak acids that may denude epithelial cells, resulting in increased mucosal permeability, ulceration, and the translocation of bacteria and toxins.

As previously mentioned, a diet low in fiber may not only predispose to the formation of diverticula but may also lead to the development of diverticulitis. By increasing stool weight and water content, fiber helps reduce colonic segmentation pressures, which may protect against perforation. Red meat intake has also been associated with diverticulitis. Heterocyclic amines are products of cooking meat and have been associated with apoptosis of colonic epithelial cells. Heme has also been shown to produce a cytotoxic factor in rat colons. These effects on the colonic epithelial cells may predispose to perforation.

Clinical Findings

A. Symptoms & Signs

Diverticulitis should be suspected in a patient presenting with lower abdominal pain, fever, and/or leukocytosis.

Table 23-1. Hinchey classification & modified Hinchey classification of acute diverticulitis.

Stage	Hinchey Classification	Stage	Modified Hinchey Classification
		0	Mild clinical diverticulitis
I	Pericolic abscess or phlegmon	Ia	Confined pericolic inflammation or phlegmon
		Ib	Confined pericolic abscess
II	Pelvic, intra-abdominal, or retroperitoneal abscess	II	Pelvic, distant intra-abdominal, or retroperitoneal abscess
III	Generalized purulent peritonitis	III	Generalized purulent peritonitis
IV	Generalized feculent peritonitis	IV	Fecal peritonitis
		Fistula	Colovesical, vaginal, enteric, cutaneous
		Obstruction	Large or small bowel obstruction, or both

Adapted with permission from Kaiser AM, Jiang JK, Lake JP, et al: The management of complicated diverticulitis and the role of computed tomography. Am J Gastroenterol. 2005;100(4):910–917.

In the West, left lower quadrant pain is the most common complaint (70%) due to sigmoid colon involvement. In patients with a large sigmoid loop or with right-sided diverticulitis, the pain may extend to the mid or right abdomen. The onset is usually gradual, and the pain may be present for several days prior to the patient seeking medical attention. The pain is constant, with intermittent exacerbations that are associated with colonic spasms and are followed by loose bowel movements. Patients may also complain of nausea and vomiting (20–62%), constipation (50%), diarrhea (25–35%), and urinary symptoms (10–15%) such as urinary urgency, frequency, or dysuria (if the abscess is near the bladder).

On examination, tenderness is usually present in the left lower quadrant, with a tender mass being present in 20%. A low-grade fever is common. An area of localized tenderness with swelling and erythema of the abdominal wall suggests an underlying abscess progressing to form a colocutaneous fistula. Diffuse tenderness suggests peritonitis. Abdominal distention and tympany on percussion may be present if an obstruction (high-pitched bowel sounds) or ileus (hypoactive bowel sounds) has developed. In cases of free perforation, hemodynamic instability may develop, along with a rigid abdomen, diffuse guarding, and rebound tenderness.

It is important to remember that patients who are immunosuppressed (eg, the elderly, those with cancer, HIV infection) or on chronic immunosuppression are much more likely to have an atypical presentation.

B. Laboratory Findings

The most common finding is leukocytosis, but it is not required to make the diagnosis. In one series, a normal white blood cell count was noted in 45% of patients. Marked leukocytosis is suggestive of peritonitis or abscess formation. Liver function tests are usually normal. If the urinary bladder is involved, pyuria or hematuria may result, and polymicrobial urinary tract infections can be seen with a colovesical fistula.

C. Imaging Studies

Plain abdominal radiographs are typically normal in patients with mild diverticulitis, but in the setting of severe disease, there may be an ileus pattern or, if obstruction is present, proximal bowel dilation. A large abscess may be associated with an air-fluid level on upright films. If there is perforation into the retroperitoneal space, the psoas shadow may be obliterated due to air diffusing along the psoas muscle. Free air under the diaphragm may be seen on upright films in the setting of intraperitoneal perforation, especially if there is feculent peritonitis.

CT scanning is currently the radiographic test of choice for diagnosing diverticulitis. Its sensitivity is as high as 97%, and specificity is reported to be as high as 100%. The following findings are seen with diverticulitis: soft tissue density of the pericolic fat (98%), diverticula (84%), bowel wall thickening of more than 4 mm (70%), and phlegmon or pericolic fluid (35%). CT scanning is also helpful in classifying patients as having mild, moderate, or severe disease; in guiding therapeutic decisions; and in diagnosing the complications of diverticulitis, such as abscess formation, fistula formation, peritonitis, or obstruction (Figure 23–4). Because CT scans cannot reliably exclude cancer, patients who have not had a recent colonoscopy within the past year should have one 6–8 weeks after the diverticulitis has resolved.

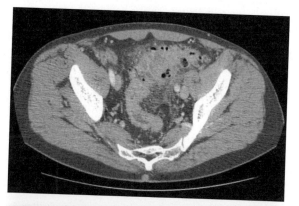

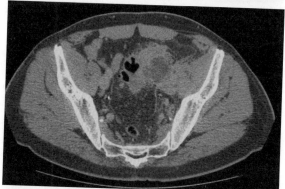

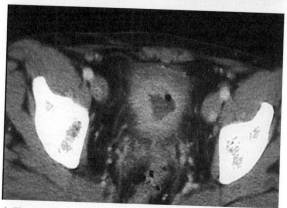

▲ **Figure 23–4.** CT scan showing uncomplicated diverticulitis (A), diverticulitis with abscess formation (B), and diverticulitis with colovesicular fistula (C).

Ultrasound is a noninvasive method with limited utility. It is highly operator dependent, and in the setting of an ileus may be limited due to distention of the bowel by gas. It may identify a phlegmon, abscess, or bowel wall thickening. It can also be helpful in guiding the drainage of intra-abdominal abscesses.

D. Endoscopy

During an acute episode of suspected diverticulitis, rigid proctoscopy, flexible sigmoidoscopy, and colonoscopy are relatively contraindicated. This is because the required air insufflation can unseal or worsen a perforation. However, as mentioned above, patients who have not recently (within the past year) had a colonoscopy should have one to exclude an underlying malignancy or other disorder, with a waiting period of 6–8 weeks following resolution of the episode of diverticulitis. If an endoscopy is to be performed in order to differentiate between acute diverticulitis and cancer or colitis prior to surgery, it should only be attempted by an experienced endoscopist, with minimal insufflation using carbon dioxide if possible. Findings of diverticulitis on endoscopy include edema, erythema, strictures, and (rarely) purulent drainage from a diverticulum. Following resolution of an episode of diverticulitis, endoscopic findings are often minimal.

▶ Differential Diagnosis

Because of the proximity of the colon to other intra-abdominal organs, and because of the varied presentations of diverticulitis, many other diagnoses need to be considered. The differential diagnosis includes inflammatory bowel disease, ischemic colitis, infectious colitis, appendicitis, colon cancer, pyelonephritis, pelvic inflammatory disease, ovarian cyst or torsion, and ectopic pregnancy. In patients with AIDS and colonic perforation, cytomegalovirus infection and Kaposi sarcoma should also be considered.

▶ Complications

Complications of acute diverticulitis are seen in approximately 25% of patients and include pericolic or pelvic abscess formation, colon obstruction, fistula formation to adjacent organs, and perforation with purulent or feculent peritonitis. Fistulas most frequently arise from the sigmoid colon and involve adjacent organs. The common fistulas are colovesical fistulas (65%) and colovaginal fistulas (25%). Peritonitis is associated with a significant mortality rate. Mortality is approximately 6% if there is purulent peritonitis and 35% if there is feculent peritonitis.

▶ Treatment

A. Medical Therapy

For patients with uncomplicated diverticulitis, medical therapy is successful in 70–100%. Patients who are candidates for outpatient therapy have pain that is mild, minimal evidence of systemic infection (eg, no higher than a low-grade fever and no concern for sepsis), ability to tolerate oral intake, and good functional status. In contrast, inpatient treatment should be considered for patients with more severe presentations, such as those who are unable to tolerate oral intake or have high fever, significant leukocytosis, or severe abdominal pain. Patients who are at higher risk of complicatons, such as the elderly, immunocompromised, or those with significant comoribidities, should also be hospitalized for treatment.

Therapy consists of bowel rest and antibiotics. Antibiotic choice is dictated by the typical bacteria associated with diverticulitis, namely gram-negative rods and anaerobes. Single antibiotic coverage using an antibiotic with activity against colonic flora is as effective as combination therapy. Examples of treatment regimens are shown in Table 23–2. The choice of antibiotics should consider medication allergies, prior antibiotic use, and local antibiotic resistance patterns. Antibiotics are typically given for 7–10 days.

Outpatients should be put on a clear liquid diet, with slow advancement of the diet once clinical improvement is seen. For patients whose symptoms resolve with outpatient management, repeat imaging studies are *not* needed to confirm resolution. Patients who fail to show signs of improvement in 2–3 days, develop increasing pain or fever, or are no longer able to tolerate fluids should be hospitalized and investigated for possible complications with repeat CT imaging (see treatment strategies below). All inpatients should receive bowel rest (clear liquid diet at most) upon admission, intravenous antibiotics, fluids, and pain medications as needed.

B. Radiologically Guided Therapy

Abscesses should be treated with IV antibiotics followed by percutaneous drainage for larger abscesses (≥4 cm), those that fail to resolve with antibiotic therapy, or if the patient's clinical status worsens. CT-guided drains are usually placed through the anterior abdominal wall, although transgluteal, transrectal, or transvaginal approaches are also used for abscesses deep within the pelvis. Catheters are left in place until the daily output drops to less than 10 mL, which may take up to 30 days. Patients who fail to improve with catheter drainage require surgery.

C. Surgical Therapy

Fifteen to 30% of patients will require surgery for their first episode of diverticulitis. Indications for surgery during an episode of diverticulitis include diffuse peritonitis, obstruction, and failure of medical therapy (including percutaneous drainage as mentioned earlier). Elective surgery is also recommended for patients with fistulas, which result from the spontaneous drainage of an abscess. Although the inflammation usually resolves, diverticular fistulas rarely close spontaneously and thus resection of the affected bowel segment is typically required (nonemergently).

Table 23-2. Common antibiotic regimens for acute diverticulitis.

Antibiotic(s)	Dose	Route of Administration
Outpatient Regimens (choose one regimen from the two listed)		
Metronidazole plus		
ciprofloxacin	500 mg three times daily	Oral
Amoxicillin–clavulanate	500 mg twice daily	Oral
	875/125 mg twice daily	Oral
Inpatient Regimens (choose one regimen from the six listed)		
Metronidazole plus		
ciprofloxacin or	500 mg every 8 hours	IV
levofloxacin or	400 mg every 12 hours	IV
ceftriaxone or	500 mg daily	IV
cefotaxime	1–2 g daily	IV
Ampicillin–sulbactam	1–2 g every 6 hours	IV
Piperacillin–tazobactam	3 g every 6 hours	IV
Ticarcillin–clavulanate	3.75 or 4.5 g every 6 hours	IV
Imipenem	3.1 g every 8 hours	IV
Meropenem	500 mg every 6 hours	IV
	1 g every 8 hours	IV

IV, intravenous.

Whether to perform elective surgery for the 16–42% of patients with recurrent episodes of diverticulitis is controversial. It was previously recommended that patients undergo elective surgery after two episodes of uncomplicated diverticulitis. However, more recent evidence showed that prior uncomplicated diverticulitis episodes do not predict a higher incidence or worse severity of recurrence. It may therefore be more appropriate to individualize recommendations about elective colectomy, instead of recommending surgery for all patients after two episodes of diverticulitis.

Prior to surgery, all patients should receive antibiotics. If possible, bowel preparation is carried out, although in emergent situations, it often is not feasible. For sigmoid diverticulitis, the proximal resection margin should be in an area of healthy (soft, nonedematous) colon. The distal resection margin is in the upper third of rectum, where the taeniae coli coalesce. Leaving the distal sigmoid colon in place doubles the risk of diverticulitis. However, it is not necessary to remove all of the diverticula, because recurrence proximal to the anastomosis is less likely.

Prognosis

Following resolution of an initial episode of diverticulitis that was managed without surgery, approximately one-third of patients will develop recurrent diverticulitis. Of note, most patients (58–84%) do not have recurrent episodes.

Patients who have recovered after having peritonitis may develop small bowel obstructions due to adhesions. Patients with colovesical fistulas may develop urosepsis, and those with coloenteric fistulas may develop malabsorption due to bacterial overgrowth or short gut syndrome (as a result of the bypassing of segments of small bowel). Local irritation of the perineum or abdominal wall skin can be seen with colovaginal and colocutaneous fistulas, respectively. These fistulas can also be associated with fluid losses.

Bharucha AE, Parthasarathy G, Ditah I, et al. Temporal trends in the incidence and natural history of diverticulitis: a population-based study. *Am J Gastroenterol.* 2015;110(11):1589–1596. [PMID 26416187]

Frattini J, Longo WE. Diagnosis and treatment of chronic and recurrent diverticulitis. *J Clin Gastroenterol.* 2006;40:S145–S149. [PMID: 16885698]

Gervaz P, Ianan I, Perneger T, et al. A prospective, randomized, single-blind comparison of laparoscopic versus open sigmoid colectomy for diverticulitis. *Ann Surg.* 2010;252:3–8. [PMID: 20505508]

Janes S, Meagher A, Frizelle FA. Elective surgery after acute diverticulitis. *Br J Surg.* 2005;92:133–142. [PMID: 15685694]

Kaiser AM, Jiang JK, Lake JP, et al. The management of complicated diverticulitis and the role of computed tomography. *Am J Gastroenterol.* 2005;100:910–917. [PMID: 15784040]

Korzenik JR. Case closed? Diverticulitis: epidemiology and fiber. *J Clin Gastroenterol.* 2006;40:S112–S116. [PMID: 16885692]

Nguyen GC, Sam J, Anand N. Epidemiological trends and geographic variation in hospital admissions for diverticulitis in the United States. *World J Gastroenterol.* 2011;17:1600–1605.

Shahedi K, Fuller G, Bolus R, et al. Long-term risk of acute diverticulitis among patients with incidental diverticulosis found during colonoscopy. *Clin Gastroenterol Hepatol.* 2013;11(12):1609. [PMID 23856358]

Strate LL, Morris AM. Epidemiology, pathophysiology, and treatment of diverticulitis. *Gastroenterology.* 2019;156(5):1282–1298. [PMID: 30660732]

Touzios JG, Dozois EJ. Diverticulosis and diverticulitis. *Gastroenterol Clin N Am.* 2009;38:513–525. [PMID: 19699411]

DIVERTICULAR HEMORRHAGE

ESSENTIALS OF DIAGNOSIS

▶ Hematochezia, maroon stool, or melena. Typically painless.

▶ Endoscopic or radiographic demonstration of diverticula.

▶ Exclusion of other bleeding sources.

General Considerations

Up to 15% of patients with diverticulosis will develop diverticular bleeding, bleeding that will be massive in approximately one-third of the patients. Mortality rates for massive hemorrhage are significant, at 10–20%, in large part because many patients with diverticular hemorrhage are elderly with comorbid illnesses.

Pathogenesis

Diverticula form at the site of penetration of the vasa recta through the muscularis propria. Thus, each diverticulum has an associated arteriole, and mucosa is all that separates the vessel from the bowel lumen. Due to recurrent exposure to injury, eccentric intimal thickening and thinning of the media may develop, which lead to segmental weakness and predispose the artery to rupture along its luminal aspect. In 50–90% of patients, the source of bleeding is right-sided diverticula (despite the fact that 75% of diverticula are located on the left). This markedly increased propensity for right-sided diverticula to bleed may occur because right-sided diverticula have wider necks and domes, so a longer portion of the vasa recta is exposed to injury. In addition, the wall of the right colon is thinner, which may also contribute.

Clinical Findings

A. Symptoms & Signs

Patients typically present with moderate to large amounts of maroon stool or hematochezia. Clots are more commonly seen with a distal source, as is bright red blood. Melena may occasionally be seen in cases of right-sided bleeding. The bleeding is typically painless, although patients may report cramping due to the cathartic effects of blood within the bowel.

On examination, pallor, tachycardia, orthostatic hypotension, or shock may be noted with massive hemorrhage. The abdomen may be mildly distended with active bowel sounds. Rectal examination shows gross blood, which can range from bright red to melenic. An upper gastrointestinal source should be ruled out with upper endoscopy if there is concern

for an upper gastrointestinal bleeding source (eg, hemodynamic instability, melena, or an elevated BUN-to-creatinine ratio above 20:1).

B. Laboratory Findings

Upon initial presentation, a normal hemoglobin is not uncommon because sufficient time may not have elapsed for hemodilution and equilibration to have occurred. Once equilibration has occurred, red cell indices should indicate a normochromic, normocytic anemia. The presence of a hypochromic, microcytic anemia suggests chronic blood loss from another source.

C. Imaging Studies

Radionuclide scanning using ^{99m}Tc pertechnetate–labeled red blood cells can be used to identify acute bleeding and to localize the site of bleeding (Figure 23–5). This technique can detect bleeding at a rate of 0.1 mL/min and can be used to detect bleeding up to 24 hours after injection. In one series, ^{99m}Tc pertechnetate-labeled red blood cell scanning demonstrated a sensitivity of 97% and a specificity of 83% for active bleeding. The major limitation of radionuclide scanning is that localization is imprecise and can only identify an area of the abdomen where the bleeding is occurring and not an exact site. The accuracy of localization ranges from 24% to 91%. Blood can move from the site of extravasation due to peristaltic or antiperistaltic motion, which can lead to inaccurate localization. In addition, because localization is to

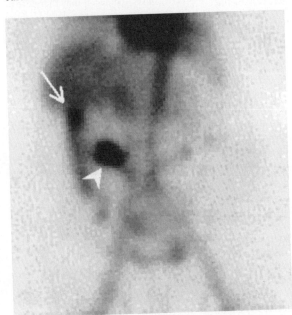

▲ **Figure 23–5.** Tagged red blood cell scan demonstrating bleeding originating in the right upper quadrant (*arrow*) along with pooling of the tagged red blood cells (*arrowhead*).

an area of the abdomen, and not an area of colon, incorrect assumptions can be made about localization. For example, bleeding from a redundant sigmoid colon may incorrectly be attributed to the right colon. Although radionuclide scanning does not allow for therapeutic maneuvers, it can aid in directing subsequent angiography.

An alternative to nuclear imaging is CT angiography, which is more widely available and produces fast results. CT angiography can detect bleeding at a rate of 0.3–0.5 mL/min. In a meta-analysis of 22 studies (672 patients), CT angiography had a sensitivity of 85% and a specificity of 92% for detecting active gastrointestinal bleeding. As with radionuclide scanning, the main disadvantage of this imaging modality is the lack of therapeutic capability. Further, CT angiography requires intravenous contrast, which carries its own risks of contrast-induced nephropathy and allergic reactions.

Mesenteric angiography, in contrast, has the advantage of being both diagnostic and therapeutic. It requires a brisker rate of bleeding than radionuclide scans of 0.5–1.0 mL/min. If a prior study has suggested a possible location for the bleed, angiography starts with the injection of the appropriate feeding vessels. However, if prior localization is not available, sequential injection of the mesenteric arteries is performed, starting with the superior mesenteric artery, as the majority of bleeds arise from the right colon. If results are negative, the inferior mesenteric artery and, finally, the celiac artery are studied. Angiography is successful in identifying a source of bleeding in 25–70% of cases. The success rate is influenced by both the timing of the study relative to an episode of active bleeding and by the expertise of the radiologist performing the study. Angiography is 100% specific, but only 47% sensitive for an acute bleed (30% for a recurrent bleed). Performing a radionuclide scan prior to angiography may decrease the rate of negative examinations, but this may be counterbalanced by an increased rate of negative tests because of the delay from performing the radionuclide scan prior to the angiography. If the initial study result is negative, the angiography catheter can be left in place for a short period to allow for rapid imaging if rebleeding occurs. Complications of angiography, which occur in 9% of patients, include arterial thrombosis, embolization, and renal failure. Angiography is thus typically resesrved for patients who cannot undergo colonoscopy due to hemodynamic instability from severe hemorrhage.

D. Endoscopy

Colonoscopy is the initial examination of choice in the evaluation of lower gastrointestinal bleeding and should be performed within 24 hours of presentation. Like angiography, it allows for both diagnosis and treatment, but also can precisely localize the size of bleeding (regardless of rate) and obtain pathology specimens as needed. Colonoscopy can be limited, however, by poor visualization due to retained blood and by the risks of sedation in an actively bleeding patient with hemodynamic instability. Although some physicians will perform a colonoscopy in an unprepared bowel, relying on the cathartic properties of blood to empty the colon, most attempt to cleanse the colon with a polyethylene glycol-based bowel preparation prior to the procedure. Urgent colonoscopy (<12 hours from admission) will lead to a definite or presumptive diagnosis in 45–90% of patients (50% of these will be diverticular), but does not reduce mortality. Although visualizing active bleeding is uncommon, a presumptive source can be identified through the visualization of an adherent clot or a mucosal lesion. Forty percent of patients with presumed diverticular bleeds demonstrate stigmata of recent hemorrhage, including a bleeding diverticulum, accumulation of fresh blood after clearing the colon, a nonbleeding visible vessel at the mouth of a diverticulum, or an adherent clot that cannot be dislodged with vigorous irrigation.

▶ Complications

Complications of diverticular hemorrhage are the result of massive blood loss, including death from exsanguination. Ischemic injuries to the heart, brain, or kidneys are the most common manifestations, especially in the elderly.

▶ Treatment

A. Medical Therapy

A general treatment algorithm is shown in Figure 23–6. In 75–90% of patients, bleeding stops spontaneously; in those with a transfusion requirement of less than 4 units/day, the rate of spontaneous resolution increases to 99%. Initial therapy focuses on resuscitation. Patients should have two large-bore peripheral intravenous lines placed and receive isotonic saline solutions while blood is cross-matched. Whether to give blood transfusions must be individualized. Blood transfusions are typically indicated in patients with massive bleeding and hemodynamic instability, since serum hemoglobin levels on presentation do not accurately reflect the degree of blood loss. For patients without massive bleeding, a more restrictive approach to transfusion may be appropriate. Studies in patients with upper gastrointestinal bleeding suggest that using a lower transfusion threshold (<7 g/dL) for patients who do not have unstable coronary artery disease is associated with better outcomes. Antiplatelet and anticoagulant agents should be discontinued, if possible. Any coagulopathies should be reversed. Patients with hemodynamic instability should receive care in an intensive care unit.

After adequate resuscitation and bowel preparation, colonoscopy should be performed within 24 hours (angiography is an alternative potential therapy if patients remain hemodynamically unstable). If a diverticular bleeding source (actively bleeding vessel) is identified endoscopically, therapy with injection of epinephrine (1:10,000 to 1:20,000) followed

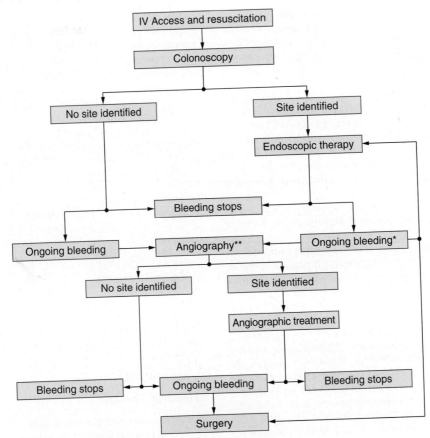

* Options include repeat endoscopy, angiography, and surgery
** Possibly preceded by tagged red blood cell scan

▲ **Figure 23–6.** Management algorithm for diverticular hemorrhage. IV, intravenous.

by thermal coagulation or hemostatic clip placement is recommended; if a nonbleeding visible vessel is seen, electrocautery or clip placement alone can be applied.

If an adherent clot is noted, it is recommended that it be removed after the base is injected with epinephrine. The clot is then shaved down using a cold guillotine technique. The pedicle of the clot, once visualized, should be treated with electrocautery or clip placement if active bleeding or a visible vessel is seen. If the bleeding vessel within a diverticulum cannot be identified, blind injection therapy with epinephrine can be carried out, or the mouth of the diverticulum can be closed with hemostatic clips. It is recommended that a tattoo or a hemoclip be placed at the site of the bleed in case there is recurrent hemorrhage requiring either repeat endoscopy or surgery.

If a bleeding source is identified with angiography, therapy can also be carried out. Vasopressin infusion will stop bleeding in 90% of patients, but 50% will rebleed when the vasopressin is stopped. Despite the significant rate of rebleeding, the use of vasopressin may allow for resuscitation and preparation for semielective surgery. Patients receiving vasopressin

should be monitored in an intensive care setting. Complications of vasopressin include cardiac ischemia and fluid and electrolyte abnormalities. Transcatheter embolization using polyvinyl alcohol particles or microcoils is a potentially more definitive method for controlling hemorrhage; however, it is complicated by intestinal infarction in up to 20% of patients.

B. Surgical Therapy

Surgery is required for patients with persistent bleeding that cannot be controlled through medical means (ie, colonoscopy or angiography), are unstable despite aggressive resuscitative measures, and/or are good surgical candidates with recurrent bleeding. For patients who lack preoperative localization, exploratory laparotomy will be successful in identifying a source in 78% of patients. During exploratory laparotomy, the small bowel should be examined, and if a significant portion of the small bowel contains blood, intraoperative enteroscopy should be performed to evaluate for a possible small bowel source. Once the source of bleeding has been localized (either preoperatively or intraoperatively), segmental colectomy is performed. A primary anastomosis is possible in most cases due to the cathartic effects of blood. It is not necessary to remove all diverticula in patients with extensive diverticular disease.

Blind segmental resection is contraindicated due to its high rebleeding rate (30–42%), morbidity (83%), and mortality (57%). Thus, if a bleeding source cannot be identified, a subtotal colectomy should be performed. Although the rebleeding rate following a subtotal colectomy is less than 10%, the morbidity and mortality rates for the procedure are high (37% and 11–33%, respectively).

▶ **Prognosis**

Seventy-five to 92% of patients will stop bleeding spontaneously. However, following an initial episode of diverticular hemorrhage, the risk of recurrent bleeding is 10–40% (often within 48 hours of the initial bleed). NSAIDs may increase the risk of early rebleeding. After a second episode, the risk of recurrent hemorrhage increases to 21–50%. Mortality is low in patients whose bleeding stops spontaneously (2% in one study). However, the overall mortality rate for those with massive hemorrhage is 10–20% and is related to comorbid illnesses.

DeBarros J, Rosas L, Cohen J, et al. The changing paradigm for the treatment of colonic hemorrhage: superselective angiographic embolization. *Dis Colon Rectum*. 2002;45:802–808. [PMID: 12072634]

Elta GH. Urgent colonoscopy for acute lower-GI bleeding. *Gastrointest Endosc*. 2004;59:402–408. [PMID: 14997144]

Garcia-Blazquez V, Vicente-Bartulos A, Olavarria-Delgado A, et al. Accuracy of CT angiography in the diagnosis of acute gastrointestinal bleeding: systemic review and meta-analysis. *Eur Radiol*. 2013;23:1181–1890. [PMID: 23192375]

Jensen DM, Machicado GA, Jutabha R, et al. Urgent colonoscopy for the diagnosis and treatment of severe diverticular hemorrhage. *N Engl J Med*. 2000;342:78–82. [PMID: 10631275]

Marti M, Artigas JM, Garzon G, et al. Acute lower intestinal bleeding: feasibility and diagnostic performance of CT angiography. *Radiology*. 2012;262(1):109–116. [PMID 22084211]

Nagata N, Niikura R, Sakurai T, et al. Safety and effectiveness of early colonoscopy in management of acute lower gastrointestinal bleeding on the basis of propensity score matching analysis. *Clin Gastroenterol Hepatol*. 2016;14(4):558. [PMID 26492844]

Strate L, Gralnek IM. ACG clinical guideline: management of patients with acute lower gastrointestinal bleeding. *Am J Gastroenterol*. 2016;111(5):755. [PMID 27151132]

Villanueva C, Colomo A, Bosch A, et al. Transfusion strategies for acute upper gastrointestinal bleeding. *N Engl J Med*. 2013;368:11–21. [PMID: 23281973]

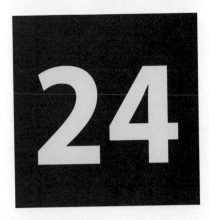

Colorectal Cancer Screening

24

Nicolette J. Rodriguez, MD, MPH

Ramona Lim, MD

Sapna Syngal, MD, MPH

Screening for colorectal cancer (CRC) can reduce disease-related morbidity and mortality. The existing evidence has led to the recommendation of CRC screening as a standard component of preventive health care.

General Considerations

CRC is the third leading cause of cancer death in the United States. The lifetime risk of CRC in the United States is approximately 5%. In 2020, it is estimated that 78,300 males and 69,650 females will be diagnosed and 53,200 individuals will die of CRC. However, overall disease survival has improved from 51% in the 1970s to 64% most recently. Increased knowledge about the pathogenesis, advances in medical and surgical care, and the increasing emphasis on CRC screening programs have contributed to these substantial gains.

CRC can be prevented through readily available screening. Prevention efforts rely on the long time interval required for a benign adenomatous polyp to progress into an invasive cancer. It is estimated that the adenoma to carcinoma sequence unfolds over a 7- to 10-year period. In addition, CRC-related deaths are preventable if the disease is detected early. When diagnosed early, the 5-year survival rate for localized stage CRC is 90%. Conversely, the 5-year survival for patients with known distant metastases is only 14%. Unfortunately, only 39% of cancers are diagnosed with localized disease and 21% of patients have distant metastases.

CRC screening is underutilized in the United States. Approximately two-thirds of the population is adherent to standard screening recommendations. Several factors contribute to the lack of adherence to CRC screening, including inappropriate perception of risk (particularly if patients are asymptomatic and without a family history of CRC), dietary restrictions or burdensome cathartic preparations, the invasiveness of procedures, perceived discomfort, embarrassment related to certain screening techniques, and logistical barriers such as time and transportation as well as financial barriers including cost and lack of insurance.

It is also critical to be aware of CRC screening health care disparities including lower screening rates among racial/ethnic populations and low SES populations. Sixty-eight percent of White individuals are up-to-date on CRC screening compared to 65% of Black, 59% of Latinx, 59% of American Indian/Alaskan Native, and 55% of Asian individuals. Moreover, only 55% of individuals at <200% the federal poverty level are up-to-date on CRC screening compared to 70% of individuals at ≥200% the federal poverty level. As a result, providers must understand that certain groups of patients have unique challenges to CRC screening and uptake.

American Cancer Society. Cancer Facts & Figures 2020. Available at: https://www.cancer.org/content/dam/cancer-org/research/cancer-facts-and-statistics/annual-cancer-facts-and-figures/2020/cancer-facts-and-figures-2020.pdf. Accessed August 2020.

American Cancer Society. Colorectal Cancer Facts & Figures 2020-2022. Available at: https://www.cancer.org/content/dam/cancer-org/research/cancer-facts-and-statistics/colorectal-cancer-facts-and-figures/colorectal-cancer-facts-and-figures-2020-2022.pdf. Accessed August 2020.

National Cancer Institute: Surveillance, Epidemiology, and End Results program. Cancer Stat Facts: Colorectal Cancer. Available at: https://seer.cancer.gov/statfacts/html/colorect.html. Accessed August 2020.

Siegel RL, Miller KD, Goding Sauer A, et al. Colorectal cancer statistics, 2020. CA Cancer J Clin. 2020;70(3):145–164. [PMID: 32133645]

Warren Andersen S, Blot WJ, Lipworth L, Steinwandel M, Murff HJ, Zheng W. Association of race and socioeconomic status with colorectal cancer screening, colorectal cancer risk, and mortality in Southern US adults. JAMA Netw Open. 2019;2(12):e1917995. Published 2019 Dec 2. [PMID: 31860105]

Pathogenesis

Three distinct molecular pathways that may lead to CRC have been recognized: the chromosomal instability (CIN), the microsatellite instability (MSI), and the CpG island methylator phenotype (CIMP) pathways.

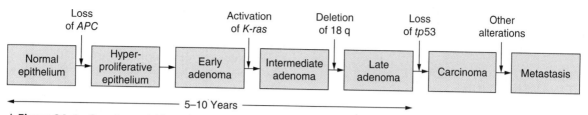

▲ Figure 24–1. Genetic model for colorectal tumorigenesis. Adapted with permission from Fearon ER, Vogelstein B. A genetic model for colorectal tumorigenesis. *Cell.* 1990;61(5):759–767.

A. Chromosomal Instability Pathway

In 1990, a stepwise, chronologic model for colorectal tumorigenesis was proposed. It outlined sequential alterations in key growth regulatory genes, such as *APC*, *K-ras*, and *tp53*, culminating in the development of a malignant neoplasm. This pathway contributes to the development of 60% of sporadic colorectal tumors that arise from preexisting adenomatous polyps. When adenomas accumulate the necessary combination of genetic mutations in the suggested stepwise manner, the end result is cancer (Figure 24–1).

The genes implicated in CRC can be divided into three categories: (1) tumor-suppressor genes, (2) proto-oncogenes, and (3) DNA repair genes.

The function of tumor-suppressor genes is to downregulate normal growth stimulatory pathways. In CRC, the genes most frequently inactivated are *APC*, *tp53*, *p16*, and chromosome 18q (*DCC*, *SMAD4*, *SMAD2*). Consistent with the Knudson "two-hit hypothesis," acquired (or somatic) mutations in both alleles of the tumor-suppressor gene are required to fully inactivate gene function and cause cancer. In autosomal-dominant CRC syndromes, a preexisting germline mutation in one allele ("first hit") is inherited and a "second hit" occurs when an acquired mutation inactivates the other allele.

Proto-oncogenes, such as *K-ras*, *SRC*, *MYC*, and *HER2* are components of signaling pathways that promote normal cellular growth and proliferation. A mutation in a proto-oncogene leads to an active gene product, known as a gain of function mutation, with a resulting tumorigenic effect.

DNA repair genes function to maintain the integrity of the genome. Individual nucleotides can be modified by biochemical reactions such as oxidation, alkylation, spontaneous deamination, and ultraviolet cross-linking. When errors occur, they are corrected through a sophisticated process known as "base excision repair."

B. Microsatellite Instability Pathway

Another manner in which errors are introduced into the genome is through mispairing of nucleotides, which can occur during normal DNA replication. These errors are corrected by a DNA "mismatch repair" (MMR) system. When either of these DNA repair processes is dysfunctional, deleterious mutations can accumulate in genes that directly control cellular growth and proliferation. Germline mutation

in MMR genes is responsible for Lynch syndrome, while somatic mutation or hypermethylation silencing of MMR genes accounts for approximately 15% of sporadic CRC.

C. CpG Island Methylator Phenotype Pathway

Epigenetic alterations which alter gene expression or function without altering the DNA sequence can occur. Aberrant hypermethylation of gene promoter regions (CpG islands) may result in gene silencing of tumor suppressor genes. CIMP-high CRCs are strongly associated with *BRAF* mutations, developing from a precursor lesion known as the sessile serrated adenoma (SSA). CRCs arising along the serrated pathway account for approximately 10–30 % of all CRC.

Fearon ER, Vogelstein B. A genetic model for colorectal tumorigenesis. *Cell.* 1990;61:759–767. [PMID: 2188735]

Hirano D, Urabe Y, Tanaka S, et al. Early-stage serrated adenocarcinomas are divided into several molecularly distinct subtypes. *PLoS One.* 2019;14(2):e0211477. Published 2019 Feb 20. [PMID: 30785889]

Koveitypour Z, Panahi F, Vakilian M, et al. Signaling pathways involved in colorectal cancer progression. *Cell Biosci.* 2019;9:97. Published 2019 Dec 2. [PMID: 31827763]

Pino MS, Chung DC. The chromosomal instability pathway in colon cancer. *Gastroenterology.* 2010;138:2059–2072. [PMID: 20420946]

RISK STRATIFICATION

The approach to CRC screening in asymptomatic individuals depends on risk stratification and the likelihood of developing the disease. Screening for CRC takes place in persons who have no personal or family history of adenomatous polyps or cancer. Surveillance takes place in persons with a personal history of either adenomatous polyps, CRC, or one of the genetic syndromes that requires more intensive monitoring. Individuals who have signs or symptoms suggestive of CRC fall outside the domain of screening and should be offered appropriate diagnostic evaluation.

CRC screening programs begin by classifying an individual's level of risk based on age, as well as personal and family medical history. This vital information helps determine when screening should be initiated, with what appropriate tests, and the frequency of subsequent examinations. CRC risk is commonly stratified into three broad categories: average risk, moderate risk, and high risk.

SCREENING & SURVEILLANCE RECOMMENDATIONS

1. Average Risk

An average-risk individual is defined as an asymptomatic person without a personal history of inflammatory bowel disease (IBD), hereditary syndromes associated with increased CRC risk or a personal or family history of CRC. The majority of the general population is considered to be at average risk for CRC. Given that age is the strongest risk factor for the development of CRC and adenomatous polyps, individuals at average risk should be offered screening beginning at age 50, except in Black populations in whom screening is recommended beginning at age 45. However, due to the increasing prevalence of early onset CRC, some recent guidelines recommend initiation of CRC screening at age 45 for all individuals.

Available screening options for average-risk individuals fall into two broad categories: (1) tests that primarily detect CRC and (2) tests that detect precancerous adenomatous polyps and CRC (Table 24–1). Tests that primarily detect cancer are fecal immunochemical tests and fecal DNA tests. These modalities provide limited opportunity for prevention because detection of premalignant adenomatous polyps is most often incidental. Tests that detect both adenomatous polyps and cancer include flexible sigmoidoscopy (FS), colonoscopy, and computed tomography colonography (CTC). Because prevention is the primary goal of CRC screening, guidelines strongly encourage clinicians to offer those tests that are designed to detect both early cancer and adenomatous polyps if resources are available and if patients are willing to undergo an invasive examination. Noninvasive tests

Table 24–1. Testing options for asymptomatic adults aged 50 & older.

Tests that detect adenomatous polyps and CRC
  Flexible sigmoidoscopy
  Colonoscopy
  Computed tomography colonography

Tests that primarily detect CRC
  Fecal immunochemical tests (FIT)
  FIT-fecal DNA test

CRC, colorectal cancer.
Adapted, with permission, from Levin B, Lieberman DA, McFarland B, et al. Screening and surveillance for the early detection of colorectal cancer and adenomatous polyps, 2008: a joint guideline from the American Cancer Society, the US Multisociety Task Force on Colorectal Cancer, and the American College of Radiology. *Gastroenterology.* 2008;134(5):1570–1595.

must be repeated at regular intervals to be effective, are less likely to prevent CRC than invasive examinations, and, if abnormal, require colonoscopy.

Health care providers are encouraged to focus on increasing screening rates through periodic use of any of the recommended CRC screening modalities. Providers should present their patients with information about the advantages and disadvantages associated with the multiple available screening tests. In turn, patients have the opportunity to select how they wish to be screened based on their own preferences. The rationale for such an approach is that it may increase the likelihood that screening will occur. Even though the currently available screening techniques are not equal in effectiveness, cost, or associated risks, they all have been demonstrated to be cost-effective compared with no screening at all.

Rex DK, Boland CR, Dominitz JA, et al. Colorectal cancer screening: recommendations for physicians and patients from the U.S. multi-society task force on colorectal cancer. *Gastroenterology.* 2017;153(1):307–323. [PMID: 28555630]

Wolf AMD, Fontham ETH, Church TR, et al. Colorectal cancer screening for average-risk adults: 2018 guideline update from the American Cancer Society. *CA Cancer J Clin.* 2018;68(4):250–281. [PMID: 29846947]

2. Moderate Risk

Individuals with a personal or family history of adenomatous polyps or CRC are considered to be at intermediate risk for the development of CRC. For these patients, colonoscopy is the recommended surveillance method. Other conventional screening modalities are not typically recommended in this setting.

A. Personal History of Adenomatous Polyps

Certain characteristics of colorectal adenomas at baseline colonoscopy are the basis for decisions about surveillance intervals. The US Multi-Society Task Force on CRC has provided detailed adenoma definitions. An advanced adenoma meets one or more of the following criteria: (1) adenoma ≥10 mm in size, (2) adenoma with tubulovillous/villous histology, and/or (3) adenoma with high-grade dysplasia. A low-risk adenoma is defined as 1–2 nonadvanced adenomas <10 mm in size. An advanced neoplasia is defined as meeting any of the advanced adenoma criteria or having CRC. Lastly, a high-risk adenoma is defined as meeting one or more of the following criteria: advanced neoplasia and/or three or more adenomas.

Patients with a history of adenoma resection may have a higher risk to develop CRC compared to the general population. Moreover, there is an increased CRC mortality in individuals with advanced adenomas compared to those without any adenoma. A proximal location of adenomas (ascending colon or cecum) may also predict metachronous advanced adenomas. However, research has yielded varying results and more studies are needed to investigate if proximal adenomas should be viewed as a modifying risk factor for CRC surveillance. In addition, there is a general consensus that individuals with adenomas with lesser findings (eg, one or two subcentimeter adenomas without high-grade dysplasia or villous features) are at lower risk for subsequent advanced adenomas.

The US Multi-Society Task Force on CRC has provided evidence-based guidelines for surveillance of postpolypectomy patients. In a randomized comparison of surveillance intervals after colonoscopic removal of newly diagnosed adenomatous polyps, there was no better detection of advanced lesions with surveillance examination 1 year after the initial colonoscopy than with follow-up examination in 3 years. This suggests that the rate of developing metachronous adenomas with advanced pathology is slow; therefore, the current recommendation for patients with adenomas of 1 cm or larger, or adenomas with tubulovillous or villous histology as well as adenomas with high-grade dysplasia, or any combination of these findings, is surveillance colonoscopy in 3 years. In addition, patients who have more than 10 adenomas removed during one endoscopic examination should be examined in a shorter time interval (1 year) based on clinical judgment and should be considered for the possibility of an underlying familial syndrome with a genetics referral. It is also important to consider genetics referral in any patient who has ten or more lifetime adenomas. The standard of care for a SSP or adenomatous polyp ≥2 cm removed by piecemeal fashion is repeat colonoscopy 6 months after the initial endoscopic resection.

The effectiveness of CRC prevention with colonoscopy assumes that the baseline examination is performed with high quality, as lesions may be missed and interval cancers can develop, notably in the proximal colon. Numerous factors may impact the detection of neoplasia in the proximal colon including the quality of the bowel preparation, time spent on visualization, size, subtle nature of flat lesions, and tumors which may be biologically different from the more prevalent neoplasia in the distal colon.

Click B, Pinsky PF, Hickey T, Doroudi M, Schoen RE. Association of colonoscopy adenoma findings with long-term colorectal cancer incidence. *JAMA.* 2018;319(19):2021–2031. [PMID: 29800214]

Gupta S, Lieberman D, Anderson JC, et al. Recommendations for follow-up after colonoscopy and polypectomy: a consensus update by the US Multi-Society Task Force on Colorectal Cancer. *Gastroenterology.* 2020;158(4):1131–1153.e5. [PMID: 32044092]

Winawer SJ, Zauber AG, Ho MN, et al. Prevention of colorectal cancer by colonoscopic polypectomy. The National Polyp Study Workgroup. *N Engl J Med.* 1993;329:1977–1981. [PMID: 8247072]

Zimmermann-Fraedrich K, Sehner S, Rex DK, et al. Right-sided location not associated with missed colorectal adenomas in an individual-level reanalysis of tandem colonoscopy studies. *Gastroenterology.* 2019;157(3):660–671.e2. [PMID: 31103625]

Zhao S, Yang X, Wang S, et al. Impact of 9-minute withdrawal time on the adenoma detection rate: a multicenter randomized controlled trial. *Clin Gastroenterol Hepatol.* 2020;S1542-3565(20)31553-6. [PMID: 33220526]

B. Personal History of CRC

Individuals with a history of CRC are at risk for recurrent cancer and metachronous neoplasms and require endoscopic surveillance after surgical resection. Between 2.3% and 12.4% of patients with CRC have one or more synchronous cancers in the colon or rectum at the time of initial diagnosis or within 6 months of initial diagnosis. It is therefore important to perform a complete colonoscopy in the preoperative period. In cases where an obstructing colonic or rectal lesion is detected and perioperative colonoscopy cannot be performed, a CT or PET should be considered perioperatively, and a complete colonoscopy should be performed 3–6 months after surgery. Once the colon is cleared of any synchronous lesions, a postoperative surveillance colonoscopy is recommended at 1 year to evaluate for any metachronous lesions. If the examination at 1 year is normal, the subsequent examination should be at 3 years. If this examination is also normal, surveillance colonoscopy can thereafter be extended to every 5 years.

Colonoscopy at 1 year after surgical resection is recommended based on reports of approximately 30% of metachronous second cancers noted within the first 2 years after resection. There is an incidence rate of 0.7% for metachronous cancers in the first 2 years after resection of the initial primary cancer with a cumulative annual incidence of metachronous cancers between 0.30% and 0.35%. Thus, colonoscopy is recommended at 1 year following surgical resection. However, this should not diminish the importance of a high-quality colonoscopic examination in the perioperative period to exclude synchronous neoplasms.

In addition, it is important to distinguish between rectal and colon cancer due to the differing rates of local recurrence. The recurrence of colon cancer at the anastomotic site occurs in only 2–4% of patients. In contrast, the local recurrence rate of rectal cancer after curative surgery is 44.6% at 5 years. High recurrence rates of rectal cancer are partly a function of surgical technique. Factors associated with local recurrence risk after curative surgery distal margin ≤2 cm, stenosis of the tumor or extracapsular invasion of lymph node metastasis. Local recurrence rates of cancer can be reduced by precise preoperative staging, using a surgical technique called mesorectal excision, as well as administering radiation and chemotherapy in the neoadjuvant, preoperative setting to patients with locally advanced disease. However, because reported local recurrence rates for rectal cancer across the United States are generally higher than those achieved in case series using total mesorectal excision, there is a rationale for performing periodic examinations of the rectum with FS or endoscopic ultrasound. Performing local surveillance at 3–6 month intervals for the first 2–3 years after surgical resection can be considered. This is performed for the detection of a surgically curable recurrence of the original rectal cancer in those patients who do not undergo mesorectal excision, receive neoadjuvant radiation and chemotherapy, undergo endoscopic submucosal dissection or local excision or undergo surgery using mesorectal excision techniques.

When colon or rectal cancer is endoscopically resected and surgery is not needed, follow-up endoscopic examination to inspect the biopsy site within 1 year is reasonable. As previously noted, colonoscopy is considered the test of choice for the detection of metachronous neoplasms in patients with a history of CRC.

Kahi CJ, Boland CR, Dominitz JA, et al. Colonoscopy surveillance after colorectal cancer resection: recommendations of the US Multi-Society Task Force on Colorectal Cancer. *Gastroenterology*. 2016;150(3):758–768.e11. [PMID: 26892199]

National Comprehensive Cancer Network. NCCN clinical practice guidelines in oncology: colon cancer. V 3.2020. Available at: http://www.nccn.org/professionals/. Accessed August 2020.

C. Family History of CRC or Adenomatous Polyps

An individual's risk of CRC is increased if there is a family history of adenomatous polyps or CRC. The screening recommendations based on familial risk are derived largely from the observed colon cancer risk in relatives of patients with CRC and adenomas diagnosed before age 60 (Table 24–2). The relative risk of developing CRC when at least one first-degree relative has CRC is 2.24. Among individuals with ≥1 first-degree relative with CRC diagnosed at less than 50 years the relative risk of CRC is 3.55. Moreover, the relative risk of CRC if ≥1 first-degree relative had an adenomatous polyp is 1.99. Pathologic features predisposing CRC risk for first-degree relatives include CRC cases that had

Table 24–2. Relative risk of colorectal cancer (CRC) based on family history.[a]

	Pooled Risk Estimate
One or more FDR with CRC	2.24
One or more FDR with CRC diagnosed at <50 years	3.55
Two or more FDR with CRC	3.97
One or more SDR with CRC	1.73
One or more FDR with an adenomatous polyp	1.99

FDR, first-degree relative; SDR, second-degree relative.
[a]Compares unaffected individuals with a family history of CRC or adenomatous polyps with unaffected individuals without a family history of CRC or adenomatous polyps.

tumors with peritumoral lymphocytes, tumor-infiltrating lymphocytes, expanding tumor margin, or a synchronous CRC. Therefore, familial risk needs to be readily identified and should prompt the early initiation of surveillance with colonoscopy.

The US Multi-society Task Force on Colorectal Cancer recommends that for patients who report one first-degree relative under 60 years or two first-degree relatives of any age with an advanced adenoma or CRC, screening colonoscopy should start at age 40 or 10 years younger than the earliest diagnosis of an affected relative (whichever one comes first) and continue every 5 years (Table 24–3). Screening should start at the same time for those patients with a single first-degree relative with CRC or an advanced adenoma diagnosed at ≥60 years, but surveillance should be performed as for average-risk individuals. The rationale for starting screening at age 40 is that the incidence of CRC in these patients resembles the risk in persons with no family history but precedes it by approximately 10 years. In addition, a patient reporting a second- or third-degree relative with adenomatous polyps or CRC has a 1.5 fold risk of developing CRC compared to the general population, and therefore, average-risk screening recommendations are sufficient.

Lowery JT, Ahnen DJ, Schroy PC 3rd, et al. Understanding the contribution of family history to colorectal cancer risk and its clinical implications: a state-of-the-science review [published correction appears in Cancer. 2017 Oct 1;123(19):3857]. *Cancer*. 2016;122(17):2633–2645. [PMID: 27258162]

Quintero E, Carrillo M, Leoz ML, et al. Risk of advanced neoplasia in first-degree relatives with colorectal cancer: a large multicenter cross-sectional study. *PLoS Med*. 2016;13(5):e1002008. Published 2016 May 3. [PMID: 27138769]

Rex DK, Boland CR, Dominitz JA, et al. Colorectal cancer screening: recommendations for physicians and patients from the U.S. Multi-Society Task Force on colorectal cancer. *Gastroenterology*. 2017;153(1):307–323. [PMID: 28555630]

3. High Risk

For individuals with a hereditary CRC syndrome, such as familial adenomatous polyposis (FAP) or Lynch syndrome, genetic counseling and special screening protocols are recommended (Table 24–4). Readily identifying these individuals is imperative given the known benefit of intensive endoscopic surveillance and prophylactic surgery on morbidity and mortality. Recognizing these syndromes also has an impact on referral for predictive genetic testing, wherein identifying gene carriers improves the efficiency of cancer surveillance and helps identify family members who require intense management versus those who can receive the standard of care. Additionally, for patients with long-standing IBD such as Crohn's disease or ulcerative colitis, surveillance colonoscopy with systematic biopsies should be performed because the risk of CRC is increased in individuals with IBD.

Table 24–3. Colorectal cancer screening recommendations.

Assessed Risk	Age to Initiate	Test	Interval
Average[a]	50 years	Colonoscopy FIT CTC FIT-fecal DNA FS	10 years or Annually or 5 years or 3 years or 10 years (or 5 years) or
Moderate			
Personal history of:			
CRC		Colonoscopy	1 year; 3 years; if normal, every 5 years
Adenomas		Colonoscopy	7–10 years
1–2 tubular adenomas <10 mm		Colonoscopy	3–5 years
3–4 tubular adenomas <10 mm		Colonoscopy	3 years
5–10 tubular adenomas <10 mm		Colonoscopy	1 year
>10 adenomas[b]		Colonoscopy	3 years
Adenoma ≥10 mm		Colonoscopy	3 years
Adenoma with tubulovillous/villous features		Colonoscopy	3 years
Adenomas with HGD complete resection			
Serrated lesions			
1–2 sessile serrated polyp(s) <10 mm		Colonoscopy	5–10 years
3–4 sessile serrated polyps <10 mm		Colonoscopy	3–5 years
5–10 sessile serrated polyps <10 mm		Colonoscopy	3 years
Sessile serrated polyp(s) ≥10 mm		Colonoscopy	3 years
Sessile serrated polyp with dysplasia		Colonoscopy	3 years
Traditional serrated adenoma		Colonoscopy	3 years
Piecemeal resection		Colonoscopy	6 months[c]
High			
FAP[d]			
Classic	10–12 years	Colonoscopy	Annually
Attenuated	Late teens	Colonoscopy	1–2 years
Serrated polyposis syndrome	No standard recommendation	Colonoscopy	Colonoscopy until all polyps ≥5 mm are resected and then every 1–3 years
Lynch syndrome[d]	20–25 for *MLH1, MSH2* or *EPCAM*	Colonoscopy	1–2 years
Crohn or ulcerative colitis	30–35 for *MSH6* or *PMS2* 8 years after diagnosis	Colonoscopy	1–2 years

CRC, colorectal cancer; CTC, computed tomography colonography; FAP, familial adenomatous polyposis; FDR, first-degree relative; HGD, high-grade dysplasia

[a]Includes those undergoing baseline/surveillance exams without a personal history of polyps or a family history of CRC, inflammatory bowel disease, or a hereditary cancer syndrome with increased CRC risk

[b]If ≥10 adenomatous polyps consider attenuated FAP diagnosis and genetics referral.

[c]Short interval of 6 months to ensure complete resection.

[d]Consider germline genetic testing.

Data from Gupta S, Lieberman D, Anderson JC, et al: Recommendations for Follow-Up After Colonoscopy and Polypectomy: A Consensus Update by the US Multi-Society Task Force on Colorectal Cancer. *Am J Gastroenterol.* 2020;115(3):415–434.

National Comprehensive Cancer Network. NCCN clinical practice guidelines in oncology: genetic/familial high-risk assessment: colorectal. V 1.2020. Available at: http://www.nccn.org/professionals/. Accessed August 2020.

Shah SC, Itzkowitz SH. Reappraising risk factors for inflammatory bowel disease-associated neoplasia: implications for colonoscopic surveillance in IBD. *J Crohns Colitis.* 2020; 14(8):1172–1177. [PMID: 32150256]

A. Familial Adenomatous Polyposis, Attenuated Familial Adenomatous Polyposis, & *MUTYH*-Associated Polyposis

FAP is an autosomal-dominant syndrome that is associated with mutations in the *adenomatous polyposis coli* (*APC*) tumor suppressor gene. Affected individuals classically develop hundreds to thousands of colorectal adenomas at

Table 24–4. Colon cancer screening recommendations for people with familial or inherited risk.

Familial Risk Category	Screening Recommendation
One first-degree relative[a] affected with colorectal cancer or an advanced adenoma at age ≥60	Same as average risk but starting at age 40
Two or more first-degree relatives[a] with colon cancer[b] or an advanced adenoma or a single first-degree relative with colon cancer or an advanced adenoma diagnosed at an age <60	Colonoscopy every 5 years, beginning at age 40 or 10 years younger than the earliest diagnosis in the family, whichever comes first

[a]First-degree relatives include parents, siblings, and children.
[b]Consider genetic evaluation for Lynch syndrome.
Adapted with permission from Winawer S, Fletcher R, Rex D, et al: Colorectal cancer screening and surveillance: clinical guidelines and rationale-Update based on new evidence. *Gastroenterology*. 2003;124(2):544–560.

a young age and have a risk of CRC approaching 100% in the absence of prophylactic colectomy. An annual sigmoidoscopy or colonoscopy (defer to colonoscopy once polyps are identified) beginning at age 10–12 with surveillance every 1–2 years is recommended for persons who have a genetic diagnosis or are at risk of having FAP in order to determine if they are expressing the genetic abnormality. These recommendations are based on data showing that only 0.2% of individuals with FAP develop CRC prior to age 15 and that the increased risk for CRC begins in the second decade of life. Germline genetic testing should be recommended in persons with an FAP phenotype and should be performed after patients (or parents of children) undergo genetic counseling. If a mutation is identified, other family members can be tested to discern the presence or absence of the same mutation with nearly 100% accuracy. Surveillance colonoscopy is performed until the polyp burden in affected individuals cannot be managed endoscopically, at which point total colectomy is recommended. Family members who test negative for the gene mutation are considered to be at average risk for CRC.

Although classic FAP can be readily identified, a subset of patients has a less obvious phenotype. Patients with 10 or more cumulative colorectal adenomas but less than 100, are at risk for a variant of FAP called attenuated FAP (AFAP). In these patients, the age of onset of adenomas is approximately 10–20 years later than with classic FAP. AFAP also has an autosomal-dominant mode of inheritance and, as with classic FAP, is due to mutations in the *APC* gene. Furthermore, the lifetime CRC risk among AFAP patients is 70% with a predisposition for right sided CRC and polyps.

The true incidence and frequency of AFAP is unknown; however, it may account for up to 10% of adenomatous polyposis families and should be considered in individuals with multiple adenomas. An attenuated form of polyposis can also be due to inheritance of biallelic mutations in the *MUTYH* gene, an autosomal recessive condition with a less striking family history of CRC. *MUTYH* associated polyposis has a right sided predilection for CRC and polyps with typical rectal sparing. The lifetime CRC risk among these patients is 80%.

For both AFAP and *MUTYH* associated polyposis, colonoscopy should be used as the initial screening modality. Surveillance should be performed with colonoscopy every 1–2 years and begin in late teens for AFAP and age 25–30 for *MUTYH* associated polyposis. As with FAP, germline genetic testing for the *APC* and *MUTYH* genes should be considered in persons presenting with the AFAP phenotype.

B. Lynch Syndrome

Lynch syndrome exhibits an autosomal-dominant pattern of inheritance, and affected individuals have between a 15% and 70% lifetime risk of developing CRC by the age of 70. It is predominantly caused by a mutation in one of four of the DNA MMR genes, *MSH2*, *MLH1*, *MSH6*, and *PMS2*, in addition to a germline mutation in the *EPCAM* gene, which causes epigenetic silencing of the *MSH2* gene. There are several classification systems for the clinical diagnosis of Lynch syndrome, including the Amsterdam Classification with recent emphasis shifting to clinical predictive models. Predictive risk assessment models (PREMM$_5$, MMRpro, MMRpredict) can be used to provide a quantitative estimate of the likelihood of Lynch syndrome to identify individuals who may benefit from genetic testing. Genetic testing is currently available for individuals suspected of having Lynch syndrome, as well as for family members who are at risk for the condition. Guidelines support universal tumor testing for evidence of MMR deficiency of all newly diagnosed CRC patients, due to greater sensitivity for identification of Lynch syndrome than use of clinical criteria.

Once Lynch syndrome has been diagnosed, an intensive screening program should be instituted. Screening colonoscopy, for individuals with *MLH1*, *MSH2*, and *EPCAM* Lynch syndrome, is recommended every 1–2 years beginning at age 20–25 or 2–5 years prior to the youngest CRC case diagnosed within the family if diagnosed before age 25. Furthermore, screening colonoscopy, for individuals with *MSH6* or *PMS2* Lynch syndrome, is recommended every 1–2 years beginning at age 30–35 or 2–5 years prior to the youngest CRC case diagnosed within the family if diagnosed before age 30.

Giardiello FM, Allen JI, Axilbund JE, et al. Guidelines on genetic evaluation and management of Lynch syndrome: a consensus statement by the US Multisociety Task Force on colorectal cancer. *Gastroenterology*. 2014;147:502–526. [PMID: 25043945]

National Comprehensive Cancer Network. NCCN clinical practice guidelines in oncology: genetic/familial high-risk assessment: colorectal. V 1.2020. Available at: http://www.nccn.org/
professionals/. Accessed August 2020.

Syngal S, Brand RE, Church JM, et al. ACG clinical guideline:
genetic testing and management of hereditary gastrointestinal
cancer syndromes. *Am J Gastroenterol.* 2015;110(2):223–263.
[PMID: 25645574]

van Leerdam ME, Roos VH, van Hooft JE, et al. Endoscopic management of Lynch syndrome and of familial risk of colorectal cancer: European Society of Gastrointestinal Endoscopy
(ESGE) Guideline. *Endoscopy.* 2019;51(11):1082–1093. [PMID:
31597170]

Yang J, Gurudu SR, Koptiuch C, et al. American Society for Gastrointestinal Endoscopy guideline on the role of endoscopy
in familial adenomatous polyposis syndromes. *Gastrointest
Endosc.* 2020;91(5):963–982.e2. [PMID: 32169282]

C. Inflammatory Bowel Disease

The CRC risk is similar in both Crohn's colitis and ulcerative colitis, with an estimated two-fold increase in the risk
of developing CRC compared to the general population. In
addition, longer IBD duration is associated with an increasing cumulative risk of CRC with a 1%, 2%, and 5% risk of
CRC development at 10, 20, and >20 years, respectively.
Furthermore, CRC accounts for 15% of all IBD deaths. Risk
factors for the development of CRC in IBD patients includes
younger age at time of IBD diagnosis, disease duration,
inflammation severity, personal history of primary sclerosing
cholangitis (PSC) or a family history of CRC. United States
based guidelines recommended initial screening colonoscopy 8 years after symptom initiation with colonoscopy surveillance every 1–2 years and yearly surveillance in patients
with PSC. The American Society for Gastrointestinal Endoscopy (ASGE) does allow extending the timing of surveillance
colonoscopy up to every 3 years in patients who have normal
endoscopic and histological findings on a minimum of two
surveillance colonoscopies.

To consider surveillance effective, an extensive biopsy
protocol during colonoscopy should be followed. Experts
recommend that biopsy specimens should be taken every
10 cm in all four quadrants and that additional biopsy specimens should be obtained from anastomotic sites (in cases
of previous colonic resections), strictures, and mass lesions
(other than pseudopolyps). The goal of a surveillance colonoscopy is for the detection of dysplasia. As a result, the
SCENIC International Consensus for the surveillance and
management of dysplasia in IBD patients recommends the
following: (1) when performing white-light colonoscopy,
high definition colonoscopy is recommended rather than
standard-definition colonoscopy, (2) when performing
standard-definition colonoscopy, chromoendoscopy is recommended rather than white-light colonoscopy, (3) when
performing high-definition colonoscopy, chromoendoscopy
is suggested rather than white-light colonoscopy, (4) when
performing standard or high-definition colonoscopy, narrow
band imaging is not recommended as an alternative to white-
light colonoscopy, and (5) when performing image enhanced
high-definition colonoscopy narrow band imaging is not recommended as an alternative to chromoendoscopy.

Dysplasia identified on surveillance colonoscopy is categorized as either visible dysplasia in the setting of targeted
biopsies with macroscopic abnormality or invisible dysplasia
in the setting of random biopsies with macroscopically normal endoscopic evaluation. If a lesion does not appear to be
endoscopically resectable, then the recommendations is to
obtain targeted biopsies and consider tattoo of the lesion with
referral to an advanced endoscopist for potential resection.
After complete resection of a dysplastic polypoid lesion, closer
surveillance colonoscopy based on lesion size and pathology
rather than colectomy is recommended. Furthermore, after
complete resection of a nondysplastic nonpolypoid lesion,
surveillance colonoscopy rather than colectomy is also suggested. For macroscopically normal appearing mucosa with
microscopic dysplasia, reviewed by a GI pathologist, referral
to an endoscopist experienced with IBD surveillance and the
use of chromoendoscopy with high-definition colonoscopy
is recommended. At this time, consensus recommendations
advise that if microscopic dysplasia correlates with a macroscopic dysplastic lesion in that same region, then surveillance
colonoscopy is recommended. However, if there is microscopic dysplasia without a macroscopic correlate lesion then
the risks and benefits of surveillance colonoscopy versus colectomy need to be discussed and individualized for each patient.
Furthermore, it is imperative that pathologic confirmation be
made by an experienced pathologist, with a specialty in IBD
dysplasia, before final management decisions are made.

4. Special Considerations: Hyperplastic & Serrated Polyps

There is no evidence to suggest that hyperplastic polyps are
at increased risk for CRC. Therefore, such patients should
undergo surveillance for CRC similar to that of average-risk
individuals.

However, literature suggests that all hyperplastic polyps
are not histologically similar and that some variants of hyperplastic polyps may evolve into a unique type of adenoma,
called a sessile serrated adenoma/polyp (SSA/P) or traditional
serrated adenoma (TSA). Serrated adenomas are linked to the
development of sporadic adenocarcinoma with MSI, felt to
arise from an alternate molecular pathway characterized by
hypermethylation of genes, known as CIMP. Polyps of this
type are often large, sessile, and located in the proximal colon.
It is important for these neoplastic lesions to be completely
removed. Current US Multi-Society Task Force guidelines
recommend repeat surveillance colonoscopy in 5–10 years if
baseline colonoscopy shows 1–2 SSPs <10 mm, 3–5 years if
there are 3–4 SSPs <10 mm, and 3 years if there are 5–10 SSPs
<10 mm, an SSP ≥10 mm or an SSP with dysplasia.

In addition, there is serrated polyposis syndrome (SPS). Patient's meeting any one of the following World Health Organization (WHO) criteria are defined as having SPS: (1) ≥5 serrated polyps proximal to the sigmoid colon, with ≥2 polyps >10 mm; (2) ≥1 serrated polyp proximal to the sigmoid colon in an individual who has a first-degree relative with SPS; or (3) ≥20 serrated polyps of any size, distributed throughout the colon. Although there seems to be an increased risk of CRC in such individuals, the exact magnitude of risk has not been determined. Surveillance colonoscopy every 1–3 years is recommended with intent to clear the colon of all serrated lesions, or all serrated lesions ≥5 mm in size if there are numerous diminutive lesions. Surgery is indicated if the size and/or number of polyps makes endoscopic control not feasible or when CRC is diagnosed.

Edelstein DL, Cruz-Correa M, Soto-Salgado M, et al. Risk of colorectal and other cancers in patients with serrated polyposis. *Clin Gastroenterol Hepatol.* 2015;13(9):1697–1699. [PMID: 25681317]

Fornaro R, Caratto M, Caratto E, et al. Colorectal cancer in patients with inflammatory bowel disease: the need for a real surveillance program. *Clin Colorectal Cancer.* 2016;15(3):204–212. [PMID: 27083409]

Laine L, Kaltenbach T, Barkun A, et al. SCENIC international consensus statement on surveillance and management of dysplasia in inflammatory bowel disease. *Gastroenterology.* 2015;148(3):639–651.e28. [PMID: 25702852]

Shah SC, Itzkowitz SH. Reappraising risk factors for inflammatory bowel disease-associated neoplasia: implications for colonoscopic surveillance in IBD. *J Crohns Colitis.* 2020;14(8): 1172–1177. [PMID: 32150256]

SCREENING MODALITIES

1. Fecal Occult Blood Testing

FOBT is a noninvasive and inexpensive test that was widely used to detect the presence of occult blood in the stool of asymptomatic persons. Available FOBT includes the standard guaiac test and immunochemical tests (see fecal immunochemical testing section). FOBT primarily detects early CRC or adenomatous polyps with the ability to remove these lesions during colonoscopy. However, FOBT is no longer a preferred CRC screening modality given its lower sensitivity for CRC and adenoma detection compared to fecal immunochemical testing (FIT). FOBT can be considered if FIT testing is not accessible.

2. Fecal Immunochemical Testing

FIT reacts with antibodies that are specific for the globin portion of the human hemoglobin molecule, and therefore, special dietary restrictions to avoid false-positive tests are not needed. Multiple studies have reported that FIT has better sensitivity and specificity than guaiac-based FOBT for the detection of CRC. The US Multi-Society Task Force recommends FIT over FOBT given evidence of higher sensitivity as well as patient adherence of FIT compared to FOBT.

A meta-analysis of FIT for the detection of CRC showed a pooled sensitivity of 75% and specificity of 94%. In addition, the effectiveness of FIT for CRC screening has been shown using "gold standard" endoscopy results for FIT-negative patients. FIT should be best regarded as an early CRC detection test. FIT is recommended annually using a 1-sample screening test. Furthermore, although the quantitative and qualitative FIT are overall similar in neoplasia detection rates, it is recommended to use quantitative tests with a ≤20 μg/g cutoff point for hemoglobin detection. Quantitative FIT has increased quality control given the automated readings and the ability to change the positive threshold value. The set threshold value should be based on multiple factors including cost effectiveness and colonoscopy availability.

Hundt S, Haug U, Brenner H, et al. Comparative evaluation of immunochemical fecal occult blood tests for colorectal adenoma detection. *Ann Intern Med.* 2009;150:162–169. [PMID: 19189905]

Morikawa T, Kato J, Yamaji Y, et al. A comparison of the immunochemical fecal occult blood test and total colonoscopy in the asymptomatic population. *Gastroenterology.* 2005;129:422–428. [PMID: 16083699]

Robertson DJ, Lee JK, Boland CR, et al. Recommendations on fecal immunochemical testing to screen for colorectal neoplasia: a consensus statement by the US Multi-Society Task Force on Colorectal Cancer. *Gastroenterology.* 2017;152(5):1217–1237.e3. [PMID: 27769517]

3. FIT-Fecal DNA Test

The food and drug administration approved FIT-fecal DNA testing as another noninvasive CRC screening modality, which is recommended every 3 years. This test is a combination of both FIT and multi-targeted stool DNA testing to detect genetic abnormalities in fecal samples. Colorectal epithelial cells are shed in stool, and stable DNA can be extracted from stool and amplified using polymerase chain reaction (PCR). This allows for the detection of mutations in numerous genes, including *K-ras*, *APC*, *BAT-26*, and *tp53*, as well as analysis of epigenetic changes such as gene methylation.

Using a fecal DNA test aimed at detecting methylated genes in CRC (Cologuard), 1187 specimens from patients with and without colorectal neoplasia were blindly evaluated. The accuracy of the fecal DNA test was 85.3% for CRC and 63.8% for adenomas greater than 1 cm, with a specificity of 88% for either. CRCs and adenomas were also detected equally in the proximal and distal colon. In addition, the sensitivity of the test was unaffected by patient gender, age, or race. Furthermore, in a more recent study of 9989 participants, multitarget fecal DNA testing demonstrated a sensitivity of 92.3% for CRC, 42.4% for advanced adenomas or SSPs ≥1 cm, and 69.2% for high-grade dysplasia lesions with a test specificity of 86.6–89.8%.

The greatest advantage of FIT-fecal DNA testing is that it has the highest one-time sensitivity among noninvasive and nonimaging CRC screening modalities. However, the greatest disadvantage is the high cost in comparison to FIT testing alone. FIT-fecal DNA testing can be up to 10 times more expensive than FIT testing. FIT-fecal DNA testing also has a decreased specificity compared to FIT testing alone. The specificity decreases with advancing age and is only 83% in individuals >65 years. However, the specificity of FIT-fecal DNA testing performed every 3 years may be comparable to the combined specificity of yearly FIT testing over 3 years.

Overall, FIT-fecal DNA tests still require careful evaluation in future studies as the substantial increased costs compared to other fecal tests remain important barriers to widespread use.

Imperiale TF, Ransohoff DF, Itzkowitz SH, et al. Multitarget stool DNA testing for colorectal-cancer screening. *N Engl J Med.* 2014;370:1287–1297. [PMID: 24645800]

Itzkowitz SH, Jandorf L, Brand R, et al. Improved fecal DNA test for colorectal cancer screening. *Clin Gastroenterol Hepatol.* 2007;5:111–117. [PMID: 17161655]

Sharma T. Analysis of the effectiveness of two noninvasive fecal tests used to screen for colorectal cancer in average-risk adults. *Public Health.* 2020;182:70–76. [PMID: 32179290]

4. Flexible Sigmoidoscopy

FS allows for direct visualization of the distal third of the colon, ideally from the rectum to the splenic flexure. Several randomized control trials have suggested that FS is associated with a 29–76% reduction in cancer incidence and/or mortality resulting from tumors found within reach of the endoscope. A multicenter, randomized controlled trial conducted in the United Kingdom found that in an 11-year follow-up of individuals undergoing a single FS for screening initiated between the ages of 55 and 64, FS substantially reduced CRC incidence and mortality by 33% and 43%, respectively. The reduction noted in this study was less compared to results from prior case-control studies and is attributed to the dominance of screen-detected prevalent cancers within the first 4 years of follow-up. Furthermore, FS had a sustained decrease in CRC incidence and mortality in the long term.

The US Multi-Society Task Force on CRC considers that screening with FS can be performed every 5–10 years for average-risk individuals. However, they ultimately favor 10-year intervals. In contrast, the American Cancer Society recommends a 5 year interval and the US Preventive Task Force recommends a 10 year interval with yearly FIT testing.

To improve the use of FS as a screening modality, certain clinical factors as well as endoscopic findings noted on FS have been considered important predictors of proximal colonic disease. These predictors include demographic factors such as older age, Black race, and female sex as well as the presence of multiple adenomas, any adenoma with villous histology or dysplasia, and a family history of CRC.

Hyperplastic polyps detected on FS are not associated with increased adenoma detection elsewhere in the colon.

The advantages cited for FS are that it is inexpensive, requires no sedation, involves a simple bowel preparation, and can be performed by primary care physicians and nonphysicians, including physician assistants and nurse practitioners. In addition, the risk of perforation is lower than that associated with colonoscopy. However, FS has a lower CRC incidence reduction compared to colonoscopy. Furthermore, the preparation used for colon cleansing prior to FS may be less than optimal, and discomfort in a nonsedated patient may interfere with the completeness of the examination.

Currently, any adenomatous polyp found on FS warrants complete colonic visualization by colonoscopy to exclude the presence of proximal lesions. Such a strategy has been associated with an increase in the adenoma detection rate. However, these findings highlight a major drawback of FS in that it can miss anywhere from 30% to 65% of proximal advanced neoplasia. This may be a particular concern for the use of FS in older patients and females, in whom higher rates of proximal neoplasia have been reported.

A second shortcoming of FS is that one-time adherence with this screening modality is less than colonoscopy. Lastly, low rates of referral for colonoscopy and colonoscopy completion have also been reported, and better measures to assure appropriate follow-up are warranted.

Holme Ø, Løberg M, Kalager M, et al. Long-term effectiveness of sigmoidoscopy screening on colorectal cancer incidence and mortality in women and men: a randomized trial. *Ann Intern Med.* 2018;168(11):775–782. [PMID: 29710125]

Miller EA, Pinsky PF, Schoen RE, Prorok PC, Church TR. Effect of flexible sigmoidoscopy screening on colorectal cancer incidence and mortality: long-term follow-up of the randomised US PLCO cancer screening trial. *Lancet Gastroenterol Hepatol.* 2019;4(2):101–110. [PMID: 30502933]

Rex DK, Boland CR, Dominitz JA, et al. Colorectal cancer screening: recommendations for physicians and patients from the U.S. Multi-Society Task Force on Colorectal Cancer. *Gastroenterology.* 2017;153(1):307–323. [PMID: 28555630]

Selby JV, Friedman GD, Quesenberry CP, et al. A case-control study of screening sigmoidoscopy and mortality from colorectal cancer. *N Engl J Med.* 1992;326:653–657. [PMID: 1736103]

5. Colonoscopy

Colonoscopy is considered by many to be the gold standard for CRC screening. Despite the lack of evidence from large-scale randomized trials of screening colonoscopy, the procedure has been shown in cohort studies to decrease the expected incidence of CRC through the removal of adenomatous polyps. The National Polyp Study (NPS) demonstrated that the removal of adenomas leads to the decreased incidence of CRC and that colonoscopy is the only single test that can provide screening, diagnosis, and treatment. In the NPS, a group of patients who underwent colonoscopy with clearing resection of colonic adenomas had a 76–90% reduction in

CRC compared with reference populations. Given the potential benefits of colonoscopy, multiple gastroenterology professional societies recommend colonoscopy as the preferred modality of screening. Not only is the risk of developing CRC reduced, but the benefits of initial screening colonoscopy are noted for up to 18 years.

Indirect evidence from several studies questions the accuracy of colonoscopy. Multiple studies reveal that 5–8% of patients with CRC have undergone screening colonoscopy within 3–5 years of diagnosis. Several studies have also demonstrated a higher rate of developing interval cancers (1.7–2.4 cases per 1000 person-years) when compared with NPS results (0.6 cases per 1000 person-years). Studies also question the effectiveness of colonoscopy in detecting proximal colonic neoplasia. A large population-based, case-control study using administrative claims data from Ontario, Canada, evaluating the association between colonoscopy and CRC deaths demonstrated that colonoscopy is associated with lower CRC mortality rates. However, the association is primarily limited to deaths from cancer developing in the left side of the colon.

Thus, the question arises whether CRCs in the proximal colon are more frequently missed due to the variability in endoscopists' performance of colonoscopy or because these lesions have different biologic features compared to distal CRCs, including higher rates of MSI and the CIMP, and perhaps these biologic features are overrepresented in interval CRCs. The performance of colonoscopy has been shown to vary by endoscopist, and the individual endoscopist may be a powerful predictor of adenomatous polyps detected during colonoscopy. To improve the accuracy (sensitivity) of colonoscopy for adenoma and CRC detection and standardize its performance among endoscopists, the ASGE and the American College of Gastroenterology Taskforce on Quality in Endoscopy proposed several measurable factors of routine colonoscopy to serve as quality indicators. They prioritize the following three quality indicators for colonoscopy: (1) adenoma detection rates for males and females undergoing screening colonoscopy, (2) adherence to screening/surveillance colonoscopy guidelines in an adequately cleansed colon, and (3) frequency of cecal visualization with photo documentation and notation of appropriate landmarks. The ultimate goal is that the accuracy of colonoscopy can be increased through quality improvement initiatives for enhanced performance of colonoscopy.

Additionally, characteristics of the baseline colonoscopy are an important predictor for subsequent neoplasia. Factors include incomplete colonic examination, polyp size ≥1 cm, any adenoma, or incomplete polyp excision in the region where a subsequent CRC is identified. A prospective study examining the incidence of advanced neoplasia within 5.5 years of screening colonoscopy revealed a strong association between baseline colonoscopy results and the rate of serious incident lesions detected during the surveillance period. It has been shown that the baseline colonoscopy is the most beneficial in that it is responsible for the major benefit of polypectomy and that subsequent examinations may not add significant benefit except in people at high risk for future advanced adenomas. This supports the need to ensure that the baseline colonoscopy is of the highest quality in order to best detect adenomas. In fact, adenoma detection rates are inversely associated with the risks of interval CRC, advanced-stage interval cancer, and fatal interval cancer.

Even though colonoscopy can fail to detect lesions, it is still considered the most sensitive of the screening methods. The advantages of this approach, in addition to the diagnosis and treatment of a lesion in a single session, include a long interval of "protection" in the setting of polypectomy and improved patient satisfaction due to the use of intravenous conscious sedation or monitored anesthesia care. However, colonoscopy involves greater cost and risk than other screening modalities. Serious complications associated with colonoscopy include bleeding and perforation and, while extremely rare, these occur at higher rates than with other screening options. Other disadvantages of colonoscopy include the need for a full bowel preparation, and risks associated with sedation.

Colonoscopy may be the "preferred" screening modality for some, but it is important to emphasize that the evidence for its efficacy is indirect and that there are no randomized controlled trials demonstrating the superiority of colonoscopy to other screening modalities. There is an ongoing randomized control trial that will ultimately evaluate the association between colonoscopy and no screening with CRC incidence and morality. This study is the The Nordic-European Initiative on Colorectal Cancer. This is a population based randomized control trial that is ongoing and assessing the effectiveness of colonoscopy screening for CRC incidence and mortality among an average risk population. The study showed similar adenoma detection rates in both the proximal and distal colon as well as a 0.5%, 10.4%, and 30.7% CRC, advanced adenoma, and all adenoma detection rate, respectively. Analysis of the primary outcome of colonoscopy versus no screening on CRC incidence and CRC mortality is planned at 15-year follow-up.

Lastly, large-scale, comparative effectiveness studies are needed to determine the impact of colonoscopy and other screening modalities on CRC incidence and mortality and whether the burden of right-sided neoplasia can be affected by colonoscopy to justify the associated extra cost and morbidity.

Bretthauer M, Kaminski MF, Løberg M, et al. Population-based colonoscopy screening for colorectal cancer: a randomized clinical trial. *JAMA Intern Med.* 2016;176(7):894–902. [PMID: 27214731]

Corley DA, Jensen CD, Marks AR, et al. Adenoma detection rate and risk of colorectal cancer and death. *N Engl J Med.* 2014;370:1298–1306. [PMID: 24693890]

Rex D. Maximizing detection of adenomas and cancers during colonoscopy. *Am J Gastroenterol.* 2006;101:2866–2877. [PMID: 17227527]

Rex DK, Boland CR, Dominitz JA, et al. Colorectal cancer screening: recommendations for physicians and patients from the U.S. Multi-Society Task Force on Colorectal Cancer. *Gastroenterology.* 2017;153(1):307–323. [PMID: 28555630]

Rex DK, Schoenfeld PS, Cohen J, et al. Quality indicators for colonoscopy. *Am J Gastroenterol.* 2015;110(1):72–90. [PMID: 25448873]

Tollivoro TA, Jensen CD, Marks AR, et al. Index colonoscopy-related risk factors for postcolonoscopy colorectal cancers. *Gastrointest Endosc.* 2019;89(1):168–176.e3. [PMID: 30144415]

ADDITIONAL SCREENING MODALITIES

Noninvasive procedures to screen for CRC are also an option to increase adherence with CRC screening strategies. The 2017 US Multi-society Task Force on Colorectal Cancer includes computed tomographic colonography (CTC) as a CRC screening modality in asymptomatic, average-risk adults aged 50 and older with consideration of video capsule endoscopy (VCE) in specific circumstances.

Rex DK, Boland CR, Dominitz JA, et al. Colorectal cancer screening: recommendations for physicians and patients from the U.S. Multi-Society Task Force on Colorectal Cancer. *Gastroenterology.* 2017;153(1):307–323. [PMID: 28555630]

1. Computed Tomographic Colonography

CTC (or virtual colonoscopy) is an alternative noninvasive test for the examination of the colon. It provides a two- and three-dimensional image of the colon using computer programming to combine data from multiple helical CT scans. CTC requires a colon preparation similar to that used for conventional colonoscopy and involves air insufflation through a rectal tube to distend the colon to enhance imaging. After the examination, a radiologist examines the scans; if an abnormality is noted, patients should undergo colonoscopy.

Results from early studies assessing the accuracy of CTC have found it to be comparable to that of conventional colonoscopy for the detection of polyps greater than 1 cm, with a high sensitivity and specificity of 94% and 96%, respectively. Two recent meta-analyses found that CTC has a pooled sensitivity of 96–97% and pooled specificity of 99–100% for the diagnosis of CRC. In terms of polyp detection, among patients at high risk for CRC, CTC has a sensitivity and specificity of 87% and 90%, respectively for detecting polyps ≥6 mm and 91% and 98%, respectively for detecting polyps ≥10 mm.

There are a number of limitations related to CTC. The false-positive rate is related to retained stool mistaken for polyps, diverticular disease that limits colon distensibility, and thickened colonic folds mistaken for lesions. CTC is also not therapeutic, as polyps cannot be removed, and masses cannot be sampled for tissue diagnosis during the procedure. Furthermore, 27–69% of patients undergoing CTC will have an incidental finding and 5–37% will have findings warranting further diagnostic evaluation. This may increase patient anxiety and lead to an increase in medical costs, given that the majority of incidental findings are expected to be benign.

CTC is an acceptable option for CRC screening in average-risk adults aged 50 and older due to the available data supporting its efficacy. The US Multi-Society Task Force recommends 5-year intervals for repeat screening in patients with normal CTC. However, patients that have one or more polyps ≥6 mm should be referred for colonoscopy. There is also a need for multidisciplinary consensus regarding the management of polyps smaller than 6 mm, particularly given the low malignancy potential for diminutive polyps. For example, a recent study analyzed the histology of small and diminutive polyps using a prospectively collected colonoscopy and polyp database. They found that among approximately 36,000 polyps that were ≤5 mm in size 2.1% had advanced histology and 0% had cancerous pathology. Furthermore, among 6523 polyps 6–9 mm in size 5.6% had advanced histology and 0% had cancerous pathology.

In terms of the safety profile for CTC, the primary disadvantage continues to be exposure to ionized radiation. However, it is estimated that for every radiation induced cancer 24–35 CRCs could be prevented with routine 5-year CTC screening. Furthermore, there is ongoing development of reduced radiation dosage CTC strategies, which will allow for decreased radiation exposure.

CTC continues to be a cost-effective approach to CRC screening compared to no screening. However, for effective implementation of CRC screening, the evolving technology needs to be standardized along with the reporting of findings. Additional information is also needed regarding the long-term follow up of extracolonic findings. Lastly, the federal Medicare program does not currently provide reimbursement for the use of CTC for routine screening but will cover diagnostic CTC reimbursement in cases of previously failed colonoscopy.

Bai W, Yu D, Zhu B, et al. Diagnostic accuracy of computed tomography colonography in patients at high risk for colorectal cancer: a meta-analysis. *Colorectal Dis.* 2020;22(11):1528–1537. [PMID: 32277562]

Chin M, Mendelson R, Edwards J, et al. Computed tomographic colonography: prevalence, nature, and clinical significance of extracolonic findings in a community screening program. *Am J Gastroenterol.* 2005;100:2271–2276. [PMID: 16393234]

Cotton PB, Durkalski VL, Pineau BC, et al. Computed tomographic colonography (virtual colonoscopy): a multicenter comparison with standard colonoscopy for detection of colorectal neoplasia. *JAMA.* 2004;291:1713–1719. [PMID: 15082698]

Gao Y, Wang J, Lv H, et al. Diagnostic value of magnetic resonance and computed tomography colonography for the diagnosis of colorectal cancer: a systematic review and meta-analysis. *Medicine (Baltimore).* 2019;98(39):e17187. [PMID: 31574825]

Lin JS, Piper MA, Perdue LA, et al. Screening for colorectal cancer: updated evidence report and systematic review for the US Preventive Services Task Force [published correction appears in JAMA. 2016 Aug 2;316(5):545] [published correction appears in JAMA. 2016 Oct 4;316(13):1412]. *JAMA.* 2016;315(23): 2576–2594. [PMID: 27305422]

Sun S, Yang C, Huang Z, et al. Diagnostic value of magnetic resonance versus computed tomography colonography for colorectal cancer: a PRISMA-compliant systematic review and meta-analysis. *Medicine (Baltimore).* 2018;97(22):e10883. [PMID: 29851808]

2. Video Capsule Endoscopy

VCE is a noninvasive modality to visualize the digestive tract and is typically utilized as a diagnostic test to further evaluate the small bowel. VCE should be considered when there is need for further evaluation of the proximal colon due to an incomplete colonoscopy or among patients that are unable to undergo a colonoscopy or obtain sedation.

CRC screening with VCE should be performed every 5 years. However, among average risk adults, VCE alone is not a recommended CRC screening option.

A video capsule is a disposable pill sized camera that is ingested by the patient and takes thousands of photographs as it travels throughout the digestive tract. All the photographs are transmitted to a wireless recording device that a patient wears. Ultimately, the patient returns the recording device 8 hours after video capsule ingestion and the images are uploaded for further review by a specialist. The patient eventually passes the VCE, which can be safely flushed.

A prospective study evaluating VCE as a screening modality among 884 patients, showed that VCE has an 88% sensitivity and 82% specificity for the detection of one or more adenomas ≥6 mm. VCE also has a 92% sensitivity and 95% specificity for the detection of one or more adenomas ≥10 mm. However, VCE SSP detection is not effective with only a 29% sensitivity for polyps ≥6 mm. Furthermore, among 9% of patients undergoing VCE, VCE was inadequate due to poor bowel preparation as well as short transit time, not allowing for complete pictographic colonic evaluation.

The largest advantage of VCE is that it is a noninvasive modality. However, disadvantages include the required bowel preparation and need for conventional colonoscopy with repeat bowel preparation if polyps are identified. It is important to note that VCE is also not reimbursed as a CRC screening option.

Rex DK, Adler SN, Aisenberg J, et al. Accuracy of capsule colonoscopy in detecting colorectal polyps in a screening population. *Gastroenterology.* 2015;148(5):948–957. [PMID: 25620668]

SUMMARY OF RECOMMENDATIONS

CRC is a preventable cancer. The appropriate identification of individuals at risk dictates the necessary screening and surveillance approach and plays an important role in decreasing CRC incidence and mortality. There are several acceptable options presently available for CRC screening, and they provide the means to improve screening adherence. High-quality colonoscopy is currently considered the preferred modality given its ability to detect and remove adenomatous polyps, which in turn decreases CRC incidence and related mortality.

Hereditary Gastrointestinal Cancer Syndromes

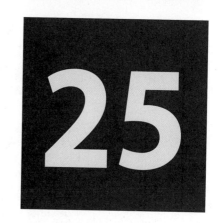

25

Nicolette J. Rodriguez, MD, MPH

Sapna Syngal, MD, MPH

Elena M. Stoffel, MD, MPH

ESSENTIALS OF DIAGNOSIS

▶ Approximately 10% of colorectal cancers (CRCs) are caused by deleterious germline variants associated with cancer predisposition.

▶ Genetic testing is clinically available for several hereditary gastrointestinal cancer syndromes and can be used to guide cancer screening recommendations.

▶ General Considerations

The majority of cases of gastrointestinal cancer are believed to be sporadic events; however, inherited factors play a role in the development of some tumors, with an estimated 10% being attributable to deleterious germline variants. Hereditary gastrointestinal cancer syndromes convey a markedly increased risk for developing cancer and require specific strategies for diagnosis and management.

Identification of hereditary gastrointestinal cancer syndromes requires a thorough evaluation of patients' personal and family history of cancer. Clinical genetic testing can be useful in confirming the diagnosis of certain hereditary cancer syndromes and guiding cancer screening for family members. Tables 25–1 and 25–2 summarize clinical characteristics and cancer screening recommendations for the hereditary gastrointestinal cancer syndromes discussed in detail in this chapter.

Robson ME, Bradbury AR, Arun B, et al. American Society of Clinical Oncology policy statement update: genetic and genomic testing for cancer susceptibility. *J Clin Oncol.* 2015;33(31): 3660–3667. [PMID: 26324357]

Syngal S, Brand RE, Church JM, et al. ACG clinical guideline: genetic testing and management of hereditary gastrointestinal cancer syndromes. *Am J Gastroenterol* 2015;110:223–262. [PMID: 25645574]

HEREDITARY COLORECTAL CANCER SYNDROMES

CRC is the most common gastrointestinal malignancy, with an estimated 147,950 new cases diagnosed in the US in 2020. Although most CRC patients do not have a striking family history of CRC, approximately 30% report having one or more family members with a diagnosis of CRC. The lifetime risk of developing CRC is approximately 4.6% among males and 4.2% among females; however, individuals who have a first-degree relative with CRC have 2–4 times the risk of developing colorectal neoplasia compared with individuals who have no family history of CRC. For individuals with numerous relatives with CRC, the cancer risk may be markedly higher; those who have deleterious germline variants in genes involved in mismatch repair (MMR) or tumor suppression have a lifetime CRC risk ranging from 20% to 100% in the absence of medical intervention.

Identification of patients at risk for hereditary CRC syndromes relies on careful family history evaluation, because many individuals may not demonstrate a characteristic phenotype. As a result, universal testing for MMR and microsatellite instability (MSI) is recommended in all newly diagnosed CRC in order to identify Lynch syndrome patients. Cancer risk stratification for every patient should involve eliciting a family history of cancers, including type of cancer and age of onset as well as family history of colorectal adenomas. Individuals whose family history includes multiple individuals with cancer, individuals diagnosed with two or more primary cancers or with tumors diagnosed at young ages, should undergo a more extensive family history evaluation of first-, second-, and third-degree relatives to determine whether there is evidence of an autosomal-dominant or autosomal-recessive pattern of inheritance. Understanding tumor/polyp genotype-phenotype allows providers to tailor surveillance and treatment options based on individual and familial risk assessment.

Table 25–1. Clinical characteristics of hereditary gastrointestinal (GI) cancer syndromes.

Syndrome	Clinical Features	Gene(s)	Genetic Testing Available
Lynch syndrome	High risk for colorectal, GI and extracolonic cancers (brain, endometrial, ovarian, urinary tract, sebaceous skin tumors) Young ages at cancer diagnosis Accelerated adenoma—carcinoma sequence CRC tumors demonstrate microsatellite instability	DNA mismatch repair (MMR) genes (*MLH1, MSH2, MSH6, PMS2, TACSTD1/EPCAM*)	Yes
Familial adenomatous polyposis (FAP)	Hundreds to thousands of colorectal adenomas appearing in second or third decade CRC risk 100% if colon is not removed Increased risk for duodenal and ampullary adenocarcinoma Risk of gastric cancer Risk of desmoid tumors	Tumor-suppressor gene *APC* Base excision repair gene *MutYH* biallelic germline variants (autosomal recessive)	Yes
Attenuated polyposis/ MutYH-associated polyposis (MAP)	10–100 colorectal adenomas High risk for CRC ± Upper gastrointestinal adenomas	Tumor -suppressor gene *APC* Base excision repair gene *MutYH* (autosomal recessive)	Yes
Peutz-Jeghers syndrome (PJS)	Hamartomatous polyps in GI tract (symptoms of abdominal pain, bleeding, intussusception) Pigmented lesions on lips Increased risk for GI cancers, breast cancer, ovarian cancer, pancreatic cancer, sex cord tumors	Tumor-suppressor gene *STK11*	Yes
Juvenile polyposis	≥5 juvenile polyps in colon and multiple in GI tract (symptoms of abdominal pain, bleeding, anemia) Family history of GI cancers Increased risk for CRC and other GI cancers Associated with congenital cardiac abnormalities	Tumor-suppressor genes *SMAD4, BMPR1A*	Yes
PTEN Hamartoma Tumor Syndrome (PHTS)	Hamartomatous polyps Increased risk for breast, endometrial, thyroid cancers and renal cell carcinoma Macrocephaly	Tumor-suppressor gene *PTEN*	Yes
Hereditary diffuse gastric cancer	Diffuse infiltrative adenocarcinoma of the stomach (linitis plastica) Increased risk for breast cancer	Tumor-suppressor gene *e-cadherin/CDH1*	Yes
Familial pancreatic cancer	Two or more family members with pancreatic cancer May be present as part of other hereditary cancer syndromes, eg, breast/ovarian cancer (HBOC), melanoma (FAMMM), or colorectal/gynecologic cancers (Lynch syndrome; Peutz-Jeghers syndrome)	*BRCA1/2* (HBOC) *STK11* (PJS) *P16/CDKN2A* (FAMMM) MMR genes (Lynch syndrome) *PRSS1, SPINK1* (hereditary pancreatitis)	Yes

CRC, colorectal cancer; FAMMM, familiar atypical multiple mole melanoma; HBOC, hereditary breast/ovarian cancer; PJS, Peutz-Jeghers syndrome.

Recent data suggest that 10% of CRCs are caused by deleterious germline variants associated with cancer predisposition.

1. Lynch Syndrome

Lynch syndrome, previously referred to as hereditary non-polyposis colorectal cancer (HNPCC), is the most common hereditary CRC syndrome and is estimated to account for approximately 3% of CRC cases. This syndrome was first described by Dr. Henry Lynch in families in which multiple cases of CRC were diagnosed at young ages. The original Lynch syndrome families were classified as having three or more cases of CRC with at least one diagnosed before age 50, as described by the Amsterdam criteria. However, additional studies have demonstrated that the cancer spectrum

Table 25–2. Cancer screening recommendations for hereditary gastrointestinal cancer syndromes.

Syndrome	Screening Test	Frequency
Lynch syndrome	1. Colonoscopy 2. Upper endoscopy 3. Pelvic exam, transvaginal ultrasound and endometrial biopsy (females)	1. Every 1–2 years beginning at age 20–25 for *MLH1*, *MSH2* or *EPCAM* Lynch syndrome; Every 1–2 years beginning at age 30–35 for *MSH6* or *PMS2* Lynch syndrome 2. Consider every 3–5 years, beginning at age 30–35 3. Annually, beginning at age 30–35
Familial adenomatous polyposis (FAP)	1. Colonoscopy until polyps are too numerous to remove, then surgical colectomy 2. Upper endoscopy with side-viewing instrument 3. Thyroid ultrasound	1. Annually, beginning at age 10–12 2. Every 3 m–4 y, depending on polyp burden, beginning when colonic polyps develop or age 20–25 years; whichever is first 3. Beginning in late teens, every 2–5 years
Attenuated polyposis (AFAP)	1. Colonoscopy 2. Upper endoscopy with side-viewing instrument 3. Thyroid ultrasound	1. Every 1–2 years, beginning in late teens, frequency varies, depending on number of polyps and rate of polyp growth 2. Every 3 m–4 y, depending on polyp burden, beginning at age 25–30 3. Beginning in late teens, every 2–5 years
MutYH-associated polyposis (MAP);	1. Colonoscopy 2. Upper endoscopy with side-viewing instrument;	1. Every 1–2 years, beginning at age 25–30 2. Every 3 m–4 y, depending on polyp burden, beginning at age 30–35
Peutz-Jeghers syndrome (PJS)	1. Upper endoscopy 2. Small bowel imaging (video capsule endoscopy, CT or MRI enterography) 3. Colonoscopy 4. Imaging of pancreas (endoscopic ultrasound or MRCP) 5. Mammogram and breast MRI 6. Pelvic exam and pap smear 7. Testicular exam	1. Every 2–3 years, beginning in late teens 2. Every 2–3 years, beginning at age 8–10 3. Every 2–3 years, beginning in late teens 4. Annually, beginning at age 30–35 5. Annually, starting at age 30 (females) with bi-annual clinical breast exam 6. Annually, starting at age 18–20 years (females) 7. Annually, starting at 10 years (males)
Juvenile polyposis	1. Colonoscopy 2. Upper endoscopy	1. Every 2–3 years, starting at age 15, with shorter intervals based one polyp number, size and pathology 2. Every 2–3 years, starting at age 15, with shorter intervals based one polyp number, size and pathology
PTEN Hamartoma Tumor Syndrome (PHTS)	1. Colonoscopy 2. Mammogram ± breast tomosynthesis or breast MRI with contrast 3. Endometrial biopsy 4. Renal ultrasound 5. Skin exam 6. Thyroid ultrasound	1. Every 5 years, starting at age 35 2. Annually for females beginning at age 30–35 with a clinical breast exam every 6–12 months beginning at age 25 3. Considered every 1–2 years beginning age 35 4. Consider every 1–2 years beginning at age 40 5. Annually 6. Beginning at age seven
Hereditary diffuse gastric cancer	1. Upper endoscopy; prophylactic gastrectomy 2. Breast MRI	1. Prophylactic gastrectomy recommended between ages 18 and 40; screening endoscopy every 6–12 months for patients who do not undergo prophylactic gastrectomy 2. Annually beginning at age 30; mammogram also recommended beginning at age 40 and can be considered beginning age 35–40
Familial pancreatic cancer	1. Endoscopic ultrasound and/or or MRI/MRCP	1. Annually; age of screening depends on clinical phenotype and/or deleterious germline variant

CT, computed tomography; MRCP, magnetic resonance cholangiopancreatography; MRI, magnetic resonance imaging.

Family History

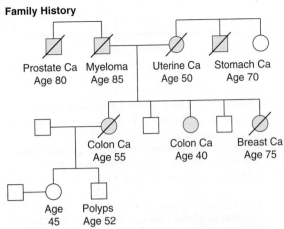

▲ **Figure 25–1.** Pedigree of a family fulfilling modified Amsterdam criteria for hereditary nonpolyposis colorectal cancer (HNPCC)/Lynch syndrome. Ca, cancer.

in these families includes other cancers, such as extra-colonic gastrointestinal, gynecologic, urinary tract, brain and sebaceous neoplasms of the skin. Because as many as 50% of families with Lynch syndrome do not meet the classic Amsterdam criteria or other clinical criteria such as the Bethesda guidelines, recent emphasis has shifted toward clinical prediction models as well as systematic screening approaches such as tumor testing for MSI, as detailed later in this chapter. Lynch syndrome should be suspected in families that have multiple relatives affected with CRC or related extracolonic tumors, or both, and in individuals who are diagnosed with CRC at a young age, have synchronous or metachronous CRCs, or develop multiple Lynch-associated tumors. Figure 25–1 shows a pedigree of a family fulfilling criteria for Lynch syndrome.

▶ Clinical Findings

A. Physical Features

CRC is usually the predominant cancer in most families with Lynch syndrome. Initial studies suggested that the mean age of onset of CRC was approximately 44 years; however, there is wide variation in ages of diagnosis among families. Although colonic tumors in Lynch syndrome are often right-sided, many patients develop tumors in the left colon and rectum. Synchronous or metachronous tumors are common, and any individual diagnosed with two primary colon cancers, or two cancers in the Lynch syndrome tumor spectrum, warrants evaluation for Lynch syndrome. Although Lynch syndrome has been referred to as HNPCC, most of the CRCs do appear to arise from adenomatous polyps, although these polyps may be few in number and can often be small and flat. The colorectal adenoma–carcinoma sequence appears to be accelerated in Lynch syndrome, with an estimated adenoma to cancer transformation time of less than 3 years. There

are also many reports of tumors arising within 3 years of a normal colonoscopy. Histopathologic features seen in colon tumors in Lynch syndrome include poorly differentiated carcinomas, tumor infiltrating lymphocytes, Crohn-like inflammatory reaction, mucinous carcinomas with signet ring cells, and most exhibit features of defective DNA mismatch repair (see Genetic Features).

Endometrial (uterine) cancer is the second most common cancer described in Lynch syndrome families; in some families, cases of endometrial cancers may outnumber CRC. In 51% of females with Lynch Syndrome endometrial or ovarian cancer is the sentinel cancer with mean age of diagnosis at 44 years old. Females with Lynch syndrome have up to a 60% lifetime risk for developing endometrial cancer compared to only 3.1% of females in the general population. The lifetime risks for developing other Lynch-associated cancers, such as urinary tract cancers, ovarian cancer, and other gastrointestinal cancers (stomach, pancreas, small intestine), are also increased for individuals with Lynch syndrome and are estimated to be between 10% and 20%. Brain tumors (eg, glioblastomas and astrocytomas) have been described in the Turcot syndrome variant of Lynch syndrome. Cutaneous sebaceous adenomas and sebaceous carcinomas are rare skin tumors seen in the Muir-Torre variant, and it is currently recommended that any individual affected with sebaceous neoplasms of the skin undergo evaluation for Lynch syndrome regardless of their family history.

However, classic Amsterdam families with multiple CRC diagnoses may include not only Lynch syndrome families, but also families with familial colorectal cancer type X (FCCTX). FCCTX is defined as families who meet Amsterdam I criteria, but whose CRC tumors are MMR proficient and no deleterious germline variant has been identified. Like Lynch syndrome, FCCTX families have multiple cases of CRC with an apparent autosomal-dominant pattern of inheritance. Affected individuals have an older mean age of first CRC diagnosis (56.1 years) and tumors occur most commonly in the rectum or sigmoid. Furthermore, there does not appear to be an increased risk for extracolonic cancers.

B. Genetic Features

The increased predisposition to developing cancer in Lynch syndrome is the result of deleterious germline variants in genes involved in DNA MMR including *MLH1, MSH2, TACSTD1/EPCAM, MSH6,* and *PMS2.* In one Icelandic study, 96% of the identified MMR alterations in Lynch syndrome families were in *MSH6* or *PMS2.*

The protein products of MMR genes are involved in identifying and repairing errors that arise during DNA replication. In the setting of defective MMR gene function, these errors accumulate in segments of DNA containing repeated sequences known as microsatellites. DNA errors that disrupt the function of genes involved in growth regulation can lead to the development of tumors. A characteristic of defective MMR gene function is MSI. Immunohistochemical (IHC) analysis of tumors for expression of MMR proteins *MLH1, MSH2, MSH6,* and *PMS2* frequently reveals loss of staining of the protein corresponding to the gene with the deleterious germline variant.

Tumors due to MSI can be divided into two MSI phenotypes: MSI-high (MSI-H) and MSI-negative (low or stable). Fifteen percent of CRC displays MSI-H and includes sporadic MSI-H CRC (12%) and Lynch syndrome (3%). CRC tumor specimens can be tested for features of defective MMR by demonstrating MSI and/or loss of staining for *MLH1, MSH2, MSH6,* and *PMS2* proteins by IHC. As a result, this pathologic testing can serve as a prescreening method to select individuals who should undergo germline testing for MMR deleterious germline variants. Tumors demonstrating loss of MLH1 expression should undergo testing for somatic *BRAF* variants and/or *MLH1* promoter hypermethylation. Universal tumor testing of newly diagnosed CRC patients for evidence of defective MMR is recommended. This approach has been shown to be cost-effective and has greater sensitivity for identification of Lynch syndrome compared with other strategies, including selective tumor testing and use of clinical criteria and prediction models.

C. Clinical Genetic Evaluation

Genetic testing for MMR deleterious germline variants associated with Lynch syndrome is available in clinical settings and provides the opportunity to confirm the diagnosis of Lynch syndrome in a family and to test other individuals in order to stratify their cancer risk. Cost-effectiveness models support the use of genetic testing for cancer risk stratification in Lynch syndrome families, and evidence suggests knowledge of a deleterious germline variant makes individuals more likely to adhere to intense cancer screening required for cancer prevention.

The most efficient strategy for genetic testing is to begin the genetic evaluation with an individual who has a cancer diagnosis. For individuals who do not have a cancer diagnosis or tumor specimens available for MSI or IHC testing, there are risk assessment models that can be used to estimate the likelihood of Lynch syndrome. The PREMM(5) model is a web-based clinical prediction algorithm that uses data from patients' personal and family history to estimate the probability that an individual carries a deleterious germline variant in the *MLH1, MSH2, MSH6, PMS2,* and *EPCAM* genes (available from the Dana-Farber Cancer Institute, at https://premm.dfci.harvard.edu). Individuals whose personal and family history produces a PREMM(5) model score of ≥2.5% should be referred for genetic evaluation for Lynch syndrome. MMRpro and MMRpredict are other web-based models that can be used for similar risk stratification to identify individuals who would benefit from genetic testing (available at http://www4.utsouthwestern.edu/breasthealth/cagene/ and http://hnpccpredict.hgu.mrc.ac.uk respectively).

Next-generation sequencing (NGS), also known as multigene testing, allows for syndrome specific panels (eg, Lynch syndrome), cancer specific panels (eg, tests for multiple genes associated with a specific cancer such as CRC or breast cancer) or comprehensive cancer panels (eg, tests for multiple genes associated with various cancers or cancer syndromes). If testing reveals a deleterious germline variant in any of these genes, then testing is considered informative, and germline-specific testing can be offered to other family members to determine who has and has not inherited the genetic predisposition to cancer. If testing in a cancer-affected individual fails to reveal a deleterious germline variant, then genetic testing is considered uninformative, and a clinical determination must be made about whether the suspicion for Lynch syndrome is sufficiently high to recommend Lynch syndrome cancer surveillance to all members of the family. Importantly, genetic testing should be performed after genetic counseling.

The difficulties in interpreting and explaining uninformative genetic testing results, the complexities of family dynamics, and concerns about genetic discrimination are challenges in clinical genetic testing. Federal legislation, the Genetic Information Nondiscrimination Act of 2008 (GINA) prohibits genetic information discrimination in health insurance and employment.

Burn J, Sheth H, Elliott F, et al. Cancer prevention with aspirin in hereditary colorectal cancer (Lynch syndrome), 10-year follow-up and registry-based 20-year data in the CAPP2 study: a double-blind, randomised, placebo-controlled trial. *Lancet.* 2020;395(10240):1855–1863. [PMID: 32534647]

Choi YH, Lakhal-Chaieb L, Król A, et al. Risks of colorectal cancer and cancer-related mortality in familial colorectal cancer type X and Lynch syndrome families. *J Natl Cancer Inst.* 2019;111(7):675-683. [PMID: 30380125]

Giardiello FM, Allen JI, Axilbund JE, et al. Guidelines on genetic evaluation and management of Lynch syndrome: a consensus statement by the US Multisociety Task Force on colorectal cancer. *Gastroenterology.* 2014;147:502–526. [PMID: 25043945]

Haraldsdottir S, Rafnar T, Frankel WL, et al. Comprehensive population-wide analysis of Lynch syndrome in Iceland reveals founder mutations in MSH6 and PMS2. *Nat Commun.* 2017;8:14755. Published 2017 May 3. [PMID: 28466842]

Kastrinos F, Uno H, Ukaegbu C, et al. Development and validation of the PREMM$_5$ Model for Comprehensive Risk Assessment of Lynch Syndrome. *J Clin Oncol.* 2017;35(19):2165–2172. [PMID: 28489507]

▶ Management

The high lifetime risk of colorectal and other extracolonic cancers, the accelerated progression of adenomas to adenocarcinomas, and the young age of onset of colorectal neoplasia require specialized strategies for cancer prevention.

A. Colorectal Cancer Screening

Individuals with *MLH1, MSH2,* and *EPCAM* Lynch syndrome should begin having colonoscopies at age 20–25, with repeat examinations every 1–2 years. However, earlier initiation of screening is recommended 2–5 years before the youngest age of diagnosis of CRC in the family if diagnosed before age 25. On the other hand, individuals with *MSH6* or *PMS2* Lynch syndrome may begin having colonoscopies at age 30–35, with repeat examinations every 1–2 years. However, earlier initiation of screening is recommended 2–5 years before the youngest age of diagnosis of CRC in the family if diagnosed before age 30. The need for a shorter interval between examinations became evident from data showing a reduction in CRC mortality for individuals who had colonoscopies every 3 years; though, cancers were still detected during that screening interval. The endoscopist should be vigilant for small or flat lesions, which may be associated with higher malignant potential in Lynch syndrome patients than in the general population.

Aspirin may be beneficial in reducing the risk of colon cancer in Lynch syndrome patients, although the mechanism of action regarding CRC reduction is unknown. Ongoing research is underway to establish the optimal dose and duration while taking into account risk of adverse events. The use of aspirin in Lynch syndrome is an individualized decision based on risks and benefits and the current evidence is not yet sufficient to make a recommendation for standard use.

B. Gynecologic Cancer Screening

Females at risk or affected by Lynch syndrome should be offered screening for gynecologic cancers beginning at age 30–35 with pelvic examination, transvaginal ultrasound, and endometrial biopsy. At present, there are no data to support the efficacy of this gynecologic screening regimen, and females who have completed childbearing (or at age 40) should be counseled to consider prophylactic hysterectomy and oophorectomy as a more definitive measure for cancer risk reduction.

C. Gastric & Small Bowel Cancer Screening

Screening for gastric cancer and small intestinal cancer using upper endoscopy with biopsy of the gastric antrum has been proposed beginning at age 30–35, with treatment of *Helicobacter pylori* infection when found. Upper endoscopy is also used to closely evaluate the duodenum. Subsequent surveillance every 3–5 years can be considered based on family history of gastric or duodenal cancer.

D. Dermatologic Screening

Individuals with Lynch syndrome from families with Muir-Torre should have annual dermatologic examinations to screen for cutaneous sebaceous neoplasms.

E. Pancreatic Cancer Screening

Annual screening with magnetic resonance imaging (MRI)/magnetic resonance cholangiopancreatography (MRCP) and/or endoscopic ultrasound (EUS) can be considered in patients with more than one first- or second-degree relative with exocrine pancreatic cancer on the same side of the family as the known deleterious germline variant. Screening should start at age 50 or 10 years prior to the youngest family member diagnosed with an exocrine pancreatic cancer.

F. Surgical Options

For Lynch syndrome patients without pathologic findings on colonoscopy or those who have endoscopically resectable adenomas, follow-up colonoscopy is recommended every 1–2 years. Based on clinical diagnosis a segmental or extended colectomy is recommended for patients with colonic adenocarcinoma or adenomas not amenable to endoscopic resection. Individuals with remaining colon or rectum after surgery should then have surveillance of their residual colonic mucosa every 1–2 years. Furthermore, a proctocolectomy or total proctocolectomy may be considered for patients with rectal adenocarcinoma.

National Comprehensive Cancer Network. NCCN clinical practice guidelines in oncology: genetic/familial high-risk assessment: colorectal. V 1.2020. Available at: http://www.nccn.org/professionals/. Accessed August 2020.

Stoffel EM, Kastrinos F. Familial colorectal cancer, beyond Lynch syndrome. *Clin Gastroenterol Hepatol.* 2014;12:1059–1068. [PMID: 23962553]

Syngal S, Brand RE, Church JM, et al. ACG clinical guideline: Genetic testing and management of hereditary gastrointestinal cancer syndromes. *Am J Gastroenterol.* 2015;110(2):223–263. [PMID: 25645574]

2. Familial Adenomatous Polyposis

FAP is the second most common inherited CRC syndrome. An individual with the classic FAP phenotype has hundreds to thousands of adenomatous polyps in the colon, with a nearly 100% risk of developing CRC by middle age if their colon is not surgically removed. FAP accounts for approximately 1% of CRC cases. The incidence of FAP is approximately one in 7000–30,000 persons. Although most cases arise in families with a known history through autosomal-dominant inheritance, approximately 20–30% of cases emerge as de novo deleterious germline variants in the *adenomatous polyposis coli* (*APC*) gene. Furthermore, biallelic germline variants in the base excision repair gene *MutYH* can produce an autosomal-recessive inheritance pattern, which accounts for less than 1% of CRC cases. Consequently, absence of a family history of polyposis does not exclude FAP.

▶ Clinical Finding

A. Physical Features

Most individuals with classic familial polyposis develop hundreds to thousands of colorectal adenomas. These adenomas are usually discovered during endoscopic evaluation for symptoms such as bleeding or diarrhea, or during routine screening in individuals with a known family history of FAP. Unfortunately, affected individuals who do not undergo early endoscopic evaluation and prophylactic colectomy often present with CRC by the fourth decade of life.

After adenocarcinoma of the colorectum, duodenal and ampullary adenocarcinoma is the second leading cause of cancer death for FAP patients. Fundic gland polyps are also seen in the majority of FAP patients and occur predominantly in the proximal stomach (gastric fundus or body). There has been a recent increase in the incidence of gastric cancer among individuals with FAP, with 40% more cases than the general population. As a result, an endoscopic classification system has been developed to identify high-risk gastric polyps in FAP patients.

Extracolonic manifestations associated with FAP include nasopharyngeal angiofibromas, dental abnormalities, papillary thyroid cancer, adrenal tumors, osteomas in any part of the skeleton, central nervous system tumors (Turcot syndrome), as well as skin and soft tissue manifestations including epidermal cysts, fibromas, and desmoid fibromatosis. Congenital hypertrophy of the retinal pigment epithelium (CHRPE) is an ophthalmologic finding that should prompt evaluation for FAP. Although not considered malignancies, desmoid tumors can result in significant morbidity when they involve the mesentery and vasculature. Desmoid tumors define the Gardner syndrome variant of FAP.

Children have an increased risk of developing hepatoblastomas. Screening can be considered every three to six months from birth until age five with α–fetoprotein and liver ultrasound.

B. Genetic Features

Approximately two-thirds of FAP cases are caused by deleterious germline variants in the *APC* gene. Although most individuals with deleterious germline variants in the *APC* gene inherited them from an affected parent, approximately one-third of patients with FAP have new deleterious germline variants in the *APC* gene and consequently do not have a family history of the disease.

The *APC* gene functions as a tumor suppressor. Loss of *APC* function in colonic epithelial cells is the first step toward neoplastic transformation, and somatic variants in *APC* can be found in 80% of sporadic colon cancer tumors. Germline variants in the *APC* gene are almost 100% penetrant and most of these patients develop hundreds to thousands of colorectal adenomas.

Deleterious germline variants in the *APC* gene are detected in more than 90% of patients with the classic FAP phenotype. Up to 30% of individuals with classic polyposis phenotypes without detectable *APC* deleterious germline variants may have biallelic germline variants in *MutYH*, a base excision repair gene.

Attenuated phenotypes include autosomal-dominant AFAP and autosomal-recessive *MutYH* associated polyposis (MAP), with patients typically developing <100 polyps.

The number of polyps associated with autosomal-recessive *NTHL* associated polyposis (NAP) and autosomal-dominant polymerase proofreading associated polyposis (PPAP) with deleterious germline variants in *POLD1* or *POLE* has not been fully elucidated.

▶ Management

A. Screening

Patients at risk of developing FAP should begin annual colorectal screening for polyps with colonoscopy beginning at age 10–12. Most affected individuals will develop colorectal adenomas during their teenage years or early 20s. Once colorectal adenomas are too numerous to be removed endoscopically, surgical removal of the colon is required. Total proctocolectomy with ileoanal anastomosis is the preferred surgical approach. Other less-extensive surgeries, such as total colectomy with ileorectal anastomosis, leave some colonic mucosa behind that is at risk for neoplastic transformation and requires frequent endoscopies. There should also be a discussion regarding the risks and benefits of chemopreventive agents, such as aspirin, to control the growth of polyps.

Once patients are found to have colorectal adenomas or are 20–25 years, whichever comes first, upper endoscopy is recommended to assess for adenomas in the duodenum and ampulla. A side-viewing upper endoscope should be used to examine the ampulla and perform biopsies. Duodenal or ampullary adenomas can be managed through endoscopic resection or medications (COX-2 inhibitors, sulindac, sulindac/erlotinib, eflornithine) to reduce polyp burden. In rare cases, extensive adenomatous involvement, severe dysplasia, or adenocarcinoma is present, which requires surgical resection of the duodenum.

Patients with FAP are at increased risk for papillary thyroid cancer, and some guidelines recommend screening with thyroid ultrasound beginning in late teens every 2–5 years.

Family members of individuals with FAP should be offered genetic testing for the deleterious germline variant identified in the family in order to stratify their risk. In cases in which an individual does not undergo genetic testing; at-risk family members should undergo colorectal screening with annual colonoscopy starting at age 10–15.

Burke CA, Dekker E, Lynch P, et al. Eflornithine plus sulindac for prevention of progression in familial adenomatous polyposis. *N Engl J Med.* 2020;383(11):1028–1039. [PMID: 32905675]

Mankaney G, Leone P, Cruise M, et al. Gastric cancer in FAP: a concerning rise in incidence. *Fam Cancer.* 2017;16(3):371–376. [PMID: 28185118]

National Comprehensive Cancer Network. NCCN clinical practice guidelines in oncology: genetic/familial high-risk assessment: colorectal. V 1.2020. Available at: http://www.nccn.org/professionals/. Accessed August 2020.

Samadder NJ, Neklason DW, Boucher KM, et al. Effect of sulindac and erlotinib vs placebo on duodenal neoplasia in familial adenomatous polyposis: a randomized clinical trial. JAMA. 2016;315(12):1266–1275. [PMID: 27002448]

Stoffel EM, Mangu PB, Gruber SB, et al. Hereditary colorectal cancer syndromes: American Society of Clinical Oncology Clinical Practice Guideline endorsement of the familial risk-colorectal cancer: European Society for Medical Oncology Clinical Practice Guidelines. J Clin Oncol. 2015;33(2):209–217. [PMID: 25452455]

B. Clinical Genetic Evaluation

Genetic testing is now part of standard of care for risk stratification of family members of patients with a clinical diagnosis of FAP. Genetic evaluation should start with the proband with the polyposis phenotype and includes testing for deleterious germline variants in both the *APC* and *MutYH* genes. In patients with classic polyposis phenotypes, full gene sequencing tests identify *APC* deleterious germline variants in 90% of patients and biallelic germline variants in the *MutYH* gene in approximately 2% of patients. *Y179C* and *G396D* are the two most common deleterious germline variants in the *MutYH* gene found in individuals of western European ancestry. When genetic testing for *APC* and *MutYH* in patients with classic polyposis fails to identify a deleterious germline variant, all family members with ≥100 polyps must be considered at risk for developing FAP and should be managed as having a personal history of FAP. Current practice guidelines recommend multi-gene panel testing for any patient with 20 or more cumulative colorectal adenomas.

Sieber OM, Lipton L, Crabtree M, et al. Multiple colorectal adenomas, classic adenomatous polyposis, and germ-line mutations in MUTYH. N Engl J Med. 2003;348:791–799. [PMID: 12606733]

Stoffel EM, Kastrinos F. Familial colorectal cancer, beyond Lynch syndrome. Clin Gastroenterol Hepatol. 2014;12:1059–1068. [PMID: 23962553]

3. Attenuated Adenomatous Polyposis: Attenuated FAP & MAP

Individuals with 10–100 cumulative colorectal adenomas are considered to have a phenotype of multiple or attenuated polyposis. These patients have an average of 30 polyps with a mean age of CRC diagnosis at >50. There is marked phenotypic and genotypic heterogeneity among patients with attenuated polyposis and estimates of the risk of CRC vary widely and can be as high as 84% among females and 94% among males. Some individuals with *APC* deleterious germline variants in the 3′ or 5′ ends of the gene or with biallelic *MutYH* germline variants present with an attenuated polyposis phenotype, rather than with classic FAP. Genetic testing for *APC* and *MutYH* germline variants is uninformative for many individuals with fewer than 100 adenomas, suggesting

that other genetic or environmental factors may be involved in the pathogenesis.

Cancer prevention in patients with attenuated polyposis focuses on frequent endoscopic surveillance with polypectomies to clear the colonic mucosa of adenomas. If adenomas are too numerous or recur too quickly to be managed endoscopically, then surgical colectomy may be indicated. Individuals with attenuated polyposis require colonoscopies every 1–2 years beginning in their late teens, with the option to increase or shorten the surveillance interval based on the rate of polyp growth. In cases of attenuated polyposis associated with an *APC* deleterious germline variant, it is recommended that at-risk individuals follow FAP screening guidelines (see earlier discussion) as phenotypes may change over time and severity of polyposis can vary among family members. For individuals with biallelic *MutYH* germline variants, it is reasonable to begin colonoscopies at age 25–30 with repeat examination every 1–2 years. Upper endoscopy can begin at age 30–35 with repeat examinations depending on the polyp burden. In cases in which genetic testing is not completed, family members of affected individuals should begin colonoscopic screening every 1–2 years beginning in their late teens as well.

HAMARTOMATOUS POLYPOSIS SYNDROMES

1. Peutz-Jeghers Syndrome

Peutz-Jeghers syndrome (PJS) is characterized by multiple intestinal hamartomatous polyps; mucocutaneous pigmentation, which characteristically involves the lips; and a high lifetime risk of gastrointestinal, pancreatic, and breast cancers.

▶ Clinical Findings

A. Physical Features

Individuals with PJS develop hamartomatous polyps throughout their gastrointestinal tract and can typically present with abdominal pain, stool that is positive for occult blood, obstruction, or intussusception. The clinical diagnosis of PJS can be made in individuals who meet any two of the following criteria: (1) two or more Peutz-Jeghers-type hamartomatous polyps in the gastrointestinal tract; (2) mucocutaneous hyperpigmentation of the eyes, nose, mouth, lips, fingers or genitalia; or (3) family history of PJS.

PJS is also associated with increased risk for gastrointestinal cancers (colorectal, small intestine, stomach, pancreas), breast cancer, ovarian cancer, cervical cancer, and sex cord tumors. Patients with PJS have up to a 93% lifetime risk of developing any cancer. Lifetime risks for gastric, colorectal, small bowel, pancreatic, and breast cancers are estimated at 29%, 12–39%, 13%, 11–36%, and 32–54%, respectively.

B. Genetic Features

PJS demonstrates an autosomal-dominant pattern of inheritance. Deleterious germline variants in *STK11*, a serene/threonine kinase gene with tumor-suppressor function, have been found in approximately 66–80% of PJS families. Research is ongoing to identify other genes that may be implicated in PJS patients.

▶ Management

Patients with PJS require careful endoscopic surveillance for removal of polyps and screening for extraintestinal cancers. Recommendations include small bowel imaging with magnetic resonance enterography (MRE), CT or video capsule endoscopy (VCE) starting at age 8–10. Earlier screening is recommended if the patient has symptoms. Follow-up interval is determined by baseline findings and repeat screening is recommended by at least 18 years with follow-up every 2–3 years. Upper endoscopy and colonoscopy are also recommended every 2–3 years beginning in late teens with removal of all polyps greater than 3 mm. The majority of polyps are located in the small bowel and should be removed if they are causing symptoms or are ≥10 mm in size. Small bowel polyps can increase the risk of intussusception, small bowel obstruction and gastrointestinal hemorrhage. These complications may require double-balloon enteroscopy in order to avoid surgery or an intraoperative enteroscopy. Furthermore, pancreatic cancer screening with annual MRCP or EUS is recommended beginning at age 30–35.

Females should also have an annual mammogram and breast MRI as well as bi-annual clinical breast exams beginning at age 30. Furthermore, an annual pelvic exam and pap smear are recommended beginning at age 18–20. It is also recommended that females have an annual physical exam with specific attention for precocious puberty beginning at age eight. Lastly, among males an annual testicular exam and physical exam with specific attention for feminizing changes should be performed beginning at age 10. If any abnormalities are noted a testicular ultrasound should be obtained.

National Comprehensive Cancer Network. NCCN clinical practice guidelines in oncology: genetic/familial high-risk assessment: colorectal. V 1.2020. Available at: http://www.nccn.org/professionals/. Accessed August 2020.

2. Juvenile Polyposis

Juvenile polyposis is characterized by the appearance of multiple juvenile polyps and increased risk for gastrointestinal cancers.

▶ Clinical Findings

A. Physical Features

The clinical diagnosis of juvenile polyposis (JPS) should be considered in any individual who meets at least one of the following criteria: (1) at least five colonic juvenile polyps; (2) multiple juvenile polyps in the gastrointestinal tract; or (3) any number of juvenile polyps in an individual with a family history of JPS. Many affected individuals present with symptoms such as anemia, bleeding, or abdominal pain during childhood. Patients with JPS often have a variable presentation of polyp distribution which may occur throughout the colon and/or stomach and the cancer risk is attributable to the presence of dysplasia in the polyps. In a longitudinal study from St. Mark's Hospital, of 44 JPS patients from 30 kindreds, a total of 787 polyps (juvenile and adenomatous) were resected. Sixty five of these 787 polyps (8.3%) contained mild/moderate architectural dysplasia, while 20 additional polyps (2.5%) were adenomatous. JPS patients are at increased risk for colorectal, gastric, small intestinal, and pancreatic cancers, many of which appear at young ages. There is also an association with cardiac abnormalities and other congenital anomalies, as well as hereditary hemorrhagic telangiectasia (HHT).

B. Genetic Features

JPS has an autosomal-dominant pattern of inheritance. Deleterious germline variants in the *SMAD4* and *BMPR1A* genes, as well as in the *ENG* and *PTEN* genes, have been identified in some patients. The combined syndrome of JPS and HHT (termed *JPS/HHT*) is present in many individuals with a *SMAD4* pathogenic variant. Clinical genetic testing is available, but is often uninformative, since as many as half of individuals who meet clinical criteria for JPS do not have detectable deleterious germline variants.

▶ Management

Patients should undergo endoscopy and colonoscopy every 2–3 years beginning at age 15 with consideration of shorter intervals based on the number, size, and pathology of resected polyps. Affected individuals should have frequent upper endoscopy and colonoscopy for removal of polyps. In some cases, surgical colectomy (or even gastrectomy) is required for management of polyp burden. Otherwise, screening for complications related to HHT (eg, cerebral and cardiopulmonary arteriovenous malformations) in all individuals with a *SMAD4* pathogenic variant is recommended within the first six months of life.

National Comprehensive Cancer Network. NCCN clinical practice guidelines in oncology: genetic/familial high-risk assessment: colorectal. V 1.2020. Available at: http://www.nccn.org/professionals/. Accessed August 2020.

3. PTEN Hamartoma Tumor Syndrome (PHTS)

PHTS includes multiple phenotypic variations including Cowden's Syndrome (CS), Bannayan-Riley-Ruvalcaba syndrome (BRRS), and Proteus syndrome. PHTS is an autosomal dominant hereditary syndrome characterized by mucocutaneous lesions including trichilemmomas, macrocephaly, and increased risk for thyroid, breast, and endometrial cancers as well as renal cell carcinoma (RCC). PHTS is associated with deleterious germline variants in the *PTEN* gene. Although hamartomas including ganglioneuromas of the gastrointestinal tract are described, the risk for gastrointestinal cancers does not appear to be as high for patients with PHTS as compared with other polyposis syndromes. However, data suggest there is an increase in risk for early-onset CRC and patients have up to an 18% risk of CRC by age 60. As a result, colonoscopy is recommended beginning at age 35 or 5–10 years prior to the youngest age of CRC diagnosis in a family member. Screening is recommended every 5 years with consideration of shorter intervals if polyps are found.

A clinical breast exam should be performed every 6–12 months starting at age 25 or 10 years prior to the youngest age of breast cancer diagnosis in a family member. An annual mammogram with consideration of breast MRI with contrast or breast tomosynthesis should also begin at age 30–35 or 5–10 years prior to the youngest age of breast cancer diagnosis in a family member. Otherwise, endometrial cancer screening with an endometrial biopsy can be considered and started by age 35 with 1–2 year intervals. Thyroid cancer screening with an annual thyroid ultrasound is recommended beginning at age seven. RCC screening with a renal ultrasound can also be considered and started at age 40 with 1–2 year intervals. Lastly, an annual skin exam for melanoma screening can be performed.

National Comprehensive Cancer Network. NCCN clinical practice guidelines in oncology: genetic/familial high-risk assessment: colorectal. V 1.2020. Available at: http://www.nccn.org/professionals/. Accessed August 2020.

Yehia L, Keel E, Eng C. The clinical spectrum of *PTEN* mutations. *Annu Rev Med.* 2020;71:103–116. [PMID: 31433956]

SERRATED POLYPOSIS SYNDROME

▶ **Clinical Findings**

A. Physical Features

Serrated polyposis syndrome (SPS) (previously described as hyperplastic polyposis syndrome) is characterized by large and/or multiple serrated lesions/polyps. Sessile serrated polyps/adenomas or traditional serrated adenomas are believed to be precursor lesions of serrated CRCs, accounting for up to 30% of CRC tumors. These polyps are typically right-sided, flat polyps, with overlying mucous cap, and indistinct borders.

SPS has been defined as a distinct entity by the World Health Organization (WHO). SPS is diagnosed if any one of the following criteria are met (at one time or cumulative): (1) ≥5 serrated lesions/polyps proximal to the rectum that are all ≥5 mm, with ≥2 polyps being ≥10 mm; (2) >20 serrated lesions/polyps of any size, distributed throughout the colon, with ≥5 located proximal to the rectum. Females, older individuals, and cigarette smokes appear to be at higher risk of SPS. There are no known extracolonic conditions associated with SPS.

B. Genetic Features

The genetic basis of SPS has not been entirely elucidated and the majority of SPS patients do not have an identified genetic cause. However, biallelic *MutYH* germline variants have been reported in individuals meeting WHO criteria for SPS. Furthermore, there has been a link to deleterious germline variants in *RNF43*, which is a gene in the WnT signaling pathway. Increased CRC risk among first-degree relatives of patients with SPS suggests a possible hereditary component.

▶ **Management**

The clinical management of SPS is similar to that of attenuated polyposis, with the goal of removal of as many polyps as feasible and 1–3 year surveillance intervals depending on the size and number of polyps removed. In cases when polyps cannot be managed endoscopically surgical resection may be considered.

Dekker E, Bleijenberg A, Balaguer F; Dutch-Spanish-British Serrated Polyposis Syndrome collaboration. Update on the World Health Organization criteria for diagnosis of serrated polyposis syndrome. *Gastroenterology.* 2020;158(6):1520–1523. [PMID: 31982410]

National Comprehensive Cancer Network. NCCN clinical practice guidelines in oncology: genetic/familial high-risk assessment: breast, ovarian and pancreatic. V 1.2020. Available at: http://www.nccn.org/professionals/. Accessed August 2020.

National Comprehensive Cancer Network. NCCN clinical practice guidelines in oncology: genetic/familial high-risk assessment: colorectal. V 1.2020. Available at: http://www.nccn.org/professionals/. Accessed August 2020.

Yan HHN, Lai JCW, Ho SL, et al. RNF43 germline and somatic mutation in serrated neoplasia pathway and its association with BRAF mutation. *Gut.* 2017;66(9):1645–1656. [PMID: 27329244]

COLORECTAL POLYPOSIS NOT OTHERWISE SPECIFIED

Advances in NGS technologies have begun to alter clinical approaches to genetic evaluation of individuals with multiple colorectal polyps. NGS has facilitated identification of novel genes. Furthermore, reports demonstrating overlap between clinical phenotypes of polyposis patients with deleterious germline variants in different genes suggest significant variability in clinical phenotype of polyposis patients and justify approaches which use multigene panels for clinical genetic testing.

Jaeger E, Leedham S, Lewis A, et al. Hereditary mixed polyposis syndrome is caused by a 40-kb upstream duplication that leads to increased and ectopic expression of the BMP antagonist GREM1. *Nat Genet.* 2012;44:699–703. [PMID: 22561515]

Ngeow J, Heald B, Rybicki LA, et al. Prevalence of germline PTEN, BMPR1A, SMAD4, STK11, and ENG mutations in patients with moderate-load colorectal polyps. *Gastroenterology.* 2013;144:1402–1409. [PMID: 23399955]

Palles C, Cazier JB, Howarth KM, et al. Germline mutations affecting the proofreading domains of POLE and POLD1 predispose to colorectal adenomas and carcinomas. *Nat Genet.* 2013;45:136–144. [PMID: 23263490]

OTHER GASTROINTESTINAL CANCER SYNDROMES

1. Hereditary Diffuse Gastric Cancer

Hereditary diffuse gastric cancer (HDGC) manifests as diffuse infiltrative adenocarcinoma of the stomach occurring in families in a pattern of autosomal-dominant inheritance, often affecting young individuals; the majority of gastric cancers occur before age 40.

▶ Clinical Findings

A. Physical Features

In contrast to most gastric cancers, which appear as ulcers or masses, diffuse gastric cancer (DGC) usually presents as diffuse thickening of the stomach wall or linitis plastica, without an obvious endoscopic lesion. The International Gastric Cancer Linkage Consortium recommends genetic testing when any of the following familial or individual criteria are met and there has been a histologic cancer diagnosis (there needs to be at least one histologic cancer diagnosis for criteria involving more than one cancer). Familial criteria include (criteria require that family members be first- or second-degree relatives of one another): (1) two or more first- or second-degree relatives with gastric cancer at any age and at least one confirmed DGC; (2) one or more first- or second-degree relatives with DGC at any age and one or more first- or second-degree relatives with lobular breast cancer (LBC) at <70 years, affecting different family members; (3) two or more first- or second-degree relatives with LBC at <50 years. Additionally, genetic testing is recommended when any of the following individual criteria is met: (1) DGC at <50 years; (2) DGC at any age in an individual of Māori descent; (3) DGC at any age in an individual with a personal or family history (first-degree relative) of cleft lip or cleft palate; (4) history of DGC and LBC with both diagnosed at <70 years; (5) bilateral LBC diagnosed at <70 years; or (6) individuals

<50 years with gastric *in situ* signet ring cells and/or pagetoid spread of signet ring cells. The estimated lifetime risk of gastric cancer in these patients is 60–80%. Studies have also demonstrated a 39–52% risk of LBC among female carriers.

B. Genetic Features

Approximately 30–50% of families who meet criteria for HDGC have deleterious germline variants in the *E-cadherin/CDH1* tumor-suppressor gene. *E-cadherin/CDH1* deleterious germline variants were first identified in Māori families with gastric cancer in New Zealand. Genetic testing for HDGC is clinically available; however, it is only informative in up to 50% of cases. If a deleterious germline variant is identified in a proband, testing can be offered to other family members.

▶ Management

Prevention of gastric cancer among individuals at increased risk is challenging because endoscopic screening has been shown to have poor sensitivity for detecting DGC. Consequently, prophylactic gastrectomy is recommended for individuals with deleterious germline variants and other patients at highest risk. Prophylactic gastrectomy carries with it considerable morbidity; however, expert panels have concluded that the cumulative lifetime risk of developing gastric cancer among individuals with a deleterious *CDH1* germline variant justifies prophylactic gastrectomy. As a result, prophylactic gastrectomy is recommended between ages 18 and 40. Although this is not recommended for patients younger than 18 years, it can be considered if a family member was diagnosed with gastric cancer at <25 years. Individuals who choose not to undergo a prophylactic gastrectomy should have a screening upper endoscopy every 6–12 months. Given the increased risk of LBC among individuals with a deleterious *CDH1* germline variant, early screening through a high-risk breast cancer clinic is recommended. An annual breast MRI, is recommended, beginning at age 30. Prophylactic mastectomy may also be considered and discussed.

Blair VR, McLeod M, Carneiro F, et al. Hereditary diffuse gastric cancer: updated clinical practice guidelines. *Lancet Oncol.* 2020;21(8):e386–e397. [PMID: 32758476]

National Comprehensive Cancer Network. NCCN clinical practice guidelines in oncology: gastric cancer. V 4.2020. Available at: http://www.nccn.org/professionals/. Accessed December 2020.

2. Familial Pancreatic Cancer

Although the vast majority of cases of pancreatic adenocarcinoma are sporadic, approximately 10% appear to have a hereditary component. Individuals with two affected first-degree relatives have a 6.4-fold risk for developing pancreatic adenocarcinoma. Risk is estimated to be 32-fold for an individual with a least three affected first-degree relatives. Familial pancreatic cancer (FPC) is most often defined as families in which there are two or more first-degree relatives with pancreatic adenocarcinoma and without another identified inherited cancer syndrome.

Studies of FPC kindreds have identified deleterious germline variants in approximately 10% of cases. Thus, for the majority of families, a genetic cause of the pancreatic cancer cannot be found. Genetic testing is recommended for all individuals with pancreatic cancer; if it is not possible to test the affected member of the family it is reasonable to test individuals that have at least one first-degree relative with pancreatic cancer.

1. Hereditary breast/ovarian cancer (HBOC; *BRCA1/BRCA2*)—Deleterious germline variants in the *BRCA1* and *BRCA2* genes account for the great majority of deleterious germline variants identified among pancreatic cancer families. Several studies have reported that prevalence of pancreatic cancer among families with HBOC is increased. The relative risk of developing pancreatic cancer for patients with a deleterious germline variant has been estimated to be 2.6 for *BRCA1* and 3.5–8 for *BRCA2*. Furthermore, the overall lifetime risk of developing pancreatic cancer is 4–8%. In some HBOC families, the pancreatic cancer history overshadows the breast cancers.

2. Familial atypical multiple mole melanoma (FAMMM; *CDKN2A* p16)—FAMMM is defined as more than 50 atypical nevi and/or malignant melanoma in one or more first- or second-degree relatives. Pancreatic cancer has been reported in nearly one-fourth of FAMMM families. Many of these FAMMM families with pancreatic cancer appear to have deleterious germline variants in the gene *CDKN2A* p16 (*cyclin dependent kinase 2A*). Carriers of a specific type of *CDKN2A* deleterious germline variant appear to have a cumulative risk of pancreatic cancer of approximately 17% by age 75.

3. Peutz-Jeghers syndrome—Individuals with PJS are most commonly characterized by their hamartomatous gastrointestinal polyps and mucocutaneous pigmentation. Up to 90% are found to have deleterious germline variants in the *LKB1/STK11* gene. In addition to conferring increased risk for breast cancer, PJS also confers an increased predisposition to pancreatic adenocarcinoma, with a lifetime risk of up to 36%.

4. Lynch syndrome—Pancreatic cancer is one of the gastrointestinal cancers that has been reported in Lynch syndrome, and lifetime risk appears to be approximately 4% for deleterious germline variants in the MMR gene.

5. Hereditary pancreatitis—Hereditary pancreatitis often presents as repeated episodes of pancreatic inflammation, ultimately resulting in chronic pancreatitis. In familial cases, there is evidence of autosomal-dominant inheritance and deleterious germline variants of the cationic trypsinogen gene (*PRSS1*) are found in up to 80% of kindreds. Deleterious germline variants in the *serene protease inhibitor Kazal*

1 (*SPINK1*) gene have also been identified in some families. These deleterious germline variants cause failure to inactivate trypsin, resulting in chronic pancreatitis, and confer a lifetime risk of pancreatic cancer of up to 40% by age 70.

6. *PALB2*—Deleterious germline variants in the *PALB2* gene have also been identified in a small number of FPC families. The PALB2 protein product binds to *BRCA2*. *PALB2* germline variants have been described in association with inherited predisposition to breast cancer.

7. *ATM*—Deleterious germline variants in the *ATM* gene, which are classically associated with an autosomal-recessive condition called ataxia–telangiectasia, have been reported in 1–2% of the general population. Among individuals diagnosed with pancreatic cancer the prevalence is higher and estimated to be 4%. However, the magnitude of risk increase for pancreatic cancer has not yet been established and the risk of pancreatic cancer among mutation carriers without a family history of pancreatic cancer also remains unclear.

8. *TP53*—Individuals carrying a deleterious *TP53* germline variant, which causes Li-Fraumeni syndrome, are at increased risk of soft tissue and osteosarcomas, breast cancer, brain tumors, and adrenocortical carcinoma. However, other cancer types have been observed, including pancreatic cancer, although the magnitude of risk has not been determined.

▶ Management

Genetic counseling in patients with a family history of pancreatic cancer should emphasize that in the majority of cases genetic testing does not reveal deleterious germline variants in any of the genes known to be associated with pancreatic cancer. Advantages of pursuing genetic testing include the potential for identifying a deleterious germline variant so that at-risk family members can undergo predisposition genetic testing and risk stratification. Also, identifying a deleterious germline variant may affect cancer screening recommendations for the affected proband, as well as for at-risk family members. Disadvantages include the fact that genetic testing may be costly and may not identify a genetic cause.

Individuals who have a deleterious germline variant in the *ATM*, *BRCA1*, *MLH1*, *MSH2*, *MSH6*, or *PALB2* gene as well as a family history of at least one first-degree relative with pancreatic cancer are eligible for pancreatic cancer surveillance. Patients are also eligible for surveillance if they have a deleterious germline variant in the *BRCA2* gene and at least one first-degree relative with pancreatic cancer or at least two relatives of any degree with pancreatic cancer. Otherwise, individuals with a deleterious germline variant in the *LKB1/STK11* or *CDKN2A* p16 gene are eligible for surveillance irrespective of family history. Lastly, regardless of gene mutation status, pancreatic cancer surveillance can be considered in individuals who have: (1) three or more relatives on the same side of the family who have/had pancreatic cancer with at least one being a first-degree relative of the person being considered for surveillance; (2) two or more relatives who are first-degree relatives to one another and have/had pancreatic cancer with at least one being a first-degree relative of the person being considered for surveillance; or (3) two or more relatives on the same side of the family who have/had pancreatic cancer with at least one being a first-degree relative of the person being considered for surveillance.

The risks and benefits of pancreatic cancer surveillance must be discussed on an individual basis. Annual surveillance can be considered with EUS and/or MRI/MRCP to try to detect abnormalities that may be precursors to pancreatic cancer, with the goal of pancreatic resection for high-risk lesions. Age of screening initiation depends on the specific deleterious germline variant and/or clinical phenotype.

Lastly, patients with a family history of pancreatic cancer should be advised to stop cigarette smoking, as this has been found consistently to be an important risk factor for pancreatic cancer.

Goggins M, Overbeek KA, Brand R, et al. Management of patients with increased risk for familial pancreatic cancer: updated recommendations from the International Cancer of the Pancreas Screening (CAPS) Consortium [published correction appears in Gut. 2020 Jun;69(6):e3]. *Gut.* 2020;69(1):7–17. [PMID: 31672839]

National Comprehensive Cancer Network. NCCN clinical practice guidelines in oncology: genetic/familial high-risk assessment: breast, ovarian and pancreatic. V 2.2021. Available at: http://www.nccn.org/professionals/. Accessed December 2020.

Stoffel EM, McKernin SE, Brand R, et al. Evaluating susceptibility to pancreatic cancer: ASCO provisional clinical opinion. *J Clin Oncol.* 2019;37(2):153–164. [PMID: 30457921]

Yurgelun MB, Chittenden AB, Morales-Oyarvide V, et al. Germline cancer susceptibility gene variants, somatic second hits, and survival outcomes in patients with resected pancreatic cancer. *Genet Med.* 2019;21(1):213–223. [PMID: 29961768]

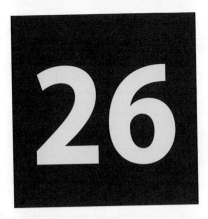

Irritable Bowel Syndrome

26

Anne F. Liu, MD

Sonia Friedman, MD

ESSENTIALS OF DIAGNOSIS

▶ In the United States, irritable bowel syndrome (IBS) is most common in young patients, predominantly between the ages of 20 and 40.

▶ IBS is more common in women with a ratio of 2:1 in the United States.

▶ Rome IV criteria include recurrent abdominal pain for more than 6 months with discomfort at least 1 day per week in the last 3 months associated with two or more of the following:

  ▶ Related to defecation.

  ▶ Associated with a change in frequency of stool.

  ▶ Associated with a change in form (appearance) of stool.

▶ Rule out "red flag" symptoms such as weight loss, rectal bleeding, family history of cancer or inflammatory bowel disease, abnormal hematological or biochemical lab results or abnormal examination findings before making a diagnosis of IBS.

▶ IBS can be mild, moderate, or severe; four different subtypes are constipation predominant, diarrhea predominant, mixed, and unclassified.

▶ The Bristol Stool Form Scale (BSFS) is helpful clinically in defining the spectrum of diarrhea to constipation.

General Considerations

IBS is the most common diagnosis made by gastroenterologists and is one of the top 10 reasons for visits to primary care physicians. IBS is the most common functional bowel disorder. Other diagnoses in the spectrum of functional bowel disorder include functional constipation, functional diarrhea, abdominal bloating/distention and unspecified functional bowel disease. IBS can cause great discomfort, sometimes intermittent or continuous, for many decades in a patient's life and can have a significantly negative impact on quality of life.

National Ambulatory Medical Care Survey (NAMCS) data from 2007 to 2015 reports 2.7 million annual ambulatory outpatient visits for IBS. In a separate meta-analysis, the prevalence of IBS in a typical primary care practice was 11.2%. The estimated total yearly cost of IBS in the United States is between $1.7 and $10 billion in direct medical costs and $20 billion in indirect costs. Direct costs include diagnostic tests, physician and emergency department visits, hospitalizations, surgeries, and medications. Indirect costs include reduced work productivity, absenteeism, travel to consultations as well as intangible costs such as human suffering and impaired quality of life.

IBS primarily affects people in the prime of their lives, predominantly between the ages of 20 and 40, with half of patients reporting their first symptoms before age 35. The prevalence of IBS between genders depends on geographic region with female-to-male ratio of 2:1 in the United States, Israel, and Canada. Of note, IBS is fairly equal among men and women in Asia. It has been suggested that hormonal differences between men and women may affect gut function and later perception of pain related to abdominal distention. Estrogen and progesterone can inhibit smooth muscle contraction and modulate peristalsis whereas testosterone can have an analgesic effect. In a recent genome-wide association study (GWAS) of a UK Biobank with 500,000 participants, variants at locus 9q31.2 were noted to increase the IBS risk in women $P = 4.29 \times 10^{-10}$. For many female patients, symptoms occur frequently and significantly impair emotional, physical, and social well-being. For instance, women with IBS were more likely to avoid domestic activities, jobs, sexual intercourse, and certain foods compared to men.

Only about 25% of IBS patients consult a physician for their symptoms. Of these, only a small percentage of these patients visit a gastroenterologist. Patients who consult a primary care physician for their IBS usually have mild symptoms and effective coping skills and social support. Of IBS patients who consult subspecialists, 60% or more may have psychological disturbances, including anxiety, somatoform or personality disorders, or chronic pain syndromes. Up to 35% of women who consult subspecialists for IBS have a history of sexual abuse.

Bonfiglio F, Zheng T, Garcia-Etxebarria K, et al. Female-specific association between variants on chromosome 9 and self-reported diagnosis of irritable bowel syndrome. *Gastroenterology*. 2018;155(1):168–179. [PMID: 29626450]

Chandar A. K. Diagnosis and treatment of irritable bowel syndrome with predominant constipation in the primary-care setting: focus on linaclotide. *Int J Gen Med*. 2017;10:385–393. [PMID: 29184433]

Ford A, Moayyedi P, Chey WD, et al. American College of Gastroenterology monograph onmanagement of irritable bowel syndrome. *Am J Gastroenterology*. 2018;113:1–18. [PMID: 29950604]

Ma C, Congly SE, Novak KL, et al. Epidemiologic burden and treatment of chronic symptomatic functional bowel disorders in the United States: a nationwide analysis. *Gastroenterology*. 2020;160(1):88–98.e4. [PMID: 33010247]

Pietrzak A, Skrzydło-Radomańska B, Mulak A, et al. Guidelines on the management of irritable bowel syndrome: in memory of Professor Witold Bartnik. *Prz Gastroenterol*. 2018;13(4):259–288. [PMID: 30581501]

▶ Pathogenesis

A. Motility

Although disturbances in small bowel motility have been reported in IBS, none appear specific for the condition. Small bowel motility shows marked diurnal variability, and hence, consistent results can only be obtained with prolonged (at least 24 hour) recordings and large numbers of subjects. Small bowel motor disturbances reported include increased frequency and duration of discrete cluster contractions (DCC), increased frequency of the migrating motor complex (MMC), more retrograde duodenal and jejunal contractions, and an exaggerated motor response to meal ingestion, ileal distention, and cholecystokinin (CCK). Corticotrophin-releasing hormone (CRH) has been reported to increase the number of DCCs. Small bowel transit is faster in IBS patients with diarrhea (IBS-D) compared with constipation (IBS-C), and unlike in healthy controls, colonic distention does not appear to reduce duodenal motility in IBS patients, suggesting an impaired intestine-intestinal inhibitory reflex. The most consistent abnormality in the colon is an exaggerated motility response to meal ingestion. Rectal compliance or increased tension, or both, has also been reported in some studies in patients with IBS. This has been proposed as a possible mechanism for enhanced visceral sensation to balloon distention in IBS.

B. Visceral Hypersensitivity

Abdominal pain causes considerable morbidity in IBS patients and are essential components of the Rome IV criteria for diagnosis of IBS. Unlike Rome III criteria, Rome IV does not have the term "discomfort" and just has "abdominal pain." Approximately two-thirds of IBS patients demonstrate heightened pain sensitivity to experimental gut stimulation, a phenomenon known as visceral hypersensitivity. Visceral hypersensitivity is thought to play an important role in the development of chronic pain and discomfort in IBS patients. It results from a combination of factors that involve both the peripheral and central nervous systems. During tissue injury, peripheral nociceptor terminals are exposed to a mixture of immune and inflammatory mediators, such as prostaglandins, leukotrienes, serotonin, histamine, cytokines, neurotrophic factors, and reactive metabolites. These inflammatory mediators act on nociceptor terminals, leading to the activation of intracellular signaling pathways, which in turn upregulate their sensitivity and excitability. This phenomenon has been termed peripheral sensitization. Peripheral sensitization is believed to cause pain hypersensitivity at the site of injury or inflammation, also known as primary hyperalgesia (increased sensitivity to painful stimuli) and allodynia (nonpainful stimuli are perceived as painful).

A secondary consequence of peripheral sensitization is the development of an area of hypersensitivity in the surrounding uninjured tissue (secondary hyperalgesia or allodynia). This phenomenon occurs due to an increase in the excitability and receptive fields of spinal neurons (with increased production of the neurotransmitters serotonin and substance P) and results in recruitment and amplification of both non-nociceptive and nociceptive inputs from the adjacent healthy tissue. There have been 30 studies showing increased mast cell counts and/or mast cell density in IBS patients compared to controls. These mast cells are located near the intrinsic and extrinsic neurons in the gastrointestinal tract where they can then release mediators such as tumor necrosis factor, histamine, prostaglandins, serotonin, leukotrienes, protease, platelet-activating factors, cytokines and chemokines. The release of histamine and protease is thought to induce visceral hypersensitivity. The release of cytokines is thought to change intestinal secretion and permeability. The release of serotonin is thought to change sensation of pain and stool caliber. Degranulated mast cells have been observed on electron microscopy on colon and rectal biopsies of patients with IBS suggesting that the mast cells are actively functioning in IBS.

Depending on the setting, about 6–17% of patients with IBS report their symptoms began with an episode of gut inflammation due to gastroenteritis. In addition, an increase in mucosal T lymphocytes, macrophages, mast cells, and enterochromatophilic cells has been reported on biopsies in patients with IBS. There is also an increase in pro-inflammatory cytokines in the serum. Therefore, the environment of nociceptor terminals in the gut of IBS patients is likely to be altered, suggesting a role for peripheral sensitization. Evidence for central sensitization as an important mechanism for the development of visceral hypersensitivity in IBS patients comes from three main observations. First, in response to colon stimulation, patients with IBS have greater radiation of pain to somatic structures in comparison to healthy subjects. Second, a proportion of IBS patients also suffer from fibromyalgia, a condition characterized by somatic hyperalgesia. Finally, patients with IBS also often demonstrate hypersensitivity of proximal areas of the gut. The innervation of the different gut organs overlaps and converges with that of the somatic structures at the level of the spinal cord, and these phenomena can be explained by central sensitization of the spinal segments that demonstrate viscerovisceral and viscerosomatic convergence.

Alterations in brain processing in IBS patients can also contribute to visceral hypersensitivity. The intestinal enterochromaffin cells play a major role in the hydroxylation of L-tryptophan to produce serotoninin, which is a critical neurotransmitter. In patients with IBS, the enterochromaffin cells have reduced levels of tryptophan hydroxylase, leading to decreased serotonin production and hence impacts on mood, cognition, and visceral hypersensitivity. There is also concurrent impaired serotonin release and reduced serotonin reuptake. Brain imaging studies have begun to address the possible neural mechanisms of hypersensitivity in IBS patients, and a common finding has been compared with healthy controls; patients with IBS exhibit altered or enhanced activation of regions involved in pain processing, such as the anterior cingulated cortex, thalamus, insula, and prefrontal cortices, in response to experimental rectal pain.

C. Postinfective IBS

The prevalence of postinfective IBS varies from 17% in primary care in the United Kingdom to as little as 6% in tertiary care in the United States. Population surveys indicate a relative risk of 11.1–11.9% of developing IBS in the year following a bout of gastroenteritis. Known risk factors include the severity of the initial illness; bacterial toxigenicity; female sex; a range of adverse psychological factors, including neuroticism, hypochondriasis, anxiety, and depression; and adverse life events. Postinfective IBS has been reported after bacterial infections (*Shigella, Salmonella, Campylobacter, Escherichia coli, Vibrio cholerae*, and *Clostroidiodes difficile*); viral infections (norovirus), and parasite infections (*Giardia lamblia* and *Trichinella brivoti*).

A systematic review of 45 studies following 21,451 individuals for the development of IBS from 1994 through 2015 discovered a pooled IBS prevalence of 10.1% at 12 months after enteritis and 14.5% at greater than 12 months after enteritis. Bacterial-associated postinfective IBS was more common than viral-associated postinfective IBS due to greater mucosal damage and inflammation. The risk factors for developing IBS were female sex (OR 2.2), antibiotic exposure (OR 1.7), anxiety (OR 2), depression (OR 1.5), somatization (OR 4.1), neuroticism (OR 3.3), and clinical indicators of enteritis severity. In general, risk of IBS was four times higher in patients after gastroenteritis compared to those without gastroenteritis. This remarkable study shows that a substantial

number of people will develop IBS after an acute episode of gastroenteritis. Specific host characteristics and acute enteritis illness can predict the long-term risk of postinfective IBS.

Histologic studies indicate that postinfective IBS is characterized by increased lymphocyte and macrophage numbers in mucosal biopsies, an effect that is seen throughout the colon. Where the terminal ileum has been biopsied, increased mast cells have also been noted. Another change following inflammation is enterochromaffin cell hyperplasia. Whereas in most subjects, these changes resolve within 3 months, in IBS patients, the levels of both lymphocytes and enteroendocrine cells remain elevated. Increased enterochromaffin cell numbers are associated with an increase in postprandial 5-HT release, an abnormality shown in both postinfective IBS and in diarrhea-predominant IBS without an obvious postinfective origin. Immediately after gastroenteritis affecting the small bowel, there may be transient lactose intolerance, which is particularly obvious in young children. However, in adults with postinfective IBS, who have had symptoms for over 6 months, the incidence of lactose malabsorption is no different from uninfected controls.

D. Stress Response

The response of an organism to external stressors is mediated through the integration of the hypothalamic-pituitary-adrenal axis (HPA) and the sympathetic branch of the autonomic nervous system with the host immune system. A recent model for the pathogenesis of IBS proposes altered stress circuits in predisposed individuals, which are triggered by external stressors resulting in the development of gut symptoms. In postinfective IBS, the persistence of chronic inflammatory mucosal changes and enterochromaffin cell hyperplasia that persists after eradication of the infectious organism are consistent with an inadequate physiologic response to gut inflammation and, in particular, an inadequate cortisol or altered sympathetic response. The key interplay between the autonomic nervous system and the HPA axis in regulating gut mucosal immunology has been explored through research looking at how the stress response, which activates both systems, may be important in IBS. Environmental stressors are important in predisposing toward IBS and in perpetuating the symptoms of IBS. Prior life stressors and a history of childhood abuse predispose toward developing IBS in later life. Psychiatric illness episodes or anxiety-provoking situations preceded the onset of bowel symptoms in two-thirds of IBS patients being treated in tertiary care centers; in addition, IBS patients report significantly more negative life events than matched peptic ulcer patients. In addition, psychological traits such as hypochondriasis, anxiety, and depression predispose previously healthy individuals who develop gastroenteritis to go on to develop symptoms of IBS. In fact, a subgroup of IBS patients has an exaggerated endocrine stress response, as shown by a heightened release of adrenocorticotropic hormone and cortisol in response to exogenous corticotropin-releasing factor administration.

This exaggerated stress response seems to be associated with mucosal immune activation.

Barbara G, Grover M, Bercik P, et al. Rome Foundation working team report on post-infection irritable bowel syndrome. *Gastroenterology*. 2019;156(1):46–58. [PMID: 30009817]

Carco C, Young W, Gearry RB, et al. Increasing evidence that irritable bowel syndrome and functional gastrointestinal disorders have a microbial pathogenesis. *Front Cell Infect Microbiol*. 2020;10:468. [PMID: 33014892]

Downs IA, Aroniadis OC, Kelly L, et al. Postinfection irritable bowel syndrome: the links between gastroenteritis, inflammation, the microbiome, and functional disease. *J Clin Gastroenterol*. 2017;51(10):869–877. [PMID: 28885302]

Klem F, Wadhwa A, Prokop L, et al. Prevalence, risk factors, and outcomes of irritable bowel syndrome after infectious enteritis: a systematic review and meta-analysis. *Gastroenterology* 2017;152:1042–1054. [PMID: 28069350]

Krammer L, Sowa AS, Lorentz A. Mast cells in irritable bowel syndrome: a systematic review. *J Gastrointestin Liver Dis*. 2019;28(4):463–472. [PMID: 31826052]

Lee KN, Lee OY. The role of mast cells in irritable bowel syndrome. *Gastroenterol Res Pract*. 2016;2016:2031480. [PMID: 28115927]

▶ Clinical Findings

IBS is a disease that can be caused by many factors. Disturbed bowel motility, visceral hypersensitivity, bacterial overgrowth, and psychological problems can all contribute to causing or exacerbating IBS. There are several important, take-home points in treating IBS. First, clinicians must take a good history and rule out "red flags." Celiac sprue, bacterial overgrowth, and microscopic colitis, among many other conditions, can masquerade as IBS. Second, clinicians should provide reassurance and close follow-up at first to make sure the diagnosis is correct. Third, despite the lack of evidence-based studies, diet plays a role in exacerbating gastrointestinal symptoms, and a good dietary history should be taken. Diaries with food intake and bowel movements spanning 14 days are recommended. Fourth, clinicians should not forget the psychological component of IBS. Many patients with IBS have coexisting depression and anxiety, and patients with severe IBS often have a history of physical and sexual abuse. Lastly, there are only a few medications with strong recommendations and high strength of evidence, considered as good data, from randomized controlled trials. Given the paucity of specific medicines with positive results in the evidence-based medical literature, treatment is often a trial and error process. However, a combination of dietary and lifestyle changes, relaxation training or psychotherapy, and individualized IBS medicines tailored to each patient's symptoms usually improves quality of life.

A. Symptoms & Signs

As the Rome IV criteria indicate (Table 26–1), the key features are abdominal pain linked to bowel function, either

Table 26–1. Rome IV diagnostic criteria[a] for irritable bowel syndrome.

Recurrent abdominal pain at least 1 day per week in the last 3 months associated with 2 or more of the following: • Related to defecation • Onset associated with a change in frequency of stool • Onset associated with a change in form (appearance) of stool

[a]Criteria fulfilled for the last 3 months with symptom onset at least 6 months prior to diagnosis.

being related to defecation or associated with a change in stool frequency or form. These symptoms are not explained by biochemical or structural abnormalities. Symptoms should be present for at least the last 3 months with symptom onset at least 6 months prior to diagnosis to clearly distinguish those from other conditions such as infections, which often pass quickly, or progressive diseases such as bowel cancer that are usually diagnosed within 6 months of symptom onset. Symptoms that are common in IBS but are not part of the Rome criteria include bloating, straining at defecation, urgency, feeling of incomplete evacuation, and the passage of mucus per rectum. Most patients experience flares intermittently, with symptoms lasting 2–4 days followed by periods of remission. In women, symptoms can be worse at the time of menstruation and can cycle with the menstrual cycle. One common symptom of IBS not part of the Rome criteria is repeated defecation in the morning (morning rush) when stool consistency changes from solid to liquid as the colon contents are evacuated. The Rome IV criteria specifically clarifies that disordered bowel habits that are constipation, diarrhea, or a mix of diarrhea and constipation are present. The IBS subtypes are based on the predominant bowel habits on the days with abnormal bowel movements.

One important exception to the Rome criteria is patients who feel abdominal pain continuously. The diagnosis in this case is likely functional abdominal pain, an unusual, particularly severe condition in which patients respond poorly to treatment and often have severe underlying psychological disturbances.

IBS is considered a painful condition with bloating and distention, whereas those with painless bowel dysfunction are labeled as having "functional constipation" or "functional diarrhea." Some of the distinguishing characteristics of IBS-C and functional constipation are detailed in Table 26–2. Patients with IBS-C rarely have a sense of anorectal obstruction or require manual maneuvers for disimpaction, unlike functional constipation. A quarter of patients with IBS-C have slow colonic transit and thus they share similarities to functional constipation in straining and feeling of incomplete evacuation. Typically, an anorectal examination is needed to also separate IBS-C and functional constipation from dyssynergic defecation.

1. IBS subtype classification—The Rome IV subclassification is based solely on predominant bowel habits on the days

Table 26–2. Comparison of irritable bowel syndrome with constipation (IBS-C) to functional constipation.

Symptom	IBS-C	Functional Constipation
Abdominal pain or discomfort	+++	±
Bloating or abdominal distention	+++	+
Sense of anorectal obstruction	–	+++
Manual maneuvers	–	+++
<3 bowel movements/week	+++	+++
Hard, lumpy stools	+++	+++
Straining	+++	+++
Feeling of incomplete evacuation	+++	+++

Table 26–4. Bristol Stool Form Scale.

Type	Description
1	Separate hard lumps, like nuts (difficult to pass)
2	Sausage shaped, but lumpy
3	Like a sausage but with cracks in its surface
4	Like a sausage or snake, smooth and soft
5	Soft blobs with clear-cut edges (passed easily)
6	Fluffy pieces with ragged edges, a mushy stool
7	Watery, no solid pieces, entirely liquid

with abnormal bowel movements and not on an average of all days which include days with normal bowel movements. The subclassifications are easy to use (Table 26–3). To better differentiate the different IBS subtypes, the Bristol Stool Form Scale (BSFS) is very helpful clinically in defining the spectrum of diarrhea to constipation (Table 26–4). Over a 14-day bowel diary, patients with hard stools more than 25% of the time and loose stools fewer than 25% of the time are classified as IBS with constipation (IBS-C), whereas patients classified as having IBS with diarrhea (IBS-D) have loose stools more than 25% of the time and hard stools fewer than 25% of the time. About one-third to one-half of patients are termed IBS-mixed (IBS-M) and have hard stools more than 25% of the time and loose stools more than 25% of the time. A small (4%) group of patients has unclassified IBS (IBS-U), with neither loose nor hard stools more than 25% of the time. Patients whose bowel habits change from one subtype to another over months or years are known as "alternators."

Table 26–3. Subtyping of irritable bowel syndrome by predominant stool pattern.

Subtype	Description
IBS with constipation (IBS-C)	Hard or lumpy stools >25% and loose (mushy) or watery stools <25% of bowel movements
IBS with diarrhea (IBS-D)	Loose (mushy) or watery stools >25% of the time and hard or lumpy stool <25% of bowel movements
Mixed IBS (IBS-M)	Hard or lumpy stools >25% and loose (mushy) or watery stools >25% of bowel movements
Unsubtyped IBS (IBS-U)	Insufficient abnormality of stool consistency to meet criteria for IBS-C, D, or M

2. IBS-associated nongastrointestinal symptoms and comorbidity with other diseases—Nongastrointestinal symptoms associated with IBS include backache; headache; urinary symptoms such as nocturia, frequency, and urgency of micturition; incomplete bladder emptying; and, in women, dyspareunia. Helpful diagnostic behavioral features of IBS in general practice include symptoms present for more than 6 months, frequent consultations for nongastrointestinal symptoms, previous medically unexplained symptoms, and patient reports that stress aggravates symptoms.

Between 20% and 50% of IBS patients also have fibromyalgia. IBS is common in several other chronic pain disorders, being found in 51% of patients with chronic fatigue syndrome, 64% of those with temporomandibular joint disorder, and 50% of those with chronic pelvic pain. The lifetime rates of IBS in patients with these syndromes are even higher: 77% in fibromyalgia, 92% in chronic fatigue syndrome, and 64% in temporomandibular joint disorder. In addition, those with overlap syndromes tend to have more severe IBS. IBS patients in primary care with numerous other somatic complaints report high levels of mood disorder, health anxiety, neuroticism, adverse life events, and reduced quality of life and increased health care seeking.

3. Psychological features—At least half of IBS patients can be described as depressed, anxious, or hypochondriacal. Studies from tertiary care centers suggest that up to two-thirds have a psychiatric disorder—most commonly depressive or anxiety disorder. The clinician should always ask the patients about any psychological problems, as well as take a history of physical and sexual abuse. Suggested questions to help assess mood include the following:

- "During the past month, have you often been bothered by feeling down, depressed, or hopeless?"
- "During the past month, have you been bothered by little interest or pleasure in doing things?"
- "Is this something with which you would like help?"

4. "Alarm" features—Certain "alarm" features indicate that the diagnosis might not be IBS. It is very important to take

Table 26–5. "Alarm" features in a patient with possible IBS.

Age >50
Short history of symptoms
Documented weight loss
Nocturnal symptoms
Male sex
Family history of colon cancer
Anemia
Rectal bleeding
Recent antibiotic usage

a careful history and perform a thorough physical examination to rule out any such red flag symptoms, which are detailed in Table 26–5. The Rome criteria in the absence of alarm symptoms were highly specific but not highly sensitive. Alarm features include age greater than 50 years at onset of symptoms, male sex, blood mixed in the stool, and blood on the toilet paper as predictors for an organic diagnosis. Characteristic features of IBS in this study were pain more than six times in the last year, pain that radiated outside the abdomen and pain that was associated with looser bowel movements, all of which were much more common in IBS than in organic disease. Other features more common in IBS included a childhood history of abdominal pain, which was found in a quarter of subjects.

5. Physical findings—Physical examination of the patient with IBS usually reveals no relevant abnormality. Important red flags to look for are thyroid abnormalities, lymphadenopathy, abdominal masses, and perianal disease such as anal fistulas, fissures, or skin tags. Abdominal wall pain originating from a hernia, local muscle injury, or a trapped nerve can be elucidated by the Carnett's test. This involves asking patients to fold their arms across their chest and raise their head off the pillow against gentle resistance from the physician's hand on the patient's abdomen. Exacerbation of pain indicates a positive Carnett's test. Painful rib syndrome is characterized by point tenderness and pain upon springing the rib cage and has a benign cause. Checking for both common musculoskeletal problems can save a lot of time and money on diagnostic testing.

B. Laboratory Findings

Diagnostic testing in patients with suspected IBS and no concerning features depends on the subtype. For all IBS subtypes, screening should include complete blood count and age-appropriate colorectal cancer screening. For IBS-D, screening includes fecal calprotectin or fecal lactoferrin, ESR or CRP, *Giardia* antigen or PCR, serologies for celiac disease, including IgA tissue transglutaminase (TTG) and a total IgA level since the celiac tests measure IgA antibodies (and if IgA deficient then test for IgG tissue transglutaminase or IgA dominated gliadin peptides), and empiric trial of bile acid binder for bile acid diarrhea. Thyroid-stimulating hormone is not recommended for all patients, only if a clinical suspicion exists.

C. Colonoscopy

The basic indications for colonoscopy in this setting are age 45 or greater, positive fecal calprotectin, frank rectal bleeding, and a family history of colon cancer. In a prospective case-control study at three US sites with 466 suspected IBS patients, colonoscopy did not change management in 98.1% of patients with presumed IBS and were negative for microscopic colitis.

▶ Differential Diagnosis

A. Lactose Intolerance

Lactose intolerance is very common and has similar symptoms to IBS. It is seen in 7–20% of Caucasians, as high as 80–95% of Native Americans, 65–75% of Africans and African Americans, and 50% of Hispanics. The prevalence is greater than 90% in some populations in East Asia. The preferred method of testing is a hydrogen breath test. For patients who are lactose intolerant, lactase preparations such as Lactaid, Lactase, and Dairy Ease may help, but many patients still have symptoms and will have to avoid all lactose-containing food products.

B. Fructose Intolerance

Fructose is another carbohydrate that is poorly absorbed in some individuals. The consumption of fructose in the United States has greatly increased over the past two decades and is due in large part to the increase of over 100% in the consumption of high-fructose corn syrup. A retrospective study of 80 IBS patients found that 38% were fructose intolerant. This same study reported that a fructose-restricted diet results in a significant improvement (P <.02) in symptoms including pain, belching, bloating, fullness, indigestion, and diarrhea. In a double-blind, randomized, placebo-controlled trial, 25 IBS patients who had responded to a change in diet (consisting of food low in free fructose and fructans) were rechallenged by graded-dose introduction of fructose or fructans (alone or in combination) or glucose. Patients who were rechallenged with fructose, fructans, or the combination had worse control over their IBS symptoms (70%, 77%, and 79%, respectively) than those rechallenged only with glucose (14%; P ≤.02). Because fructose intolerance or malabsorption can occur simultaneously with IBS, fructose should be restricted over a trial period to see if IBS patients respond.

C. Carbohydrate Intolerance

Because of the evidence of carbohydrate intolerance in patients with IBS-D, a trial of a very low carbohydrate diet (VLCD) in 17 IBS patients was initiated. All patients had moderate to severe IBS-D and were provided a 2-week standard diet and then 4 weeks of a VLCD (20 g of carbohydrate). Thirteen of 17 patients completed the study, with 10 patients (77%) reporting adequate relief for all 4 VLCD weeks.

Stool frequency decreased (2.6 ± 0.8 to 1.4 ± 1.2 stools per day; P <.001), stool consistency improved from diarrheal to normal form (Bristol Stool Scale score: 5.3 ± 0.7 to 3.8 ± 1.2; P <.001), and pain scores and quality of life measures significantly improved. Outcomes were independent of weight loss.

D. Bile Acid Malabsorption

Idiopathic adult-onset bile acid malabsorption is not rare and could contribute to the watery diarrhea of patients with IBS-D. In a pooled analysis of 18 relevant studies in IBS patients, bile acid malabsorption was determined by excessive secretion of an artificial bile salt, selenium homocholic acid taurine (SeHCAT), at 7 days. Five studies (429 patients) indicated that 10% of patients (95% confidence interval [CI], 7–13%) had severe bile acid malabsorption (SeHCAT <5%). Seventeen studies (1073 patients) indicated that 32% of patients (95% CI, 29–35%) had moderate bile acid malabsorption (SeHCAT <10%), and seven studies (618 patients) indicated that 26% of patients (95% CI, 23–30%) had mild bile acid malabsorption (SeHCAT <15%). Pooled data from 15 studies showed a dose-response relationship according to severity of malabsorption to treatment with a bile acid binder. A response to cholestyramine occurred in 96% of severe patients, 80% of moderate patients, and 70% of mild patients. One of the mechanisms for bile acid diarrhea may be defective feedback inhibition of bile acid biosynthesis via fibroblast growth factor-19.

E. Food Intolerances

There have been 12 randomized controlled trials and two systemic reviews and meta-analyses on the efficacy of a low fermentable oligo-, di-, monosaccharides, and polyols (low FODMAP) diet to reduce IBS symptoms. The overall recommendation is for a 6-week trial of low FODMAP diet and if no improvement, the recommendation is to not repeat the diet. These compounds in food are poorly absorbed, highly osmotic, and rapidly fermented by GI bacteria, leading to increased water and gas in the GI tract, which then leads to GI tract distention that causes changes in GI motility, bloating, discomfort, and flatulence. This diet limits but does not eliminate foods that contain lactose, fructose, fructans, galactans, and sugar alcohols (polyols). Common high FODMAP foods to avoid are shown in Table 26–6. Additional foods

Table 26–6. The low FODMAP diet.

The FODMAPs in the diet are:
Fructose (fruits, honey, high-fructose corn syrup [HFCS], etc)
Lactose (dairy)
Fructans (wheat, garlic, onion, inulin, etc)
Galactans (legumes such as beans, lentils, soybeans, etc)
Polyols (sweeteners containing isomalt, mannitol, sorbitol, xylitol, stone fruits such as avocado, apricots, cherries, nectarines, peaches, plums, etc)

Table 26–7. Foods likely to cause loose bowel movements & excessive gas.

All caffeine-containing beverages especially coffee with chicory
Peaches, pears, cherries, apples
Fruit juices, orange, cranberry, apple
Cola beverages that are not caffeine-free, sugar-free
Brassica vegetables such as broccoli, asparagus, cauliflower, cabbage, Brussels sprouts
Bran cereal, whole-wheat bread, high-fiber foods
Pastries, candy, chocolate
Waffle syrup, donuts
Wine (>3 glasses in susceptible individuals)
Milk and milk products if one is sensitive to lactose

likely to cause loose bowel movements and excessive gas and foods likely to cause constipation are detailed in Tables 24–7 and 24–8, respectively. True food allergies are rare in adults, and in particular patients in whom there is a high suspicion should be referred to an allergist. There is also support for a diet rich in soluble fiber at 10–25 g daily and peppermint oil at 180–225 mg twice a day for 2–12 weeks. There is no recommendation favoring a gluten-free diet, an elimination diet nor cannabinoids in relieving IBS symptoms. In the Nutri-NetSante Cohort published in 2018 with 33,343 participants, the more highly processed the diet, the greater the symptom severity.

F. Infections

Most bowel infections should be transient, and symptoms will not be present for 6 months in order to meet the Rome criteria. Broad-spectrum antibiotics lead to transient diarrhea in 10% of cases which, if severe and persistent, should lead to consideration of testing for *Clostriodies difficile* toxin or sigmoidoscopy to exclude pseudomembranous colitis. Chronic giardiasis can last for months and manifest with bloating, abdominal pain, and diarrhea. Stool enzyme-linked immunosorbent assay testing for *Giardia* antigen and polymerase chain reaction testing for *Giardia* small subunit ribosomal RNA are sensitive (90–100%) and specific (95–100%) methods to test for *Giardia* and should be considered in patients presenting with chronic diarrhea. If the patients also have histories of exposure to poor sanitary conditions during their travels or immigration from these areas, then testing the stool for ova and parasites may also be considered.

Table 26–8. Foods likely to cause constipation or at least help control bowel movements.

Rice, bread
Potatoes, pasta
Meat, veal, poultry, fish
Cooked vegetables
Bananas

G. Celiac Disease

Celiac disease occurs in about 1 in 250 people in the United States. It can be identified through blood analysis of immunoglobulin A (IgA) level, antiendomysial antibody, and anti-transglutaminase antibody. IgA level should be checked, because IgA deficiency is more common in patients with celiac disease. Patients who are antibody positive or in whom there is a high suspicion should undergo upper endoscopy and biopsy. Genetic testing is helpful in certain cases. More than 99% of patients with celiac disease have HLA-DQ2, -DQ8, or both, compared with about 40% of the general population. Thus, celiac disease is highly unlikely in patients without these haplotypes. The treatment of celiac disease is a strict gluten-free diet.

Celiac disease may present with symptoms of IBS. In a study by Sanders et al., 66 of 300 IBS patients have antigliadin (IgA) or IgG antibodies and/or antiendomysial antibodies and 14 (4.7%) had celiac disease confirmed by duodenal biopsy. Three of these 14 patients were antiendomysial antibody negative (21.4%). In another study with 105 IBS patients and 105 controls, celiac disease was diagnosed in 12 IBS patients and no controls. All 12 had positive tests for antiendomysial antibody, and all had compatible histologic findings. Of the 12 patients, 3 presented with diarrhea, 4 with constipation, and 5 with alternating diarrhea and constipation. The current serologic test most commonly used in the diagnosis of celiac disease is the tissue transglutaminase antibody, which has a sensitivity of greater than 90% and specificity of greater than 95%.

H. Tropical Sprue

The key diagnostic test in tropical sprue is small intestinal mucosal biopsy, which is usually obtained at esophagogastroduodenoscopy. Gross findings at endoscopy include flattening of duodenal folds and so-called scalloping. The latter finding was originally thought to be pathognomonic of celiac disease but also occurs in tropical sprue and other small bowel diseases. The major histologic findings are shortened, blunted villi, and elongated crypts with increased inflammatory cells in the lamina propria. These histologic changes are similar but not identical to those occurring in patients with untreated celiac disease. Most authorities recommend tetracycline (250 mg orally, four times daily) plus folic acid (5 mg/day) for 3–6 months for the treatment of tropical sprue. Even on this regimen, relapses or reinfection occur in up to 20% of patients living in the tropics.

I. Small Intesintal Bacterial Overgrowth

Small intestinal bacterial overgrowth (SIBO) is characterized by nutrient malabsorption associated with an increased number or type of bacteria in the upper gastrointestinal tract. Affected patients can have abdominal pain, watery diarrhea, dyspepsia, and weight loss. The most frequent presenting symptoms in one series of 100 adult patients were diarrhea, weight loss, bloating, and excess flatulence. A $[^{14}C]$-D-xylose breath test is helpful in making the diagnosis. Xylose is a pentose sugar that is catabolized by gram-negative aerobes, which are invariably part of the microflora implicated in bacterial overgrowth. Bacterial action on the sugar releases the radioactive isotope $^{14}CO_2$, which, after absorption, is detectable in breath samples. Breath hydrogen testing is performed by administering a test dose of carbohydrate (usually lactose or glucose), which, in patients with bacterial overgrowth, is associated with a rise in breath hydrogen levels. It is possible to have no rise in hydrogen production during a lactulose breath hydrogen test if hydrogen is converted to methane or hydrogen sulfide by hydrogen consumptive microbes. Concurrent testing with methane may enhance sensitivity.

Most patients with bacterial overgrowth require treatment with antibiotics. Effective antibiotic treatment should cover both aerobic and anaerobic enteric bacteria, and adequate antimicrobial coverage can be achieved with the following: a 14-day course of rifaximin for IBS-D, IBS-M or IBS-U. In the event of first and second recurrences, a 4-week interval followed by repeat 14-day course of rifaximin is recommended. Some patients may require prolonged therapy (eg, 1–2 months) before a response is seen. It is usually unnecessary to repeat diagnostic testing if symptoms or objective measures of malabsorption respond to treatment. Studies show that patients on rifaximin reported decreased bloating and flatulence after 10 days ($P = .03$) and 20 days ($P = .02$). There was decreased hydrogen breath excretion among responders ($P = .01$).

There have been over 55 trials on the efficacy of probiotics for IBS. Thirteen studies showed improvement in parameters such as quality of life, reduced bloating, decreased abdominal circumference and/or less pain. It is currently recommended to use certain strains rather than probiotics as a group, in patients with IBS. The monostrains include: *Bifidobacterium bifidum*, *Bifidobacterium infantis*, *Bifidobacterium lactis*, *Escherichia coli*, *Lactobacillus acidophilus*, *Lactobacillus plantarum*, *Bacillus coagulans*, *Bifidobacterium animalis*, and *Saccharomyces boulardii*.

J. Inflammatory Bowel Disease

Crohn's disease and ulcerative colitis are easy to distinguish from IBS with modern diagnostic testing. Most patients with inflammatory bowel disease present with weight loss, bleeding, and abdominal pain. Laboratory studies often reveal anemia, increased sedimentation rate, and sometimes leukocytosis. Fecal calprotein or fecal lactoferrin are typically elevated. Colonoscopy in patients with colitis reveals inflammation, erythema, exudates, and sometimes ulcerations. Pathologic examination shows chronic changes in the mucosa. Subtle Crohn's disease of the small bowel can be found by computed tomographic enterography, magnetic resonance (MR) enterography, or capsule endoscopy in cases that are difficult to diagnose.

K. Microscopic Colitis

Two atypical colitides—collagenous colitis and lymphocytic colitis—have completely normal endoscopic appearances.

Collagenous colitis has two main histologic components: increased subepithelial collagen deposition and colitis with increased intraepithelial lymphocytes. The female to male ratio is 9:1, and most patients present in the sixth or seventh decades of life. The main symptom is chronic watery diarrhea. Treatments include sulfasalazine, mesalamine, Lomotil, bismuth, budesonide, prednisone, and azathioprine/6-mercaptopurine for refractory disease. Risk factors include smoking; use of nonsteroidal anti-inflammatory diseases (NSAIDs), proton pump inhibitors, or β-blockers; and a history of autoimmune disease.

Lymphocytic colitis has features like collagenous colitis, including age at onset and clinical presentation, but it has almost equal incidence in men and women and no subepithelial collagen deposition on pathologic section. Use of sertraline (but not β-blockers) is an additional risk factor. However, intraepithelial lymphocytes are increased. The frequency of celiac disease is increased in lymphocytic colitis and ranges from 9% to 27%. Celiac disease should be excluded in all patients with lymphocytic colitis, particularly if diarrhea does not respond to conventional therapy. Treatment is like that of collagenous colitis with the exception of a gluten-free diet for those who have celiac disease.

L. Fecal Incontinence

Fecal incontinence with involuntary loss of solid stool, liquid stool, flatus or a combination may masquerade as diarrhea and patients are often reluctant to report fecal incontinence because it is embarrassing. In a study of symptomatic pelvic floor disorders in US, 5–15% reported fecal incontinence with a female predominance. The prevalence of fecal incontinence increases with age, cigarette smoking, multiparity, and cholecystectomy. Obesity and poverty increased the likelihood of symptoms. Other causes of fecal incontinence are a history of a forceps delivery, a total abdominal hysterectomy, diabetes, pelvic radiation, an errant episiotomy, and a perianal fistula repair. Pelvic floor muscle training with repeated voluntary pelvic floor muscle contractions performed several days of the week for at least eight weeks has been found to be beneficial for incontinence. Training is to be followed by maintenance exercises.

M. Endometriosis

Patients with IBS appear to be more symptomatic during their menstruations, notably with increased gastrointestinal smooth muscle contractions in line with prostaglandin release. Endometriosis also appears with similar symptoms to IBS. A questionnaire sent to 50 women with IBS and 51 women with gynecological disorders found that dyspareunia was similar in both groups and that the two disorders can coexist.

The differential diagnosis of IBS-D is detailed in Table 26–9.

Table 26–9. Differential diagnosis of irritable bowel syndrome with diarrhea (IBS-D).

Lactose, fructose, carbohydrate and/or food intolerance
Bile acid malabsorption
Infections
Celiac disease
Tropical sprue
Small bowel bacterial overgrowth
Inflammatory bowel disease
Microscopic colitis
Fecal incontinence
Endometriosis

Austin GL, Dalton CB, Hu Y, et al. A very low carbohydrate diet improves symptoms and quality of life in diarrhea predominant irritable bowel syndrome. *Clin Gastroenterol Hepatol*. 2009;7:706–708. [PMID: 19281859]

Chey WD, Nojkov B, Rubenstein JH, et al. The yield of colonoscopy in patients with non-constipated irritable bowel syndrome: results from prospective, controlled US trial. *Am J Gastroenterol*. 2010;105(4):859–865. [PMID: 20179696]

De Roest RH, Dobbs BR, Chapman BA, et al. The low FODMAP diet improves gastrointestinal symptoms in patients with irritable bowel syndrome: a prospective study. *Int J Clin Pract*. 2013;67:895–903. [PMID: 23701141]

Halmos EP, Power VA, Sheperd SJ, et al. A diet low in FODMAPs reduces symptoms of irritable bowel syndrome. *Gastroenterology*. 2014;146:67–75. [PMID: 24076059]

Kumar D. Irritable bowel syndrome, chronic pelvic inflammatory disease and endometriosis. *Eur J Gastroenterol Hepatol*. 2004;16(12):1251–1252. [PMID: 15618826]

Lacy BE, Patel NK. Rome criteria and a diagnostic approach to irritable bowel syndrome. *J Clin Med*. 2017;11:99. [PMID: 29072609]

Nygaard I, Barber MD, Burgio KL, et al. Prevalence of symptomatic pelvic floor disorders in US women. *JAMA*. 2008;300:1311–1316. [PMID: 18799443]

Pimentel M, Park S, Mirocha J, et al. The effect of a nonabsorbed oral antibiotic (rifaximin) on the symptoms of the irritable bowel syndrome. *Ann Intern Med*. 2006;145:557–563. [PMID: 17043337]

Philpott H, Nandurkar S, Lubel J, et al. Food, fibre, bile acids and the pelvic floor: an integrated low risk low cost approach to managing irritable bowel syndrome. *World J Gastroenterol*. 2015;21(40):11379–11386. [PMID: 26525925]

Posserud I, Stotzer PO, Björnsson ES, et al. Small intestinal bacterial overgrowth in patients with irritable bowel syndrome. *Gut*. 2007;56:802–808. [PMID: 17148502]

Sanders DS, Carter MJ, Hurlstone DP, et al. Association of adult coeliac disease with irritable bowel syndrome: a case-control study in patients fulfilling ROME II criteria referred to secondary care. *Lancet*. 2001;358:1504–1508. [PMID: 11705563]

Scarpellini E, Gabrielli M, Lauritano CE, et al. High dosage rifaximin for the treatment of small intestinal bacterial overgrowth. *Aliment Pharmacol Ther*. 2007;25:781–786. [PMID: 17373916]

Schnabel L, Buscail C, Sabate JM, et al. Association between ultra-processed food consumption and functional gastrointestinal disorders: results from the French NutriNet-Santé Cohort. *Am J Gastroenterol*. 2018;113(8):1217–1228. [PMID: 29904158]

Shahbazkhani B, Forootan M, Merat S, et al. Coeliac disease presenting with symptoms of irritable bowel syndrome. *Aliment Pharmacol Ther.* 2003;18:231–235. [PMID: 12869084]

Sharara AI, Aoun E, Adbul-Baki H, et al. A randomized double-blind placebo-controlled trial of rifaximin in patients with abdominal bloating and flatulence. *Am J Gastroenterol.* 2006;101:326–333. [PMID: 16454838]

Shepherd SJ, Parker FC, Muir JG, et al. Dietary triggers of abdominal symptoms in patients with irritable bowel syndrome; randomized placebo-controlled evidence. *Clin Gastroenterol Hepatol.* 2008;6:765–771. [PMID: 18456565]

Smally W, Falck-Ytter C, Carrasco-Labra A, et al. AGA Clinical Practice Guidelines on the laboratory evaluation of functional diarrhea and diarrhea-predominant irritable bowel syndrome in adults (IBS-D). *AGA* 2019;157(3):851–854. [PMID: 31378676]

Walters JR, Tasleem AM, Omer OS, et al. A new mechanism for bile acid diarrhea: defective feedback inhibition of bile acid biosynthesis. *Clin Gastroenterol Hepatol.* 2009;7:1189–1194. [PMID: 19426836]

Wedlake L, A'Hern R, Russell D, et al. Systematic review: the prevalence of idiopathic bile acid malabsorption as diagnosed by SeHCAT scanning in patients with diarrhea-predominant irritable bowel syndrome. *Aliment Pharmacol Ther.* 2009;30:707–717. [PMID: 19570102]

► Complications

The complications of IBS are decreased quality of life, time off from work and school, personal expenses of medications and physician visits, and psychological problems such as depression and anxiety. It is commonplace for IBS patients to undergo unnecessary procedures and surgeries, and it is the role of the treating physician to avoid these complications. Comprehensive patient appointments, close follow-up, and much reassurance by the physician are recommended. When asked what they want from their health care professional, IBS patients in England offered their 10 top requests, which are listed in Table 26–10.

Table 26–10. Top 10 patient requests compiled by the IBS Network in the United Kingdom.

"When I visit my health professional about my IBS I would like them to give me …"
1. A clear knowledgeable explanation of what IBS is
2. A statement there is no miracle cure
3. A clear indication that it is my body, my illness, and that it is up to me to take control
4. A clear explanation that there will be good days and bad days but there will be light at the end of the tunnel
5. An explanation of the different treatment options
6. Recognition that IBS is an illness
7. Consider and discuss complementary/alternative therapies
8. Offer at least one complementary/alternative therapy
9. Offer support and understanding
10. Be aware of conflicting emotion in someone who is newly diagnosed

► Treatment

Current treatment options for IBS are limited and include dietary modification, fiber supplements, pharmacologic agents (Table 26–11), and psychotherapy.

A. Fiber

Poorly fermentable, soluble fiber found in whole grains, fruits, nuts, seeds, and vegetables and also in the form of fiber supplements containing psyllium (Metamucil), guar gum (Benefiber), calcium polycarbophil (FiberCon), and methylcellulose (Citrucel) helps to regulate bowel movements and improve stool consistency, especially in IBS-C. Insoluble fiber such as wheat bran may exacerbate pain and bloating, thus is to be avoided. Although it may help individual patients and is used commonly for patients with IBS-M disease or alternators, there is no high-quality evidence-based literature supporting the benefits of fiber in treating IBS.

B. Antidiarrheal Agents

Loperamide (Imodium) is no longer recommended for IBS patients given lack of statistically significant effect compared to placebo in two trials involving 42 patients. Diphenoxylate hydrochloride–atropine sulfate (Lomotil) may decrease diarrhea but has no effect on bloating or abdominal pain.

Up to 50% of patients with IBS-D have concurrent bile acid diarrhea. Bile acids increase mucosal permeability and accelerate transit by triggering colonic contractions. Frequently IBS-D patients are placed on bile acid sequestrants such as cholestyramine, colestipol, or colesevelam. Cholestyramine resin binds bile salts and slows down diarrhea but similarly to loperamide has no effect on abdominal pain or bloating. In one study, the bile acid sequestrants improved IBS symptoms in 56% of the patients. A limiting factor is the poor palatability leading to low medication adherence. These agents can be helpful for IBS in combination with other antispasmodics or can be used to provide as-needed therapy for diarrhea.

C. Enemas & Suppositories

Among patients who need these agents for intractable constipation, the majority will use them only occasionally. The safest suppository to use is a glycerin suppository because it is not a stimulant laxative and has no lasting ill effects on the gut. Fleets, tap water, or mineral oil enemas can be used occasionally for refractory constipation but insertion of air that comes with the enema fluid will only exacerbate bloating and abdominal pain.

D. Laxatives

Various laxatives are available for the constipation component of IBS. They include the stimulant laxatives (senna, bisacodyl, cascara) and the osmotic laxatives (polyethylene glycol, lactulose, sorbitol). The stimulant laxatives may

Table 26–11. Possible drugs for dominant symptoms in irritable bowel syndrome.

Symptom	Drug Class	Dose
Diarrhea	Cholestyramine resin 5-HT$_3$ antagonist (alosetron) u-opid and k-opioid receptor agonist and δ-opioid receptor antagonist (eluxadoline)	4 g with meals 0.5–1 mg twice daily (for severe IBS in women) 75–100 mg twice a day
Constipation	Psyllium husk Methylcellulose Calcium polycarbophil Lactulose syrup 70% Sorbitol Polyethylene glycol Lubiprostone Linaclotide Plecanatide Magnesium hydroxide 5-HT$_4$ agonist (tegaserod) 5-HT$_4$ agonist (prucalopride)	3.4 g twice daily with meals, then adjust 2 g twice daily with meals, then adjust 1 g daily to 4 times daily 10–20 g twice daily 15 mL twice daily 17 g in 8 oz water daily 24 µg twice daily (for chronic constipation), 8 µg twice daily (for IBS-C) 145 µg once daily for chronic constipation 290 µg once daily for IBS-C 3 mg once a day 2–4 tbsp daily 6 mg twice a day before meals for 4–6 weeks for initial dosing, if effective can extend to 12 weeks (efficacy beyond 12 weeks not established) 2 mg once a day
Abdominal pain	Smooth muscle relaxant Tricyclic antidepressant Selective serotonin reuptake inhibitors Peppermint oil	4 times daily before meals Start 25–50 mg at bedtime, then adjust Begin small dose, increase as needed Depends on brand
Bloating	Rifaximin Probiotics Fecal microbiota transplant	400 mg three times a day for 10 days Depends on brand Capsules, upper endoscopy, or colonoscopy with instillation in cecum

cause permanent damage to the myenteric plexus but studies are conflicting. In any case, they do exacerbate abdominal cramps and bloating when used chronically. Abdominal cramps and excess gas and bloating are seen with the osmotic laxative, but MiraLax was deemed effective for chronic constipation in one long-term study.

E. Antispasmodics

There is only minimal evidence-based literature that antispasmodics are effective in treating the pain component of IBS. Antispasmodics relax the smooth muscle of the gut and include dicyclomine hydrochloride (Bentyl), hyoscyamine sulfate (Levsin), scopolamine and phenobarbital (Donnatal), and clidinium bromide with chlordiazepoxide (Librax). These medicines are usually given before meals to inhibit abdominal pain and immediate, uncontrolled bowel movements.

F. Tricyclic Antidepressants

Tricyclic antidepressants, such as amitriptyline hydrochloride (Elavil) and nortriptyline hydrochloride (Pamelor), prescribed at low doses, are beneficial in patients with and without diagnosed depression and anxiety because their benefit derives more from pain reduction than depression.

There is some evidence-based literature favoring amitriptyline in treating visceral hypersensitivity. Side effects of both antispasmodics and tricyclics include dry mouth, dry eyes, and fatigue. Weight gain is a side effect particular to tricyclics.

G. Selective Serotonin Reuptake Inhibitors

Citalopram hydrobromide (Celexa) has been tested in patients with IBS. One study found that this selective serotonin reuptake inhibitor (SSRI), which is commonly used for depression, was effective in patients with IBS. Citalopram significantly improved symptoms of abdominal pain and bloating and improved quality of life and overall well-being. Fluoxetine hydrochloride (Prozac), an SSRI commonly used in the treatment of depression, is also effective in treating IBS. In a recent study in patients with IBS-C, fluoxetine decreased abdominal discomfort and bloating and increased bowel movements.

H. Psychological Therapies

Through a review of 36 separate randomized control trials, provider-directed cognitive behavioral therapy, relaxation therapy, hypnotherapy, and dynamic psychotherapy were shown with some weak evidence to improve overall symptom control in IBS patients.

I. Newer Medical Therapies for IBS

A few newer medical therapies for inflammatory bowel disease focus on the serotonin receptor in the gut. Alosetron (Lotronex) is a 5-HT$_3$ antagonist approved for use in women with severe IBS-D who have failed conventional therapy. Alosetron slows colonic transit, decreases rectal urgency and abdominal pain. The drug was launched in February 2000 and temporarily withdrawn from the market in November of that year due to isolated reports of constipation and ischemic colitis. There were 3 deaths and 77 hospitalizations. Public outcry resulted in approval by the US Food and Drug Administration (FDA) to allow the reintroduction of alosetron on a limited basis, and the drug was reintroduced in November 2002 under a new risk-management program. Restrictions on the use of alosetron include updated warnings in the complete Prescribing Information; including a Medication Guide for patients that explains what to do if they become constipated or have signs of ischemic colitis; a lower starting dose (0.5 mg twice a day) than previously approved; and a prescribing program for physicians to be enrolled in, based on self-attestation of qualifications and acceptance of certain responsibilities in prescribing alosetron. There is significant evidence-based literature which recommend use of alosetron in women with severe IBS-D, and it is an important drug in the IBS armamentarium. Studies show a statistically significant increase in global improvement in IBS symptoms, adequate relief of IBS pain and discomfort, and improvement in bowel symptoms.

Tegaserod (Zelnorm) is a selective serotonin-4 (5-HT$_4$) agonist approved for use in women with IBS-C. Tegaserod targets 5-HT$_4$ receptors of smooth muscle cells and neurons in the GI tract to decrease pain signals and induce contraction and relaxation. There are three double blind placebo controlled randomized control trials in 2470 woman who had demonstrated improvement in constipation, gastric emptying, and dyspeptic symptoms. It was originally approved in 2002 but was pulled off the market in US in 2007 for concerns for cardiac related side effects. After a complete safety review by the FDA that negated the side effects, tegaserod is now reintroduced in 2019.

Prucalopride (Montegrity) is also a selective serotonin-4 (5-HT$_4$) agonist approved for use in women with chronic idiopathic constipation but has been extended for use in IBS-C with refractory constipation. A meta-analysis of nine clinical trials revealed that prucalopride was effective for eliciting at least three bowel movements weekly with improvement in stool consistency and quality of life compared to placebo. There are also potential roles for chronic intestinal pseudo-obstruction, but data is still limited. Side effects include diarrhea, headaches, nausea, and abdominal pain. Caution is advised in impaired liver and renal function. It is not recommended during pregnancy or breastfeeding (Category C).

Eluxadoline (Viberzi or Truberzi) was approved in 2015 for the use of IBS-D. It is a u-opid and k-opioid receptor agonist and δ-opioid receptor antagonist, thus acting on the intestinal nervous system to reduce diarrhea. There are three randomized and placebo-trials on eluxadoline 100 mg twice a day compared to placebo that showed a positive effect on global symptoms and stool consistency. Adverse effects include acute pancreatitis and sphincter of Oddi spasm. Therefore patients with pancreatitis, sphincter of Oddi spasms, cholecystectomy, alcohol use disorder, or have liver or pancreas conditions are not recommended to take eluxadoline.

J. Prosecretory Agents

The three prosecretory agents are Lubiprostone, Linaclotide, and Plecanatide. They are currently indicated for the treatment of chronic constipation and IBS-C.

Lubiprostone (Amitiza) is a specific chloride channel-2 activator that enhances intestinal fluid secretion with efflux of chloride and water to facilitate increased motility. Lubiprostone increases weekly spontaneous bowel movements, and a significant number of patients respond within 24 hours. It is the only medicine for constipation with an indication for patients of age 65 and older. There is one high-quality study published on lubiprostone in chronic constipation, and the rest of the data are in abstract form only. The main side effect is nausea, which can be alleviated by taking the medicine with food.

Linaclotide is a minimally absorbed 14-amino acid peptide agonist of the guanylate cyclase C receptor that improves symptoms of chronic constipation and constipation predominant IBS. In two 12-week double-blind, placebo-controlled trials of 1276 patients, linaclotide significantly reduced bowel and abdominal symptoms in patients with chronic constipation. In another double-blind, placebo-controlled trial of 804 patients with IBS-C, linaclotide improved symptoms of abdominal pain, bloating, and constipation. The dose of linaclotide for IBS-C is 290 μg once a day and the dose for chronic constipation is 145 μg/day.

Plecanatide is a 16-amino acid peptide that is like uroguanylin. There are three randomized control trials that show higher rates of diarrhea with plecanatide compared to placebo. Thus, plecanatide was approved by the FDA for IBS-C and chronic idiopathic constipation.

K. Rifaximin

Rifaximin (Xifaxan) is a nonsystemic (<0.4%) semisynthetic antibiotic whose spectrum includes most gram-positive and gram-negative bacteria, both aerobes and anaerobes. In one questionnaire study in patients with IBS, there was a statistically significant improvement in overall symptoms and less bloating ($P = .020$) over placebo. There was no difference in pain, diarrhea, or constipation. The dosage of rifaximin used in this study (400 mg orally, three times daily for 10 days) is higher than that approved by the FDA for traveler's diarrhea.

L. Probiotics

In a recent study, *Bifidobacterium infantis* 35624 was shown to alleviate abdominal pain and bloating and bowel movement difficulty. Another probiotic, which contains eight different strains of bacteria including lactobacillus and bifidobacterial, alleviated flatulence and slowed down stools in IBS patients. On the other hand, prebiotics and synbiotics are not recommended for IBS patients. These are food or dietary supplements that change the GI microbiota, in contrast to liver microorganisms in probiotics.

M. Peppermint Oil

There are a very small number of trials regarding peppermint oil for IBS. Nevertheless, peppermint oil is suggested as helpful in symptom improvement. Of note, there are adverse reports of heartburn.

N. Fecal Microbiota Transplant

Fecal microbiota transplant (FMT) has been successful in treating *Clostridioides difficile* infections by changing the intestinal microbiota. Given that IBS patient have significant bloating, likely with associated disrupted microbial compositions, there has been strong interest in applying FMT to the treatment of IBS. There have been mixed results in randomized double blinded placebo-controlled studies. In one study with 52 adults with IBS randomized to FMT or placebo capsules for 6 months, there was no difference in symptom relief between the two groups. In another study with 83 adults with IBS randomized 2:1 to active or placebo FMT with colonoscopy to the cecum, there was significant symptom relief in the patients with FMT compared to placebo. In a third study with 62 patients with treatment refractory IBS with bloating symptoms randomized to FMT with donor stool versus autologous transplant, the patients undergoing FMT had symptom relief although the effects slowly wore off over 1 year and lead to FMT being repeated.

Camilleri M. Bile acid diarrhea: prevalence, pathogenesis, and therapy. *Gut Liver*. 2015;9(3):332–339. [PMID: 25918262]

Chey WD, Chey WY, Heath AT, et al. Long-term safety and efficacy of alosetron in women with severe diarrhea-predominant irritable bowel syndrome. *Am J Gastroenterol*. 2004;99:2195–2203. [PMID: 15555002]

Chey WD, Lembo AJ, Lavins BJ, Shiff SJ. Linaclotide for irritable bowel syndrome with constipation: a 26-week, randomized, double-blind, placebo-controlled trial to evaluate efficacy and safety. *Am J Gastroenterol*. 2012;107:1702–1712. [PMID: 22986437]

Daniali M, Nikfar S, Abdollahi M. An overview of the efficacy and safety of prucalopride for the treatment of chronic idiopathic constipation. *Expert Opin Pharmacother*. 2019;20(17): 2073–2080. [PMID: 31557072]

DiPalma JA, Cleveland MB, McGowan J, et al. A randomized, multicenter, placebo-controlled trial of polyethylene glycol laxative for chronic treatment of chronic constipation. *Am J Gastroenterol*. 2007;102:1436–1441. [PMID: 17984738]

Ford A, Moayyedi P, Chey WD, et al. American College of Gastroenterology monograph on management of irritable bowel syndrome. *Am J Gastroenterology*. 2018;113:1–18. [PMID: 29950604]

Halkjær SI, Christensen AH, Lo BZS, et al. Faecal microbiota transplantation alters gut microbiota in patients with irritable bowel syndrome: results from a randomised, double-blind placebo-controlled study. *Gut*. 2018;67(12):2107–2115. [PMID: 29980607]

Holvoet T, Joossens M, Vázquez-Castellanos JF, et al. Fecal microbiota transplantation reduces symptoms in some patients with irritable bowel syndrome with predominant abdominal bloating: short- and long-term results from a placebo-controlled randomized trial. *Gastroenterology*. 2020;S0016-5085(20)34937-4. [PMID: 32681922]

Johanson JF, Ueno R. Lubiprostone, a locally acting chloride channel activator, in adult patients with chronic constipation: a double-blind, placebo-controlled, dose-ranging study to evaluate efficacy and safety. *Aliment Pharmacol Ther*. 2007;25: 1351–1361. [PMID: 17509103]

Johnsen PH, Hilpüsch F, Cavanagh JP, et al. Faecal microbiota transplantation versus placebo for moderate-to-severe irritable bowel syndrome: a double-blind, randomised, placebo-controlled, parallel-group, single-centre trial. *Lancet Gastroenterol Hepatol*. 2018;3(1):17–24. [PMID: 29100842]

Krause R, Ameen V, Gordon SH, et al. A randomized, double-blind, placebo-controlled study to assess efficacy and safety of 0.5 mg and 1 mg alosetron in women with severe diarrhea-predominant IBS. *Am J Gastroenterol*. 2007;102:1709–1719. [PMID: 17509028]

Lembo A, Schneier HA, Schiff SJ, et al. Two randomized trials of linaclotide for chronic constipation. *N Engl J Med*. 2011; 365:527–536. [PMID: 21830967]

Mearin F, Ciriza C, Mínguez M, et al. Clinical Practice Guideline: irritable bowel syndrome with constipation and functional constipation in the adult. *Rev Esp Enferm Dig*. 2016;108(6):332–363. [PMID: 27230827]

Pimentel M, Lembo A, Chey WD, et al; TARGET Study Group. Rifaximin therapy for patients with irritable bowel syndrome without constipation. *N Engl J Med*. 2011;364:22–32. [PMID: 21208106]

Rao SS, Quigley EM, Shiff SJ. Effect of linaclotide on severe abdominal symptoms in patients with irritable bowel syndrome with constipation. *Clin Gastroenterol Hepatol*. 2014;12:616–623. [PMID: 24075889]

Acute Lower Gastrointestinal Bleeding

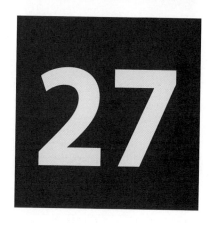

John R. Saltzman, MD

▶ Diverticulosis, angioectasias, ischemic colitis, neoplasms, and hemorrhoids are the most common causes of lower gastrointestinal bleeding (LGIB).

▶ Clinical presentation ranges from occult to overt bleeding.

▶ Endoscopic and radiologic tests are diagnostic and can provide therapy.

▶ Early colonoscopy within 24 hours of hospital admission after hemodynamic resuscitation and a bowel preparation is recommended.

General Considerations

Lower gastrointestinal bleeding (LGIB) is defined as bleeding that occurs from a source in the colon, rectum, or anus. It accounts for about 30% of major gastrointestinal (GI) bleeding (requiring hospitalization) and is less common than upper GI bleeding. In 2018, LGIB was responsible for 370,000 annual visits to the emergency department, and approximately 144,000 hospitalizations per year in adults in the United States. LGIB generally occurs in older adults between ages 63 and 77 years. Nearly 80% of LGIB stops spontaneously, similar to upper GI bleeding. The overall mortality rate of LGIB is about 1.5%. Similar to upper GI bleeding, patients who develop LGIB as outpatients have a significantly lower mortality rate than those who develop LGIB as inpatients.

Peery AF, Crockett SD, Murphy CC, et al. Burden and cost of gastrointestinal, liver, and pancreatic diseases in the United States: update 2018. *Gastroenterology.* 2019;156(1):254–272. [PMID: 30315778]

EVALUATION OF LOWER GI BLEEDING

Definition of Bleeding

Hematochezia is defined as bright red blood per rectum and usually implies a left colonic source, although it can be caused by a brisk, more proximal source of bleeding. Maroon stools are maroon-colored blood mixed with stool and are often associated with a right colonic source of bleeding; however, they also can result from a brisk, source of bleeding proximal to the colon. Melena refers to black, tarry, foul-smelling stool that results from the bacterial degradation of hemoglobin over a period of at least 14 hours. It usually implies an upper GI source of bleeding although it may be associated with right colonic or cecal bleeding. Ingestion of iron, bismuth, charcoal, and licorice all can turn stool black and should be specifically asked for on history. Occult blood refers to the presence of small quantities of blood in the stool that does not change the stool color and can only be detected by performing a stool guaiac (or similar) test. Blood loss of at least 5–10 mL/day can be detected by stool guaiac card tests. The GI tract normally loses about 0.5–1.5 mL of blood per day, which is not usually detected by guaiac tests.

Diagnostic Approach

When patients initially present with LGIB, they should be triaged and managed based on the severity of the hemorrhage (Figure 27–1). Initial management should include fluid resuscitation and support with blood transfusions if needed. Transfusions recommendation for packed red blood cells (PRBCs) are similar to those for upper GI bleeding, with transfusions given to keep the hemoglobin level >7 g/dL in most patients, with higher transfusion threshold of 8 g/dL in patients with significant coexisting illness such as massive active bleeding, acute coronary syndromes, symptomatic peripheral vascular disease, or a history of cerebrovascular disease.

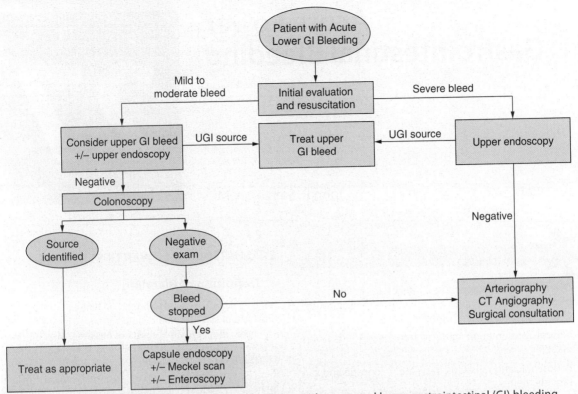

▲ **Figure 27–1.** Algorithm for the management of patients with suspected lower gastrointestinal (GI) bleeding. UGI, upper gastrointestinal.

The strongest risk factors identified for mortality in LGIB include hemodynamic instability (hypotension, tachycardia or syncope), age >60 years, creatinine >1.7 g/dL, ongoing bleeding, and the presence of multiple comorbidities. Prognostic risk scores are helpful in triage and can help define patients at low-risk and high-risk for need for intervention and mortality. Patients at lowest risk can be managed as outpatients with semi-elective evaluation by a gastroenterologist and colonoscopy examination. The Oakland score predicts low-risk LGIB patients and was originally derived in the United Kingdom but recently validated in the United States. A score of ≤8 can predict a low-risk LGIB with an accuracy of 98%, although specificity is 16%. Patients at high-risk may best be identified by the Strate score. This score includes 7 discrete predictors of outcomes (hypotension [<115 mmHg], tachycardia [>100 bpm], syncope, nontender abdomen, bleeding within 4 hours of presentation, aspirin use, and >2 comorbid conditions); the number of positive predictors is totaled to determine the score. The rate of severe bleeding with 0 predictors is 9%, with 1–3 predictors is 43% and with >3 predictors is 84%. Incorporation of prognostic risk score calculation in clinical practice should be used as an evidence-based adjunct to clinical judgment.

Patients who have minor bleeding with scant hematochezia represent 75–90% of all patients with LGIB and may be evaluated as outpatients. In patients with "outlet-type bleeding," defined as blood seen during or after defecation on the toilet paper or in the toilet bowl without symptoms or special risk factors for colorectal neoplasia, most causes would be in the distal colon and detected by flexible sigmoidoscopy. However, several studies demonstrate that 10–30% of patients with rectal bleeding have more proximal lesions, which would be missed by flexible sigmoidoscopy. Patients who initially undergo sigmoidoscopy without a definitive source of bleeding detected need to undergo a colonoscopy. Furthermore, physicians are unable to reliably predict on history which patients with rectal bleeding will have significant pathology. As there has recently been a rapid increase in young patients diagnosed with colon cancer, most patients with LGIB, even with outlet-type bleeding, should be evaluated with a colonoscopy.

Another category of patients presents with chronic intermittent bleeding that manifests as guaiac-positive stool or iron deficiency anemia (which may be asymptomatic), or both. Although evaluation of these patients is usually appropriate in the outpatient setting, if patients are severely anemic or with cardiopulmonary symptoms, inpatient admission should be considered. All of these patients must be evaluated with colonoscopy. However, if no source is identified on colonoscopy or if the patient has upper gastrointestinal symptoms, an upper endoscopy should also be performed.

Patients with LGIB that have episodic severe bleeding or continuous active bleeding must be managed in the hospital. It is important to be aware that 10–15% of hospitalized cases initially thought to have a LGIB ultimately have an upper GI source. Clues to the presence of a possible upper GI source include hematochezia with hemodynamic instability, a BUN/creatinine of >30, and a history of upper GI bleeding. Obtaining a prompt upper endoscopy examination should be done to rule out an upper GI source in patients with severe LGIB.

Pasha SF, Shergil A, Acosta RD, et al. ASGE Guideline: the role of endoscopy in the patient with lower GI bleeding. *Gastrointest Endosc.* 2014;79:875–885. [PMID: 24703084]

Strate LL, Naumann CR. The role of colonoscopy and radiological procedures in the management of acute lower intestinal bleeding. *Clin Gastroenterol Hepatol.* 2010;8:333–343. [PMID: 20036757]

▶ Initial Clinical Assessment

During the initial clinical assessment of patients with suspected acute LGIB, resuscitation should proceed simultaneously with placement of two large-bore peripheral catheters (18 gauge or larger) followed by administration of intravenous fluids (normal saline or lactated Ringer solution) and if needed PRBCs.

A. Symptoms & Signs

1. History—The history in patients with LGIB should focus on factors that could be associated with potential causes: blood coating the stool suggests hemorrhoidal bleeding while blood mixed in the stool implies a more proximal source; bloody diarrhea and tenesmus is associated with inflammatory bowel disease while bloody diarrhea with fever and abdominal pain especially with recent travel history suggests infectious colitis; pain with defecation occurs with hemorrhoids and anal fissure; change in stool caliber and weight loss is concerning for colon cancer; abdominal pain can be associated with inflammatory bowel disease, infectious colitis, or ischemic colitis; painless bleeding is characteristic of bleeding from diverticulosis, angioectasia, and radiation proctitis; use of antiplatelet agents including aspirin and nonsteroidal anti-inflammatory drug (NSAID) is a risk factor for diverticular bleeding; and recent colonoscopy with polypectomy suggests postpolypectomy bleeding. Patients should be asked about symptoms from hemodynamic compromise including dyspnea, chest pain, lightheadedness, and fatigue.

2. Physical findings—The physical examination should focus on the following areas:

A. Vital signs—Orthostatic hypotension implies at least a 15% loss of blood volume.

B. Abdominal examination—Evaluate for tenderness, masses, hepatomegaly, and splenomegaly.

C. Rectal examination—Key elements include inspection of the anus, palpation for anal or rectal masses, and characterization of the stool color.

B. Laboratory Findings

Among the blood tests that should be performed are a complete blood count, blood urea nitrogen (BUN) and creatinine, international normalized ratio (INR), partial thromboplastin time, and type and crossmatch for blood products.

Coagulopathy and thrombocytopenia should be corrected if there is evidence of active bleeding or hemodynamic compromise. Platelets should be maintained above 50,000/mL and coagulopathy should be corrected to an INR of <2.5 in order to safely perform endoscopic therapy with prothrombin concentrate complex (rapid, low-volume reversal) or fresh frozen plasma. The effects of fresh frozen plasma last about 3–5 hours and large volumes (>2–3 L) may be required to completely reverse a coagulopathy. Patients on antithrombotics should be managed in a multidisciplinary manner with cardiology/neurology and gastroenterology to optimally balance the risk of further bleeding with the risk of thromboembolic events. In the setting of acute bleeding the antithrombotic medications may be temporarily held, but if given for secondary prophylaxis should either be continued or restarted as soon as the bleeding has been stabilized. The management of antithrombotics in LGIB is similar to that for upper GI bleeding (detailed in Chapter 20).

C. Diagnostic Tests

Diagnostic evaluation must be performed after patients have been adequately resuscitated. If an upper GI source is suspected, an upper endoscopy should first be performed. Lower GI evaluation can be performed with anoscopy, flexible sigmoidoscopy, colonoscopy, and various radiologic studies.

1. Anoscopy—Anoscopy is useful only for diagnosing bleeding sources at the anorectal junction and anal canal, including internal hemorrhoids and anal fissures. It is superior to flexible sigmoidoscopy for detecting hemorrhoids and can be performed quickly in the office or at the bedside. In patients with small volume outlet-type bleeding, anoscopy is useful if a definite source of bleeding is identified, otherwise further testing will be required.

2. Flexible sigmoidoscopy—Flexible sigmoidoscopy allows for visualization of the left colon. It can be performed with or without sedation and requires a preparation using enemas. However, the diagnostic yield of sigmoidoscopy in acute LGIB is about 10%. The role of sigmoidoscopy in patients with acute LGIB is extremely limited, as most patients will need to undergo colonoscopy.

3. Colonoscopy—Colonoscopy is the test of choice in the vast majority of patients with acute LGIB since it can be both diagnostic and therapeutic. The diagnostic accuracy of colonoscopy in LGIB ranges from 48% to 90%, and some studies suggest urgent colonoscopy may increase diagnostic yield. The presence of fresh blood in the terminal ileum without a source in the colon indicates a more proximal source of bleeding.

The overall complication rate of colonoscopy in acute LGIB is 0.3–1.3%. A bowel preparation is required but is safe and tolerated by most patients, however, up to 10% of colonoscopy preparations in patients hospitalized with acute LGIB are inadequate. A polyethylene glycol prep solution (4–6 liters) or similarly effective preparation should be administered orally (or via nasogastric tube) until the effluence is clear of stool, clots, and old blood. Antiemetics and prokinetics such as metoclopramide may be needed during the preparation, especially if a rapid or large volume of the prep solution is given. In patients at risk of aspiration (older and debilitated patients) or fluid overload the preparation must be cautiously administered.

Colonoscopy can provide therapy if the bleeding source is localized. Diverticulosis, angioectasias, and postpolypectomy bleeding are the most likely sources of LGIB to benefit from endoscopic hemostasis. The therapies for LGIB are similar to those in UGIB and include injection of dilute epinephrine (1:10,00–1:20,00 dilution), bipolar coagulation, argon plasma coagulation (APC), hemostatic clip placement, over-the-scope clips, and hemostatic spray. The choice of treatment depends on the nature of the bleeding lesion and the stigmata of recent hemorrhage (active bleeding, nonbleeding visible vessel, or adherent clot). Combination treatment with epinephrine injection and bipolar coagulation or hemostatic clips is effective in most patients. In patients with bleeding angioectasias APC is commonly used, whereas in patients with diverticular and postpolypectomy bleeding, hemostatic clips are recommended. Hemostatic spray is effective in patients with active LGIB and often is used as a rescue therapy when other treatment modalities fail to control bleeding.

Early rebleeding following urgent colonoscopy (rebleeding prior to hospital discharge) occurs in 22% and late rebleeding in 16% (rebleeding after hospital discharge). For most patients with recurrent bleeding a repeat colonoscopy should be performed, with endoscopic hemostasis if indicated.

4. Emergent colonoscopy—Overall aggressive evaluation with emergent colonoscopy has not been shown to improve outcome in patients with severe LGIB. There are three prospective randomized trials to date of patients with significant LGIB who were randomized to standard care or emergent colonoscopy. Although some studies found a higher diagnostic yield in the emergent colonoscopy group, overall there was no difference in patient outcomes including further bleeding,

length of hospital stay, surgery, mortality, or complications. Colonoscopy within 24 hours is associated with a decreased hospital length of stay and costs. Therefore, urgent colonoscopy does not improve patient outcomes and is not recommended, whereas early colonoscopy decreases costs and length of stay, and should be done where logistically feasible.

Gralnek IM, Neeman Z, Strate LL. Acute lower gastrointestinal bleeding. *N Engl J Med.* 2017;376(11):1054–1063. [PMID: 28296600]

Hookey L, Barkun A, Sultanian R, Bailey R. Successful hemostasis of active lower GI bleeding using a hemostatic powder as monotherapy, combination therapy, or rescue therapy. *Gastrointest Endosc.* 2019;89(4):865–871. [PMID: 30612959]

Kherad O, Restellini S, Almadi M, et al. Systematic review with meta-analysis: limited benefits from early colonoscopy in acute lower gastrointestinal bleeding. *Aliment Pharmacol Ther.* 2020;52(5):774–788. [PMID: 32697886]

Niikura R, Nagata N, Yamada A, et al. Efficacy and safety of early vs elective colonoscopy for acute lower gastrointestinal bleeding. *Gastroenterology.* 2020;158(1):168–175. [PMID: 31563627]

Oakland K, Kothiwale S, Forehand T, et al. External validation of the Oakland score to assess safe hospital discharge among adult patients with acute lower gastrointestinal bleeding in the US. *JAMA Netw Open.* 2020;3(7):e209630. [PMID: 32633766]

Strate LL, Ayanian JZ, Kotler G, Syngal S. Risk factors for mortality in lower intestinal bleeding. *Clin Gastroenterol Hepatol.* 2008;6:1004–1010. [PMID: 18558513]

Strate LL, Gralnek IM. ACG Clinical Guideline: management of patients with acute lower gastrointestinal bleeding. *Am J Gastroenterol.* 2016;111(4):459–474. [PMID: 26925883]

5. Radiologic studies—Tagged RBC scans, CT angiography (CTA) and angiography are often performed in unstable patients with massive LGIB (often along with an upper endoscopy to exclude a massive upper GI bleed), in those with ongoing bleeding and a negative colonoscopy, or in patients who are unlikely to tolerate a bowel preparation and colonoscopy. Tagged RBC scans and CTAs are solely diagnostic examinations whereas angiography can be both diagnostic and therapeutic.

6. Tagged red blood cell scans—A low bleeding rate of 0.1–0.5 mL/min is required for detection by tagged RBC scans. A ^{99m}Tc-labeled RBC radiotracer is commonly used and involves labeling the patient's RBCs *in vitro* and then reinjecting them back into the patient. The labeled RBCs persist in the circulation for at least 24 hours. This allows for repeated imaging if the patient rebleeds during this time window (if the initial scan is negative). The radiotracer circulates in the blood and extravasation of blood into the GI lumen can be identified on a series of static images captured after injection or on multiple sequential dynamic images (Figures 27–2A and 27–2B).

About 45% of tagged RBC scans for LGIB are positive. Accuracy of localization of the bleeding site is poor and

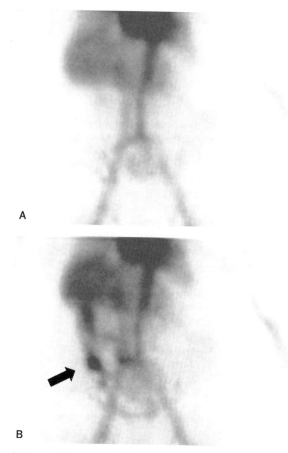

A

B

▲ **Figure 27–2. A.** Baseline tagged red blood cell scan. **B.** Tagged red blood cell scan with active bleeding from the right colon (arrow).

ranges from 24% to 80%. The main role of tagged RBC scan is before angiography because it selects patients who are bleeding sufficiently for an angiogram to detect and allows more targeted angiography with a decreased contrast load. It is important that following a positive tagged RBC scan, urgent angiography be performed (within 90 minutes if feasible). Delaying angiography may lead to increased negative results because LGIB is often episodic and intermittent. Surgery should not be performed using localization information only obtained at tagged RBC scan. Overall CTA is now preferred at most institutions over tagged RBC scans.

7. CT angiography—CTA allows for the rapid noninvasive diagnosis of LGIB by with enhanced delineation of mesenteric vessels, fast scanning time, and accurate acquisition of images in arterial and venous phases. Patients do not ingest oral contrast material and, after an initial unenhanced CT scan, images using intravenous contrast are obtained during

the arterial phase to identify extravasation of contrast into the bowel lumen. Studies demonstrate a sensitivity of >90% and specificity of 99% for detecting acute GI bleeding with CTA, with nearly 100% accuracy in localization of the bleeding site. CTA may approach the detection ability of tagged RBC scans as bleeding rate of 0.3–0.5 mL/min is required for detection by CTA.

CTA is now recommended as the initial test to perform in unstable patients with LGIB by the British Society of Gastroenterology. CTA has several advantages over tagged RBC scans including the ability to promptly obtain in most emergency departments, the use of IV contrast instead of labeled RBC's, and the ability to accurately localize a bleeding source. CTA examinations are preferred prior to angiography unless an angiographer specifically requests a tagged RBC scan.

Oakland K, Chadwick G, East JE, et al. Diagnosis and management of acute lower gastrointestinal bleeding: guidelines from the British Society of Gastroenterology. *Gut.* 2019;68(5):776–789. [PMID: 30792244]

8. Angiography—Angiography offers both the ability to localize a bleeding site and provide therapy. However, a more rapid rate of bleeding of at least 0.5–1.5 mL/min is necessary for detection during angiography (Figure 27–3) compared with a tagged RBC scan or CTA. Patients who are massively bleeding and hemodynamically unstable should be resuscitated and proceed directly to angiography, with a CTA first if feasible. The diagnostic yield of angiography ranges from

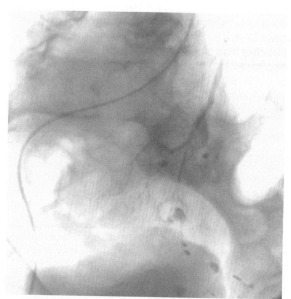

▲ *Figure 27–3.* Angiography with active bleeding from the right colon.

27% to 77% with a mean of 47%; sensitivity and specificity are 47% and 100%, respectively. Provocative angiography given to induce active bleeding using heparin, urokinase, or, tissue plasminogen activator increases the likelihood of identifying a bleeding site, but confers a risk of uncontrollable bleeding and death. Complications of angiography are not infrequent occurring in 10–20% of patients and include renal failure from the intravenous dye load, hematoma, and artery injury at the puncture site, and ischemia and infarction from the therapy.

Jacovides CL, Nadolski G, Allen SR, et al. Arteriography for lower gastrointestinal hemorrhage: role of preceding abdominal computed tomographic angiogram in diagnosis and localization. *JAMA Surg.* 2015;150:650–656. [PMID: 25992504]

Koh FH, Soong J, Lieske B, et al. Does the timing of an invasive mesenteric angiography following a positive CT mesenteric angiography make a difference? *Int J Colorectal Dis.* 2015;30: 57–61. [PMID: 25367183]

Maleux G, Roeflaer F, Heye S, et al. Long-term outcome of transcatheter embolotherapy for acute lower gastrointestinal hemorrhage. *Am J Gastroenterol.* 2009;104:2042–2046. [PMID: 19455109]

▶ Differential Diagnosis

The differential diagnosis of acute LGIB is broad, although the vast majority of bleeding is due to diverticulosis, ischemic colitis, angioectasias, polyps or neoplasia, and hemorrhoids (Table 27–1). Following evaluation, the cause of LGIB remains uncertain in about 10–15% of cases.

Table 27–1. Common sources and prevalence of lower gastrointestinal bleeding.

Source	Prevalence %
Diverticulosis	20–65
Ischemia	1–19
Malignancy	1–17
Colonic angiodysplasia	3–15
Hemorrhoids/anorectal	5–10
Postpolypectomy	2–6
Unknown	8–12

Data from Longstreth GF. Epidemiology and outcome of patients hospitalized with acute lower gastrointestinal hemorrhage a population-based study. *Am J Gastroenterol.* 1997,92:419; Pasha SF, Shergil A, Acosta RD, et al. ASGE. Guideline: the role of endoscopy in the patient with lower GI bleeding. *Gastrointest Endosc.* 2014;79:875-85; Hreinsson JP, Guomundsson S, Kalaitzakis E, Bjornsson ES. Lower gastrointestinal bleeding: incidence, etiology, and outcomes in a population-based setting. *Eur J Gastroenterol and Hepatol.* 2013;25:37-43.

SPECIFIC CAUSES OF ACUTE LOWER GI BLEEDING

1. Diverticulosis

Diverticulosis is the most common cause of LGIB in patients requiring hospitalization. A detailed discussion of diverticular disease appears in Chapter 23.

Most people with diverticulosis are asymptomatic; however up to 15% will experience diverticular bleeding. Massive bleeding occurs in 3–5% of patients. Abrupt painless bleeding characterizes diverticular bleeding; mild lower abdominal cramping may occur due to passage of bright red or maroon blood.

The vast majority of diverticular bleeding will spontaneously stop. Colonoscopy is the initial diagnostic procedure of choice performed to rule out other lesions and to localize the bleeding site. If bleeding without a clear source persists or recurs, a colonoscopy can be repeated or a CTA or tagged RBC scan can be performed rapidly followed by angiography if positive. Angiography is a treatment option that is usually performed if there is ongoing bleeding and the source cannot be defined and/or controlled during colonoscopy. An algorithm for management of diverticular bleeding is included in Chapter 23 (see Figure 23–6).

There are multiple endoscopic treatment options if a bleeding diverticulum is identified including epinephrine injection, bipolar coagulation, mechanical therapy, and combination therapy. Thermal therapy should generally be avoided due to risk of perforation. Bleeding diverticula may best be treated using mechanical therapy with endoscopic hemostatic clips, although over-the-scope clips or endoscopic band ligation may also be selectively used (Plates 42 and 43). Once a bleeding diverticulum is identified, the location should be marked with submucosal injection of ink or application of a hemostatic clip. This allows for precise localization of the bleeding area if further endoscopic, angiographic, or surgical therapy is needed.

Persistent massive hemorrhage and recurrent diverticular bleeding are indications for surgery. Surgeons should be consulted early in the hospital course of patients with high-risk clinical features and severe bleeding.

Niikura R, Nagata N, Aoki T, et al. Predictors for identification of stigmata of recent hemorrhage on colonic diverticula in lower gastrointestinal bleeding. *J Clin Gastroenterol.* 2015;49:e24–e30. [PMID: 24859714]

Pham T, Tran BA, Ooi K, et al. Super-selective mesenteric embolization provides effective control of lower GI bleeding. *Radiol Res Pract.* 2017;2017:1074804. [PMID: 28210507]

Song LWK, Baron TH. Endoscopic management of acute lower gastrointestinal bleeding. *Am J Gastroenterol.* 2008;103: 1881–1887. [PMID: 18796089]

2. Angiodysplasia

Angiodysplasias are the source of LGIB in 3–15% of patients and are common in the elderly. They may be congenital but usually are acquired and found in 1–2% of colon autopsy specimens. Angiodysplasia, arteriovenous malformation, angioectasia, and vascular ectasia are terms often used synonymously. Telangiectasia, which is anatomically similar, is the term used in the context of systemic or congenital diseases. Over half are located in the right colon, and patients experience painless hematochezia similar to diverticular hemorrhage. Patients with bleeding angiodysplasias can present with chronic, intermittent bleeding. Risk factors for bleeding include advanced age (older than 60), use of antiplatelets or anticoagulants, end-stage kidney disease, von Willebrand disease, and possibly aortic stenosis.

The diagnostic sensitivity of colonoscopy is 80–90% with the characteristic finding of a 2–10-mm red, fern-like flat lesion with ectatic vessels radiating from a central vessel. Poor bowel preparation and use of meperidine, which transiently decreases mucosal blood flow, can potentially hinder the identification of angiodysplasias. Use of naloxone may enhance colonic vasculature and angiodysplasia identification. Angiography is considered the gold standard in diagnosing angiodysplasias, although rarely performed clinically. Findings include ectatic slowly emptying veins, vascular tufts, or early filling veins.

Bleeding angiodysplasias discovered during colonoscopy can be treated with a variety of therapies. The noncontact method APC is the most commonly used endoscopic treatment. Treatment should begin with treating the outer feeder vessels and progressing toward the central vessel (Plates 44 and 45). Nonbleeding angiodysplasias without evidence of GI incidentally found during colonoscopy performed for other reasons bleeding should not be treated. However, if there is a history of guaiac-positive stool or iron deficiency anemia, angiodysplasias should be treated, even if not actively bleeding at the time of the procedure.

There is a potential role for medical treatment of angiodysplasias, although the quality of the available data is limited. Case series and reports have suggested a possible benefit of octreotide administered subcutaneously in doses ranging from 50 to 100 μg two times a day by (or intramuscularly with long-acting somatostatin analogues) with decreased need for transfusions. A randomized study supported the role of thalidomide taken orally at 100 mg daily for 4 months in decreasing bleeding from angiodysplasias. However, side effects with thalidomide therapy are not uncommon and this medication cannot be used in women of childbearing potential due severe birth defects. Bevacizumab is a humanized monoclonal antibody against vascular endothelial growth factor that has been used in case reports and small case series to treat refractory bleeding from angiodysplasia with some success. However data is extremely limited in the treatment of colonic angiodysplasia. Long-term estrogen–progesterone treatment has been evaluated as a possible treatment, however, is not recommended, as a randomized trial with 1-year follow-up did not decrease rebleeding.

Brown C, Subramanian V, Wilcox CM, Peter S. Somatostatin analogues in the treatment of recurrent bleeding from gastrointestinal vascular malformations: an overview and systematic review of prospective observational studies. Dig Dis Sci. 2010;55(8):2129–2134. [PMID: 20393879]

Sami SS, Al-Araji A, Ragunath K. Review article: gastrointestinal angiodysplasia—pathogenesis, diagnosis, and management. Alim Pharmacol Ther. 2014;39:15–34. [PMID: 24138285]

3. Ischemic Colitis

The diagnosis of colonic ischemia is established by a combination of clinical setting, physical diagnosis, and diagnostic studies. The differential diagnosis includes infectious colitis, inflammatory bowel disease, diverticulitis, radiation enteritis, and colon cancer. In hospitalized patients *Clostridium difficile* infection must be excluded. Patients often present with bloody bowel movements associated with crampy abdominal pain. A typical patient is elderly woman in warm or hot weather with evidence of dehydration. Although there are no specific blood tests for colonic ischemia, elevations may be noted in the white blood cell count, amylase, creatine phosphokinase, and serum lactate levels. Most plain radiographs in colonic ischemia have nonspecific findings, although thumbprinting due to submucosal edema and pneumatosis coli may be seen typically in patients with more advanced disease.

CT scans may reveal segmental thickening of the involved colon. Endoscopic evaluation with colonoscopy can confirm the diagnosis and exclude other disease in patients who do not have signs of perforation. Care must be taken to avoid overdistention during the colonoscopic examination to prevent worsening of ischemic damage. Endoscopic findings typically occur in a segmental distribution and vary depending on the degree of damage, ranging from pale mucosa with petechial bleeding to cyanotic, necrotic bowel. Angiography is usually not indicated in colonic ischemia as the interrupted blood flow is typically in a watershed distribution in the colon and flow often returns to normal by the time of clinical presentation. An exception to this is in thromboembolic disease, which typically involves embolism along the ileocolic artery and affects the cecum and proximal right colon.

Demetriou G, Nassar A, Subramonia S. The pathophysiology, presentation and management of ischaemic colitis: a systematic review. World J Surg. 2020;44(3):927–938. [PMID: 31646369]

4. Neoplasm

Neoplasms of the colon may present with GI bleeding. In patients over the age of 50, rectal bleeding is due to a neoplasm in about 10% of cases; however, neoplasms are an increasingly common source of rectal bleeding in persons younger than age 50. Although most bleeding from colonic neoplasms tends to be low grade and occult, bleeding may be brisk and overt at times. Bleeding occurs due to erosion or ulceration of the lesion. Distal lesions (left colon and rectum) are more likely to present with bright red blood per rectum whereas more proximal lesions tend to present with maroon stool, melena, or occult blood.

The diagnosis of a neoplasm as the source of LGIB is typically established by colonoscopy, with biopsies performed to confirm the diagnosis. Larger neoplasms may be detected on a CT scan. The therapeutic options for those patients with bleeding neoplasms are limited. Standard endoscopic therapies have marginal effectiveness. The use of hemostatic sprays has been reported to be effective in small studies (Plates 46 and 47). The treatment for most patients with bleeding colonic neoplasms is surgical resection.

5. Hemorrhoids

Hemorrhoids and other anorectal disorders (solitary rectal ulcers and anal fissures) are an important source of LGIB, responsible for ≤20% of LGIB. Hemorrhoids are dilated submucosal vessels in the anus, which are considered internal if above the dentate line (Plate 48) and external if below. Hemorrhoids are extremely common and usually asymptomatic but can present with thrombosis or hematochezia. Bleeding from hemorrhoids occurs when there is rupture of a blood vessel.

The clinical manifestations of bleeding hemorrhoids include painless hematochezia with the stool being coated with bright red blood. Further bleeding may occur, with blood dripping into the toilet bowl or staining underwear. Although bleeding from hemorrhoids is usually low grade, high-volume or massive bleeding may rarely occur. Severe bleeding from hemorrhoids is more common in patients with a coagulopathy or on antithrombotic medications. Acute treatment for most patients with bleeding hemorrhoids is not needed since most episodes are mild and resolve spontaneously. Topical medical treatments help decrease inflammation and surgery is rarely needed, except for those with persistent or massive bleeding.

6. Postpolypectomy Bleeding

Postpolypectomy bleeding occurs after 2–6% of polypectomies and is the leading major complication following colonoscopy with polypectomy. Acute hemorrhage occurring at the time of polypectomy is usually easily treatable. Therapeutic options include resnaring the stalk of the polypectomy site to apply pressure, injection therapy with epinephrine, thermal treatment with bipolar coagulation or APC, and hemostatic clip application (Plates 49 and 50). Hemostatic clip placement is the preferred treatment option as it avoids further tissue injury that occurs with thermal methods of coagulation therapy. Hemostatic sprays can be used to control active bleeding, although generally is reserved for cases refractory to other methods of hemostasis. Although postpolypectomy bleeding usually occurs within 7 days, delayed bleeding can occur up to 29 days following polypectomy when the eschar falls off the site. Postpolypectomy bleeding is usually self-limited and over 70% of cases resolve with supportive care.

Risk factors for postpolypectomy bleeding include removal of large polyps (>2 cm in diameter), proximal location of polyps, thick stalk, and use of antithrombotic medications. Avoidance of cautery techniques to remove polyps decreases the risk of postpolypectomy bleeding and is recommended for polyps <1 cm. Placement of prophylactic hemostatic clips following removal of large (>2 cm) polyps, especially on the right side of the colon, has been shown in some (but not all) studies to decrease delayed postpolypectomy bleeding.

Inoue T, Ishihara R, Nishida T, et al. Prophylactic clipping not effective in preventing post-polypectomy bleeding for < 20-mm colon polyps: a multicenter, open-label, randomized controlled trial. *J Gastroenterol Hepatol.* 2021;36(2):383–390. [PMID: 32511792]

Pohl H, Grimm IS, Moyer MT, et al. Clip closure prevents bleeding after endoscopic resection of large colon polyps in a randomized trial. *Gastroenterology.* 2019;157(4):977–984. [PMID: 30885778]

7. Radiation Proctitis

Pelvic radiation such as given for prostate cancer can cause both acute and chronic radiation proctitis. Acute damage presents within 3 months of radiation therapy with diarrhea, tenesmus, and rarely bleeding. Chronic radiation proctitis typically presents 9–14 months following radiation in up to 20% of patients but can occur years later (Plate 51). Bleeding is a prominent symptom caused by mucosal atrophy and fibrosis, which result in chronic mucosal ischemia.

There are no standardized recommendations for treatment of bleeding from radiation proctitis. Endoscopic therapy is superior to medical treatment in reducing severe bleeding. APC is the most commonly used endoscopic treatment method and has an 85–100% success rate in reducing or stopping bleeding after two to three treatments every 1–2 months. Visualized telangiectasias are obliterated at each session, while persistent rectal ulcers resulting from previous treatments are avoided. Short-term complications occur in 7% of patients and include rectal pain and fever. Rare major complications include rectovaginal fistula, anal, or rectal stricture, and acute perforation secondary to accumulation of combustible gas and explosion with APC use. A full bowel preparation is necessary for APC treatment since there have been multiple reports of explosions causing perforation when an enema preparation was used. During long-term follow-up over 1–5 years, recurrent bleeding occurs in up to 10% of patients. Most patients refractory to treatment with APC can be successfully treatment with radiofrequency ablation or cryoablation.

Hyperbaric oxygen is a possible therapeutic option and promotes angiogenesis and collagen formation, leading to reepithelialization. In select patients who failed previous medical or endoscopic therapy for hyperbaric oxygen treatment, success has been reported in 75–100% with a decrease or cessation of bleeding. The treatment regimen is rigorous; for example, one study placed patients in a hyperbaric chamber with 100% oxygen for 90 minutes for 5–7 days per week for an average of 36 sessions. Hyperbaric oxygen therapy is usually only considered in the rare patient refractory to endoscopic treatment. Surgery is reserved for refractory or severe cases.

Tabaja L, Sidani SM. Management of radiation proctitis. *Dig Dis Sci.* 2018;63(9):2180–2188. [PMID: 29948565]

Acute Pancreatitis

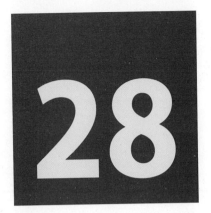

David X. Jin, MD, MPH

Darwin Conwell, MD

Peter A. Banks, MD

ESSENTIALS OF DIAGNOSIS

▶ Gallstone disease and alcohol are the most common causes of acute pancreatitis; other causes include hyper-triglyceridemia, drugs, and specific disorders of the biliary tree and pancreas.

▶ Diagnosis is made when at least two of the following three criteria are fulfilled: characteristic abdominal pain; threefold elevation in serum amylase and/or lipase; abnormal radiographic imaging showing changes of acute pancreatitis.

▶ Severe acute pancreatitis is characterized by persistent (>48 hours) organ failure (systemic blood pressure <90 mm Hg, PaO_2 <60 mm Hg, and/or creatinine >2.0 mg/dL).

▶ Diagnosis of necrotizing pancreatitis is confirmed by contrast-enhanced abdominal computed tomography (CT) scan or MRI scan.

▶ General Considerations

Acute pancreatitis is an acute inflammatory disorder of the pancreas characterized by severe abdominal pain and often the development of regional and systemic complications. With a mortality <1% in mild cases but up to 30% in severe cases, an early assessment of severity is critical to guiding subsequent care.

A. Incidence

Acute pancreatitis is the third most common inpatient gastrointestinal diagnosis in the United States, accounting for >275,000 admissions annually with hospital costs exceeding $2.7 billion. Worldwide, the annual incidence rate is 13–45 cases per 100,000 individuals and appears to be increasing.

B. Causes & Risk Factors

The most common causes of acute pancreatitis in the United States are gallstones and alcohol, accounting for approximately 70% of cases. Table 28–1 lists other etiologies, including cigarette smoking, hypertriglyceridemia, drug reactions, iatrogenic causes (eg, postsurgical or endoscopic retrograde cholangiopancreatography [ERCP]), and hereditary factors, among others.

Gallstone-induced pancreatitis occurs in the setting of choledocholithiasis and is believed to be related to transient or complete obstruction of pancreatic ductal flow or reflux of bile into the pancreatic duct. The first episode of alcohol-induced acute pancreatitis typically occurs after many (eg, 8–10 years) years of heavy alcohol consumption. Independent of alcohol, cigarette smoking is a risk factor for not to only acute pancreatitis, but also recurrent acute pancreatitis and chronic pancreatitis. Hypertriglyceridemia-associated acute pancreatitis does not typically occur unless the triglyceride level exceeds 1000 mg/dL with severity that is level dependent.

Although many drugs have been associated with acute pancreatitis, the strength of association between the use of a particular drug and the development of acute pancreatitis warrants careful scrutiny. Table 28–2 lists drugs that have a reported association with acute pancreatitis.

Post ERCP pancreatitis is the most common iatrogenic cause, with rates of 4–6% at most centers. The use of rectal indomethacin, prophylactic pancreatic duct stenting, and aggressive intravenous hydration with lactated ringers has been shown to be protective, particularly in high risk patients, such as those with minor papilla sphincterotomy, sphincter of Oddi dysfunction, prior history of post-ERCP pancreatitis, age <60 years, more than two contrast injections into the pancreatic duct, and involvement of endoscopic trainees in the procedure.

Several germline mutations are associated with increased risk. Hereditary pancreatitis is an autosomal-dominant disease most commonly associated with mutations in the

Table 28–1. Causes of acute pancreatitis.

Alcohol
Autoimmune (type 1 and type 2)
Biliary (eg, gallstones, gallbladder microlithiasis/sludge)
Drug-induced (see Table 28–2)
Iatrogenic
    Surgery (eg, common bile duct exploration, sphincterotomy,
        splenectomy, distal gastrectomy)
    ERCP
Idiopathic
Infectious (eg, ascariasis, clonorchiasis, mumps, toxoplasmosis,
    coxsackievirus, cytomegalovirus, tuberculosis, *Mycobacterium
    avium* complex)
Inherited
    PRSS1 (cationic trypsinogen) mutations
    CFTR (cystic fibrosis transmembrane conductance regulator)
    mutations
    SPINK1 (serine protease inhibitor, Kazal type 1) mutations
Metabolic (eg, hypercalcemia, hypertriglyceridemia)
Neoplastic (eg, pancreatic or ampullary tumors)
Structural (eg, pancreatic divisum, annular pancreas, sphincter of
    Oddi dysfunction, periampullary diverticula, duodenal duplication
    cysts, choledochocele, anomalous pancreaticobiliary junction,
    regional enteritis)
Smoking
Toxic (eg, organophosphates, scorpion venom)
Traumatic (especially motor vehicle accidents)
Vascular

cationic trypsinogen (*PRSS1*) gene that leads to the inability of prematurely activated intracellular trypsin to undergo autocatalytic degradation. Hereditary pancreatitis should be suspected in patients with early-onset (before 20 years of age) acute pancreatitis or those with a strong family history of idiopathic acute pancreatitis in first- or second-degree relatives. Mutations in the protease inhibitor (*SPINK1*) gene interferes with its ability to inhibit intracellular trypsin during an acute inflammatory process, in turn leading to acinar cell injury. The inheritance pattern of *SPINK1* mutations is autosomal-recessive. Mutations in the cystic fibrosis transmembrane conductance regulator (*CFTR*) gene are recognized as a cause of both acute and chronic pancreatitis. The mechanism of injury is not completely known but is most likely related to decreased pancreatic juice flow due to duct cell secretory dysfunction. Patients with a family history of cystic fibrosis or a history of recurrent pulmonary symptoms (eg, bronchitis, asthma), nasal polyps, or sterility among males should be considered for genetic testing.

ASGE Standards of Practice Committee. Adverse events associated with ERCP. *Gastrointest Endosc.* 2017;85:32–47. [PMID: 27546389]

Peery AF, Crockett SD, Murphy CC, et al. Burden and cost of gastrointestinal, liver, and pancreatic diseases in the United States: update 2018. *Gastroenterology.* 2019;156:254–272. [PMID: 30315778]

Setiawan VW, Pandol SJ, Porcel J, et al. Prospective study of alcohol drinking, smoking, and pancreatitis: the multiethnic cohort. *Pancreas.* 2016;45:819–825. [PMID: 27171516]

Shelton CA, Whitcomb DC. Genetics and treatment options for recurrent acute and chronic pancreatitis. *Curr Treat Options Gastroenterol.* 2014;12:359–371. [PMID: 24954874]

Simons-Linares CR, Elkhouly MA, Salazar MJ. Drug-induced acute pancreatitis: an update. *Pancreas.* 2019;48:1263–1273. [PMID: 31688589]

Pathogenesis

The pathogenesis of acute pancreatitis continues to be elucidated, but generally thought to develop in response to premature activation of intracellular trypsinogen (which causes acinar cell injury) and the release of chemokines and cytokines (which results in the recruitment of neutrophils and macrophages). Factors that lead to an imbalance of proteases and their inhibitors within pancreatic acinar cells result in inappropriate activation of pancreatic zymogens with subsequent autodigestion and inflammation.

The exact mechanisms leading to gallstone and alcohol-induced pancreatitis remain to be defined. Acute gallstone pancreatitis is most commonly caused by the passage of a stone from the gallbladder through the cystic duct into the common bile duct; impaction at the ampulla of Vater causes either reflux of bile into the pancreatic duct or outflow obstruction of the pancreatic duct.

Only a small proportion of patients who abuse alcohol will develop pancreatitis. Alcohol metabolism is governed by both oxidative and nonoxidative processes. The oxidative pathway lies primarily within the liver while the nonoxidative pathway lies primarily in the pancreas. The nonoxidative pathway leads to the formation of fatty acid ethanol esters (FAEEs). It is postulated that accumulation of FAEEs may result in alcohol-induced pancreatitis.

Clinical Findings

A. Symptoms & Signs

Abdominal pain is the most common symptom in patients presenting with acute pancreatitis. The pain is typically severe, persistent, located in the epigastrium, and may radiate to the back. Patients often develop nausea and vomiting. In patients with severe acute pancreatitis, signs and symptoms parallel the presence of a systemic inflammatory response and organ dysfunction. Patients with systemic inflammatory response syndrome (SIRS) (temperature >38°C, respiratory rate >24 per minute, heart rate >90 per minute, white blood count >12,000, or >10% bands), which arises in response to proinflammatory mediators, can present with fever, tachycardia, tachypnea, or a combination of these findings. Other examination findings include respiratory distress, crackles or absent breath sounds on lung auscultation, cool extremities, impaired mental status, decreased bowel sounds, abdominal

Table 28–2. Drugs implicated in acute pancreatitis based on class.

Class IA[a]	Class IB[b]	Class II[c]
Acetaminophen	Azathioprine	*All-trans* retinoic acid
Acetaminophen-codeine	Bortezomib	L-Asparaginase/peg asparaginase
5-Aminosalicylate	Carbamazepine	Canagliflozin
Amiodarone	Clonidine	Chlorothiazide
Androgenic Anabolic steroids	Clozapine	Codeine
Arsenic trioxide	Cytosine arabinoside	Dideoxy inosine
Cannabis	Dapsone	Gold therapy
Carbimazole	Dexamethasone	Hydrochlorothiazide
Cimetidine	Fenofibrate	Interferon α2b/ribavirin
Clomiphene	Hydrocortisone	Lisinopril
Enalapril	6-Mercaptopurine	Meglumine antimonate
Estrogen and related products	Methimazole	Nilotinib
Furosemide	Mirtazapine	Olanzapine
In vitro fertilization	Nelfinavir	Prednisolone
Isoniazid	Nitrofurantoin	Riluzole
Losartan	Omeprazole	Sitagliptin
Methyldopa	Paclitaxel	
Metronidazole	Pentamidine	
Nadolol	Prednisone	
Pravastatin	Propofol	
Perindopril	Quetiapine	
Procainamide	Sodium stibogluconate	
Pyritinol	Sorafenib	
Ranitidine	Tigecycline	
Rosuvastatin	Valproic acid	
Saxagliptin	Valsartan	
Simvastatin		
Sulindac		
Tamoxifen		
Telaprevir		
Tetracycline		
Trimethoprim–sulfamethoxazole		

[a]Class IA: at least one case report with positive rechallenge, excluding all other causes of acute pancreatitis.
[b]Class IB: at least one case report with positive rechallenge; however, other causes of acute pancreatitis not ruled out.
[c]Class II: at least four cases in the literature, consistent latency in ≥75% of cases (period between initiation of drug and development of acute pancreatitis).
Adapted with permission from Simons-Linares CR, Elkhouly MA, Salazar MJ. Drug-Induced Acute Pancreatitis in Adults: An Update. *Pancreas.* 2019;48(10):1263–1273.

distention, oliguria, and anuria. Cullen sign (periumbilical ecchymoses) and Grey Turner sign (flank ecchymoses) are rare but can be seen in cases of acute pancreatitis with hemorrhage and are associated with increased mortality.

B. Laboratory Findings

Serum amylase and lipase are the principal laboratory tests that aid in the diagnosis of acute pancreatitis. Elevations greater than three times the upper limit of normal are typically used to aid in diagnoses. However, serum levels of both enzymes can be elevated in other disease states. Amylase is also produced by nonpancreatic organs such as salivary glands, ovaries, and fallopian tubes; thus, diseases of these organs can increase the serum amylase level. Both serum amylase and lipase can be elevated by other intra-abdominal disease states (eg, perforated ulcers, intestinal obstruction, mesenteric infarction) as well as with renal insufficiency, critical illness, or with manipulation of the pancreas (eg, ERCP) in the absence of pancreatitis.

Serum amylase has rapid clearance and a short half-life and therefore is best measured soon after symptom onset. Serum lipase rises later and its longer half-life makes it useful to measure when there has been a delay in seeking care. Because serum lipase is a more sensitive and specific indicator of acute pancreatitis than serum amylase, and because the combination of both does not increase the accuracy of diagnosis, checking only serum lipase is typically required. The degree of elevation of both serum amylase and lipase does not correlate with severity of acute pancreatitis, nor does the daily assessment of serum pancreatic enzymes help to determine clinical deterioration or resolution.

Elevated findings on liver biochemical tests in a patient with suspected acute pancreatitis usually signify a biliary cause. A threefold elevation in alanine aminotransferase in the setting of acute pancreatitis has been shown to have a 95% positive predictive value for gallstone pancreatitis.

C. Imaging Studies

Transabdominal ultrasound is recommended to evaluate for cholelithiasis as a potential etiology and for common bile duct dilation which may suggest choledocholithiasis. Contrast-enhanced abdominal computed tomography (CT) is not recommended for the initial evaluation of acute pancreatitis unless the diagnosis is uncertain. By contrast, in the setting of persistent abdominal pain or clinical deterioration after 48–72 hours, a contrast-enhanced CT can be useful to evaluate for local complications such as necrosis or development of an acute fluid collection. Findings of interstitial acute pancreatitis that are typically seen on CT scan include enlargement of the pancreas with edema, heterogeneous pancreatic parenchyma, peripancreatic fat stranding, and peripancreatic fluid collections (Figure 28–1). Acute pancreatic necrosis typically appears as focal or diffuse areas of nonenhanced pancreatic parenchyma (Figure 28–2).

Magnetic resonance cholangiopancreatography (MRCP) can be a helpful modality for further evaluation of a biliary etiology or detection of a retained stone in the bile duct.

The timing of CT or MRI studies is important. If an admission diagnosis of acute pancreatitis can be made on the basis of history, physical examination, and elevated pancreatic enzymes, these studies should generally be deferred. Given that some patients will present with or develop acute

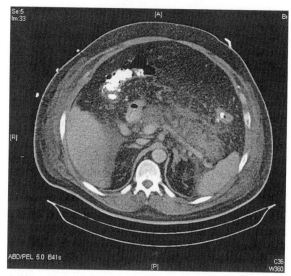

▲ **Figure 28–2.** CT scan showing necrotizing acute pancreatitis. Pancreatic perfusion is diminished on contrast enhancement.

kidney injury, aggressive fluid resuscitation with correction of renal function (until estimated glomerular filtration rate exceeds at least 30 mL/min/1.73 m^2) should take place prior to administration of iodinated or gadolinium contrast due to the risk of contrast-induced acute kidney injury or nephrogenic systemic fibrosis, respectively. Alternatively, a non–contrast-enhanced study can be performed.

D. Diagnostic Approach

1. Confirmation of the diagnosis—The diagnosis of acute pancreatitis is made when at least two of the following three criteria are fulfilled: (1) characteristic acute abdominal pain; (2) at least threefold elevation in serum amylase and/or lipase; and (3) abnormal imaging (typically abdominal CT) demonstrating changes consistent with acute pancreatitis.

2. Indications for more extensive evaluation—Even after a careful history and physical examination, laboratory evaluation, and imaging, the cause of 15–20% of cases of acute pancreatitis remains idiopathic. Recent reports suggest that nearly 70% of patients with a single or recurrent episode of idiopathic acute pancreatitis have biliary microlithiasis or sludge from cholesterol monohydrate crystals or calcium bilirubinate granules. Repeating an abdominal ultrasound after symptom resolution evaluates for biliary pathology that can be missed in the acute setting.

There is considerable debate regarding which subgroup of patients requires even more extensive evaluation after being diagnosed with idiopathic acute pancreatitis. It has been suggested that patients younger than age 40, who have had only a single episode of acute pancreatitis, need no further evaluation as the recurrence rate is low. However, in patients older

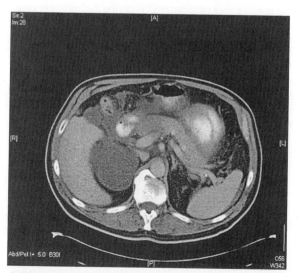

▲ **Figure 28–1.** CT scan showing interstitial acute pancreatitis. There is uniform enhancement of the pancreatic parenchyma, indicating that pancreatic perfusion is preserved.

Table 28–3. Causes of idiopathic or unexplained acute pancreatitis diagnosed by endoscopic evaluation.[a]

Ampullary lesions
Choledocholithiasis
Chronic pancreatitis
Gallbladder microlithiasis or sludge
Pancreas divisum
Pancreatic cancer
Sphincter of Oddi dysfunction

[a]Exclusion of hyperlipidemia and medications.

than 40 or patients who have had 2+ episodes of idiopathic pancreatitis, more extensive evaluation in recommended. In these patients, a contrast-enhanced CT, MRCP, or endoscopic ultrasound (EUS) following resolution of acute pancreatitis is recommended to evaluate for underlying neoplastic or anatomical abnormalities which may prompt appropriate endoscopic or surgical therapy. Causes of idiopathic acute pancreatitis commonly found during endoscopic evaluation are listed in Table 28–3.

E. Classification of Severity

Assessment of severity in patients with acute pancreatitis is essential for appropriate triage and management. The basis for the classification, severity, and complications of acute pancreatitis was established at the International Symposium held in Atlanta in 1992, and subsequently revised in 2012. It stratifies severity as mild, moderately severe, or severe acute pancreatitis. Though severity varies worldwide, the majority of patients (70–80%) will develop mild acute pancreatitis, which is characterized by the absence of organ failure and the absence of local or systemic complications. Moderately severe acute pancreatitis is characterized by transient organ failure (lasting <48 hours) and/or local and/or systemic complications. Local complications typically refer to fluid collections which develop in the acute setting (acute peripancreatic fluid collections [APFC] and acute necrotic collections [ANC]), as well as those that develop after 4 weeks (pancreatic pseudocysts and walled-off necrosis [WON]). Systemic complications are defined as exacerbations of pre-existing comorbidities, including congestive heart failure or chronic lung disease. Severe acute pancreatitis is characterized by persistent organ failure (lasting >48 hours).

The assessment of severity is important due to stark differences in morbidity and mortality. While patients who develop mild or moderately severe acute pancreatitis typically recover within 1–2 weeks and have low mortality (0–3%), those who develop severe acute pancreatitis often develop pancreatic necrosis, are hospitalized for weeks to months, and have mortality rates reaching 30–60%. The high mortality rate in severe pancreatitis is driven not just by the presence of persistent organ failure, but also by how many organ systems (cardiovascular, respiratory, renal) are involved. Persistent single organ failure has a lower mortality (20%) than persistent double (40%) or triple (60%) organ failure.

F. Clinical Severity Indices

Traditional severity indices such as APACHE II and Ranson criteria have not been as useful clinically because they are cumbersome, require collection of a large number of clinical and laboratory variables over 48 hours, and do not have acceptable positive and negative predictive values for severe acute pancreatitis. Moreover, the vast majority of patients with acute pancreatitis who require admission to an intensive care unit experience clinical deterioration within the first 24 hours of hospitalization. A more parsimonious severity index is the BISAP score, which assigns one point for the presence of each of the following, either at admission or during the initial 24 hours of hospitalization: **B**UN >25 mg/dL, **I**mpaired mental status, **S**IRS, **A**ge >60, and a **P**leural effusion. A score of ≥3 points has been associated with increased risk of mortality and complications such as necrosis or organ dysfunction. More recently, the pancreatitis activity scoring system (PASS) was developed in an effort to provide daily measurements of pancreatitis disease activity using the presence of organ failure, SIRS, abdominal pain, analgesic requirements, and ability to tolerate a solid diet as weighted parameters. An elevated PASS score at admission is associated with severe acute pancreatitis, while an elevated PASS score at discharge is associated with early (<30 day) readmission.

Apart from the severity indices, patient-related risk factors for severe acute pancreatitis include older age (>60 years), obesity (body mass index ≥30 kg/m²), and comorbid disease. Additionally, the presence of hemoconcentration at admission (hematocrit >44%), persistence of SIRS for >48 hours, or rise in blood urea nitrogen (BUN) during the initial period of resuscitation indicate a poor prognosis marked by increased risk of organ failure and in-hospital mortality.

CT scoring systems, such as the modified CT Severity Index, predict severity by assessing the degree of necrosis, pancreatic inflammation, and extra-pancreatic complications. Because the extent of necrosis may only become apparent 72–96 hours after symptom onset, CT scoring systems should typically be utilized thereafter.

Banks PA, Bollen TL, Dervenis C, et al. Classification of acute pancreatitis—2012: revision of the Atlanta classification and definitions by international consensus. *Gut*. 2013;62:102–111. [PMID: 23100216]

Jin DX, Lacson R, Cochon LR, et al. A clinical model for the early diagnosis of acute pancreatitis in the emergency department. *Pancreas*. 2018;47:871–879.

Koutroumpakis E, Wu BU, Bakker OJ, et al. Admission hematocrit and rise in blood urea nitrogen at 24 h outperform other laboratory markers in predicting persistent organ failure and pancreatic necrosis in acute pancreatitis: a post hoc analysis of three large prospective databases. *Am J Gastroenterol*. 2015;110: 1707–1716. [PMID: 26553208]

Matta B, Gougol A, Gao X, et al. Worldwide variations in demographics, management, and outcomes of acute pancreatitis. *Clin Gastroenterol Hepatol.* 2020;18:1567–1575. [PMID: 31712075]

Schepers NJ, Bakker OJ, Besselink MG, et al. Impact of characteristics of organ failure and infected necrosis on mortality in necrotising pancreatitis. *Gut.* 2019;68:1044–1051. [PMID: 29950344]

Wu BU, Batech M, Quezada M, et al. Dynamic measure of disease activity in acute pancreatitis: the pancreatitis activity scoring system. *Am J Gastroenterol.* 2017;112:1144–1152. [PMID: 28462914]

Differential Diagnosis

It is important to exclude other intra-abdominal conditions in patients for whom the diagnosis of acute pancreatitis is not certain, especially when management calls for potential surgical intervention. Table 28–4 lists conditions of which the clinician should be particularly aware.

Treatment

A. Mild Acute Pancreatitis

The majority of patients with mild acute pancreatitis respond to supportive care measures that include intravenous hydration with crystalloid, analgesic, and antiemetics. The use of lactated Ringer's solution is preferred to normal saline due to reduced rates of SIRS after 24 hours. While traditionally patients were made nil per os, oral intake can be resumed once the patient is hungry and free from severe pain or vomiting, often within the initial 24 hours. A recent systematic review showed that initiating oral nutrition with a low-fat solid diet is safe, and does not increase risk of necrosis, persistent organ failure, or mortality. Patients discharged with continued pain or tolerating less than a solid diet are at increased risk for early readmission for pancreatitis.

Patients with gallstone pancreatitis are also at increased risk of recurrent biliary complications. A cholecystectomy during the same admission is recommended as a cost-effective intervention which reduces risk for readmission. In patients who are not surgical candidates based on comorbid disease or local complications (Figure 28–3) an endoscopic biliary sphincterotomy or interval cholecystectomy are alternative approaches to mitigate risk of recurrent biliary complications.

Table 28–4. Differential diagnosis of acute pancreatitis.

Perforated viscus
Cholecystitis
Bowel obstruction
Vascular occlusion (especially mesentery venous disease)
Renal colic
Inferior myocardial infarction
Diabetic ketoacidosis
Duodenal ulcer

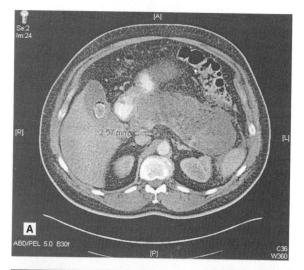
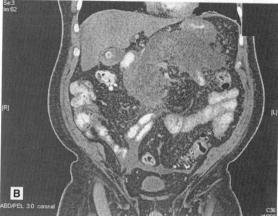

▲ **Figure 28–3.** CT scan in a patient with gallstone pancreatitis. **A.** Axial image with walled-off necrosis and gallbladder stone. **B.** Coronal image showing extent of necrosis and presence of a calcified gallstone.

B. Severe Acute Pancreatitis

In addition to the aforementioned supportive measures, patients at increased risk of severe acute pancreatitis at admission based on obesity, hemoconcentration, or azotemia should receive vigorous fluid resuscitation, typically starting with bolus of 20 cc/kg, followed by maintenance infusion of 3cc/kg/hr. A decrease in hematocrit and/or fall in the BUN by at least 5 mg/dL during the initial 12–24 hours suggest a favorable response to fluid resuscitation. If the hematocrit remains elevated or the BUN rises during resuscitation, the patient may require further hemodynamic monitoring to facilitate adequate resuscitation.

Patients who are elderly, who have severe comorbidities, or who develop persistent organ failure not responding to increased fluids (to counteract hypotension and increased serum creatinine) or supplemental oxygen (to overcome hypoxemia), should be transferred to an intensive care unit for close monitoring as these patients may require intubation with mechanical ventilation, hemodialysis, and support of blood pressure.

Once it is clear that a patient will not be able to tolerate oral feeding due to pain (rather than gastroparesis or ileus), enteral nutrition (rather than total parenteral nutrition) should be considered. Enteral nutrition maintains gut barrier integrity, thereby preventing bacterial translocation, is less expensive, and is associated with fewer complications than parenteral nutrition. When choosing enteral feeding, administration via either a nasogastric or nasojejunal route is acceptable. When patients with necrotizing pancreatitis begin oral intake of food, consideration should also be given to the addition of pancreatic enzyme supplementation to assist with fat digestion, and proton pump inhibitor therapy to reduce gastric acid because of reduced pancreatic bicarbonate secretion.

C. Role of Antibiotics & ERCP

There is no role for prophylactic antibiotics in either interstitial or necrotizing pancreatitis. Multiple randomized controlled trials have demonstrated no reduction in rates of infected necrosis, nonpancreatic infections, or mortality with use of prophylactic antibiotics. In the absence of cholangitis or infected necrosis, antibiotics should be avoided.

Urgent ERCP (within 24 hours) is indicated in patients who have concomitant cholangitis. Otherwise, there is no role for urgent ERCP or biliary sphincterotomy in patients with acute biliary pancreatitis. Elective ERCP with sphincterotomy can be considered in patients with persistent or incipient biliary obstruction for >24 hours, those deemed to be poor candidates for cholecystectomy, and those in whom there is strong suspicion of bile duct stones before or after cholecystectomy.

D. Management of Pancreatic Fluid Collections/Necrosis

The majority of patients with peripancreatic fluid collections including sterile necrotic collections can be managed without intervention as many will remain asymptomatic or resolve spontaneously. Sterile collections may require intervention when causing pain, nausea, or anorexia, typically a result of mass effect causing gastric-outlet, intestinal, or biliary obstruction. When drainage is indicated, it should ideally be deferred for at least 4 weeks until acute peripancreatic fluid collections (APFC) and ANC have consolidated into pseudocysts or WON, respectively. A step-up approach beginning with direct endoscopic necrosectomy results in better outcomes compared to both minimally-invasive surgical necrosectomy and an open surgical approach.

Infected pancreatic necrosis should be suspected when SIRS or organ failure persist, or newly develop, >7 days after presentation, with incidence peaking 2–4 weeks from onset of necrotizing pancreatitis. Infected pancreatic necrosis is confirmed by the presence of gas within a fluid collection on imaging or with positive gram stain/culture via percutaneous aspiration. Once the diagnosis of infected necrosis is established, appropriate antibiotics should be initiated and temporizing measures such as percutaneous catheter drainage should be utilized until the collection organizes into WON that is amenable to endoscopic drainage. Surgical debridement should be considered for symptomatic collections that are refractory or inaccessible to endoscopic drainage.

Bang JY, Arnoletti JP, Holt BA, et al. An endoscopic transluminal approach, compared with minimally invasive surgery, reduced complications and costs for patients with necrotizing pancreatitis. *Gastroenterology.* 2019;156:1027–1040.

Baron TH, DiMaio CJ, Wang AY, et al. American Gastroenterological Association clinical practice update: management of pancreatic necrosis. *Gastroenterology.* 2020;158:67–75. [PMID: 31479658]

Crockett SD, Wani S, Gardner TB, et al. American Gastroenterological Association Institute Guideline on Initial Management of Acute Pancreatitis. *Gastroenterology.* 2018;154:1096–1101. [PMID: 29409760]

Da Costa DW, Bouwense SA, Schepers NJ, et al. Same-admission versus interval cholecystectomy for mild gallstone pancreatitis (PONCHO): a multicenter randomised controlled trial. *Lancet.* 2015;386:1261–1268. [PMID: 26460661]

Schepers NJ, Hallensleben ND, Besselink MG, et al. Urgent endoscopic retrograde cholangiopancreatography with sphincterotomy versus conservative treatment in predicted severe acute gallstone pancreatitis (APEC): a multicenter randomised controlled trial. *Lancet.* 2020;396:167–176. [PMID: 32682482]

▶ Prognosis

Recent studies have shown increased long-term rates of both endocrine and exocrine pancreatic insufficiency following acute pancreatitis. The prevalence of newly diagnosed prediabetes or diabetes mellitus following a first episode of acute pancreatitis is nearly 40%, and the risk of diabetes mellitus doubles over 5 years. This risk appears to be minimally impacted by age, etiology, or severity. The prevalence of exocrine pancreatic insufficiency following an episode of acute pancreatitis exceeds 25%, particularly in those with alcohol induced and/or severe disease. Screening for both endocrine and exocrine pancreatic insufficiency is therefore warranted after even one episode of acute pancreatitis.

Following an initial episode of acute pancreatitis, approximately 17% of patients will develop recurrent episodes and 8% will develop chronic pancreatitis. The risk of progression is highest among smokers, alcoholics, and those with necrosis. Notably, the risk of progression to chronic pancreatitis in patients who smoke and abuse alcohol is 30%. As both smoking and alcohol cessation have been shown to decrease risk of recurrent acute pancreatitis, appropriate counseling remains essential.

An association between acute pancreatitis and pancreatic cancer has been observed. In a large, population based, matched cohort study, the two- and five-year risk of pancreatic cancer following an episode of acute pancreatitis was 0.70% and 0.87%, respectively, compared to a five-year risk of 0.13% in matched controls.

Ahmed Ali U, Issa Y, Hagenaars JC, et al. Risk of recurrent pancreatitis and progression to chronic pancreatitis after a first episode of acute pancreatitis. *Clin Gastroenterol Hepatol.* 2016;14: 738–746. [PMID: 26772149]

Das SL, Singh PP, Phillips AR, et al. Newly diagnosed diabetes mellitus after acute pancreatitis: a systematic review and meta-analysis. *Gut.* 2014;63:818–831. [PMID: 23929695]

Hollemans RA, Hallensleben ND, Mager DJ, et al. Pancreatic exocrine insufficiency following acute pancreatitis: systematic review and study level meta-analysis. *Pancreatology.* 2018;18:253–262. [PMID: 29482892]

Kirkegård J, Cronin-Fenton D, Heide-Jørgensen U, et al. Acute pancreatitis and pancreatic cancer risk: a nationwide matched-cohort study in Denmark. *Gastroenterology.* 2018;154: 1729–1736. [PMID: 29432727]

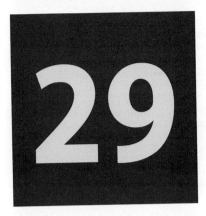

Chronic Pancreatitis

Julia McNabb-Baltar MD, MPH

Peter A. Banks, MD

ESSENTIALS OF DIAGNOSIS

▸ Diagnosis relies on a combination of clinical findings, imaging tests, and pancreatic function testing.

▸ Pancreatic calcifications, irregular and dilated pancreatic duct, diabetes mellitus, and maldigestion characterize advanced disease.

▸ Early-stage diagnosis and overdiagnosis remains a clinical challenge, especially in patients with chronic or episodic abdominal pain and no imaging abnormalities.

General Considerations

Although several risk factors of chronic pancreatitis have been identified, the cause remains uncertain in some cases. Among established risk factors, alcohol ingestion is associated with up to 60–70% of cases of chronic pancreatitis. In addition, ductal obstruction, autoimmune disease, tropical disease, and an association with further systemic illnesses such as scleroderma and hypertriglyceridemia have been described. Recently new insights have been gained into the genetic and molecular basis associated with hereditary forms of chronic pancreatitis. Recent epidemiologic studies clearly demonstrate that smoking is emerging as an independent risk factor for chronic pancreatitis development. The most widely accepted system of etiologic classification for chronic pancreatitis is the TIGAR-O system, which categorizes risk factors according to mechanism and prevalence (Table 29–1). M-ANNHEIM a multiple risk factor classification system incorporates etiology, different stages of the disease, and various degrees of clinical severity. This system will be helpful for research studies investigating the impact and interaction of various risk factors on the course of the disease and will facilitate the comparison and combination of interinstitutional data.

Conwell DL, Banks PA, Sandhu BS, et al. Validation of demographics, etiology, and risk factors for chronic pancreatitis in the USA: a report of the North American Pancreas Study (NAPS) Group. *Dig Dis Sci.* 2017;62(8):2133–2140. [PMID: 28600657]

Hegyi P, Párniczky A, Lerch MM, et al. International Consensus Guidelines for risk factors in chronic pancreatitis. recommendations from the working group for the international consensus guidelines for chronic pancreatitis in collaboration with the International Association of Pancreatology, the American Pancreatic Association, the Japan Pancreas Society, and European Pancreatic Club. *Pancreatology.* 2020;20(4):579–585. [PMID: 32376198]

Singhvi A, Yadav D. Myths and realities about alcohol and smoking in chronic pancreatitis. *Curr Opin Gastroenterol.* 2018;34(5):355–361. [PMID: 29965868]

Tjora E, Dimcevski G, Haas SL, et al. Patient reported exposure to smoking and alcohol abuse are associated with pain and other complications in patients with chronic pancreatitis. *Pancreatology.* 2020;20(5):844–851. [PMID: 32507681]

Pathogenesis

Morphologic changes associated with chronic pancreatitis include ductal, parenchymal, and nerve changes. Pancreatic ducts may become dilated, irregular, or strictured. Meanwhile, the glandular tissue itself is often characterized by irregular and patchy replacement of normal acinar cell architecture with fibrosis. Morphologic features of neuritis and hypertrophy of nerves may account for part of the pain syndrome.

Acute recurrent pancreatitis may lead to chronic pancreatitis in up to 35% of cases. Several hypotheses have been proposed to explain the mechanisms underlying the pathogenesis of chronic pancreatitis. These focus on (1) the role of oxidative stress, (2) toxic-metabolic causes, (3) obstructive causes, and (4) necrosis-fibrosis (also referred to as the *Sentinel Acute Pancreatitis Event* [SAPE] hypothesis) (Table 29–2). The oxidative-stress hypothesis attributes pancreatic damage to reflux of bile rich in reactive oxidation byproducts. The toxic-metabolic theory involves direct damage to pancreatic acinar

Table 29–1. TIGAR-O classification of chronic pancreatitis.

Toxic-Metabolic
Alcoholic
Tobacco smoking
Hypercalcemia (hyperparathyroidism)
Hyperlipidemia (rare and controversial)
Chronic renal failure
Idiopathic
Cause unknown, likely genetic origin
Tropical
Genetic
Autosomal dominant
Cationic trypsinogen
Autosomal-recessive/modifier genes
CFTR mutations
SPINK1 mutations
α_1-Antitrypsin deficiency (possible)
Autoimmune
Isolated autoimmune chronic pancreatitis
Associated with:
• Primary sclerosing cholangitis
• Sjögren syndrome
• Primary biliary cirrhosis
• Type 1 diabetes mellitus
Recurrent and Severe Acute Pancreatitis
Post necrotic (severe acute pancreatitis)
Vascular diseases/ischemia
Post radiation exposure
Obstructive
Pancreas divisum (controversial)
Sphincter of Oddi dysfunction (controversial)
Duct obstruction (tumors, post-traumatic)

Table 29–2. Sentinel Acute Pancreatitis Event (SAPE) hypothesis.

Step 1: Acinar cell stimulation
—Alcohol, gallstone, elevated triglyceride, oxidative stress, smoking, genetic mutations
Step 2: Sentinel event
—Early: proinflammatory response
—Late: stellate cells, profibrotic response
Step 3: Removal of stimulus
—Abstinence from alcohol
—Cholecystectomy
—Lipid lowering agents
Step 4: Recurrent stimulation
—Stellate cell-mediated periacinar fibrosis
• TGFβ, PDGF, procollagen, matrix proteins

PDGF, platelet-derived growth factor; TGFβ, transforming growth factor-β.
Data from Stevens T, Conwell DL, Zuccaro G: Pathogenesis of chronic pancreatitis: an evidence-based review of past theories and recent developments, *Am J Gastroenterol* 2004;99(11):2256–2270.

cells from noxious stimuli such as alcohol. The obstructive theory attributes the majority of injury to pancreatic ductal injury resulting from obstruction related to increased lithogenicity, the latter, in turn, caused by either genetic or environmental exposures (eg, alcohol). Finally, the necrosis-fibrosis hypothesis describes chronic pancreatitis as a continuum that is initiated early by an attack of acute pancreatitis; the subsequent recurrent injury and remodeling lead to pancreatic fibrosis. This hypothesis has gained further support with the observation of progression to chronic pancreatitis from childhood through adulthood of patients with a rare disorder known as hereditary pancreatitis. This disorder, which is caused by a gain of function mutation in cationic trypsinogen, leads to recurrent bouts of acute pancreatitis with later onset of chronic pancreatitis. These explanations are not necessarily mutually exclusive, and a unifying model explaining the precise mechanisms leading to impaired ductal bicarbonate secretion and the patchy inflammatory changes seen on histopathologic examination remains to be further elucidated. The additive effect of alcohol and smoking on pancreatic injury appear to be related to increased endoplasmic reticulum stress in the pancreatic acinar cells.

Recent characterization of pancreatic stellate cells (PSCs) has added insight to the underlying cellular responses behind the development of chronic pancreatitis. Specifically, PSCs are believed to play a role in maintaining normal pancreatic architecture, which can shift toward fibrogenesis in the case of chronic pancreatitis. It is believed that alcohol or additional stimuli lead to matrix metalloproteinase–mediated destruction of normal collagen in pancreatic parenchyma that later allows for pancreatic remodeling. Proinflammatory cytokines tumor necrosis factor-α (TNF-α), interleukin (IL)-1, and IL-6, as well as oxidant complexes, are able to induce PSC activity with subsequent new collagen synthesis. In addition to being stimulated by cytokines, oxidants, or growth factors, PSCs also possess transforming growth factor-β (TGFβ)–mediated self-activating autocrine pathways, which may explain disease progression in chronic pancreatitis even after removal of noxious stimuli.

Lugea A, Gerloff A, SuHY, et al. The combination of alcohol and cigarette smoke induces endoplasmic reticulum stress and cell death in pancreatic acinar cells. *Gastroenterology.* 2017;153(6):1674. [PMID: 28847752]

Mayerle J, Sendler M, Hegyi E, et al. Genetics, cell biology, and pathophysiology of pancreatitis. *Gastronterology.* 2019;156(7):1951–1968. [PMID: 30660731]

Pang TCY, Wilson JS, Apte MV. Pancreatic stellate cells: what's new? *Curr Opin Gastroenterol.* 2017;33(5):366–373. [PMID: 28590306]

► Clinical Findings

A. Symptoms & Signs

The hallmark features of chronic pancreatitis are abdominal pain and pancreatic insufficiency. Advanced disease can also be associated with weight loss and diabetes

(Diabetes Mellitus Type 3c). The possibility of chronic pancreatitis should be entertained in any patient with symptoms of chronic abdominal pain, bloating, and gas. Further supporting features on history include postprandial pain triggered by high-fat or protein-rich meals. In addition, predisposing etiologic factors according to the TIGAR-O classification should be actively sought with attention paid to indicators of possible inherited pancreatic disease such as family history of pancreatitis, pancreatic cancer, or cystic fibrosis.

1. Abdominal pain—The pain associated with chronic pancreatitis is described as epigastric, often with radiation to the back. Pain is often unrelenting and difficult to treat. Pain may be postprandial, associated with nausea and vomiting. The pain pattern varies significantly ranging from intermittent pain (mild, moderate, or severe), constant (mild, moderate, or severe) and of variable intensity. The pain pattern is poorly correlated with the severity of imaging findings, but constant pain is correlated with worse quality of life. Ultimately, the pattern and course of pain symptoms is highly variable among patients with chronic pancreatitis. Up to 20–45% of patients having objective evidence of pancreatic endocrine or exocrine dysfunction may never have pain. Thus, pain is not a prerequisite for the diagnosis of chronic pancreatitis.

2. Pancreatic insufficiency—The second cardinal feature of chronic pancreatitis is the development of pancreatic exocrine and endocrine dysfunction with advanced disease. By comparison to the pain of chronic pancreatitis, the symptoms of pancreatic insufficiency are relatively easily managed. Clinically significant protein malabsorption and fat deficiency does not occur until over 90% of pancreatic function is lost. Typically, steatorrhea precedes the onset of protein malabsorption. Fat malabsorption can manifest clinically as poorly formed greasy, malodorous stools that stick to the side of the toilet bowl. Although absorption of fat-soluble vitamins may be reduced, clinically significant vitamin deficiency is rarely reported. There have been numerous small reports of metabolic bone disease in patients with pancreas insufficiency. Multiple studies have reported a high prevalence of low-trauma fracture in chronic pancreatitis. In fact, the odds of fracture in chronic pancreatitis approached that of other high-risk gastrointestinal illnesses such as inflammatory bowel disease for which osteoporosis screening guidelines exist. Further studies are needed to explore the strength of this association.

Pancreatic endocrine insufficiency presenting as diabetes is a distinctly late occurrence. Patients with chronic calcific pancreatitis, history of pancreatic surgery, or with a family history of diabetes have been observed to be at increased risk of developing this complication.

Bang UC, Benfield T, Bendtsen F, et al. The risk of fractures among patients with cirrhosis or chronic pancreatitis. *Clin Gastroenterol Hepatol.* 2014;12:320–326. [PMID: 23644391]

Machicado JD, Amann ST, Anderson MA, et al. Quality of Life in chronic pancreatitis is determined by constant pain, disability/unemployment, current smoking, and associated co-morbidities. *Am J Gastroenterol.* 2017;112(4):633–642. [PMID: 28244497]

Steinkohl E, Olesen SS, Drewes AM, et al. Progression of pancreatic morphology in chronic pancreatitis is not associated with changes in quality of life and pain. *Scand J Gastroenterol.* 2020;55(9):1099–1107. [PMID: 32672476]

Srivoleti P, Yang AL, Jin DX, et al. Does provider type affect bone health surveillance in chronic pancreatitis? *Dig Dis Sci.* 2021 Jul;66(7):2235–2239. [PMID: 32816216]

Wilcox MC, Yadav D, Ye T, et al. Chronic pancreatitis pain pattern and severity are independent of abdominal imaging findings. *Clin Gastroenterol Hepatol.* 2015;13(3):552–560. [PMID: 25424572]

B. Laboratory Findings

Initial evaluation of chronic pancreatitis should begin with relatively simple and inexpensive testing. Amylase and lipase are often elevated during acute pain episodes early in the natural history of the disease. By contrast, normal or even low levels of amylase or lipase can be found in patients with moderate to advanced chronic pancreatitis. Fecal pancreatic elastase-1 (FPE-1) is a marker of exocrine pancreatic function. FPE-1 is assessed by an enzyme-linked immunosorbent assay (ELISA) performed on stool specimens. A level >200 µg/g of stool is considered normal, and FPE-1 levels <100 µg/g of stool correlate with severe exocrine pancreatic insufficiency. Of note, pancreatic enzyme supplementation does not interfere with interpretation of test results. Liquid stool can lead to a false positive result. The widespread availability of FPE-1 testing has reduced the need for 24-hour fecal fat quantitation as a means of evaluating steatorrhea. A subset of patients with diarrhea-predominant irritable bowel syndrome (D-IBS) has abnormal fecal elastase levels suggesting the presence of pancreas exocrine insufficiency. Pancreatic exocrine insufficiency was detected in 6.1% of patients who fulfilled the Rome II criteria for D-IBS in one study. In these patients, pancreatic enzyme therapy might reduce diarrhea and abdominal pain. The authors conclude that pancreatic exocrine insufficiency should be considered in patients with D-IBS. However, diarrhea can cause a falsely low (abnormal) fecal elastase and caution must be taken when interpreting results in this setting.

Additional tests that may be useful in evaluating chronic pancreatitis include hemoglobin A_{1c} (to investigate glucose intolerance) and markers of autoimmune chronic pancreatitis, including immunoglobulin G_4. Elevation of liver function tests may signal compression of the pancreatic portion of the bile duct from fibrosis, edema, or tumor development.

Domínguez-Muñoz JE, D Hardt P, Lerch MM, et al. Potential for screening for pancreatic exocrine insufficiency using the Fecal Elastase-1 Test. *Dig Dis Sci.* 2017;62(5):1119–1130. [PMID: 28315028]

C. Imaging Studies

Plain abdominal radiographs may reveal calcifications within the pancreas (common in alcoholic and tropical pancreatitis). In general, transabdominal ultrasound has been associated with low sensitivity in diagnosing chronic pancreatitis except in patients with severe disease. Contrast-enhanced computed tomography (CT) and magnetic resonance imaging (MRI) offer enhanced visualization of the pancreas and adjoining structures. These latter two imaging modalities have increasingly become the mainstay of noninvasive imaging techniques for the diagnosis of chronic pancreatitis.

In addition to visualizing calcifications, contrast-enhanced CT allows evaluation of the parenchymal architecture (Figure 29–1). Complications such as pseudocysts (Figure 29–2), pseudoaneurysms, and venous thromboses are well characterized by CT. CT can identify pancreatic atrophy which can be seen in chronic pancreatitis, other conditions and normal aging, but is not a good predictor of histologic fibrosis.

MRI technology, specifically magnetic resonance cholangiopancreatography (MRCP), has the ability to visualize fluid-filled structures allowing characterization of the pancreatic duct. When compared with endoscopic retrograde cholangiopancreatography (ERCP), MRI demonstrates similar ability to detect main duct abnormalities but is not as accurate in evaluating side branch disease. Administration of secretin has been demonstrated to enhance visualization of both the main pancreatic duct and side branches, which may be particularly useful in patients with early disease prior to the onset of clear ductal dilation but has not been universally accepted yet (Figure 29–3). Standardization of reports

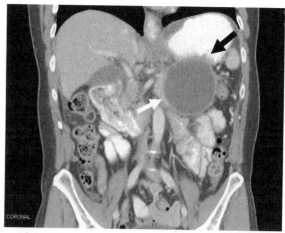

▲ **Figure 29–2.** CT scan: Chronic symptomatic pseudocyst. Coronal CT scan with large pancreatic pseudocyst with visible compression of stomach (*black arrow*) and distal pancreas parenchyma (*white arrow*).

and prospective studies are warranted to determine the diagnostic accuracy of MRI in the assessment of early chronic pancreatitis.

Faghih M, Noe M, Mannan R, et al. Pancreatic volume does not correlate with histologic fibrosis in adult patients with recurrent acute and chronic pancreatitis *Pancreatology.* 2020;20(6): 1078–1084. [PMID: 32819846]

Sainani NI, Kadiyala V, Mortele K, et al. Evaluation of qualitative magnetic resonance imaging features for diagnosis of chronic pancreatitis. *Pancreas.* 2015;44(8):1280–1289. [PMID: 26465953]

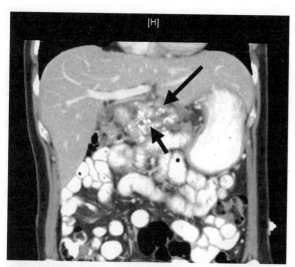

▲ **Figure 29–1.** CT scan: Chronic calcific p. coronal view of CT scan with visible calcifications throughout pancreas in a dilated main duct filled with stones.

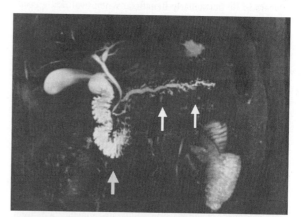

▲ **Figure 29–3.** Secretin-enhanced MRCP (sMRCP): Chronic pancreatitis. MRCP/sMRCP with abnormal pancreatic duct with visible side branches (*white arrows*) and fluid-filled duodenum (*gray arrow*) after secretin stimulation.

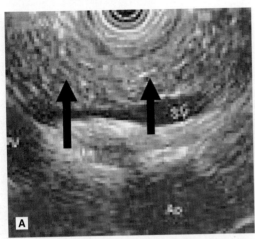 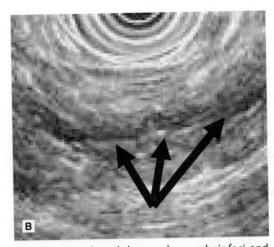

▲ **Figure 29–4.** Endoscopic ultrasound: Chronic pancreatitis features. **A.** Parenchymal changes, hyperechoic foci, and strands. **B.** Ductal changes, dilated and irregular duct with hyperechoic margins. (Reproduced with permission of Linda S. Lee, MD.)

D. Endoscopy

1. Endoscopic ultrasound—One of the challenges for noninvasive testing remains the diagnosis of early chronic pancreatitis. Increasingly endoscopic ultrasound (EUS) has played a role in this disease group. Previously established endosonographic criteria for the diagnosis of chronic pancreatitis include parenchymal features (atrophy, hyperechoic foci, stranding, cysts, and lobularity) and ductal features (narrowing, dilation, irregularity, calculi, side branch dilation, and hyperechoic walls) (Figure 29–4). The diagnosis usually requires identification of five (or more) of nine criteria. The diagnostic significance of some features may be more important (major criteria) than other (minor criteria) but is an area of active research investigation. EUS also appears to be particularly beneficial when evaluating cystic lesions or neoplasms believed to be arising in the background of chronic pancreatitis as well as examining parenchyma when presence of disease is equivocal. New variations of EUS imaging including elastography, contrast-enhanced EUS may decrease the subjectivity of image interpretation for early diagnosis and help differentiate chronic pancreatitis from pancreatic ductal adenocarcinoma.

Dominguez-Muñoz JE, Iglesias-Garcia J, Castiñeira Alvariño M, et al. EUS elastography to predict pancreatic exocrine insufficiency in patients with chronic pancreatitis. *Gastrointest Endosc.* 2015;81:136–142. [PMID: 25088920]

Wilcox CM, Gress T, Boermeester M, et al. International consensus guidelines on the role of diagnostic endoscopic ultrasound in the management of chronic pancreatitis. Recommendations from the working group for the international consensus guidelines for chronic pancreatitis in collaboration with the International Association of Pancreatology, the American Pancreatic Association, the Japan Pancreas Society, and European Pancreatic Club. *Pancreatology.* 2020;20(5):822–827. [PMID: 32631791]

2. Endoscopic retrograde cholangiopancreatography—While providing excellent views of the pancreatic main duct and side branches, ERCP also offers the possibility of therapeutic intervention such as removal of pancreatic duct stones with extracorporeal shock wave lithotripsy (ESWL) assistance (Figure 29–5) or per-oral pancreatoscopy-guided lithotripsy. However, given the associated risks of inducing acute pancreatitis, ERCP is generally reserved for situations in which therapeutic intervention is likely. Combining EUS with MRI/MRCP is a practical, less invasive, and safe alternative to evaluating the pancreaticobiliary anatomy before attempting ERCP in chronic pancreatitis.

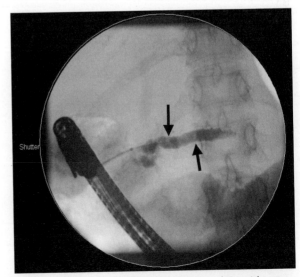

▲ **Figure 29–5.** ERCP: Dilated pancreatic duct with stones. Arrows point to filling defects.

E. Special Tests

1. Gene testing—The role of genetic testing for patients with suspected hereditary forms of chronic pancreatitis continues to evolve. Hereditary and idiopathic forms of chronic pancreatitis account for up to 20–30% of cases. Genetic alterations associated with chronic pancreatitis include mutations in the cationic trypsinogen gene *PRSS1* (carriers bear a markedly increased lifetime risk of pancreatic cancer), the cystic fibrosis transmembrane conductance regulator (*CFTR*, an apical membrane chloride channel), the serine protease inhibitor, Kazal type 1 (*SPINK1*), the digestive enzyme chymotrypsin C (CTRC), and the calcium-sensing receptor gene (CASR). Although widespread screening has yet to come into routine practice, it is indicated in patients with otherwise unexplained onset of chronic pancreatitis or suggestive family history.

Gardner TB, Adler DG, Forsmark CE, et al. ACG Clinical Guideline: chronic pancreatitis. *Am J Gastroenterol.* 2020;115(3): 322–339. [PMID: 32022720]

2. Pancreatic function testing—Sampling of secretin-stimulated pancreatic fluid from duodenal aspirates theoretically allows detection of impaired pancreatic function prior to the onset of structural abnormalities. The technique originally described consists of aspiration of duodenal juice through a dual lumen (Dreiling tube) every 15 minutes for a total of 60 minutes following administration of secretin. A peak bicarbonate concentration <80 mEq/L is consistent with the diagnosis of chronic pancreatitis. More recently endoscopic pancreatic function testing has emerged at specialized centers as an alternative modality for direct sampling of duodenal aspirates. Endoscopic pancreas function testing is very helpful in evaluating patients with chronic pain syndromes and equivocal imaging for early chronic pancreatitis. It can also be combined with EUS to simultaneously assess both structure and secretory physiology (Figure 29–6). Furthermore, breath testing using ^{13}C-labeled mixed triglyceride has recently been shown to be equivalent to fecal fat measurements and may allow a noninvasive means of monitoring therapy but is not available in the United States.

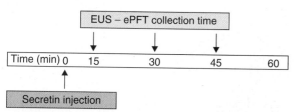

▲ **Figure 29–6.** Combined EUS-ePFT procedure. Timeline of secretin administration and pancreatic fluid collection with endoscopic view of duodenum at selected time points.

Dominguez-Muñoz JE. Diagnosis and treatment of pancreatic exocrine insufficiency. *Curr Opin Gastroenterol.* 2018;34(5): 349–354. [PMID: 29889111]

F. Diagnostic Challenges

The diagnosis of early chronic pancreatitis can be challenging due to overlap with several other chronic pain syndromes and in many cases the late occurrence of objective laboratory or radiographic abnormalities. Moreover, repeated instrumentation (pancreas duct stenting) of the pancreas itself can often lead to significant pathologic changes in the pancreatic parenchyma and duct architecture. Ultimately, a rational approach to diagnosing chronic pancreatitis requires the appropriate use of clinical history, laboratory testing, and radiographic and endoscopic investigation. The role of genetic testing continues to be defined. Molecular biology techniques, such as proteomics analysis, and cytokine or miRNA profiling of biofluids, may provide insight into the pathogenesis of chronic pancreatitis and identify molecular targets for drug therapy.

Conwell DL, Lee LS, Longnecker DS, et al. American pancreatic association practice guidelines in chronic pancreatitis: evidence-based report on diagnostic guidelines. *Pancreas.* 2014;43: 1143–1162. [PMID: 25333398]

Hart PA, Conwell DL. Chronic pancreatitis: managing a difficult disease. *Am J Gastroenterol.* 2020;115(1):49–55. [PMID: 31764092]

▶ Differential Diagnosis

The differential diagnosis of patients presenting with pain from chronic pancreatitis often includes peptic ulcer disease, inflammatory bowel disease, gastric dysmotility, and irritable bowel syndrome in addition to psychogenic or factitious/drug-seeking disorders. These must be further discriminated through careful clinical evaluation. The maldigestion associated with chronic pancreatitis must be distinguished from other malabsorptive disorders such as carbohydrate malabsorption and celiac disease. It may help to ask about a history of "sticky" or greasy stools as well as the presence of oil drops separating from the main stool. These are features often associated with significant steatorrhea and strongly suggest the diagnosis of pancreatic insufficiency.

▶ Complications

Complications associated with chronic pancreatitis include pseudocyst, biliary ductal, or duodenal obstruction, pancreatic ascites or pleural effusion, splenic vein thrombosis, pancreatic fistulae, pseudoaneurysms, and an increased risk of pancreatic cancer.

▶ Treatment

Treatment for chronic pancreatitis begins with lifestyle modifications, including cessation of alcohol, consumption of smaller meals, and quitting smoking. Further therapy should be directed toward treatment of symptoms and guided by the underlying suspected cause.

A. Pain

By far the most difficult aspect of treatment of chronic pancreatitis relates to management of chronic pain. Treatment should be aimed at analgesia, reducing inflammation, and overcoming intrapancreatic pressure. In addition, investigations are currently underway to evaluate means of altering neural transmission in order to improve analgesia. Increasingly, it has become recognized that many patients labeled with the diagnosis of chronic pancreatitis may not actually have visceral pain. These patients are much less likely to respond to therapy. Another common cause of pain that can be seen in chronic pancreatitis is narcotic bowel syndrome. This is an underrecognized source of abdominal discomfort seen in patients on high dosages of narcotics in whom the character or activity of the disease process is not sufficient to fully explain the pain syndrome.

The mechanisms causing pain in pancreatitis have been the focus of intense study due to their enigmatic nature. Likely multifactorial, previously reported factors contributing to pain in chronic pancreatitis have included recurrent tissue inflammation, necrosis, pancreatic ductal hypertension, increased interstitial fluid pressure, pancreatic ischemia, and fibrotic encasement of sensory nerves (Figure 29–7). More recently, attention has focused on pain in chronic pancreatitis as a neurobiologic phenomenon. Researchers have reported increased changes in the brain cortex of patients with chronic pancreatitis when compared with controls. Recent studies have also demonstrated upregulation of the pain mediator substance P and calcitonin gene–related peptide in tissue samples from patients with chronic pancreatitis, as well as nerve growth factor–dependent nociceptors. TrkA, a high-affinity receptor for a nerve growth receptor, has been found to be overexpressed in acinar cells in chronic pancreatitis and may serve as a link between inflammation and hyperalgesia. Additional nociceptive pathways implicated in chronic pancreatitis include brain-derived neurotrophic factor as well as proteinase-activated receptor-2 (PAR-2)–mediated stimulation of nociceptive neurons by trypsin activation. Two emerging concepts with respect to pain mediation in chronic pancreatitis include "mechanical allodynia," whereby pain is sensed even in the absence of noxious stimuli given prior sensitization of the nociceptive system, and "inflammatory hyperalgesia," in which relatively minor episodes of inflammation may trigger increased pain response due to already "primed" pancreatic nociceptors.

Alcohol and smoking cessation may help decrease pain in patients with chronic pancreatitis and should be strongly recommended. Analgesics should be administered in conjunction with pain service with emphasis on alternative nonnarcotic management of the abdominal pain syndrome. The WHO has a suggested stepwise approach to chronic pain management.

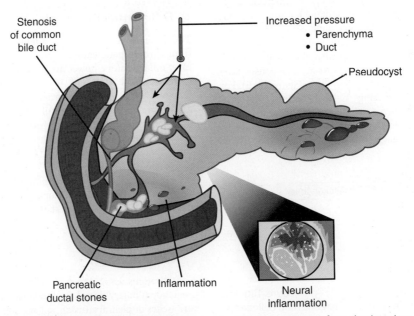

▲ **Figure 29–7.** Sources of pain in chronic pancreatitis. (Reproduced with permission from the American Gastroenterological Association Gastroenterology Teaching Project.)

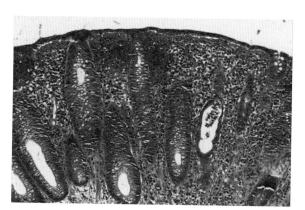

▲ **Plate 1.** Rectal mucosal biopsy specimen from a patient with dysentery caused by shigellosis. There is considerable mucosal inflammation caused by infiltration with polymorphonuclear leukocytes and mononuclear cells, as well as substantial damage to surface epithelial cells. However, mucosal architecture is generally preserved with straight, closely adjacent crypts. A crypt microabscess is seen on the right.

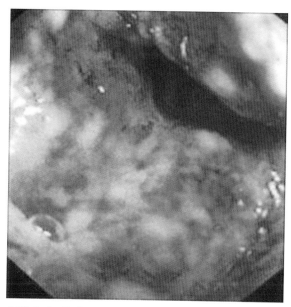

▲ **Plate 3.** Endoscopic appearance of colonic ischemia. (Reproduced with permission from David Stockwell, MD.)

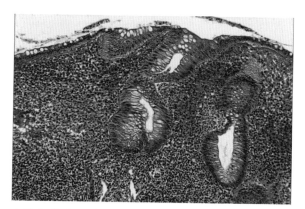

▲ **Plate 2.** Rectal mucosal biopsy specimen from a patient with dysenteric stools caused by a flare of chronic ulcerative colitis. The mucosa is heavily infiltrated with polymorphonuclear leukocytes and mononuclear cells. In contrast to Plate 1, mucosal architecture is markedly distorted, with substantial reduction in crypts and distortion of those that remain.

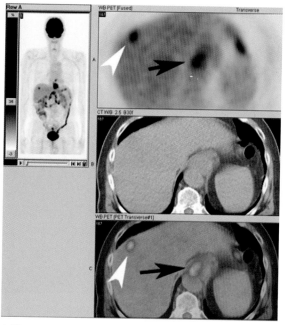

▲ **Plate 4.** Esophageal carcinoma. Fused PET-CT image shows a "hot spot" (*black arrow*) at the level of the distal esophagus corresponding to squamous cell carcinoma. Note the hepatic metastasis (*white arrowhead*).

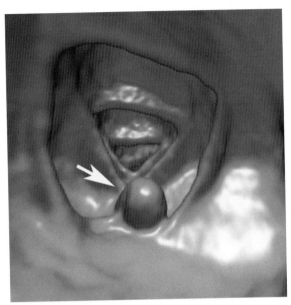

▲ **Plate 5.** Colonic polyp. Three-dimensional endoluminal reconstructed image confirms the presence of a colonic polyp (*arrow*). (For corresponding axial MDCT image, see Figure 9–19 in the text.)

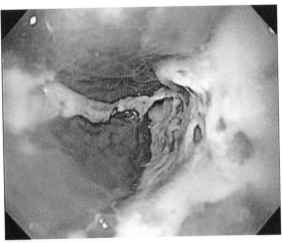

▲ **Plate 6.** Severe erosive esophagitis with peptic stricture.

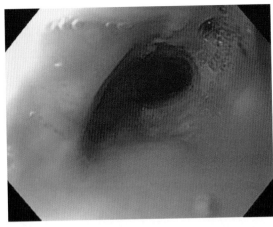

▲ **Plate 7.** Esophageal stricture prior to dilation.

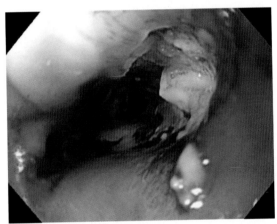

▲ **Plate 8.** Postdilation appearance of esophageal stricture shown in Plate 7.

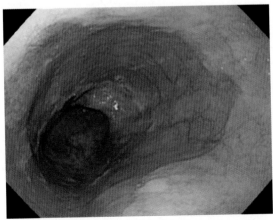

▲ **Plate 9.** Endoscopic appearance of Barrett esophagus.

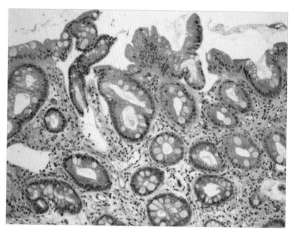

▲ **Plate 10.** Histopathologic findings in nondysplastic Barrett esophagus. Note the glandular epithelium containing goblet cells. (Reproduced with permission from Jason Hornick, MD, PhD, Brigham and Women's Hospital.)

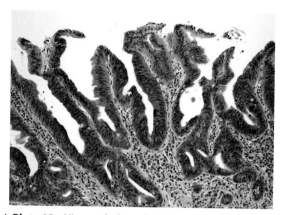

▲ **Plate 12.** Histopathologic findings of high-grade dysplasia in Barrett esophagus. There is full-thickness nuclear stratification and the mucosa has a villous appearance. (Reproduced with permission from Jason Hornick, MD, PhD, Brigham and Women's Hospital.)

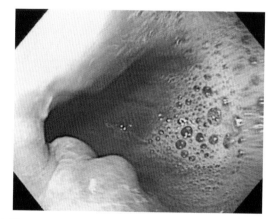

▲ **Plate 13.** Nodule of high-grade dysplasia in Barrett esophagus.

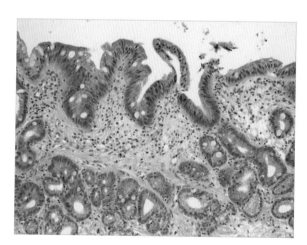

▲ **Plate 11.** Histopathologic findings of low-grade dysplasia in Barrett esophagus. The surface epithelium displays nuclear stratification, limited to the lower half of the cytoplasm. (Reproduced with permission from Jason Hornick, MD, PhD, Brigham and Women's Hospital.)

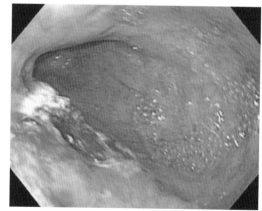

▲ **Plate 14.** Same area shown in Plate 13 after endoscopic mucosal resection.

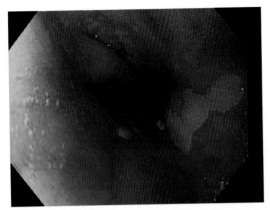

▲ **Plate 15.** Endoscopic view of circumferential long segment Barrett esophagus with a few islands of normal pale pink squamous mucosa where prior surveillance biopsies have healed.

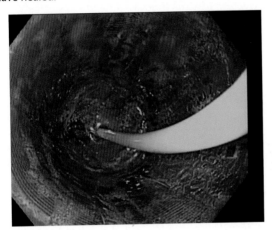

▲ **Plate 16.** Endoscopic view of the radiofrequency balloon catheter inflated to treat circumferential Barrett esophagus.

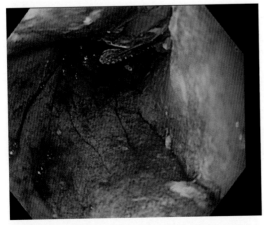

▲ **Plate 17.** Immediate post-ablation appearance.

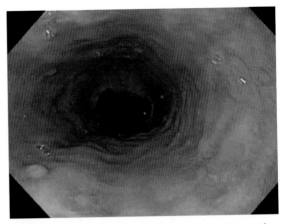

▲ **Plate 18.** Endoscopic findings in eosinophilic esophagitis. Note trachea-like mucosal rings.

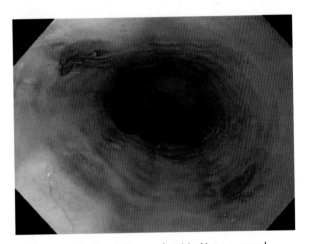

▲ **Plate 19.** Eosinophilic esophagitis. Note mucosal lacerations.

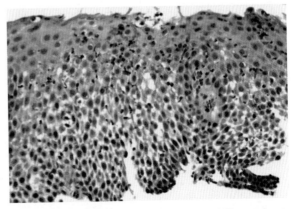

▲ **Plate 20.** Histologic findings in eosinophilic esophagitis. Note increased eosinophils in the squamous mucosa.

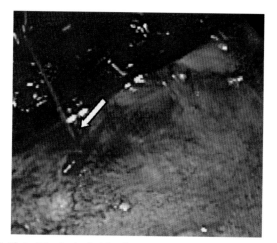

▲ **Plate 21.** Actively bleeding gastric ulcer.

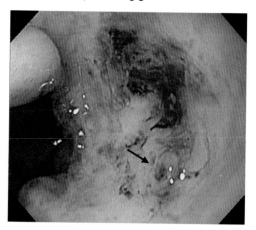

▲ **Plate 22.** Nonbleeding visible vessels. Giant duodenal ulcer occupying the entire duodenal bulb, with a non-bleeding visible vessel at bottom right (*arrow*).

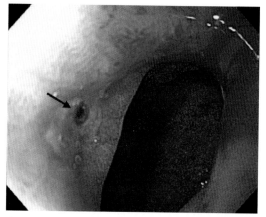

▲ **Plate 23.** Nonbleeding visible vessels. A pyloric channel ulcer with a pigmented, nonbleeding visible vessel (*arrow*).

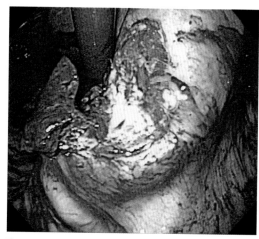

▲ **Plate 24.** Adherent clot on a gastric ulcer.

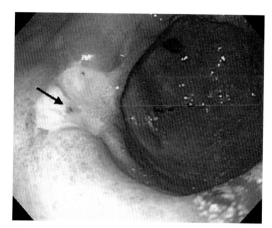

▲ **Plate 25.** Flat spot on a gastric ulcer (*arrow*).

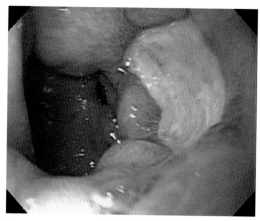

▲ **Plate 26.** Clean based prepyloric ulcer.

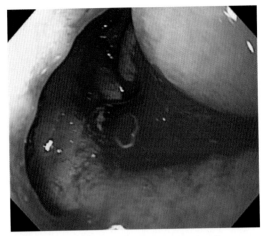

▲ **Plate 27.** Duodenal ulcer with active bleeding.

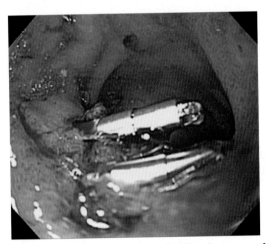

▲ **Plate 28.** Duodenal ulcer controlled by placement of two hemoclips.

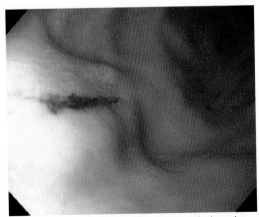

▲ **Plate 29.** Linear Mallory-Weiss tear just below the gastroesophageal junction.

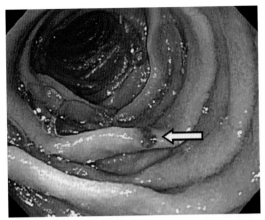

▲ **Plate 30.** Vascular malformation in the duodenum (*arrow*).

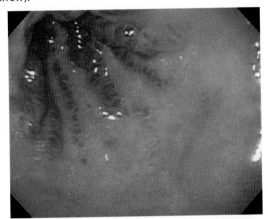

▲ **Plate 31.** Watermelon stomach.

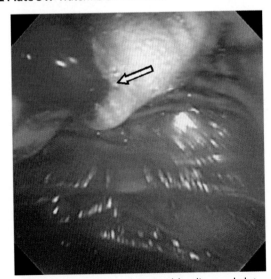

▲ **Plate 32.** Hemobilia with active bleeding and clots coming from ampullary orifice (*arrow*).

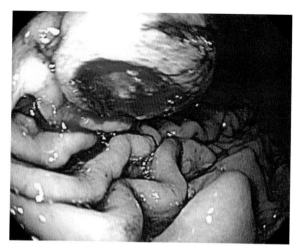

▲ **Plate 33.** Metastatic sarcoma to the stomach with active bleeding.

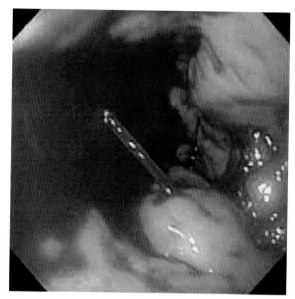

▲ **Plate 35.** Esophageal varices. Actively bleeding esophageal varix.

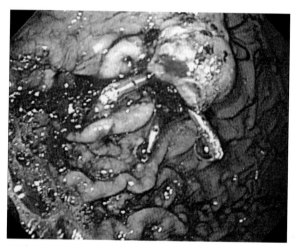

▲ **Plate 34.** Metastatic sarcoma treated by placement of hemoclips.

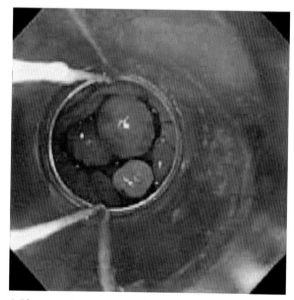

▲ **Plate 36.** Esophageal varices post–band ligation therapy.

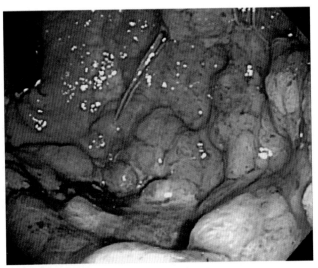

▲ **Plate 37.** Gastric varices in the body and fundus.

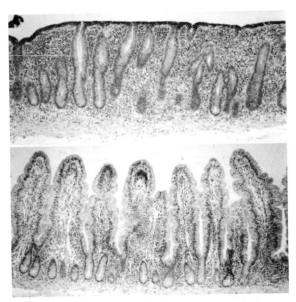

▲ **Plate 38.** The upper panel shows a characteristic severe lesion from a patient with untreated celiac sprue. Villi are absent, crypts are hyperplastic, and the lamina propria is infiltrated with many mononuclear cells. For comparison, the lower panel shows a biopsy sample from a normal volunteer showing normal mucosal architecture with tall villi and shallow crypts and just a few mononuclear cells in the lamina propria.

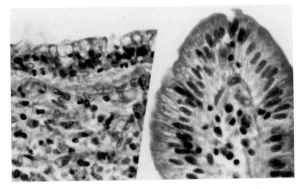

▲ **Plate 39.** The left panel shows at higher magnification the absorptive surface of the biopsy sample from the patient with celiac sprue shown in the upper panel of Plate 38. The surface absorptive cells are decreased in height and vacuolated, and the nuclei have lost their polarity. Numerous intraepithelial lymphocytes (IELs) can be seen between adjacent epithelial cells. The underlying lamina propria is heavily infiltrated with lymphocytes and plasma cells. For comparison, in the panel on the right is the tip of a villus from the biopsy sample shown in upper panel of Plate 40 from a normal individual. In contrast to the panel on the left, the absorptive cells are tall and have a well-developed brush border, with only occasional IELs evident between epithelial cells.

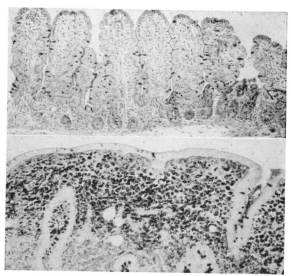

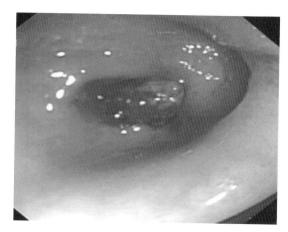

▲ **Plate 42.** Diverticulum with a large, oozing visible vessel.

▲ **Plate 40.** Upper panel shows a biopsy sample obtained from a normal volunteer and stained with periodic acid–Schiff (PAS) stain. The glycoprotein-rich epithelial cell brush border and the goblet cell mucous are PAS-positive. The biopsy sample in the lower panel was obtained from a patient with untreated Whipple disease. The villus architecture is markedly distorted and the lamina propria is packed with large PAS-positive macrophages that virtually replace the lymphocytes and plasma cells that would normally be seen. Additionally, profiles of dilated lymphatics are evident in the lamina propria.

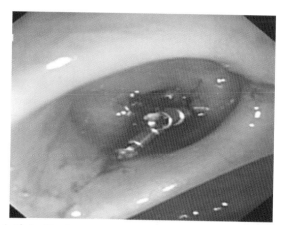

▲ **Plate 43.** Post-treatment of diverticulum with two endoclips.

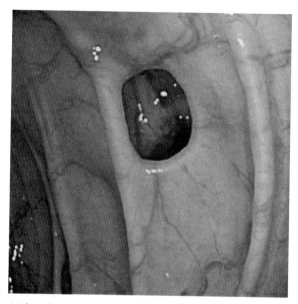

▲ **Plate 41.** Diverticulum.

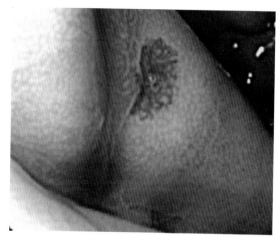

▲ **Plate 44.** Arteriovenous malformation in a patient with lower gastrointestinal bleeding.

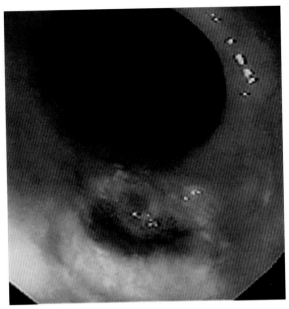

▲ **Plate 45.** Post-treatment of arteriovenous malformation with bipolar cautery.

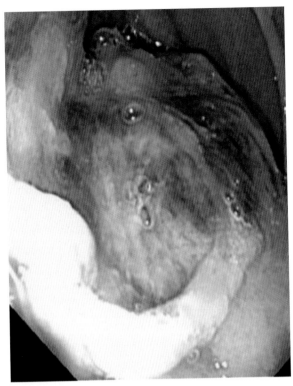

▲ **Plate 47.** Post-treatment of bleeding.

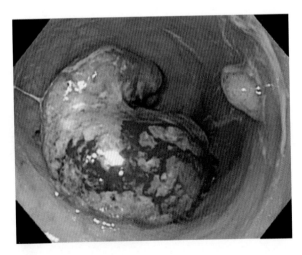

▲ **Plate 46.** Colon cancer.

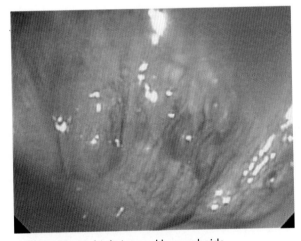

▲ **Plate 48.** Multiple internal hemorrhoids.

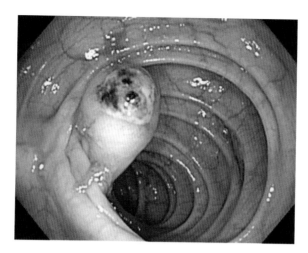

▲ **Plate 49.** Visible vessels at polypectomy site.

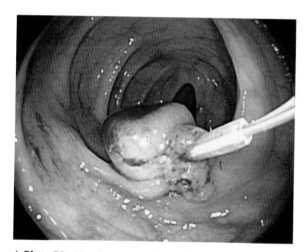

▲ **Plate 50.** Bleeding controlled with placement of an endoloop.

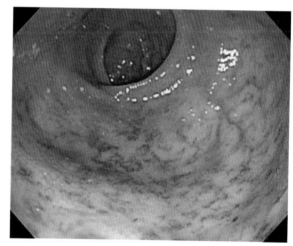

▲ **Plate 51.** Chronic radiation proctitis.

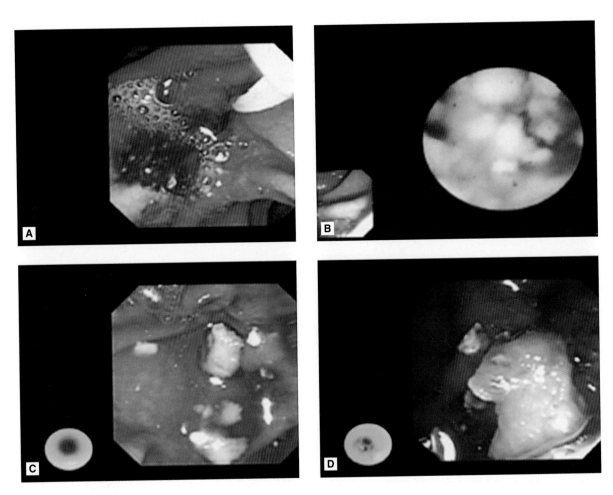

▲ **Plate 52.** ERCP + ESWL: symptomatic pancreatic duct stones. **A.** area of papilla in the duodenum, **B–D.** stones. (Reproduced with permission from David Leslie Carr-Locke, MD.)

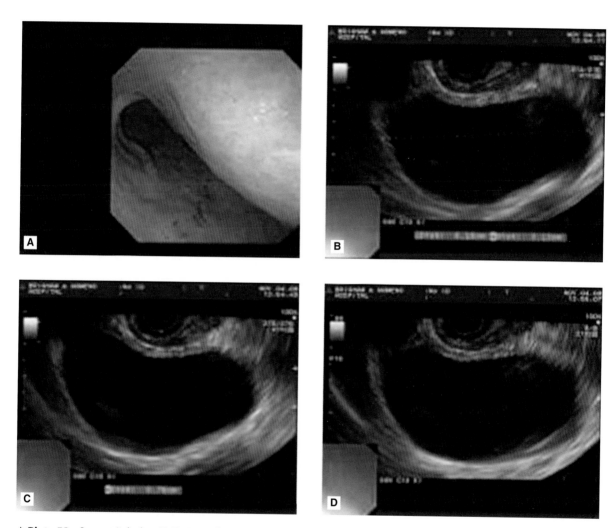

▲ **Plate 53.** **A.** gastric bulge, **B–D.** EUS of pseudocyst. (Reproduced with permission from Christopher Thompson, MD.)

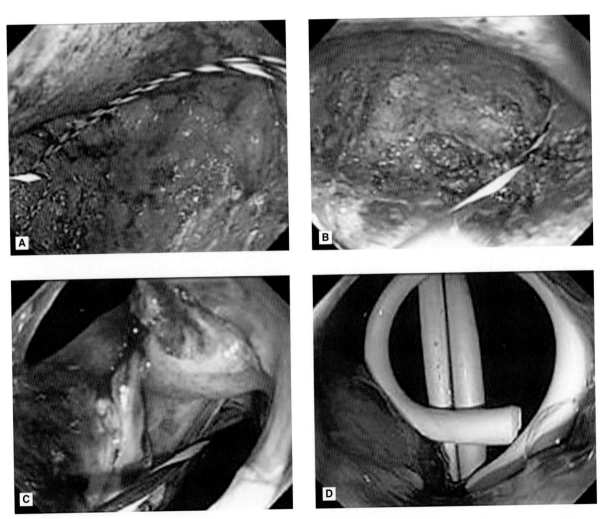

▲ **Plate 54.** Stepwise images (Plates 53, A–D and 54, A–D) of endoscopic drainage of symptomatic pancreas. **A.** pseudo-cyst, **B.** wire in cyst cavity, **C.** cystogastrostomy site with wire, **D.** residual pigtail catheters. (Reproduced with permission from Christopher Thompson, MD.)

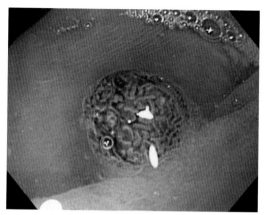

▲ **Plate 55.** Endoscopic view of a diminutive adenomatous polyp before cold snare excision (narrow-band imaging mode).

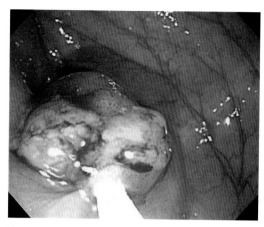

▲ **Plate 58.** Sessile adenomatous polyp undergoing hot snare polypectomy without mucosal injection. Same patient as in Plate 57.

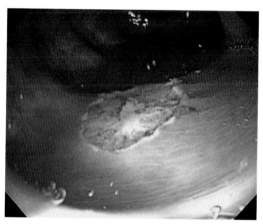

▲ **Plate 56.** Diminutive adenomatous polyp after cold snare excision. Same patient as in Plate 55.

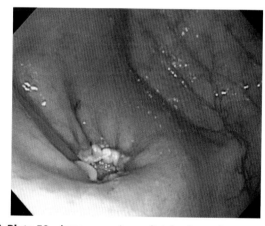

▲ **Plate 59.** Appearance immediately after polypectomy. Same patient as in Plate 57.

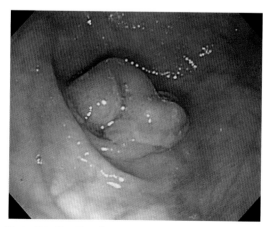

▲ **Plate 57.** Sessile adenomatous polyp.

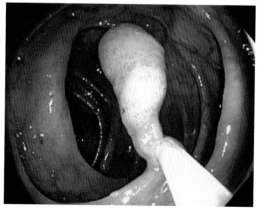

▲ **Plate 60.** Endoscopic view of a standard snare polypectomy for a pedunculated polyp.

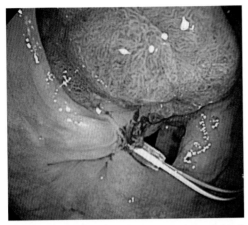

▲ **Plate 61.** Snare polypectomy for a large pedunculated polyp, with endoloop in place prior to snare resection.

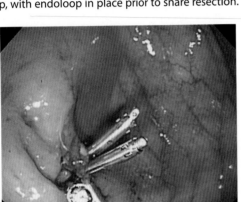

▲ **Plate 62.** Hemostatic clips applied after polypectomy for hemostasis and suspected perforation. Same patient as in Plate 57.

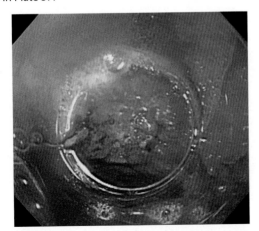

▲ **Plate 63.** Endoscopic mucosal resection: cap method with transparent cap positioned over irregular nodule in Barrett mucosa.

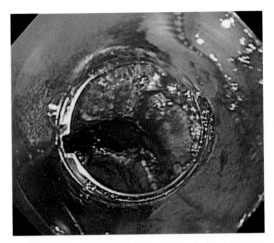

▲ **Plate 64.** Barrett nodule after suction and snare resection (snare not shown). Same patient as in Plate 63.

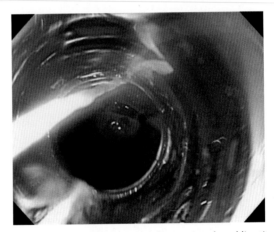

▲ **Plate 65.** Endoscopic mucosal resection: band ligation method with Barrett nodule ligated.

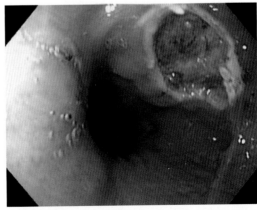

▲ **Plate 66.** Barrett nodule after snare resection. Same patient as in Plate 65. (Reproduced with permission from Dr John R. Saltzman, Brigham and Women's Hospital.)

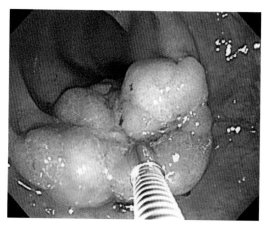

▲ **Plate 67.** Endoscopic mucosal resection: needle injection method.

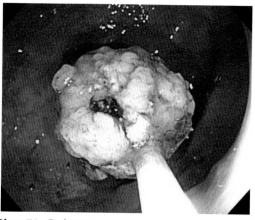

▲ **Plate 70.** Endoscopic mucosal resection: net retrieval of specimens.

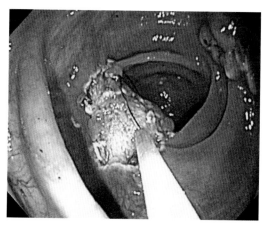

▲ **Plate 68.** Endoscopic mucosal resection: piecemeal snare polypectomy.

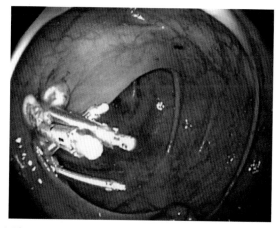

▲ **Plate 71.** Endoscopic mucosal resection: closure of the mucosal defect with clips.

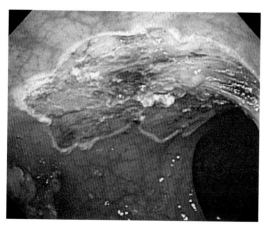

▲ **Plate 69.** Appearance after snare resection. Same patient as in Plate 68.

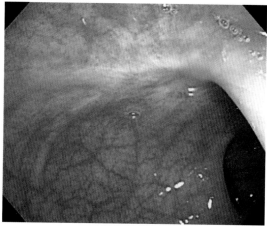

▲ **Plate 72.** Endoscopic mucosal resection: scar after 3 months.

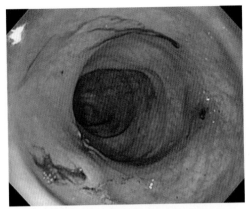

▲ **Plate 73.** Ink marking a polypectomy site.

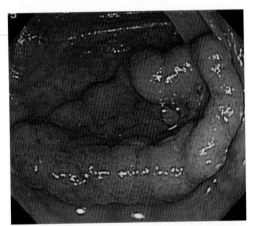

▲ **Plate 74.** Endoscopic submucosal dissection: large sessile polyp. (Reproduced with permission from Professor Yutaka Saito, National Cancer Center Hospital, Tokyo, Japan.)

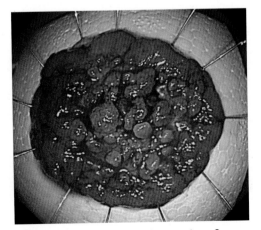

▲ **Plate 75.** Resected specimen in one piece. Same patient as in Plate 74. (Reproduced with permission from Professor Yutaka Saito, National Cancer Center Hospital, Tokyo, Japan.)

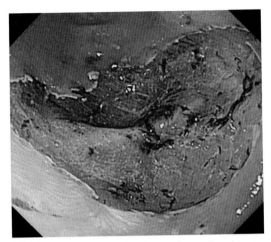

▲ **Plate 76.** Mucosal defect after endoscopic submucosal dissection. Same patient as in Plate 74. (Reproduced with permission from Professor Yutaka Saito, National Cancer Center Hospital, Tokyo, Japan.)

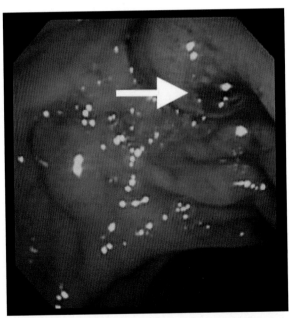

▲ **Plate 77.** Endoscopic view of bleeding from the minor papilla in a patient with pancreatic cancer (*arrow*).

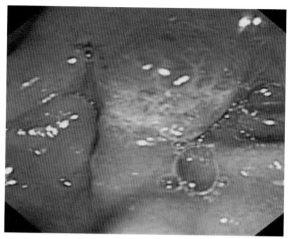

▲ **Plate 78.** Adenoma of the papilla.

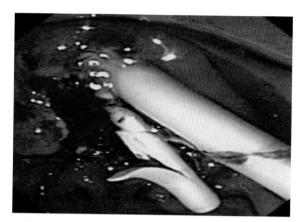

▲ **Plate 80.** Biliary and pancreatic stents in place.

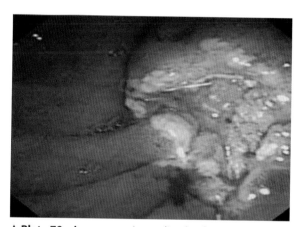

▲ **Plate 79.** Appearance immediately after papillectomy.

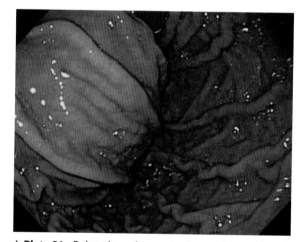

▲ **Plate 81.** Bulge along the proximal posterior gastric wall.

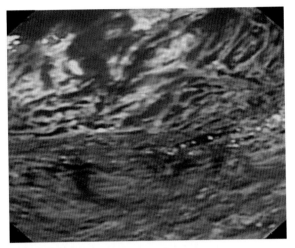

▲ **Plate 82.** View inside a pseudocyst.

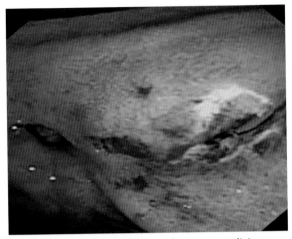

▲ **Plate 84.** Endoscopic therapy for pancreas divisum showing minor papillotomy.

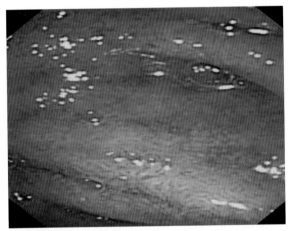

▲ **Plate 83.** Endoscopic therapy for pancreas divisum showing minor papilla.

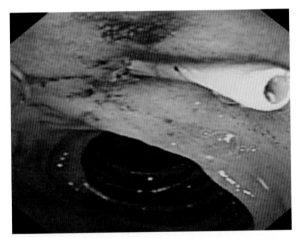

▲ **Plate 85.** Endoscopic therapy for pancreas divisum showing stent placed across papillotomy.

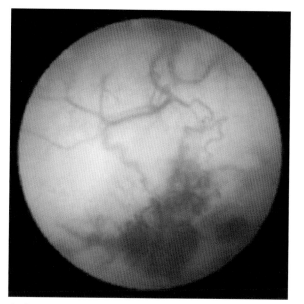

▲ **Plate 86.** Small bowel angioectasia.

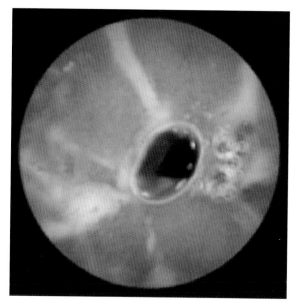

▲ **Plate 88.** Small bowel Crohn disease.

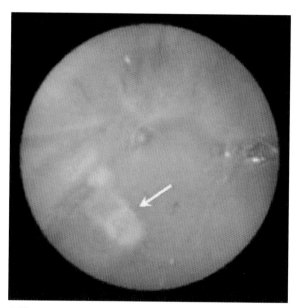

▲ **Plate 87.** Small bowel ulcer (NSAID associated).

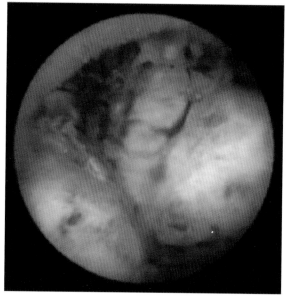

▲ **Plate 89.** Metastatic melanoma.

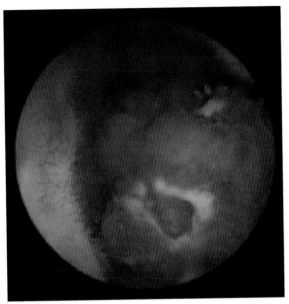

▲ **Plate 90.** Peutz-Jeghers polyp.

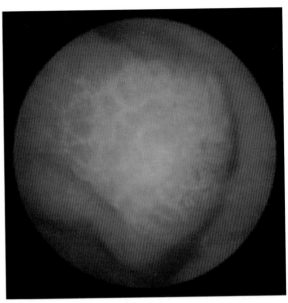

▲ **Plate 92.** Mosaic pattern of mucosa in celiac disease.

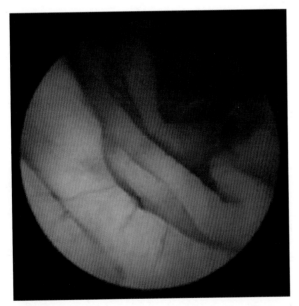

▲ **Plate 91.** Scalloping and mucosal fissures in celiac disease.

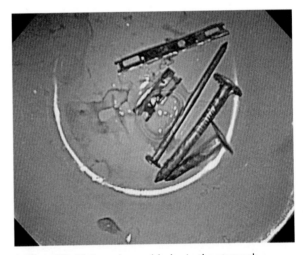

▲ **Plate 93.** Nails and razor blades in the stomach.

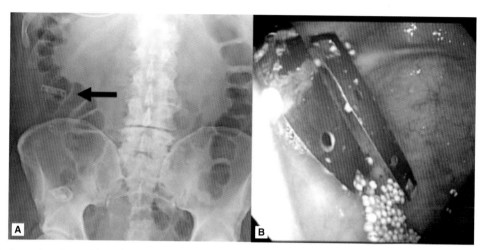

▲ **Plate 94.** Intentionally swallowed razor blades are seen on abdominal x-ray (**A**, *arrow*) and on colonoscopic view in the cecum (**B**). These were retrieved successfully with use of a Roth net and overtube to protect the tortuous sigmoid colon.

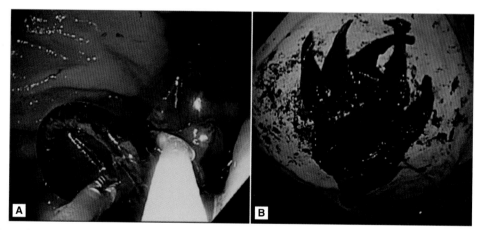

▲ **Plate 95.** A plastic-appearing bezoar was found in a patient's stomach (**A**) which had hardened and was very difficult to remove. After retrieval, with difficulty the object was unfolded and discovered to be a vulcanized latex glove (**B**).

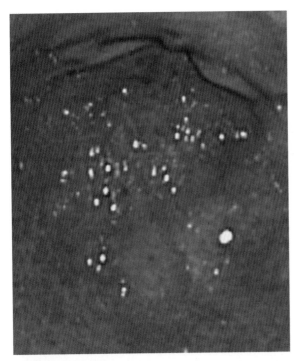

▲ **Plate 96.** Lipoma.

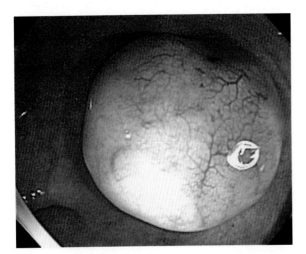

▲ **Plate 97.** Rectal carcinoid.

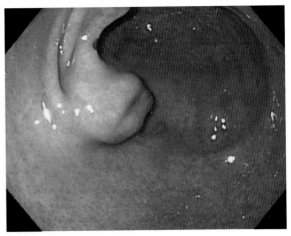

▲ **Plate 98.** Pancreatic rest.

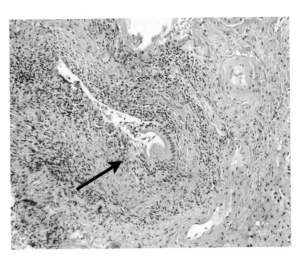

▲ **Plate 99.** Nonsuppurative destructive cholangitis. A large bile duct (*arrow*) shows lymphocytic inflammation and periductal ("onion-skin") fibrosis. (Reproduced with permission from Jason Hornick, MD, PhD, Brigham and Women's Hospital.)

Singh VK, Yadav D, Garg PK. Diagnosis and management of chronic pancreatitis: a review. *JAMA*. 2019;322(24):2422–2434. [PMID: 3186005]

1. Inflammation and pancreatic pressure—Attempts to reduce pancreatic inflammation should include smoking and alcohol cessation, smaller meals, trial of total parenteral nutrition or enteral feeding, surgery for obstructive pancreatitis, and corticosteroids for autoimmune chronic pancreatitis. Methods of reducing pancreatic pressure include suppression of secretion via administration of a proton pump inhibitor and pancreatic enzymes. In the rare but now increasingly recognized instance where autoimmune pancreatitis is suspected, therapy with corticosteroids has also been found to be beneficial (see Chapter 30).

2. Obstruction—If ductal obstruction is present due to stricture, stone, or pseudocyst with mass effect, invasive therapy may be necessary. In the case of ductal stones, endoscopic clearance (Plate 52), surgical therapy, or ESWL may be attempted although evidence for individual treatment modalities is limited. Symptomatic pseudocysts may be drained percutaneously, endoscopically (Plates 53 and 54), or surgically. For pancreatic duct obstruction drainage, recent data from randomized head-to-head trials indicate somewhat improved outcomes with surgical drainage over endoscopic therapy. Surgical options for chronic pancreatitis include lateral pancreaticojejunostomy for decompression of a dilated main duct, removal of localized disease by either a Whipple procedure or tail resection, and, finally, total pancreatectomy and total pancreatectomy with islet cell autotransplantation which is offered in specialized centers for very selected patients.

3. Modification of neural transmission—Chronic pain in chronic pancreatitis is complex and may have several origins. Methods of modifying the nociceptive process involved in chronic pancreatitis include EUS-guided celiac plexus block, bilateral thoracoscopic splanchnicectomy, transcranial magnetic stimulation, as well as additional investigational techniques including medications. One study examining celiac plexus block via EUS found that 55% of subjects had decreased pain after 8 weeks (Figure 29–8), with only 10% experiencing decreased pain after 24 weeks. For the most part, all of these modalities have achieved success only in producing moderate short-term pain relief, with high rates of relapse after long-term follow-up.

Abu-El-Haija M, Anazawa T, Beilman GJ, et al. The role of total pancreatectomy with islet autotransplantation in the treatment of chronic pancreatitis: a report from the International Consensus Guidelines in chronic pancreatitis. *Pancreatology*. 2020;20(4):762–771. [PMID: 32327370]

Issa Y, Kempeneers MA, Bruno MJ, et al. Effect of early surgery vs endoscopy-first approach on pain in patients with chronic pancreatitis: the ESCAPE randomized clinical trial. *JAMA*. 2020;323(3):237–247. [PMID: 31961419]

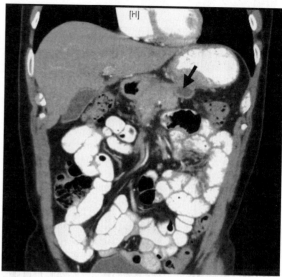

▲ **Figure 29–8.** CT scan: Residual asymptomatic pseudocyst 6–8 weeks after endoscopic drainage (*arrow*).

Kitano M, Gress TM, Garg PK, et al. International consensus guidelines on interventional endoscopy in chronicpancreatitis. Recommendations from the working group for the international consensus guidelines for chronic pancreatitis in collaboration with the International Association of Pancreatology, the American Pancreatic Association, the Japan Pancreas Society, and European Pancreatic Club. *Pancreatology*. 2020;20(6): 1045–1055. [PMID: 32792253]

B. Exocrine Insufficiency

Pancreatic enzyme supplementation can aid in addressing the difficulty in digesting protein and lipid products in patients with severe chronic pancreatitis. Typically, these enzymes should be given with each meal and snacks. We usually start with 50,000–75,000 units of lipase per meal and 25,000–35,000 units of lipase per snacks and titrate according to symptoms. Dietary modifications are not usually necessary. Enzyme supplementation to reduce pain in chronic pancreatitis, mediated through reduced duodenal cholecystokinin release, has also been evaluated but has not been proven.

de la Iglesia-García D, Huang W, Szatmary P, et al. Efficacy of pancreatic enzyme replacement therapy in chronic pancreatitis: systematic review and meta-analysis. *Gut*. 2017;66(8):1354–1355. [PMID: 27941156]

Forsmark CE, Tang G, Xu H, et al. The use of pancreatic enzyme replacement therapy in patients with a diagnosis of chronic pancreatitis and pancreatic cancer in the US is infrequent and inconsistent. *Aliment Pharmacol Ther*. 2020;51(10):958–967. [PMID: 32249970]

Yaghoobi M, McNabb-Baltar J, Bijarchi R, et al. Pancreatic enzyme supplements are not effective for relieving abdominal pain in patients with chronic pancreatitis: meta-analysis and systematic review of randomized controlled trials. *Can J Gastroenterol Hepatol.* 2016;2016:8541839. [PMID: 27446871]

C. Endocrine Insufficiency

The treatment of pancreatogenic diabetes (type 3c) is complex and complicated by concomitent maldigestion and malnutrition. Diabetes associated with chronic pancreatitis is often insulin-requiring, but patients taking insulin are also at increased risk of hypoglycemia due to impaired glucagon synthesis resulting from pancreatic α-cell destruction leading to brittle diabetes.

Johnston PC, Thompson J, Mckee A, et al. Diabetes and chronic pancreatitis: considerations in the holistic management of an often neglected disease. *J Diabetes Res.* 2019;2019:2487804. [PMID: 31687406]

▶ Course & Prognosis

The natural history of chronic pancreatitis remains poorly defined in part because of its highly variable nature. The relationship between etiologic factors, genetic predisposition, and the pace of disease progression requires further clarification. Modifiable risk factors need to be identified and treated. It appears that discontinuance of alcohol, cessation of smoking, and early administration of corticosteroids in autoimmune disease may affect the natural history and prognosis of the disease. A French report on the natural history of hereditary pancreatitis has provided insight that can be extrapolated to chronic pancreatitis of other etiologies. This study documents the timeline of initial episodes of abdominal pain and recurrent pancreatitis in childhood that later develop into pancreas insufficiency, diabetes, and, in some, pancreas cancer later as an adult. Patients with PRSS1 mutation, chronic calcific pancreatitis, smokers, and those with a family history of pancreatic cancer are at higher risk of developing pancreatic cancer. Furthermore, establishing the diagnosis of pancreatic cancer can be difficult especially in patients with pancreatic head expansion caused by chronic pancreatitis.

Agarwal S, Sharma S, Gunjan D, et al. Natural course of chronic pancreatitis and predictors of its progression. *Pancreatology.* 2020;20(3):347–355. [PMID: 32107194]

Hao L, Zeng XP, Xin L, et al. Incidence of and risk factors for pancreatic cancer in chronic pancreatitis: a cohort of 1656 patients. *Dig Liver Dis.* 2017;49(11):1249–1256. [PMID: 28756974]

Shelton CA, Umapathy C, Stello K, et al. Hereditary pancreatitis in the United States: survival and rates of pancreatic cancer. *Am J Gastroenterol.* 2018;113(9):1376. [PMID: 30018304]

Autoimmune Pancreatitis

30

Alice A. Lee, MD
David X. Jin, MD, MPH

ESSENTIALS OF DIAGNOSIS

- ▶ Two forms: type 1 autoimmune pancreatitis (AIP) and type 2 AIP.

- ▶ Presentation with obstructive jaundice in up to 75% of patients.

- ▶ Histopathology reveals periductal lymphoplasmacytic infiltration, obliterative phlebitis, and storiform fibrosis (type 1 autoimmune pancreatitis [AIP]) versus granulocytic epithelial lesions (GELs) (type 2 AIP).

- ▶ Imaging shows diffuse enlargement of the pancreas or focal enlargement mimicking pancreatic adenocarcinoma.

- ▶ Elevated serum immunoglobulin G_4 (IgG_4) levels and extrapancreatic organ involvement seen in type 1 AIP.

- ▶ Association with inflammatory bowel disease observed in type 2 AIP.

- ▶ Resolution or marked improvement after corticosteroid treatment.

General Considerations

Autoimmune pancreatitis (AIP) is a rare disorder with characteristic clinical, serologic, histologic, and morphologic findings. It is classically described as a fibroinflammatory form of chronic pancreatitis that typically presents with painless, obstructive jaundice, lymphoplasmacytic infiltrates with fibrosis on histology, and dramatic therapeutic response to corticosteroids.

Knowledge of AIP has grown rapidly in the past 10–15 years. There are two distinct subtypes of autoimmune pancreatitis, referred to as type 1 AIP, or Lymphoplasmacytic Sclerosing Pancreatitis (LPSP), and type 2 AIP, or Idiopathic Duct-centric Chronic Pancreatitis (IDCP). While the two subtypes share similarities including presenting symptoms,

certain histologic features, and dramatic therapeutic response to corticosteroids, they are considered distinct entities with significant differences in epidemiologic patterns and natural course.

Type 1 Autoimmune Pancreatitis

Type 1 AIP is the subtype often equated with the term "autoimmune pancreatitis." It is considered the pancreatic manifestation of IgG_4-related disease, a systemic disease process marked by tumefactive lesions, dense lymphoplasmacytic infiltration of IgG_4-positive plasma cells, and often the elevation of serum IgG_4 levels.

Epidemiology

The estimated annual incidence of type 1 AIP is 1–3 per 100,000. It most commonly presents in older men, with a 3:1 male to female predominance, and mean age of diagnosis >60 years. Risk factors for developing type 1 AIP remain unclear.

Clinical Findings

A. Symptoms & Signs

Painless jaundice is the most common presenting symptom, seen in up to 75% of patients. Other symptoms include mild abdominal pain and symptoms of pancreatic exocrine and endocrine dysfunction including malabsorption, diarrhea, weight loss, and glucose intolerance. Despite its name, attacks of acute pancreatitis are unusual and type 1 AIP is not a common cause of idiopathic recurrent pancreatitis. Patients may also present with symptoms related to extrapancreatic manifestations of IgG_4-related disease, including retroperitoneal fibrosis, proximal bile duct strictures, and salivary gland enlargement.

B. Diagnostic Criteria

The HISORt criteria is a widely utilized diagnostic tool that helps characterize the many important histologic, imaging,

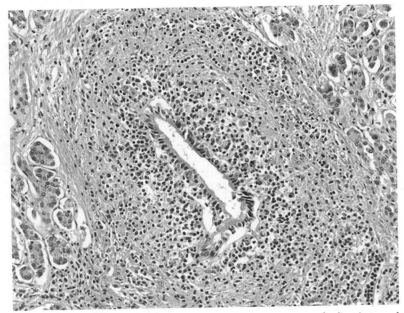

▲ **Figure 30–1.** Periductal lymphoplasmacytic infiltrates are the hallmark histologic finding in type 1 AIP.

serologic, other organ involvement, and response to therapy features of type 1 AIP.

C. Histologic Findings

Pancreatic periductal lymphoplasmacytic infiltrates (Figure 30–1) are the hallmark histologic finding in type 1 AIP. Additional histologic features include obliterative phlebitis or venulitis with lymphocytes and plasma cells, a swirling or "storiform" pattern of fibrosis, and abundant infiltration of IgG_4 plasma cells on immunostaining (>10 cells per high-power field). Varying degrees of pancreatic parenchymal atrophy may be present, and islets may be encased with intralobular fibrosis.

Despite the common association of IgG_4 plasma cells with type 1 AIP, it is important to note that IgG_4 infiltration can be seen in other conditions including pancreatic adenocarcinoma and chronic pancreatitis. A ratio of IgG_4/IgG-staining plasma cells of >40% may help distinguish type 1 AIP from other IgG_4 infiltrative diseases. The diagnosis of AIP can be missed because of inadequate sampling area or patchy involvement of the pancreatic parenchyma. Endoscopic ultrasound (EUS) guided core needle biopsies or surgical biopsies are often necessary for diagnosis.

D. Imaging Studies

Computed tomography (CT) and magnetic resonance imaging (MRI) findings in type 1 AIP include diffuse pancreatic enlargement sometimes referred to as "sausage pancreas" (Figure 30–2), a low-attenuating rim around the affected pancreas ("halo sign") and focal mass-like enlargement of one, or multiple, parts of the pancreas (Figure 30–3). Noteworthy is the lack of vascular encasement, calcifications, or peripancreatic fluid.

Endoscopic retrograde cholangiopancreatography (ERCP) or magnetic resonance cholangiopancreatography (MRCP) findings include long or multifocal strictures in the pancreatic duct without significant upstream dilation (Figure 30–4). There may also be strictures in the common bile duct (CBD) or intrahepatic ducts (Figure 30–5) due to concurrent IgG_4-associated cholangitis. EUS is increasingly being used to support a diagnosis of autoimmune pancreatitis, with characteristic findings of diffuse pancreatic enlargement and focal irregular hypoechoic masses. EUS-guided

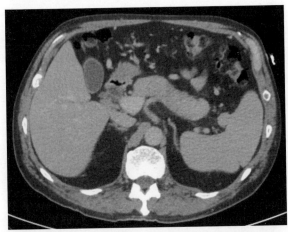

▲ **Figure 30–2.** CT finding of a diffusely enlarged pancreas ("sausage pancreas").

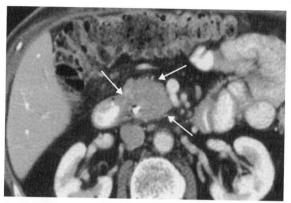

▲ **Figure 30–3.** Focal enlargement of the pancreatic head and uncinate (*arrows*), and lack of vascular invasion and peripancreatic changes in all segments. (Reproduced with permission of Dr. Dushyant V. Sahani, Massachusetts General Hospital.)

biopsies are often necessary to provide diagnostic histology and exclude underlying malignancy.

E. Serologic Findings

While elevated serum IgG_4 levels can also be found in other pancreaticobiliary diseases including chronic pancreatitis and pancreatic adenocarcinoma, it has been suggested that levels >2 times the upper limit of normal is strongly suggestive of type 1 AIP (53% sensitive and 99% specific).

Various other serologic abnormalities have also been reported, including elevated levels of total immunoglobulin G (IgG), immunoglobulin E (IgE), eosinophilia, antinuclear antibodies (ANA), gamma-globulins, rheumatoid factor antibody, antilactoferrin antibody, anti-carbonic anhydrase antibody, anti-plasminogen binding peptide, CRP, and low complement levels, though none with high specificity or sensitivity. A cholestatic pattern of liver injury is also commonly observed (ie, disproportionately elevated serum alkaline phosphatase with minimally elevated serum aminotransferases), particularly with concurrent IgG_4 biliary involvement.

F. Other Organ Involvement

IgG_4 disease can affect virtually any organ. Besides the pancreas, the most commonly involved organ is the biliary tree. Termed IgG_4-associated cholangitis, it often manifests as long strictures in the intrahepatic or extrahepatic bile ducts. Other extrapancreatic manifestations include retroperitoneal fibrosis, submandibular gland enlargement, mediastinal lymph node involvement, and tubulointerstitial nephritis (Table 30–1).

G. Response to Steroid Therapy

Dramatic response to corticosteroid therapy is a characteristic feature of both type 1 and type 2 AIP. Corticosteroid

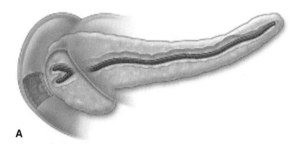

A

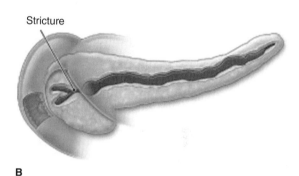

B

C

D

▲ **Figure 30–4.** Pancreatic ductal change in autoimmune pancreatitis. **A.** Normal pancreatic duct. **B.** Focal pancreatic duct stricture. **C.** Segmental pancreatic duct strictures. **D.** Diffuse pancreatic duct narrowing.

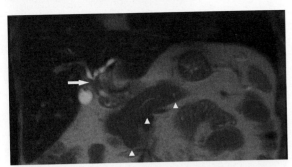

▲ Figure 30–5. MRI showing a diffusely enlarged pancreas consistent with type 1 AIP (*arrowheads*) and a common hepatic duct stricture (*arrow*) which can be found in IgG$_4$-associated cholangitis.

therapy often leads to marked improvement in clinical symptoms, resolution of radiologic findings, and reduction in serum IgG$_4$ levels. While a diagnostic trial of steroids should not be used under most scenarios, significant clinical improvement following corticosteroid therapy does provide useful support for distinguishing AIP from other mimicking conditions such as pancreatic adenocarcinoma or primary sclerosing cholangitis. Additional treatment options and recommendations are discussed in the following sections.

Hart PA, Zen Y, Chari ST. Recent advances in autoimmune pancreatitis. *Gastroenterology.* 2015;149:39–51. [PMID: 25770706]

Kurita A, Yasukawa S, Zen Y, et al. Comparison of a 22-gauge Franseen-tip needle with a 20-gauge forward-bevel needle for the diagnosis of type 1 autoimmune pancreatitis: a prospective, randomized, controlled, multicenter study (COMPAS study). *Gastrointest Endosc.* 2020;91:373–381. [PMID: 31654634]

Majumder S, Takahashi N, Chari ST. Autoimmune pancreatitis. *Dig Dis Sci.* 2017;62:1762–1769. [PMID: 28365915]

Table 30–1. Characteristic extrapancreatic & histopathologic features in type 1 autoimmune pancreatitis.

Extrapancreatic Findings	Histopathologic Findings
Bile duct strictures (IgG$_4^-$ associated cholangitis)	Extensive periductal lymphoplasmacytic infiltrate
Lung nodules, adenopathy, and infiltrates	Inflammatory cells clustered in walls of small veins and nerves
Salivary gland involvement	PMN infiltrate extending transmurally → obliterative phlebitis
Retroperitoneal fibrosis	Islet cell encasement with intralobular "storiform" fibrosis
Interstitial nephritis	>40% plasma cells staining positive for IgG$_4$
Autoimmune thyroiditis	Varying degrees of pancreatic parenchymal atrophy

PMN, polymorphonuclear neutrophil.

Masamune A, Kikuta k, Hamada S, et al. Nationwide epidemiological survey of autoimmune pancreatitis in Japan in 2016. *J Gastroenterol.* 2019;55:462–470. [PMID: 31872350]

Shimosegawa T, Chari ST, Frulloni L, et al. International consensus diagnostic criteria for autoimmune pancreatitis. *Pancreas.* 2011;40:352–358. [PMID: 21412117]

Stone JH, Brito-Zeron P, Bosch X, Ramos-Casals, M. Diagnostic approach to the complexity of IgG4-related disease. *Mayo Clin Proc.* 2015;90:927–939. [PMID: 26141331]

▶ Type 2 Autoimmune Pancreatitis

Much less is known about type 2 AIP (IDCP). This is due, in part, to the challenge in diagnoses. As opposed to type 1 AIP, IDCP is more commonly diagnosed at a younger mean age of 40–50 years old (typically a decade younger than type 1 AIP) and without a predilection for either sex. Clinical presentation can include painless jaundice or acute pancreatitis. There are no extra-pancreatic manifestations of IDCP, as it is not a systemic disease. However, IDCP is associated with inflammatory bowel disease, particularly ulcerative colitis, in up to 40% of patients. Unlike type 1 AIP, IDCP has no known serologic marker and IgG$_4$ infiltrates are either absent or scarce (<10 cells per high-power field). Thus, histology remains the only method for obtaining a definitive diagnosis. Like type 1 AIP, IDCP can also have periductal lymphoplasmacytic infiltrates and storiform fibrosis. However, the pathognomonic histologic finding in IDCP is a neutrophilic infiltration of small and medium-sized pancreatic ducts, which when severe, leads to obliteration of the duct lumen. For this reason, IDCP is sometimes referred to as AIP with granulocytic epithelial lesions (GEL).

Khandelwal A, Inoue D, Takahashi N. Autoimmune pancreatitis: an update. *Abdom Radiol.* 2020;45:1359–1370. [PMID: 31650376]

Lorenzo D, Maire F, Stefanescu C, et al. Features of autoimmune pancreatitis associated with inflammatory bowel disease. *Clin Gastroenterol Hepatol.* 2018;16:59–67. [PMID: 28782667]

▶ Diagnosis & Differential Diagnoses

AIP should be considered in the differential diagnosis of patients presenting with obstructive jaundice, particularly in conjunction with characteristic imaging and serologic findings. In 2009, Chari et al. proposed the now widely accepted revised HISORt criteria, which suggested that in addition to (1) diagnostic histology, a diagnosis of type 1 AIP may be based upon (2) typical imaging findings (ie, diffuse sausage-shaped pancreas) with elevated serum IgG$_4$ levels and/or other organ involvement; or (3) response to corticosteroid therapy in patients in whom typical imaging features of AIP are lacking, cancer is excluded, and additional supportive features of AIP are present (Table 30–2). However, there remains variability in diagnostic criteria around the world. The 2011 international consensus diagnostic criteria for autoimmune pancreatitis (ICDC) provides an additional diagnostic framework that is commonly used.

Table 30–2. Diagnosis of type 1 autoimmune pancreatitis based on revised HISORT criteria.

Autoimmune pancreatitis can be diagnosed by one of the following:
A. Diagnostic histology: (H)
   - On resection specimen or
   - On pancreatic core biopsy (indicated in a patient with pancreatic mass and/or obstructive jaundice due to distal bile duct obstruction with a negative workup for cancer)
B. Typical imaging (I) + any one of the following:
   - Elevated IgG$_4$ (S)
   - Other organ involvement (O)
   - Compatible histology
C. Response to steroids (Rt): Resolution/marked improvement in pancreatic/extrapancreatic manifestations in patients meeting criteria for steroid use:
   - Patients in groups A and B
   - Patients without typical imaging findings with negative workup for cancer and suggestive feature of autoimmune pancreatitis or definitive other organ involvement
   - A steroid trial in the absence of adequate or no collateral evidence of autoimmune pancreatitis must be used with caution

Data from Chari ST, Takahashi N, Levy MJ, et al. A diagnostic strategy to distinguish autoimmune pancreatitis from pancreatic cancer. *Clin Gastroenterol Hepatol.* 2009;7(10):1097–1103.

The most important condition to exclude when considering AIP is pancreatic adenocarcinoma. Both conditions often present with painless jaundice and focal mass-like enlargement of the pancreas on imaging. Because the prevalence of AIP is much lower than that of pancreatic adenocarcinoma, ruling out malignancy is imperative and should be considered an initial priority. Symptoms such as cachexia, PO intolerance, and severe pain requiring narcotics are less characteristic of AIP. Imaging differences between AIP and pancreatic adenocarcinoma are detailed in Table 30–3. The aforementioned rim-like enhancement of the pancreas is a characteristic feature of AIP, while characteristic features more suggestive of pancreatic adenocarcinoma (eg, focal low-density mass, vascular encasement, peripancreatic changes, ductal dilatation/cutoff with or without pancreatic atrophy) are usually lacking in AIP.

Table 30–3. Differences between autoimmune pancreatitis & pancreatic cancer on computed tomography scan.

Structure	Autoimmune Pancreatitis	Pancreatic Cancer
Pancreas	Diffuse enlargement or focal mass	Focal mass lesion
Pancreatic rim halo	Yes	No
Ducts	Narrow	Dilated
Vessel encasement	No	May be present
Lymphadenopathy	May be present	May be present

Other conditions to consider on the differential diagnoses include pancreatitis of other etiology, primary sclerosing cholangitis, and cholangiocarcinoma. Unlike other types of pancreatitis, AIP does not typically present with abdominal pain as the predominant symptom.

Treatment

A. Corticosteroid Therapy

In type 1 AIP, the goal of treatment involves induction and maintenance of remission. Maintenance therapy is not typically required in type 2 AIP, given low rates of relapse. Prednisone is commonly administered for induction therapy at an initial high dose of 40 mg/day for 4 weeks followed by a taper of the daily dosage by 5 mg/week until discontinued, based on monitoring of clinical parameters. Relief of symptoms, resolution of imaging abnormalities, decreasing serum IgG$_4$ levels, and improvements in liver tests are suggested parameters to follow.

A dramatic therapeutic response to corticosteroids, often within a brief 2–4 week period, is a distinct characteristic of both type 1 and type 2 AIP. On the other hand, a poor therapeutic response should trigger consideration of alternative diagnoses, including pancreatic adenocarcinoma. In a prospective cohort trial of 22 patients who had atypical imaging findings for AIP but in whom initial malignancy workup was negative, a therapeutic response to 2 weeks of corticosteroids helped to differentiate all 15 patients who were ultimately diagnosed with AIP from the 7 nonresponders who were ultimately confirmed to have pancreatic adenocarcinoma.

Relapse following initial remission is observed in 20–60% of patients with type 1 AIP. Patients at risk for relapse (involvement of the proximal bile duct, diffuse pancreatic enlargement, persistently elevated serum IgG$_4$ levels after corticosteroid treatment, involvement of extrapancreatic organs) may benefit from maintenance therapy after initial induction of remission. In cases of relapse, treatment options include (1) repeating a pulse of high dose corticosteroids followed by gradual taper to discontinuation, (2) pulse of high dose corticosteroids followed by gradual taper to low-dose maintenance corticosteroids, (3) pulse of high dose corticosteroids while transitioning to steroid-sparing agents, or (4) rituximab induction therapy, with or without maintenance (discussed in the following section). Data regarding the optimal treatment of relapsing AIP is lacking. In the only randomized controlled trial to date comparing treatment regimen, patients who were maintained on low dose corticosteroids after initial steroid-induced remission had lower relapse-free survival rates after 3 years versus those randomized to steroid withdrawal (23% vs 58%, $P = 0.011$).

Hirano K, Tada M, Isayama H, et al. Outcome of long-term maintenance steroid therapy cessation in patients with autoimmune pancreatitis: a prospective study. *J Clin Gastroenterol.* 2016;50:331–337. [PMID: 26565969]

Madhani K, Farrell JJ. Autoimmune pancreatitis: an update on diagnosis and management. *Gastroenterol Clin North Am.* 2016;45:29–43. [PMID: 26895679]

Masamune A, Nishimor I, Kikuta K, et al. Randomised controlled trial of long-term maintenance corticosteroid therapy in patients with autoimmune pancreatitis. *Gut.* 2017;66:487–494. [PMID: 27543430]

Moon SH, Kim MH, Park DH, et al. Is a 2-week steroid trial after initial negative investigation for malignancy useful in differentiating autoimmune pancreatitis from pancreatic cancer? A prospective outcome study. *Gut.* 2008;57:1704–1712. [PMID: 18583399]

Okazaki K, Chari ST, Frulloni L, et al. International consensus for the treatment of autoimmune pancreatitis. *Pancreatology.* 2017;17:1–6. [PMID: 28027896]

Tacelli M, Celsa C, Magro B, et al. Risk factors for rate of relapse and effects of steroid maintenance therapy in patients with autoimmune pancreatitis: systematic review and meta-analysis. *Clin Gastroenterol Hepatol.* 2019;17:1061–1072. [PMID: 30312787]

B. Immunomodulatory Drugs & Rituximab

Several studies have reported on the use of immunomodulatory drugs (azathioprine, 6-mercaptopurine, mycophenolate mofetil, cyclophosphamide) for maintenance of remission in AIP. While azathioprine is most commonly used, the other agents have comparable results. Further studies aimed at identifying the optimal dosing of immunomodulators for maintenance treatment are necessary.

Rituximab (RTX), a monoclonal CD20 antibody, is the only nonsteroid agent shown to be effective for both inducing and maintaining AIP remission. Two dosing protocols have been described for RTX induction: (1) 375 mg/m^2 BSA IV weekly for 4 weeks and (2) two 1000 mg IV doses spaced 2 weeks apart. A prospective trial evaluating the efficacy of the second dosing protocol on 30 patients with IgG$_4$-related disease (18 with type 1 AIP) found disease response in 77% at 6 months, with subsequent relapse in 23%. The addition of maintenance RTX therapy (375 mg/m^2 BSA every 2–3 months) may lower relapse rates compared to receiving RTX induction therapy only. However, adverse events including infections may occur more frequently in those receiving maintenance RTX therapy and relapse has been observed following discontinuation.

Carruthers MN, Topazian MD, Khosroshahi A, et al. Rituximab for IgG4-related disease: a prospective open-label trial. *Ann Rheum Dis.* 2015;74:1171–1177. [PMID: 25667206]

Hart PA, Topazian MD, Witzig TE, et al. Treatment of relapsing autoimmune pancreatitis with immunomodulators and rituximab: the Mayo Clinic experience. *Gut.* 2013;62:1607–1615. [PMID: 22936672]

Majumder S, Mohapatra S, Lennon RJ, et al. Rituximab maintenance therapy reduces rate of relapse of pancreaticobilliary immunoglobulin G4-related disease. *Clin Gastroenterol Hepatol.* 2018;16:1947–1953. [PMID: 29526692]

Course & Prognosis

Patients with AIP can develop pancreatic atrophy with resultant exocrine and endocrine insufficiency. Pancreatic exocrine insufficiency, defined as a fecal elastase-1 <200 µg/g, has been observed in 82% of patients, while diabetes has been observed in 57%. The high prevalence of both suggests a role for active screening for these sequelae.

Data regarding risk of malignancy in patients with AIP is conflicting. One study observed an increased risk of various extrapancreatic malignancies, primarily within the first year of diagnosis. A recent prospective study of 107 AIP patients observed no cases of pancreatic cancer and extrapancreatic malignancy rates comparable to an age- and sex-matched reference population over a median follow up period of 75 months. AIP has not been shown to increase mortality.

Buijs J, Cahen DL, van Heerde MJ, et al. The long-term impact of autoimmune pancreatitis on pancreatic function, quality of life, and life expectancy. *Pancreas.* 2015;44:1065–1071. [PMID: 26355549]

Hart PA, Kamisawa T, Brugge WR, et al. Long-term outcomes of autoimmune pancreatitis: a multicentre, international analysis. *Gut.* 2013;62:1771–1776. [PMID: 23232048]

Masuda A, Shiomi H, Matsuda T, et al. The relationship between pancreatic atrophy after steroid therapy and diabetes mellitus in patients with autoimmune pancreatitis. *Pancreatology.* 2014;14:361–365. [PMID: 25278305]

Shiokawa M, Kodama Y, Yoshimura K, et al. Risk of cancer in patients with autoimmune pancreatitis. *Am J Gastroenterol.* 2013;108:610–617. [PMID: 23318486]

Vujasinovic M, Valente R, Maier P, et al. Diagnosis, treatment, and long-term outcome of autoimmune pancreatitis in Sweden. *Pancreatology.* 2018;18:900–904. [PMID: 30236651]

Tumors of the Pancreas

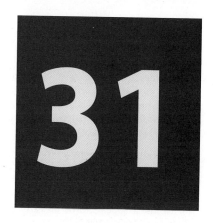

Julia McNabb-Baltar, MD, MPH

ESSENTIALS OF DIAGNOSIS

▶ Abdominal protocol computed tomography (CT) with arterial and venous phases is generally the best initial modality for diagnosis and staging.

▶ Endoscopic ultrasound (EUS) is superior to CT in diagnosing small tumors, and can be used to obtain pathologic confirmation of the diagnosis.

▶ Fewer than 20% of tumors are resectable at the time of diagnosis.

▶ Carbohydrate antigen 19-9 (CA 19-9) and carcinoembryonic antigen (CEA) have a low specificity and sensitivity but can be followed for treatment response if initially elevated.

PANCREATIC CANCER

General Considerations

Pancreatic cancer is a challenging disease with fewer than 20% of the tumors resectable at diagnosis. After resection the overall 5-year survival is still below 25% with negative margins and 10% if there were regional lymph node metastasis. The overall 5-year survival is still only 9%. It is the second most common gastrointestinal malignancy, and the fourth leading cause of cancer-related deaths in the United States. In 2018, the age-standardized rate was 7.6 per 100,000 people in North America.

The disease is more common in men than in women (1.3:1) and in certain ethnic and racial groups (eg, African Americans). It is rare before the age of 40, but the incidence increases sharply after the seventh decade.

Rawla P, Sunkara T, Gaduputi V. Epidemiology of pancreatic cancer: global trends, etiology and risk factors. *World J Oncol.* 2019;10(1):10–27. [PMID: 30834048]

Pathogenesis & Risk Factors

Most pancreatic neoplasms arise from the three different types of the epithelial cells found in the pancreas. Acinar cells account for 80% of the volume of the gland but constitute 1% of exocrine tumors. Ductal cells constitute 10–15% of the volume but give rise to 85% of all tumors. Other malignant pancreatic tumors from the exocrine pancreas include intraductal papillary mucinous neoplasms (IPMNs) with invasive carcinoma (2–3%), mucinous cystic neoplasms (MCNs) with invasive carcinoma (1%), solid pseudopapillary neoplasms (SPNs) (<1%), acinar cell carcinoma (<1%), and serous cystadenocarcinoma (<1%). Endocrine cells are 1–2% of volume and account for 1–2% of the tumors. These tumors are known as pancreatic neuroendocrine tumors (PNETs) or islet cell tumors. Nonepithelial tumors are very rare.

Approximately 70% of ductal tumors are localized to the head of the pancreas, 5–10% to the body, and 10–15% to the tail. These tumors appear as scirrhous whitish irregular tumor with a desmoplastic reaction that can mimic chronic pancreatitis particularly at the time of surgical resection. The desmoplastic reaction can make it impossible to evaluate radiologically the response to preoperative treatment.

These tumors are often associated with pancreatic intraepithelial neoplasia (PanIN), which is metaplasia and proliferation of the ductal epithelium. PanIN is associated with varying degrees of dysplasia ranging from mild (PanIN-1), moderate (PanIN-2), to severe (PanIN-3), which was previously known as carcinoma in situ. In general, a surgeon will resect to remove invasive carcinoma and PanIN-3, but not PanIN-1 or PanIN-2.

A. Molecular Pathogenesis

It has been proposed that pancreatic cancer develops from PanIN following an evolution similar to the adenoma–carcinoma sequence seen in colorectal tumors with accumulating genetic alterations with progression of low to high grade in PanIN-1 to -3. Although the precise mechanism and sequence of genetic mutations responsible for the development of pancreatic cancer remains unclear, genetic alterations found in these tumors can be classified into three categories: (1) activation of oncogenes; (2) inactivation of tumor suppressor genes; and (3) defects in DNA mismatch repair genes. The sonic hedgehog signaling pathway also appears to play a role. The sonic hedgehog gene, which is involved with embryonic development, appears to be unregulated in early and late stages of pancreatic carcinogenesis.

1. Activation of oncogenes—Mutations of the *K-ras* oncogene are seen in more than 90% of tumors and are the hallmark of pancreatic adenocarcinoma. Although this mutation may be seen in nonmalignant conditions such as chronic pancreatitis, it appears to be an early genetic alteration in pancreatic carcinogenesis.

2. Inactivation of tumor suppressor genes—Inactivation and loss of function of tumor suppressor genes results in critical disruption of the cell cycle involving cellular differentiation, growth inhibition, regulation of transcription, DNA repair, and apoptosis. The genes most frequently involved are *CDKN2A* (95%), *P53* (60%), *DPC4* (50%), *BRCA2*, and *STK11*. About 10% of patients with hereditary pancreatic cancer harbor germline mutations of the *BRCA2* gene.

3. Defect of DNA mismatch repair gene—Mutations of mismatch repair genes, such as *MLH1* and *MSH2*, have been found in 4% of pancreatic tumors.

B. Hereditary Risk Factors

1. Family history of pancreatic cancer—Genetic predisposition is the greatest risk factor for the development of pancreatic cancer. About 5–10% of patients with pancreatic cancer have a first-degree relative with the disease. The risk of pancreatic cancer increases according to the number of family members with the disease; the risk of developing cancer is twofold for a patient with one family member compared to the general population, and the risk increases to 6- and 30-folds with two and three family members, respectively. These patients present at an earlier age, and smoking appears to contribute to the development of the cancer.

2. Hereditary pancreatitis—This autosomal-dominant condition caused by a *PRSS1* gene mutation is strongly associated with pancreatic cancer although it accounts for only a small fraction of the total number of cases. Patients presents with recurrent attacks of acute pancreatitis early in life that may progress to chronic pancreatitis. The risk of an affected family member developing cancer is as high as 40% by age 70 and is highest among those who smoke.

3. Other conditions—Several hereditary syndromes are associated with an increased risk of developing endocrine or exocrine pancreatic cancer. These include familial atypical multiple-mole melanoma (FAMMM) syndrome, multiple endocrine neoplasia type I syndrome, Lynch syndrome II, von Hippel Lindau syndrome, and ataxia–telangiectasia.

C. Environmental Risk Factors

The best-established environmental risk factor associated with pancreatic cancer is cigarette smoking. It is estimated that 30% of pancreatic cancer is due to cigarette smoking. The relative risk of pancreatic cancer among current smokers is two- to threefold compared to the general population. The risk increases with the number of cigarettes consumed and returns to baseline 10–15 years after the patient stops smoking.

Diet appears to be another important environmental factor. Diets high in fat, meat, total energy, and carbohydrates appear to be linked to the development of pancreatic cancer, while consumption of citrus fruits, vegetables, fiber, and vitamin C seem to have a protective effect. Low levels of selenium and lycopene have been associated with the development of pancreatic cancer.

Data on coffee and alcohol consumption, use of aspirin and other nonsteroidal anti-inflammatory drugs, and the development of pancreatic cancer have been conflicting, and recent studies show no definite relationship. Some studies have shown an association between *Helicobacter pylori* infection and pancreatic cancer, as well as hepatitis B virus, although the exact mechanism is still unclear.

D. Nonhereditary Risk Factors

The cumulative 20-year risk of pancreatic adenocarcinoma is 4% in patients with nonhereditary chronic pancreatitis. Diabetes mellitus is associated with pancreatic cancer, especially with new-onset diabetes after the age of 50. In most patients, the diagnosis of pancreatic cancer is made within 2 years of the onset of diabetes mellitus. Obesity is associated with increased risk of pancreatic cancer and decreased survival after diagnosis. Gastrectomy for peptic ulcer disease increases the risk of pancreatic cancer; the mechanism is unknown but might be related to the relative achlorhydria.

Goggins M, Overbeek KA, Brand R, et al. Management of patients with increased risk for familial pancreatic cancer: updated recommendations from the International Cancer of the Pancreas Screening (CAPS) Consortium. *Gut.* 2020;69(1):7–17. [PMID: 31672839]

Mizrahi JD, Surana R, Valle JW, et al. Pancreatic cancer. *Lancet.* 2020;395(10242):2008–2020. [PMID: 3259333]

▶ Clinical Findings

A. Symptoms & Signs

Owing to the lack of characteristic signs and symptoms, most patients with pancreatic tumors present late in the course of the disease. As a result, fewer than 20% of tumors are resectable at the time of diagnosis. Patients may present with vague, low-intensity, dull abdominal discomfort, or pain that radiates to the back and may be associated with weight loss, anorexia, weakness, fatigue, diarrhea, and vomiting (Table 31–1).

Table 31–1. Clinical manifestations that may be associated with pancreatic cancer.

Symptoms and Signs	Laboratory Findings
Abdominal pain or discomfort	↑ Serum alkaline phosphatase
Weight loss	↑ Bilirubin
Anorexia	↑ Transaminases
Weakness	↑ Erythrocyte sedimentation rate
Jaundice	↑ Serum CA 19-9
Irritable bowel syndrome (diarrhea)	
New-onset diabetes after age 50	
New onset mood changes	

The pain is primarily due to the invasion of the celiac and superior mesenteric plexus but may rarely be due to acute pancreatitis due to occlusion of the main pancreatic duct by tumor.

Location of the tumor also defines the symptoms and the prognosis. Tumors of the head of the pancreas produce symptoms early, and painless jaundice is seen in more than 50% of cases due to obstruction of the extrahepatic bile duct. In fewer than one-third of patients, obstruction of the bile duct by pancreatic neoplasm is accompanied by a palpable, nontender gallbladder referred to as *Courvoisier sign*. This finding also may be seen in bile duct obstruction by cholangiocarcinoma, duodenal carcinoma, and carcinoma of the ampulla of Vater.

Tumors of the body and tail are either "asymptomatic" or manifest with nonspecific symptoms, such as abdominal discomfort, and the diagnosis is mostly made after metastatic disease has developed. They can also present with jaundice, caused by liver metastasis.

Obstruction of the pancreatic duct may lead to pancreatic exocrine insufficiency in the form of steatorrhea and malabsorption. New-onset diabetes mellitus after the age of 50 has been associated with the development of pancreatic cancer, especially in the absence of a family history of diabetes. Other uncommon manifestations of pancreatic neoplasm include thrombophlebitis, specifically migratory superficial thrombophlebitis first described as Trousseau syndrome, psychiatric disturbances, signs and symptoms of gastrointestinal bleeding, and obstruction due to erosion and growth of the pancreatic neoplasm into the duodenal lumen. In patients older than age 50, pancreatic cancer can present with features of irritable bowel syndrome. Paraneoplastic syndrome includes cicatricial and bullous pemphigoid and pancreatic panniculitis presenting as erythematous subcutaneous nodular fat necrosis classically located in the lower extremities.

PNETs are rare, accounting for less than 5% of pancreatic neoplasm. Between 50% and 70% are functioning, producing hormones including insulin, glucagon, gastrin, and vasoactive intestinal peptide. Gastrinomas and nonfunctioning PNETs are the most frequent malignant PNET; insulinomas are the most frequent benign PNET. Nonfunctioning PNETs present with symptoms related to the mass. Functioning PNETs present with symptoms related to the active secreted hormone.

With the widespread use of abdominal CT imaging, incidental asymptomatic small pancreatic lesions are being detected in increasing frequency. Most incidental pancreatic lesions are benign and cystic, but adenocarcinomas and PNETs can also be found incidentally.

B. Laboratory Findings

Malignant obstruction of the distal bile duct by a neoplasm of the pancreatic head characteristically produces cholestatic liver enzyme elevations with elevated alkaline phosphatase level and direct bilirubin (see Table 31–1). The rise in transaminases is usually mild. Despite biliary stasis, cholangitis is uncommon. Lipase and amylase are elevated in tumors that cause pancreatic duct obstruction and can present as acute pancreatitis.

1. Tumor markers—CA 19-9 is a sialylated Lewis antigen that has been found in the biliary cells. It can be elevated with pancreatic cancer but also biliary obstruction of other etiology. It has a poor sensitivity for early-stage pancreatic cancer and is not recommended for screening purposes. When elevated, it can be useful to monitor treatment response. A level above 1000 units/mL is considered more specific for pancreatic cancer, although any level may be seen with benign conditions.

Luo G, Jin K, Deng S, et al. Roles of CA19-9 in pancreatic cancer: biomarker, predictor and promoter. *Biochim Biophys Acta Rev Cancer.* 2021;1875(2):188409. [PMID: 32827580]

C. Imaging & Other Diagnostic Studies

Pancreatic adenocarcinoma is staged using a TNM classification (Table 31–2). It consists of evaluating the characteristics of the primary tumor, namely tumor size and infiltration into major vessels (T stage), regional lymph node involvement (N stage), and the presence and absence of distant metastasis (M stage). Various modalities are available for the diagnosis and staging of pancreatic tumors (see Chapter 9), including those described in the following text.

1. Computed tomography scan—The best initial imaging study is a high-quality three-phase helical CT scan of the abdomen and pelvis. This study will assess possible metastases to the liver, lung bases, regional lymph nodes, and peritoneal cavity (carcinomatosis). If there is no evidence of metastasis, the study will assess resectability from the standpoint of vascular invasion. A high-quality CT scan is quite accurate in assessing vascular invasion with a sensitivity of 85% and specificity of 82%. A chest CT is also performed to assess for lung metastasis.

2. Endoscopic ultrasound—EUS has a diagnostic sensitivity similar to CT scan but may be superior in diagnosing small pancreatic tumors. EUS-guided fine-needle aspiration (EUS–FNA) has a diagnostic sensitivity of about 85–90%

Table 31–2. Staging of pancreatic exocrine cancer.

Definition of TNM	
Primary Tumor (T)	
TX	Primary tumor cannot be assessed
T0	No evidence of primary tumor
Tis	In situ carcinoma
T1	Tumor limited to the pancreas, ≤2 cm in greatest dimension
T1a	Tumor limited to the pancreas, ≤0.5 cm in greatest dimension
T1b	Tumor limited to the pancreas, >0.5 cm but <1 cm in greatest dimension
T1c	Tumor limited to the pancreas, 1–2 cm in greatest dimension
T2	Tumor limited to the pancreas, >2 cm in greatest dimension
T3	Tumor extends beyond pancreas but without involvement of celiac axis or superior mesenteric artery
T4	Tumor involves celiac axis or superior mesenteric artery (unresectable primary tumor)
Regional Lymph Nodes (N)	
NX	Regional lymph nodes cannot be assessed
N0	No regional lymph node metastasis
N1	Metastasis in 1–3 regional lymph node
N2	Metastasis in 4 or more regional lymph node.
Distant Metastasis (M)	
MX	Distant metastasis cannot be assessed
M0	No distant metastasis
M1	Distant metastasis
Stage Grouping	
Stage 0	Tis, N0, M0
Stage IA	T1, N0, M0
Stage IB	T2, N0, M0
Stage IIA	T3, N0, M0
Stage IIB	T1–3, N1, M0
Stage III	T1–3 N2, M0 or T4, any N, M0
Stage IV	Any T, any N, M1

Used with permission of the American College of Surgeons, Chicago, Illinois. The original source for this information is the AJCC Cancer Staging System (2020).

with a false-negative rate of 10–15%. It is a safe procedure with minimal risk of tumor seeding. EUS is less accurate in predicting superior mesenteric vein (SMV) and superior mesenteric artery involvement by the tumor.

3. Endoscopic retrograde cholangiopancreatography—Pancreatic tumors appear as strictures of the pancreatic duct or the bile duct on endoscopic retrograde cholangiopancreatography (ERCP). This stricturing of both the bile duct and the pancreatic duct is referred to as the "double duct sign." Advances in pancreatic imaging such as helical CT and magnetic resonance imaging (MRI) have made ERCP unnecessary as an initial diagnostic test. Major limitations of ERCP are the limited ability to obtain a tissue diagnosis in malignant bile duct obstruction (positive in <50% of cases); limited utility for pancreatic tumor staging, as it provides no information about tumor extent, vascular invasion, or involvement of the lymph nodes; and risk of complications such as pancreatitis and perforation.

4. Magnetic resonance imaging—Accuracy of MRI to determine resectability appears comparable to the three-phase helical CT scan. Magnetic resonance cholangiopancreatography (MRCP) is as sensitive as ERCP in the diagnosis of pancreatic tumors.

5. Positron emission tomography—Positron emission tomography (PET) scanning is not routinely used in diagnosis of pancreatic cancers. It can be useful in diagnosing tumor reoccurrence after pancreatic resection.

6. Laparoscopy—Staging laparoscopy can detect <2 mm in diameter foci of metastatic disease to the peritoneal cavity or surface of the liver. These deposits are too small to be detected by a CT scan or PET. Some surgeons use staging laparoscopy prior to a planned resection while others do not as they feel the yield is too small. In select patients, staging laparoscopy along with peritoneal cytologic examination can detect unsuspected metastasis and prevent unwarranted laparotomy. Such an approach can be considered in patients with tumors localized to the body and tail of the pancreas, that appear resectable by helical CT criteria, given the high frequency of unsuspected spread to the peritoneum (as high as 50%) and patients with CA 19-9 level above 100 units/mL.

D. Diagnostic Approach

Figure 31–1 presents an algorithm for the diagnosis and treatment of suspected pancreatic cancer. The need for tissue to establish a diagnosis in a suspected pancreatic cancer remains controversial. Although consensus on an optimal approach is lacking, any diagnostic strategy should aim to reliably and safely establish a diagnosis; determine resectability; and avoid morbidity and mortality associated with unnecessary surgical intervention.

Comparing imaging modalities (such as EUS, MRI, and CT) has methodological limitations, such as patient selection,

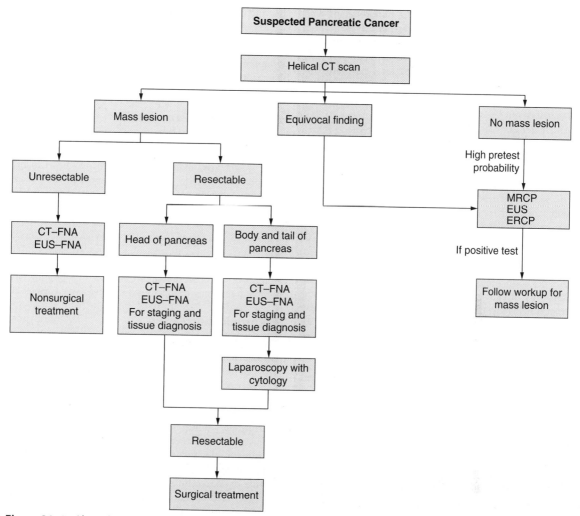

▲ **Figure 31–1.** Algorithm for the diagnosis and treatment of suspected pancreatic carcinoma. CT, computed tomography; ERCP, endoscopic retrograde cholangiopancreatography; EUS, endoscopic ultrasound; FNA, fine-needle aspiration; MRCP, magnetic resonance cholangiopancreatography.

study design, and quality. EUS has been generally found to be superior to CT and MRI in detection and characterization of smaller lesions. It has been found to be superior to helical CT scan and MRI for tumor and nodal staging, with a sensitivity of >90%. EUS does not offer any advantage over helical CT in determining resectability of preoperatively suspected pancreatic adenocarcinoma, and the two modalities are considered complementary.

High-quality three-phase helical CT scan is usually the preferred initial test for locoregional staging and detection of distant metastasis. Based on the CT scan findings, pancreatic masses fall into one of the following four broad categories: (1) no mass, (2) unresectable mass, (3) resectable mass, and (4) equivocal findings.

Based on clinical suspicion and pretest probability, further imaging by MRCP, EUS, ERCP, or a combination of these methods may be necessary, even if the initial CT findings are negative for any mass lesion. EUS can identify lesions not seen on CT or MRI.

If a clearly unresectable mass is identified on CT scan, a tissue diagnosis is indicated prior to starting any palliative chemotherapy or radiotherapy. EUS–FNA, or a percutaneous approach using a CT or transabdominal ultrasound, can be used. In patients with pancreatic cancer who experience pain, EUS can be used to perform celiac plexus neurolysis during the initial diagnostic and staging examination.

Patients identified as having a resectable mass on CT scan should be considered for EUS as a complementary test because it is more accurate for local tumor staging and possibly more accurate in predicting vascular invasion. The need to obtain a tissue diagnosis in this group is controversial. Beyond the patient's desire for a tissue diagnosis, pretest probability of a tumor, and available local expertise, the major consideration determining whether to obtain a tissue diagnosis should be its impact on clinical decision making and management.

The major drawback of pursuing a tissue diagnosis is that the sensitivity of EUS–FNA is 85–90%, giving it a false-negative rate of 10–15%. If the pretest probability based on the clinical presentation laboratory data and radiologic findings for cancer is high, then a negative tissue diagnosis should not influence the decision to proceed with surgery. Although minimal, the potential for complications such as bleeding, pancreatitis, and tumor seeding during fine-needle aspiration should also be considered. If EUS-FNA is nondiagnostic or further molecular testing is required, fine needle biopsy (FNB) can be obtained which can increase the diagnostic yield (99% vs 92%).

Besides confirming the diagnosis of pancreatic cancer in the majority of patients, the advantages of obtaining tissue are that it helps identify other malignancies, such as neuroendocrine tumors, lymphoma, and small-cell carcinoma, as well as nonmalignant conditions such as autoimmune pancreatitis and chronic pancreatitis, resulting in changes in treatment and prognosis.

Complications from surgery are another major concern. Pancreatoduodenectomy is associated with significant morbidity, and the mortality rate can range from less than 1% in a large-volume center to about 15% in centers performing few such surgeries per year. This must be taken into account by the physicians and the patient prior to surgical resection of the pancreas.

In patients whose CT findings are equivocal regarding the presence of a mass or potential for resectability, EUS is indicated, as it is the most sensitive method to detect small tumors of the pancreas and evaluate for vascular invasion.

Allen VB, Gurusamy KS, Takwoingi Y, et al. Diagnostic accuracy of laparoscopy following computed tomography (CT) scanning for assessing the resectability with curative intent in pancreatic and periampullary cancer. *Cochrane Database Syst Rev* 2016;7(7):CD009323. [PMID: 27383694]

Pereira SP, Oldfield L, Ney A, et al. Early detection of pancreatic cancer. *Lancet Gastroenterol Hepatol.* 2020;5(7):698–710. [PMID: 32135127]

Swanson R, Pezzy C, Mallin K, et al. The 90-day mortality after pancreatectomy for cancer is double the 30-day mortality: more than 20,000 resections from the National Cancer Data Base. *J Surg Oncol.* 2014;21:4059–4067. [PMID: 25190121]

E. Staging

When the diagnosis of pancreatic cancer is suspected, staging studies are done to determine which of three clinical stages are appropriate: resectable, locally advanced and unresectable, or metastatic.

Differential Diagnosis

Pancreatic adenocarcinoma must be differentiated from the following conditions of the pancreas that can mimic its symptoms: autoimmune pancreatitis, chronic pancreatitis, pancreatic lymphoma, neuroendocrine tumors of the pancreas, and cystic lesions of the pancreas.

A. Autoimmune Pancreatitis

Autoimmune pancreatitis is a rare disorder of presumed autoimmune etiology that can manifest with obstructive jaundice, weight loss, abdominal pain, and new-onset diabetes. Imaging studies show diffuse enlargement of the pancreas, irregular narrowing of the pancreatic duct, strictures of the common bile duct, and stricture of the intrahepatic radicals similar to that seen in primary sclerosing cholangitis (refer to Table 30–3). Increased levels of serum γ-globulins, especially immunoglobulin G_4, are present. Lymphoplasmacytic infiltration with fibrosis and obliterative phlebitis is seen on histologic examination. Corticosteroids are effective in alleviating symptoms and reversing histopathologic changes (see Chapter 30).

B. Chronic Pancreatitis

The incidence of pancreatic adenocarcinoma in patients with chronic pancreatitis increases about 2% per decade after onset of the disease. Abdominal pain, weight loss, and jaundice may occur in patients with chronic pancreatitis, making it difficult to differentiate chronic pancreatitis complicated by adenocarcinoma.

Imaging studies are not always useful as patients with chronic pancreatitis can present with strictures of the pancreatic and bile duct on ERCP, a mass lesion on CT (variant of autoimmune pancreatitis), or with changes in the echo texture of pancreatic tissue, making EUS images difficult to interpret. EUS appears to be superior to CT scan for detection of coexistent malignancy.

Although CA 19-9 is elevated in about 80% of patients with adenocarcinoma, it can also be elevated in patients with chronic pancreatitis, though not usually above 500, and very high values may occur in patients with obstructive jaundice and cholangitis.

K-ras mutations do not seem to be clinically useful in differentiating chronic pancreatitis and pancreatic cancer.

Treatment

Patients with pancreatic cancer can be subdivided into three categories based on the extent of tumor spread: (1) tumor confined to the pancreas (resectable disease at diagnosis), representing approximately 15–20% of patients; (2) locally advanced disease (unresectable), 40%; and (3) metastatic disease, 40%.

A. Resectable Disease

Surgical resection is the only curative treatment for pancreatic cancer. Owing to the characteristically late presentation, only 15% of patients are candidates for pancreatectomy. Pancreatectomy is appropriate for patients with no distant metastasis, a good performance status, few comorbidities and without evidence of interface between the primary tumor and the mesenteric vessels. The most common surgery is the Whipple pancreaticoduodenectomy, used in patients with cancers located in the head of the pancreas. The procedure involves en bloc removal of the gastric antrum, pancreas, gallbladder, and duodenum. A modified pylorus-sparing pancreaticoduodenectomy can also be performed with low rates of delayed gastric emptying. Removal of regional lymph nodes has not been shown to be associated with improved survival. Mortality rates for this procedure are about 1–3% at centers that perform a large number of these surgeries.

As noted earlier, even after surgical resection with negative margins, patients have a 5-year survival rate of 10–25%, with median survival of 10–20 months. Involvement of the lymph nodes in resected patients is the most important prognostic factor; 5-year survival after the Whipple procedure is 10% for patients with node-positive disease and 25–30% for those with node-negative disease. Tumor size <3 cm, well-differentiated tumors, negative surgical margins, and absence of lymph node metastasis are associated with improved survival. After resection, most patients would receive adjuvant chemotherapy. Trials are currently evaluating the benefit of neoadjuvant chemotherapy in these patients.

Surgical resection of tumors located on the body and the tail consists of distal pancreatectomy with splenectomy.

Endoscopic stent placement in patients with resectable tumors to relieve jaundice prior to surgery does not alter postoperative morbidity and mortality and is not recommended. If the surgery is scheduled for several weeks later, a stent can be placed to relieve jaundice and reduce the risk of cholangitis.

B. Borderline Resectable Disease

The definition of borderline resectable disease is variable and optimal treatment remains controversial. Borderline resectable disease may include patients with a potentially resectable tumor but have a low performance status or comorbidities preventing surgery or have focal tumor abutment of the visceral arteries, a short-segment occlusion of the superior mesenteric vein or venous narrowing without occlusion. In this group, given the high rate of lymph node involvement, neoadjuvant treatment should be considered including neoadjuvant chemotherapy and radiationtherapy. The optimal neoadjuvant therapy is still controversial and will vary according to the performance status of the patient and include FOLFIRINOX, gemcitabine with nabpaclitaxel. Disease burden should be reassessed at 2 and 4 months for distant metastasis, if there is no metastasis, neoadjuvant radiation therapy should be considered followed when possible with surgical resection.

C. Locally Advanced Unresectable Disease

Locally advanced unresectable disease is defined as tumor encasement of the vessel (more than one-half of the vessel circumference) or occlusion/thrombus of the superior mesenteric artery, unreconstructable SMV or SMV/ portal vein confluence occlusion, direct involvement of the inferior vena cana, aorta, or celiac axis or absence of fat plane between the tumor and the vascular structures. Optimal treatment in these patients remains controversial. The combination of chemotherapy and radiation is associated with modest improvements in median survival but may produce significant side effects. Survival is approximately 12 months with palliative therapy. When staging studies do not show metastasis, then preoperative chemotherapy or chemoradiotherapy with a view toward shrinking the tumor ("downstaging") to make it resectable may be appropriate. If the tumor shrinks and becomes resectable, then results will correspond to the resectable group. If the tumor does not become resectable, then survival will mimic the locally advanced unresectable group noted earlier.

Symptom palliation is an essential component of care for patients with locally advanced disease. Patients with tumors localized to the pancreatic head can develop obstructive jaundice and gastric outlet obstruction; severe abdominal pain is more common with tumors involving the body and tail of the pancreas.

Ghanch P, Kleeff J, Halloran CM, et al. The impact of positive resection margins on survival and recurrence following resection and adjuvant chemotherapy for pancreatic ductal adenocarcinoma. *Ann Surg.* 2019;269(3):520–529. [PMID: 29068800]

Mizrahi JD, Surana R, Valle JW, et al. Pancreatic cancer. *Lancet.* 2020;395(10242):2008–2020. [PMID: 3259333]

1. Obstructive jaundice—Compression or invasion of the bile duct by the tumor can cause obstructive jaundice. Endoscopic stent placement is the most effective approach to relieve malignant bile duct obstruction. Metal stents are preferred over plastic ones for palliation once the patient is no longer considered a surgical candidate. Unlike plastic stents, which require frequent periodic changes due to occlusion, metal stents have a significantly higher patency rate. The stents may be placed percutaneously if an endoscopic approach is not possible as a result of tumor in-growth or previous surgery. Rarely, a surgical biliary enteric bypass is required to relieve the obstruction.

2. Gastric outlet obstruction—Obstruction of the gastric outlet is caused by extension of the pancreatic cancer and can be treated by gastrojejunostomy (surgically or by new EUS-directed techniques using expandable stents) or by endoscopically placed expanding metal stents.

3. Pain—Narcotic medications are usually required to control pain associated with pancreatic cancers. Celiac plexus block or neurolysis can be achieved through a percutaneous approach, or the block can be performed using EUS. Radiation can be used to control intractable pain.

Wyse JM, Carone M, Paquin SC, et al. Randomized, double-blind, controlled trial of early endoscopic ultrasound-guided celiac plexus neurolysis to prevent pain progression in patients with newly diagnosed, painful, inoperable pancreatic cancer. *J Clin Oncol.* 2011;29:3541–3546. [PMID: 21844506]

D. Metastatic Disease

When staging studies determine that a cancer has metastasized, then chemotherapy or supportive care is appropriate. FOLFIRINOX is a multidrug regimen that uses fluorouracil (5-FU), leucovorin, oxaliplatin, and irinotecan. It was shown to be superior to gemcitabine for metastatic pancreatic cancer. This regimen is associated with more toxicity and patients with lower performance status may not tolerate it. Alternatives include FOLFOX (5-FU, leucovorin, and oxaliplatin) gemcitabine plus cisplatin, gemcitabine plus nabpaclitaxel. Multiple treatment regimens are currently being studied. Patient survival without chemotherapy is 4-months.

Nevala-Plagemann C, Hidalgo M, Garrido-Laguna I. From state-of-the-art treatments to novel therapies for advanced-stage pancreatic cancer. *Nat Rev Clin Oncol.* 2020;17(2):108–123. [PMID: 31705130]

Schizas D, Charalampakis N, Kole C, et al. Immunotherapy for pancreatic cancer: a 2020 update. *Cancer Treat Rev.* 2020;86:102016. [PMID: 32247999]

CYSTIC NEOPLASMS OF THE PANCREAS

These lesions represent a spectrum of benign and malignant tumors and are found in 2–19% of the general population undergoing abdominal imaging for unrelated reasons. The most common—intraductal papillary mucinous neoplasms, MCNs, serous cyst adenomas, and SPNs (rare)—are described in detail later in this section. Table 31–3 contrasts epidemiologic and biologic characteristics of these and other pancreatic cystic neoplasms.

▶ Clinical Findings

A. Symptoms & Signs

Characteristic manifestations for each lesion are described in detail later in this section.

B. Imaging Studies

CT and MRI are excellent tests for initial detection and characterization of cystic lesions of the pancreas, but differentiation of benign and malignant disease on the basis of imaging alone is difficult (see Figures 9–46 to 9–48). Besides providing better characterization of the cystic lesion, MRCP may also be able to show the communication between the cyst and the pancreatic duct. EUS findings alone are not accurate to determine the type of cystic lesion or its malignant potential. EUS–FNA has emerged as the technique of choice for obtaining cyst fluid for evaluation of tumor makers and cells. It also assists in detecting malignant transformation by

Table 31–3. Epidemiologic & biologic characteristics of pancreatic cystic neoplasms.

Type	Sex Predilection	Peak Decade of Life	% of Cystic Neoplasms	Malignant Potential and Natural History
Mucinous cystic neoplasm	Female	5th	10–45	Resection curative, regardless of degree of epithelial dysplasia; poor prognosis when invasive adenocarcinoma present
Serous cyst adenoma (Figure 9–46)	Female	7th	32–39	Resection curative; serous cystadenocarcinoma extremely rare
Intraductal papillary mucinous neoplasm (Figures 9–47, 9–48)	Equal distribution	6th–7th	21–33	Excellent prognosis for lesions showing only adenomatous and borderline cytologic atypia; poor prognosis when invasive carcinoma present
Solid pseudopapillary neoplasm	Female	4th	<10	Indolent neoplasm with rare nodal and extranodal metastases; excellent prognosis when completely resected
Cystic endocrine neoplasm	Equal distribution	5th–6th	<10	Similar to solid neuroendocrine neoplasm
Ductal adenocarcinoma with cystic degeneration	Slight male predominance	6th–7th	<1	Dismal prognosis, similar to solid adenocarcinoma
Acinar cell cystadenocarcinoma	Male	6th–7th	<1	Similar to solid type; aggressive neoplasm with slightly better prognosis than ductal adenocarcinoma

Table 31–4. Fluid analysis in cystic lesions of the pancreas.

	Mucinous Cystic Neoplasm	Serous Cyst Adenoma	IPMN	Pseudocyst
Viscosity	High	Low	High	Low
CEA	High (>200 ng/mL)	Low (5–20 ng/mL)	High (>250 ng/mL)	Low
Lipase/amylase	Low	Low	High	High
Cytology	Mucinous epithelial cells ± Malignant cells if adenocarcinoma	Cuboidal cells ± High glycogen content	Mucinous epithelial cells ± Malignant cells if adenocarcinoma	Histiocytes or acellular
DNA analysis	*K-ras* mutations High DNA amount or high-amplitude allelic loss in malignancy	Rare abnormalities	*K-ras* mutations High DNA amount or high amplitude allelic loss in malignancy	No abnormalities

CEA, carcinoembryonic antigen; IPMN, intraductal papillary mucinous neoplasm.

providing cells from the cyst walls. EUS–FNA carries a 2–3% risk of pancreatitis. ERCP is useful in detecting intraductal neoplasms, especially IPMN, but its role has become limited by advances in pancreatic imaging.

C. Cytology & Tumor Markers

Cytologic analysis of the cyst fluid has high specificity for mucinous lesions as well as presence of malignancy, but its sensitivity is low (Table 31–4). The yield of cells obtained from EUS–FNA can be insufficient to make a definitive diagnosis or confirm malignant transformation as the lining of the cystic lesions is often denuded. Tumor markers have been shown to improve diagnostic accuracy and differentiation of cystic lesions. Level of CEA is usually high in mucinous lesions. A CEA cutoff level of 192 ng/mL was found to be most accurate for differentiating between mucinous and nonmucinous cystic lesions with a sensitivity of 73% and specificity of 84%.

Molecular markers, cyst fluid DNA, cyst fluid glucose levels, and proteomic mucin profiling are other methods that have been used to differentiate mucinous from nonmucinous lesions. K-ras mutation can be seen in mucinous lesions and GNAS mutation are seen in IPMNs. Low cyst glucose appears to have similar test characteristics as CEA in identifying mucinous lesions.

Serous cyst adenomas can contain high numbers of glycogen cells whereas mucinous lesions can have fluid high in mucin. The presence of mucin-like antigen as a marker for mucinous tumors has also been used.

Amylase levels are high in both pseudocysts and IPMN, and low in serous cyst adenomas and most mucinous cyst adenomas. CA 19-9 is not elevated in cystic lesions of the pancreas.

Puppa G, Christinat Y, McKee TA. Towards optimal pancreatic cyst fluid management: the need for standardisation. *Gut.* 2019;68(10):1906. [PMID: 30301772]

Differential Diagnosis

True cystic neoplasms of the pancreas must be differentiated from inflammatory pseudocysts, which are the most common cystic lesions of the pancreas. Pseudocysts are collections of pancreatic secretions without an epithelial lining that occur as a result of inflammation of the pancreas, or obstruction or disruption of the pancreatic duct. Clinical history and associated radiologic findings of acute or chronic pancreatitis, gland atrophy, ductal dilation, and calcification help differentiate pseudocysts from cystic neoplasms. High levels of amylase and low CEA are usually noted in the pseudocyst fluid.

1. Mucinous Cystic Neoplasms

MCNs are common cystic tumors of the pancreas, comprising 20% of these neoplasms. They occur predominantly in middle-aged women (>80%) and are mostly localized to the body or tail of the pancreas.

Pathogenesis

These tumors are premalignant lesions and are classified as benign (adenomatous), low-grade malignant (borderline), or malignant (carcinoma in situ and invasive cancer) based on the degree of tissue dysplasia. The presence of malignancy in these tumors as estimated in published reports is estimated to be between 10% and 37%.

These tumors are filled with ovarian-type stroma with high viscosity and generally elevated CEA levels. Unlike IPMNs, these tumors do not communicate with the pancreatic ductal system. Larger size, presence of peripheral eggshell calcification on imaging, and association of a solid component with the cystic lesion are features suggestive of malignant progression.

Clinical Findings

A. Symptoms & Signs

Mucinous cystic tumors are most commonly incidental findings on abdominal imaging or can manifest with abdominal pain, palpable mass, recurrent pancreatitis, and vomiting due to gastric outlet obstruction. Jaundice and weight loss are more common with malignant transformation.

B. Imaging Studies

These tumors appear unilocular or multilocular on CT and MRI, with few discrete compartments. EUS can be helpful to further characterize the lesion and obtain cells for evaluation of malignant transformation.

C. Cyst Fluid Analysis, Cytology & Tumor Markers

The cyst fluid has high viscosity, with high CEA levels (>192 ng/mL). Cytology may show columnar cells with variable atypia.

▶ Treatment

Surgical resection is recommended in patients with acceptable surgical risk, because of the significant potential for malignant transformation. Resection is associated with an excellent 5-year survival rate (>95% for benign and borderline tumors and 50–75% for malignant tumors with negative margins). As most of these lesions are localized to the tail of the pancreas, distal pancreatectomy is the most common surgery performed.

2. Serous Cyst Adenomas

These tumors, seen mostly in women, are the second most common cystic tumors of the pancreas. About 50% of serous cyst adenomas occur in the body or tail of the pancreas and have a very low potential for malignant transformation.

▶ Clinical Findings

A. Symptoms & Signs

Serous cyst adenomas are usually asymptomatic, but patients can present with abdominal discomfort, a palpable mass, and, if the tumor is large, with bile duct and gastric outlet obstruction.

B. Imaging Studies

On CT scan the tumor consists of multiple tiny cysts separated by delicate fibrous septa arranged around a central stellate scar that may be calcified, giving them a honeycomb appearance. The pathognomonic CT finding of a "sunburst" due to the central scar is seen in 20% of patients.

C. Cyst Fluid Analysis, Cytology & Tumor Markers

The cyst fluid has low viscosity (clear and watery), with low CEA levels (<5 ng/mL). Cytology can show cuboidal cells with positive glycogen stain.

▶ Treatment

Surgery is indicated in symptomatic patients and in those with rapidly enlarging serous cystadenomas. In asymptomatic patients, observation with serial imaging is a valid strategy because of the low risk of malignant transformation.

3. Intraductal Papillary Mucinous Neoplasms

IPMNs are papillary tumors that arise from the pancreatic duct and are associated with mucin hypersecretion; they are the most common cystic neoplasms comprising 38% of resected pancreatic cystic neoplasms. They occur equally in men and women, and the median age at presentation is 65. These tumors occur predominantly in the head of the pancreas. IPMNs may involve the main pancreatic duct, a side branch, or both.

▶ Pathogenesis

The role of smoking, alcohol, and genetic predisposition in the development of IPMN remains unclear. Although genetic alterations such as *P53* overexpression, *K-ras* mutations, and *DPC4* overexpression have been identified, their role in the development of IPMN is not understood. Unlike pancreatic cancers, where *DPC4* inactivation is seen in most tumors, *DPC4* is expressed in almost all IPMNs. In 30% of cases IPMNs are associated with extrapancreatic tumors, adenocarcinoma of the colon and stomach being the most common.

Kromrey ML, Bülow R, Hübner J, et al. Prospective study on the incidence, prevalence and 5-year pancreatic-related mortality of pancreatic cysts in a population-based study. *Gut.* 2018;67:138. [PMID: 28877981]

A. Classification

IPMNs are classified into three types, based on the involvement of the main pancreatic duct (main duct IPMN) or the side branches (branch duct IPMN) or both (mixed IPMN). Side branch IPMNs are multifocal in 40% of cases. The main duct type IPMN is more aggressive and has a higher incidence of malignancy.

The World Health Organization (WHO) has histologically classified IPMN into three categories:

- IPMN adenoma: The cystic lesion is lined by mucin-containing columnar cells with no dysplasia.
- IPMN borderline: Lining cells show moderate dysplasia.
- Intraductal papillary mucinous carcinoma: Presence of severe dysplasia.

The malignant tumors are further classified as noninvasive (carcinoma in situ) or invasive, based on the absence or presence of extension beyond the basement membrane. The location of the IPMN predicts its malignant potential. The risk of malignancy was found to be 57–92% in main duct IPMN, 6–46% in a side branch IPMN, and 35–40% in a mixed IPMN in surgically resected specimen. While the prognosis for a benign, borderline, and carcinoma in situ is good, the 5-year survival rate for an invasive malignant lesion is between 30% and 75%.

Clinical Findings

A. Symptoms & Signs

About 30% of IPMN are diagnosed on routine imaging studies and are asymptomatic. In symptomatic patients, abdominal pain is the most common presenting complaint and is seen in 50–70% patients. About 25% of patients present with acute pancreatitis. Many patients have a history of recurrent bouts of acute pancreatitis, or features of chronic pancreatitis such as diarrhea, new-onset diabetes, weight loss, as a result of obstruction of the pancreatic duct by mucus plugs. Weight loss, jaundice, and shorter duration of symptoms are associated with malignant IPMN, though about 40% of malignant IPMN are asymptomatic at presentation.

B. Imaging Studies

Cystic lesions in the pancreas in communication with a dilated pancreatic duct can be seen on CT scan, EUS, and MRI. The sensitivity and specificity of MRCP in diagnosing malignancy in IPMN have been reported to be 70% and 92%, respectively. The presence of mural nodules, segmental or diffuse dilation of the main pancreatic duct >15 mm in diameter, presence of solid component in the cyst is associated with malignant disease. EUS–FNA is also useful in detecting the presence of mucin and provides cells to evaluate for malignant transformation. The cyst fluid aspirate can be useful in distinguishing mucinous lesions from nonmucinous cystic lesions of the pancreas. A CEA level of 192 g/mL was 79% sensitive in differentiating mucinous tumors from nonmucinous tumors. ERCP is rarely used in the diagnosis of IPMN. The pathognomonic sign on ERCP is a patulous ampulla of Vater with extruding mucus, or fish mouth appearance. Pancreatography may also show filling defects due to mucus and communication between the pancreatic duct and cystic areas. Peroral pancreatoscopy can also help assess IPMN and clarify main duct involvement.

While both IPMN and MCN contain mucin and have high CEA levels, MCN does not communicate with the pancreatic duct, and is seen mostly in females in the fourth to fifth decade of life. Unlike IPMN, which predominantly occurs in the head of the pancreas, the MCN are seen mostly in the body and tail of the pancreas.

Treatment

Main duct IPMN and mixed IPMN have a significant risk for malignant transformation. About 30–40% of malignant IPMN can be asymptomatic and have a negative cytology on FNA. Surgical resection is recommended in these patients while the prognosis for nonmalignant IPMN is good, reoccurrence rate of 50–60% is noted in patients with invasive IPMN with a 5-year survival of 35–75%.

During surgery the resected margins must be examined by frozen section to confirm clearance of the tumor as IPMNs tend to grow longitudinally along the pancreatic ducts rather than radially into the parenchyma.

The risk of malignancy in the side branch IPMN is about 3% at 5 years. In asymptomatic patients with side branch IPMN of size <3 cm and no radiologic features worrisome for malignancy surveillance is recommended. EUS with FNA or FNB is recommended in side branch IPMN with 2 of the following features: mural nodule, cyst size ≥3 cm, dilated main pancreatic duct or velocity of growth ≥5 mm per year. Surgical resection is indicated in obstructive jaundice, ≥5 mm enhancing mural nodule, main pancreatic duct dilation ≥10 mm or cytology with high grade dysplasia or carcinoma

Surveillance with periodic imaging is recommended in patients with invasive IPMN, as reoccurrence (most often within the first 3 years) occurs in 50–65% of cases. Patients with carcinoma in situ have a low but significant reoccurrence rate of about 8% and should be followed by yearly CT scan or MRI.

Elta GH, Enestvedt BK, Sauer BG, et al. ACG clinical guideline: diagnosis and management of pancreatic cysts. *Am J Gastroenterol.* 2018;113(4):464–479. [PMID: 29485131]

European Study Group on Cystic Tumours of the Pancreas. European evidence-based guidelines on pancreatic cystic neoplasms. *Gut.* 2018;67(5):789–804. [PMID: 29574408]

Hasan A, Visrodia K, Farrell JJ, et al. Overview and comparison of guidelines for management of pancreatic cystic neoplasms. *World J Gastroenterol.* 2019;25(31):4405–4413. [PMID: 31496620]

Tanaka M, Fernández-Del Castillo C, Kamisawa T, et al. Revisions of international consensus Fukuoka guidelines for the management of IPMN of the pancreas. *Pancreatology.* 2017;17(5): 738–753. [PMID: 28735806]

van Huijgevoort NCM, Del Chiaro M, Wolfgang CL, et al. Diagnosis and management of pancreatic cystic neoplasms: current evidence and guidelines. *Nat Rev Gastroenterol Hepatol.* 2019;16(11):676–689. [PMID: 31527862]

Vege SS, Ziring B, Jain R, et al. American gastroenterological association institute guideline on the diagnosis and management of asymptomatic neoplastic pancreatic cysts. *Gastroenterology.* 2015;148(4):819–822; quize12-3. [PMID: 25805375]

4. Solid Pseudopapillary Neoplasms

SPNs are rare neoplasms with low, malignant potential. They are seen almost exclusively in young women. They account for approximately 5% of cystic tumors of the pancreas and are more often located in the body or tail of the pancreas. The diagnosis is usually made when a patient presents with obstructive symptoms such as jaundice or abdominal pain but can also be found incidentally on abdominal imaging. Diagnosis confirmation is usually achieved using cytology. Surgical resection is usually curative.

PANCREATIC LYMPHOMA

Pancreatic lymphoma represents 1–2% of all pancreatic tumors. It presents as large mass, usually without bile duct obstruction, pain, or weight loss. Treatment consists of combination of chemotherapy and radiation and is associated with good 5-year survival rates.

Polypectomy

32

Sanchit Gupta, MD, MS
Kunal Jajoo, MD

► General Considerations

Many epithelial tumors of the gastrointestinal tract develop as benign polyps before becoming malignant, as discussed in detail in earlier chapters of this book. These may be symptomatic or asymptomatic, pedunculated or sessile, and range in size from millimeters to many centimeters in diameter. If confined to the mucosa or superficial submucosa, they are nearly all amenable to endoscopic removal by one of a variety of polypectomy techniques, endoscopic mucosal resection (EMR), or endoscopic submucosal dissection (ESD).

The principles of endoscopic polypectomy have evolved to a standardized set of techniques since their introduction almost 40 years ago. EMR and ESD techniques continue to be developed as more recent innovations. Endoscopic resection aims to remove a tumor in its entirety for cure, for complete pathologic assessment, and to reduce or eradicate the risk of recurrence while maintaining the integrity of the wall of the gastrointestinal tract and avoiding procedure-related morbidity.

Bleeding is the most common complication of polypectomy, occurring in 9.8/1000 (95% CI 7.7–12.1) or 0.1–0.6% of cases. Postpolypectomy hemorrhage can occur immediately (within 12 hours) or can be delayed (up to 30 days) and is more likely to occur with larger polyps, polyps with thick stalks, right-sided lesions, laterally-spreading tumors; hemorrhage may be influenced by patient factors, such as cardiovascular or renal disease or use of anticoagulation. Using epinephrine injection with or without combination therapy using a mechanical device during polypectomy may reduce rates of early postpolypectomy bleeding. Perforation, the most feared complication of polypectomy, remains rare but relatively unchanged in incidence since the introduction of these techniques. Perforation occurs in 0.8/1000 (95% CI 0.6–1.0) or 0.7–0.9% of cases and is more likely to occur with piecemeal cautery polypectomy of sessile polyps, cecal polyps, nonpolypoid lesions, impaired lifting, and with ESD. Postpolypectomy coagulation syndrome may occur hours to days after the procedure. It is thought to be a consequence of thermal injury to the bowel after cautery, leading to localized inflammation and peritonitis without bowel perforation. This can present with fever, abdominal tenderness, leukocytosis, with radiographic studies showing air in the bowel wall but not free air in the abdomen, and should be managed with bowel rest, antibiotics, intravenous fluids, and close observation. Postpolypectomy syndrome may occur in 1–3/100,000 cases, and is associated with lesions >10 mm, nonpolypoid lesions, and hypertension.

Polypectomy, EMR, and ESD can all be accomplished in the sedated patient as there are no pain receptors in the mucosa and submucosa. The muscularis propria and serosa together with the mesentery are capable of generating pain sensation caused by mechanical forces (eg, stretching) and the thermal effects of electrosurgery. A wide range of accessories is now available for endoscopic polypectomy and the last decade has also seen improvements in electrosurgical generators with respect to ease of use, safety, and efficacy. All endoscopists should be equipped to remove small- to medium-sized sessile polyps and nearly all pedunculated polyps in the colon. Larger sessile polyps (>2 cm in diameter), very large pedunculated polyps in the colon, and polyps of all types in the esophagus, stomach, duodenum, and small bowel require additional expertise and technology and are usually referred to centers with experience in these areas. Such tertiary referral has been demonstrated to be safe and effective and to avoid the risk of unnecessary surgery. It is also cost-effective.

EQUIPMENT

Removal of polyps throughout the gastrointestinal tract requires appropriate access with an endoscope bearing an instrumentation channel diameter adequate to take standard accessories. Most of these will pass through a 2.8-mm channel but some may require 3.2 mm or greater. Accessories include biopsy forceps, snares, injection needles, combination devices marrying more than one function in a single instrument, hemostatic clips and loops, bipolar and multipolar probes, and EMR sets providing a spray catheter, injector needle, special snare, and transparent cap, which comes in many shapes and diameters. Additional ESD accessories include an endoscopic knife, cap and hood, and coagulator probe or hemostatic forceps. Most accessories designed for colonoscopy will also be long enough for some enteroscopes when therapy in the small bowel is being planned.

Special stains for surface chromoendoscopy (eg, indigo carmine, Lugol iodine, methylene blue, and cresyl violet) may be needed prior to resection in order to optimize visualization of a polyp and its margins. A variety of fluids can be used for submucosal injection during EMR or ESD. Epinephrine can be added to augment immediate hemostasis and methylene blue can be added to enhance visualization. Some experts prefer to inject a fluid of higher viscosity (eg, hyaluronic acid, hydroxyethyl starch, and commercially available premixed gels), which dissipates less rapidly during resection allowing for a more sustained submucosal cushion during difficult polypectomy. Many endoscopes are capable of imaging with restricted wavelengths of light (eg, narrow-band imaging or multiband imaging), which allows visualization of morphology and vasculature in the submucosa, enhancing the endoscopist's ability to recognize the edges of polyps and any malignant features. Marking agents, which are prefilled vials of a sterile suspension of very fine carbon particles (Spot; GI Supply, Camp Hill, PA); can be used for permanent documentation of a tumor resection site for future endoscopic or surgical reference. With the increasing use of laparoscopic colorectal surgery and the fact that 10–20% of endoscopically identified tumors can be incorrectly localized, endoscopic tattoo marking is essential for subsequent identification.

Many electrosurgical generators are manufactured specifically for endoscopic applications. Most incorporate computer-controlled outputs modified by feedback through the accessory to achieve the desired tissue effect with the least power necessary. They also incorporate menus for specific endoscopic procedures with defaults set by the manufacturer. All endoscopists and assistants performing electrosurgery should have a thorough knowledge of monopolar high-frequency circuits and their properties in order to understand the safe principles of cutting and coagulation, and to troubleshoot any problems that occur during polypectomy. The concept of current density (power per unit area) is essential to comprehend because this is how snare polypectomy cuts and coagulates tissue as it is being mechanically cut by the closing snare. Bowel preparation must be good to excellent both for visibility and to reduce the risk of ignition of bowel gases such as hydrogen and methane. All fluid must be removed from around the polyp to be resected in order to maximize the current density where it is desired at the point of resection.

POLYPECTOMY FOR SESSILE POLYPS

Small polyps less than 5 mm in diameter are often referred to as "diminutive." Irrespective of their site in the gastrointestinal tract, they can usually be removed by any of a number of simple methods that include "cold" biopsy forceps with standard or so-called jumbo forceps, "hot" (ie, combined with electrocautery) biopsy forceps, "cold" snare, and "hot" snare. A common practice is to place a small diameter snare (eg, 1-cm oval) over the polyp, including a small cuff of normal surrounding mucosa, and then close the snare handle and mechanically cut through the trapped tissue, which will excise the polyp. Because the bleeding risk of simple mechanical cutting and avulsion with cold techniques is minimal, these are favored for such small lesions, which can usually be removed by one pass of the forceps or snare. Such methods are quick and effective and provide the necessary specimen for histopathologic evaluation (Plates 55 and 56) with almost no risk. Resected tissue can be aspirated into the endoscope suction system, to which a specimen trap can be added. In the United States, cold snare polypectomy is recommended for diminutive (≤5 mm) and small (6–9 mm) poylps, and cold forceps polypectomy is not recommended for these lesions but may be considered for polyps ≤2 mm.

Sessile polyps larger than 10 mm and up to a diameter of 2 cm can usually be removed using a cold snare or hot snare with electrocautery (Plates 57, 58, and 59). Snares are available in many sizes and shapes, with choice being determined by personal or endoscopy unit preference. The principle is to place the snare over the entire polyp and either (1) close it as a cutting or combined cutting and coagulation current is applied until the polyp is detached from the submucosa, or, more commonly or (2) close it as far as possible before applying a pure coagulating current, and then continue closing until the polyp is removed. In both sequences, it is important to lift the entrapped tissue away from the wall of the gastrointestinal tract to minimize any deep injury to the gastrointestinal wall. It is particularly important to maintain a minimal cuff of normal tissue around sessile polyps. A prospective study of over 1,400 patients with 5–20 mm nonpedunculated polyps demonstrated a 10% incomplete resection rate when biopsies were taken from the resection site after what was deemed endoscopically complete polypectomy. Specimen retrieval is accomplished by suction through the endoscope into a specimen trap. Multiple polyps or those too large for aspiration-retrieval can be collected by a retrieval net.

Several safe methods are available to achieve hemostasis when excessive bleeding occurs immediately after cold or hot snare polypectomy or, very rarely, after forceps removal. Placement of one or more hemostatic clips, injection of diluted epinephrine 1:10,000, application of monopolar coagulation with the snare tip or by argon plasma coagulation, bipolar or multipolar coagulation with a dedicated probe, and band ligation are all used. Endoscopic clips can be readily utilized for immediate hemostasis and for prophylaxis of delayed hemorrhage, due to their ease of use. However, there are no studies directly comparing the efficacy of hemoclips and thermal techniques.

Suspected perforation or inadvertent deep submucosal injury can be promptly closed by placing clips to appose the mucosa on either side of the defect. In addition, endoscopic suturing devices can be considered but this requires additional training and expertise.

POLYPECTOMY FOR PEDUNCULATED POLYPS

Pedunculated polyps are so-called because the tumor is situated at the end of a stalk or pedicle and protrudes into the gastrointestinal tract lumen. The principle of polypectomy with these lesions is to resect through the stalk at a sufficient distance from the tumor to ensure its complete removal but not so close to the gut wall as to risk deep thermal injury. A point approximately one-third to one-half way along the stalk from the polyp head is usually chosen for placement of the snare loop (Plate 60); electrocautery is then applied while the snare loop is closed, until the stalk is completely severed. The polyp is then retrieved using either the aspiration method, if small enough, or by snare or net capture.

In contrast to sessile polyps, pedunculated polyps may be so large that the proximal side of the lesion may not be visible endoscopically during snare placement and polypectomy (Plate 61). The endoscopist must then take special precautions (1) to avoid inadvertently trapping normal mucosa in the snare and (2) to avoid injury to the opposite bowel wall if the polyp is touching it. Safe snare position can be confirmed by securing the snare tip on the proximal (further) side first by pulling it toward the endoscope and confirming that the polyp stalk, only, is ensnared before closing it prior to applying cautery. The large polyp extending across the bowel lumen can be removed safely by moving the snare back and forth to prevent any stray current from passing through an undesired site with enough current density to cause injury. This also reduces the power required to achieve the polypectomy. For very large stalks with vessels presumed to be larger than usual, some experts pretreat the stalk with an injection of diluted epinephrine or place an additional mechanical device such as a clip or endoloop before proceeding with polypectomy.

Bleeding from the cut polyp stalk is most readily controlled by resnaring it immediately for tamponade, without applying further cautery, and waiting for natural hemostasis to occur. If this fails, or if the snare has already been removed, any of the methods mentioned earlier can be used. Clips have become popular because of their ease of use and mechanical mechanism of action, which does not risk deep injury to the bowel wall after polypectomy (Plate 62).

ENDOSCOPIC MUCOSAL RESECTION

For sessile polyps larger than 2 cm in the colon or duodenum and almost any sized sessile polyp or early cancer in certain anatomic locations, such as the esophagus or stomach, a different set of techniques has been developed, collectively known as EMR. Although there are many technical variations and accessories, the principle of EMR is the same for all.

The lesion is lifted or separated from the underlying submucosa before resection is performed either by physical traction or by injecting fluid. One technique employs a two-channel endoscope to lift the lesion first with a grasping device, such as a biopsy forceps passed through one channel of the endoscope, over which is placed a snare, passed through the second channel, to complete the removal. This method, however, has never gained popularity in the United States. A second technique, originally developed in Japan, employs a transparent cap fitted to the tip of an endoscope into which, after submucosal injection of fluid, the lesion is aspirated, and a specially designed ultra-flexible snare placed around the "pseudopolyp" so created. Suction is then released and the polyp resected using the same electrocautery settings as for standard polypectomy (Plates 63 and 64). This method is particularly applicable in the esophagus, stomach, and rectum but is rarely used elsewhere in the gastrointestinal tract.

A third technique employs a band ligation system to raise the lesion into a pseudopolyp before snare resection; this has become popular for small sessile lesions in the upper gastrointestinal tract (Plates 65 and 66). A fourth method, which has become the dominant technique for EMR, is the use of an injection needle to instill fluid around and deep to the polyp to lift it away from the submucosa (Plate 67). Alternative needleless methods for elevation with fluid are also becoming available. This not only ensures that the lesion is safe to resect, as it is not invading deep to the mucosa, but also provides a cushion of safety, protecting the bowel wall from thermal injury. The nonlifting sign after such an attempted injection is an accurate indication of submucosal invasion of carcinoma. After injection, the polyp is snared piecemeal (Plate 68) until the entire area of mucosa has been removed (Plate 69). The specimens are retrieved by aspiration if they are small enough or by a net (Plate 70), and should be mounted on a paraffin wax block before fixation to aid in pathologic evaluation. The site may be left to heal, or this can be accelerated and possible complications reduced by closing the defect with clips (Plate 71). Although the scar may be visible for follow-up examinations (Plate 72), the site may also be marked with an injection of permanent ink for future endoscopic surveillance or surgical resection (Plate 73). Underwater EMR is a more recently developed approach, in which air is suctioned and instead, water is instilled to fill the lumen. This immersion allows the mucosa and submucosa to involute and the lesion to float away from the mucularis propria layer in the absence of gas distension, potentially making grasping easier for en block resection and avoiding submucosal injection.

Injection solutions vary, and include normal saline, hypertonic sodium chloride, hyaluronic acid, hydroxypropyl methylcellulose, succinylated gelatin, hydroxyethyl starch, dextrose, glycerol, ORISE gel, and Eleview. Injection agents made with normal saline dissipate faster, and other agents have been shown to increase the length of time of lifting and reduce the volume of injectant necessary. Thus, viscous injectant solutions are preferred (eg, hydroxyethyl starch, Eleview, ORISE gel). Additionally, contrast agents such as indigo carmine or methylene blue should be used in the submucosal injection to distinguish submucosa from mucosa and muscularis propria layers, and can help identify a potential injury or perforation.

Injection-assisted EMR should be used for nonpolypoid and serrated lesions 10–19 mm and ≥20 mm nonpedunculated colorectal lesions. Local recurrence after EMR occurs in 20% of cases with piecemeal removal and 3% of cases with *en bloc* resection and can be retreated with endoscopic therapy. Resection of the lesion in a single endoscopy session is preferred, as previous failed attempts are associated with risk of recurrence or incomplete resection. Thermal ablation of visible residual tissue should be avoided in favor of complete resection, as there is an increased risk of recurrence. However, adjuvant ablation can be used in the resection margins after no endoscopically visible residual lesion remains. Tattooing these lesions can lead to submucosal fibrosis and hamper the success of a future endoscopic resection, and thus is recommended against. Intraprocedural bleeding rates are estimated to be 11–22% for colorectal EMR of lesions >20 mm and can be treated with soft coagulation with a snare tip, or with the methods already outlined. Postprocedural bleeding rates from colorectal EMR range from 2% to 11%. Perforation rates after EMR of colonic lesions are <1%, and small peforations can be managed using endoscopic clips as described.

ENDOSCOPIC SUBMUCOSAL DISSECTION

An extension of EMR developed in Japan is ESD. This collection of techniques aims to remove the lesion as one piece by marking the perimeter of the lesion with cautery, injecting a lifting agent into the submucosa deep to the lesion, using an endoscopic knife to incise the perimeter of the polyp with a small margin of normal mucosa in a circumferential fashion, followed by careful dissection in the superficial submucosal plane until the resection is complete (Plates 74, 75, and 76). Several accessories are available worldwide. Although originally intended for removing early gastric cancers, ESD has been successfully applied to the colon and is increasingly becoming available in the United States, though there is not yet a current procedural terminology code for billing and reimbursement purposes.

ESD devices are designed for single use only, and most can be used with a 2.8 mm endoscopic instrument channel. Multiple electrosurgical knives are available with varying shapes, blade lengths, and electrodes (ITKnife, HookKnife, Triangle Tip Knife, DualKnife, FlexKnife, HybridKnife). Additionally, monopolar and bipolar forceps have been developed for both hemostasis and grasping or cutting, with varying availability. A cap on the tip of the endoscope holds the flap of resected mucosa away from the endoscope lens, maintaining visualization during dissection. Additional devices for tissue retraction include weighted clips, clips with thread traction, external forceps, among others. Spray chromoendoscopy can better demarcate lesion borders and tissue planes, and, similar to EMR, be used in conjunction with the injectant for lifting. CO_2 gas for luminal insufflation is more appropriate than air insufflation in ESD, due to the more rapid absorption and theoretical reduction in tension pneumoperitoneum if there is a perforation, which is estimated to occur in 4–10% of cases. Bleeding during ESD can be managed with coagulation using hemostatic forceps or electrosurgical knife.

ESD can be considered for lesions >20 mm under consideration for endoscopic rather than surgical resection and in which en block resection with EMR may not be possible. Factors to consider include suspicion for submucosal invasion, residual early carcinoma after endoscopic resection, fibrotic mucosal lesions, and local nonpolypoid colorectal dysplasia in patients with inflammatory bowel disease. Similarly, due to the extent of submucosal fibrosis in colitis-associated dysplasia, ESD may be considered preferentially over EMR in these situations.

R0 or curative resections are defined by the Japanese Society for Cancer of the Colon and Rectum as *lacking*: depth of submucosal invasion greater than 1000 μm, lymphovascular invasion, poor differentiation, and grade 2 or 3 tumor budding at deepest invasion. Compared to EMR, ESD has been shown to resect larger lesions, with higher en block resection rates, and possibly less local recurrence. ESD can obviate the need for surgery for appropriate lesions.

ENDOSCOPIC FULL-THICKNESS RESECTION

Endoscopic full-thickness resection (EFTR) is a recently developed technique that removes all layers of the colon wall. This allows for resection of lesions involving muscularis propria, such as subepithelial tumors or those with significant fibrosis. EFTR may be indicated for lesions <30 mm, nonlifting lesions, or lesions involving a diverticulum and requires closure of the defect after resection. In "exposed" EFTR, the resection is conducted first with defect closure afterwards, and can use tunneled and nontunneled techniques. In "nonexposed" EFTR, closure is effectively conducted prior to resection by making a serosa-to-serosa apposition with invagination of the involved bowel segment prior to full-thickness resection. This technique can be conducted using needle-knife catheters and ESD knives, through the scope clips, cap-mounted clips, endoscopic stapling devices, and endoscopic plicating and suturing devices. Ovesco has developed an FDA-approved full-thickness resection and closer device based on an over-the-scope clip system with a mounted clip and snare at the tip. The cap has a diameter of 20 mm which limits the size of lesion that can be resected. Further studies on techniques and outcomes will better define indications for EFTR.

Aslanian HR, Sethi A, Bhutani MS, et al. ASGE Technology Committee. ASGE guideline for endoscopic full-thickness resection and submucosal tunnel endoscopic resection. *VideoGIE.* 2019;4(8):343–350. [PMID: 31388606

Carpenter S, Petersen BT, Chuttani R, et al. Polypectomy devices. *Gastrointest Endosc.* 2007;65:741–749. [PMID: 17397841]

Choi HS, Chun HJ. Accessory devices frequently used for endoscopic submucosal dissection. *Clin Endosc.* 2017;50(3):224–233. [PMID: 28609818]

Hewett DG. Cold snare polypectomy: optimizing technique and technology (with videos). *Gastrointest Endosc.* 2015;82(4): 693–696. [PMID: 26385278]

Hirasawa K, Sato C, Makazu M, et al. Coagulation syndrome: delayed perforation after colorectal endoscopic treatments. *World J Gastrointest Endosc.* 2015;7(12):1055–1061. [PMID: 26380051]

Hwang JH, Konda V, Abu Dayyeh BK, et al. ASGE Technology Committee. Endoscopic mucosal resection. *Gastrointest Endosc.* 2015;82(2):215–226. [PMID: 26077453]

Kaltenbach T, Anderson JC, Burke CA, et al. Endoscopic removal of colorectal lesions: recommendations by the US Multi-Society Task Force on Colorectal Cancer. *Am J Gastroenterol.* 2020;115(3):435–464. [PMID: 32058340]

Kethu SR, Banerjee S, Desilets D, et al; ASGE Technology Committee. Endoscopic tattooing. *Gastrointest Endosc.* 2010;72: 681–685. [PMID: 20883844]

Kim JS, Lee BI, Choi H, et al. Cold snare polypectomy versus cold forceps polypectomy for diminutive and small colorectal polyps: a randomized controlled trial. *Gastrointest Endosc.* 2015;81(3):741–747. [PMID: 25708763]

Lo SK, Fujii-Lau LL, Enestvedt BK, et al. ASGE Technology Committee. The use of carbon dioxide in gastrointestinal endoscopy. *Gastrointest Endosc.* 2016;83(5):857–865. [PMID: 26946413]

Manfredi MA, Abu Dayyeh BK, Bhat YM, et al. ASGE Technology Committee. Electronic chromoendoscopy. *Gastrointest Endosc.* 2015;81(2):249–261. [PMID: 25484330]

Maple JT, Abu Dayyeh BK, Chauhan SS, et al. ASGE Technical Committee. Endoscopic submucosal dissection. *Gastrointest Endosc.* 2015;81(6):1311–1325.

Park HJ. Endoscopic instruments and electrosurgical unit for colonoscopic polypectomy. *Clin Endosc.* 2016;49(4):350–354. [PMID: 27399313]

Pohl H, Srivastava A, Bensen SP, et al. Incomplete polyp resection during colonoscopy-results of the complete adenoma resection (CARE) study. *Gastroenterology.* 2013;144:74–80. [PMID: 23022496]

Reumkens A, Rondagh EJ, Bakker CM, Winkens B, Masclee AA, Sanduleanu S. Post-colonoscopy complications: a systematic review, time trends, and meta-analysis of population-based studies. *Am J Gastroenterol.* 2016;111(8):1092–1101. [PMID 27296945]

Rutter MD, Jover R. Personalizing polypectomy techniques based on polyp characteristics. *Clin Gastroenterol Hepatol.* 2020;18(13):2859–2867. [PMID: 31563558]

Singh R, Chiam KH, Leiria F, Pu LZCT, Choi KC, Militz M. Chromoendoscopy: role in modern endoscopic imaging. *Transl Gastroenterol Hepatol.* 2020;5:39. [PMID: 32632390]

Thirumurthi S, Raju GS. Management of polypectomy complications. *Gastrointest Endosc Clin N Am.* 2015;25(2):335–357. [PMID: 25839689]

Tokar JL, Barth BA, Banerjee S, et al. ASGE Technology Committee. Electrosurgical generators. *Gastrointest Endosc.* 2013;78(2): 197–208. [PMID: 23867369]

Yang M, Pepe D, Schlachta CM, Alkhamesi NA. Endoscopic tattoo: the importance and need for standardised guidelines and protocol. *J R Soc Med.* 2017;110(7):287–291. [PMID: 28537104]

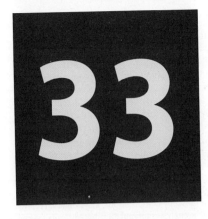

Endoscopic Management of Acute Biliary & Pancreatic Conditions

Russell D. Dolan, MD

Andrew C. Storm, MD

Christopher C. Thompson, MD

General Considerations

Since the introduction of endoscopic retrograde cholangio-pancreatography (ERCP) in 1968 and endoscopic sphincterotomy in 1974, the management of various biliary and pancreatic illnesses has evolved from surgical to endoscopic methods with substantial improvements in patient outcomes. Additionally, development of custom accessories has improved procedural efficiency and success rates; these include balloons and baskets for stone extraction, lithotripsy devices, stents, drains, and duodenoscope-assisted cholangiopancreatoscopy. Success rates for many therapeutic endoscopic pancreaticobiliary interventions exceed 90% technical success in expert centers.

Several acute biliary and pancreatic conditions are amenable to endoscopic diagnosis and therapy. ERCP has been shown to have better outcomes than surgery when dealing with most ductal obstructions and leaks. Additionally, ERCP may have a limited role in the diagnosis of bleeding conditions and the treatment of associated complications. This chapter details endoscopic treatment options for these conditions.

ACUTE CHOLANGITIS

ESSENTIALS OF DIAGNOSIS

► Diagnosis of acute biliary obstruction with cholangitis relies on clinical findings, blood cell counts, chemistries, biochemical profile, and imaging studies such as MRI with MRCP.

► Endoscopic biliary drainage is the standard of care, with emergent drainage for patients not responding to antibiotics and supportive measures or showing signs of clinical deterioration (ie, hypotension, altered mental states, and signs of continuing infection such as persistent fever).

Acute cholangitis is characterized by biliary stasis and infection of the bile ducts. In 1877, Charcot defined the clinical triad of fever, right upper quadrant pain, and jaundice that is present in up to 70% of patients with acute cholangitis. The spectrum of clinical presentation ranges from mild pain and low-grade fever, to a fulminate course with septic shock or death. In 1959, the Charcot triad was modified to include hypotension and mental status changes, subsequently known as the Reynolds pentad. Clinical presentation is, however, not useful in differentiating between suppurative and nonsuppurative cholangitis, which can only be determined at the time of endoscopic therapy. In the latter form, bacteria are still present in bile, but without the formation of pus. Suppurative cholangitis has a more acute course and is less likely to respond to antibiotics; however, either form is potentially life threatening, and when acute cholangitis is suspected, urgent diagnosis and treatment are critical.

Pathogenesis

Bile duct obstruction and infection are requisite for the development of cholangitis. Over 90% of cases are attributed to common bile duct stones. Other causes of obstruction include iatrogenic biliary instrumentation and endoprostheses. Less common causes include malignant biliary obstruction, benign bile duct strictures, ampullary adenomas, periductal adenopathy, choledochal cysts, parasites, and blood clots.

Following bile duct obstruction and biliary stasis, infection may occur either by direct ascent from the bowel, or via the lymphatics or portal vein. The latter assumes translocation of bacteria from the bowel into the portal circulation and subsequent clearance of bacteria by the reticuloendothelial system with excretion into bile. Although the origin of infecting organisms is questionable, the most common organisms are enteric and often polymicrobial. *Escherichia coli*, *Klebsiella*, *Enterobacter*, and *Proteus* are most common, while *Enterococcus* and anaerobes are less frequent. Positive bile cultures are seen in approximately one third of patients with bacteremia.

Clinical Findings

Initial studies include blood cultures, a complete blood count, and a full biochemical profile. Several noninvasive imaging studies are available to diagnose biliary obstruction. Abdominal ultrasound is sensitive for intrahepatic biliary dilation; however, it is poor at identifying choledocholithiasis, with a sensitivity of less than 30%. Additionally, up to one-third of patients with choledocholithiasis do not have evidence of biliary dilation, and cholangitis can occur before the bile duct becomes dilated. Nuclear hepatobiliary imaging can detect biliary obstruction earlier than ultrasound, with higher sensitivity. However, magnetic resonance imaging (MRI) with magnetic resonance cholangiopancreatography (MRCP) is most accurate, with a sensitivity of 97%. ERCP is no longer viewed as an initial diagnostic option and is reserved for therapy.

Treatment

A. Supportive Care

Supportive care for sepsis with volume resuscitation and broad-spectrum antibiotics, including gram-negative coverage, should be promptly instituted. Additionally, anaerobic and pseudomonal coverage should be considered if there is a history of prior instrumentation. Up to 85% of patients will respond to these conservative measures allowing for semielective biliary drainage within 48 hours. Emergent drainage is indicated in those patients who do not respond to conservative measures or when clinical deterioration occurs, particularly with the development of hypotension or alteration of mental status.

B. Endoscopic Biliary Drainage

Endoscopic biliary drainage is the standard of care for most causes of cholangitis. Definitive therapy typically involves endoscopic sphincterotomy with removal of stones or other obstructions, which has proven to be safer than surgical options. Complete clearance of gallstones is possible in up to 90% of cases on the initial procedure, with morbidity and mortality rates of 6% and nearly 0%, respectively.

It is important to avoid excess contrast injection, as this may precipitate cholangiovenous reflux and sepsis. Bile should initially be aspirated to decompress the collecting system, with samples sent for culture which may aid in tailoring of antibiotics for a specific pathogen. The amount of contrast injected should be half that of the bile removed to reduce elevating the pressure within the biliary system that may increase the risk of liver abscess and/or hematologic seeding.

If the patient is particularly ill or requiring anticoagulation, a two-step approach may be preferred, consisting

of ERCP with stent placement alone followed by definitive endoscopic sphincterotomy and stone removal when the patient is optimized. Additionally, when stones are too large to remove, stents may be placed as a temporizing measure to ensure adequate drainage and potential reduce stone number and/or size as a result of continuous friction to facilitate disintegration.

Mechanical or electrohydraulic lithotripsy may be necessary for the complete removal of large common duct stones (over 2 cm), however this should not be attempted during the initial treatment of acute cholangitis.

C. Percutaneous Transhepatic Cholangiography & Rendezvous Procedures

When endoscopic drainage is not possible, percutaneous transhepatic cholangiography (PTC) with drainage is indicated. The degree of urgency similarly depends on the clinical situation; however, emergent drainage should be performed if partial injection occurred on attempted ERCP. Since its introduction in 1974, PTC has evolved into numerous therapeutic interventions including stenting, stone removal, and in rare cases, even sphincterotomy. In the setting of acute cholangitis, the initial procedure is limited to drainage of the obstructed system. Definitive therapy with stone removal can be achieved on subsequent procedures. A wire may be placed through the transhepatic access and into the duodenum allowing for endoscopic stone removal; this is referred to as a rendezvous procedure. If endoscopic access to the biliary system is not possible, a series of procedures is typically required involving upsizing of drains and various methods of lithotripsy.

Endoscopic ultrasound (EUS) may also be used to access the biliary system and perform a rendezvous procedure, and is becoming more widely performed. In this procedure, a 19-gauge FNA needle is used to access the bile duct via a transduodenal or transgastric approach. Following aspiration, contrast may be injected through the needle and a wire passed. If the wire is placed successfully through the papilla and into the duodenum, it may be used to guide retrograde access and perform a rendezvous procedure. If the wire is unable to pass from the duct and into the duodenum, a stent may be placed antegrade into the bile duct (choledochoduodenostomy) as a temporary measure.

D. The Pregnant Patient with Cholangitis

Gallstones and their complications occur at increased rates during pregnancy because of decreased gallbladder motility and increased concentration of cholesterol in bile. Acute cholecystitis is the second most common indication for surgery in the pregnant patient, following appendicitis. If the diagnosis of choldedocholithiasis is unclear, MRCP is considered safe and does not require gadolinium, which is known to cross the placenta. In general, the management of pregnant patients with choledocholithiasis and cholangitis is the same as nonpregnant patients. Goal directed management of sepsis, including antibiotics, and ERCP are considered standard of care. However, the choice of antibiotic regimen, as well as radiation exposure and lead uterus shielding during ERCP should be carefully considered to prevent toxicity to the fetus. ERCP without fluoroscopy may be considered especially in the first trimester, when the fetus is most susceptible to defects in organogenesis.

E. Endoscopic Retrograde Cholangiopancreatography in the Gastric Bypass Patient

The Roux-en-Y Gastric Bypass is a commonly performed bariatric procedure and is efficacious at treating obesity and its associated comorbid conditions, such as diabetes mellitus. Owing to the extended distance between the gastric pouch and biliary system, which requires scope advancement through both the Roux and pancreaticobiliary limbs, ERCP scope lengths are typically unable to access the ampulla without device assistance. This has traditionally required surgical assistance in the operative room, where a laparoscopic approach guides endoscope insertion through a surgical enterotomy within the pancreaticobiliary limb. Since the development and evolution of lumen apposing metal stents (LAMS), however, an entirely endoscopic approach has become available via either the Gastric Access Temporary for Endoscopy (GATE) or EUS-directed transgastric ERCP (EDGE) procedures. This involves placing a LAMS to communicate the gastric pouch and remnant stomach, after which a duodenoscope can be passed for antegrade access to the pancreaticobiliary system. Although well-studied in the setting of nonurgent ERCP, the role of these approaches in the setting of cholangitis has not been evaluated to date.

Cappell MS, Stavropoulos SN, Friedel D. Systematic review of safety and efficacy of therapeutic endoscopic-retrograde-cholangiopancreatography during pregnancy including studies of radiation-free therapeutic endoscopic-retrograde-cholangiopancreatography. *World J Gastrointest Endosc.* 2018; 10(10):308–321. [PMID: 30364767]

Iwashita T, Yasuda I, Mukai T, et al. EUS-guided rendezvous for difficult biliary cannulation using a standardized algorithm: a multicenter prospective pilot study (with videos). *Gastrointest Endosc.* 2016;83(2):394–400. [PMID: 26089103]

Kedia P, Tyberg A, Kumta NA, et al. EUS-directed transgastric ERCP for Roux-en-Y gastric bypass anatomy: a minimally invasive approach. *Gastrointest Endosc.* 2015;82(3):560–565. [PMID: 25952086]

Manes G, Paspatis G, Aabakken L, et al. Endoscopic management of common bile duct stones: European Society of Gastrointestinal Endoscopy (ESGE) guideline. *Endoscopy.* 2019;51(5): 472–491. [PMID: 30943551]

Mayumi T, Okamoto K, Takada T, et al. Guidelines 2018: management bundles for acute cholangitis and cholecystitis. *J Hepatobiliary Pancreat Sci.* 2018;25(1):96–100. [PMID: 29090868]

Wang TJ, Thompson CC, Ryou M. Gastric access temporary for endoscopy (GATE): a proposed algorithm for EUS-directed transgastric ERCP in gastric bypass patients. *Surg Endosc.* 2019;33(6):2024–2033. [PMID: 30805786]

Surgical Drainage

Surgical biliary drainage carries significant risk of morbidity and a mortality rate as high as 40%. A surgical choledochotomy and T-tube drain placement has lower mortality than cholecystectomy with common bile duct exploration, however the risk is still greater than nonoperative biliary drainage. Operative management should be strictly reserved for cases in which endoscopic or percutaneous methods fail.

Arshad SA, Phuoc VH. Surgical palliation of biliary obstruction: bypass in the era of drainage. *J Surg Oncol.* 2019;120(1):65–66. [PMID: 30825212]

GALLSTONE PANCREATITIS

 ESSENTIALS OF DIAGNOSIS

► Diagnosis is guided by clinical evaluation and imaging studies (eg, MRCP).

► Endoscopic drainage and papillotomy is reserved for suspected ascending cholangitis, established choledocholithiasis, or deteriorating course.

Gallstone pancreatitis is defined as acute pancreatitis with clinical evidence of gallstones, in the absence of other causes of pancreatitis. A clinical definition is needed for this condition, since calculi are often challenging to demonstrate by abdominal imaging during an acute episode, and frequently pass spontaneously into the small bowel lumen. Although this is the most common cause of acute pancreatitis, the exact pathogenesis remains unclear, and in up to 30% of patients with acute pancreatitis, the cause is considered idiopathic.

Pathogenesis

Several theories have been proposed to explain the development of gallstone pancreatitis.

Gallstones can be identified in the stool of up to 94% of patients with acute gallstone pancreatitis compared with only 10% in patients with symptomatic cholelithiasis and no history of pancreatitis. The bile reflux theory, first postulated by Lancereaux in 1899, suggests that as stones pass through the ampulla it is disrupted allowing reflux of bile, and other duodenal contents, into the pancreatic duct with subsequent intraglandular pancreatic enzyme activation.

The association of an impacted gallstone at the ampulla of Vater and fatal acute pancreatitis, first described by Opie in 1901, prompted the development of the common channel theory. This theory suggests that impaction of a stone at the ampulla of Vater leads to increased biliary pressures that exceed pancreatic duct pressure, with secondary reflux of bile into the pancreatic duct. This theory is weakened by the fact that some patients do not have common channels, and by studies that have shown sterile bile does not activate proteolytic enzymes. Nevertheless, infected bile is a potent stimulator of these enzymes due to the presence of bacterial amidase and the theory remains popular.

A third theory, the obstructive theory, suggests an increase in pancreatic duct pressure alone due to complete pancreatic duct obstruction is sufficient to trigger gallstone pancreatitis. This has been suggested by various animal models and remains a favored concept.

The true pathogenesis is likely multifactorial and depending on patient anatomy and stone size, any one of these theories may be more applicable.

Clinical Findings

A. Symptoms & Signs

Although the diagnosis of acute gallstone pancreatitis is a clinical one, there are no signs or symptoms that are specific for the condition. A thorough history excluding other potential causes of pancreatitis is essential. Alcohol, elevated triglyceride or calcium levels, infectious agents, autoimmune disease, medications and hereditary etiologies should be considered.

B. Laboratory Findings

Once other etiologies have been excluded, the likelihood of gallstone pancreatitis must be determined. Several biochemical parameters have been evaluated with conflicting results.

Various studies have shown aspartate aminotransferase (AST), bilirubin, alkaline phosphatase, or γ-glutamyl transpeptidase (GGT) to be most sensitive at predicting gallstone pancreatitis; however, there is no consensus and none of these parameters are specific.

C. Imaging Studies

Several abdominal imaging modalities are available, and some are more useful than others at assisting with the diagnosis.

Abdominal ultrasound is capable of identifying gallstones with 92% accuracy, and has the advantages of being widely available, inexpensive, and noninvasive. However, as 10% of the adult population have gallstones, this is not adequate for the diagnosis of gallstone pancreatitis. Ultrasonography has a sensitivity between 55% and 91% for identifying bile duct dilation, which is associated with a higher prevalence of choledocholithiasis; however, this is highly operator-dependant and is not sensitive at detecting common duct stones.

Computed tomography (CT) is good at identifying cholelithiasis and can be used to measure common bile duct diameter. Additionally, helical CT cholangiography is an evolving technique that has sensitivities as high as 95% in diagnosing choledocholithiasis; however, the contrast agents required cause significant nausea, and the technique is not highly utilized.

MRCP is an accurate and noninvasive modality, with a sensitivity and specificity for detecting choledocholithiasis of 81–100% and 92–100%, respectively. Although MRCP is expensive and may not detect stones smaller than 5 mm, the technique is comparable to diagnostic ERCP and intraoperative cholangiography and has emerged as the noninvasive diagnostic modality of choice.

EUS also has sensitivity and specificity of 88–97% and 96–100%, respectively; however, the technique is invasive and requires sedation. Thus, the role of EUS is not well established in most centers where MRCP is available.

ERCP was historically the diagnostic procedure of choice with accuracy similar to MRCP; however, it is associated with complication rates as high as 15% that include cholangitis, pancreatitis, perforation, and bleeding. With improved accuracy and increased availability of less invasive modalities, ERCP is no longer considered to be a first-line diagnostic procedure.

Treatment

The management of acute gallstone pancreatitis has been controversial. Supportive care with aggressive intravenous hydration, nothing by mouth, and pain control is similar to the management of pancreatitis due to other etiologies; however, timing and method of common bile duct exploration for possible gallstone removal have been the focus of many studies. It is clear that ERCP is favored over surgery due to significantly better patient outcomes, with lower morbidity and mortality (Figure 33–1). The exact timing of ERCP has been more difficult to establish and depends on severity of illness. What appears to be consistent across most studies is that in patients with biliary pancreatitis and associated cholangitis, early drainage is indicated, typically within 48 hours of onset and after initial stabilization. Additionally, patients with clinical deterioration, as indicated by fever, increasing pain, and confusion, are likely to benefit from urgent ERCP. In patients without obstructive jaundice, early ERCP does not appear to be beneficial. Also, in patients with a mild course of biliary pancreatitis, up to 80% will have already passed the culprit stone and urgent ERCP is not recommended. A meta-analysis evaluated the role of early ERCP in patients with predicted severe acute pancreatitis, without cholangitis, which included three randomized trials, consisting of a total 450 patients. Subgroup analyses showed that early ERCP was not associated with improvement in overall complications or mortality from acute pancreatitis, regardless of predicted severity of pancreatitis. This was further supported by a more recent large randomized trial that demonstrated no benefit in early ERCP versus conservative management.

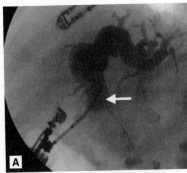 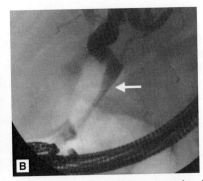

▲ **Figure 33–1. A.** Wire and stent deployment catheter within the common bile duct via transduodenal puncture (arrow). **B.** Palliative stent placed from the duodenum into the common bile duct to allow for decompression of the biliary system (arrow).

Additionally, although endoscopic sphincterotomy has been shown to be protective regarding future episodes of gallstone pancreatitis, cholecystectomy remains the standard of care. More than 25% of patients who do not undergo cholecystectomy will have a recurrent episode, or related biliary complication, within 6 weeks following an initial episode. Early cholecystectomy is safe, and the preferred timing is upon resolution of pancreatitis and prior to hospital discharge.

D. The Pregnant Patient with Gallstone Pancreatitis

While uncommon, acute biliary pancreatitis in the pregnant patient may occur and generally, as with nonpregnant patients, requires endoscopic intervention. Recurrence of pancreatitis during pregnancy is reported to occur in up to 70% of patients managed conservatively (ie, without intervention) and is associated with increased maternal and fetal mortality. Endoscopic sphincterotomy is recommended to protect against a recurrent event of pancreatitis and is generally considered safe in pregnancy.

ASGE Standards of Practice Committee, Buxbaum JL, Abbas Fehmi SM, Sultan S, et al. ASGE guideline on the role of endoscopy in the evaluation and management of choledocholithiasis. *Gastrointest Endosc.* 2019;89(6):1075–1105. [PMID: 30979521]

García de la Filia Molina I, García García de Paredes A, Martínez Ortega A, et al. Biliary sphincterotomy reduces the risk of acute gallstone pancreatitis recurrence in non-candidates for cholecystectomy. *Dig Liver Dis.* 2019;51(11):1567–1573. [PMID: 31151894]

Hernandez V, Pascual I, Almela P, et al. Recurrence of acute gallstone pancreatitis and relationship with cholecystectomy or endoscopic sphincterotomy. *Am J Gastroenterol.* 2004;99: 2417–2423. [PMID: 15571590]

Luthra AK, Patel KP, Li F, et al. Endoscopic intervention and cholecystectomy in pregnant women with acute biliary pancreatitis decrease early readmissions. *Gastrointest Endosc.* 2019;89(6):1169–1177. [PMID: 30503844]

Petrov MS, van Santvoort HC, Besselink MG, et al. Early endoscopic retrograde cholangiopancreatography versus conservative management in acute biliary pancreatitis without cholangitis a meta-analysis of randomized trials. *Ann Surg.* 2008;247:250–257. [PMID: 18216529]

Schepers NJ, Hallensleben NDL, Besselink MG, et al. Dutch Pancreatitis Study Group. Urgent endoscopic retrograde cholangiopancreatography with sphincterotomy versus conservative treatment in predicted severe acute gallstone pancreatitis (APEC): a multicentre randomised controlled trial. *Lancet.* 2020;396(10245):167–176. [PMID: 32682482]

BILE DUCT INJURIES

 ESSENTIALS OF DIAGNOSIS

► Bile duct leaks, transection, and occlusion from ligature or strictures occur most often after cholecystectomy.

► Diagnosis can be established by imaging, including ultrasound to identify fluid accumulations and hepatoiminodiacetic acid derivative (HIDA) scan to detect occlusion or active leakage.

Types of bile duct injuries include leaks, transection, occlusion (ligation or stricture), or a combination. The majority of bile duct injuries are iatrogenic, most commonly following laparoscopic cholecystectomy, with an incidence of 0.3–2%. Common reasons for injury include aberrant anatomy, inadequate exposure, and otherwise difficult cases. Additional causes of bile duct injury include other biliary surgery, liver biopsy, penetrating or blunt abdominal trauma, and, rarely, spontaneous perforation.

► **Clinical Findings**

Patients usually present with abdominal pain that may be diffuse or localized. Nausea, anorexia, and abdominal distention due to ileus may also be seen. Clinically apparent ascites and bile peritonitis are less common. Fever is often absent, and laboratory evaluation typically reveals leukocytosis and nonspecific liver function test abnormalities. Initial imaging studies should involve abdominal ultrasound to assess for fluid collections or abnormalities in the biliary tree such as focal dilation, and radionuclide biliary scintigraphy to assess for ongoing leakage. Technetium-99m–labeled HIDA scanning is most accurate, approaching 100%.

Treatment

Bile duct injuries were historically managed surgically, but with significant morbidity and mortality. Endoscopic intervention has replaced surgery in the majority of cases. The flow of bile is pressure dependent, and it will follow the path of least resistance. The objective of endoscopic therapy is to make the path to the duodenum that of lowest resistance. This requires stenting the sphincter of Oddi or sphincterotomy. The procedure reduces the leakage of bile and allows healing of the defect. Additionally, drainage of large fluid collections either surgically or percutaneously is important for prompt resolution of pain and prevention of infection.

The Bergman classification system is useful for grading severity and prognosticating response to therapy. Type A injuries are leaks from the cystic duct or the ducts of Luschka. They are typically mild and have a near-100% response rate to ERCP with sphincterotomy or stent placement (Figure 33–2). Type B lesions are of the common bile duct or main hepatic ducts, with or without stricturing. These may be amenable

to endoscopic therapy, with a 71% response rate to stenting. Bridging the defect with the stent is important for resolution of type B defects. Type C injuries consist of strictures without leak. Endoscopic stent placement is now considered the standard of care for these lesions. Costamagna and others have shown that upsizing and the use of multiple stents are critical to success. Type D injuries are complete transections of the biliary system. Diagnosis is best made by MRCP, and surgical hepaticojejunostomy is standard of care.

Boraschi P, Donati F, Pacciardi F, Ghinolfi D, Falaschi F. Biliary complications after liver transplantation: assessment with MR cholangiopancreatography and MR imaging at 3T device. *Eur J Radiol.* 2018;106:46–55. [PMID: 30150050]

Haidar H, Manasa E, Yassin K, Suissa A, Kluger Y, Khamaysi I. Endoscopic treatment of post-cholecystectomy bile leaks: a tertiary center experience. *Surg Endosc.* 2021;35(3):1088–1092. [PMID: 32107631]

Shin M, Joh JW. Advances in endoscopic management of biliary complications after living donor liver transplantation: comprehensive review of the literature. *World J Gastroenterol.* 2016;22(27):6173–6191. [PMID: 27468208]

Vlaemynck K, Lahousse L, Vanlander A, Piessevaux H, Hindryckx P. Endoscopic management of biliary leaks: a systematic review with meta-analysis. *Endoscopy.* 2019; 51(11):1074–1081. [PMID: 30759468]

Yang Q, Liu J, Ma W, et al. Efficacy of different endoscopic stents in the management of postoperative biliary strictures: a systematic review and meta-analysis. *J Clin Gastroenterol.* 2019;53(6):418–426. [PMID: 30807403]

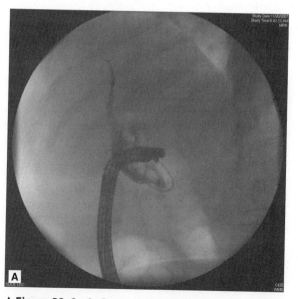
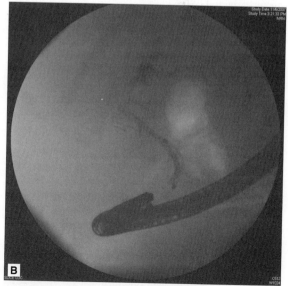

▲ **Figure 33–2.** **A.** Common bile duct stones in a patient with cholangitis. **B.** Stent placement adjacent to stones for temporary drainage.

PANCREATIC DUCT INJURIES

ESSENTIALS OF DIAGNOSIS

▶ Pancreatic duct injuries may be iatrogenic or occur after trauma or necrotizing pancreatitis.

▶ Diagnosis may be suspected on computed tomographic (CT) examination; however, MRCP is more specific.

The reported incidence of pancreatic injury is relatively low, ranging from 0.2% to 6% following abdominal trauma. However, the exact incidence is difficult to determine as many patients with significant abdominal trauma never have a laparotomy. Additionally, while the retroperitoneal location affords some degree of protection to the gland, it can also mask signs of significant injury.

The majority of affected patients are men under 40 years of age. Penetrating trauma is responsible for over 70% of traumatic injuries, with gunshot wounds and stabbings being most common. Location of injury following penetrating trauma is uniform among head and neck, body, and tail, with less than 5% having an injury at multiple sites. Blunt trauma is responsible for roughly 20% of injuries, with motor vehicle accidents accounting for the majority of cases. The distribution is similar to that of penetrating trauma, with a slight preponderance for pancreatic body injuries due to compression of the gland against the underlying spine at this location. Iatrogenic causes are also notable and are more commonly seen after pancreatic surgery, splenectomy, and ERCP.

Irrespective of the method of injury, the degree of injury ranges from simple contusion to complete transection, and typically results in local inflammation and fluid collections. Additionally, associated injury is typical and varies depending on location of injury. Penetrating injuries to the head are associated with major vascular injury in over 50% of cases. Hollow viscus injuries are also common, occurring nearly in 40% of cases, with liver and spleen injuries in less than 20% of cases. Overall mortality rates are between 10% and 31%, with over 50% of deaths occurring within 48 hours of presentation. Early mortality is typically due to associated injuries, with less than 10% due to pancreatic injury.

The majority of patients managed nonoperatively will develop a complication related to the pancreatic injury. Pseudocysts occur in up to 75% of patients who survive beyond 48 hours. Pancreatic fistula, pancreatitis, and peripancreatic abscess are also seen in roughly 30%. Although several organ injury grading systems exist, the most important factor in predicting clinical course and guiding therapy is the integrity of the main pancreatic duct. This is a key element of the diagnostic and management strategy.

▶ Clinical Findings

Presenting symptoms vary from minimal pain or nausea to frank peritonitis and hemodynamic instability. With severe presentations and penetrating wounds, imaging or laparotomy is requisite and diagnosis is relatively straightforward. Diagnosis is more challenging and often delayed with more subtle presentations or when other injuries serve as confounders.

A. Symptoms & Signs

Epigastric pain is the most common symptom following blunt pancreatic trauma, with a pattern of initial abatement followed by escalation over the subsequent 6–8 hours. Physical examination is neither sensitive nor specific, and even profound pancreatic injury may not be detected on initial examination. If pain is present, it is often out of proportion to tenderness, and guarding is unusual.

B. Laboratory Findings

No single laboratory test is adequate for early detection. Serum amylase at time of admission is unreliable. Elevation of serum amylase may be seen due to causes other than pancreatic trauma, including bowel injury, head trauma, alcohol ingestion, profound hypotension, and salivary gland damage. Early reports showed that only 8% of patients with elevated serum amylase at the time of admission were found to have pancreatic injury. In other series, only 14% of patients with confirmed pancreatic gland injury had elevated amylase at the time of admission. Additionally, isoenzymes were not found to significantly improve diagnostic accuracy in this setting. Serial amylase levels have, however, been found to be useful in identifying pancreatic injury and guiding management. As such, consistently normal serum amylase levels have a negative predictive value of 93–98%, and persistently abnormal or rising levels have sensitivity as high as 89%. Nevertheless, additional diagnostic modalities are typically needed.

C. Imaging Studies

Plain film radiographs and ultrasound are of limited value. Loss of a distinct psoas margin or a halo of air surrounding the kidney or psoas may suggest a retroperitoneal process, however, this is nonspecific.

Abdominal CT scan is useful and may have findings specific to the diagnosis, including pancreatic transaction, local hematoma, fluid separating the pancreas and splenic vein, pancreatic enlargement, and increased attenuation of the peripancreatic fat. In lieu of these, the admission CT scan may hold signs suggestive of pancreatic injury, including fluid in the lesser sac, thickening of the anterior renal fascia, and associated injuries to local structures. CT rarely shows ductal disruption. Sensitivity for detecting pancreatic injury by initial CT scan alone ranges from 60% to 80%, and repeat imaging may be helpful. Specificity is high, ranging from 80% to 100%, although CT tends to underestimate degree of injury.

MRCP is particularly reliable at identifying pancreatic injury and at characterizing type and degree of damage. Complete visualization of normal size main ducts occurs in 97% of patients. MRCP is excellent at clarifying ductal status and at detailing parenchymal injury. ERCP is no longer considered a first-line diagnostic option, due to its invasive nature.

Treatment

Management is dependent on type and degree of injury. Severe cases with associated injury to local structures usually require emergent surgery. In such cases, the first priority is control of hemorrhage followed by complete pancreatic evaluation. This requires significant tissue dissection and mobilization. If parenchymal damage is seen, the integrity of the main pancreatic duct must be assessed. Intraoperative pancreatography may be performed in a variety of ways and is effective at identifying ductal disruption. If ductal injury is not present, typical management involves debridement and wide external drainage. If ductal injury is identified, choice of procedure depends on location of the injury. For distal injuries, distal pancreatectomy is preferred. The surgical approach to proximal ductal injuries is more varied and duodenal diversion may be necessary.

ERCP with pancreatic stent placement is a less invasive alternative that should be considered when emergent surgery is not required and when disruption is suggested on imaging (Figure 33–3). Stent insertion is technically possible in 95% of cases, and outcomes appear to vary depending on the degree and location of disruption. Partial disruptions in the body and head appear to have the highest response rates. Additionally, placement of a stent that bridges the disruption is associated with better outcomes. In a recent series of 43 patients described by Telford and colleagues, multivariable analysis found that only bridging stent position was correlated with successful outcome. In this series bridging position was associated with a 92% success rate, compared with a 44% success rate for stents that merely cross the papilla. This is unlike the treatment of bile duct leaks, where elimination of the biliary duodenal pressure gradient by stenting across the papilla is sufficient. Patients with complete duct disruptions do not fare as well with endoscopic treatment; however, data are limited. Pancreatic duct stent placement is relatively safe and complications are well defined, including occlusion, migration, stricture formation, infection, and duodenal erosion. In a study by Varadarajulu and associates, a complication rate of 7.1% was seen for stent placement in the treatment of pancreatic duct disruption. Finally, pancreatic cyst drainage may be required and may be performed via a transgastric approach; however, fluid collection encapsulation takes several weeks and must occur before it is safe to proceed with endoscopic therapy.

Chen Y, Jiang Y, Qian W, et al. Endoscopic transpapillary drainage in disconnected pancreatic duct syndrome after acute pancreatitis and trauma: long-term outcomes in 31 patients. *BMC Gastroenterol.* 2019;19(1):54. [PMID: 30991953]

Das R, Papachristou GI, Slivka A, et al. Endotherapy is effective for pancreatic ductal disruption: a dual center experience. *Pancreatology.* 2016;16(2):278–283. [PMID: 26774205]

Varadarajulu S, Noone TC, Tutuian R, et al. Predictors of outcome in pancreatic duct disruption managed by endoscopic transpapillary stent placement. *Gastrointest Endosc.* 2005;61:568–575. [PMID: 15812410]

HEMORRHAGIC BILIARY & PANCREATIC CONDITIONS

Hemobilia and hemosuccus pancreaticus are rare and potentially life-threatening conditions that are typically considered late in the diagnostic evaluation of the bleeding patient. Each condition has specific etiologies, requiring a unique approach to diagnosis and management.

1. Hemobilia

 ESSENTIALS OF DIAGNOSIS

▶ Hemobilia can occur after trauma, gallstones, tumor, and vascular disorders and should be suspected in patients with hemorrhage, biliary colic, and jaundice.

▶ Diagnosis may be suggested by MRI with MRCP; however, selective arteriography is most accurate.

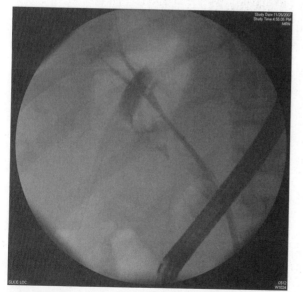

▲ **Figure 33–3.** Type A bile duct injury with extravasation of contrast from the cystic duct.

Hemobilia is an abnormal communication between blood vessels and bile ducts either within the liver or the extra-hepatic biliary tree. Clinical manifestations are due to blood loss and biliary obstruction from blood clots. Symptoms include melena in 90% and hematemesis in 60%, biliary colic in 70%, and jaundice in 60%. Simultaneous presence of the cardinal symptoms of melena, jaundice and abdominal pain is known as the Quincke triad, which is uncommonly present. The spectrum of hemobilia spans massive exsanguination precipitating hemorrhagic shock and minor recurrent hemobilia resulting in chronic anemia. Whenever biliary symptoms are present in the setting of gastrointestinal bleeding or anemia, the diagnosis should be considered.

Pathogenesis

Common causes of biliary-vascular fistula that lead to hemobilia include blunt or penetrating trauma, iatrogenic etiologies (especially after transjuguar or percutaneous liver biopsy), gallstones, tumors, and vascular disorders. Presentation may be immediate or several months after the inciting event. Additionally, parasites, choledochal cysts, portal hypertension, and blood coagulation defects may be implicated. Of these, iatrogenic causes are most common, with liver biopsy and PTC the most frequent.

When a communication is formed by one of these mechanisms, blood follows the path of least resistance and results in hemobilia. Blood clots may form leading to symptoms of biliary obstruction; however, bile has fibrinolytic properties that serve to dissolve clots and clear the duct of fibrin deposits. Clots are more likely to cause obstruction when they are sheltered from the bile stream as is the case with T-tubes or other biliary drains. Additionally, continuous hemorrhage with clot formation may exceed the rate of fibrinolysis leading to jaundice. The clots typically mold to the form of a luminal cast, and the consistency may vary from soft to well defined and firm.

In rare cases where the pressure in the biliary tree is greater than that of the vascular system, bilhemia occurs. This is typically seen with distal bile duct obstruction and low hepatic vein pressure. Symptoms include rapidly worsening jaundice and elevated direct bilirubin without increase in liver transaminases. Mortality rates in this rare condition are as high as 50 and ERCP with drainage is the initial therapy of choice, with surgery reserved for failed cases.

Clinical Findings

The diagnosis of hemobilia is typically readily made when considered in the differential. Upper endoscopy is essential to rule out other sources of bleeding, and use of a side-viewing duodenoscope for proper evaluation of the papilla is recommended. Biliary imaging to evaluate for clotted blood is also helpful. Ultrasonography has been used with success; however, MRI with MRCP is more sensitive and can show active bleeding. Selective arteriography is most accurate for verifying suspected hemobilia and specifically identifying the source. Blood clots may be seen at ERCP; however, endoscopic therapy is not a long-term solution for hemostasis.

Treatment

Treatment of hemobilia is dependent on the cause. Transarterial embolization is the preferred method for hepatic artery sources. Surgical ligature or resection is reserved for embolization failure and hemorrhage from the gallbladder. Liver resection may also be required for central liver rupture and some tumors. At the present time, ERCP is not an accepted therapeutic option for the treatment of hemobilia; however, ERCP is the preferred alternative for restoring biliary patency when the bile duct is obstructed with clots (Figure 33–4). If

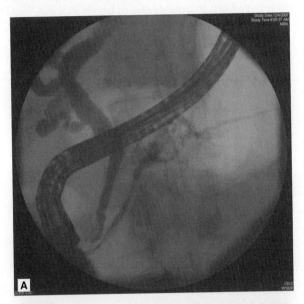

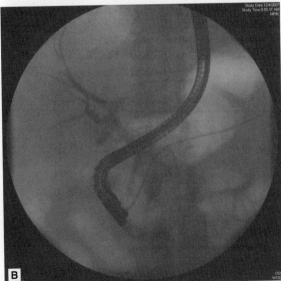

▲ **Figure 33–4. A.** Pancreatic duct disruption at genu. **B.** Stent bridging disruption.

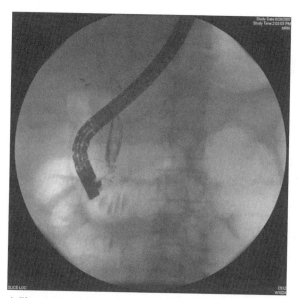

▲ **Figure 33–5.** Blood clot in bile duct seen in a patient with hemobilia.

bleeding stops spontaneously and treatment of obstruction is required prior to definitive bleeding therapy, stent placement may be preferable to sphincterotomy and clot extraction as the latter may lead to recurrent hemorrhage (Figure 33–5).

Cathcart S, Birk JW, Tadros M, Schuster M. Hemobilia: an uncommon but notable cause of upper gastrointestinal bleeding. *J Clin Gastroenterol.* 2017;51(9):796–804. [PMID: 28644311]

Feng W, Yue D, ZaiMing L, et al. Iatrogenic hemobilia: imaging features and management with transcatheter arterial embolization in 30 patients. *Diagn Interv Radiol.* 2016;22(4):371–377. [PMID: 27328719]

2. Hemosuccus Pancreaticus

Hemosuccus pancreaticus, or hemorrhage from the pancreatic duct, is also rare and management depends on the underlying cause. Episodic bleeding and sharp epigastric pain are the most common presenting symptoms. Anemia may be the only sign in up to 10% of patients. Endoscopy to evaluate for a clotted papilla is unreliable for diagnosis, and there is no endoscopic therapeutic option. Common etiologies include splenic artery aneurysm and chronic pancreatitis with pseudoaneurysm. Other less common causes include malignancy (Plate 77), acute pancreatitis, and pseudocyst. CT angiography is the diagnostic modality of choice and can make the diagnosis with high accuracy even in patients without active bleeding. Transarterial coil embolization is the suggested treatment for primary splenic artery aneurysms, whereas surgical arterial ligation and targeted pancreatectomy, pseudocyst resection or pancreaticoduodenectomy is indicated with persistent or massive bleeding.

Kitano M, Gress TM, Garg PK, et al. International consensus guidelines on interventional endoscopy in chronic pancreatitis. Recommendations from the working group for the international consensus guidelines for chronic pancreatitis in collaboration with the International Association of Pancreatology, the American Pancreatic Association, the Japan Pancreas Society, and European Pancreatic Club. *Pancreatology.* 2020;20(6): 1045–1055. [PMID: 32792253]

Mohan SC, Srinivasan S, Paul SPL, Chung R, Natarajan SK. Hemosuccus pancreatitis due to a ruptured splenic artery pseudoaneurysm - diagnosis and endovascular management. *J Radiol Case Rep.* 2020;14(5):7–15. [PMID: 33082922]

Yashavanth HS, Jagtap N, Singh JR, et al. Hemosuccus pancreaticus: a systematic approach. *J Gastroenterol Hepatol.* 2021;36(8): 2101–2106. [PMID: 33445212]

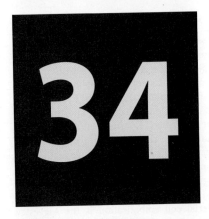

34

Endoscopic Retrograde Cholangiopancreatography (ERCP)

Russell D. Dolan, MD

David L. Carr-Locke, MA, MD

Christopher C. Thompson, MD

ESSENTIALS OF DIAGNOSIS

▶ Endoscopic Retrograde Cholangiopancreatography (ERCP) is a highly successful diagnostic and therapeutic modality, however, carries the risk of adverse events in up to 7% of cases.

▶ Functional Gallbladder Disorder and Functional Biliary Disorder have eclipsed prior definitions of Sphincter of Oddi disorders, for which ERCP is now uncommonly performed.

▶ ERCP remains an option for choledocholithiasis, bile leak, biliary strictures (both benign and malignant), and pancreatic duct strictures or stones.

General Considerations

ERCP is a combined endoscopic and fluoroscopic procedure introduced in the early 1970s to allow access to the biliary and pancreatic ductal systems and their openings at the major and minor duodenal papillae (Figure 34–1). ERCP has evolved from a purely diagnostic modality, performed by few, into a complex set of procedures offered in all major medical centers integrating diagnosis and therapy for a wide variety of pancreatobiliary disorders. For many of these, ERCP has become the minimally invasive treatment of choice when supported by prospective studies comparing it with the standard alternatives which, in the past, often involved open surgery. ERCP requires dedicated training in order to acquire the range of techniques that include endoscopic papillectomy, sphincter of Oddi manometry, biliary sphincterotomy, pancreatic sphincterotomy, stone removal, tissue sampling, placement of plastic and metallic stents, and drainage of pancreatic fluid collections. Although it has become a highly successful therapeutic modality, ERCP also carries a risk of adverse events of 7% or less that includes pancreatitis (4%), hemorrhage (1%), cholangitis (1%), perforation (0.5%), and

death (0.1%). Since the advent of magnetic resonance cholangiopancreatography (MRCP) (Figure 34–2) with dedicated ability to image the pancreatic and biliary tracts noninvasively and without risk, the need for purely diagnostic ERCP has appropriately diminished considerably and the demands for therapy have grown.

Cotton PB. Fifty years of ERCP: a personal review. *Gastrointest Endosc.* 2018;88(2):393–396. [PMID: 29654739]

Johnson KD, Perisetti A, Tharian B, et al. Endoscopic retrograde cholangiopancreatography-related complications and their management strategies: a "Scoping" literature review. *Dig Dis Sci.* 2020;65(2):361–375. [PMID: 31792671]

Welle CL, Miller FH, Yeh BM. Advances in MR imaging of the biliary tract. *Magn Reson Imaging Clin N Am.* 2020;28(3): 341–352. [PMID: 32624153]

DISORDERS OF THE MAJOR DUODENAL PAPILLA

1. Adenoma & Carcinoma

Small intestinal tumors represent 2.4% of all gastrointestinal malignancies and more than half of these are found in the duodenum. Duodenal adenomas occur in 50–100% of patients with familial adenomatous polyposis (FAP) and are most commonly in the periampullary location. Sporadic adenomas of the papilla also occur; like their genetic counterpart, they may be detected as an incidental finding during upper endoscopy performed for another indication or may manifest with recurrent pancreatitis, weight loss, or biliary obstruction. The frequency of carcinoma in papillary adenomas ranges from 30% to 65%.

Adenomas of the papilla follow the adenoma–carcinoma sequence similar to that seen in the colon; thus, resection of these lesions is recommended. Traditionally, the approach was wide radical resection by pancreaticoduodenectomy,

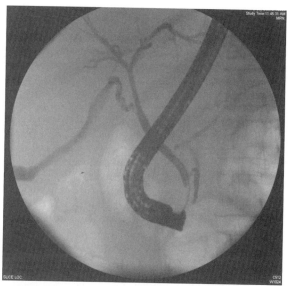

▲ **Figure 34–1.** ERCP radiograph showing standard endoscope position and normal biliary and pancreatic ductal systems.

because the presence of malignancy could not be completely excluded based on evaluation of preoperative biopsies. This resection was accompanied by significant morbidity and, even with improvements in surgery, local resection is currently the method of choice. Since the first reports of endoscopic resection of the papilla in the early 1990s, endoscopic papillectomy or ampullectomy has gained wider acceptance

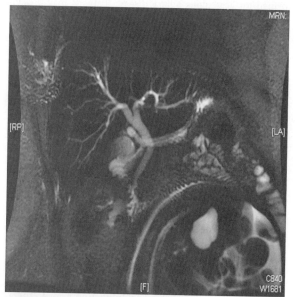

▲ **Figure 34–2.** MRCP image showing small distal common bile duct stones during late pregnancy.

as a less invasive treatment modality, particularly for patients with adenomas, small neuroendocrine tumors, and T1 cancers in poor operative candidates.

The technique involves inspection of the papilla with a side-viewing duodenoscope, and ERCP to define any intraductal tumor extension and to opacify the ducts with contrast to aid in identifying the ductal orifices after the procedure is completed. Most experts resect the papilla and surrounding normal mucosa en bloc with an electrocautery polypectomy snare and retrieve the specimen for histopathologic examination. Residual adenomatous tissue at the margins of the resection site can be ablated with contact thermal or noncontact argon plasma coagulation. After resection, a short polyethylene pancreatic stent is placed to minimize the risk of postprocedural pancreatitis, and many endoscopists also place a biliary stent if a sphincterotomy has not been performed (Plates 78, 79, and 80). The stents are endoscopically removed after 1 month, when the site is additionally inspected for residual adenoma. Surveillance endoscopy with a duodenoscope is offered every 6–12 months.

Accurate preoperative diagnosis and staging of papillary malignancies is essential. ERCP with biopsies and endoscopic ultrasound is the current accepted approach for diagnosis and staging of local invasion and assessment of lymph node status. Inoperable ampullary cancer causing biliary obstruction is best treated by sphincterotomy into the unaffected bile duct if feasible, or by placement of a self-expanding metal stent.

Kawashima H, Ohno E, Ishikawa T, et al. Endoscopic papillectomy for ampullary adenoma and early adenocarcinoma: analysis of factors related to treatment outcome and long-term prognosis. *Dig Endosc.* 2021;33(5):858–869. [PMID: 33107134]

Sulbaran M, Campos FG, Ribeiro U Jr, et al. Risk factors for advanced duodenal and ampullary adenomatosis in familial adenomatous polyposis: a prospective, single-center study. *Endosc Int Open.* 2018;6(5):E531–E540. [PMID: 29713679]

2. Functional Gallbladder & Biliary Disorders

The sphincter of Oddi is a complex muscular structure that surrounds the distal pancreatic duct, bile duct, and ampulla of Vater. This sphincter mechanism lies mostly within the duodenal wall and measures 6–10 mm in length. Functionally, the sphincter of Oddi is independent from the duodenal smooth muscle system. It serves to prevent reflux of duodenal contents into the ductal system and controls the flow of bile and pancreatic secretions into the duodenum.

Sphincter of Oddi dysfunction (SOD) had previously encapsulated a series of diagnoses to describe an abnormality within the sphincter, either motility related (dyskinesia or spasm) or structural (stenosis), which can involve the biliary sphincter, the pancreatic sphincter, or both. Whereas prior renditions of the Rome consensus criteria stratified between SOD types I–III depending on the presence of serologic abnormalities, onset of pancreatitis and biliary duct dilatation, definitions of functional pancreaticobiliary disorders have altered more recently. A major criterion is the presence of biliary-type pain, which is characterized by a crescendo in intensity to a steady level that lasts 30 minutes or greater, occurring at varying intervals (not daily), not significantly related to either bowel movements, postural change or change with acid suppression and severe enough to disrupt daily activities.

Functional Gallbladder Disorder

Functional gallbladder disorder requires the presence of biliary-type pain in the absence of gallstones or other structural pathology. The diagnosis is further supported by a reduced gallbladder ejection fraction on scintigraphy and normal liver enzymes, bilirubin or pancreas enzymes, however these are not required for the diagnosis. Evaluation with abdominal ultrasound, potentially complemented with EUS, should be considered to evaluate for gallstones, polyps or alternative organic etiologies. It is important to distinguish functional gallbladder disorder from other functional pancreaticobiliary disorders, as there is currently no role for ERCP in its management.

Functional Biliary Sphincter Disorder

Suspected functional biliary sphincter disorder has eclipsed prior definitions of SOD, which differentiated between types I–III depending on serologic and imaging abnormalities, in part to differentiate between therapeutic approaches. The updated Rome IV criteria now suggest that patients with formerly type I SOD truly have organic stenosis and therefore benefit from sphincterotomy. Contrarily, individuals with postcholecystectomy pain and objective findings of either elevated liver enzymes or dilated CBD on imaging and exclusion of organic causes are now considered as "suspected functional biliary sphincter disorder," whereas the formerly termed type III SOD is abandoned. Suspected FBSD patients may be considered for ERCP if noninvasive imaging has exonerated organic causes. Sphincter function can be evaluated by noninvasive methods that include hepatobiliary scintigraphy, ultrasound assessment of pancreatic and bile duct after secretin or cholecystokinin stimulation, and secretin stimulated MRCP. In general, although manometry had been a prior gold standard and can be considered in these patients, it is uncommonly performed in favor of empiric ERCP sphincterotomy. This approach must be pursued in caution, however, as the rate of complications is high in patients undergoing endoscopic sphincterotomy for sphincter of Oddi-related pain and can vary between 10% and 22%, with pancreatitis as the most common. Subsequently, there remains no consensus to management and further studies are required to guide management.

Pancreatic Sphincter of Oddi Disorder

The concept of sphincter hypertension precipitating increased pressures within the pancreatic duct, and subsequently causing pancreatic pain is an attractive theory, however currently speculative in terms of diagnosis and management. This entity exists within the Rome IV criteria for gallbladder and sphincter of Oddi disorders, with defining criteria including all of recurrent pancreatitis without alternative etiology, negative EUS, and abnormal sphincter manometry. However, this is a challenging diagnosis to confirm given risks associated with sphincter manometry. Whether abnormal sphincter function exists as an etiology to pancreatitis remains uncertain, however, as an additional theory poses that sphincter dysfunction is rather an epiphenomenon in response to prior episodes of pancreatitis. Further research is required to define this entity and provide further guidance on approach and management.

Cotton PB, Elta GH, Carter CR, Pasricha PJ, Corazziari ES. Rome IV. Gallbladder and sphincter of oddi disorders. *Gastroenterology.* 2016:S0016-5085(16)00224-9. [PMID: 27144629]

Cotton PB, Pauls Q, Keith J, et al. The EPISOD study: long-term outcomes. *Gastrointest Endosc.* 2018;87(1):205–210. [PMID: 28455162]

BILIARY SYSTEM

1. Bile Duct Stones

Bile duct stones occur in up to 15% of symptomatic patients with cholelithiasis and in up to 2% of cholecystectomies performed for acalculous biliary disease. Patients may present with abdominal pain of biliary origin (erroneously termed biliary colic), cholangitis, jaundice, pancreatitis, transient elevation of transaminases, or filling defect with or without biliary ductal dilation on imaging studies such as transabdominal ultrasound, computed tomography (CT), and MRCP. When choledocholithiasis is suspected, therapy is directed toward extraction of the stones from the biliary tree to minimize serious complications such as severe pancreatitis, sepsis, and death. Stone extraction can be achieved endoscopically, surgically, or by the transhepatic approach radiologically.

Endoscopic removal of bile duct stones is the first-line therapy of choice in centers that have expertise in this technique (Figure 34–3). Since the first descriptions of endoscopic sphincterotomy in 1974, the role of ERCP in the management of bile duct stones has undergone tremendous growth. The standard techniques of stone extraction can achieve success in up to 90% of bile duct stones. The remaining 10% of cases require more advanced techniques. Patients generally receive monitored anesthesia care or general anesthesia with endotracheal intubation prior to therapeutic ERCP. Access to the bile duct by deep cannulation is

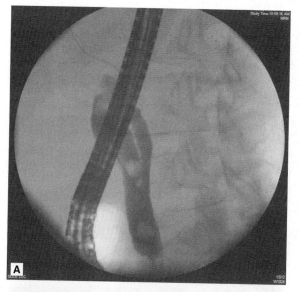

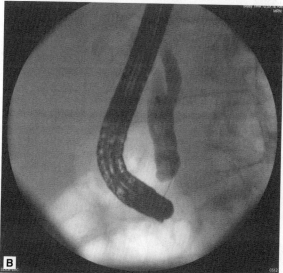

▲ **Figure 34–3.** ERCP images showing (**A**) bile duct stones being extracted by (**B**) basket.

Multivariate analysis of large series of sphincterotomies has shown that five risk factors for complications are significant: suspected SOD, cirrhosis, difficult bile duct cannulation, precut (access) papillotomy, and use of a combined percutaneous-endoscopic procedure. The rate of complications was highest when the indication for the procedure was suspected SOD (22%) and lowest when the indication was removal of bile duct stones within 30 days of laparoscopic cholecystectomy (5%). Endoscopists who performed more than one sphincterotomy per week had lower rates of all complications (8.4% vs 11.1%, $P = 0.03$) and severe complications (0.9% vs 2.3%, $P = 0.01$) than those who did less than one per week.

As an alternative to sphincterotomy, endoscopic balloon dilation of the papilla was introduced in the 1980s. This involves the use of a hydrostatic balloon positioned across the papilla and inflated under high pressure while dilation is monitored fluoroscopically. The potential advantages over endoscopic sphincterotomy are preservation of the sphincter and possible reduction of long-term complications.

When comparing endoscopic balloon dilation with sphincterotomy in the treatment of bile duct stones, there are similar outcomes in overall complications and success rates. Although there was a prior concern for higher rates of post-procedural pancreatitis with balloon dilation (7.4% vs 4.3%), more recently studies have subsequently alleyed this concern and shown risk of postprocedural pancreatitis is similar between sphincterotomy and balloon dilation. Mechanical lithotripsy may also be required for large stones, generally when greater than 1.5–2 cm. Most recently, however, evidence suggests balloon dilation following sphincterotomy is associated with increased success at stone removal, significant reduction in adverse events, reduced need for mechanical lithotripsy and shorter procedural times compared to endoscopic sphincterotomy alone.

Unless temporary drainage, only, is considered expedient, an attempt at stone extraction should always be made after a biliary sphincterotomy. The most commonly used accessories for this purpose are balloon catheters and metal wire baskets (see Figure 34–3). Stones larger than 15 mm present a challenge and often require additional endoscopic techniques such as mechanical, electrohydraulic, or laser lithotripsy. When complete stone removal fails, insertion of a biliary stent provides temporary drainage, minimizing the risk of biliary sepsis before further endoscopic attempts at duct clearance can be made. Long-term biliary drainage in the old or frail patient has now been questioned as a safe alternative to clearance because the cholangitis and cholecystitis rates are unacceptably high.

Hepatolithiasis, the presence of stones in the intrahepatic biliary tree above the hepatic duct confluence, is difficult to treat and poses a major challenge to the endoscopist in countries where this is common. Surgery is often required but rarely solves the problem as stone recurrence is high.

mandatory in order to achieve endoscopic therapy. When biliary access is difficult there are several technical options to gain entry to the bile duct, including access papillotomy. Once stones are identified on a cholangiogram, a biliary sphincterotomy (incision of the intraduodenal portion of the common bile duct sphincter muscle) is usually performed to the maximum extent of endoscopic landmarks and under direct endoscopic guidance and is achieved with a bow-type sphincterotome, a catheter carrying a cutting electrosurgical wire at its distal end.

Dong SQ, Singh TP, Zhao Q, Li JJ, Wang HL. Sphincterotomy plus balloon dilation versus sphincterotomy alone for choledocholithiasis: a meta-analysis. *Endoscopy.* 2019;51(8):763–771. [PMID: 30786316]

Karsenti D, Coron E, Vanbiervliet G, et al. Complete endoscopic sphincterotomy with vs. without large-balloon dilation for the removal of large bile duct stones: randomized multicenter study. *Endoscopy.* 2017;49(10):968–976. [PMID: 28753698]

Park JS, Jeong S, Lee DK, et al. Comparison of endoscopic papillary large balloon dilation with or without endoscopic sphincterotomy for the treatment of large bile duct stones. *Endoscopy.* 2019;51(2):125–132. [PMID: 29969808]

2. Cholelithiasis with Choledocholithiasis

When patients present with the combined problem of gallstones in the gallbladder and bile duct simultaneously, there are two questions to answer: (1) what is the best method for clearing the bile duct and (2) what should be done with the gallbladder? The sequential options are (1) laparoscopic cholecystectomy with laparoscopic bile duct exploration, (2) laparoscopic or open cholecystectomy followed by postoperative ERCP, (3) preoperative ERCP followed by cholecystectomy (laparoscopic or open), (4) open cholecystectomy with open exploration of the bile duct, (5) ERCP and no cholecystectomy, and, in special circumstances, (6) a range of additional and much less commonly used surgical and nonsurgical techniques such as percutaneous cholecystostomy, percutaneous access to the bile duct (including percutaneous cholangioscopy), techniques for Mirizzi syndrome, management of hepatolithiasis, and approaches to recurrent stones after biliary and nonbiliary upper gastrointestinal surgery. It is unlikely that one option will be appropriate for all clinical circumstances in all centers in all countries because the variables of disease states, patient demographics, and risk stratifications; available endoscopic, radiologic, and surgical expertise; patient preferences; and health care economics will all have significant influences on practice.

In patients with contemporaneous cholelithiasis and choledocholithiasis, it is usually the latter that dominates the acute clinical presentation and leads to intervention for pain, obstructive jaundice, cholangitis, pancreatitis, or any combination thereof. Less commonly, asymptomatic bile duct stones are discovered incidentally on noninvasive imaging for nonbiliary indications, during evaluation of symptomatic cholelithiasis, or intraoperatively during cholecystectomy. Since the universal adoption of laparoscopic cholecystectomy as the primary method for treating cholelithiasis in the early 1990s, only a minority of surgeons have mastered the techniques required for laparoscopic transcystic or direct choledochal exploration to treat choledocholithiasis and there has been some reluctance to convert to open bile duct exploration for this indication. Since ERCP has become the standard approach for acute presentations of choledocholithiasis in the 1980s and with the overall success of endoscopic bile duct clearance, the question of treating choledocholithiasis surgically has become a secondary issue.

Although there is evidence that elective and emergent clearance of the bile duct by ERCP had advantages over open bile duct exploration, the comparison of ERCP therapy with laparoscopic bile duct clearance is much more equivalent for most stones in the elective setting. Unfortunately, this surgical option is not always available, and the evidence is therefore tempered by local expertise. Following endoscopic bile duct clearance, the decision to leave the gallbladder in situ and follow the patient expectantly (option 5, earlier) compared with routine laparoscopic cholecystectomy has been questioned as there is an unacceptably high incidence of cholecystitis unless the gallbladder is empty. Where the expertise is available, elective management of cholelithiasis and choledocholithiasis by the laparoscopic approach is optimal. The role for ERCP in acute calculous disease remains central to the management of biliary disease.

ASGE Standards of Practice Committee, Buxbaum JL, Abbas Fehmi SM, Sultan S, et al. ASGE guideline on the role of endoscopy in the evaluation and management of choledocholithiasis. *Gastrointest Endosc.* 2019;89(6):1075–1105.e15. [PMID: 30979521]

3. Mirizzi Syndrome

First described by Mirizzi in 1948, this syndrome is a rare complication of gallstone disease and refers to stone impaction in the neck of the gallbladder or the cystic duct, with subsequent inflammation and extrinsic compression of the main bile duct leading to obstructive jaundice and cholangitis (Figure 34–4). Type I refers to extrinsic compression of the main bile duct secondary to a stone in the cystic duct or

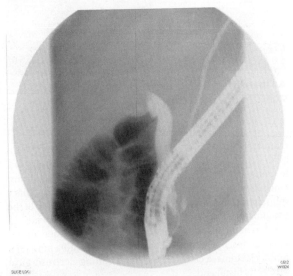

▲ **Figure 34–4.** ERCP image of Mirizzi syndrome.

gallbladder, and type II occurs when there is cholecystocho-ledochal fistula.

Treatment of Mirizzi syndrome has traditionally been surgical. Endoscopic management consists of drainage and decompression of the bile duct or gallbladder, or both, prior to surgical intervention but can be definitive if the impacted stone can be fragmented and removed.

ASGE Standards of Practice Committee, Buxbaum JL, Abbas Fehmi SM, Sultan S, et al. ASGE guideline on the role of endoscopy in the evaluation and management of choledocholithiasis. *Gastrointest Endosc.* 2019;89(6):1075–1105.e15. [PMID: 30979521]

4. Benign Bile Duct Strictures

Benign biliary strictures have many causes, with the most common being anastomosis, operative injury, and chronic pancreatitis. Patients present with cholestasis, cholangitis, or, rarely, secondary biliary cirrhosis. In the past, surgical management was the standard approach, with an associated morbidity and mortality, but currently endoscopic therapy with dilation and stenting offers a less invasive and an effective line of therapy (Figure 34–5). The insertion of multiple biliary stents, to achieve maximum dilation for the diameter of the bile duct distal to the stricture, has gained increasing acceptance and carries a 90% success rate in the short term with a less than 10% complication rate. The use of self-expanding metal stents in benign bile duct strictures had not been advocated until availability of covered stents, which are potentially removable.

Bill JG, Mullady DK. Stenting for Benign and Malignant Biliary Strictures. *Gastrointest Endosc Clin N Am.* 2019;29(2):215–235. [PMID: 30846150]

Ma MX, Jayasekeran V, Chong AK. Benign biliary strictures: prevalence, impact, and management strategies. *Clin Exp Gastroenterol.* 2019;12:83–92. [PMID: 30858721]

5. Malignant Bile Duct Strictures

Biliary obstruction secondary to malignant bile duct stricture of pancreatic, biliary, or metastatic origin is now usually palliated by stent placement. Polyethylene plastic stents are placed into the bile duct of patients with tumors that may be surgically resectable, and during initial evaluation when histologic or cytologic findings are not yet available. Patients with locally advanced and metastatic tumors of biliopancreatic origin and those who are poor surgical candidates are suitable candidates for metal stents (Figure 34–6). Self-expandable metal stents (SEMS) are commonly used for their ease of deployment, high patency rate, and cost-effectiveness despite the high cost of individual stents, because the reintervention rate is drastically reduced compared with plastic stents. Metal stents remain patent twice as long as polyethylene stents, a median of about 270 days versus 125 days. Unlike plastic stents, SEMS occlude not from a bacterial biofilm but from tumor ingrowth or over-growth, tissue hyperplasia at the ends of the stent, and migration. Uncovered SEMS have a higher occlusion rate, but lower migration rate compared with covered ones.

Tissue sampling of bile duct strictures is important in defining their nature (benign vs malignant) and can be achieved by forceps biopsy, brush cytology, and needle aspiration. Biliary brush cytology is the most common method of sampling and has low sensitivity of 30–60% but a specificity of over 90%. The sensitivity for brush cytology is higher for primary bile duct tumors (80–86%) and when combined with biopsies of the stricture (63%). Additional molecular

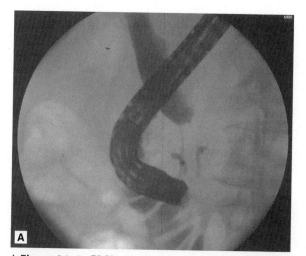 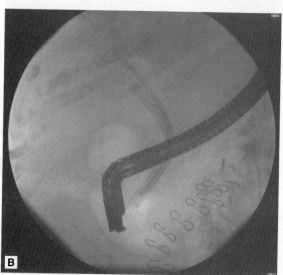

▲ **Figure 34–5.** ERCP sequence showing **(A)** benign biliary stricture and **(B)** placement of multiple plastic stents.

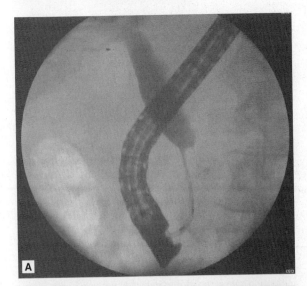

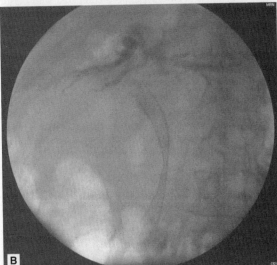

▲ **Figure 34–6.** ERCP images showing (**A**) malignant biliary obstruction and (**B**) placement of a self-expanding metallic stent.

techniques such as fluorescence in situ hybridization, digital image analysis, flow cytometry, and next generation sequencing may improve accuracy.

Bill JG, Mullady DK. Stenting for benign and malignant biliary strictures. *Gastrointest Endosc Clin N Am.* 2019;29(2):215–235. [PMID: 30846150]

Dumonceau JM, Tringali A, Papanikolaou IS, et al. Endoscopic biliary stenting: indications, choice of stents, and results: European Society of Gastrointestinal Endoscopy (ESGE) Clinical Guideline - Updated October 2017. *Endoscopy.* 2018;50(9):910–930. [PMID: 30086596]

Singhi AD, Nikiforova MN, Chennat J, et al. Integrating next-generation sequencing to endoscopic retrograde cholangio-pancreatography (ERCP)-obtained biliary specimens improves the detection and management of patients with malignant bile duct strictures. *Gut.* 2020;69(1):52–61. [PMID: 30971436]

6. Bile Leak

Injury to the bile duct is a well-recognized complication of cholecystectomy. Postoperative bile leak occurs in up to 0.5% of patients after open cholecystectomy and up to 1% after laparoscopic cholecystectomy, and cystic duct leaks are the most common type. Patients may present with abdominal pain, abdominal tenderness, fever, and continued drainage through a drain when present. ERCP is the most accurate technique in defining the biliary anatomy, delineating the site of the leak, and providing definitive therapy (Figure 34–7), which is highly successful. Endoscopic therapy is most commonly achieved by stent placement to decrease the pressure gradient between the bile duct and duodenum, allowing preferential flow of bile through the transpapillary route and sealing of the leak site. The stent does not have to cross the leak site unless there is a major bile duct injury.

Haidar H, Manasa E, Yassin K, Suissa A, Kluger Y, Khamaysi I. Endoscopic treatment of post-cholecystectomy bile leaks: a tertiary center experience. *Surg Endosc.* 2021;35(3):1088–1092. [PMID: 32107631]

Vlaemynck K, Lahousse L, Vanlander A, Piessevaux H, Hindryckx P. Endoscopic management of biliary leaks: a systematic review with meta-analysis. *Endoscopy.* 2019;51(11):1074–1081. [PMID: 30759468]

7. Bile Duct Cysts

Choledochal cysts are congenital anomalies typically seen in children and young adults but can be diagnosed at any age. They may affect the intrahepatic biliary tree, extrahepatic biliary tree, or both. They occur in 1 in 13,000 to 1 in 2,000,000 live births and are three times more common in females than in males.

The cysts are commonly classified into five types, with type I the most common and type V the least. Type I (80–90%) involves the extrahepatic bile duct and is subclassified into IA (common type), IB (segmental dilation), and IC (diffuse dilation). Type II (2%) is a diverticulum in the main bile duct. Type III cysts (1.4–5%) involve the intraduodenal portion of the bile duct and are also referred to as choledochoceles. Type IV (13%) is the second most common type and more frequently seen in adults. It is subclassified into IVA (multiple intrahepatic and extrahepatic cysts) and IVB (multiple extrahepatic cysts). Type V (<1%), or Caroli disease, refers to single or multiple dilations of intrahepatic bile ducts (Figure 34–8).

Anomalous pancreatobiliary union (APBU) is frequently associated with a long common channel (>15 mm). The risk of biliary malignancy (gallbladder and bile duct) is increased

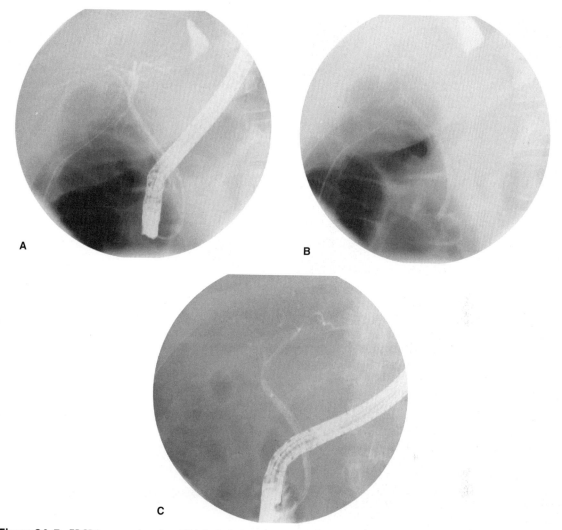

▲ **Figure 34–7.** ERCP images showing (**A**) bile leak after partial left hepatectomy, (**B**) treatment by a short 10-French plastic stent, and (**C**) no leak present at the time of stent removal.

when APBU is present, with an overall risk of 14% in patients with choledochal cysts and 50% in those without. The classic presenting symptoms and signs of jaundice, abdominal mass, and pain are more common in children than adults (82% vs 25%, respectively). Adults often present with vague abdominal pain, cholecystitis, cholangitis, and pancreatitis.

Many choledochal cysts are detected on imaging studies such as abdominal ultrasonography and CT scan done for other reasons. ERCP usually establishes the diagnosis, classifies bile duct cysts, and detects the presence of APBU, but MRCP is increasingly being used as a noninvasive imaging modality as it has an accuracy rate of 96% for choledochal cyst detection.

Surgical management (cyst excision and biliary reconstruction) is the recommended approach for all except type III cysts to avoid the risk of biliary tract malignancy.

Management of choledochocele by biliary sphincterotomy has been recommended.

Ronnekleiv-Kelly SM, Soares KC, Ejaz A, Pawlik TM. Management of choledochal cysts. *Curr Opin Gastroenterol.* 2016;32(3):225–231. [PMID: 26885950]

PANCREAS

1. Gallstone Pancreatitis

The goal of therapeutic ERCP in the setting of acute gallstone pancreatitis is to clear the bile duct of stones that, if left in place, may worsen the severity of pancreatitis and increase

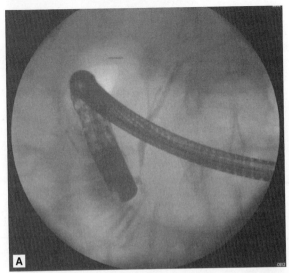
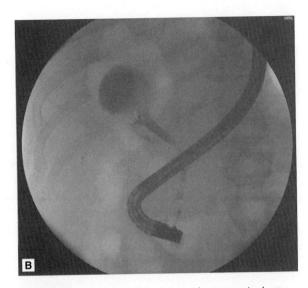

A Figure 34–8. ERCP images of choledochal cysts. **A.** Type 1 with anomalous union of the bile and pancreatic ducts. **B.** Type 5 with a single large intrahepatic cyst.

the risk of further attacks. The role of urgent ERCP and sphincterotomy in gallstone pancreatitis has clearly been shown to improve morbidity and mortality in patients with severe attacks but has little or no benefit in patients with mild pancreatitis as the majority of these patients pass the stones spontaneously and recover with supportive care. Meta-analyses of all randomized prospective studies have shown that ERCP with endoscopic sphincterotomy reduces morbidity and mortality of patients with acute biliary pancreatitis and treating 26 such patients is predicted to save one life. Tables 34–1 and 34–2 summarize the results. Cholecystectomy should be planned for the same admission, if possible, but can be delayed after

sphincterotomy as this confers a degree of protection from further pancreatitis.

Acosta JM, Katkhouda N, Debian KA, et al. Early ductal decompression versus conservative management for gallstone pancreatitis with ampullary obstruction: a prospective randomized clinical trial. *Ann Surg.* 2006;243:33–40. [PMID: 16371734]

Schepers NJ, Hallensleben NDL, Besselink MG, et al.; Dutch Pancreatitis Study Group. Urgent endoscopic retrograde cholangiopancreatography with sphincterotomy versus conservative treatment in predicted severe acute gallstone pancreatitis (APEC): a multicentre randomised controlled trial. *Lancet.* 2020;396(10245):167–176. [PMID: 32682482]

Table 34–1. ERCP in mild biliary pancreatitis.

Country	N	Morbidity (%)		Mortality (%)	
		ERCP	Conventional	ERCP	Conventional
United Kingdom[a]	68	11.8	11.8	0	0
Hong Kong[b]	69	17.6	17.1	0	0
Poland[c]	155	10.0[e]	25.3	0	5.3
Germany[d]	160	41.7	47.4	2.4	0

[a]Data from Neoptolemos JP, Carr-Locke DL, London NJ, et al. Controlled trial of urgent endoscopic retrograde cholangiopancreatography and endoscopic sphincterotomy versus conservative treatment for acute pancreatitis due to gallstones. *Lancet.* 1988;2:979–983.
[b]Data from Fan ST, Lai EC, Mok FP, et al. Early treatment of acute biliary pancreatitis by endoscopic papillotomy. *N Engl J Med.* 1993;328:228–232.
[c]Data from Nowak A, Marek TA, Nowakowska-Dulawa E, et al. Biliary pancreatitis needs endoscopic retrograde cholangiopancreatography with endoscopic sphincterotomy for cure. *Endoscopy.* 1998;30:A256–A259.
[d]Data from Folsch UR, Nitsche R, Ludtke R, et al. Early ERCP and papillotomy compared with conservative treatment for acute biliary pancreatitis. The German Study Group on Acute Biliary Pancreatitis. *N Engl J Med.* 1997;336:237–242.
[e]$P < 05$ compared with conventional treatment.

Table 34–2. ERCP in severe biliary pancreatitis.

Country	N	Morbidity (%)		Mortality (%)	
		ERCP	Conventional	ERCP	Conventional
United Kingdom[a]	53	24.0[e]	60.7	4.0	17.9
Hong Kong[b]	58	13.3	53.6	0	17.9
Poland[c]	50	39.1[e]	74.0	4.3[a]	33.3
Germany[d]	46	65.4	70.0	23.1	14.3

[a]Data from Neoptolemos JP, Carr-Locke DL, London NJ, et al. Controlled trial of urgent endoscopic retrograde cholangiopancreatography and endoscopic sphincterotomy versus conservative treatment for acute pancreatitis due to gallstones. *Lancet.* 1988;2:979–983.
[b]Data from Fan ST, Lai EC, Mok FP, et al. Early treatment of acute biliary pancreatitis by endoscopic papillotomy. *N Engl J Med.* 1993;328:228–232.
[c]Data from Nowak A, Marek TA, Nowakowska-Dulawa E, et al. Biliary pancreatitis needs endoscopic retrograde cholangiopancreatography with endoscopic sphincterotomy for cure. *Endoscopy.* 1998;30:A256–A259.
[d]Data from Folsch UR, Nitsche R, Ludtke R, et al. Early ERCP and papillotomy compared with conservative treatment for acute biliary pancreatitis. The German Study Group on Acute Biliary Pancreatitis. *N Engl J Med.* 1997;336:237–242.
[e]P <05 compared with conventional treatment.

2. Nonbiliary Acute Pancreatitis

ERCP plays a role in delineating and treating rare causes of pancreatitis, such as ampullary adenoma, pancreas divisum, autoimmune disease, rare tumors, and helminths if not detected by noninvasive imaging.

3. Chronic Pancreatitis

Chronic pancreatitis is a progressive disease characterized by persistent inflammation, fibrosis, atrophy of the gland, and ductal abnormalities. Chronic pancreatitis causes significant morbidity related to chronic abdominal pain, loss of exocrine and endocrine function, and complications such as pancreatic stones, strictures, and fluid collections.

Pancreatic duct pressure may be elevated secondary to strictures, stones, or outflow obstruction at the level of the major papilla. The goal of therapeutic ERCP is to decompress the pancreatic ductal system and relieve the obstruction with the hope of minimizing attacks of recurrent pancreatitis and alleviating chronic abdominal pain.

Benign strictures and stone disease of the main pancreatic duct (Figure 34–9) can result in ductal hypertension, which may be the basis of relapsing pain and recurrent pancreatitis. Strictures are treated by balloon or catheter dilation and insertion of one or more plastic stents that are exchanged every 2–4 months for up to 1 year. Stone extraction is technically feasible if the stones are small, few in number, located in the head of the pancreas, and not impacted. A pancreatic sphincterotomy is usually required, and the stones are removed with a basket or balloon. Stones located in the upstream duct proximal to a stricture require stricture dilation prior to extraction. Direct pancreatoscopy and electrohydraulic lithotripsy of pancreatic duct stones has been advocated as an additional option, and extracorporeal shock wave lithotripsy in treatment of refractory stones has also been used successfully. Most studies have shown an overall long-term improvement in about 67% of patients who undergo endoscopic therapy.

Dumonceau JM, Delhaye M, Tringali A, et al. Endoscopic treatment of chronic pancreatitis: European Society of Gastrointestinal Endoscopy (ESGE) Guideline - Updated August 2018. *Endoscopy.* 2019;51(2):179–193. [PMID: 30654394]

4. Pancreatic Ductal Disruption & Fluid Collection

Pancreatic duct disruption and fluid collections can be the result of acute or chronic pancreatitis. A pseudocyst is

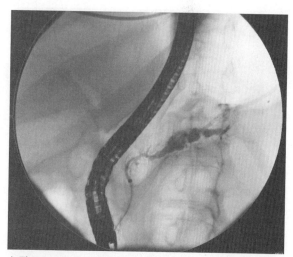

▲ **Figure 34–9.** ERCP showing chronic pancreatitis with narrowed main duct in the head, ectatic side branches, and an irregular dilated main pancreatic duct in the body and tail. A transgastric stent is in place.

a collection of amylase-rich pancreatic juice enclosed by a wall of nonepithelialized, fibrous, or granulation tissue. Symptomatic pseudocysts may be drained percutaneously (radiologically), surgically, or endoscopically. Endoscopic drainage of pancreatic pseudocysts and pancreatic necrosis can be performed by using transpapillary or transmural (transgastric, transduodenal) placement of endoprostheses. The transpapillary approach is utilized for pseudocysts communicating with the main pancreatic duct, with the tip of the stent positioned in the cyst cavity after a pancreatic sphincterotomy. Fluid collections not clearly communicating with the pancreatic duct are drained using the transmural approach. The goal is to establish a communication between the cyst cavity and gastric or duodenal lumen for continuous drainage of pancreatic juice. The major prerequisite for such a procedure is a distance between the cyst and gastrointestinal tract of 10 mm or less and an obvious bulge on endoscopy or a "window" for needle puncture demonstrated on endoscopic ultrasound (Figure 34–10, Plates 81 and 82), which also permits detection of varices or other vascular structures (eg, pseudoaneurysm) that may impede access or create a complication.

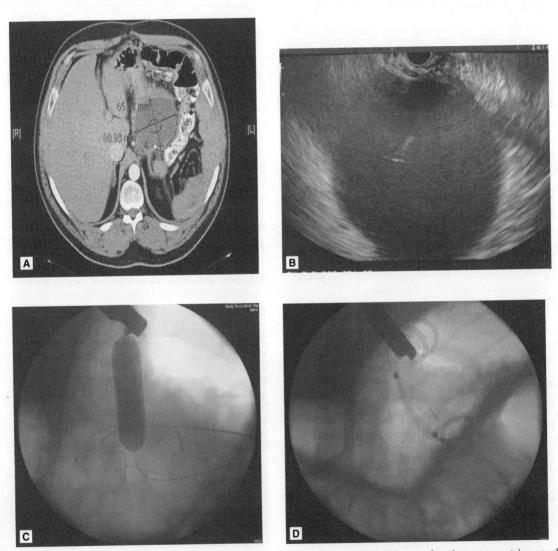

▲ **Figure 34–10.** Sequence of pseudocyst drainage: (**A**) computed tomographic (CT) scan showing retrogastric pseudocyst, (**B**) endoscopic ultrasound image with needle inside cyst, (**C**) balloon dilation of the cystgastrostomy track, (**D**) double pigtail stents across cystgastrostomy stoma, and (**E**) follow-up CT scan showing resolution. See also Plates 81 and 82.

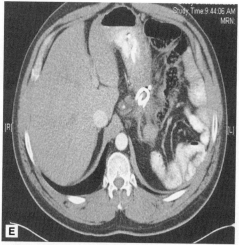

▲ **Figure 34–10.** (Continued)

pancreatitis" (AIP) was not proposed until 1995. The epidemiology of AIP is not well known but a prevalence of 5% has been reported among patients with chronic pancreatitis. The disease is more common in men in their late 50s. The coexistence and association of AIP with other autoimmune diseases, such as primary sclerosing cholangitis, Sjögren syndrome, and diabetes mellitus, has been reported (see Chapter 29). Diagnostic criteria include (1) pancreatic imaging studies showing diffuse narrowing of the main pancreatic duct with irregular walls and diffuse enlargement of the pancreas, (2) laboratory data demonstrating abnormally elevated levels of serum γ-globulin, or immunoglobulin G, or the presence of autoantibodies, and (3) histopathologic examination of the pancreas showing fibrotic changes with lymphocyte and plasma cell infiltration. For diagnosis of AIP, criterion 1 must be present along with 2 or 3. There is currently no therapeutic role for ERCP in this condition unless there is concomitant biliary obstruction, in which case ERCP appears feasible and safe in the setting of AIP.

Hammad T, Khan MA, Alastal Y, et al. Efficacy and safety of lumen-apposing metal stents in management of pancreatic fluid collections: are they better than plastic stents? A systematic review and meta-analysis. *Dig Dis Sci*. 2018;63(2):289–301. [PMID: 29282638]

Naitoh I, Nakazawa T, Okumura F, et al. Endoscopic retrograde cholangiopancreatography-related adverse events in patients with type 1 autoimmune pancreatitis. *Pancreatology*. 2016;16(1):78–82. [PMID: 26626204]

5. Pancreas Divisum

Pancreas divisum, the failure of fusion of dorsal and ventral pancreatic ductal systems during embryogenesis, is the most common variant of pancreatic ductal anatomy and occurs in about 10% of individuals (Plates 83, 84, and 85). The relationship between pancreas divisum and pancreatitis remains controversial, but endoscopic therapy in patients with recurrent pancreatitis and a normal dorsal duct aims at decompressing the dorsal pancreatic duct by minor papillotomy and temporary stent insertion with greater than 80% long-term success. These patients were the first group shown to develop ductal changes resulting from stent therapy, and care must be taken to avoid this complication by not leaving stents in place longer than necessary.

Hammad T, Khan MA, Alastal Y, et al. Efficacy and safety of lumen-apposing metal stents in management of pancreatic fluid collections: are they better than plastic stents? A systematic review and meta-analysis. *Dig Dis Sci*. 2018;63(2):289–301. [PMID: 29282638]

6. Autoimmune Pancreatitis

The first case of chronic inflammatory sclerosis of the pancreas with possible underlying autoimmune mechanism was reported in 1961, but the terminology of "autoimmune

7. Intraductal Papillary Mucinous Neoplasm

Intraductal papillary mucinous neoplasm (IPMN) is a cystic neoplasm of the pancreas that involves the main pancreatic duct, side branches, or both. It is characterized by intraductal growth of mucin-producing epithelium, segmental or diffuse ductal dilation, and, when the tumor is in the head of the pancreas, a gaping or "fish-mouth" papilla from which large amounts of mucus flow (Figure 34–11). Approximately 75% of IPMNs arise from the main pancreatic duct in the head of the pancreas, whereas the branch duct type most commonly arises from the uncinate process or, less commonly, from the tail of the pancreas. IPMN occurs more commonly in elderly men who may present with recurrent pancreatitis and/or diabetes. Jaundice and weight loss can be the presenting symptoms in cases with malignant transformation.

Several imaging modalities are used to diagnose IPMN, including CT, endoscopic ultrasound, magnetic resonance imaging, and ERCP. A pancreatogram is usually remarkable for dilated pancreatic ducts, intraluminal filling defects, and mural nodules. During ERCP, pancreatic juice can be aspirated for cytology, and transpapillary brushings and biopsies can be obtained from suspicious lesions seen on pancreatography. Direct pancreatoscopy involves the use of an ultrathin endoscope of 10-French diameter or less introduced through the working channel of a duodenoscope and advanced into the pancreatic duct through the major papilla. The ductal epithelium can be examined and directed biopsies of suspicious mural nodules or masses can be performed.

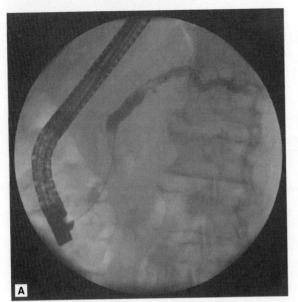 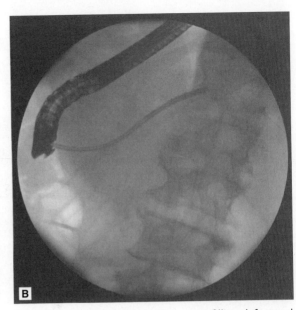

▲ **Figure 34–11.** ERCP in a patient with IPMN showing (**A**) a dilated main pancreatic duct with a mucus filling defect and (**B**) direct pancreatoscopy, which demonstrated the ductal tumor.

Pancreatoscopy has been increasingly used as an adjunct to other imaging modalities for diagnosis and determining the extent of IPMN, because the tumor is easily seen as a "cluster of eggs" appearance when it affects the main duct and surgical resection currently aims to be as conservative as possible.

Trindade AJ, Benias PC, Kurupathi P, et al. Digital pancreatoscopy in the evaluation of main duct intraductal papillary mucinous neoplasm: a multicenter study. *Endoscopy.* 2018;50(11): 1095–1098. [PMID: 29698989]

Video Capsule Endoscopy & Deep Small Bowel Enteroscopy

Daniel J. Stein, MD, MPH

Ramona M. Lim, MD

ESSENTIAL CONCEPTS

▶ Multiple systems are available for capsule endoscopy with targeted visualization ranging from upper gastrointestinal tract to the colon.

▶ Common indications are suspected small bowel bleeding, Crohn's assessment, and surveillance for polyposis syndromes.

▶ Most capsules are swallowed, but endoscopic placement is possible for patients with dysphagia or stricture.

▶ The most common complication is capsule retention; if suspicion is high for retention, a dissolvable patency capsule can be used first.

▶ Small bowel capsule yield is dependent on the indication; for bleeding, the highest yield is in overt bleeding and capsule examination at the time of the index bleed.

▶ For small bowel interventions, balloon-assisted (single or double) or spiral enteroscopy provide access to most or all of the small bowel.

▶ Therapeutic deep endoscopy yield is dependent on indication but generally high (34–80%), especially in bleeding and with a known lesion from capsule endoscopy.

▶ Complications from deep enteroscopy include abdominal pain, sore throat, performation, pancreatitis, and ileus.

VIDEO CAPSULE ENDOSCOPY

General Considerations

The first human ingestion of a video capsule endoscope occurred in 1999, and high-quality images from healthy human volunteers were described in 2000. In August 2001, the US Food and Drug Administration (FDA) approved a commercially available capsule for use in the United States. The capsule had been approved for use in Europe earlier that year.

Several video capsules are available for use in the United States. Four capsules are used for small bowel visualization, the PillCam SB3 (Medtronic, Minneapolis, MN), the EndoCapsule EC-10 (Olympus Corporation, Allentown, PA), the MiRoCam (IntroMedic Co, Ltd, Seoul, South Korea), and the CapsoCam Plus (CapsoVision US, Saratoga, CA). While PillCam and EndoCapsule EC-10 capsules transmit images using ultrahigh frequency band radio telemetry, the MiRoCam instead uses electric field propagation to transmit the images, using the human body as conductive medium. In further contrast, the CapsoCam Plus is the only device without a sensing system; because of the large amount of data generated, it cannot transmit data by radiofrequency but instead must be retrieved from the fecal stream using a magnetic wand for subsequent download and processing. A fifth capsule, the PillCam UGI (formerly PillCam ESO, Medtronic), is used for visualization of the upper GI system including esophagus through duodenum. Finally, there is a capsule used for visualization of the colon with or without small bowel imaging (PillCam COLON or PillCam Crohn's, Medtronic) that has FDA approval for examination of the colon in patients who have undergone incomplete colonoscopy (with adequate preparation) or who have lower GI bleeding and are at high risk for standard colonoscopy, whereas PillCam Crohn's is specifically marketed for the assessment of Crohn's disease activity in both the small bowel and colon within a single examination. All systems have a corresponding software package, which include features such as localization data, progress of capsule transit within the GI tract, quick reference image atlases, bleeding indicators and report generation capabilities. Numerous efforts are underway to introduce artificial intelligence to supplement manual physician review (generally 30–90 minutes for a small bowel capsule), but none are yet commercially available.

The small bowel and esophageal radiofrequency capsules are approximately 11×26 mm in size, whereas the colon capsule is 11×32 mm. The PillCam SB3 and EndoCapsule EC-10 small bowel capsules have fields of view that vary from 156 to 160 degrees. The capsules' resolution have higher magnification (1:8) than that of conventional endoscopes, which allows for visualization of individual villi. These radiofrequency capsules acquire between two and six frames per second, with battery lives of 8, 12, and up to 20 hours. The MiRoCam capsule technology was approved by the FDA in 2013 and has a battery life of more than 12 hours. The CapsoCam Plus, approved by the FDA in 2016, has four side-viewing cameras providing 360 degrees field of view and variable frame rate, with a battery life up to 15 hours.

The upper GI capsule has cameras at both ends and acquires images at a variable frame rate (35 frames per second for the first 10 minutes and 18 frames per second for the last 80 minutes), with a battery life of 90 minutes. Finally, like the upper GI capsule, the colon capsule has cameras at both ends with 172 degree field of view. It acquires images at an adaptive frame rate (ranging from four frames per second to 35 frames per second, depending on when the system detects a change in image or when the capsule is in motion), with a battery life of about 10 hours. The colon capsule initially records for 5 minutes and then enters a "sleep mode," reactivating after 2 hours. This is done to maximize colon visualization. The PillCam Crohn's has similar adaptive frame technology as the PillCam Colon, but instead begins immediately on duodenal recognition, and enables direct visualization of both the small bowel and colon in one exam.

Arnott ID, Lo SK. The clinical utility of wireless capsule endoscopy. *Dig Dis Sci.* 2004;49:893–901. [PMID: 15309874]

ASGE Technology Committee. Technology Status Evaluation Report: video capsule endoscopy. *Gastrointest Endosc.* 2021;93: 784–796. [PMID: 33642034]

Swain P. Wireless capsule endoscopy. *Gut.* 2003;52(suppl IV): iv48–iv50. [PMID: 12746269]

▶ Indications

The indications for small bowel, upper GI, and colonic capsule endoscopy are summarized in Table 35–1.

A. Suspected Small Bowel Bleeding

Suspected small bowel bleeding (formerly known as obscure gastrointestinal bleeding) refers to bleeding that persists or recurs, without a source identified after standard endoscopic evaluation with upper endoscopy and colonoscopy. Suspected small bowel bleeding can be subdivided into overt and occult gastrointestinal bleeding. Patients with overt gastrointestinal bleeding present with visual evidence of bleeding, such as hematemesis, melena, or hematochezia. Occult bleeding is manifested by stool that is positive for occult blood, frequently with iron deficiency anemia, without evidence of

Table 35–1. Indications for small bowel, upper GI, & colon capsule endoscopy.

Indications for small bowel capsule endoscopy
Suspected small bowel bleeding (formerly obscure gastrointestinal bleeding)
Diagnosis of Crohn's disease
Evaluation of disease activity in established Crohn's disease
Small bowel tumors
Diagnosis of celiac disease
Evaluation of refractory celiac disease
Polyp surveillance in polyposis syndromes
Surveillance for graft rejection after small bowel transplant
Detection of graft-versus-host disease
Evaluation of unexplained abdominal pain
Evaluation of unexplained diarrhea
Indications for upper GI capsule endoscopy
Screening for esophageal varices
Screening for Barrett esophagus
Detection of esophagitis
Indications for colon capsule endoscopy
Screening for colorectal cancer
Incomplete colonoscopy
Evaluation of GI bleeding in those at high risk of undergoing colonoscopy

visible blood loss to the patient or clinician. Suspected small bowel bleeding accounts for approximately 5–10% of patients with gastrointestinal bleeding, and the source of bleeding is frequently from the small bowel (approximately 75%), between the ligament of Treitz and the ileocecal valve, with the remainder due to missed pathology in the upper gastrointestinal and lower gastrointestinal tracts. Common causes of small bowel bleeding include vascular ectasias, small bowel tumors, Crohn disease, and nonsteroidal anti-inflammatory drug (NSAID) enteropathy (Table 35–2; see also Plates 86 and 87). Vascular ectasias are the most common cause of suspected small bowel bleeding, accounting for 30–40% overall, and are responsible for the majority of suspected small bowel bleeds in older patients. Patients between the ages of 30 and 50 are more likely to have a small bowel tumor as the source of their bleeding. Young patients are more commonly found to have an ulcerated Meckel diverticulum as the source. While rare, bleeding from a Meckel diverticulum may occur at any age.

ASGE Standards of Practice Committee. The role of endoscopy in the management of suspected small-bowel bleeding. *Gastrointest Endosc.* 2017;85:22–31. [PMID: 27374798]

Gerson LB, Fidler JL, Cave DR, et al. ACG clinical guideline: diagnosis and management of small bowel bleeding. *Am J Gastroenterol.* 2015;110:1265–1287. [PMID: 26303132]

B. Crohn's Disease

In patients with Crohn's disease limited to the small bowel, or in those with indeterminate colitis, arriving at a correct

Table 35–2. Sources of small bowel bleeding.

Vascular ectasias, often associated with:
  Advanced age
  Chronic renal failure
  Valvular heart disease
  Left ventricular assist devices
  von Willebrand disease
  Scleroderma with CREST syndrome (calcinosis cutis, Raynaud phenomenon, esophageal dysmotility, sclerodactyly, telangiectasias)
  Hereditary hemorrhagic telangiectasia syndrome (Osler-Weber-Rendu syndrome)
Small bowel tumors
  Small bowel gastrointestinal stromal tumors (eg, leiomyoma, leiomyosarcoma, GIST)
  Adenocarcinoma
  Lymphoma
  Carcinoid
  Kaposi sarcoma
  Metastatic cancer (eg, melanoma)
Crohn's disease
NSAID enteropathy
Pelvic radiotherapy
Dieulafoy lesions
Aortoenteric fistulas
Meckel diverticula
Small bowel polyps
Small bowel varices
Hemosuccus pancreaticus
Strongyloides stercoralis
Pseudoxanthoma elasticum

NSAID, nonsteroidal anti-inflammatory drug.

Table 35–3. Differential diagnosis of small bowel erosions & ulcerations.

Inflammatory
  Crohn's disease
  Sarcoidosis
  Behçet syndrome
Drugs and medications
  Antibiotics
  Aspirin
  Cocaine
  Chemotherapy
  NSAIDs
  Potassium supplements
  Methamphetamine
Infections
  Bacterial
    Mycobacterium tuberculosis
    Mycobacterium avium–intracellulare complex
    Yersinia enterocolitica
    Yersinia pseudotuberculosis
    Typhlitis
    Salmonella
    Actinomycosis israelii
  Viral
    Cytomegalovirus
  Fungal and yeast
    Histoplasma capsulatum
    Cryptococcosis
  Parasitic
  Protozoan
  Helminthic
    Anisakiasis
Neoplastic
  Adenocarcinoma
  Carcinoid tumor
  Lymphoma
  Lymphosarcoma
  Metastatic disease
Collagen vascular disease
  Churg-Strauss syndrome
  Dermatomyositis
  Giant cell arteritis
  Henoch-Schönlein purpura
  Lymphomatoid granulomatosis
  Mixed connective tissue disease
  Polyarteritis nodosum
  Polymyositis
  Rheumatoid arthritis vasculitis
  Systemic lupus erythematosus
  Takayasu arteritis
  Thromboangiitis obliterans
  Thrombotic thrombocytopenic purpura
  Wegener granulomatosis
Trauma
  Intussusception
  Foreign body
  Incarcerated hernia
Celiac disease

(Continued)

diagnosis can be difficult. Video capsule endoscopy (VCE) also can be used in patients with known Crohn's disease to assess for small bowel involvement or degree of disease activity. VCE can help diagnose suspected small bowel Crohn's disease by providing mucosal detail that is not available radiologically (Plate 88). It also provides the opportunity to visualize areas of the bowel not accessible by standard endoscopy. Because VCE has a resolution of 0.1 mm, it is able to detect small, superficial defects, such as aphthous ulcers. It is important to note, however, that mucosal ulcerations occur not due to Crohn's disease (Table 35–3). Ten to 23% of normal volunteers who are not taking NSAIDs will have mucosal breaks and other lesions seen on VCE, and 50–71% of NSAID users will have evidence of small bowel injury (red spots, erosions, and ulcerations). Therefore, it is important to use VCE findings in combination with other clinical information to arrive at the correct diagnosis.

C. Small Bowel Tumors & Polyposis Syndromes

VCE may be able to detect malignant small bowel tumors years before they would be detected by other imaging modalities, potentially increasing the chance to remove them while still localized and small (Plate 89).

Table 35–3. Differential diagnosis of small bowel erosions & ulcerations. (Continued)

Chronic idiopathic enterocolitis
Eosinophilic gastroenteritis
Food allergies
Graft-versus-host disease
Heavy metal poisoning
Hypogammaglobulinemia
Ischemia
Lymphocytic enteritis
Malnutrition
Meckel diverticulum with heterotopic gastric mucosa
Radiation
Uremia
Zollinger-Ellison syndrome

NSAID, nonsteroidal anti-inflammatory drug.

VCE can also detect small bowel polyps in patients with hereditary polyposis syndromes. Peutz-Jeghers syndrome and familial adenomatous polyposis (FAP) are two of the hereditary polyposis syndromes that are associated with small bowel polyps and malignancies. Patients with Peutz-Jeghers syndrome form hamartomatous polyps throughout the gastrointestinal tract, along with mucocutaneous pigmentation. The polyps have a predilection for the small bowel and will develop in more than 90% of patients (Plate 90). Complications from the polyps include gastrointestinal bleeding, anemia, intestinal obstruction, intussusception, and development of cancer. Patients with Peutz-Jeghers syndrome have a 13% lifetime risk of developing small bowel cancer, so surveillance of the small intestine is recommended. Traditionally, patients underwent radiographic imaging with a small bowel series or enteroclysis every 2 years, starting at age 10 years. This approach exposes a patient to significant amounts of ionizing radiation. In addition, radiologic evaluation with small bowel follow-through, computed tomography (CT) enterography, or magnetic resonance enterography (MRE) lacks sensitivity for detecting small polyps. Push enteroscopy has also been employed, but is only able to visualize a portion of the upper small bowel. VCE on the other hand, is capable of detecting small polyps throughout the small bowel and may help guide the need for deep enteroscopy or other therapeutic interventions.

D. Celiac Disease

The role of VCE in celiac disease is evolving. Celiac disease affects up to 0.3–1% of Caucasians. Celiac disease has traditionally been diagnosed by detection of antibodies (eg, antiendomysial and tissue transglutaminase antibodies), followed by endoscopy with biopsies of the small bowel to confirm the diagnosis. VCE has been proposed as a possible alternative to endoscopy for the diagnosis of celiac disease. VCE findings of celiac disease include scalloping, a mosaic mucosal pattern, loss of mucosal folds, visible vessels, and micronodularity (Plates 91 and 92). An advantage of VCE is

that it allows for visualization of the entire small bowel, and symptom severity in celiac disease is more closely related to the length of small bowel involved and not to the severity of the villous atrophy seen on biopsy.

VCE may have an even more important role in the evaluation of refractory celiac disease. Celiac disease can be complicated by small bowel adenocarcinoma, lymphoma (including enteropathy-associated T-cell lymphoma), and ulcerative jejunitis. In patients who fail to respond to a gluten-free diet or who have a recurrence of symptoms while on a gluten-free diet, further evaluation is needed to differentiate between refractory celiac disease (ie, celiac disease that does not respond to a gluten-free diet), ongoing gluten ingestion (intentional or unintentional), or a complication of celiac disease.

E. Other Applications

VCE has also been used to evaluate for evidence of small bowel graft-versus-host disease in patients following bone marrow transplantation, to look for evidence of rejection following small intestinal transplantation, and to evaluate for radiation enteritis. However, in the case of suspected radiation enteritis, the risk of capsule retention is increased. In addition, VCE may detect small intestinal varices or portal hypertensive enteropathy in patients with portal hypertension.

Upper GI VCE can be used to detect esophageal varices, erosive esophagitis, and Barrett esophagus. Finally, colon capsule endoscopy is used for colorectal cancer screening.

▶ Contraindications

VCE is contraindicated in some patients. Because cooperation is required, demented patients are not good candidates for VCE. VCE is also contraindicated in pregnant women (due to a lack of data on the effects of VCE in pregnancy). Although cardiac devices are still cited as a contraindication to VCE, the most recent guidelines from the American Gastroenterological Association and the European Society of Gastrointestinal Endoscopy advocate that patients with pacemakers may undergo VCE without special precautions. In patients with cardiac pacemakers or defibrillators, many centers perform VCE since studies suggest that the capsules do not interfere with the cardiac devices. In addition, cardiac devices have only rarely been shown to disrupt the capsule study (with the exception of one instance of images being lost as a capsule passed the pulse generator of an abdominally implanted pacemaker, as well as potential interference of image acquisition by left ventricular assist devices and wireless telemetry). If cardiac monitoring is necessary during VCE, wired systems should be used. Patients should be instructed not to undergo magnetic resonance imaging until passage of the capsule has been confirmed, which can be done with a plain abdominal radiograph if the capsule was not seen to pass in the stool.

Patients with gastrointestinal tract obstructions, strictures, or fistulas (either suspected or demonstrated on imaging studies) should not undergo VCE because of an increased risk of capsule retention or obstruction, and patients who are inoperable or refuse surgery are not good candidates for VCE. A patency capsule (PillCam Patency Capsule, Medtronic) is available to confirm small bowel patency in patients with suspected strictures or obstructions. The capsule is a dissolvable dummy capsule with a transmitter, which is used to assess the small bowel patency prior to undergoing VCE (see Procedure). The patient swallows the capsule, and then after 30 hours a hand-held scanner or a plain abdominal film is used to determine if the capsule is still present in the small bowel. If it is not, then it is safe to proceed with the VCE study. Patency capsules retained due to a stricture or obstruction will begin to dissolve after 30 hours, and typically do not present with symptomatic obstructions.

In patients with swallowing disorders, such as achalasia, esophageal strictures, esophageal diverticula, or gastroparesis, the capsule may need to be delivered using a special delivery device to ensure that it enters and traverses the small bowel during its recording time. The AdvanCE capsule endoscope delivery device (Steris, Mentor, Ohio) allows for direct endoscopic placement of video capsules directly into the stomach or duodenum. It is composed of a catheter that is passed through the channel of a gastroscope. A specialized capsule cap that holds the capsule is then screwed onto the end of the catheter and the activated video capsule is inserted into the cap. The scope is then advanced blindly into the esophagus (the cap obscures visualization). Once in the esophagus, the catheter can be advanced slightly to allow for limited visualization. The scope is then advanced to the small bowel, where the capsule is deployed, ideally after endoscopic gastric loop reduction. A standard upper endoscopy examination should be carried out before using the device to detect any abnormalities that could complicate capsule delivery. Alternative delivery methods include placing the capsule in the stomach by inserting it through an overtube and then advancing it to the small bowel using snares or nets.

Bandorski D, Hölgen R, Stunder D, et al. Capsule endoscopy in patients with cardiac pacemakers, implantable cardioverter defibrillators and left heart assist devices. *Ann Gastroenterol.* 2014;27:3–8. [PMID: 24714370]

Bandorski D, Kurniawan N, Baltes P, et al. Contraindications for video capsule endoscopy. *World J Gastroenterol.* 2016;22: 9898–9908. [PMID: 28018097]

Enns RA, Hookey L, Armstrong D, et al. Clinical practice guidelines for use of video capsule endoscopy. *Gastroenterology.* 2017;152:497–514. [PMID: 28063287]

Pennazio M, Spada C, Eliakim R, et al. Small-bowel capsule endoscopy and device-assisted enteroscopy for diagnosis and treatment of small-bowel disorders: European Society of Gastrointestinal Endoscopy (ESGE) clinical guideline. *Endoscopy.* 2015;47:352–376. [PMID: 25826168]

▶ Procedure

A. Small Bowel Examination

1. Patient preparation—Studies can be performed on both inpatients and outpatients. For a small bowel study, a patient fasts for 8–12 hours before the examination. Some centers also have the patient consume only clear liquids for up to 24 hours prior to the examination. Data are conflicting, but some studies suggest that preparing the small bowel with 2–4 L of a polyethylene glycol (PEG) solution may improve visualization. In a 2018 meta-analysis of 12 randomized trials of 1221 patients, the use of a purgative bowel preparation did not improve diagnostic yield, quality of small bowel mucosal visualization, nor VCE completion rate, though there was significant heterogeneity among the studies. In cases where there is concern for slowed gastric transit, such as in diabetic patients, a prokinetic agent such as metoclopramide or erythromycin can be given approximately 30–60 minutes prior to the study, though there is minimal data to support the utility of this approach. Some centers give patients simethicone prior to the study in an attempt to decrease air bubbles that can obscure the view of the mucosa. The most recent AGA guidelines (2017) strongly recommend the use of bowel preparation on the basis of low quality evidence. No specific preparation was recommended. Some centers routinely utilize bowel preparations for inpatients.

2. Techniques—Prior to capsule ingestion, a sensor belt containing a three-lead sensor array is placed around the patient's abdomen. This sensor belt has largely replaced PillCam's original eight-lead sensor array which requires adhesives but may still be utilized for patients unable to wear the sensor belt or who have a large pannus. EndoCapsule EC-10 has similar eight-lead sensor array and belt-type sensor array as an alternative, and MiroCam uses a sensor array attached to the abdomen. For these three systems, the sensor array is connected to a solid-state recorder, battery pack, and real-time viewer, worn on a belt. CapsoCam does not require a sensor array or external recording system as the data are stored directly in the capsule, necessitating recovery from fecal stream prior to image processing.

Removing the magnet that is packaged with the capsule activates the capsule. The patient then swallows the capsule in an upright position, or the capsule is placed endoscopically (see preceding text), and images are transmitted to a recording device worn around the patient's waist. During the study, patients are instructed to avoid activities that could lead to sensor detachment, such as exercise. After 2 hours, the patient is permitted to have clear liquids, and a light meal can be consumed after 4 hours. An exception to these dietary restrictions is with the MiRoCam system, where patients are permitted to drink water immediately after capsule ingestion and throughout the duration of the entire study. At the end of the study, the images are downloaded to a computer workstation equipped with proprietary software. With the exception of CapsoCam, the capsules are disposable and are excreted with bowel movements. A physician can then read the study and generate a report, a process that takes on average 40–60 minutes. To aid in reading the study, the software has features such as a blood indicator that marks areas with suspected bleeding.

To allow real-time viewing of the images, hand-held devices have been developed. A possible disadvantage is that reading a study in real time takes significantly longer than reviewing downloaded images (the average small bowel transit time is ~4 hours). However, in certain situations, real-time imaging may have a role. For example, the capsule could be administered in the emergency department with immediate viewing to help guide further evaluation and management.

Enns RA, Hookey L, Armstrong D, et al. Clinical practice guidelines for use of video capsule endoscopy. *Gastroenterology.* 2017;152:497–514. [PMID: 28063287]

Gkolfakis P, Tziatzios G, Dimitriadis GD, et al. Meta-analysis of randomized controlled trials challenging the usefulness of purgative preparation before small-bowel video capsule endoscopy. *Endoscopy.* 2018;50:671–683. [PMID: 29409067]

B. Patency Capsule

1. Patient preparation—For the patency capsule, patients are instructed to ingest a liquid diet starting at noon and to fast for 8–12 hours beginning the evening before the examination.

2. Techniques—The patient ingests the capsule the following morning (suggested 7 or 8 am). Following capsule ingestion, liquids may be taken after 2 hours, and food may be taken after 4 hours. The patient is assessed the next day at as close to, but not exceeding, 30 hours (eg, if the capsule is ingested at 8 am, the assessment should be done before 2 pm the next day) by the use of a handheld scanning device or a plain abdominal film. Evaluation beyond 30 hours is not reliable, as the biodegradable plugs at each end allow the capsule to start to dissolve after 30 hours, and to fully dissolve by 40 to 80 hours after ingestion, allowing the capsule to pass even in the presence of a stricture.

Patency is suggested if at or before 30 hours: the capsule is no longer present in the abdomen; the capsule is in the abdomen, but imaging indicates its location in the colon; or the patient is a reliable historian and reports that the capsule passed fully intact. The patency capsule does not have the ability to acquire images.

C. Upper GI Examination

1. Patient preparation—For the upper GI examination, patients need to fast for 2 hours prior to ingesting the capsule.

2. Techniques—A three-element sensor array is attached to the patient's chest in a designated pattern, and the patient consumes 100 mL of water with simethicone while standing. The patient then lies supine and the capsule is swallowed with a 10-mL sip of water. The patient remains supine for 2 minutes, and then progressively moves into an upright position (30 degrees for 2 minutes, 60 degrees for 1 minute, then upright for the remainder of the study). The images are then downloaded to the workstation and reviewed. The upper GI examination is designed to include views of the esophagus, stomach, and duodenum.

Due to difficulty with adherence to the ingestion protocol, an alternative simplified ingestion protocol has been developed for the esophageal examination. The patient lies in the right lateral decubitus position with their head on a pillow. The patient then swallows the capsule with a sip (~15 mL) of water. The patient remains on the right side and takes an additional sip of water every 30 seconds for a total of 7 minutes. After 7 minutes, the patient sits upright and takes an additional sip of water. The patient may then get up and walk for the remainder of the study. The images are then downloaded to the computer workstation for review.

D. Colon Examination

1. Patient preparation—The patient needs to take a bowel preparation prior to colon capsule examination. One approach is for the patient to consume a clear liquid diet the day prior to the examination (with the exception of a light breakfast). The evening prior to the examination, the patient consumes 3 L of PEG and then consumes another liter of PEG the morning of the examination, 1 to 2 hours prior to capsule ingestion.

2. Techniques—The patient wears a sensor belt during the procedure. The patient swallows the capsule in an upright position with a small amount of water. After 10 hours, the images are downloaded to the workstation and reviewed.

▶ Efficacy

A. Suspected Small Bowel Bleeding

Suspected small bowel bleeding is the most common indication for performing a VCE. The overall yield of VCE is 55–70%, and leads to alterations in management in approximately one-third of patients (range, 25–71%). Compared with intraoperative enteroscopy as a gold standard, VCE has a sensitivity of 95%, a specificity of 75%, a positive predictive value of 95%, and a negative predictive value of 86% for detecting a bleeding source.

The yield of VCE is highly dependent on the indication for the study and the timing of the examination. In obscure GI bleeding, approximately 56–61% yield is seen in appropriately selected patients. When the study is performed relative to the bleeding affects the yield of VCE given the tendency of bleeding sources to intermittently resolve. A study from 2013 divided hospitalized patients with obscure bleeding into two groups based on when they underwent VCE (<3 days after admission or 3 or more days after admission). Performance of VCE within 3 days of admission was associated with a higher diagnostic yield than either later VCE as an inpatient or outpatient VCE (44% vs 28% and 26%, respectively).

VCE has been compared with push enteroscopy, small bowel barium radiography (small bowel follow-through or enteroclysis), CT angiography, and mesenteric angiography in the evaluation of obscure gastrointestinal bleeding. Overall yield for VCE is approximately 2–3 times that of push enteroscopy alone, with meta-analyses showing approximately 56–71% yield in comparison to 26–29% for push enteroscopy (although other studies have estimated the yield of push enteroscopy to be higher, at 40–65%). A small prospective study that compared VCE with both CT angiography and mesenteric angiography in 25 patients who were able to complete all three studies found that VCE was superior to both for sensitivity, detecting a bleeding source in 72% of patients compared with 24% for CT angiography and 56% for mesenteric angiography, although the difference between the two studies did not reach statistical significance.

Repeat VCE in patients with an initial negative study should be considered, but generally only in the context of recurrent bleeding. One small study found that 18 of 24 patients (75%) undergoing repeat VCE for the evaluation of obscure-overt or obscure-occult gastrointestinal bleeding had new findings, and in 15 patients (62.5%), the findings resulted in a change in management. However, in the absence of recurrent bleeding, the role of repeat capsule is generally minimal; a meta-analysis of 3657 patients evaluating VCE in both overt and occult suspected small bowel bleeding, found pooled rate of rebleeding after negative VCE was 19% and not different for overt versus occult bleeding. It is therefore reasonable to wait for evidence of rebleeding before repeating a VCE.

Gerson LB. Small bowel bleeding: updated algorithm and outcomes. *Gastrointest Endosc Clin North Am.* 2017;27:171–180. [PMID: 27908516]

Lepileur L, Dray X, Antonietti M, et al. Factors associated with diagnosis of obscure gastrointestinal bleeding by video capsule enteroscopy. *Clin Gastroenterol Hepatol.* 2012;10:1376–1380. [PMID: 22677574]

Liao Z, Gao R, Xu C, Li ZS. Indications and detection, completion, and retention rates of small-bowel capsule endoscopy: a systematic review. *Gastrointest Endosc.* 2010;71:208–286. [PMID: 20152309]

Rondonotti E, Spada C, Adler S, et al. Small-bowel capsule endoscopy and device-assisted enteroscopy for diagnosis and treatment of small-bowel disorders: European Society of Gastrointestinal Endoscopy (ESGE) technical review. *Endoscopy.* 2018;50:423–446. [PMID: 29539652]

Singh A, Marshall C, Chaudhuri B, et al. Timing of video capsule endoscopy relative to overt obscure GI bleeding: implications from a retrospective study. *Gastrointest Endosc.* 2013;77:761–766. [PMID: 23375526]

Yung DE, Koulaouzidis A, Avni T, et al. Clinical outcomes of negative small-bowel capsule endoscopy for small-bowel bleeding: a systematic review and meta-analysis. *Gastrointest Endosc.* 2017;85:305–317. [PMID: 27594338]

Table 35–4. Factors associated with positive capsule endoscopy studies in patients with suspected small bowel Crohn's disease.

Abdominal pain
Diarrhea
Weight loss
Nonspecific abnormalities on small bowel imaging
Elevated erythrocyte sedimentation rate
Anemia
Low serum albumin
Elevated fecal calprotectin

B. Crohn's Disease

VCE is superior to other diagnostic modalities in detecting small bowel disease when the suspicion for Crohn's disease is high (Table 35–4). A meta-analysis demonstrated that VCE is superior to small bowel radiography, colonoscopy with ileoscopy, CT enterography or enteroclysis, and push enteroscopy for the detection of nonstricturing small bowel Crohn's disease (incremental yields of 40%, 15%, 38%, and 38%, respectively). Overall, VCE had a yield of 46–72% for detecting small bowel Crohn's disease. It had a yield of 33–70% in patients with suspected Crohn's disease, and a yield of 68–86% in patients with established Crohn's disease. In a second meta-analysis, VCE detected evidence of small bowel Crohn's disease in 55% of patients with known or suspected Crohn's disease.

It is possible, however, that the yield of VCE for suspected Crohn's disease is significantly lower in practice because patients being evaluated for possible Crohn's disease do not always fulfill the selection criteria used in studies. In a study of patients being evaluated for abdominal pain who had undergone previous endoscopic or radiographic evaluations, a cause was detected by VCE in only 6% of those with abdominal pain alone, and in 13% of those with abdominal pain and diarrhea. VCE can also help in the evaluation of indeterminate colitis. In patients with indeterminate colitis, two retrospective studies of VCE have demonstrated small bowel ulcerations in 33–49% of patients, suggesting (but not proving) a diagnosis of Crohn's disease.

In addition to detecting small bowel Crohn's disease, VCE can help in defining the extent of disease, diagnosing a Crohn's flare, or detecting a postoperative recurrence in patients with established disease. In one study, patients who were suspected of having a Crohn's flare underwent VCE. In 20% of the patients there was no active disease, suggesting that the symptoms may have been due to other causes, such as a superimposed functional disorder. An evolving indication for VCE is in the assessment of mucosal healing in established Crohn's disease. Careful consideration is important prior to pursuing VCE in patients with known or suspected Crohn's strictures, as capsule retention has been described in up to 13% of patients undergoing a VCE for known Crohn's disease, even after performing an initial small bowel study (see Complications).

Dionisio PM, Gurudu SR, Leighton JA, et al. Capsule endoscopy has a significantly higher diagnostic yield in patients with suspected and established small-bowel Crohn's disease: a meta-analysis. *Am J Gastroenterol.* 2010;105:1240–1248. [PMID: 20029412]

Gomollon F, Dignass A, Annese V, et al. 3rd European evidence-based consensus on the diagnosis and management of Crohn's disease 2016. Part 1: diagnosis and medical management. *J Crohns Colitis.* 2017;11:3–25. [PMID: 27660341]

Kopylov U, Yablecovitch D, Lahat A, et al. Detection of small bowel mucosal healing and deep remission in patients with known small bowel Crohn's disease using biomarkers, capsule endoscopy, and imaging. *Am J Gastroenterol.* 2015;110:1316–1323. [PMID: 26215531]

Melmed GY, Dubinsky MC, Rubin DR, et al. Utility of video capsule endoscopy for longitudinal monitoring of Crohn's disease activity in the small bowel: a prospective study. *Gastrointest Endosc.* 2018;88:947–955. [PMID: 30086261]

C. Small Bowel Tumors & Polyposis Syndromes

VCE is capable of detecting tumors and polyps of all sizes throughout the small bowel; however, because many of the tumors are subepithelial, it can be difficult to differentiate a tumor from the transient bulges that are frequently seen during VCE. In addition, a tumor may only be seen tangentially on one frame of the study, making characterization of the mass difficult, especially when it comes to size. Because VCE lacks biopsy capability, arriving at a definitive diagnosis is rarely possible using VCE alone. However, a presumptive diagnosis can be made in some cases, such as in a patient with a small bowel mass and known metastatic melanoma (see Plate 89).

In a study of patients with polyposis syndromes, VCE detected polyps in 10 of 11 patients (91%) with Peutz-Jeghers syndrome. That study also examined patients with FAP. It found that 24% of FAP patients (5 of 12 patients) with duodenal adenomas had distal jejunal or ileal polyps detected on VCE. In patients without duodenal adenomas, however, more distal polyps occurred in only 12%. Of note, VCE often failed to achieve adequate visualization of the ampulla of Vater, an area of frequent polyp and adenocarcinoma development in patients with FAP. Therefore, VCE is not a substitute for standard surveillance using a side-viewing duodenoscope with ampullary biopsies. The American College of Gastroenterology guideline on management of FAP does not recommend routine VCE or small bowel surveillance distal to the ligament of Treitz unless clinically indicated, but the American Society of Gastrointestinal Endoscopy has recommended an optimal strategy to consider screening the subset of FAP patients with Spigelman stage 4 or advanced duodenal polyposis, as they are at increased risk for distal adenomas either by VCE or MRE. VCE has been shown to have efficacy in polyp detection for FAP.

VCE is routinely used in surveillance of Peutz-Jeghers syndrome (PJS). When compared to MRE, VCE is more sensitive for detection of small polyp (<5 mm), and VCE and MRE have similar detection rates for polyps >10 mm, but MRE appears to be more sensitive for polyps >15 mm. In a multicenter study evaluating PJS patients undergoing VCE followed by double balloon enteroscopy (DBE), there was strong agreement for polyp size and location between VCE and DBE.

VCE has also been proposed for small bowel surveillance in Lynch syndrome, but the majority of small bowel neoplasms detected are within reach of a standard upper endoscopy. There are no clear guidelines supporting the use of VCE in surveillance of patients with *MUTYH*-associated polyposis syndrome, juvenile polyposis syndrome, and Cowden syndrome as the prevalence of distal small bowel polyps is quite low.

Haanstra JF, Al-Toma A, Dekker E, et al. Prevalence of small-bowel neoplasia in Lynch syndrome assessed by video capsule endoscopy. *Gut.* 2015;64:1578–1583. [PMID: 25209657]

Syngal S, Brand RE, Church JM, et al. ACG clinical guideline: genetic testing and management of hereditary gastrointestinal syndromes. *Am J Gastroenterol.* 2015;110:223–262. [PMID: 25645574]

Yamada A, Watabe H, Iwama T, et al. The prevalence of small intestinal polyps in patients with familial adenomatous polyposis: a prospective capsule endoscopy study. *Fam Cancer.* 2014;13:23–28. [PMID: 23743563]

Yang J, Gurudu SR, Koptiuch C, et al. American society for gastrointestinal endoscopy guideline on the role of endoscopy in familial adenomatous polyposis syndromes. *Gastrointest Endosc.* 2020;91:963–982. [PMID: 32169282]

D. Celiac Disease

Studies suggest that VCE has a sensitivity of 56–88% and a specificity of 85–100% for diagnosing celiac disease. As an example, in a small, blinded study of 20 patients (10 with celiac disease and 10 with controls), VCE had a sensitivity of 70%, a specificity of 100%, a positive predictive value of 100%, and a negative predictive value of 77% for the diagnosis of celiac disease. Interobserver agreement for experienced capsule endoscopists was perfect ($\kappa = 1.0$). Patients with extensive small bowel involvement were more likely to have classic celiac disease symptoms, including diarrhea and weight loss, whereas those with only proximal involvement had mild, nonspecific symptoms.

Studies have examined the role of VCE in management of patients with refractory celiac disease. In a study of 47 patients with celiac disease and persistent abdominal pain, occult blood loss, or refractory iron deficiency anemia, VCE identified lesions in 87% (41 of 47 patients). The VCE studies detected findings consistent with celiac disease in a majority of patients (32 with villous atrophy, 29 with scalloping and fissuring, and 9 with a mosaic pattern). Additional findings included ulcerations (21 patients), nodularity (6 patients), an adenocarcinoma (1 patient), a polyp (1 patient), a stricture (1 patient), intussusception (1 patient), and a submucosal mass (1 patient). This study suggests that in patients with ongoing symptoms, despite the report of adherence to a gluten-free diet, VCE has a high yield for identifying abnormalities. In a meta-analysis of 10 studies and 439 patients with refractory celiac disease, the diagnostic yield of VCE for clinically significant findings of ulcerative jejunitis or neoplasia was 13%. Similarly, a retrospective multicenter study of 189 patients with either refractory celiac disease or alarm features, VCE detected ulcerative jejunitis or neoplasia in 29 patients (15.3%), with findings which changed the treatment plan in 112 patients (59.3%).

Atlas DS, Rubio-Tapia A, Van Dyke CT, et al. Capsule endoscopy in nonresponsive celiac disease. *Gastrointest Endosc.* 2011;74:1315–1322. [PMID: 21835400]

Elli L, Casazza G, Locatelli M, et al. Use of enteroscopy for the detections of malignant and premalignant lesions of the small bowel in complicated celiac disease: a meta-analysis. *Gastrointest Endosc.* 2017;86:264–273. [PMID: 28433612]

Perez-Cuadrado-Robles E, Lujan-Sanchis M, Elli L, et al. Role of capsule endoscopy in alarm features and non-responsive celiac disease: a European multicenter study. *Dig Endosc.* 2018;30: 461–466. [PMID: 29253321]

Rondonotti E, Spada C, Cave D, et al. Video capsule enteroscopy in the diagnosis of celiac disease: a multicenter study. *Am J Gastroenterol.* 2007;102:1624–1631. [PMID: 17459022]

E. Upper GI Capsule Endoscopy

Initially validated for esophagus only, the most current version of the Pillcam UGI is designed to include the esophagus, stomach, and duodenum. There is only one system clinically available. This is a two-sided capsule with more frequent sampling (approximately 10x compared to the small bowel capsule) to improve detection in areas of rapid transit. In a study of 32 patients, there was 97% concordance between capsule endoscopy and upper endoscopy for the detection of varices, and 91% concordance for the diagnosis of portal hypertensive gastropathy. While capsule endoscopy can screen for the presence of erosive esophagitis, its role in the evaluation of Barrett's esophagus is less clear, since it does not have the ability to sample tissue. Two cost-benefit analysis studies concluded that screening for Barrett's esophagus with PillCam ESO was not cost-effective compared with standard screening with upper endoscopy. The most common indication is evaluation of bleeding in stable patients.

Emergency department usage has been demonstrated for acute upper gastrointestinal bleeding but has seen limited clinical usage. In a study of 83 patients presenting with suspected upper gastrointestinal bleeding, capsule endoscopy was performed prior to upper endoscopy. The yield for identifying a bleeding source using capsule endoscopy was 66% (41/62). Failure to visualize the duodenum was an important contributing factor in 7 of 21 patients (33%) with bleeding missed by capsule endoscopy. In a randomized trial of 71 patients presenting with acute upper gastrointestinal bleeding undergoing VCE (n=37) versus standard care (n=34), 7 patients were admitted to the hospital, compared with all 34

patients in the standard of care group (19 vs 100%). There were similar outcomes with regard to recurrent bleeding and 30-day mortality in both groups. Currently, UGI VCE might be utilized as an initial triage tool prior to standard conventional endoscopy, but cannot be considered an alternative to EGD in the setting of GI bleeding.

Chandran S, Testro A, Urquhart P, et al. Risk stratification of upper GI bleeding with an esophageal capsule. *Gastrointest Endosc.* 2013;77:891–898. [PMID: 23453185]

Meltzer AC, Ali MA, Kresiberg RB, et al. Video capsule endoscopy in the emergency department: a prospective study of acute upper gastrointestinal hemorrhage. *Ann Emerg Med.* 2013;61:438–443. [PMID: 23398660]

Sung JJ, Tang RS, Ching JY, et al. Use of capsule endoscopy in the emergency department as a triage of patients with GI bleeding. *Gastrointest Endosc.* 2016;84:907–913. [PMID: 27156655]

F. Colon Capsule Endoscopy

Colonic capsule endoscopy has been introduced as an alternative method for performing screening colonoscopy. Initial studies looking at the ability of colon capsule endoscopy to detect polyps have had variable results. In a meta-analysis of 7 studies of 1292 patients, the sensitivity for polyps ≥6 mm was 86% and specificity was 88%, whereas the sensitivity for polyps ≥10 mm was 87% and specificity was 95%. A more recent randomized trial of 349 patients compared capsule endoscopy versus CT colonography in randomized fashion for patients with occult positive screening tests and sensitivity of capsule to be 96.1% versus 79.3% for CT when using colonoscopy as the gold standard. No cancers were missed. Some of the improvement seems to have come from improved preparation and capsule technology.

In the United States, colon capsule endoscopy is approved for use in patients who have undergone incomplete colonoscopy. Currently, the U.S. Multisociety Task Force has designated colon capsule endoscopy as a lower tiered (tier 3) alternative screening method for colorectal cancer. In a 2020 update to its 2014 guideline, the European Society for Gastrointestinal Endoscopy (ESGE) suggests that colon capsule endoscopy is a reasonable alternative to CT colonography for those patients who undergo incomplete colonoscopy.

González-Suárez B, Pagés M, Araujo IK, et al. Colon capsule endoscopy versus CT colonography in FIT-positive colorectal cancer screening subjects: a prospective randomised trial - the VICOCA study. *BMC Med.* 2020;18:255. [PMID: 32943059]

Rex DK, Boland CR, Dominitz JA, et al. Colorectal cancer screening: recommendations for physician and patients from the U.S. Multi-Society Task Force on Colorectal Cancer. *Gastroenterology.* 2017;153:307–323. [PMID: 28600072]

Spada C, Hassan C, Bellini D, et al. Imaging alternatives to colonoscopy: CT colonography and colon capsule. European Society of Gastrointestinal Endoscopy (ESGE) and European Society of Gastrointestinal and Abdominal Radiology (ESGAR) Guideline - update 2020. *Endoscopy.* 2020;52:1127–1141. [PMID: 33104846]

Spada C, Pasha SF, Gross SA, et al. Accuracy of first- and second-generation colon capsules in endoscopic detection of colorectal polyps: a systematic review and meta-analysis. *Clin Gastroenterol Hepatol.* 2016;14:1533–1543. [PMID: 27165469]

Limitations

An advantage of VCE is that it has the potential to image the entire length of the small bowel. However, in many instances there is poor visualization of areas of mucosa due to quick passage, inability to insufflate, tangential views, and debris. Additionally, in approximately 15% of cases, the capsule does not reach the colon prior to the battery running out using standard 8 hour capsules, but this may be substantially reduced with prolonged battery life capsules. A significant limitation is that VCE lacks biopsy capability. This can be a problem because findings such as erythema, aphthous ulcerations, or frank ulcerations are seen in multiple disorders (see Table 34–3). In addition, nodules cannot be biopsied to determine if there is an underlying malignancy. Some of these limitations can now be addressed using deep small bowel enteroscopy if an abnormality is found on VCE (see "Deep Small Bowel Enteroscopy," later in this chapter).

Complications

The most important complication related to VCE is capsule retention. Overall, the risk of retention is 1–2%. Many of the disorders for which VCE is being employed, such as Crohn's disease or radiation enteritis, can increase the risk of retention. Patients with Crohn's disease are at increased risk because of possible small bowel strictures (which may be missed on conventional imaging). In the setting of established Crohn's disease, the risk or retention increases to 4–13%. In patients with established Crohn's disease, small bowel radiographic imaging (small bowel follow-through or CT or MRE) should be performed prior to VCE to decrease the risk of retention. The use of a patency capsule (PillCam Patency Capsule, Medtronic) can also decrease the risk of retention (see "Contraindications" discussed earlier).

Capsule retention rarely causes obstruction and is often associated with the identification of significant pathologic findings that require further surgical or endoscopic intervention. In a study of 733 cases, capsule retention occurred in 1.9% (14 patients). Of these, all occurred at a site of pathology (Crohn's disease [5], small bowel stenosis [5], small bowel neoplasm [3], and mesenteric ischemia [1]). Eleven patients underwent surgery for capsule removal, two had the capsule removed endoscopically, and one (with mesenteric ischemia) did not have the capsule removed. Deep small bowel enteroscopy is one option for retrieving capsules that are retained in the mid or distal small bowel and are thus out of reach of a standard enteroscopy (see the section on "Deep Small Bowel Enteroscopy").

In a meta-analysis of patients undergoing VCE, capsule retention occurred in 2.1% of 5876 studies done for suspected small bowel bleeding, 3.6% of 968 studies done for suspected IBD, 8.2% of 558 studies done for established IBD, and 2.2% of studies done for abdominal pain and/or diarrhea. In subgroup analysis of those studies done for established IBD, the retention rate was reduced to 2.7% if the patient underwent a patency capsule study or CT enterography to assess patency before performing capsule study. The most common reasons for retention were small bowel strictures (77% of retentions), but etiology was not provided in all studies.

Uncommon complications of VCE include aspiration of the capsule, impaction at the cricopharyngeus, or retention in a Zenker or Meckel diverticulum. A case of aspiration was noted in a patient who was part of the study of 733 VCE examinations. In that case, the patient was able to expel the capsule by coughing. These complications reinforce the need to evaluate patients carefully for swallowing disorders prior to performing a VCE study.

Cheifetz AS, Kornbluth AA, Legnani P, et al. The risk of retention of the capsule endoscope in patients with known or suspected Crohn's disease. *Am J Gastroenterol.* 2006;101:2218–2222. [PMID: 16848804]

Rezapour M, Amadi C, Gerson LB. Retention associated with video capsule endoscopy: systematic review and meta-analysis. *Gastrointest Endosc.* 2017;85:1157–1168. [PMID: 28069475]

Rondonotti E, Herrerias JM, Pennazio M, et al. Complications, limitations, and failures of capsule endoscopy: a review of 733 cases. *Gastrointest Endosc.* 2005;62:712–716. [PMID: 16246685]

DEEP SMALL BOWEL ENTEROSCOPY

General Considerations

The small bowel is 500 +/− 100 cm (16 ft) long on average. Push enteroscopy, however, can at most be advanced to 160 cm beyond the ligament of Treitz. With the advent of VCE, it is now possible to visualize the entire length of the small bowel, but VCE lacks biopsy and therapeutic capability. Lesions detected by VCE that are beyond the reach of a push enteroscope can be evaluated using deep small bowel enteroscopy. Total enteroscopy is possible in some cases with balloon- or spiral-assisted enteroscopy and has the advantage of allowing for biopsies and for therapeutic interventions. Yamamoto and colleagues first described double balloon enteroscopy in 2001, and it was FDA approved for use in the United States in the fall of 2004 (Double balloon endoscope, FUJIFILM Medical Systems U.S.A., Lexington, MA). Two additional systems using single balloon enteroscopy (Single Balloon Enteroscope System, Olympus, Tokyo, Japan) and manual spiral enteroscopy (Spirus Endo-Ease Discovery SB System, Spirus Medical, Stoughton, MA) have become available. Powered spiral enteroscopy is not yet available in the United States.

ASGE Technology Committee. Enteroscopy. *Gastrointest Endosc.* 2015;82:975–990. [PMID: 26388546]

Jonnalagadda S. Double balloon enteroscopy: wired technology meets wireless. *Gastroenterology* 2006;131:327–329. [PMID: 16831620]

Teitelbaum EN, Vaziri K, Zettervall S, et al. Intraoperative small bowel length measurements and analysis of demographic predictors of increased length. *Clin Anat.* 2013;26:827–832. [PMID: 23519889]

Yamamoto H, Sekine Y, Sato Y, et al. Total enteroscopy with a nonsurgical steerable double balloon method. *Gastrointest Endosc.* 2001;53:216–220. [PMID: 1174299]

Indications

Deep small bowel enteroscopy is used most often for the evaluation of obscure gastrointestinal bleeding, small bowel radiographic abnormalities, abnormalities identified on VCE, chronic diarrhea and malabsorption, and in polyposis syndromes to detect and remove polyps (Table 35–5). It has also been used to biopsy and dilate small bowel strictures, to screen for disease recurrence in patients with a history of small bowel malignancies, to evaluate patients with refractory celiac disease, and to retrieve foreign bodies (eg, video capsules). In patients who have undergone Roux-en-Y gastric bypass, it can visualize the defunctionalized stomach and gain access to the bile and pancreatic ducts.

ASGE Technology Committee. Enteroscopy. *Gastrointest Endosc.* 2015;82:975–990. [PMID: 26388546]

Shah RJ, Smolkin M, Yen R, et al. A multicenter, U.S. experience of single-balloon, double-balloon, and rotational overtube-assisted enteroscopy ERCP in patients with surgically altered pancreaticobiliary anatomy (with video). *Gastrointest Endosc.* 2013;77:593–600. [PMID: 23290720]

Table 35–5. Indications for deep small bowel enteroscopy.

Suspected small bowel bleeding
Small bowel radiographic abnormalities
Abnormalities seen on capsule endoscopy
Chronic diarrhea and malabsorption
Detection and removal of polyps in polyposis syndromes
Dilation and biopsy of small bowel strictures
Screening for recurrence of small bowel malignancy
Refractory celiac disease
Visualization of the defunctionalized stomach after Roux-en-Y gastric bypass
Access to the bile and pancreatic ducts after Roux-en-Y gastric bypass or Roux-en-Y hepaticojejunostomy
Small bowel foreign body retrieval (including video capsules)

Procedure

A. Patient Preparation

Patients who are undergoing an antegrade (per os) study fast for 8 hours prior to the study. For a retrograde (per anus) study, a standard colonoscopy preparation is employed.

B. Techniques

1. Double balloon enteroscopy—The double balloon enteroscopy system is composed of an enteroscope, an overtube, and a balloon pump controller. The system uses two latex balloons, one on the end of the enteroscope and one on the end of the overtube (Figure 35–1). Through a combination of antegrade and retrograde approaches, the entire small bowel can be examined in 4–86% of patients, depending on the population studied.

The examination is typically performed with anesthesia assistance most commonly with deep sedation eg, propofol, although some centers prefer general anesthesia due to the length of the study and the potential for patient discomfort. During an antegrade study, the scope and overtube are advanced until both are within the duodenum past the ampulla. The balloon on the end of the overtube is then inflated to anchor the small bowel. The scope is then advanced. When the scope can no longer be advanced, the balloon at the tip of the scope is inflated, again anchoring the small bowel. The balloon on the overtube is then deflated and the overtube is advanced until it reaches the end of the scope. At this point, the balloon on the end of the overtube is again inflated. With both balloons inflated, the scope and the overtube are gently withdrawn until resistance is met. In so doing, the small bowel is pleated onto the overtube and loops are reduced. The balloon on the scope is then deflated and the scope is again advanced. This sequence is repeated until the lesion of interest is reached or until the scope can

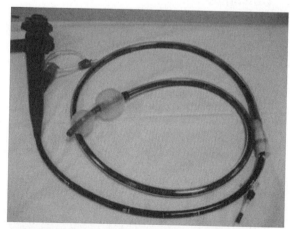

▲ **Figure 35–1.** Double balloon enteroscope.

no longer be advanced. Fluoroscopic guidance may be used to aid with scope advancement and reductions. When a retrograde approach is employed, the scope and overtube are advanced until they are both within the terminal ileum, and the same sequence is then carried out.

Using the antegrade approach, an average of 220–360 cm of small bowel can be examined. With the retrograde approach, an average of 120–180 cm of small bowel can be visualized. The reported rates of complete small bowel visualization (often through a combination of antegrade and retrograde examinations) vary widely (4–86%), with higher rates being reported in Japan and lower rates in Europe and the United States.

The double balloon enteroscope has an accessory channel that will accommodate biopsy forceps, argon plasma coagulation probes, bipolar hemostasis probes, cytology brushes, Roth nets, snares, and injection needles.

2. Single balloon enteroscopy—The single balloon enteroscopy system is similar to the double balloon system except that instead of employing a balloon on the end of the enteroscope, the tip of the enteroscope is angulated sharply to anchor the scope. Average depths of small bowel insertion are 130–270 cm for antegrade studies and 70–200 cm for retrograde studies.

3. Spiral enteroscopy—Spiral enteroscopy uses an enteroscope and an overtube with a soft, raised helical spiral. The enteroscope is advanced into the small bowel along with the overtube. As the overtube is rotated, the small bowel is pulled onto it. Reported insertion depths are similar to those seen with antegrade studies performed using balloon-assisted enteroscopy. Current availability is limited as the device is no longer active development. A powered spiral system now in use in Europe is currently undergoing testing in the United States.

▶ Outcomes

The data available on outcomes come primarily from research on double balloon enteroscopy, although results reported for single balloon and spiral enteroscopy are similar. The diagnostic yield for double balloon enteroscopy ranges from 34% to 80%, with a therapeutic yield of 18–55%. The indication for the procedure is an important predictor of diagnostic yield. In a study of 1765 patients undergoing double balloon enteroscopy, the diagnostic yield overall was 48%. The yield was highest for patients with an indication of Peutz-Jeghers syndrome (82%), followed by mid-gastrointestinal bleeding (53%), and Crohn's disease (47%). It was lowest for patients with an indication of abdominal pain (19%) or diarrhea (16%). A therapeutic procedure was carried out during double balloon enteroscopy in 529 patients (30%). Argon plasma coagulation was the most common intervention (23% of patient). Other interventions included polypectomy (4%),

dilation of small bowel stenoses (2%), and injection therapy at bleeding sites (2%).

A second study of 353 patients found a similar diagnostic yield of 75% for small bowel lesions. Sixty percent of the patients were being evaluated for suspected small bowel bleeding, 10% had chronic abdominal pain, 9% had a polyposis syndrome, 8% had Crohn's disease, and 13% underwent the study for other indications, including foreign body extraction. The findings influenced subsequent therapy in 67%. Endoscopic therapy was performed in 59%, and medical therapy was initiated or changed in 19%. Twenty-two percent of the patients required surgery. Not surprisingly, the majority of patients who received endoscopic therapy suffered from small bowel bleeding (74%).

Baniya R, Upadhaya S, Subedi SC, et al. Balloon enteroscopy versus spiral enteroscopy for small-bowel disorders: a systematic review and meta-analysis. *Gastrointest Endosc.* 2017;86: 997–1005. [PMID: 28652176]

Beyna T, Arvanitakis M, Schneider M, et al. Motorised spiral enteroscopy: first prospective clinical feasibility study. *Gut.* 2021;70:261–267. [PMID: 32332141]

Khashab MA, Lennon AM, Dunbar KB, et al. A comparative evaluation of single balloon enteroscopy and spiral enteroscopy for patients with mid-gut disorders. *Gastrointest Endosc.* 2010;71:766–772. [PMID: 20619404]

May A, Nachbar L, Pohl J, et al. Endoscopic interventions in the small bowel using double balloon enteroscopy: feasibility and limitations. *Am J Gastroenterol.* 2007;102:527–535. [PMID: 17222315]

Moschler O, May A, Muller MK, et al. Complications and performance of double-balloon enteroscopy (DBE): results from a large prospective DBE database in Germany. *Endoscopy.* 2011;43:484–489. [PMID: 21370220]

▶ Limitations

The primary limitation of deep small bowel enteroscopy is incomplete mucosal visualization. As noted in the preceding discussion, the entire small bowel can be examined in 4–86% of patients using a combined antegrade and retrograde approach with double balloon enteroscopy, leaving a significant percentage of patients with incomplete small bowel visualization. Most commonly, this occurs due to inability to advance the scope through the entire length of small bowel. Deep small bowel enteroscopy is also limited by the fact that it typically requires two operators (at least one of whom is a physician), and it is time consuming, with an average procedure time of 73–115 minutes for balloon-assisted enteroscopy, though the time required for spiral-assisted enteroscopy may be less. In addition, because of potential patient discomfort, some centers use general anesthesia, which can make procedures logistically more difficult to arrange and expensive.

▶ Complications

The most common adverse event is abdominal pain, the day of or the day after the procedure. This occurs in up to 20% of patients, though may be less pronounced with the use of carbon dioxide insufflation. Patients also may report a sore throat. Perforations have been reported, including multiple perforations following chemotherapy for lymphoma and following small bowel polypectomy. Perforation is also associated with surgically altered gastrointestinal tract anatomy (eg, ileoanal anastomosis or an ileostomy), with a perforation rate in one study of 3% in this setting. Postprocedure paralytic ileus and pancreatitis have also been reported. Bleeding has been seen following polypectomies.

The overall major complication rate in the study discussed above of 1765 patients undergoing double balloon enteroscopy was 1.2%. There were 6 bleeding complications (0.3%), 3 perforations (0.13%), 4 cases of pancreatitis (0.3% of antegrade procedures), and 11 sedation-related complications (0.5%). A higher (though still low) complication rate of 3.4% was seen in the study of 353 patients. Bleeding occurred in 1.1%, perforation in 1.7%, and enteritis in 0.6%. This, however, underestimates the risk associated with individual interventions. Of the 46 patients who underwent polypectomies, 5 (10.8%) suffered complications. Bleeding occurred in 2 (4.3%) and perforation occurred in 3 (6.5%). All of the complications in patients undergoing polypectomy occurred after the removal of polyps that were larger than 3 cm. Argon plasma coagulation had a lower complication rate of 1 in 108 (0.9%).

Thus, while the overall rate of complications is low, patients undergoing polypectomy should be advised that there is a significant complication rate associated with the removal of large polyps, as are often seen in Peutz-Jeghers syndrome, approaching 5–10%. However, given that the alternative in these patients is intraoperative enteroscopy, which has a morbidity rate up to 30% and a mortality rate of 2%, deep small bowel enteroscopy is still preferable in most situations when feasible.

Gastrointestinal Foreign Bodies

Russell D. Dolan, MD

Andrew C. Storm, MD

Christopher C. Thompson, MD

ESSENTIALS OF FOREIGN BODIES

▶ Plain films (radiographies) should be the initial diagnostic study; obtain both lateral and posteroanterior films of the neck, chest, and abdomen as indicated.

▶ Avoid oral contrast as this may obscure endoscopic visualization.

▶ Endoscopic evaluation may be required for objects that are potentially radiolucent in patients with a compelling history but negative imaging findings.

▶ Impacted meat is typically radiolucent and is the most common esophageal foreign body in adults; perform endoscopy promptly in all cases with clinical evidence of obstruction and failure to spontaneously pass with initial medical management.

▶ Consider endotracheal intubation prior to foreign body extraction to protect the airway from both secretions and risk of aspiration of the foreign body upon retrieval.

▶ Many foreign bodies pass spontaneously, but some objects (eg, sharp objects and batteries) require urgent intervention.

General Considerations

Gastrointestinal (GI) foreign bodies occur in all age groups and are commonly seen by the gastroenterologist, as well as by those in various surgical disciplines. The endoscopic removal of foreign bodies dates back to the early 1900s, with more widespread adoption following the advent of the fiberscope in 1957. Methods of diagnosis and treatment have continued to evolve since that time with the development of enhanced imaging, specialized accessories, and improved procedural efficacy.

Foreign body ingestion, including dietary foreign bodies or food bolus impaction, currently represents the second most common indication for emergent GI endoscopy, after GI hemorrhage. Patients with foreign body ingestion typically present to their primary care physician or the emergency department, and the majority of foreign bodies pass spontaneously. Nevertheless, significant complications may arise resulting in approximately 1500–1600 deaths in the United States annually. Therefore, it is essential for the endoscopist to efficiently determine which patients require therapeutic intervention, and to be comfortable with proper methods of extraction. This chapter reviews indications for foreign body removal, the typical diagnostic evaluation, and endoscopic techniques for foreign body management.

Clinical Findings

A. Symptoms & Signs

Following foreign body ingestion patients may present in a variety of manners, ranging from asymptomatic to having signs and symptoms of complete esophageal obstruction or frank perforation. In the majority of cases, a careful clinical history provides the correct diagnosis. Clinical history may be less reliable in children younger than age 5, individuals with mental illness, and in otherwise uncooperative patients. In such populations, symptoms and diagnostic studies are more critical to clarifying the diagnosis.

Most true foreign body ingestions occur in children between the ages of 1 and 5 who swallow small household items or toys. Fortunately, most of these objects are small and blunt, and they typically pass spontaneously. Adults who ingest true foreign bodies often have psychiatric disturbance, mental retardation, alcoholism, or identifiable reasons for secondary gain, such as incarceration. Dietary foreign bodies and food bolus impactions typically occur in older adults, denture wearers, and those with underlying esophageal disorders.

Presenting symptoms are determined by the type of ingested foreign body and its location.

1. Esophageal foreign bodies—Esophageal foreign bodies may result in symptoms of dysphagia, odynophagia, or signs of complete esophageal obstruction, including inability to swallow secretions, sialorrhea, and regurgitation. Sudden onset of odynophagia following eating suggests impaction of a bone, sharp food fragment, toothpick, or similar object in the esophagus. Respiratory symptoms such as coughing and stridor are common in younger children as their compliant tracheal rings are more easily compressed by an adjacent esophageal foreign body. Upper airway obstruction is a rare presentation for adults with an esophageal foreign body; however, meat bolus impaction at the level of the cricopharyngeus can result in respiratory obstruction, which has been referred to as "steak house syndrome."

Plain films of the neck may demonstrate the location of a radiopaque object in the esophagus (Figure 36–1). Subcutaneous emphysema in the supraclavicular area or the neck suggests perforation of the esophagus or hypopharynx. Esophageal perforation by sharp objects at the level of the aortic arch may also result in an aortoesophageal fistula, which typically presents with a herald bleed, followed by massive hemorrhage. Fortunately, these presentations are rare.

2. Gastric foreign bodies—Gastric foreign bodies are generally asymptomatic, except when they are large enough to be associated with postprandial emesis and early satiety. Long-standing foreign bodies or those that are sharp and pointed may become impacted in the gastric wall and result in inflammation, ulceration, hemorrhage, or perforation. These patients often present with pain or bleeding.

3. Small bowel foreign bodies—Foreign bodies that have made their way to the small bowel typically remain asymptomatic if they are able to pass the fixed bend of the retroperitoneal duodenum (ie, Ligament of Treitz). However, foreign bodies are also at risk of failed passage beyond the ileocecal valve into the colon if greater than 2 cm in dimeter. Symptoms of small bowel foreign bodies are typically those of perforation or obstruction.

4. Colorectal foreign bodies—Once beyond the ileocecal valve, foreign bodies typically pass spontaneously, however rarely may be associated with obstruction or perforation of the colon or rectum. In the event of perforation, injury to intra-abdominal structures including the liver, pancreas, spleen, kidneys, aorta and iliac arteries, bladder and reproductive organs may occur.

B. Physical Findings

Physical examination may yield important clues to identifying complications due to ingested foreign bodies. Crepitus in the supraclavicular and cervical areas suggests perforation of the hypopharynx or esophagus. Large gastric foreign bodies may occasionally be palpable on abdominal examination. Peritoneal signs often suggest gastric or intestinal perforation, and physical findings typical of bowel obstruction may occur with small bowel foreign bodies.

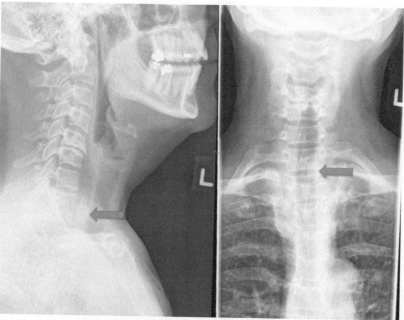

▲ **Figure 36–1.** Plain film radiographs. Anteroposterior and lateral neck films showing large calcium pill impacted in the proximal esophagus (*arrow*).

C. Imaging Studies

The plain film radiograph should be the initial diagnostic study. Both lateral and posteroanterior films should be obtained of the neck, chest, and abdomen. This is important in identifying small or flat objects that may overlie the spine, and in determining the exact location of a foreign body. The lateral film is often essential in differentiating between tracheobronchial and esophageal locations. Perforation may also be identified if the object is seen extending beyond the lumen wall, or if a soft tissue mass is seen adjacent to the object. Plain films should also be obtained to evaluate food bolus impactions, as the presence of bone fragments may alter the endoscopic management. If precise localization within the GI tract using plain films is difficult, computed tomography may aid in localization of a foreign body by adding a degree of dimensionality from plain film radiographs.

Objects that are relatively radiolucent, such as plastic, wood, most glass, and small bones, may not be seen on plain film, in which case xeroradiography or computed tomography may be helpful in making the diagnosis.

Contrast studies should be avoided. Gastrografin is contraindicated as it is hypertonic resulting in a severe chemical pneumonitis if aspirated, and barium can obscure endoscopic visualization, thereby complicating therapy.

Endoscopic evaluation may also be required, even in the absence of imaging findings, for a suspected radiolucent foreign body and compelling history. Additionally, endoscopy is often the therapeutic method of choice.

▶ Treatment

Although the majority of foreign bodies pass spontaneously, certain objects need urgent intervention. The type of foreign body and its location determine management. In general, the following should be removed: all esophageal foreign bodies, elongated and sharp gastric foreign bodies, and blunt foreign bodies persisting for 2 weeks in the stomach. Endoscopic removal may be technically challenging depending on the object's shape, quantity and material, and several accessories are available to enhance procedural success. Details of management are as follows:

A. Foreign Body Classification & Management

A wide variety of ingested foreign bodies may be encountered by the GI endoscopist. Roughly 75% of all foreign bodies pass spontaneously, with 1% resulting in serious complication or need for surgery.

Foreign bodies may be broadly classified as true foreign bodies or dietary foreign bodies. They may be further categorized as dull or sharp, blunt or pointed, long or short, toxic or nontoxic, and as food bolus impactions. These features are associated with prognosis and depending on anatomic location, may indicate when urgent removal is necessary.

1. Sharp and pointed objects—The most common sharp objects include fish or chicken bones and toothpicks; however, razor blades, hat pins, nails, and fragments of glass may also be seen (Figure 36–2; Plates 93–95). Although the

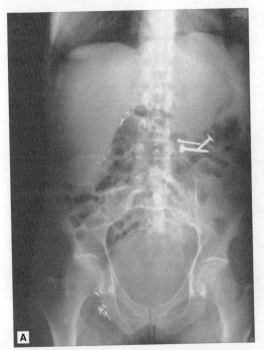 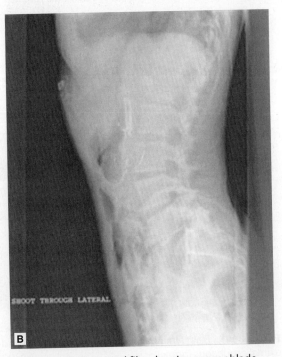

▲ **Figure 36–2.** Plain film radiographs. **A.** Posteroanterior film showing nails. **B.** Lateral film showing a razor blade.

majority of such objects can pass safely through the GI tract, perforation rates are as high as 35%. Thus, endoscopic removal is necessary if the object is within reach of the endoscope. When the object is above the cricopharyngeus, referral to an otolaryngologist for direct laryngoscopy is indicated. Otherwise, urgent flexible endoscopy should be considered. If the object has passed beyond the duodenum, daily radiographs should be obtained to determine its location and detect free air or other evidence of complications. If the object fails to progress for three consecutive days, then surgical intervention should be considered.

2. Long objects—Long and narrow foreign bodies such as toothbrushes and stiff wires are associated with a high incidence of perforation as they have difficulty passing the fixed curves of the duodenum. Objects 6 cm in length or longer are particularly problematic, and early endoscopic intervention is recommended.

3. Blunt foreign bodies—This is perhaps the most diverse class of ingested foreign bodies and is the most common in the pediatric population. In a review describing the management of 242 foreign bodies, coins were the most common foreign body ingested by children. Other objects in this class include marbles, small toys, and disc batteries. Conservative outpatient management is indicated for the vast majority of blunt foreign bodies that have passed into the stomach. Rounded objects larger than 2.5 cm are less likely to pass the pylorus, and endoscopic removal should be considered if the object fails to pass the stomach within 2–3 weeks. If the object successfully passes through the stomach, a radiograph should be obtained every 3–4 days to assess passage. Surgical removal should be considered if the object remains in the same location for more than 1 week.

Button batteries or disc batteries require special consideration. The most common disc battery systems include silver oxide, manganese dioxide, and mercuric oxide. These typically contain alkaline solutions of either sodium hydroxide or potassium, which can cause direct corrosive effects or low-voltage burns. Liquefaction necrosis and perforation can also occur. Urgent endoscopic evaluation with battery removal is thus indicated. If battery disruption is noted, heavy metal levels should be monitored in the blood and urine. Mercury poisoning is a rare complication of battery disruption. Copper, nickel, and lead poisoning have also been reported after prolonged retention of various metallic foreign objects. If a disc battery successfully passes into the stomach, it will typically pass the GI tract without consequence. Forceps should be avoided if endoscopic removal is attempted as they can lead to battery disruption. Cathartics and acid suppression have no proven role and should also be avoided.

Magnets are another blunt object prone to causing mischief after ingestion. Particularly in the case of magnets swallowed in succession over time, opposite poles of two (or more) separate magnets may meet across the walls of separate lumens, which can lead to compression necrosis and formation of fistulas between segments of the GI tract

(ie, gastrojejunal, enteroenteral, and enterocolonic). These fistulae can lead to calorie malabsorption, internal herniation, and other negative consequences. For this reason, close follow-up of patient's symptoms and serial abdominal images should be used to follow magnets through the GI, when endoscopic removal is not possible.

Finally, it is important to note that some foreign bodies may remain undigested in the stomach for long periods of time and can be encountered incidentally. Materials may change over time with long-term exposure to stomach acid making them especially difficult to remove (see Plate 95).

4. Toxic foreign bodies—Internal concealment of illicit drugs wrapped in plastic or latex packages, also known as "body packing," is seen with higher frequency in regions of drug trafficking. Package rupture or leakage can be fatal, and such foreign bodies require special consideration. Endoscopic removal should not be attempted.

Drug packages can be subdivided into three types. Type 1 includes condoms and balloons. These typically appear as a density with surrounding halo of gas on radiography. Each condom can contain 3–5 g of cocaine, and ingestion of 1–3 g may be lethal. As these packages are very susceptible to breakage, early surgical removal should be considered.

Type 2 and type 3 packages consist of layers of tubular latex or plastic, with or without aluminum foil. Type 2 packages may appear similar to type 1 on radiography. Type 3 packages are typically smaller and may not be seen on radiographs. These packages are less susceptible to breakage and, if identified, they may be followed with daily radiographs. Indications for surgery include failure of the package to progress on the daily radiograph, evidence of intestinal obstruction, visualization of broken packages on radiograph, passage of broken packages, or development of symptoms.

5. Food bolus impaction—Impacted meat is the most common esophageal foreign body in adults. Total esophageal obstruction is implied by drooling and inability to swallow secretions. This is an indication for urgent endoscopic intervention. Ideally all meat boluses should be extracted or advanced into the stomach urgently (within a few hours of ingestion) as patients are at risk for aspiration. Additionally, with prolonged bolus impaction there is risk for local esophageal ischemia and pressure ulceration, and with time the bolus may be partially digested, requiring piecemeal removal. In adults, the administration of glucagon (1 mg intravenously) may be attempted prior to endoscopy to encourage spontaneous passage. This may be repeated at 10 minutes; however, if this is not effective further doses are not recommended. Glucagon has little effect on the proximal esophagus but causes substantial relaxation of the smooth muscle of the lower esophageal sphincter, allowing spontaneous passage of a distal impaction in up to 50% of cases. Patients with structural abnormalities are less likely to respond to this form of medical therapy. In children, small randomized trials have shown no benefit of glucagon over placebo, and because nausea and vomiting are major side effects of the medication, it is not recommended for use in this age group. Glucagon is contraindicated in patients with underlying pheochromocytoma, insulinoma, and Zollinger-Ellison syndrome. Papain and other meat tenderizers should be strictly avoided. Many impactions occur in the proximal esophagus, for instance at the level of cervical spine bone spurs, and careful attention must be paid to this area on initial esophageal intubation. Additionally, many patients with food bolus impactions have underlying esophageal disease, such as peptic stricture, Schatzki ring, or eosinophilic esophagitis. Local trauma and edema often preclude an accurate diagnosis of such conditions at the initial endoscopic evaluation, and subsequent studies are typically required. This may include repeat upper endoscopy with biopsy several weeks after resolution of the food bolus impaction.

6. Rectal foreign bodies—Numerous objects, including bottles, vibrators, various fruits and vegetables, flashlights, light bulbs, and a propane tank, have been reported in the literature. Because of this wide variety of objects and the varying degree of trauma that may be seen, it is important to have a systematic approach to the diagnosis and management of retained rectal foreign bodies. Additionally, delayed presentations are common, due to embarrassment and reluctance to seek medical attention, and patients are often not entirely truthful regarding important details, further complicating management. Manual or surgical removal is commonly required, and colorectal surgeons are typically asked to manage these cases. It is important to exclude perforation in all patients with abdominal imaging prior to considering endoscopy. Surgery is indicated in all cases of perforation. In addition, objects that are 10 cm in diameter, have been in place for more than 2 days, and that are proximal to the rectum, typically require surgical removal. If a transanal approach is feasible, anal sphincter relaxation is critical. Perianal nerve block, and/or spinal anesthetic, should be considered in addition to intravenous conscious sedation. Perforation may only be noticed after extraction, and imaging post foreign body removal is also important.

B. Methods of Removal

The removal of esophageal foreign bodies dates back to the early 1900s and since that time, endoscopes and through-the-scope tools have evolved to assist in the removal of ingested foreign bodies. Methods of removal in current use are detailed in this section.

Prior to removal, a complete history and physical examination are essential to determine the need for removal and to assess the safety of the procedure. This will also help in selection of the correct instruments based on the type of foreign body and its location.

1. Sedation—When planning foreign body extraction, the first decision involves determining the most appropriate form of sedation for the patient. Many patients who have ingested foreign material are poor candidates for conscious sedation because of baseline characteristics. History of alcoholism, drug abuse, and psychiatric conditions may render a patient difficult to sedate and increase the associated procedural risk. General anesthesia with endotracheal intubation provides deeper sedation and additional airway protection that may be desirable in certain circumstances.

2. Choice of endoscope—The second decision involves which type of endoscope to use. Forward-viewing (single-channel or double-channel) or side-viewing endoscopes may each have a role, and selection should not be arbitrary. The forward-viewing endoscopes have an advantage over side-viewing endoscopes in visualizing the esophagus and most parts of the stomach and small bowel. Dual-channel endoscopes are also particularly useful for removing elongated objects as accessories may be passed through both channels, which may be helpful in positioning an object for capture or to hold it in a straight position for extraction. The double-channel endoscope, however, is larger in diameter than the single-channel endoscope and may not be compatible with all accessories, such as a hood or some overtubes. Additionally, the double-channel endoscope may be too large for use in infants or small children due to concern for tracheal compression. The side-viewing endoscope provides better visualization of the medial aspect of the lesser curve and the periampullary area in the small bowel and may be useful in addressing foreign bodies lodged in these areas.

3. Choice of accessories—Several accessories may facilitate the endoscopic management of foreign bodies. Various devices are available to protect the GI tract or airway during extraction, and to grasp objects of different sizes and shapes.

A. FORCEPS AND SNARES—Different types of forceps or graspers are available, and certain varieties may be more or less useful for specific materials. Rat-toothed forceps and alligator forceps are more effective than standard biopsy forceps at grasping various foreign materials, including plastics and metal (Figure 36–3). Snares, biliary stone retrieval baskets, and snares fitted with netting may also be useful for contending with certain objects. Netted snares are particularly useful for dealing with objects that are prone to crumbling and button batteries.

The orientation of which the objects are grasped is important to consider. For elongated objects, it is important to grasp them at one end and keep the long axis in line with the esophagus. For sharp objects, it is critical to grasp the object such that the sharp end is trailing. Additionally, when planning a procedure, it is recommended that various instruments be tested on a similar object external to the patient, as this will reduce procedure time and could lead to improved outcomes.

B. OVERTUBES—An overtube is a plastic sheath with an inner diameter large enough to accommodate an endoscope, and several varieties are available (Figure 36–4). Use of an overtube should be considered if multiple intubations are anticipated, if airway protection is desired, or if sharp objects have been ingested.

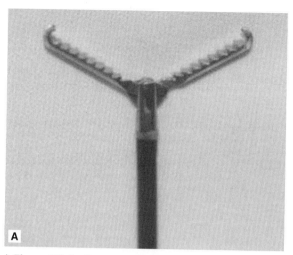
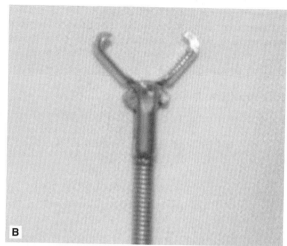

▲ **Figure 36–3.** Graspers. **A.** Alligator forceps. **B.** Rat-toothed forceps.

Overtubes come in various lengths and may extend to the midesophagus or into the proximal stomach. There are two methods for placing overtubes. Reusable overtubes may be introduced over a snug fitting wire-guided Savary dilator, and single-use overtubes may be preloaded over the endoscope with the matching tapered-tip introducer. It is not acceptable to place a reusable overtube by preloading it over an endoscope as the resulting gap between the endoscope and the overtube could result in perforation of the hypopharynx. The inner diameter of the overtube varies depending on the specific product but is typically less than 14 mm in diameter. This feature can be limiting when dealing with large objects.

C. FOLEY CATHETERS AND MAGNET-ATTACHED NASOGASTRIC TUBE—Although less commonly used today, utilization of a foley catheter or magnet-attached nasogastric tube can be attempted and may be helpful in specific situations. Attempting prior to endoscopy may obviate the need for sedation, particularly in children, or serve as an alternative when endoscopy is not immediately available. Although there are benefits, including that specific training is not required and this technique is comparatively inexpensive, retrieval is typically limited to magnetic foreign bodies.

D. HOODS—The foreign body hood is an alternative to the overtube and is particularly useful when dealing with sharp foreign objects (Figure 36–5). The protective hood is attached to the bending segment of the endoscope and is folded back to avoid compromising endoscopic visualization. After the object is grasped using the appropriate endoscopic

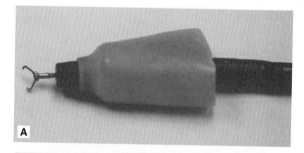
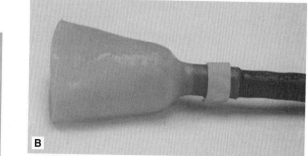

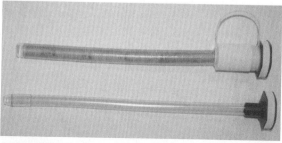

▲ **Figure 36–4.** Overtube and internal introducer with tapered tip.

▲ **Figure 36–5.** Foreign body hood protector. **A.** Open configuration. **B.** Closed hood, following acquisition of a foreign body and withdrawal of the endoscope.

accessories, the endoscope is withdrawn. As the hood passes through the lower esophageal sphincter, it is folded forward covering the object and protecting the gastric cardia and esophagus from contact with the object. Unlike the overtube, the hood does not provide additional airway protection.

C. Alternatives to Removal

For food bolus impactions, it may be safer to push the object into the stomach rather than attempt removal. This must be done with care. It is essential to first evaluate the area beyond the foreign body, to make certain there is no stricture, or other anatomic defect. Gentle pressure may then be applied to the object to facilitate passage. This is typically not acceptable for large true foreign bodies.

Bekkerman M, Sachdev AH, Andrade J, Twersky Y, Iqbal S. Endoscopic management of foreign bodies in the gastrointestinal tract: a review of the literature. *Gastroenterol Res Pract.* 2016;2016:8520767. [PMID: 27807447]

Birk M, Bauerfeind P, Deprez PH, et al. Removal of foreign bodies in the upper gastrointestinal tract in adults: European Society of Gastrointestinal Endoscopy (ESGE) Clinical Guideline. *Endoscopy.* 2016;48(5):489–496. [PMID: 26862844]

Choe JY, Choe BH. Foreign body removal in children using Foley catheter or magnet tube from gastrointestinal tract. *Pediatr Gastroenterol Hepatol Nutr.* 2019;22(2):132–141. [PMID: 30899689]

Lee CY, Kao BZ, Wu CS, et al. Retrospective analysis of endoscopic management of foreign bodies in the upper gastrointestinal tract of adults. *J Chin Med Assoc.* 2019;82(2):105–109. [PMID: 30839499]

Shields HM, Scheid FJ, Pierce TT, et al. Case 4-2019: an 18-year-old man with abdominal pain and hematochezia. *N Engl J Med.* 2019;380(5):473–485. [PMID: 30699318]

Tringali A, Thomson M, Dumonceau JM, et al. Pediatric gastrointestinal endoscopy: European Society of Gastrointestinal Endoscopy (ESGE) and European Society for Paediatric Gastroenterology Hepatology and Nutrition (ESPGHAN) Guideline Executive summary. *Endoscopy.* 2017;49(1):83–91. [PMID: 27617420]

Endoscopic Ultrasound

37

Russell D. Dolan, MD
Linda Lee, MD

ESSENTIALS OF DIAGNOSIS

▶ Endoscopic ultrasound (EUS) is a critical tool in cancer staging and is superior to computed tomography (CT) and positron emission tomography (PET), in locoregional esophageal cancer staging.

▶ EUS-guided fine-needle aspiration (EUS-FNA) and more recently fine needle biopsy (FNB) is the most sensitive method for diagnosing pancreatic cancer; overall accuracy of EUS is similar to CT for assessing vascular invasion.

▶ EUS helps evaluate subepithelial lesions, although the yield of EUS-FNA/FNB is lower for subepithelial than for extraluminal lesions.

▶ EUS is an important tool in diagnosing chronic pancreatitis.

▶ Diagnostic yield for EUS is similar to magnetic resonance cholangiopancreatography (MRCP) in detecting choledocholithiasis with the choice of modality guided by local availability.

▶ Newer imaging modalities and tools including elastography, contrast-enhanced EUS, needle-based confocal endomicroscopy and microforceps may enhance EUS diagnosis of pancreatic masses and cysts.

▶ Therapeutic EUS offers many potential opportunities to replace percutaneous or surgical management including celiac plexus block (CPB) or neurolysis, drainage of pseudocysts and walled-off necrosis, and creation of gastroenterostomies.

General Considerations

EUS is the premier tool for staging gastrointestinal cancers and has revolutionized the role of gastrointestinal endoscopy in diagnostic imaging inside and outside the gastrointestinal tract. EUS merges endoscopy, which is limited to visualizing the lumen of the gastrointestinal tract, with ultrasonography, which allows imaging of the layers of the gastrointestinal wall and surrounding structures. Tissue diagnosis can be obtained with EUS-FNA or FNB, which uses a catheter with a retractable needle that can be advanced into visualized tissue. Advances in the therapeutic application of EUS began with CPB and neurolysis for pain control in chronic pancreatitis and pancreatic cancer and have expanded to include endoscopic pseudocyst and walled off necrosis drainage, biliary and pancreatic duct access, EUS-guided fine-needle injection (EUS-FNI) therapy, EUS-guided gastroenterostomy to bypass malignant gastric outlet obstructions, EUS-guided gallbladder drainage, and EUS-guided gastric varix coil embolization.

A. Equipment

Radial scanning echoendoscopes were the first instruments used with the advent of EUS in the 1980s (Figure 37–1). The ultrasound transducer is mounted on the tip of the endoscope and provides 360-degree cross-sectional images perpendicular to the long axis of the endoscope (Figure 37–2). The endoscopic viewing optic is located proximal to the ultrasound transducer and provides an oblique view of the lumen. Later, the linear echoendoscope was developed which enabled biopsy (Figure 37–3). To overcome the problem of ultrasound waves traveling through an air-filled lumen, a balloon that can be filled with water surrounds the ultrasound transducer. Various ultrasonic frequencies between 5 and 20 MHz are used.

Linear array echoendoscopes provide ultrasound images along the long axis of the endoscope usually in a 120- to 180-degree arc (see Figure 37–2). This is critical to allow simultaneous imaging of the needle and target lesion during EUS-FNA/FNB. A variety of needles, including 19-, 22-, and 25-gauge, can be passed through the endoscopic working channel. The linear array echoendoscope has enabled the development of therapeutic EUS.

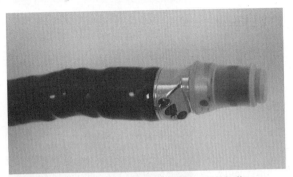

▲ **Figure 37–1.** Radial echoendoscope with balloon inflated.

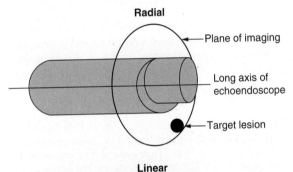

▲ **Figure 37–2.** Imaging planes for radial and linear echoendoscopes. The radial echoendoscope provides images in a plane perpendicular to the long axis. The linear echoendoscope provides images along the long axis in an 80–105-degree arc with fine-needle aspiration capability.

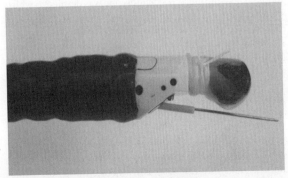

▲ **Figure 37–3.** Linear echoendoscope.

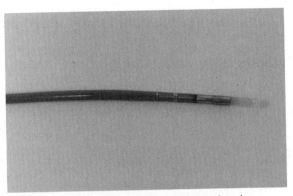

▲ **Figure 37–4.** High-frequency ultrasound probe.

In high-frequency ultrasound probe sonography, a catheter with a tiny mechanically rotating ultrasound transducer at the tip is inserted through the endoscopic working channel (Figure 37–4). The probe images with frequencies between 12 and 30 MHz with higher resolution allowing for more detailed imaging at the cost of decreased depth of penetration. Wire-guided probes can be introduced into the biliary and pancreatic ducts to perform intraductal ultrasound (IDUS).

B. Technique

Typically, a standard upper endoscopy or flexible sigmoidoscopy for rectal EUS is performed before the EUS to identify the area of interest and to ensure the echoendoscope can be safely advanced in the gastrointestinal tract. Most echoendoscopes are passed in a "blind" manner similar to the duodenoscope due to the oblique endoscopic optics. There is a forward viewing echoendoscope that can accomplish standard endoscopy and EUS using the echoendoscope. After advancing the echoendoscope to the area to be imaged, a water interface is established between the ultrasound transducer and the gastrointestinal wall. This can be accomplished by inflating the balloon on the tip of the transducer, by filling the gastrointestinal lumen with water, or by using both techniques. Once a sufficient water interface has been established, EUS images should be obtained perpendicular to the lesion of interest as oblique images commonly distort the gastrointestinal wall and lead to false interpretations.

EUS-FNA/FNB is performed with the linear echoendoscope. The needle is advanced under endosonographic guidance into the lesion of interest, the stylet may be withdrawn, and suction may be applied using a 10- to 25-cc syringe while advancing the needle back and forth within the lesion.

C. Normal EUS Anatomy

EUS imaging of the gastrointestinal wall layer typically reveals five layers alternating in bright and dark bands (Figure 37–5). The first bright or hyperechoic layer closest to the probe represents the superficial mucosa; the second dark or hypoechoic layer corresponds to the deep mucosa or

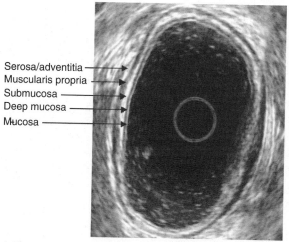

Serosa/adventitia
Muscularis propria
Submucosa
Deep mucosa
Mucosa

▲ **Figure 37–5.** EUS image of normal gastrointestinal wall layers.

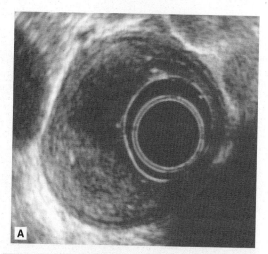

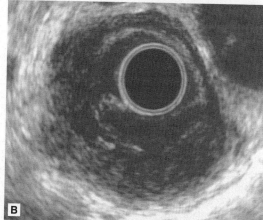

▲ **Figure 37–6.** EUS images of esophageal cancer. **A.** Stage T2. **B.** Stage T3.

muscularis mucosa; the third hyperechoic layer is the submucosa; the fourth hypoechoic layer is the muscularis propria; and the fifth hyperechoic layer represents the serosa or adventitia. The normal thickness of the gastrointestinal wall varies from 2 to 4 mm.

CANCER STAGING

Most cancers are staged according to the TNM system of the American Joint Commission on Cancer. Depth or extent of tumor invasion (T), presence or absence of locoregional lymph nodes (N), and presence or absence of distant metastases (M) are captured by the TNM system. The stages of tumor invasion are defined as Tis, limited to mucosa, lamina propria intact; T1, invades lamina propria or submucosa; T2, invades muscularis propria; T3, invades adventitia or serosa; and T4, invades surrounding structures.

1. Esophageal Cancer

As with many cancers, the prognosis of esophageal cancer correlates with stage at diagnosis. Although the optimal management of patients with locally advanced esophageal cancer remains controversial, preoperative chemoradiation likely improves survival compared with surgery alone. In addition, endoscopic resection provides curative therapy for select T1 tumors. Thus, accurate staging is important to select the appropriate treatment for patients.

The TNM staging includes tumors at the gastroesophageal (GE) junction and the proximal 5 cm of the stomach extending into the GE junction or esophagus. Multiple studies have confirmed the superiority of EUS over CT in T and N staging of esophageal cancer (Figure 37–6 and Table 37–1). Both CT and fluorodeoxyglucose–positron emission tomography (FDG-PET) identify more distant metastases than EUS, and FDG-PET appears superior to CT.

With the high-frequency ultrasound probes, T1 stage can be subdivided into T1m (tumor confined to mucosa) and T1sm (tumor invading submucosa) more accurately than using a conventional echoendoscope. About 8–50% of T1sm tumors have local lymph node metastases. Patients with stage T1sm cancer have a lower 5-year overall survival rate of 58% compared with 91% for T1m; therefore, local endoscopic therapy should not be performed for T1sm lesions.

For each T stage, presence of positive nodes increases the overall tumor stage and predicts a worse prognosis. EUS characteristics suggestive of a malignant lymph node include size greater than 1 cm, round, well-defined, and hypoechoic. Presence of all four features predicts malignancy in 80–100% of cases, but only 20–40% of all malignant lymph nodes have all four findings. FNA of lymph nodes improves accuracy of nodal staging compared with EUS alone. If FNA is not possible, the number of lymph nodes correlates with 5-year survival, and the staging system incorporates number of metastatic regional lymph nodes in nodal staging. In addition,

Table 37–1. Accuracy of imaging modalities for T & N staging of gastrointestinal cancers.

Modality	T Stage	N Stage
Esophageal Cancer		
CT	50%	50–60%
PET	71%	60–74%
EUS	61–90%	75%
EUS-FNA	—	87%
Gastric Cancer		
Multidetector-row CT	77–89%	50–75%
MRI	71–83%	52%
EUS	65–92%	50–87%
Rectal Cancer		
CT	65–75%	54–70%
Endorectal coil MRI	75–85%	65–76%
EUS	80–95%	70–75%

CT, computed tomography; EUS, endoscopic ultrasound; FNA, fine-needle aspiration; MRI, magnetic resonance imaging; PET, positron emission tomography.

celiac axis lymph nodes as well as lymph nodes in the chest and around the esophagus are all considered regional nodes.

Restaging of esophageal cancer following chemoradiation with EUS is significantly less accurate than pretreatment staging. Accuracy of T staging is about 29–60%, and the majority of tumors are over staged presumably due to peritumor inflammation and fibrosis being mistaken for tumor. Reduction in the cross-sectional area or thickness of the tumor by more than 50% has been associated with response to treatment and possibly improved survival.

The clinical impact of EUS on management of esophageal cancer has been demonstrated in several studies. Treatment strategy was changed in about 75% of patients following EUS-FNA, and performance of EUS was associated with increased recurrence-free and overall survival. This was attributed to greater use of chemoradiation following more accurate preoperative staging with EUS.

Dumonceau JM, Deprez PH, Jenssen C, et al. Indications, results, and clinical impact of endoscopic ultrasound (EUS)-guided sampling in gastroenterology: European Society of Gastrointestinal Endoscopy (ESGE) Clinical Guideline - Updated January 2017. *Endoscopy.* 2017;49(7):695–714. [PMID: 28511234]

Heinzow HS, Seifert H, Tsepetonidis S, et al. Endoscopic ultrasound in staging esophageal cancer after neoadjuvant chemotherapy—results of a multicenter cohort analysis. *J Gastrointest Surg.* 2013; 17:1050–1057. [PMID: 23546561]

Liu L, Hofstetter WL, Rashid A, et al. Significance of the depth of tumor invasion and lymph node metastasis in superficially invasive (T1) esophageal adenocarcinoma. *Am J Surg Pathol.* 2005;29:1079–1085. [PMID: 16006804]

Luo LN, He LJ, Gao XY, et al. Endoscopic ultrasound for preoperative esophageal squamous cell carcinoma: a meta-analysis. *PLoS One.* 2016;11(7):e0158373. [PMID: 27387830]

Pfau PR, Perlman SB, Stanko P, et al. The role and clinical value of EUS in a multimodality esophageal carcinoma staging program with CT and positron emission tomography. *Gastrointest Endosc.* 2007;65:377–384. [PMID: 17321235]

2. Gastric Cancer

Similar to esophageal cancer, perioperative chemotherapy may improve survival in specific patients with operable gastric adenocarcinoma, while endoscopic resection is also indicated for early-stage gastric cancers. Therefore, accurate pretreatment staging is important in determining appropriate management. Sensitivity of EUS for T1 and N staging of gastric cancer appears significantly greater than multidetector-row CT (MDCT) although specificity remains similarly modest with either modality. EUS and MDCT performed comparably in T2–4 staging. EUS-FNA of lymph nodes likely increases accuracy for N staging. As with esophageal cancer, EUS can identify superficial mucosal tumors, which may be amenable to endoscopic mucosal resection or endoscopic submucosal dissection. Limitations in accuracy of EUS staging in gastric cancer include early cancers, large or ulcerated lesions, and lesions at the cardia or incisura.

EUS-staging of gastric mucosa–associated lymphoid tissue (MALT) lymphomas is 95% accurate for T staging and seems to predict response to *Helicobacter pylori* treatment. Complete remission occurs in 78% of patients with T1m disease compared with 12.5% of patients with T1sm tumor. Therefore, EUS may allow early selection of patients with higher T stage disease for consideration of other treatments.

Caletti G, Fusaroli P, Togliani T. EUS in MALT lymphoma. *Gastrointest Endosc.* 2002;56(suppl 4):21–26. [PMID: 12269963]

Nie RC, Yuan SQ, Chen XJ, et al. Endoscopic ultrasonography compared with multidetector computed tomography for the preoperative staging of gastric cancer: a meta-analysis. *World J Surg Oncol.* 2017;15(1):113. [PMID: 28577563]

3. Rectal Cancer

Preoperative chemoradiation followed by radical resection for rectal cancers that have extended into the perirectal fat or have local lymph nodes (T3/T4, N1, or both) decreases local recurrence by about half to less than 10% and possibly improves survival. There are limited data on the benefits of neoadjuvant chemoradiation in patients with node positive

T1 or T2 tumors although some experts suggest neoadjuvant therapy for these patients as well. On the other hand, local excision, which does not remove the mesorectum containing lymph nodes, rather than radical resection should be performed in only select patients with favorable T1 tumors. Local recurrence can be as high as 11–29% for T1 tumors and 25–62% for T2 tumors, which most likely reflects lymph node involvement occurring in 0–12% of T1 and 12–28% of T2 tumors. Tumor size greater than 3 cm, poorly differentiated histology, and lymphovascular invasion are associated with increased risk of lymph node metastases.

Accurate staging of rectal cancer is thus critical for correct patient selection for the appropriate preoperative and operative treatment. EUS remains superior to CT and MRI (without endorectal coil) for both overall T and N staging; however, the accuracy of EUS appears comparable to endorectal coil MRI for both T and N staging. The modest accuracy of EUS for staging rectal cancer is attributed to several factors, including inflammation surrounding the tumor leading to overstaging; operator experience; and level of tumor in the rectum, with distal lesions being staged less accurately. The National Comprehensive Cancer Network guideline suggests MRI for staging, however EUS should be considered if MRI is contraindicated.

Similar to esophageal cancer, EUS-FNA of regional lymph nodes in rectal cancer may improve accuracy of N staging although data are conflicting with one study demonstrating similar accuracy for N staging with EUS and EUS-FNA while another study suggested improved staging and outcomes with EUS-FNA. EUS imaging alone found that presence of malignant EUS features (size ≥10 mm, hypoechoic, round, smooth border) was not predictive of malignant lymph nodes unless all four criteria were present. In addition, preoperative EUS-FNA of extramesenteric lymph node metastases upstages 7% of rectal cancers. Therefore, EUS-FNA of lymph nodes in rectal cancer is recommended to determine nodal status. Prophylactic antibiotics are not necessary for transrectal EUS-FNA procedures of solid lesions due to low risk for infectious complications.

EUS-FNA may offer a powerful method to survey for local recurrence of rectal cancer, which often occurs extraluminally following surgical resection. Standard endoscopy is inadequate for detecting these recurrences, and CT scan is limited due to artifacts from surgical metal clips and the inability to differentiate between postoperative changes and recurrence. Sensitivity of EUS for detecting recurrence is 91–100% compared with 82–85% for CT scan and 83% for MRI, with limited specificity for EUS of 57% that improves to 93% with EUS-FNA. There is no standard recommendation for surveillance with EUS following surgical resection; however, the patients who may benefit most include those with more advanced stage tumors at diagnosis and those who underwent local excision. The greatest risk of recurrence occurs in the first 2 years following surgery; therefore, EUS may be performed at some interval during this time in select patients.

Benson AB, Venook AP, Al-Hawary MM, et al. Rectal Cancer, Version 2.2018, NCCN Clinical Practice Guidelines in Oncology. *J Natl Compr Canc Netw.* 2018;16(7):874–901. [PMID: 30006429]

Chan BPH, Patel R, Mbuagbaw L, Thabane L, Yaghoobi M. EUS versus magnetic resonance imaging in staging rectal adenocarcinoma: a diagnostic test accuracy meta-analysis. *Gastrointest Endosc.* 2019;90(2):196–203. [PMID: 31004599]

Gleeson FC, Clain JE, Papachristou GI, et al. Prospective assessment of EUS criteria for lymphadenopathy associated with rectal cancer. *Gastrointest Endosc.* 2009;69:896–903. [PMID: 18718586]

Puli SR, Bechtold ML, Reddy JB, Choudhary A, Antillon MR, Brugge WR. How good is endoscopic ultrasound in differentiating various T stages of rectal cancer? Meta-analysis and systematic review. *Ann Surg Oncol.* 2009;16:254–265. [PMID: 19018597]

4. Pancreatic Cancer

The role of EUS in pancreatic cancer includes diagnosis (Figure 37–7) and staging. Tissue diagnosis is important to confirm malignancy and rule out metastatic lesions to the pancreas, which comprised 11% of masses referred for EUS-FNA in one study. About 5–11% of patients who underwent surgical resection for presumed malignant pancreatic lesions were proven to have benign pathology. EUS-FNA is the most accurate diagnostic modality, with 80–95% sensitivity and near 100% specificity compared with CT- or ultrasound-guided FNA, which have sensitivity ranging from 62% to 81%. Diagnostic sensitivity diminishes to 73% in the setting of chronic pancreatitis. Presence of a rapid onsite evaluation (ROSE) with a cytopathologist increases diagnostic accuracy while reducing procedure time, number of needles used, and overall procedure cost although randomized studies have confirmed the noninferiority of 7 EUS-FNA passes without ROSE compared to EUS-FNA guided by ROSE. EUS-FNA is favored because of its accurate detection of small lesions less than 1.5 cm, and because the needle tract along which seeding can theoretically occur is resected for lesions in the

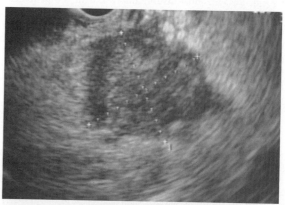

▲ **Figure 37–7.** EUS image of a pancreatic mass.

pancreatic head. Case reports have documented tumor spread along the needle tract. Therefore, for potentially resectable tumors located in the pancreatic body or tail, the options of proceeding directly to surgery without a tissue diagnosis versus EUS-FNA should be considered if there is no concern for other diagnoses including autoimmune pancreatitis. FNB has recently replaced FNA due to greater histologic specimens that procure tissue amenable for molecular analyses in the era of personalized medicine, fewer passes needed for diagnosis and possible improved diagnostic accuracy.

The best outcome in pancreatic cancer occurs in patients without nodal, vascular, or systemic metastases (5-year survival up to 25%). More accurate patient selection could reduce unnecessary surgeries in patients with unresectable tumors. A review of studies comparing EUS and CT for preoperative staging of pancreatic cancer concluded that it is unclear which modality is superior for both tumor and nodal staging.

EUS criteria for vascular invasion are not standardized and criteria with the highest specificity are most helpful for optimizing patients most likely to benefit from surgery. These criteria include irregular vascular wall, presence of venous collaterals, and visible tumor within the vessel. Presence of any one of these criteria indicates vascular invasion. A meta-analysis examining the accuracy of EUS criteria for assessing vascular invasion demonstrated 73% sensitivity and 90% specificity. EUS is more reliable for evaluating invasion into the portal vein and splenic confluence than the superior mesenteric artery or vein. With recent advances in helical CT and MRI, these modalities will most likely surpass EUS for vascular staging. Initial staging should be performed with pancreatic protocol CT scan. EUS will still have a potentially important impact on staging through identifying and sampling lymph nodes, ascites, and hepatic lesions.

Pancreatic neuroendocrine tumors are notoriously difficult to diagnose, and EUS is particularly helpful in evaluating these tumors (Figure 37–8). EUS is superior to CT for detecting these lesions, especially those smaller than 2.5 cm. Because most insulinomas occur in the pancreas, sensitivity of EUS is highest for these neuroendocrine tumors at 83%. Gastrinomas and glucagonomas more commonly occur in extrapancreatic sites leading to decreased diagnostic sensitivity for EUS and a more important role in diagnosis for somatostatin receptor scintigraphy, functional PET, CT, and MRI.

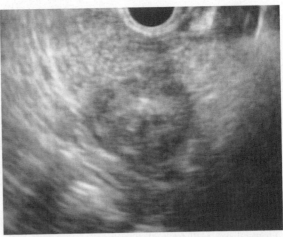

▲ **Figure 37–8.** EUS image of a pancreatic neuroendocrine tumor.

Soriano A, Castells A, Ayuso C, et al. Preoperative staging and tumor resectability assessment of pancreatic cancer: prospective study comparing endoscopic ultrasonography, helical computed tomography, magnetic resonance imaging, and angiography. *Am J Gastroenterol.* 2004;99:492–501. [PMID: 15056091]

Lee LS, Nieto J, Watson RR, et al. Randomized noninferiority trial comparing diagnostic yield of cytopathologist-guided versus 7 passes for EUS-FNA of pancreatic masses. *Dig Endosc.* 2016;28(4):469–475. [PMID: 26694852]

5. Other Gastrointestinal Malignancies

Early detection of small hepatocellular carcinomas remains problematic, with over 70% of lesions smaller than 1 cm missed by MRI. In one study, patients with cirrhosis and at high risk for hepatocellular carcinoma because of elevated α-fetoprotein levels or abnormal radiologic findings underwent ultrasound, CT, MRI, and EUS or EUS-FNA, and diagnostic accuracy was statistically similar (38%, 69%, 92%, and 94%, respectively). EUS alone had a lower accuracy of 65% mainly due to poor specificity. Complications following EUS-FNA of hepatic lesions occurred in about 4% of patients and included bleeding, fever, and abdominal pain, and death in one patient with obstructive jaundice who developed cholangitis. Case reports have documented safe diagnosis of HCC by EUS-FNA of portal vein thrombus. Determining tumor invasion into the portal vein is important because this makes the patient ineligible for surgical resection or transplant.

Cholangiocarcinoma remains a difficult diagnostic dilemma. Several small studies suggest EUS-FNA is safe and useful in diagnosing biliary strictures following negative endoscopic retrograde cholangiopancreatography (ERCP) brush cytology, with sensitivity ranging from 43% to 86% and 100% specificity based on surgical pathology. EUS finding of

Hewitt MJ, McPhail MJ, Possamai L, Dhar A, Vlavianos P, Monahan KJ. EUS-guided FNA for diagnosis of solid pancreatic neoplasms: a meta-analysis. *Gastrointest Endosc.* 2012;75: 319–331. [PMID: 22248600]

Kitano M, Yoshida T, Itonaga M, Tamura T, Hatamaru K, Yamashita Y. Impact of endoscopic ultrasonography on diagnosis of pancreatic cancer. *J Gastroenterol.* 2019;54(1):19–32. [PMID: 30406288]

bile duct wall thickness of 3 mm or greater or an irregular edge to the outer wall of the bile duct is suggestive but not diagnostic of malignancy. Similarly, diffuse bile duct wall thickening over a long segment suggests a benign process although may occur in cholangiocarcinoma as well. One caution about EUS-FNA in cholangiocarcinoma is the potential for malignant seeding along the needle track. Because liver transplantation is potentially curative for unresectable cholangiocarcinoma confined to the liver and biliary system, EUS-FNA of perihilar strictures is contraindicated in a potential transplant candidate. IDUS offers data about depth of tumor invasion and invasion into the pancreas and portal vein, with accuracies greater than 85%. Another imaging tool that maybe helpful is probe-based confocal endomicroscopy (pCLE). In addition, cholangioscopy allows potential tissue diagnosis with targeted biopsies of the stricture. Therefore, EUS-FNA is helpful in initial diagnosis of distal biliary strictures, but should not be performed in perihilar strictures in potential transplant candidates. ERCP with brush cytology, fluoroscopic-guided biopsies, cholangioscopy with biopsies, pCLE, and IDUS are included in the armamentarium for evaluating potentially malignant biliary strictures.

Koduru P, Suzuki R, Lakhtakia S, Ramchandani M, Makmun D, Bhutani MS. Role of endoscopic ultrasound in diagnosis and management of hepatocellular carcinoma. *J Hepatocell Carcinoma.* 2015;2:143–149. [PMID: 27508203]

Nguyen NQ, Schoeman MN, Ruszkiewicz A. Clinical utility of EUS before cholangioscopy in the evaluation of difficult biliary strictures. *Gastrointest Endosc.* 2013;78(6):868–874. [PMID: 23800700]

Tabibian JH, Visrodia KH, Levy MJ, Gostout CJ. Advanced endoscopic imaging of indeterminate biliary strictures. *World J Gastrointest Endosc.* 2015;7(18):1268–1278. [PMID: 26675379]

6. Lung Cancer

The scope of EUS is not limited to the gastrointestinal tract, and it can have a major impact on staging in lung cancer, which remains the leading cause of cancer-related mortality in the United States. As with gastrointestinal cancers, accurate staging is critical in determining prognosis and appropriate treatment for patients with lung cancer. Standard staging methods include CT, PET, transbronchial FNA, mediastinoscopy, and thoracoscopy. EUS-FNA can safely access areas complementary to the other techniques, and approximately 14% of thoracotomies can be avoided by performing EUS-FNA in addition to mediastinoscopy.

Korevaar DA, Colella S, Spijker R, et al. Esophageal endosonography for the diagnosis of intrapulmonary tumors: a Systematic Review and Meta-Analysis. *Respiration.* 2017;93(2):126–137. [PMID: 27926910]

NONMALIGNANT LESIONS

1. Subepithelial Lesions

For subepithelial lesions, accurate preoperative diagnosis can prevent unnecessary surgical resection of benign lesions. Before EUS, this was difficult because subepithelial lesions grow underneath the mucosa and cannot be readily diagnosed by endoscopy and biopsy. EUS appears most useful for differentiating subepithelial lesions from extrinsic compression and for characterizing the subepithelial lesion. Extrinsic compression from adjacent organs or blood vessels is correctly differentiated from a subepithelial lesion in 94% of cases. Using EUS, the size, layer of origin, margins, and echo pattern of the subepithelial lesion are determined; the layer of origin and echotexture are most useful in suggesting a diagnosis (Table 37–2) although imaging alone is only 45.5% accurate for diagnosis. Malignancy can be inferred from larger lesions (>3 cm) with irregular margins. EUS-guided FNA has limited diagnostic yield with definitive diagnosis possible in only 43–68% of cases. FNB appears to improve diagnostic accuracy.

The most common subepithelial lesion is a gastrointestinal stromal tumor (GIST), which has a mesenchymal cell of origin. On EUS, GISTs are hypoechoic and typically arise from the fourth muscularis propria layer although occasionally from the second muscularis mucosa layer (Figure 37–9). Presence of an irregular border, cystic spaces, echogenic foci, and size greater than 3 cm are suggestive of malignancy.

Lipoma is the second most common subepithelial lesion and may be readily diagnosed during endoscopy by its yellowish hue and soft texture. If the diagnosis is unclear, EUS should be performed; it will reveal a hyperechoic lesion arising from the third submucosal layer (Figure 37–10 and Plate 96). Cysts are also easily diagnosed by EUS as anechoic structures lying within the second, third, or fourth layer.

Carcinoid tumors are mildly hypoechoic, homogeneous, and typically arise from the second or third layer (Figure 37–11 and Plate 97). Size is usually predictive of malignancy, and

Table 37–2. Endoscopic ultrasound (EUS) characteristics of subepithelial lesions.

Lesion	EUS Characteristic
GIST	Hypoechoic, 2nd or 4th layer
Lipoma	Hyperechoic, 3rd layer
Carcinoid	Mildly hypoechoic, 2nd or 3rd layer
Cyst	Anechoic, 2nd, 3rd or 4th layer
Pancreatic rest	Hypoechoic or heterogeneous; 2nd, 3rd, 4th layer; ductal structures
Granular cell tumor	Heterogeneous, 2nd or 3rd layer

GIST, gastrointestinal stromal tumor.

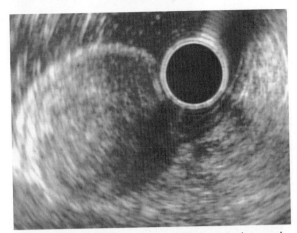

▲ **Figure 37–9.** EUS image of a gastrointestinal stromal tumor.

they are usually benign if less than 2 cm. Other malignant subepithelial tumors include metastases, which are rare, and lymphomas, which may appear as hypoechoic heterogeneous masses within the gastrointestinal wall.

Other benign subepithelial lesions include pancreatic rests and granular cell tumors. Pancreatic rests are subepithelial deposits of ectopic pancreatic tissue that typically occur in the antrum and have a characteristic umbilicated appearance on endoscopy. On EUS, they appear hypoechoic or heterogeneous, arise from the second, third, or fourth layer and may contain ductal structures (Figure 37–12 and Plate 98). Granular cell tumors are believed to arise from neural tissue (Schwann cells) and appear heterogeneous within the third submucosal layer.

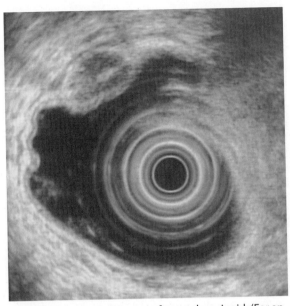

▲ **Figure 37–11.** EUS image of a rectal carcinoid. (For an endoscopic view, see Plate 97.)

Management of these subepithelial lesions is guided by their diagnosis, size, location, presence of symptoms and potential for malignancy. GISTs containing several EUS features raising concern for malignancy should be removed surgically. Smaller benign-appearing GISTs may be observed. The appropriate follow-up interval is unknown although 6–12-month intervals are generally accepted. Lipomas should only be removed if symptomatic. Carcinoids smaller than 2 cm confined to the first three layers can be removed

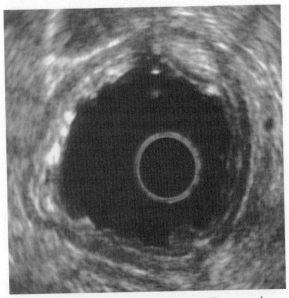

▲ **Figure 37–10.** EUS image of a lipoma. (For an endoscopic view, see Plate 96.)

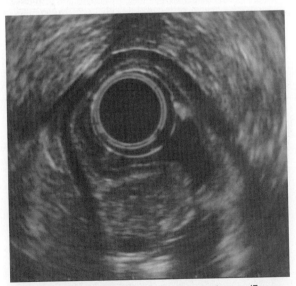

▲ **Figure 37–12.** EUS image of a pancreatic rest. (For an endoscopic view, see Plate 98.)

endoscopically, whereas larger lesions growing into the fourth muscularis propria layer should be surgically resected.

Mekky MA, Yamao K, Sawaki A, et al. Diagnostic utility of EUS-guided FNA in patients with gastric submucosal tumors. *Gastrointest Endosc.* 2010;71:913–919. [PMID: 20226456]

Philipper M, Hollerbach S, Gabbert HE, et al. Prospective comparison of endoscopic ultrasound-guided fine-needle aspiration and surgical histology in upper gastrointestinal submucosal tumors. *Endoscopy.* 2010;42:300–305. [PMID: 20306384]

2. Thickened Gastric Folds

Large gastric folds present a diagnostic dilemma that often necessitates multiple diagnostic studies. The differential diagnosis is broad and includes malignant and benign conditions (Table 37–3). Endoscopic appearance does not usually enable differentiation between malignant and benign conditions, and superficial mucosal biopsies may miss malignancy. Snare resection or cap-assisted endoscopic mucosal resection increases diagnostic yield from 17% to 87% but carries increased risk of complications from bleeding and potentially perforation.

Few studies exist examining the utility of EUS in evaluating a thickened gastric wall (Figure 37–13). The main predictor of malignancy is thickening of the deep gastric layers, in particular the muscularis propria, whereas enlargement of the superficial mucosal layers is associated with benign conditions or MALT lymphoma, which is usually readily diagnosed with biopsies. Gastric wall thickening at least 10 mm is also associated with malignancy. Ascites and lymph nodes are present in over 60% of patients with gastric wall thickening from malignancy.

Ginès A, Pellise M, Fernández-Esparrach G, et al. Endoscopic ultrasonography in patients with large gastric folds at endoscopy and biopsies negative for malignancy: predictors of malignant disease and clinical impact. *Am J Gastroenterol.* 2006;101:64–69. [PMID: 16405535]

Table 37–3. Causes of thickened gastric folds.

Malignant	Benign
Adenocarcinoma	Ménétrier disease
Lymphoma metastasis	Zollinger-Ellison syndrome
	Gastric varices
	Benign hyperrugosity
	Granulomatous disease (Crohn's, sarcoidosis, secondary syphilis)
	Amyloidosis
	Eosinophilic gastritis
	Lymphocytic gastritis
	Acute *Helicobacter pylori* gastritis

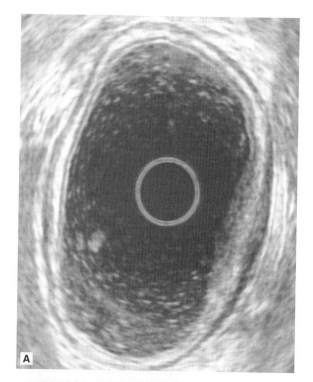

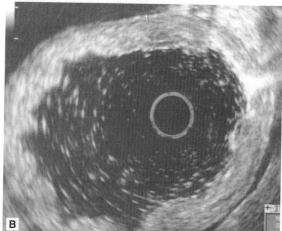

▲ **Figure 37–13.** EUS images of the gastric wall. **A.** Normal gastric wall. **B.** Thickened gastric wall.

3. Pancreatic Cysts

Pancreatic cysts are increasingly discovered with improved and frequently utilized abdominal imaging studies. These lesions are often of unclear clinical significance and pose a diagnostic dilemma. Pancreatic cysts may be categorized as nonneoplastic cysts, cystic neoplasms, and necrotic degeneration of solid tumors. Cystic neoplasms account for two-thirds of all pancreatic cysts and include nonmucinous lesions (serous cystadenoma [SCA], solid pseudopapillary neoplasm [SPN]) and mucinous cysts (mucinous cystic neoplasm [MCN], intraductal papillary mucinous neoplasm [IPMN]). Mucinous lesions and SPNs are premalignant or malignant. Therefore, it is important to differentiate among these different cysts and in particular, to identify mucinous cysts.

SCAs occur anywhere throughout the pancreas, typically in women over the age of 60. On radiology or EUS imaging, they usually appear microcystic and less commonly macrocystic or solid due to the presence of numerous microcysts that give the appearance of a homogeneous hypoechoic mass. A central calcification is pathognomonic but is only seen in about 10–20% of SCAs. Malignant transformation is very rare, and these cysts do not need to be followed.

MCNs are premalignant lesions that nearly exclusively occur in women between 40 and 50 years old. They typically appear macrocystic in the body and tail of the pancreas with a rare, peripheral eccentric calcification. IPMN is also a mucinous cystic lesion that arises from the pancreatic ductal epithelium of the main duct, side branches, or both (Figure 37–14), which leads to the subtypes of main duct IPMN (MD-IPMN), branch duct IPMN (BD-IPMN), and mixed type IPMN. It occurs more commonly in men between the ages of 50 and 60. About 40–70% of main duct and mixed type IPMNs contain malignancy, which informs the recommendations for surgical resection of these lesions in surgically fit patients. Features suggestive of malignancy in BD-IPMNs include presence of symptoms, a mass, mural nodule, dilated main pancreatic duct, cyst size greater than 3 cm, and rapid rate of growth at least 2.5 mm annually.

MRI of the pancreas with MRCP is the preferred imaging modality to evaluate pancreatic cystic lesions with likely higher accuracy compared to CT for identifying mucinous lesions and superior ability to detect nodules, ductal communication, and main duct involvement. EUS may help not only to characterize high-risk cysts, but also differentiate mucinous from nonmucinous cysts when radiology is indeterminate.

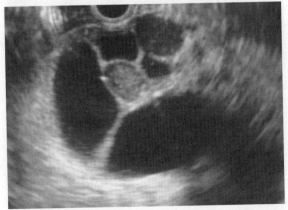

▲ **Figure 37–14.** EUS image of intraductal papillary mucinous neoplasm.

Table 37–4. Diagnostic markers for pancreatic cysts.

Marker	Sensitivity	Specificity
CEA <5 ng/mL (serous cystadenoma, pseudocyst, cystic neuroendocrine tumor)	54%	94%
CEA >192 ng/mL (mucinous cyst)	75%	84%
Cyst fluid cytology (mucinous cyst)	35–63%	83%
Amylase <250 units/L (excludes pseudocyst)	44%	98%
KRAS mutation (mucinous cyst)	45%	96%
KRAS/GNAS mutation (mucinous cyst)	89%	100%
Glucose <50 mg/dL (mucinous cyst)	89%	78%

CEA, carcinoembryonic antigen.

EUS imaging alone is not sufficient to diagnose pancreatic cystic lesions with about 50% accuracy. EUS-FNA probably improves diagnostic yield for pancreatic cystic lesions and FNB may be superior to FNA; however, the optimal cyst fluid markers remain unknown. Elevated carcinoembryonic antigen (CEA), low glucose and presence of KRAS and GNAS mutations appear most useful for identifying mucinous cysts while cyst fluid cytology has poor sensitivity and accuracy in differentiating mucinous from nonmucinous lesions as well as benign from malignant or premalignant lesions (Table 37–4). These cyst fluid markers do not appear to improve identification of malignant cystic lesions. FNA of the cyst wall for cytology and FNB may improve diagnostic yield. Other EUS-guided tools that may help diagnose pancreatic cysts include needle-based confocal endomicroscopy and microforceps. However, further study is required to understand the incremental benefit of these technologies beyond cyst fluid markers and confirm safety of these devices. A death has been reported in Europe following use of the microforceps.

Further work is necessary to discover new and more accurate markers of malignancy and mucinous cystic lesions as pancreatic cystic lesions are increasingly uncovered on incidental imaging studies. American Gastroenterological Association (AGA) guideline suggests performing EUS in patients with incidental pancreatic cysts who have at least 2 high risk features (solid component, size >3 cm, dilated pancreatic duct). The International Association of Pancreatology guidelines broaden the recommendations for EUS by including those with pancreatitis, nodule, thick cyst wall, and change in pancreatic duct caliber with upstream atrophy.

Chiang AL, Lee LS. Clinical approach to incidental pancreatic cysts. *World J Gastroenterol.* 2016;22(3):1236–1245. [PMID: 26811661]

Tanaka M, Fernández-Del Castillo C, Kamisawa T, et al. Revisions of international consensus Fukuoka guidelines for the management of IPMN of the pancreas. *Pancreatology.* 2017; 17(5):738–753. [PMID: 28735806]

Vege SS, Ziring B, Jain R, Moayyedi P. American gastroenterological association institute guideline on the diagnosis and management of asymptomatic neoplastic pancreatic cysts. *Gastroenterology.* 2015;148:819–822. [PMID: 25805375]

4. Chronic Pancreatitis

Diagnosis of chronic pancreatitis remains challenging, especially because there is no defined gold standard. Histology may be considered the true gold standard; however, it is available in a minority of patients, sampling error may occur if only a core biopsy specimen is obtained, and there is no consensus on a histologic grading scale for severity of chronic pancreatitis. Endoscopic retrograde pancreatography (ERP) is less attractive as a diagnostic modality due to its potential complications and decreased sensitivity for early-stage chronic pancreatitis. In addition, the Cambridge classification for ERP changes in chronic pancreatitis was based on expert consensus and has not been validated.

EUS is an attractive alternative diagnostic possibility due to its relatively low morbidity and ability to assess both parenchymal and ductal features. EUS criteria for chronic pancreatitis include the following parenchymal and ductal changes: hyperechoic foci, hyperechoic strands, lobulation, cysts, calcifications, main duct dilation, main duct irregularity, hyperechoic walls of the main duct, and visible side branches (Figure 37–15). A retrospective study noted that the

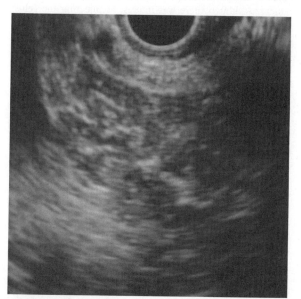

▲ **Figure 37–15.** EUS image of chronic pancreatitis demonstrating lobularity.

presence of four or more EUS criteria had 91% sensitivity and 86% specificity for diagnosing chronic pancreatitis using histology as the gold standard. The threshold for diagnosing chronic pancreatitis can be varied depending on whether one is trying to establish or exclude the diagnosis. In the previous study, presence of five or more criteria had 100% specificity. In a population at low to moderate risk of chronic pancreatitis, EUS is most accurate when unambiguously normal with two or fewer criteria or abnormal with five or more criteria present. This is especially true in elderly patients, in whom up to three EUS criteria for chronic pancreatitis may be present without actual pancreatic disease. International consensus guidelines support five or more criteria as strongly supportive of chronic pancreatitis while two or fewer criteria strongly counter the diagnosis. Certain features including calcification and lobulation are more indicative of chronic pancreatitis, and a weighted scoring system termed the Rosemont classification accounting for these factors has been proposed based on expert opinion. The Rosemont classification appears highly specific but not sensitive for chronic pancreatitis.

The clinical significance of the presence of three or four EUS criteria for chronic pancreatitis is unclear. The addition of FNA/FNB may improve negative predictive value for chronic pancreatitis, but studies are scarce in support of this. A study comparing EUS and MRCP using the gold standards of ERP, histology, or long-term clinical follow-up of median 15 months demonstrated higher sensitivity of 93% for EUS compared with 65% sensitivity for MRCP, and similar specificity of 90–93%. The combination of both studies yielded higher sensitivity and specificity of 98% and 83%. Therefore, the less invasive modalities of EUS and MRCP have largely supplanted ERCP in the diagnosis of chronic pancreatitis. Furthermore, secretin-stimulated MRCP has higher sensitivity than MRCP alone for the pancreatic duct and may enable diagnosis of early chronic pancreatitis. CT is particularly helpful for detecting calcifications, parenchymal atrophy, and inflammatory pancreatic masses, but does not allow accurate diagnosis of early chronic pancreatitis. Some studies suggest that the addition of endoscopic pancreatic function testing, which can be performed during routine endoscopy or EUS, may facilitate earlier diagnosis of chronic pancreatitis. Only one study has compared secretin-stimulated functional studies with histology, which found accuracy of the functional test to be 81%.

Kitano M, Gress TM, Garg PK, et al. International consensus guidelines on interventional endoscopy in chronic pancreatitis. Recommendations from the working group for the international consensus guidelines for chronic pancreatitis in collaboration with the International Association of Pancreatology, the American Pancreatic Association, the Japan Pancreas Society, and European Pancreatic Club. *Pancreatology.* 2020;20(6): 1045–1055. [PMID: 32792253]

Lee LS, Tabak YP, Kadiyala V, et al. Diagnosis of chronic pancreatitis incorporating endosonographic features, demographics,
and behavioral risk. *Pancreas.* 2017;46(3):405–409. [PMID:
28099256]

Trikudanathan G, Munigala S, Barlass U, et al. Evaluation of Rosemont criteria for non-calcific chronic pancreatitis (NCCP)
based on histopathology - a retrospective study. *Pancreatology.*
2017;17(1):63–69. [PMID: 27836330]

5. Autoimmune Pancreatitis

Autoimmune pancreatitis (AIP) can be extremely difficult
to diagnose and often mimics pancreatic cancer in presentation with a pancreatic mass. Observation of a diffusely
hypoechoic, enlarged pancreas with chronic inflammatory
cells on cytology should raise concern for AIP. EUS-FNA
findings are often nonspecific and histology is required,
where three of the four following features are consistent with
a diagnosis of AIP: storiform fibrosis, obliterative phlebitis,
lymphoplasmacytic infiltrate and >10 IgG4-positive cells per
high-power field. International consensus guidelines recommend pancreatic core biopsy when trying to diagnose AIP. As
expected, EUS-FNB is superior to EUS-FNA for diagnosis of
AIP (63% vs 46%, respectively), but overall diagnostic yield
is lower than biopsy of solid pancreatic masses. Most studies have focused on type 1 AIP with few type 2 AIP patients
included. Early study of artificial intelligence with EUS
reported 90% sensitivity and 93% specificity for distinguishing AIP from pancreatic ductal adenocarcinoma.

Facciorusso A, Barresi L, Cannizzaro R, et al. Diagnostic yield
of endoscopic ultrasound-guided tissue acquisition in autoimmune pancreatitis: a systematic review and meta-analysis.
Endosc Int Open. 2021;9(1):E66–E75. [PMID: 33403238]

Marya NB, Powers PD, Chari ST, et al. Utilisation of artificial intelligence for the development of an EUS-convolutional neural
network model trained to enhance the diagnosis of autoimmune
pancrcatitis. *Gut.* 2021;70(7):1335–1344. [PMID: 33028668]

6. Bile Duct Stones

EUS has proven to be a powerfully accurate and safe
method for detecting choledocholithiasis. A meta-analysis
of randomized controlled blinded trials comparing EUS and
MRCP with the gold standard of ERCP or intraoperative
cholangiography in patients with suspected bile duct stones
demonstrated sensitivity for EUS and MRCP of 97% and
87%, with similar specificities of 90% and 92%, respectively.
MRCP is less sensitive for diagnosing small stones and choledocholithiasis near the ampulla. A prior cost-analysis study
indicated that initial EUS rather than MRCP had the greatest
cost-utility by reducing unnecessary ERCP procedures. For
patients with intermediate probability of choledocholithiasis,
EUS or MRCP should be performed based on the test that is
readily available at different institutions.

Meeralam Y, Al-Shammari K, Yaghoobi M. Diagnostic accuracy of
EUS compared with MRCP in detecting choledocholithiasis: a
meta-analysis of diagnostic test accuracy in head-to-head studies. *Gastrointest Endosc.* 2017;86(6):986–993. [PMID: 28645544]

Verma D, Kapadia A, Eisen G, Adler D. EUS vs. MRCP for detection of choledocholithiasis. *Gastrointest Endosc.* 2006;64:
248–254. [PMID: 16860077]

THERAPEUTIC ENDOSCOPIC ULTRASOUND

With the advent of EUS-FNA, a new realm of diagnostic possibilities was discovered, followed more recently by various
innovative therapeutic techniques. The following sections
discuss both well-established and more novel therapeutic
uses of EUS.

1. Celiac Plexus Neurolysis & Block

Celiac plexus neurolysis (CPN) refers to the permanent
destruction of the celiac plexus using absolute ethanol. Temporary block of the plexus with corticosteroid injection is
termed CPB. Pancreatic pain is predominantly controlled
by the celiac plexus. CPN using surgical and transcutaneous
approaches has been used for many years; however, major
complications including paralysis occur in about 1% of cases.
Case reports of paralysis following EUS-CPN/CPB have also
been published.

The EUS technique involves first flushing a 22-gauge
needle with normal saline to clear the needle of air followed
by insertion of the needle 1 cm cranial and anterior to the
take-off of the celiac artery and aspiration to ensure no blood
returns. Although there was interest in injecting the celiac
ganglia visible during EUS with a small randomized trial suggesting improved short-term response with this approach, a
recent randomized trial of patients with pain from pancreatic
cancer found significantly lower survival for patients undergoing celiac ganglion neurolysis (5.59 months) compared to
CPN (10.46 months). Therefore, celiac ganglion neurolysis
cannot be recommended at this time.

For CPN, 10 mL of 0.25% bupivacaine is injected followed by 20 mL of 98% absolute ethanol. For CPB, 20 mL
of 0.25% bupivacaine is injected followed by 80 mg of triam-
cinolone. Minor complications include transient diarrhea
in 4–15% of patients, transient increase in pain in 9%, and
transient orthostasis in 1%. Normal saline is administered
during the procedure, and patients should be monitored for
2 hours postprocedure for orthostasis. Major complications
include retroperitoneal bleed, peripancreatic abscess, and
rare reports of paralysis.

A meta-analysis suggested that EUS-CPN offers safe
and effective pain relief for patients with pancreatic cancer.
Over 70% of patients with pancreatic cancer experienced
pain relief while the response rate and durability are lower
in chronic pancreatitis, with initial 55% response rate that
decreased to 10% at 24 weeks. Pain reduction lasted about

20 weeks following EUS-CPN in pancreatic cancer compared with 2 weeks for chronic pancreatitis with EUS-CPB. A recent randomized controlled trial including metastatic pancreatic adenocarcinoma patients evaluated EUS-guided radiofrequency ablation (EUS-RFA), which significantly decreased pain scores with fewer GI symptoms compared to EUS-CPN. RFA therefore may be a promising alternative that requires further study.

Bang JY, Sutton B, Hawes RH, Varadarajulu S. EUS-guided celiac ganglion radiofrequency ablation versus celiac plexus neurolysis for palliation of pain in pancreatic cancer: a randomized controlled trial (with videos). *Gastrointest Endosc.* 2019;89(1):58–66. [PMID: 30120957]

Levy MJ, Gleeson FC, Topazian MD, et al. Combined celiac ganglia and plexus neurolysis shortens survival, without benefit, vs plexus neurolysis alone. *Clin Gastroenterol Hepatol.* 2019;17(4):728–738. [PMID: 30217513]

Puli SR, Reddy JBK, Bechtold ML, Antillon MR, Brugge WR. EUS-guided celiac plexus neurolysis for pain due to chronic pancreatitis or pancreatic cancer pain: a meta-analysis and systematic review. *Dig Dis Sci.* 2009;54:2330–2337. [PMID: 19137428]

2. Pseudocyst Drainage & Endoscopic Necrosectomy

Pancreatic pseudocysts and pancreatic necrosis may complicate acute and chronic pancreatitis, and both may be managed endoscopically. Studies suggest that even large pseudocysts greater than 6 cm can be followed conservatively until symptoms develop or the cyst increases in size. Surgical drainage had been the standard of care but carries a 10% morbidity rate and a 1% mortality rate; therefore, radiologic and endoscopic drainage have replaced surgical drainage as initial treatment. Complications of endoscopic pseudocyst drainage include early bleeding, perforation of adjacent structures, and infection. Traditionally, endoscopic pseudocyst drainage was performed by piercing the endoscopically visible bulge. Access to the pseudocyst can be achieved by using a needle-knife with electrocautery or the Seldinger technique, which advances a guidewire through a 19-gauge needle. Retrospective studies suggest that the rate of bleeding is reduced to 4.6% using the Seldinger technique compared with 15.7% using the needle-knife. After establishing access to the cavity, the opening is dilated with a balloon followed by placement of several pigtail stents.

EUS allows drainage of pseudocysts that do not create a visible bulge and has changed the management of about 25% of patients undergoing endoscopic pseudocyst drainage. EUS is helpful for several reasons, including detecting blood vessels in the wall of the pseudocyst or path of drainage, confirming that the distance between the wall of the pseudocyst and the gastric wall is less than 1 cm, and characterizing the pseudocyst and its contents. Two randomized trials comparing EUS-guided pseudocyst drainage with non–EUS-guided

techniques both suggest that the technical success rate is higher for EUS-guided drainage although complication rates were similar. Presence of necrotic debris within the pseudocyst necessitates endoscopic necrosectomy, which involves entering the cavity with the endoscope and removing necrotic debris with a variety of accessories. Two recent randomized trials comparing surgical to endoscopic necrosectomy for infected necrosis reported similar mortality rates while the US study found significantly lower rate of major complications including organ failure, fistulae, and bleeding with the endoscopic approach (12% vs 41%, $P = .007$). The Dutch study did not find significant differences in complications between the two groups, but reported lower rates of pancreatic fistulae and length of hospital stay with endoscopic necrosectomy. Therefore, the endoscopic approach should be the initial treatment of choice. Further studies are needed to define optimal patient selection, the most efficacious methodology of debridement including how much to debride initially and agents used during debridement, when to use plastic stents versus lumen apposing metal stents (LAMS), and how long to leave various stents although LAMS should be removed no later than 4 weeks after placement due to concern for increased, potential massive bleeding when left in too long.

Bang JY, Arnoletti JP, Holt BA, et al. An endoscopic transluminal approach, compared with minimally invasive surgery, reduces complications and costs for patients with necrotizing pancreatitis. *Gastroenterology.* 2019;156(4):1027–1040. [PMID: 30452918]

Park DH, Lee SS, Moon SH, et al. Endoscopic ultrasound-guided versus conventional transmural drainage for pancreatic pseudocysts: a prospective randomized trial. *Endoscopy.* 2009;41:842–848. [PMID: 19798610]

van Brunschot S, van Grinsven J, van Santvoort HC, et al.; Dutch Pancreatitis Study Group. Endoscopic or surgical step-up approach for infected necrotising pancreatitis: a multicentre randomised trial. *Lancet.* 2018;391(10115):51–58. [PMID: 29108721]

3. EUS-Guided Biliary & Pancreatic Drainage

Endoscopic decompression of biliary and pancreatic obstruction has been traditionally performed via ERCP, with greater than 90% success in biliary drainage by skilled endoscopists. For ERCP of native anatomy, failure to cannulate by expert endoscopists should be <1%. Unsuccessful endoscopic drainage results from surgically altered anatomy, tumor invasion, periampullary diverticulum, endoscopist inexperience, or other causes. Alternative therapeutic options include percutaneous transhepatic drainage or surgery. Morbidity from percutaneous transhepatic drainage is not insignificant, ranging from 4% to 32% with a mortality rate up to 5.6%. Therefore, EUS-guided decompression offers a potentially attractive endoscopic alternative for failed ERCP procedures.

A randomized study demonstrated similar efficacy for EUS-guided biliary drainage (EUS-BD) compared with percutaneous biliary drain and significantly lower complications with the EUS approach (9% vs 31%) and decreased frequency of needing reintervention (0.34 vs 0.93). A meta-analysis of six randomized trials comparing EUS-BD to ERCP reported similar success rates over 90% and adverse events up to 20% although EUS-BD had lower risk of pancreatitis and tumor in/overgrowth. EUS-BD certainly seems reasonable to offer in lieu of percutaneous biliary drain. Whether it should replace ERCP for primary biliary drainage requires further study.

The technique of EUS-guided biliary and pancreatic drainage involves either a rendezvous procedure with ERCP or the creation of an EUS-guided enterobiliary or enteropancreatic fistula. During a rendezvous procedure, a 19- or 22-gauge needle is used to access the bile duct or pancreatic duct under EUS guidance. A guidewire is then advanced into the duodenum, followed by exchange of the echoendoscope for a duodenoscope to complete the procedure. One study suggested that puncture of the bile duct closest to the point of obstruction may increase technical success whereas another suggested that entering the extrahepatic bile duct may lead to greater complications. Success with rendezvous is typically lower ranging 74% to 80% with 11% complications including bile leak, peritonitis, bleeding, and pneumoperitoneum.

Another EUS-guided technique involves creating an enterobiliary or enteropancreatic fistula. For biliary access, it is unclear whether a hepaticogastrostomy is superior to choledochoduodenostomy. EUS-choledochoduodenostomy has been demonstrated as a safe procedure prior to pancreaticoduodenctomy and should not preclude surgery if indicated. Overall complications range from 9% to 30%. The intrahepatic or extrahepatic bile duct or pancreatic duct is punctured with a 19-gauge needle followed by guidewire placement, dilation of the puncture tract to 4–6 mm, and placement of metal or plastic pigtail stents. A meta-analysis suggested significantly lower complications with metal compared with plastic stents. However, the optimal metal stent remains unclear with choices among covered metal stent, LAMS, and hybrid stents designed for these procedures. Finally, there is an antegrade approach which involves puncturing into dilated left intrahepatic bile ducts and advancing a stent across the papilla without creating a transgastric anastomosis. This approach is not commonly used with lower success rates.

EUS-guided access to the pancreatic duct is even more challenging with lower technical success rates (70–85%) and complications in approximately 18% with 4% considered severe. Similar to EUS-guided biliary access, approaches include rendezvous and antegrade approach with stent placement across the papilla or surgical anastomosis or creation of a pancreaticogastrostomy. Particularly challenging parts of the procedure include creation of the pancreaticogastrostomy and stent placement. Better tools, stents and techniques are needed to address these issues.

Gaujoux S, Jacques J, Bourdariat R, et al. Pancreaticoduodenectomy following endoscopic ultrasound-guided choledochoduodenostomy with electrocautery-enhanced lumen-apposing stents an ACHBT - SFED study. *HPB (Oxford)*. 2021;23(1): 154–160. [PMID: 32646808]

Lee TH, Choi JH, Park do H, et al. Similar efficacies of endoscopic ultrasound-guided transmural and percutaneous drainage for malignant distal biliary obstruction. *Clin Gastroenterol Hepatol*. 2016;14(7):1011–1019. [PMID: 26748220]

Miller CS, Barkun AN, Martel M, Chen YI. Endoscopic ultrasound-guided biliary drainage for distal malignant obstruction: a systematic review and meta-analysis of randomized trials. *Endosc Int Open*. 2019;7(11):E1563–E1573. [PMID: 31723579]

Tyberg A, Bodiwala V, Kedia P, et al. EUS-guided pancreatic drainage: a steep learning curve. *Endosc Ultrasound*. 2020;9(3): 175–179. [PMID: 32584312]

4. EUS-Guided Fiducial Placement

Inactive radiographic markers termed fiducials serve as targets for stereotactic radiation therapy and can be placed under EUS guidance. Stereotactic radiation therapy delivers high doses of precisely targeted, small beams of radiation using real-time image guidance. This technique reduces radiation exposure of surrounding organs, the total time of radiation treatment, and side effects compared with conventional radiotherapy. Fiducials have traditionally been placed surgically or percutaneously; however, safe EUS-guided delivery of fiducials into abdominal (predominantly pancreatic cancer) and mediastinal tumors has been demonstrated. Whether this translates into improved patient outcomes remains unclear.

Coronel E, Cazacu IM, Sakuraba A, et al. EUS-guided fiducial placement for GI malignancies: a systematic review and meta-analysis. *Gastrointest Endosc*. 2019;89(4):659–670. [PMID: 30445001]

FUTURE DIRECTIONS

EUS continues to grow as a diagnostic and therapeutic modality. In the future, EUS will be coupled with other imaging modalities to allow more accurate diagnosis of both benign and malignant lesions. The realm of therapeutic EUS will require ongoing development of innovative devices and accessories and perhaps new echoendoscopes to allow many potential procedures to become a reality.

1. New Diagnostics with EUS

Recent development of three-dimensional (3D) software to allow rendering of two-dimensional (2D) EUS images into 3D images may allow more accurate tumor staging. A study of rectal cancer staging using 2D and 3D radial EUS demonstrated no difference in staging for T1 and T2 tumors. However, 40% of patients with tumors identified as T3N0 by 2D EUS were upstaged to T3N1 using 3D EUS. Overall accuracy of staging for 2D and 3D EUS was 71.4% and 88.6%, respectively.

Combining EUS with CT images and a real-time guidance system called the image-registered gastroscopic ultrasound (IRGUS) system may improve the diagnostic capability of EUS. The system uses a miniaturized tracking sensor that is attached to the tip of an echoendoscope and allows real-time displays of the position of the echoendoscope within a previously obtained CT scan. In a porcine model, endosonographers were more efficient and effective, identifying 25% more basic structures in a timed trial using the IRGUS system compared with standard EUS, and 90% of the users preferred the IRGUS system.

Techniques using contrast agents, elastography, and digital image analysis (DIA) with fluorescence in situ hybridization (FISH) appear promising in their ability to detect malignancies (Table 37–5).

Elastography is based on the principle that cancer changes the elastic properties or the hardness of tissue. Slight compression of tissue by an ultrasound transducer displaces the tissue, and the stiffness of tissue can be measured qualitatively and quantitatively. Studies have suggested EUS elastography is highly sensitive (>90%) but not very specific (~65%) for diagnosing pancreatic cancer. It may help in identifying chronic pancreatitis with studies suggesting correlation between quantitative elastography values and Rosemont criteria, histology and pancreatic exocrine insufficiency. Further studies are needed to assess the value of EUS-elastography in liver disease.

Contrast-enhanced EUS relies on intravenous injection of contrast agents which enhance the microvasculature differences between normal and abnormal tissue. Contrast agents available in the United States include perflutren (Definity or Optison) for echocardiograms and sulfur hexafluoride (Lumason) for liver imaging as well. Therefore, use in the pancreas is off label in the United States and patients should be informed of the very low risk of adverse reactions including back pain, headache, and allergic reaction to perflutren. Following contrast injection, benign lesions such as inflammatory changes from chronic pancreatitis enhance to appear hyperechoic whereas malignant tumors are under-perfused and hypoechoic. Meta-analyses suggest high sensitivity over 90% and slightly lower specificity (85–89%) for diagnosing pancreatic adenocarcinoma. The combination of elastography and contrast enhanced EUS may be more accurate. Contrast-enhanced EUS also appears helpful in distinguishing nodules from mucus globules in pancreatic cysts.

Needle-based confocal laser endomicroscopy (nCLE) through a 19-gauge EUS needle into pancreatic cystic lesions may aid in the diagnosis of pancreatic cysts. The identification of a superficial vascular network pattern was 100% specific and 69% sensitive for the diagnosis of SCA. Papillary patterns are consistent with IPMN. While some studies suggest EUS-nCLE may improve differentiation between mucinous and nonmucinous cysts beyond CEA and cytology, further studies are needed to understand the role of nCLE with the many cyst fluid markers available.

A microforceps that can be advanced through the 19G EUS needle to biopsy the cyst wall may hold promise for increasing diagnostic yield of pancreatic cysts, however, this too requires further study to ensure the safety of the technique as 10% of adverse events have been reported including one death.

Portal pressure gradient measurement is possible using a linear array echoendoscope and 22-gauge FNA needle preloaded with a digital pressure wire to obtain pre- and post-hepatic portal pressures. Access is confirmed with portal venography. This technique appears safe and accurate when compared with transjugular hepatic venous pressure gradient in preliminary studies.

Kovacevic B, Klausen P, Rift CV, et al. Clinical impact of endoscopic ultrasound-guided through-the-needle microbiopsy in patients with pancreatic cysts. *Endoscopy*. 2021;53(1):44–52. [PMID: 32693411]

Napoleon B, Palazzo M, Lemaistre AI, et al. Needle-based confocal laser endomicroscopy of pancreatic cystic lesions: a prospective multicenter validation study in patients with definite diagnosis. *Endoscopy*. 2019;51(9):825–835. [PMID: 30347425]

Obstein KL, Estépar RS, Jayender J, et al. Image Registered Gastroscopic Ultrasound (IRGUS) in human subjects: a pilot study to assess feasibility. *Endoscopy*. 2011;43(5):394–399. [PMID: 21425041]

Vosburgh KG, Stylopoulos N, Estepar RS, Ellis RE, Samset E, Thompson CC. EUS with CT improves efficiency and structure identification over conventional EUS. *Gastrointest Endosc*. 2007;65(6):866–870. [PMID: 17466206]

Zhang W, Peng C, Zhang S, et al. EUS-guided portal pressure gradient measurement in patients with acute or subacute portal hypertension. *Gastrointest Endosc*. 2021;93(3):565–572. [PMID: 32615178]

Table 37–5. Diagnostic techniques for detecting malignancies.

Diagnostic Technique	Sensitivity	Specificity
Contrast agents	94%	89–100%
Elastography (pancreatic mass)	80.6–100%	92.9%
DIA/FISH (various malignancies)	97%	100%
Standard cytology	87%	100%

DIA, digital image analysis; FISH, fluorescence in situ hybridization.

2. Future Therapeutic Uses of EUS

The realm of therapeutic EUS has developed slowly given a relatively limited number of endosonographers and the lack of incentive for instrument manufacturers to invest time and resources in this area, however, it has gained more attention recently. EUS-fine needle injection (FNI) encompasses injection of any material through the needle. It may allow more directed and potentially more efficacious anticancer treatments such as brachytherapy and local injection of antitumor therapy. A few small case series have demonstrated the feasibility of placing radioactive seeds into head and neck cancer, lymph nodes, and pancreatic cancer. The technique involves withdrawing the stylet about 1 cm and backloading the radioactive seed into a 19-gauge needle.

Targeted local injection of antitumor therapy under EUS-guidance is feasible. EUS has been used to deliver allogenic mixed lymphocyte culture (cytoimplant), antitumor viral therapy, and dendritic cells into pancreatic adenocarcinoma and a novel gene therapy agent, TNFerade, which is a replication-deficient adenovector containing human tumor necrosis factor-α gene, into pancreatic and esophageal adenocarcinoma. A phase I trial using cytoimplant in patients with pancreatic cancer was halted early because patients in the control arm receiving gemcitabine therapy had better outcomes. Another trial using the antitumor viral therapy was also stopped early due to poor response and a high rate of complications, including sepsis and duodenal perforation. Studies with EUS-FNI of TNFerade injected into pancreatic cancer failed to demonstrate improved survival. Similarly, a phase 2b study in esophageal cancer demonstrated no survival benefit when EUS-FNI of paclitaxel was added to standard of care compared to standard of care alone.

Expanding on the premise of EUS-FNI, EUS-guided radiofrequency ablation for pancreatic masses, in particular neuroendocrine tumors, has shown promise. EUS-guided photodynamic therapy seems feasible with the photosensitizer found in greater concentrations in malignant pancreatic tissue compared with normal tissue. EUS-guided pancreatic cyst ablation with alcohol and/or chemotherapeutics has been studied with complete or partial resolution of cysts occurring in approximately two-thirds of patients with significantly lower complications in alcohol free paclitaxel-gemcitabine ablations. Finally, there are a few case reports of successful treatment of splenic and superior mesenteric artery pseudoaneurysms using thrombin injected into the vessels under EUS guidance.

Gastric variceal bleeding is associated with high morbidity and mortality. Endoscopic treatment has evolved from endoscopic injection of cyanoacrylate glue into gastric varices to EUS-guided treatments. EUS-guided glue or coil injection is believed to be superior to endoscopic-guided injection although a recent metanalysis suggested treatment efficacy and rebleeding rates were comparable for both techniques. EUS-guided treatment did have higher rates of obliterating the gastric varices (84% vs 63%, $P = 0.02$). Regarding EUS-technique, combination therapy with injecting glue and coil appears superior to either alone for obliterating gastric varices and need for reintervention. Case series have reported injection of thrombin and absorbable gelatin sponge with or without coils. Adverse events were lower when coil is injected with or without glue. One of the feared complications of glue injection is embolization with reports of this occurring asymptomatically in up to 50% of patients. While an exciting technique, most of the literature in this area relies on case series and larger, randomized studies are needed.

The advent of LAMS has ushered in fistulae creation between the GI tract and multiple adjacent organs and collections. One of the widest experiences exists for palliation of malignant gastric outlet obstruction through creation of an EUS-guided gastroenterostomy. This is performed by distending a jejunal loop with fluid and contrast under EUS-guidance to create a target loop of bowel into which the distal flange of the LAMS is deployed while the proximal flange is deployed within the stomach. Compared to enteral stenting, EUS-gastroenterostomy offers a durable option with fewer reinterventions needed for stent ingrowth or migration. Technical and clinical success, symptom recurrence, and reintervention appear comparable to surgical gastrojejunostomy with faster resumption of oral intake and decrease length of hospital stay in the endoscopic group.

LAMS has opened up a novel way to access the defunctionalized remnant stomach in order to perform ERCP in patients with Roux-en-Y gastric bypass anatomy in whom ERCP is otherwise incredibly challenging. A temporary fistula is created using LAMS between the gastric pouch and remnant stomach to permit an antegrade approach to access the ampulla for ERCP. Some call this procedure a gastric access temporary for endoscopy (GATE) procedure while others refer to it as EDGE (EUS-directed transgastric ERCP).

EUS-guided gallbladder drainage for acute cholecystitis is also possible with LAMS. Technical success has been very high approaching 90%, however, early trials demonstrated high adverse event rates of 50%, including overall mortality of 27%. As the technique has evolved, safety has improved, and a subsequent larger trial of 76 patients achieved a technical success of 99.3% with adverse event rate of 7.1%. Potential risks of this approach include stent obstruction causing recurrent acute cholecystitis, bleeding, infection, perforation and stent migration although this risk is low using LAMS.

Ge PS, Young JY, Dong W, Thompson CC. EUS-guided gastroenterostomy versus enteral stent placement for palliation of malignant gastric outlet obstruction. *Surg Endosc.* 2019;33(10):3404–3411. [PMID: 30725254]

Krishnamoorthi R, Dasari CS, Thoguluva Chandrasekar V, et al. Effectiveness and safety of EUS-guided choledochoduodenostomy using lumen-apposing metal stents (LAMS): a systematic review and meta-analysis. *Surg Endosc.* 2020;34(7):2866–2877. [PMID: 32140862]

Mohan BP, Chandan S, Khan SR, et al. Efficacy and safety of endoscopic ultrasound-guided therapy versus direct endoscopic glue injection therapy for gastric varices: systematic review and meta-analysis. *Endoscopy.* 2020;52(4):259–267. [PMID: 32028533]

Moyer MT, Sharzehi S, Mathew A, et al. The safety and efficacy of an alcohol-free pancreatic cyst ablation protocol. *Gastroenterology.* 2017;153(5):1295–1303. [PMID: 28802565]

Walter D, Teoh AY, Itoi T, et al. EUS-guided gall bladder drainage with a lumen-apposing metal stent: a prospective long-term evaluation. *Gut.* 2016;65(1):6–8. [PMID: 26041748]

Wang TJ, Thompson CC, Ryou M. Gastric access temporary for endoscopy (GATE): a proposed algorithm for EUS-directed transgastric ERCP in gastric bypass patients. *Surg Endosc.* 2019;33(6):2024–2033. [PMID: 30805786]

Endoscopic & Surgical Treatment of Obesity

Pichamol Jirapinyo, MD, MPH

Colston Edgerton, MD

Malcolm K. Robinson, MD

ESSENTIAL CONCEPTS

▶ Body mass index (BMI) ≥25 kg/m² is considered overweight; ≥30 kg/m², class I obesity; ≥35 kg/m², class II obesity; ≥40 kg/m², class III obesity; and ≥50 kg/m², "super obesity."

▶ In Asians and other high-risk ethnic groups, these BMI criteria are reduced by 2.5 kg/m².

▶ Using these criteria, two-thirds of Americans are overweight or have obesity.

▶ Lifestyle modification (LM) and pharmacotherapy are noninvasive treatment options for obesity; however, they are of limited efficacy with the majority of patients not being able to achieve sustained clinically significant weight loss, defined as ≥5% total weight loss (TWL).

▶ Patients with a BMI ≥30 kg/m² may qualify for endoscopic bariatric and metabolic therapies (EBMTs).

▶ Currently, there are several EBMTs that are approved by the Food and Drug Administration (FDA) and commercially available, such as intragastric balloons (IGBs), endoscopic sleeve gastroplasty (ESG), primary obesity surgery endoluminal (POSE), and aspiration therapy (AT).

▶ Several studies have demonstrated the efficacy of EBMTs at inducing clinically significant weight loss with medium-term data up to 5 years as well as an improvement obesity-related comorbidities.

▶ Patients with a BMI ≥35 kg/m² can be considered for metabolic/bariatric surgery if they have severe weight-related comorbid conditions (eg, diabetes, hypertension, disabling arthritis, or sleep apnea).

▶ Patients with a BMI ≥40 kg/m² may qualify for metabolic surgery, with or without weight-related comorbid conditions.

▶ A recent meta-analysis showed a reduction in all-cause mortality of metabolic surgery patients compared to matched nonsurgery controls by 41%. This and other studies have shown this to be due to decreased mortality from coronary artery disease, stroke, diabetes, and cancer.

▶ Several randomized studies have documented the profound effects that bariatric surgical procedures have in the treatment of diabetes. The American Diabetes Association (ADA) and the International Diabetes Federation (IDF) now recommend that bariatric surgery be considered for individuals with BMI ≥30 kg/m² who have poorly controlled type 2 diabetes with optimal medical therapy.

General Considerations

Obesity is pandemic and is associated with a high burden of disease. It is second only to cigarette smoking as a preventable cause of death and deaths attributable to obesity far outnumber that of colon cancer. Obesity has been the single greatest contributor to the reduced rate of improvement in life expectancy seen in the United States compared to other developed countries. If current trends continue, the annual health care costs attributable to obesity will exceed $850 billion by 2030, which represents a 16% of all US healthcare expenditures. By this time, 1 in 2 Americans are projected to meet criteria for obesity while 1 in 4 will have a BMI ≥35 kg/m². There will be 29 states with the prevalence of obesity exceeding 50%. In short, obesity is a major public health problem that requires aggressive prevention and treatment.

EBMT is a minimally invasive treatment approach for patients with obesity. To date, there are several EBMT devices and procedures that are approved and/or cleared by the FDA, including IGBs, ESG, POSE, and AT. Studies have shown that EBMTs are effective at inducing greater than 10% TWL at 1 year with sustained results up to at least 5 years. Given an increasing prevalence of obesity and the number of patients who are not eligible for bariatric surgery, such as those with class I obesity or class II obesity without comorbidities, the number of EBMTs being performed has been rising over the past decade.

Metabolic surgery is an effective treatment for patients with class III obesity or class II obesity with related comorbidities. More recently, the benefits of surgery for patients with class I obesity and uncontrolled type 2 diabetes mellitus (T2DM) has been recognized. It is now recommended that surgery be considered for this group of patients due to the increased percent of patients who achieve complete or partial remission of T2DM and have a greater reduction in hemoglobin A1c values following metabolic surgery compared to medical controls. The number of bariatric procedures performed per year continues to increase. In 2018, there were 252,000 bariatric procedures performed in the United States. This represents a 60% increase from 2011. The sleeve gastrectomy (SG) has become the most commonly performed procedure, while others such as the adjustable gastric band (AGB) have decreased significantly in popularity. These changes are predicated on consistent analysis and publication of patient outcomes. In the modern era of bariatric surgery, excluding AGB procedures, percent excess weight loss (%EWL) has been found to be between 56% and 74% with the peak weight loss experienced 12–24 months after surgery. This degree of weight loss is associated with substantial amelioration of co-morbid conditions, the pathophysiology of which is continuing to be elucidated.

This chapter will review the currently available EBMTs and metabolic surgery procedures, as well as their safety and efficacy outcomes.

ASGE Bariatric Endoscopy Task Force, Sullivan S, Kumar N, Edmudowicz SA, et al. ASGE position statement on endoscopic bariatric therapies in clinical practice. *Gastrointest Endosc.* 2015;82(5):767–772. [PMID: 26282949]

Buchwald H, Oien DM. Metabolic/bariatric surgery worldwide 2011. *Obese Surg.* 2013;23:427–436. [PMID: 23338049]

English WJ, DeMaria EJ, Hutter MM, et al. American Society for Metabolic and Bariatric Surgery 2018 estimate of metabolic and bariatric procedures performed in the United States. *Surg Obes Relat Dis.* 2020;16(4):457–463. [PMID: 32029370]

Flegal KM, Carroll MD, Kit BK, Ogden CL. Prevalence of obesity and trends in the distribution of body mass index among US adults, 1999-2010. *JAMA.* 2012;307:491–497. [PMID: 22253363]

Jirapinyo P, Thompson CC. Endoscopic bariatric and metabolic therapies: surgical analogues and mechanisms of action. *Clin Gastroenterol Hepatol.* 2017;15(5):619–630. [PMID: 27989851]

Maggard MA, Shugarman LR, Suttorp M, et al. Meta-analysis: surgical treatment of obesity. *Ann Intern Med.* 2005;142:547–559. [PMID: 15809466]

Mokdad AH, Marks JS, Stroup DF, et al. Actual causes of death in the United States. *JAMA.* 2000;291:1238–1245. [PMID: 15010446]

O'Brien PE, Hindle A, Brennan L, et al. Long-term outcomes after bariatric surgery: a systematic review and meta-analysis of weight loss at 10 or more years for all bariatric procedures and a single-centre review of 20-year outcomes after adjustable gastric banding. *Obes Surg.* 2019;29(1):3–14. [PMID: 30293134]

Preston SH, Vierboom YC, Stokes A. The role of obesity in exceptionally slow US mortality improvement. *Proc Natl Acad Sci.* 2018;115(5):957–961. [PMID: 29339511]

Sullivan S, Edmundowicz S, Thompson CC. Endoscopic bariatric and metabolic therapies: new and emerging technologies. *Gastroenterology.* 2017;152(7):1791–1801. [PMID: 28192103]

Wang Y, Beydoun MA, Liang L, et al. Will all Americans become overweight or obese? Estimating the progression and cost of the US obesity epidemic. *Obesity.* 2008;16(10):2323–2330. [PMID: 18719634]

Ward ZJ, Bleich SN, Cradock, AL, et al. Projected US state-level prevalence of adult obesity and severe obesity. *N Engl J Med.* 2019;381(25):2440–2450. [PMID: 31851800]

TREATMENT OF OBESITY

Treatment of obesity is based on the degree of excess body weight and the presence or absence of weight-related conditions. The degree and categorization of excess body weight is routinely based on BMI. A patient's BMI is calculated by dividing weight in kilograms by the height in meters squared. This index normalizes weight for a given height and is independent of gender. The BMI is generally considered a better classification scheme of excess body weight than the outdated Metropolitan Life tables, which are gender-dependent and require a rough estimate of body frame size.

A BMI of 18.5–24.9 kg/m² is considered "normal." A BMI of 25 kg/m² or greater is considered "overweight" (Table 38–1). Based on these criteria two-thirds of adult Americans are overweight or have obesity. Obesity is defined as when a BMI of 30 kg/m² or higher, and is divided into at least three categories, classes I (BMI 30–34.9 kg/m²), II (BMI 35–39.9 kg/m²), and III (BMI of 40 kg/m² or higher). Bariatric surgeons have defined an additional "super obese" category, which is a BMI of 50 kg/m² or greater. This extra surgical category has been used in clinical studies when analyzing data and correlating outcomes with preoperative weight class. Furthermore, certain ethnicities demonstrate a higher burden of disease at lower BMI's for the same medical comorbidities of metabolic syndrome. In

Table 38–1. Classification and health risks of overweight individuals.[a]

Category	Body Mass Index (BMI)	Health Risk	Risk with Comorbidities
Normal	18.5–25	Minimal	Low
Overweight	25–26.9	Low	Moderate
	27–29.9	Moderate	High
Obese			
Class I	30–34.9	High	Very high
Class II	35–39.9	Very high	Extremely high
Class III	>40	Extremely high	Extremely high

[a]Based on NIH recommendations for the treatment of overweight and obesity in adults.

particular, Asians manifest greater severity of T2DM related complications at a lower BMI than white patients. For this reason, weight categorization is reduced in Asians by 2.5 kg/m^2 such that class I obesity ranges from 27.5 to 32.4 kg/m^2, class II from 32.5 to 37.4 kg/m^2, and class III ≥37.5 kg/m^2. Outcomes for metabolic surgery in these lower BMI ranges have been studied more extensively in Asian countries with promising results, including the remission of comorbid conditions such as T2DM.

Although BMI correlates with excess body fat, it is possible for a highly trained, muscular athlete who in fact is quite lean to have a high BMI. In addition, the association between obesity and mortality appears to be weaker for African Americans as compared with Anglo-Americans. Although the validity of BMI may vary in some patient populations according to their demographic characteristics, including ethnicity, the index has proven to be a clinically relevant measure of obesity that can be linked to disease and mortality risk. For example, the BMI associated with the lowest risk of death is within the normal range for most men and lies within the normal to overweight range for most women (see Table 38–1).

Weight related health risk is based on the BMI classification and the presence or absence of associated comorbid conditions. The National Institutes of Health (NIH) treatment recommendations start with "healthy eating, exercise, and lifestyle changes" for those with minimal and low health risks and then recommend the addition of pharmacotherapy, EBMT or bariatric surgery as health risk increases to the "extremely high health risk" category (Table 38–2). These weight loss treatment recommendations are theoretically based on three parameters: (1) the risk of not treating individuals who are overweight or have obesity; (2) the risk of a particular weight loss treatment; and (3) the likelihood and degree of benefit from the treatment.

LM and pharmacotherapy are available noninvasive treatment options for obesity. LM, which consists of diet, exercise and behavior therapy, is the most common self- and primary care provider–prescribed therapy. To date, there are two landmark studies on LM: the Diabetes Prevention Program (DPP) and Look AHEAD studies. Both evaluated the efficacy of intensive lifestyle intervention, which consisted of 22 and 42 LM sessions in 12 months, respectively. The studies demonstrated that with this frequency of contacts, patients lost up to 8.6% TWL at 1 year. Nevertheless, at 5 and 10 years, patients gained almost all of their lost weight, although the incidence of newly developed T2DM remained lower in the LM group compared to the control. Regarding pharmacotherapy, as of 2021, there are four medications that are approved by the FDA for the treatment of obesity, which include orlistat (Xenical), phentermine/topiramate (Qsymia), bupropion/naltrexone (Contrave), and liraglutide (Saxenda). With the exception of orlistat, which blocks absorption of 25–30% of fat calories, these medications target appetite mechanisms specifically by working in the arcuate nucleus to stimulate POMC neurons to promote satiety. Previous studies have demonstrated the efficacy of pharmacotherapy to range between 6% and 8% TWL at 1 year. Nevertheless, it is important to discuss both potential benefits and adverse events (AEs) with the patient as well as checking for drug-drug interactions prior to initiation. Furthermore, if the patient experiences lower than 5% TWL at 3 months, it is recommended that the medication be discontinued and/or switched to an alternative medication or treatment approach.

Apovian CM, Aronne LJ, Bessessen DH, et al. Pharmacological management of obesity: an endocrine Society clinical practice guideline. *J Clin Endocrinol Metab.* 2015;100(2):342–362. [PMID: 25590212]

Christiansen T, Bruun JM, Madsen EL, et al. Weight loss maintenance in severely obese adults after an intensive lifestyle intervention: 2- to 4-year follow-up. *Obesity (Silver Spring).* 2007;15:413–420. [PMID: 17299115]

Clinical guidelines on the identification, evaluation, and treatment of overweight and obesity in adults—the evidence report. National Institutes of Health. *Obes Res.* 1998;6(suppl 2): S51–S209. [PMID: 9813653]

Fontaine KR, Redden DT, Wang C, et al. Years of life lost due to obesity. *JAMA.* 2003;289:187–193. [PMID: 12517229]

Jensen MD, Ryan DH, Apovian CM, et al. 2013 AHA/ACC/TOS guideline for the management of overweight and obesity in adults: a report of the American College of Cardiology/American Heart Association Task Force on Practice Guidelines and The Obesity Society. *Circulation.* 2014;129:S102–S138. [PMID: 24222017]

Jirapinyo P, Thompson CC. Obesity primer for the practicing gastroenterologist. *Am J Gastroenterol.* 2021;116(5):918–934.

Knowler WC, Barrett-Connor E, Fowler SE, et al. Reduction in the incidence of type 2 diabetes with lifestyle intervention or metformin. *N Engl J Med.* 2002;346(6):393–403. [PMID: 11832527]

Look AHEAD Research Group, Pi-Sunyer X, Blackburn G, Brancati FL, et al. Reduction in weight and cardiovascular disease risk factors in individuals with type 2 diabetes: one-year results of the look AHEAD trial. *Diabetes Care.* 2007;30: 1374–1383. [PMID: 17363746]

McTigue KM, Harris R, Hemphill B, et al. Screening and interventions for obesity in adults: summary of the evidence for the U.S. preventive services task force. *Ann Intern Med.* 2003;139: 933–949. [PMID: 14644897]

Table 38–2. Risk-based treatment in obese individuals.[a]

Health Risk[b]	Treatment
Minimal or low	Healthy eating, exercise, and lifestyle changes
Moderate	All of the above, plus low-calorie diet
High or very high	All of the above, plus pharmacotherapy or very low–calorie diet
Extremely high	All of the above, plus bariatric surgery

[a]Based on NIH recommendations for the treatment of overweight and obesity in adults.
[b]See Table 38–1.

Waden TA, Volger S, Sarwer DB, et al. A two-year randomized trial of obesity treatment in primary care practice. *N Engl J Med.* 2011;365:1969–1979. [PMID: 22082239]

Yanovski SZ, Yanosski JA. Long-term drug treatment for obesity: a systematic and clinical review. *JAMA.* 2014;311:74–86. [PMID: 24231879]

ENDOSCOPIC BARIATRIC & METABOLIC THERAPIES

EBMTs may be considered in patients with a BMI of 30 kg/m^2 or higher, who have failed LM and/or pharmacotherapy or are not eligible for bariatric surgery. It may be divided into gastric and small bowel interventions. In general, gastric interventions primarily induce weight loss with secondary effects on metabolic conditions. In contrast, small bowel interventions have direct effects on metabolic conditions with or without weight loss. As of 2021, all of the currently-FDA approved devices are gastric interventions. Small bowel interventions are under investigation only.

IGBs occupy space in the stomach and have been shown to delay gastric emptying. As of 2021, there are two IGBs that are available in the United States—Orbera (Apollo Endosurgery, Austin, TX) and Obalon (Obalon Therapeutics, Carlsbad, CA). Orbera is a single fluid-filled balloon that is placed and removed endoscopically at 6 months. It is filled with saline with a fill volume ranging between 400 and 700 cc. Once filled, the volume is not adjustable. Obalon is a 3-balloon system, filled with 250 cc nitrogen gas each. This system does not require endoscopic insertion; however, it is removed endoscopically at 6 months. For placement, the balloon, which is enclosed in a capsule that is attached to a slender tube, is swallowed and the position is confirmed via x-ray or magnetic resonance before the removal of the tube. If the first balloon is tolerated, a second and third balloon can be swallowed at 4 and 8 weeks, respectively. In the US Orbera pivotal study (ORBERA trial), which was an open-label, randomized non-sham-controlled trial including 255 patients, TWL was 10.5% at 6 months in the Orbera group, compared to 4.7% in the control group. A meta-analysis of Orbera studies, including 17 studies and 1638 patients, demonstrated an 11.3% TWL at 12 months. The most common AEs were pain and nausea (33.7%). The serious adverse event (SAE) rate was 1.6%, which included migration (1.4%), perforation (0.1%), and death (0.08%). For Obalon, the US pivotal trial (SMART trial), which was a double-blind, randomized sham-controlled trial including 387 patients, revealed a 6.9% TWL at 12 months with an SAE rate of 0.4%. However, an open label real world experience study including 1343 patients demonstrated a 10% TWL with an SAE rate of 0.15% including severe abdominal pain and gastric perforation.

Endoscopic gastric remodeling may be performed via suturing or plication and dates back to as early as 2008. As of 2021, there are two devices that are cleared by the FDA for tissue approximation and are used for this purpose, although they do not have specific weight loss claims. These include

Overstitch (Apollo Endosrugery), which is an endoscopic suturing device, and Incisionless Operating Platform (IOP) (USGI Medical, San Clemente, CA), which is an endoscopic plication device. ESG is currently the most common gastric remodeling procedure that utilizes the Overstitch suturing device to place several sutures in a running fashion along the greater curvature. A second layer of sutures may also be placed medically for reinforcement. A multicenter trial (Primary Obesity Multicenter Incisionless Suturing Evaluation: the PROMISE trial) was recently completed. Twenty patients were included and lost 48.2% EWL at 12 months with no SAEs. A meta-analysis of 8 ESG studies with 1772 patients demonstrated the efficacy of the procedure to be 16.5% TWL at 12 months with an SAE rate of 2.2% including pain/nausea, bleeding, per-gastric leak and fluid collection. At 5 years, a single center study revealed a 15.9% TWL (compared to 15.6% TWL at 1 year). In contrast, endoscopic gastric plication, also known POSE, utilizes the IOP plication device to place tissue plications in the stomach. In contrast to ESG which may be endoscopically reversible, POSE focuses on serosal apposition and is not reversible. The traditional POSE procedure involves placement of plications primarily in the fundus. A more recent pattern, also known as distal POSE or POSE2, however, involves placing plications solely in the gastric body. A US pivotal sham-controlled study (ESSENTIAL trial) including 332 patients demonstrated that at 12 months, POSE patients experienced 4.95% TWL (compared to 1.38% in the sham group). A meta-analysis of 5 POSE studies demonstrated that traditional POSE was associated with 12.1% and 13.2% TWL at 6 and 12–15 months, respectively with an SAE rate of 3.2% including chest pain, low grade fever, extragastric bleeding, and hepatic abscess. With the new plication pattern, the efficacy appeared to be higher with approximately 15% and 17.5% TWL at 6 and 9 months, respectively. From a mechanistic standpoint, ESG and POSE have been shown in small studies to be associated with delayed gastric emptying, which may contribute to weight loss.

AT removes a portion of food from the stomach approximately 20–30 minutes after ingestion. The system consists of a large fenestrated gastrostomy tube (A-tube), an external port at the skin for aspiration, and a portable device to perform aspiration. A-tube placement is performed via a standard pull percutaneous gastrostomy tube placement technique and the port is attached at 1–2 weeks. In a US pivtotal randomized non-sham controlled study (PATHWAY trial), which included 171 patients, the EWL in the AT group was 31.5% compared to 9.8% in the control group at 1 year. A meta-analysis including 5 AT studies with 590 patients demonstrated a 17.8% TWL at 1 year with an SAE rate of 4.1% including buried bumper, peritonitis, abdominal pain, and product malfunction.

Other gastric devices including the Spatz balloon, which is an adjustable balloon, and Elipse balloon, which is a procedureless swallowable balloon that self-dissolves, are currently undergoing FDA review. At the time of this writing, all small bowel interventions are under investigation only with duodenal-jejunal bypass liner and duodenal mucosal resurfacing currently undergoing US clinical trials. According to the American Society of Gastrointestinal Endoscopy (ASGE)/American Society of Metabolic and Bariatric Surgery (ASMBS), a new endoscopic procedure intended as a primary obesity intervention should achieve at least 25% EWL at 1 year with a minimum of 15% EWL over control with an SAE rate less than 5%.

Overall, EMBTs should be considered in patients with a BMI of 30–34.9 kg/m^2 and 35–39.9 kg/m^2 without a comorbidity who fail to achieve clinically significant weight loss with LM, as they are not a candidate for bariatric surgery. Other considerations for offering EBMTs include (1) primary therapy for patients who do not wish to undergo bariatric surgery despite a qualifying BMI, (2) bridge therapy for patients who are deemed too high risk for a variety of surgery, such as primary bariatric surgery, transplant surgery, and orthopedic surgery, and (3) AT, which is approved by the FDA for patients with a BMI of 35–55 kg/m^2. Contraindications for EBMTs include history of severe acid reflux (for IGB), large hiatal hernia (for IGB), prior fundoplication (for IGB), being on anticoagulation (relative contraindication for ESG), and eating disorder (for AT).

To date, there have been no head-to-head prospective comparison between EBMTs and other treatment approaches, such as LM or bariatric surgery. However, there have been a few retrospective studies. Specifically, a retrospective single-center matched-cohort study compared 105 patients who underwent ESG + low intensity LM with 281 patients who underwent high intensity LM, defined as 800–1200 kcal/day with biweekly to monthly visits. The study showed superiority of ESG compared to high intensity LM at 12 months (20.6% TWL vs 14.3% TWL, respectively, P <0.001). Another single-center study retrospectively evaluated 278 patients, who underwent ESG (n = 91), SG (n = 120), and AGB (n = 67). The study demonstrated that at 12 months, LSG patients experienced greater weight loss than those who underwent ESG or AGB (29.3% TWL vs 17.6% TWL vs 13.3% TWL, P <0.0001, for SG, ESG, and AGB, respectively). However, ESG was associated with lower AE rate and length of stay compared to SG and AGB (2.2% vs 9.2% vs 9.0% AE rate, P <0.05; 0.3 vs 3.1 vs 1.7 days, P <0.01, for ESG, SG, and AGB, respectively).

ASGE Bariatric Endoscopy Task Force and ASGE Technology Committee, Abu Dayyeh BK, Kumar N, Edmundowicz SA, et al. ASGE Bariatric Endoscopy Task Force systematic review and meta-analysis assessing the ASGE PIVI thresholds for adopting endoscopic bariatric therapies. *Gastrointest Endosc.* 2015;82:425–438. [PMID: 26232362]

Cheskin LJ, Hill C, Adam A, et al. Endoscopic sleeve gastroplasty versus high-intensity diet and lifestyle therapy: a case-matched study. *Gastrointest Endosc.* 2020;91:342–349. [PMID: 31568769]

Courcoulas A, Abu Dayyeh BK, Eaton L, et al. Intragastric balloon as an adjunct to livestyle intervention: a randomized controlled trial. *Int J Obes.* 2017;41(3):427–433. [PMID: 28017964]

Hedjoudje A, Abu Dayyeh BK, Cheskin LJ, et al. Efficacy and safety of endoscopic sleeve gastroplasty: a systematic review and meta-analysis. *Clin Gastroenterol Hepatol.* 2020;18(5):1043–1053. [PMID: 31442601]

Jirapinyo P, Kumar N, Saumoy M, Copland A, Sullivan S. Association for bariatric endoscopy systematic review and meta-analysis assessing the American Society for Gastrointestinal Endoscopy Preservation and Incorporation of Valuable Endoscopic Innovations thresholds for aspiration therapy. *Gastrointest Endosc.* 2021;93(2):334–342. [PMID: 33218669]

Jirapinyo P, Thompson CC. Endoscopic bariatric and metabolic therapies: surgical analogues and mechanisms of action. *Clin Gastroenterol Hepatol.* 2017;15(5):619–630. [PMID: 27989851]

Jirapinyo P, Thompson CC. Endoscopic gastric body plication for the treatment of obesity: technical success and safety of a novel technique (with video). *Gastrointest Endosc.* 2020;91(6):1388–1394.

Lopez-Nava G, Asokkumar R, Laster J, et al. Primary obesity surgery endoluminal (POSE-2) procedure for treatment of obesity in clinical practice. *Endoscopy.* 2021;53(11):1169–1173. [PMID: 33246352]

Moore RL, Seger MV, Garber SM, et al. Clinical safety and effectiveness of a swalloable gas-filled intragastric balloon system for weight loss: consecutively treated patients in the initial year of U.S. commercialization. *Surg Obes Relat Dis.* 2019;15:417–423. [PMID: 30797717]

Novikov AA, Afneh C, Saumoy M, et al. Endoscopic sleeve gastroplasty, laparoscopic sleeve gastrectomy, and laparoscopic band for weight loss: how do they compare? *J Gastrointest Surg.* 2018;22:267–273. [PMID: 29110192]

Sharaiha RZ, Hajifathalian K, Kumar R, et al. Five-year outcomes of endoscopic sleeve gastroplasty for the treatment of obesity. *Clin Gastroenterol Hepatol.* 2021;19(5):1051–1057. [PMID: 33011292]

Sullivan S, Edmundowicz SA, Thompson CC. Endoscopic bariatric and metabolic therapies: new and emerging technologies. *Gastroenterology.* 2017;152:1791–1801. [PMID: 28192103]

Sullivan S, Swain JM, Woodman G, et al. Randomized sham-controlled trial evaluating efficacy and safety of endoscopic gastric plication for primary obesity: The ESSENTIAL trial. *Obesity.* 2017;25(2):294–301. [PMID: 28000425]

Sullivan S, Swain J, Woodman G, et al. Randomized sham-controlled trial of the 6-month swallowable gas-filled intragastric balloon system for weight loss. *Surg Obes Relat Dis.* 2018;14:1876–1889. [PMID: 30545596]

Thompson CC, Abu Dayyeh BK, Kushner R, et al. Percutaneous gastrostomy device for the treatment of Class II and Class III obesity: results of a randomized controlled trial. *Am J Gastroenterol.* 2017;112(3):447–457. [PMID: 27922026]

METABOLIC SURGERY

The indications for surgical treatment of severe obesity are based on the recommendations of the NIH Consensus Development Conference on Gastrointestinal Surgery for Severe Obesity. The first criterion that must be met before considering a patient for bariatric surgery is weight as assessed by BMI. Patients with a BMI of 35–39.9 kg/m^2 (ie, class II obesity) can be considered for surgical intervention if they have severe weight-related conditions such as diabetes, hypertension, debilitating osteoarthritis, or sleep apnea. Those with a BMI of 40 kg/m^2 or greater (ie, class III obesity) may be appropriate candidates for bariatric surgery with or without weight-related comorbid conditions. Approval for surgery based on the preceding BMI criteria assumes there are no contraindications to surgery. In addition, the panel stated that "patients seeking therapy for severe obesity for the first time should be considered for treatment in a nonsurgical program with integrated components of a dietary regimen, appropriate exercise, and behavioral modification and support." While intended to establish a framework for proper patient selection and to optimize outcomes, there was little guidance or specific recommendations included for this portion of the work-up for patients who may be candidates for surgery. It is also important to recognize that these guidelines were published in the 1990's, based largely off data from open bariatric surgery. With the wide adoption of laparoscopic techniques and significantly improved safety profile, there has been much discussion within bariatric societies if a strict BMI cutoff should be revisited. In practice, this is largely driven by the insurance company payers who have used this outdated metric to benchmark coverage decisions and have also widely implemented inconsistent requirements for preoperative supervised medical weight loss prior to surgery. This heterogeneity between different health insurance plans has led to variable access to a potentially life saving procedure for patients. Perhaps most importantly, it has removed much of the preoperative decision-making capabilities from the clinician treating the patient. This has been the subject of much debate. In 2004 the ASMBS produced a position statement that discouraged participation in insurance mandated medical weight loss programs as a prerequisite for surgery. These conclusions have been driven by numerous studies that show no improvement of outcomes between patients who have not only participated in these programs, but also in patients who have lost a certain amount of weight before surgery. While very low calorie diets have been shown to have a favorable effect on shrinking the liver before surgery and may make the procedure technically easier in patients with severe obesity, there is a paucity of evidence that weight loss before surgery consistently improves outcomes and therefore has been unable to be recommended by national and international societies. For example, while weight loss may facilitate an anastomotic case in a patient with a large BMI, a patient with comorbidities addressed with bariatric surgery at the lower range of the BMI cutoff who has unsuccessfully attempted medical wight loss in the past may be forced to undergo an unnecessary and time consuming process of proving they have met their insurance mandate with little accomplished to change their intraoperative technical considerations, or postoperative outcomes. As such, these decisions should be individualized by the clinician caring for patients with obesity. In response to this, an FDA advisory panel voted to lower the acceptable weight limits for certain types of weight loss surgery in December of 2010.

The FDA now recommends that patients with a BMI of 30–35 kg/m^2 with weight-related comorbid conditions may be acceptable for adjustable gastric banding. Because this procedure has largely fallen out of favor, even this attempt to expand the pool of patients who meet criteria have been relatively ineffective. Some Asian countries are moving to expand the selection criteria for more popular procedures such as the SG as it has been shown that the burden of diabetes and other comorbidities may be more significant in patients with lower BMIs than Caucasias. However, despite these somewhat restrictive criteria, in 2018, only 1.1% of patients who qualified for bariatric surgery in the United States underwent surgery.

The IDF and the ADA now recommend that metabolic surgery be considered for patients with class I obesity (BMI 30–34.9 kg/m^2) to treat T2DM that is not uncontrolled with optimal medical therapy. This recommendation was published as a joint statement of international diabetes organizations from the 2nd Diabetes Surgery Summit in 2016. Hsu et al. examined T2DM remission in patients with BMI <35 kg/m^2 and found that at 5 years, 68% of patients in the surgery cohort to have at least partial remission of diabetes compared to 2.8% in the medical management group. The STAMPEDE trial randomized 150 patients to surgical vs medical management with BMI's ranging from 27 to 43 kg/m^2 and an average of 37 kg/m^2. Five-year outcomes demonstrated a sustained significant benefit of surgery in reduction of hemoglobin A1c and complete or partial remission of T2DM. A meta-analysis that included five randomized controlled trials and six observational clinical studies found that in patients with BMI <35 kg/m^2 with uncontrolled T2DM, metabolic surgery was associate with a higher remission rate of T2DM (OR 14.1, 95% [confidence interval] CI 6.7–29.9) than best medical therapy.

The Metabolic and Bariatric Surgery Accreditation and Quality Improvement Program (MBSAQIP) is an accreditation body created in 2012 by the American College of Surgeons (ACS) and the ASMBS. If a patient satisfies the BMI criteria for bariatric surgery, he or she is more fully evaluated according to criteria established by MBSAQIP. Two core components of this are nutrition counseling and psychiatric assessment. Patients must demonstrate understanding of the risk of nutritional and micronutrient deficiencies following bariatric surgery, as well as a commitment to be compliant with vitamin supplementation. Patients undergoing bariatric surgery may have a higher rate of psychiatric diagnoses and several studies have shown that the only cause of death that is high in certain bariatric surgery populations compared to controls is accidents and suicide. The anatomic changes made by surgery also increases the absorption rate of alcohol and may place patients already at risk for alcohol or substance abuse at even higher risk post-operatively. For these reasons a complete preoperative psychiatric evaluation is essential for proper patient selection. Many surgeons operate on patients with depression, but decline to operate on those with unstable conditions. For example, a recent suicide attempt may preclude surgery for at least 1 year or more depending on the ability to demonstrate psychological stability.

Additional consideration is given to the status of major organs. The bariatric surgical patient should not have severe organ dysfunction, which would make perioperative morbidity and mortality risk unacceptably high. Patients with unstable angina, end-stage pulmonary disease, or cirrhosis may have relative or absolute contraindications to bariatric surgery. However, optimization of treatment of such conditions may improve a patient to the point where he or she may become a bariatric surgical candidate. There is growing evidence that bariatric surgery improves hepatic steatosis, and may even improve or reverse fibrosis in 30% of patients. In addition, patients with end stage renal disease have been shown to have improved all cause mortality and a higher percentage of transplantation following bariatric surgery compared to matched controls. Generally speaking, there are no contraindications regarding bariatric surgery in those with chronic conditions such as HIV/AIDS or a history of treated cancer.

The appropriate age limit for patients considering bariatric surgery is an area of controversy. Adults in the age range of 21–60 years are generally deemed appropriate candidates assuming they have no contraindications to surgery. Several articles have explored operative risk in individuals older than 55 years who undergo bariatric surgery. Although it is generally accepted that operative risk is higher in older compared with younger individuals, it does not seem prohibitive. Accordingly, some surgeons believe that operating on severely obese patients up to age 70 to induce weight loss may be appropriate. In general, a firm age cutoff is not necessary if patients are selected carefully and comorbid medical conditions are brought under optimal control before surgical intervention for weight loss. It should be recognized, however, that older patients require a more extensive evaluation looking for silent organ disease, such as asymptomatic atherosclerotic heart disease. Although such a workup may not prevent a bariatric surgical complication, it will theoretically select for those who have the physiologic reserve to better tolerate and survive a complication if one were to occur. In short, the ultimate decision to proceed in older patients should be based on the specific individual's risks relative to the potential benefits, and not just age alone.

Adolescent bariatric surgery is being studied as well, given the rise in type 2 diabetes and other weight-related comorbidities in this age group. Initial studies indicate significant benefits in this age group, which is slowly increasing the medical community's comfort level with having adolescents being considered for bariatric surgery. As with operating in individuals at the other end of the age spectrum, there are special considerations. The Teen-LABS study was a landmark prospective assessment of outcomes in adolescents following bariatric surgery published in 2017.

This demonstrated that surgery is safe and effective, with significant and durable weight loss at 3 years and higher T2DM remission compared to adults. The ASMBS Pediatric Committee updated their evidence-based guidelines for indications for metabolic and bariatric surgery in patients <19 years old in 2018. Unlike a strict BMI cutoff in adults, class II obesity in adolescents is defined as either 120% of the 95th percentile or BMI ≥35 kg/m², whichever is lowest, and class III obesity as 140% of the 95th percentile or BMI ≥40 kg/m² by the Center for Disease Control and Prevention. Patients should be considered for surgery with class III obesity, or class II obesity with one or more of the following comorbidities: hyperlipidemia, HTN, T2DM, insulin resistance, depressed health related quality of life scores, gastroesophageal reflux disease (GERD), obstructive sleep apnea, nonalcoholic fatty liver disease, orthopedic disease, or idiopathic intracranial hypertension. Puberty status as defined by Tanner stages or growth status as defined by linear height and bone age, as well as developmental delay, autism spectrum, and syndromic obesity are not contraindications for surgery. SG has become the most popular procedure in the adolescent population and has been demonstrated to have similar weight loss and comorbidity resolution as Roux en Y gastric bypass (RYGB). It is associated with a lower incidence of iron deficiency, and presumably less risk for complications such as internal hernia and marginal ulceration across the life of the patient, as well as future difficulty with endoscopic evaluation. Because most of the published long-term data is in outcomes following RYGB, recommendations for one over the other cannot be formalized. Furthermore, the long-term risks of GERD and Barrett's esophagus in adolescents following SG has not been well studied. The family support system takes on an especially important role when operating on younger individuals. It is the extremely rare individual who at so young age does not absolutely require the full support of family. Thus, patient evaluation in the very young essentially mandates extensive evaluation of the patient's family and support network as well.

In general, the decision to proceed with bariatric surgery requires careful evaluation of the patient and analysis of both physical and psychological well-being of the patient. This usually requires a multidisciplinary team with a comprehensive program to support patients preoperatively, during hospitalization, and for a lifetime postoperatively. Procedures available for the treatment of obesity are outlined next.

Adams TD, Gress RE, Smith SC, et al. Long-term mortality after gastric bypass surgery. N Engl J Med. 2007;357(8):753–761. [PMID: 17715409]

Blackledge C, Graham LA, Gullick AA, et al. Outcomes associated with preoperative weight loss after laparoscopic Roux-en-Y gastric bypass. Surg Endosc. 2016;30(11):5077–5083. [PMID: 26969666]

Davidson LE, Adams TD, Kim J, et al. Association of patient age at gastric bypass surgery with long-term all-cause and cause-specific mortality. *JAMA Surg*. 2016;151(7):631–637. [PMID: 26864395]

English WJ, DeMaria EJ, Hutter MM, et al. American Society for Metabolic and Bariatric Surgery 2018 estimate of metabolic and bariatric procedures performed in the United States. *Surg Obes Relat Dis*. 2020;16(4):457–463. [PMID: 32029370]

Fakhry TK, Mhaskar R, Schwitalla T, et al. Bariatric surgery improves nonalcoholic fatty liver disease: a contemporary systematic review and meta-analysis. *Surg Obes Relat Dis*. 2019;15(3):502–511. [PMID: 30683512]

Holderbaum M, Casagrande DS, Sussenbach S, Buss C. Effects of very low calorie diets on liver size and weight loss in the preoperative period of bariatric surgery: a systematic review. *Surg Obes Relat Dis*. 2018;14(2):237–244. [PMID: 29239795]

Hsu CC, Almulaifi A, Chen JC, et al. Effect of bariatric surgery vs medical treatment on type 2 diabetes in patients with body mass index lower than 35: five-year outcomes. *JAMA Surg*. 2015;150(12):1117–1124. [PMID: 26374954]

Hubbard VS, Hall WH. Gastrointestinal surgery for severe obesity. *Obes Surgery*. 1991;1(3):257–265. [PMID: 10775921]

Inge TH, Courcoulas AP, Jenkins TM, et al. Weight loss and health status 3 years after bariatric surgery in adolescents. *N Engl J Med*. 2016;374(2):113–123. [PMID: 26544725]

Müller-Stich BP, Senft JD, Warschkow R, et al. Surgical versus medical treatment of type 2 diabetes mellitus in nonseverely obese patients: a systematic review and meta-analysis. *Ann Surg*. 201;261(3):421–429. [PMID: 25405560]

National Heart, Lung, Blood Institute, National Institute of Diabetes, Digestive and Kidney Diseases (US), 1998. *Clinical guidelines on the identification, evaluation, and treatment of overweight and obesity in adults: the evidence report* (No. 98). National Heart, Lung, and Blood Institute.

Papasavas PK, Gagne DJ, Kelly J, et al. Laparoscopic Roux-en-Y gastric bypass is a safe and effective operation for the treatment of morbid obesity in patients older than 55 years. *Obes Surg*. 2004;14:1056–1061. [PMID: 15479593]

Pratt JSA, Browne A, Browne NT, et al. ASMBS pediatric metabolic and bariatric surgery guidelines, 2018. *Surg Obes Relat Dis*. 2018;14(7):882–901. [PMID: 30077361]

Rubino F, Nathan DM, Eckel RH, et al. Delegates of the 2nd Diabetes Surgery Summit. Metabolic surgery in the treatment algorithm for type 2 diabetes: a joint statement by International Diabetes Organizations. *Diabetes Care*. 2016;39(6):861–877. [PMID: 27222544]

Schauer PR, Bhatt DL, Kirwan JP, et al. STAMPEDE Investigators. Bariatric surgery versus intensive medical therapy for diabetes - 5-year outcomes. *N Engl J Med*. 2017;376(7):641–651. [PMID: 28199805]

Schneider A, Hutcheon DA, Hale A, et al. Postoperative outcomes in bariatric surgical patients participating in an insurance-mandated preoperative weight management program. *Surg Obes Relat Dis*. 2018;14(5):623–630. [PMID: 29525261]

Sheetz KH, Gerhardinger L, Dimick JB, et al. Bariatric surgery and long-term survival in patients with obesity and end-stage kidney disease. *JAMA Surg*. 2020;155(7):581–588. [PMID: 32459318]

Sjöström L, Narbro K, Sjöström CD, et al. Swedish Obese Subjects Study. Effects of bariatric surgery on mortality in Swedish obese subjects. *N Engl J Med*. 2007;357:741–752. [PMID: 17715408]

Sugerman HJ, DeMaria EJ, Kellum JM, et al. Effects of bariatric surgery in older patients. *Ann Surg*. 2004;240:243–247. [PMID: 15273547]

METABOLIC SURGICAL PROCEDURES

Surgical treatment of obesity began in the early 1950s when several groups proposed shortening the intestinal tract via "bypass" procedures to produce substantial decreases in absorptive area. This proposal was based on the observation that massive small bowel resections for treatment of other pathologic conditions resulted in weight loss followed by weight stabilization. Since that time, more than 30 different surgical techniques have been described for treating obesity. The field underwent a recent revolution with the introduction of minimally invasive laparoscopic techniques to produce surgical weight loss. In general, the surgical approach to obesity treatment is designed to create negative energy balance by (1) reducing caloric absorption by way of a small intestinal bypass; (2) reducing caloric consumption by severely restricting gastric capacity; or (3) producing weight loss through a procedure that combines both malabsorption and restriction of caloric intake. Although restriction and malabsorption are the traditional mechanistic ways to categorize weight loss procedures, there has been much research into better understanding the neuroendocrine and microbiological basis for weight loss and metabolic changes. Neuroendocrine mechanisms, particularly the changes observed in gut hormone profiles, are thought to be a significant cause of weight loss after bariatric surgery. The description of every type of bariatric procedure and proposed mechanisms for metabolic changes is beyond the scope of this chapter. However, the commonly used, well-known, and emerging procedures are described below with discussion of outcomes and postoperative complications in subsequent sections.

Akkary E. Bariatric surgery evolution from the malabsorptive to the hormonal era. *Obes Surg*. 2012;22:827–831. [PMID: 22434197]

Kim JJ, Tarnoff ME, Shikora SA. Surgical treatment for extreme obesity: evolution of a rapidly growing field. *Nutr Clin Pract*. 2003;18:109–123. [PMID: 16215028]

1. Roux-en-Y Gastric Bypass

RYGB has been replaced by SG as the most popular bariatric procedure in the world, but largely remains the gold standard for durable long-term weight loss and comorbidity resolution. In 2018, RYGB comprised 17% of all bariatric procedures in the US compared to 42.7% in 2011. While this is due to a decline in the number of RYGB procedures done annually (approximately 60,000 in 2011 compared to 42,945 in 2018), this has largely been driven by the increase in the number of sleeve gastrectomies performed. There has been a slight increase in the number of RYGB procedures done over the past several years (Figure 38–1).

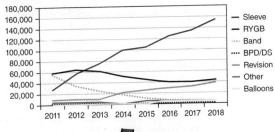

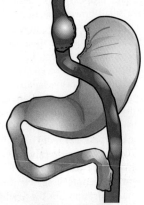

▲ **Figure 38–1.** Metabolic and bariatric procedure trend in the United States, 2011–2018. BPD/DS 5 biliopancreatic diversion-duodenal switch; RYGB 5 Roux-en-Y gastric bypass. (Reproduced with permission from English WJ, DeMaria EJ, Hutter MM, et al: American Society for Metabolic and Bariatric Surgery 2018 estimate of metabolic and bariatric procedures performed in the United States, *Surg Obes Relat Dis.* 2020;16(4):457–463.)

In the RYGB procedure, a 30-mL pouch is constructed to which a Roux loop of jejunum is anastomosed. This creates a short "biliopancreatic limb" through which bile and pancreatic secretions flow; an "alimentary limb" of 100–200 cm, depending on a patient's preoperative weight, through which food from the gastric pouch travels; and a "common limb" that consists of the remainder of the small bowel just distal to the anastomosis of the alimentary and biliopancreatic limbs.

The majority of the stomach, the duodenum, and several centimeters of proximal jejunum are bypassed in this configuration. Thus, the procedure is traditionally said to combine both restrictive and malabsorptive features. The small gastric pouch created as part of the RYGB procedure does in fact limit the amount of food that one can eat to approximately 1 oz. However, there is no macronutrient (ie, fat, carbohydrate, or protein) malabsorption following RYGB and as such malabsorption is not a significant component of weight loss following RYGB. Other neuroendocrine alterations, such as changes in "incretin" levels and other gut hormones are thought to play an important role in weight loss following RYGB. These changes are thought to be due to bypass of the duodenum or the faster transit of food to the distal ileum following RYGB.

The RYGB procedure was one of the first bariatric surgeries to be pioneered in the field. As such, much of the preliminary outcomes came from data series of open surgeries. With the advent and wide adoption of advanced laparoscopic and minimally invasive techniques, the safety profile has seen significant improvements over time without compromising the metabolic effects of the procedure.

Akkary E. Bariatric surgery evolution from the malabsorptive to the hormonal era. *Obes Surg.* 2012;22:827–831. [PMID: 22434197]

Buchwald H, Oien DM. Metabolic/bariatric surgery worldwide 2011. *Obese Surg.* 2013;23:427–436. [PMID: 23338049]

English WJ, DeMaria EJ, Hutter MM, et al. American Society for Metabolic and Bariatric Surgery 2018 estimate of metabolic and bariatric procedures performed in the United States. *Surg Obes Relat Dis.* 2020;16(4):457–463. [PMID: 32029370]

Karamanakos SM, Vagenas K, Kalfarentos F, Alexandride TK. Weight loss, appetite suppression, and changes in fasting and postprandial ghrelin and peptide-YY levels after Roux-en-Y gastric bypass and sleeve gastrectomy: a prospective, double blind study. *Ann Surg.* 2008;247:401–407. [PMID: 18376181]

Le Roux CW, Aylwin SJB, Batterham LM, et al. Gut hormone profiles following bariatric surgery favor an anorectic state, facilitate weight loss, and improve metabolic parameters. *Ann Surg.* 2006;243:108–114. [PMID: 16371744]

Nguyen NT, Hinojosa M, Fayad C, et al. Use and outcomes of laparoscopic versus open gastric bypass at academic medical centers. *J Am Coll Surg.* 2007;205:248–255. [PMID: 17660071]

Youssieff A, Emmanuel J, Karra E et al. Differential effects of laparoscopic sleeve gastrectomy and laparoscopic gastric bypass on appetite, circulating acyl-ghrelin, peptide YY3-36 and active GLP-1 levels in non-diabetic humans. *Obes Surg.* 2014;24:241–252.

2. Sleeve Gastrectomy

SG was first performed in 1990 by Marceau as a modification of the biliopancreatic diversion (BPD) which was popularized by Scopinaro in the late 1970's and early 1980's. In this modification, a longitudinal gastrectomy was performed over a transesophageal bougie and a gastric "sleeve" was created as a first stage of the operation (Figure 38–2) followed later by the bypassing of the proximal duodenum to the ileum to create a long biliopancreatic limb and shorter common channel in the second stage. This theoretically decreased the morbidity of the more complex anastomotic portion of the second stage procedure after the patient had experienced some degree of weight loss. However, the early experience of this technique showed that the resulting weight loss of the first SG stage was sufficient without proceeding with the second stage. There was also an appreciable effect of comorbidity resolution. The first laparoscopic application of this technique was performed in 1999. Over time, the relative technical ease of performing the longitudinal gastrectomy along with the avoidance of an anastomosis or creating mesenteric defects which can lead to internal hernias in RYGB and BPD has caused this to become the most popular bariatric surgical procedure performed in the world today. In 2018, sleeve gastrectomies comprised 61.4% of all bariatric surgeries in the United States.

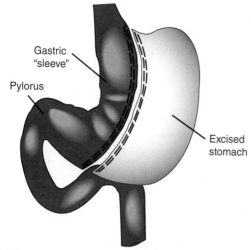

▲ Figure 38–2. Sleeve gastrectomy.

This evidence includes a, double-blind study in which SG was compared with RYGB. The authors found that weight loss for the sleeve was better than the RYGB (69.7% vs 60.5% EWL at 1 year, $P = .05$ SG vs RYGB). This result was associated with the finding that the orexigenic gastric peptide, ghrelin, was significantly lower in the sleeve group, as was appetite, compared with that of the RYGB group. While there is a restrictive component to the operation, this has fallen out of favor as the sole explanation for the profound metabolic benefits seen with this procedure. Ghrelin is an orexigenic hormone that is produced in the fundus of the stomach. By removing the fundus during the gastrectomy, it is theorized that one of the central hunger mechanism is removed. More recent data have shown a change in the microbiome of patients undergoing SG which influences bile acid metabolism and has been correlated with weight loss.

Bellanger DE, Greenway FL. Laparoscopic sleeve gastrectomy, 529 cases without a leak: short-term results and technical considerations. *Obes Surg.* 2011;21:146–150. [PMID: 21132397]

Bohdjalian A, Langer FB, Shakeri-Leidenmuler S, et al. Sleeve gastrectomy as sole and definitive bariatric procedure: 5-year results for weight loss and ghrelin. *Obes Surg.* 2010;20:535–540. [PMID: 20094819]

Buchwald H, Oien DM. Metabolic/bariatric surgery worldwide 2011. *Obese Surg.* 2013;23:427–436. [PMID: 23338049]

Huang R, Ding X, Fu H, Cai Q. Potential mechanisms of sleeve gastrectomy for reducing weight and improving metabolism in patients with obesity. *Surg Obes Relat Dis.* 2019;15(10):1861–1871. [PMID: 31375442]

Karamanakos SN, Vagenas K, Kalfarentzos F, et al. Weight loss, appetite suppression, and changes in fasting and postprandial ghrelin and peptide-YY levels after Roux-en-Y gastric bypass and sleeve gastrectomy. *Ann Surg.* 2008;247:401–407. [PMID: 18376181]

Marceau P, Biron S, Bourque RA, et al. Biliopancreatic diversion with a new type of gastrectomy. *Obes Surg.* 1993;3(1):29–35. [PMID: 10757900]

McCarty TR, Jirapinyo P, Thompson CC. Effect of sleeve gastrectomy on ghrelin, GLP-1, PYY, and GIP gut hormones: a systematic review and meta-analysis. *Ann Surg.* 2020;272(1):72–80. [PMID: 31592891]

Myronovych A, Kirby M, Ryan KK, et al. Vertical sleeve gastrectomy reduces hepatic steatosis while increasing serum bile acids in a weight-loss-independent manner. *Obesity (Silver Spring).* 2014;22(2):390–400. [PMID: 23804416]

Nguyen NT, Nguyen B, Gebhart A, Hohmann S. Changes in the makeup of bariatric surgery: a national increase in use of laparoscopic sleeve gastrectomy. *J Am Coll Surg.* 2013;216:252–257. [PMID: 23177371]

Scopinaro N, Gianetta E, Gianetta E, et al. Bilio-pancreatic bypass for obesity: II. Initial experience in man. *Br J Surg.* 1979;66:618–620. [PMID: 497645]

3. Adjustable Gastric Band

AGB is a purely restrictive procedure which was approved by the FDA for use in the United States in 2001. In the AGB procedure, a silicone-jacketed, belt-like device (ie, the band) is wrapped around the upper part of the stomach near the angle of His. This results in partitioning of the stomach into a small 30-mL proximal pouch and a larger distal stomach remnant in continuity with the pouch. The inner part of the band has an inflatable fluid-filled sack to which a catheter is attached. The catheter, in turn, is attached to a port, which sits just beneath the skin of the abdominal wall. The port can be accessed through the skin with a syringe and a needle to either add or remove saline from the sack, thereby tightening or loosening the band, respectively. Thus, the band is "adjustable." Patients have their bands adjusted depending on adequacy of weight loss or symptoms suggesting that it is too tight.

The advantage of the AGB is that it is a fast and relatively safe. The major downside of the laparoscopic adjustable silicone gastric banding (LASGB) is that weight loss is significantly slower and frequently less than that achieved using any of the other bariatric procedures. In addition, long-term LAGB data have demonstrated a troubling incidence of the band slipping out of position, esophageal dilations, or debilitating GERD. Up to 60% of the time, the band will need to be revised or completely removed because of these and other issues. As a result the popularity of the band has plummeted worldwide and is used less than 5% of the time as a bariatric procedure in the United States.

Buchwald H, Oien DM. Metabolic/bariatric surgery worldwide 2011. *Obese Surg.* 2013;23:427–436. [PMID: 23338049]

Jan JC, Hong D, Pereira N, et al. Laparoscopic adjustable gastric banding versus laparoscopic gastric bypass for morbid obesity: a single-institution comparison study of early results. *J Gastrointest Surg.* 2005;9:30–39. [PMID: 15623442]

Nguyen NT, Nguyen B, Gebhart A, Hohmann S. Changes in the makeup of bariatric surgery: a national increase in use of laparoscopic sleeve gastrectomy. *J Am Coll Surg.* 2013;216:252–257. [PMID: 23177371]

O'Brien PE, MacDonald L, Anderson M, et al. Long-term outcomes after bariatric surgery: fifteen year follow up of adjustable gastric banding and systematic review of the bariatric surgical literature. *Ann Surg*. 2013;257:87–94. [PMID: 23235396]

4. Biliopancreatic Diversion

BPD is a true malabsorptive procedure in which SG is performed followed by a duodenoileostomy and ileoileostomy to result in a longer bioliopancreatic limb and shorter common channel than the RYGB. As mentioned above, it has undergone several modifications to its currently accepted form (Figure 38–3). There has been debate as to the length of each of the bowel limbs. Historically, the BPD was first described as having a common channel of only 50 cm. More recently authors endorse the common channel between 100 and 200 cm in which food and biliopancreatic secretions mix and most of the digestion and absorption of consumed food occurs. This is performed by first dividing the small bowel 250–300 cm proximal to the ileocecal valve and anastomosing the distal small bowel to the first portion of the duodenum that was divided after dissecting over the gastroduodenal artery. The end of the proximal small bowel limb is anastomosed to the side of the distal small bowel limb to give an alimentary limb of approximately 100–150 cm.

The mechanisms through which the BPD produces weight loss are quite distinct from that observed for the RYGB. The BPD operation does produce weight loss by inducing malabsorption, which is not the mechanism through which RYGB effects weight loss. However, the relatively large gastric remnant in the BPD does little to restrict food intake. Similar to the RYGB, the BPD can be done open or laparoscopically. This procedure is popular in certain parts of Europe, although only 2% of bariatric procedures done worldwide are of this type. Some believe that the malabsorption induced by the BPD can be overly harsh and lead to debilitating diarrhea as a result of the typical, high-fat American diet compared with the high-in-complex-carbohydrate diet characteristic of Italy. Some surgeons have modified to make a longer common channel in an effort to reduce the incidence of malabsorption and diarrhea.

The single anastomosis duodenoiliostomy or "SADI" has become more popular in recent years. The proposed benefit is one less anastomosis and less chance of internal hernias. Traditionally, a roux or alimentary limb has been thought to be necessary to avoid bile reflux as can be seen in a bilroth II reconstruction, but the preservation of the pylorus in a SADI helps to prevent this. In this modification, the same SG and division of the proximal duodenum is performed. A loop of ileum is then brought up to the duodenum and anastomosed in an end to side fashion. This anastomosis is often more proximal on the ileum between 300 and 400 cm. Since this represents the total alimentary limb length as well as the common channel, it is longer than in a standard two anastomosis duodenal switch to prevent nutritional deficiencies and steatorrhea. The SADI has also been proposed as a revisional surgery for inadequate weight loss following SG. Proponents of this argue that it is less morbid than conversion to RYGB in that the original sleeve is not manipulated to create a gastric pouch and there is one anastomosis rather than two.

Brown WA, Ooi G, Higa K, et al. IFSO-appointed task force reviewing the literature on SADI-S/OADS. Single Anastomosis Duodenal-Ileal Bypass with Sleeve Gastrectomy/One Anastomosis Duodenal Switch (SADI-S/OADS) IFSO Position Statement. *Obes Surg*. 2018;28(5):1207–1216. [PMID: 29572769]

Buchwald H, Oien DM. Metabolic/bariatric surgery worldwide 2011. *Obes Surg*. 2013;23:427–436. [PMID: 23338049]

Lee Y, Ellenbogen Y, Doumouras AG, et al. Single- or double-anastomosis duodenal switch versus Roux-en-Y gastric bypass as a revisional procedure for sleeve gastrectomy: a systematic review and meta-analysis. *Surg Obes Relat Dis*. 2019;15(4):556–566. [PMID: 3083711]

Ren CJ, Patterson E, Gagner M. Early results of laparoscopic biliopancreatic diversion with duodenal switch: a case series of 40 consecutive patients. *Obes Surg*. 2000;10:514–523. [PMID: 11175958]

Roslin M, Tugertimur B, Zarabi S, et al. Is there a better design for a bariatric procedure? The case for a single anastomosis duodenal switch. *Obes Surg*. 2018;28(12):4077–4086. [PMID: 30288670]

POSTOPERATIVE CARE & COMPLICATIONS

In high-volume centers, hospital stay for bariatric surgery patients varies from 1 to 3 days depending on the type of procedure performed. RYGB patients who have surgery

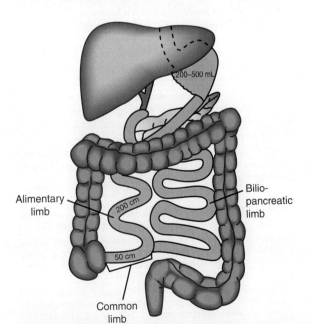

200–500 mL

Alimentary limb

200 cm

Biliopancreatic limb

50 cm

Common limb

▲ **Figure 38–3.** Biliopancreatic diversion procedure.

performed laparoscopically are generally discharged from the hospital in 2–3 days. Routine care during hospitalization focuses on providing adequate pain control and ensuring adequate oral intake. Once these are achieved, the patient can be safely discharged to home. The diet is advanced through various "stages" over several weeks, and patients receive extensive education about maintaining hydration status and consuming adequate protein.

The most common "complication" in bariatric surgical patients is nausea and vomiting, which may occur in as many as 30–40% of patients. This can lead to rehospitalization to treat dehydration, despite no identifiable anatomic obstruction of the gastrointestinal tract. Patients usually receive intravenous hydration and are discharged to home in 24–48 hours in good condition. Complications specific to RYGB include marginal ulcers at the gastrojejunal anastomosis and internal hernias. The wide adoption of laparoscopic techniques has greatly reduced the incidence of incisional hernias and adhesive small bowel obstruction. Wound infections may affect 1–2% of patients undergoing laparoscopic procedures to as high as 10–15% of those undergoing open procedures.

The most common life-threatening complications from bariatric surgery include peritonitis and intra-abdominal abscess associated with an anastomotic leak or iatrogenic, unrecognized perforation of a viscus. Bariatric patients are notorious for having a paucity of classic signs of peritonitis. Instead of abdominal pain and rebound tenderness, these patients may complain of back and left shoulder pain and have a relatively "benign" abdominal examination until impending clinical deterioration. The first manifestation is often tachycardia and less often tachypnea and hypoxia. The surgeon should have a low threshold for obtaining radiologic evaluation with water-soluble contrast agents if any of these symptoms should occur without clear explanation. However, radiologic studies may be falsely negative given the patient's body habitus and technical difficulties associated with obtaining and interpreting radiographs patients with morbid obesity. Thus, a patient requires surgical reexploration even in the face of negative studies if he or she is clinically unstable and without an identifiable source of pathology. As the volume of laparoscopic bariatric procedures has increased, the incidence of anastomotic leaks has decreased and is currently less than 1% in most published series in experienced hands.

Pulmonary embolism, although feared and often discussed, is relatively uncommon in bariatric surgery patients. It occurs fewer than 1% of the time in those who receive appropriate prophylaxis against pulmonary embolism. Recommendations by the ASMSBS are for all bariatric surgery patients to have both mechanical (pneumatic compression boots) and chemical venothromboembolism prophylaxis. There conflicting data in the literature regarding the use of low molecular weight versus unfractionated heparin and at what dose. Pulmonary embolism can be hard to diagnose in patients with morbid obesity. Persistent tachypnea and hypoxia may be suggestive, but many patients with obesity have a preoperative history of pulmonary issues with such symptoms, which may lull practitioners into a false sense of security. Hence, there should be a low threshold to work up bariatric patients with ventilation-perfusion scans or spiral chest computed tomography (CT) for even subtle changes in pulmonary status. Most venous thromboembolism (VTE) events have been shown to occur after hospital discharge within the first 4 weeks after surgery. As such, patients with higher than average risk such as high BMI, personal or family history of clotting disorders or VTE events are recommended to be discharged with extended dose chemoprophylaxis.

On the contrary, bleeding was shown in one review to be the most common complication following bariatric surgery at 0.7%. While it can lead to extended length of stays or reoperation, it was one of the lowest contributors to more serious outcomes such as death and end organ dysfunction. This is a particular concern in SG in which a long, well vascularized staple line is created. Methods to minimize postoperative bleeding and leaks include oversewing the staple line and using buttress reinforcement material. Commonly used materials include bovine pericardium and biocompatible glycolide copolymer. Several studies have shown a decrease in bleeding events using staple line reinforcement with conflicting data regarding leaks.

Several complications specific to RYGB warrant discussion. Because the jejunal mucosa is exposed to acid secreted by the gastric pouch, bypass patients are at risk for ulcers at this location termed "marginal" ulcers. Modifiable risk factors are the most significant etiologies for this to occur which includes smoking and the use of non-steroid anti-inflammatory drugs (NSAID). The most feared complication from this is a perforation of the ulcer which can progress to peritonitis and sepsis if left untreated. Internal hernias are unique to any anastomotic bariatric surgery and can occur in several locations. These include the mesenteric defect created during division of the small bowel and mesentery, "Peterson's space" which is created when a roux limb is brought up adjacent to the transverse mesocolon, an additional space in a retrocolic RYGB where the roux limb is passed through the mesenteric defect. Studies have demonstrated reduction in the incidence of internal hernias by suturing closed these defects at the time of surgery. Like perforated ulcers, an internal hernia represents a surgical emergency over concern that the herniated bowel may have compromised blood flow and become ischemic. The most common presentation is central abdominal pain and anyone managing these patients in the outpatient setting should have a low threshold to obtain cross-sectional imaging in a patient with a history of anastomotic bariatric surgery and unexplained abdominal symptoms. However, internal hernias have been shown to be missed on anywhere from ½ to ¾ of CT scans reviewed by radiologist specifically looking for this finding, and the consequences of missing or delaying this diagnosis could be catastrophic. As such, there should be a low threshold for diagnostic laparoscopy to rule this out. Because the biliopancreatic limb may be obstructed, elevated serum pancreatic enzymes amylase and lipase may also be elevated and could alert the clinician to an occult presentation. Finally, intussusception at the small bowel anastomosis can also cause bowel obstruction in RYGB and BPD patients. This can have a wide range of clinical presentations from an incidental finding on cross-sectional imaging to complete bowel obstruction. The management of this finding therefore depends on the presentation and evidence of bowel obstruction or an intussusception that does not resolve on subsequent imaging should be managed with either laparoscopic or open exploration and reduction.

It has been observed that some patients following SG are at risk for de novo GERD. A review of the literature cites an increase in reflux symptoms after SG in four studies, while six studies reported a reduction in GERD symptoms postoperatively. This discrepancy may be due to anatomic considerations before and after surgery. Some authors endorse the repair of a concomitant hiatal hernia at the time of sleeve. De novo postoperative GERD may be due to destruction of the phrenoesophageal membrane, the section of the sling fibers at the cardial region and the disappearance of the angle of His. Creation of the gastric sleeve and preservation of the pylorus also causes a high pressure system that may be exacerbated by narrowing the angularis incisura. Barrett's esophagus has been noted in as high as 17% of patients after SG with the severity of reflux symptoms not correlating to histologic findings. The International Federation for the Surgery of Obesity and Metabolic Disorders (IFSO) has therefore recommended routine postoperative surveillance following SG at 1, 3, and 5 years postoperatively.

Bariatric surgical training fellowships and multidisciplinary teams have been introduced in order to improve outcomes from bariatric surgery procedures. This has been associated with a dramatic decrease in morbidity and mortality following bariatric surgery. Mortality rates are now less than 1%, regardless of the type of bariatric surgical procedure performed and down from 4% to 5% observed in previous years.

Amor IB, Kassir R, Debs T, et al. Impact of mesenteric defect closure during Laparoscopic Roux-en-Y Gastric Bypass (LRYGB): a Retrospective Study for a Total of 2093 LRYGB. Obes Surg. 2019;29(10):3342-3347. [PMID: 31175588]

Bellanger DE, Greenway FL. Laparoscopic sleeve gastrectomy, 529 cases without a leak: short-term results and technical considerations. Obes Surg. 2011;21:146–150. [PMID: 21132397]

Birkmeyer NJ, Dimick JB, Share D, et al. Hospital complication rates with bariatric surgery in Michigan. JAMA. 2010;304:435–442. [PMID: 20664044]

Bohdjalian A, Langer FB, Shakeri-Leidenmuler S, et al. Sleeve gastrectomy as sole and definitive bariatric procedure: 5-year results for weight loss and ghrelin. Obes Surg. 2010;20:535–540. [PMID: 20094819]

Chiu S, Birch DW, Shi X, et al. Effect of sleeve gastrectomy on gastroesophageal reflux disease: a systematic review. Surg Obes Relat Dis. 2011;7:510–515.[PMID: 21130052]

Cunningham-Hill M, Mazzei M, Zhao H, et al. The impact of staple line reinforcement utilization on bleeding and leak rates following sleeve gastrectomy for severe obesity: a propensity and case-control matched analysis. Obes Surg. 2019;29(8):2449–2463. [PMID: 30989567]

Daigle CR, Brethauer SA, Tu C, et al. Which postoperative complications matter most after bariatric surgery? Prioritizing quality improvement efforts to improve national outcomes. Surg Obes Relat Dis. 2018;14(5):652–657. [PMID: 29503096]

Dittrich L, Schwenninger MV, Dittrich K, et al. Marginal ulcers after laparoscopic Roux-en-Y gastric bypass: analysis of the amount of daily and lifetime smoking on postoperative risk. Surg Obes Relat Dis. 2020;16(3):389–396. [PMID: 31956065]

Melissas J, Braghetto I, Molina JC, et al. Gastroesophageal reflux disease and sleeve gastrectomy. Obes Surg. 2015;25(12):2430–2435 [PMID: 26428250]

Nguyen NT, Nguyen B, Gebhart A, et al. Changes in the makeup of bariatric surgery: a national increase in use of laparoscopic sleeve gastrectomy. J Am Coll Surg. 2013;216:252–257. [PMID: 23177371]

Pyke O, Yang J, Cohn T, et al. Marginal ulcer continues to be a major source of morbidity over time following gastric bypass. Surg Endosc. 2019;33(10):3451–3456. [PMID: 30543040]

Robinson MK. Surgical treatment of obesity–weighing the facts. N Engl J Med. 2009;361:520–521. [PMID: 19641209]

Sapala JA, Wood MH, Schuhknecht MP, et al. Fatal pulmonary embolism after bariatric operations for morbid obesity: a 24-year retrospective analysis. Obes Surg. 2003;13:819–825. [PMID: 14738663]

Shikora SA, Kim JJ, Tarnoff ME, et al. Laparoscopic Roux-en-Y gastric bypass: results and learning curve of a high-volume academic program. Arch Surg. 2005;140:362–367. [PMID: 15837887]

Shikora SA, Mahoney CB. Clinical benefit of gastric staple line reinforcement (SLR) in gastrointestinal surgery: a meta-analysis. Obes Surg. 2015;25(7):1133–1141. [PMID: 25968078]

Spector D, Perry Z, Shah S, Kim JJ, et al. Roux-en-Y gastric bypass: hyperamylasemia is associated with small bowel obstruction. Surg Obes Relat Dis. 2015;11(1):38–43. [PMID: 25264325]

Smith SC, Edwards CB, Goodman GN, et al. Open vs laparoscopic Roux-en-Y gastric bypass: comparison of operative morbidity and mortality. Obes Surg. 2004;14:73–76. [PMID: 14980037]

Stephenson D, Moon RC, Teixeira AF, et al. Intussusception after Roux-en-Y gastric bypass. Surg Obes Relat Dis. 2014;10(4):666–670. [PMID: 24935180]

The Longitudinal Assessment of Bariatric Surgery Consortium. Perioperative safety in the longitudinal assessment of bariatric surgery. N Engl J Med. 2009;361:445–454. [PMID: 19641201]

GASTROENTEROLOGY EVALUATION & TREATMENT

1. Nausea & Vomiting

Nausea and vomiting with or without abdominal pain is a common complaint after bariatric surgery. Hence, it is not uncommon for gastroenterologists, particularly those based at bariatric surgical centers, to be asked to evaluate patients with these symptoms. The most common cause of nausea and vomiting in the early postoperative period is dehydration and dietary noncompliance, as previously noted. Red meat, bread (particularly doughy breads such as bagels), pasta, and dry chicken are poorly tolerated and can lead to nausea, vomiting, and subsequent dehydration. Patients may also be lactose intolerant, and the consumption of milk-based liquid supplements, which are frequently prescribed in the immediate postoperative period, can precipitate symptoms. Nausea and vomiting purely related to dehydration and dietary indiscretion quickly resolve with rehydration and consultation with a knowledgeable bariatric dietitian. However, one must be on guard when evaluating nausea and vomiting in bariatric surgical patients; the list of differential diagnoses is long and varies from the self-limited to the life threatening.

The first step in evaluating the bariatric surgery patient with nausea and vomiting is determining the type of procedure the patient had. Nomenclature of procedures is variable around the country, and those unfamiliar with bariatric surgical procedures (eg, patients and primary care providers) may use terms incorrectly to convey what procedure was performed. Hence, it is advisable to obtain an operative report if possible and time permits.

The most common patient population that the gastroenterologist will be called to evaluate is one who has had RYGB or SG, as these are the most commonly performed procedures. Although dehydration and dietary noncompliance may be immediately evident, it is possible that there are other concomitant problems that need to be ruled out. Regurgitation of food and epigastric pain that occur when eating, are absent when not eating, and may be described as the sensation of a "knot" or "ball" in the epigastrium, all suggest a problem with the gastrojejunal anastomosis or stricture within the sleeve usually at angularis incisura. Initial evaluation usually includes an upper gastrointestinal (UGI) radiocontrast series to rule out an anastomotic stricture and gastro-gastric fistula with or without an anastomotic ulcer in the case of the RYGB or a strictured sleeve. If the UGI series rules in one of these findings, or the patient has persistent epigastric pain without a known etiology, an upper endoscopy (esophagogastroduodenoscopy [EGD]) is indicated.

The EGD will identify a stricture, ulcer, and possible gastrogastric fistula if present virtually 100% of the time. Strictures can successfully be dilated endoscopically to avoid revisional surgery greater than 95% of the time by an experienced gastroenterologist. Some strictures may require serial dilation at planned intervals to achieve durable results. Narrow strictures (eg, 5 mm or less) should be redilated two times at 2-week intervals for a total of three successive dilations to ensure long-term relief of the stricture. Although dilation may be attempted up to six times, the average number of dilations required for durable success is two to three. Furthermore, in addition to balloon dilation, a temporary placement of a lumen-apposing metal stent (LAMS) up to 8 weeks may be considered and has been shown to be effective at treating gastrojejunal anastomotic stricture. Ulcers are treated with standard medical therapy and must be treated aggressively, particularly if associated with a stricture or UGI bleeding. Due to a rapid gastric emptying physiology in patients with RYGB or SG anatomy, open proton pump inhibitor (PPI) should be prescribed as it has been shown to be associated with more rapid time to ulcer healing compared to intact PPI. Similarly, gastrogastric fistulae (ie, a connection between the gastric pouch and remnant stomach) should be treated for symptoms such as ulcer formation, acid reflux, diabetes recurrence, and weight regain.

A new subspecialty within gastroenterology is emerging in which the preceding complications and others are being treated endoscopically by gastroenterologists who specialize in the treatment and evaluation of the postoperative bariatric surgical patient. Conditions that formerly were thought to mandate surgical exploration and revision are now being treated successfully with outpatient, low-morbidity—although complex—endoscopic procedures. For example, patients who have weight regain or nonhealing ulcers associated with gastrogastric fistulae have been treated successfully with endoscopic suturing to close the orifice leading to the bypassed stomach pouch. Similarly, patients who have weight gain secondary to a dilated gastrojejunal anastomosis and pouch dilation may benefit from an attempt at endoscopic suturing to reduce anastomotic and pouch size (see Weight Regain section). Finally, patients, with acute or chronic anastomotic or sleeve leaks may be treated endoscopically using a variety of techniques depending on the nature of the leak. Available endoscopic techniques include fully-covered metal stent placement, plastic pigtail stent placement, septotomy and suturing. These procedures should be done only by advanced endoscopists, ideally who specialize in caring for bariatric patients, in a bariatric multidisciplinary center.

Nausea and vomiting may also occur with more distal pathology such as jejunojejunal anastomotic stricture, jejunal intussusception, and an internal hernia. Usually patients present with abdominal pain as well as vomiting with these conditions, and the initial evaluation includes abdominal CT scanning. The CT scan may miss the diagnosis, in which case persistent symptoms may prompt EGD interrogation down to the jejuno-jejunal anastomosis. Pathology may be identified by endoscopic interrogation and may identify a diagnosis missed on CT scan. Chronic vomiting, particularly with abdominal pain and unknown etiology or in the acutely ill patient, should prompt exploratory laparotomy to rule out internal hernias, intussusception, or jejunojejunal stricture. Such diagnoses can be hard to make short of surgery, and missing an internal hernia, for example, can be fatal in the postoperative bariatric surgical patient.

The causes of nausea and vomiting in the lap band patient include dehydration and dietary indiscretion, similar to that observed in the RYGB or SG patient. Band-related causes include overtightening of the band and band slippage. Patients may find they can tolerate liquids but not solids immediately after band tightening. This suggests overtightening of the band and can be relieved by simple withdrawal of saline from the port. In contrast, acute or slowly progressive dysphagia to solid and liquids in a patient in whom band tightening has not recently occurred should prompt a UGI study to rule out band slippage. Band slippage is the anterior or posterior herniation of the stomach through the band ring. Pain and inability to swallow food and liquids should prompt urgent evaluation to rule out band slip. Withdrawal of saline from the port may alleviate the pain associated with this complication and should be done to alleviate any stomach ischemia even before obtaining a UGI to confirm the diagnosis. The acute onset of pain and inability to swallow food and liquids should be evaluated urgently to rule out band slip. An acute slip with pain is indicative of stomach ischemia and can lead to frank stomach necrosis if not treated promptly. For a subgroup of patients with band slippage and/or erosion, endoscopic removal of the band may be achieved if the buckle is seen endoscopically. Described techniques include the use of a mechanical lithotripter or endoscissors to cut and remove the band transorally, followed by port removal percutaneously. Finally, AGB port site infection, which does not occur in the immediate postoperative period, should prompt local treatment of the port site as well as EGD to rule out band erosion. Band erosion may allow tracking of gastric bacteria along the catheter retrograde to the port.

2. Cholelithiasis & Cholecystitis

It is well known that rapid weight loss is associated with the development of cholelithiasis and cholecystitis. Controversy still exists among bariatric surgeons regarding whether the gallbladder, if present, should be removed in all bariatric surgical patients. It is clear, however, that the gastroenterologist will occasionally be asked to assist with treatment of those patients who have choledocholithiasis. This is generally straightforward in band and sleeve patients, although one should consider complete deflation of the band to assist with endoscopic retrograde cholangiopancreatography (ERCP) if indicated.

In contrast, ERCP in the RYGB patient can be quite challenging, although possible. Traditionally, balloon enteroscopy-assisted ERCP can be performed, where single balloon, double balloon, or spiral enteroscopy is carried out down to the jejunojejunal anastomosis and going retrograde up the biliopancreatic limb to access the duodenal ampulla of Vater to perform ERCP. More recently, gastric access temporary for endoscopy (GATE), also known as endoscopic ultrasound-directed transgastric ERCP (EDGE), has been described where a LAMS is placed under an endoscopic ultrasound (EUS) guidance to gain access into the remnant stomach to facilitate standard ERCP. If peroral ERCP is unsuccessful, laparoscopic gastrostomy and transabdominal passage of a sterile duodenoscope into the remnant stomach and antegrade down the duodenum to the ampulla can be done. This procedure requires general anesthesia but generally causes less morbidity than an open or laparoscopic common bile duct exploration,

and the gallbladder can be removed at the same time if appropriate. A recent meta-analysis including 24 studies and 1268 patients demonstrated that the technical and clinical success of GATE is comparable to that of laparoscopic ERCP (technical success: 95.9% for GATE and 95.3% for laparoscopic ERCP; clinical success: 95.9% for GATE and 92.9% for laparoscopic ERCP), but is better than balloon ERCP (technical success: 71.4%; clinical success: 58.7%). Pooled rates of all AEs with GATE were 21.9%, compared to 17.4% for laparoscopic ERCP and 8.4% for balloon ERCP. Most common AEs for GATE were stent migration (13.3%) followed by bleeding (6.6%). At our institution, GATE is usually performed in two stages with the first stage involving LAMS placement to gain access into the remnant stomach without passage of a duodenoscope through the LAMS to minimize risk of stent migration. The patient is then brought back 4–6 weeks later when ERCP is performed through the LAMS.

Dhindsa BS, Dhaliwal A, Mohan BP, et al. EDGE in Roux-en-Y gastric bypass: how does it compare to laparoscopy-assisted and balloon enteroscopy ERCP: a systematic review and meta-analysis. *Endosc Int Open.* 2020;8(2):E163–E171. [PMID: 32010749]

Go MR, Muscarella P, Needleman BJ, et al. Endoscopic management of stomal stenosis after Roux-en-Y gastric bypass. *Surg Endosc.* 2004;18:56–59. [PMID: 14625732]

Merrifield BF, Lautz D, Thompson CC. Endoscopic repair of gastric leaks after Roux-en-Y gastric bypass: a less invasive approach. *Gastrointest Endosc.* 2006;63:710–714. [PMID: 16564884]

Moore KA, Ouyang DW, Whang EE. Maternal and fetal deaths after gastric bypass surgery for treatment of morbid obesity. *N Engl J Med.* 2004;351:721–722. [PMID: 15306679]

Nguyen NT, Hinojosa MW, Slone J, et al. Laparoscopic transgastric access to the biliary tree after Roux-en-Y gastric bypass. *Obes Surg.* 2007;17:416–419. [PMID: 17546853]

Pai RD, Carr-Locke DL, Thompson CC. Endoscopic evaluation of the defunctionalized stomach by using ShapeLock technology (with video). *Gastrointest Endosc.* 2007;66:578–581. [PMID: 17725949]

Schulman AR, Chan WW, Devery A, et al. Opened proton pump inhibitor capsules reduce time to healing compared with itact capsules for marginal ulceration following Roux-en-Y gastric bypass. *Clin Gastroenterol Hepatol.* 2017;15(4):494–500. [PMID: 27773764]

Schulman AR, Thompson CC. Complications of bariatric surgery: what you can expect to see in your GI practice. *Am J Gastroenterol.* 2017;112(11):1640–1655. [PMID: 28809386]

Thompson CC, Carr-Locke DL, Saltzman J, et al. Per oral repair of staple-line dehiscence in Roux-en-Y gastric bypass: a less invasive approach. Presented at the 45th annual meeting of the Society for Surgery of the Alimentary Tract, 2004.

Thompson C, Robinson MK, Lautz D. FACS. Enteroscopic diagnosis of internal hernia after Roux-en gastric bypass, a case study. Presented at the annual meeting of the Society of American Gastrointestinal and Endoscopic Surgeons, 2006.

Thompson CC, Slattery J, Bundga ME, et al. Peroral endoscopic reduction of dilated gastrojejunal anastomosis after Roux-en-Y gastric bypass: a possible new option for patients with weight regain. *Surg Endosc.* 2006;20:1744–1748. [PMID: 17024527]

Wang TJ, Cortes P, Jirapinyo P, et al. A comparison of clinical outcomes and cost utility among laparoscopy, enteroscopy, and temporary gastric access-assisted ERCP in patients with Roux-en-Y gastric bypass anatomy. *Surg Endosc.* 2021;35(8):4469–4477. [PMID: 32886240]

Want TJ, Thompson CC, Ryou M. Gastric access temporary for endoscopy (GATE): a proposed algorithm for EUS-directed transgastric ERCP in gastric bypass patients. *Surg Endosc.* 2019;33(6):2024–2033. [PMID: 30805786]

LONG-TERM OUTCOMES OF METABOLIC SURGERY

Metabolic surgery is associated with significant weight loss and resolution of weight-related conditions. The Swedish Obese Subjects (SOS) study, which examined weight reduction, reduction in cardiovascular risk factors, and mortality over a 10-year period, is probably the best-known study of long-term bariatric surgery outcomes. In this study, 2010 subjects with obesity who underwent bariatric surgery were contemporaneously matched with 2037 control subjects with obesity who received nonsurgical treatment. Patients were followed for up to 15 years, and the investigators found that weight loss for all patients undergoing surgery was significantly greater compared with that observed in the control patients (Figure 38–4).

RYGB patients lost 32% of initial body weight at 1 year, which was maintained at a level of 28% loss of initial body weight at 15 years. Band patients lost less than the GBP patients but still a significant amount: 21% of initial body weight at the 1-year mark and 13% at the 15-year mark after surgical intervention. In contrast, conventionally treated patients essentially had no change in weight over the 15 years of study.

When the surgical patients in the SOS study were compared with the control patients, a marked, statistically significant improvement was seen in lipid profile, diabetes, hypertension, and hyperuricemia, as well as a decrease in the risk of developing these conditions if not present at the time of surgery. The authors concluded that, as compared with conventional, nonsurgical treatment, bariatric surgery results in long-term weight loss, improved lifestyle, and amelioration of a variety of cardiovascular risk factors.

The SOS study notably did not analyze outcomes of SG which has become the most popular bariatric procedure in the world. A recent review of randomized studies comparing outcomes of RYGB and SG included five studies and found a greater %EWL in RYGB compared to SG (65.7% vs 57.3%) as well as greater resolution in diabetes (37.4% vs 27.5%). Another review of 33 randomized trials found RYGB patients to lose 1.25 kg/m² more BMI than SG at 3 years but insufficient evidence of 5-year outcomes.

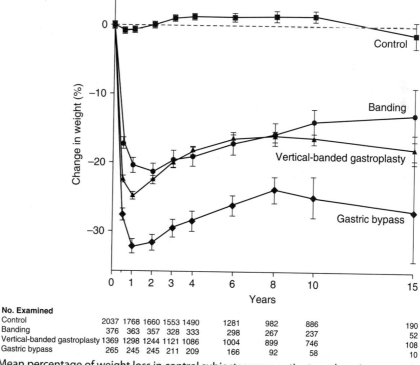

▲ **Figure 38–4.** Mean percentage of weight loss in control subjects versus patients undergoing gastric bypass, vertical banded gastroplasty, and adjustable gastric banding in the Swedish Obese Subjects (SOS) study. (Data from Sjöström L, Narbro K, Sjöström CD, et al. Effects of bariatric surgery on mortality in Swedish obese subjects. *N Engl J Med.*2007;357(8):741–752.)

Dyslipidemia was improved at 5 years with no difference in diabetes remission.

There have been several high-quality studies examining the effects of bariatric surgical procedures on patients with obesity with concomitant T2DM. The results can be summarized as follows: (1) bariatric surgery procedures, particularly the RYGB, can provide durable glycemic control in patients with obesity with concomitant T2DM; (2) bariatric surgical procedures are more effective in controlling T2DM in individuals with obesity compared to intensive medical therapy; and (3) gastric bypass may uniquely restore pancreatic B-cell function and reduces truncal fat, thus reversing the core defects in diabetes—findings that have never been demonstrated with medical therapy. Generally speaking, RYGB appears to be more effective than SG which in turn is more effective than AGB in controlling T2DM in the individuals with obesity.

The impact of surgical treatment of individuals with obesity is not just limited to weight loss and alleviation of comorbid conditions. The SOS study found a statistically significant (29%) reduction in death in patients undergoing surgery compared with conventionally treated individuals. In another study, Adams and colleagues assessed mortality risk in 7925 gastric bypass patients compared with 7925 control patients matched for age, gender, and BMI. The adjusted long-term mortality in the surgery group decreased by 40% compared with that in the control group.

A final question regarding use of surgery to treat morbid obesity is the financial cost. Can we as a nation afford to offer such treatment given the high number of patients who potentially qualify for surgery? It is clear that initial health care costs for individuals with obesity who undergo surgery are higher than the costs for individuals with obesity who receive nonsurgical treatments or go untreated. However, 3 years after surgery, the health care costs of surgical patients are less than those of patients who do not undergo obesity surgery. Over a 5-year period, the number of hospitalizations, total hospital days, physician visits, and prescription costs are less in surgically treated individuals. This is associated with up to a 25% reduction in health care costs in these individuals compared with patients with obesity who receive nonsurgical or no treatment for their weight condition. Hence, bariatric surgery is also cost-effective compared with nonsurgical treatments.

Although it makes intuitive sense that massive weight loss leads to improved health and decreased mortality, the mechanism through which surgery exerts its salubrious effects has yet to be fully identified. One theory is that surgery has a beneficial effect on the inflammatory mediators associated with obesity. Initial work has suggested that inflammatory mediators such as angiotensinogen, transforming growth factor-β, tumor necrosis factor-α, and interleukin-6 are all elevated in obesity. These mediators may in part lead to the development of several cardiovascular risk factors, such as hypertension, diabetes, dyslipidemia, and thromboembolic phenomena. Weight loss surgery is associated with reduction of these factors, possibly through reduction of adipocyte mass, and therefore may be the mechanism through which weight loss surgery so effectively reduces cardiovascular risk and prolongs life. Clearly, much more study is needed to examine how weight loss in general, and obesity surgery in particular, improves outcome. However, at this time, the evidence is quite strong in favor of surgery for treatment of individuals with severe obesity compared with prolonged efforts at nonsurgical treatment.

Adams TD, Gress RE, Smith SC, et al. Long-term mortality after gastric bypass surgery. N Engl J Med. 2007;357:753–761. [PMID: 17715409]

Brethauer SA, Aminian A, Romero-Talamas H, et al. Can diabetes be surgically cured? Long-term metabolic effects of bariatric surgery in obese patients with type 2 diabetes mellitus. Ann Surg. 2013;258:628–637.

Cottam DR, Mattar SG, Barinas-Mitchell E, et al. The chronic inflammatory hypothesis for the morbidity associated with morbid obesity: implications and effects of weight loss. Obes Surg. 2004;14:589–600. [PMID: 15186624]

Dixon JB, Dixon ME, O'Brien PE. Birth outcomes in obese women after laparoscopic adjustable gastric banding. Obstet Gynecol. 2005;106:965–972. [PMID: 1626013]

Dixon JB, O'Brien PE, Playfair J, et al. Adjustable gastric banding and conventional therapy for type 2 diabetes: a randomized controlled trial. JAMA. 2008;299:316–323. [PMID: 18212316]

Ikramuddin S, Korner J, Lee WJ, et al. Roux-en-Y gastric bypass vs intensive medical management for the control of type 2 diabetes, hypertension, and hyperlipidemia: the Diabetes Surgery Study randomized clinical trial. JAMA. 2013;309:2240–2249.

Kashyap SR, Bhatt DL, Wolski K, et al. Metabolic effects of bariatric surgery in patients with moderate obesity with type 2 diabetes: analysis of a randomized control trial comparing surgery with intensive medical therapy. Diabetes Care. 2013;36:2175–2182.

Lee Y, Doumouras AG, Yu J, et al. Laparoscopic sleeve gastrectomy versus laparoscopic Roux-en-Y gastric bypass: a systematic review and meta-analysis of weight loss, comorbidities, and biochemical outcomes from randomized controlled trials. Ann Surg. 2021;273(1):66–74. [PMID: 31693504]

Maggard MA, Shugarman LR, Suttorp M, et al. Meta-analysis: surgical treatment of obesity. Ann Intern Med. 2005;142:547–559. [PMID: 15809466]

Patel JA, Colella JJ, Esaka E, et al. Improvement in infertility and pregnancy outcomes after weight loss surgery. Med Clin North Am. 2007;91:515–528. [PMID: 17509393]

Ramos EJ, Xu Y, Romanova I, et al. Is obesity an inflammatory disease? Surgery. 2003;134:329–335. [PMID: 12947337]

Sampalis JS, Liberman M, Auger S, et al. The impact of weight reduction surgery on health-care costs in morbidly obese patients. Obes Surg. 2004;14:939–947. [PMID: 15329183]

Schauer PR, Bhatt DL, Kirwan JP, et al. Bariatric surgery versus intensive medical therapy for diabetes—3-year outcomes. N Engl J Med. 2014;370:2002–2013.

Sharples AJ, Mahawar K. Systematic review and meta-analysis of randomised controlled trials comparing long-term outcomes of Roux-En-Y gastric bypass and sleeve gastrectomy. Obes Surg. 2020;30(2):664–672. [PMID: 31724116]

Sjöström L, Lindroos AK, Peltonen M, et al. Lifestyle, diabetes, and cardiovascular risk factors 10 years after bariatric surgery. *N Engl J Med.* 2004;351:2683–2693. [PMID: 15616203]

Sjöström L, Narbro K, Sjöström D, et al; Swedish Obese Subjects Study. Effects of bariatric surgery on mortality in Swedish obese subjects. *N Engl J Med.* 2007;357:741–752. [PMID: 17715408]

WEIGHT REGAIN

Weight nadir typically occurs 12–24 months following bariatric surgery. After this time anywhere from 15% to 35% of patients will regain >15% of lost weight. Weight regain after RYGB has been shown to be as high as 30%, which can also lead to relapse of comorbidities such as diabetes and hypertension. There are several possible etiologies for this phenomenon including dietary noncompliance, physical inactivity, presence of gastrogastric fistula, enlarged pouch or dilated gastrojejunal anastomosis in the case of RYGB or dilated sleeve, as well as psychiatric or metabolic factors. As such, there are several different management approaches depending on the presumed cause. Traditionally, weight regain has been treated with revisional surgery, although it has been shown to have a higher rate of complications and morbidity than primary surgery. Weight loss medications have been approved since the 1950's and recently have been used off-label to treat weight regain following bariatric surgery. Studies have demonstrated between 37% and 57% of patients will achieve at least 5% TWL using medications with the amount of weight loss ranging between 3% and 8%. Common weight loss medications include Phentermine, Topiramate, Bupropion/Naltrexone, and Liraglutide. Alternatively, weight regain may also be treated endoscopically. For RYGB patients, an endoscopic approach may be considered especially in those with a gastrojejunal anastomosis greater than 15 mm and/or pouch longer than 5 cm. Options include argon plasma coagulation (APC), transoral outlet reduction (TORe) using the Overstitch endoscopic suturing device (Apollo Endosurgery) and restorative obesity surgery endoscopic (ROSE) using the IOP endoscopic plication device (USGI). Studies demonstrated the efficacy of endoscopic revision of RYGB to be ranging between 9% and 12% TWL at 12 months with its durability up to at least 5 years. Similar to RYGB, SG may be revised endoscopically using the Overstitch or IOP device with reported efficacy of 16% to 18% at 12 months.

Bastos EC, Barbosa EM, Soriano GM, et al. Determinants of weight regain after bariatric surgery. *Arq Bras Cir Dig.* 2013;26(suppl 1):26–32. [PMID: 24463895]

Cooper TC, Simmons EB, Webb K, et al. Trends in weight regain following Roux-en-Y gastric bypass (RYGB) bariatric surgery. *Obes Surg.* 2015;25(8):1474–1481. [PMID: 25595383]

Dayyeh BKA, Lautz DB, Thompson CC. Gastrojejunal stoma diameter predicts weight regain after Roux-en-Y gastric bypass. *Clin Gastroenterol Hepatol.* 2011;9(3):228–233. [PMID: 21092760]

de Moura DTH, Barrichello S, de Moura EGH, et al. Endoscopic sleeve gastroplsty in the management of weight regain after sleeve gastrectomy. *Endoscopy.* 2020;52(3):202–210. [PMID: 31940667]

Hanipah ZN, Nasr EC, Bucak E, et al. Efficacy of adjuvant weight loss medication after bariatric surgery. *Surg Obes Relat Dis.* 2018;14(1):93–98. [PMID:29287757]

Jirapinyo P, de Moura DTH, Dong WY, Farias G, Thompson CC. Dose response for argon plasma coagulation in the treatment of weight regain after Roux-en-Y gastric bypass. *Gastrointest Endosc.* 2020;91(5):1078–1084. [PMIE: 31904378]

Jirapinyo P, de Moura DTH, Thompson CC. Endoscopic submucosal dissection with suturing for the treatment of weight regain after gastric bypass: outcomes and comparison with traditional transoral outlet reduction (with video). *Gastrointest Endosc.* 2020;91(6):1282–1288. [PMID: 32007520]

Jirapinyo P, Kroner PT, Thompson CC. Purse-string transoral outlet reduction (TORe) is effective at inducing weight loss and improvement in metabolic comorbidities after Roux-en-Y gastric bypass. *Endoscopy.* 2018;50(4):371–377. [PMID: 29253919]

Jirapinyo P, Kumar N, AlSamman MA, et al. Five-year outcomes of transoral outlet reduction for the treatment of weight regain after Roux-en-Y gastric bypass. *Gastrointest Endosc.* 2020;91(5):1067–1073. [PMID: 31816315]

Maselli DB, Alqahtani AR, Abu Dayyeh BK, et al. Revisional endoscopic sleeve gastroplasty of laparoscopic sleeve gastrectomy: an international, multicenter study. *Gastrointest Endosc.* 2021;93(1):122–130. [PMID: 32473252]

Odom J, Zalesin KC, Washington TL, et al. Behavioral predictors of weight regain after bariatric surgery. *Obes Surg.* 2010;20(3):349–356. [PMID: 19554382]

Stanford FC, Alfaris N, Gomez G, et al. The utility of weight loss medications after bariatric surgery for weight regain or inadequate weight loss: a multi-center study. *Surg Obes Relat Dis.* 2017;13(3):491–500. [PMID: 27986587]

RECOMMENDATIONS & CAVEATS

Weight loss surgery is the treatment of choice for appropriately selected individuals who have class II obesity with weight-related comorbid conditions and patients with class III obesity with or without comorbid conditions. Several surgical procedures designed to treat individuals with obesity and current procedures are quite effective in inducing long-term weight loss. However, patients require a careful, comprehensive evaluation before proceeding with such treatment to minimize surgical risks and justify such an invasive treatment. In appropriately selected individuals, bariatric surgery is associated with reduced cardiovascular and other weight-related risks, reduced mortality, and reduced health care costs, making such surgery appropriate in this group of individuals until equally or more effective weight loss treatments are developed.

Approach to Abnormal Liver Tests

Jordan Sack, MD, MPH

Gyorgy Baffy, MD, PhD

ESSENTIALS OF DIAGNOSIS

▶ Abnormal liver tests (serum assays for ALT, AST, alkaline phosphatase, and bilirubin) can be characterized by pattern, severity, and duration which help guide the differential and workup.

▶ Liver tests should not be mistaken for liver function, which is assessed using INR and serum albumin.

▶ Most causes of abnormal liver tests can be determined from a careful history and exam in conjunction with selective noninvasive testing.

▶ Information should be elicited on history of abnormal liver tests; temporal correlation with hypotension, medications, antibiotics, supplements, alcohol, viral exposures, travel, pregnancy; diagnosis of metabolic syndrome, autoimmune disorder, hematologic disease, heart failure, or inflammatory bowel disease; family history of liver disease; and nonhepatic causes of assay abnormalities.

▶ Liver test values do not correlate with the degree of hepatic fibrosis.

General Considerations

Routine liver chemistries consist of serum assays for the level of alanine aminotransferase (ALT), aspartate aminotransferase (AST), alkaline phosphatase, and bilirubin (direct and indirect). These tests can assess and characterize liver injury but they are not markers of liver function which is measured using international normalized ratio (INR) and albumin. The presence of an INR ≥1.5 and encephalopathy in a patient without chronic liver disease should prompt urgent evaluation for acute liver failure.

It is important to be aware that many laboratories will provide varying reference ranges for a normal ALT and AST based on their prevalence in the tested population. The upper limit of normal (ULN) values is considered an ALT or AST of 19–25 IU/L for females and 29–33 IU/L for males and values higher than this should be considered abnormal. Furthermore, any predominant isolated liver enzyme elevation should prompt consideration of nonhepatic causes as these enzymes can also be found outside of the liver.

In general, the pattern, severity, and duration of abnormal liver tests can inform the differential and diagnostic workup. Careful history taking and physical exam are paramount to promptly identify the cause of these abnormalities and to prioritize laboratory testing. Not all causes of liver disease can be identified by testing alone (eg, drug-induced liver injury) and causes that can be tested are not always considered (eg, hepatitis E or celiac disease) or may not be sought by the right test (eg, obtaining hepatitis C antibody instead of hepatitis C viral load for acute liver injury).

The initial evaluation should encompass detailed information on any history of abnormal liver tests; any temporal association with hypotension, medications (particularly prescriptions, antibiotics, supplements, herbals), alcohol use, viral exposures, travel, pregnancy; any diagnoses of metabolic syndrome, autoimmune disorders, hematologic disease, heart failure, or inflammatory bowel disease; any family history of liver diseases; and any potential nonhepatic etiology. Patients should also be assessed for chronic liver disease on physical exam.

As most causes of abnormal liver tests can be identified with careful history-taking along with noninvasive workup, it is rare for a liver biopsy to be needed urgently. A biopsy should be obtained after discussion with a hepatologist and is usually reserved for cases with persistent abnormalities where noninvasive testing is unable to confirm or rule out a specific diagnosis and the biopsy would affect the patient's management (eg, autoimmune hepatitis, Wilson disease, and infiltrative diseases).

An assessment of hepatic fibrosis should be considered in patients who have chronic liver test abnormalities and/or have evidence of chronic liver disease on history, exam, or laboratory testing. This evaluation of hepatic fibrosis is typically done non-invasively with vibration controlled transient elastography (VCTE). In centers without access to VCTE, several noninvasive scoring systems for advanced hepatic fibrosis can be utilized as a first step but their sensitivity and specificity are lower than VCTE. No assumptions should be made regarding underlying hepatic fibrosis solely based on the absence, presence, or severity of liver test abnormalities.

Pathogenesis

Within the hepatocyte, ALT is found in the cytoplasm, AST is localized to the mitochondria, while alkaline phosphatase is bound to the canalicular membrane. These enzymes can rise depending on the type and degree of injury to the hepatocyte. As these enzymes can be found outside of the liver, a nonhepatic source should be considered when there is an isolated elevation in one of these enzymes. Specifically, ALT can be found in the kidney, AST can be found in the muscle, kidney, heart, and brain, while alkaline phosphatase can be found in the bone, placenta, and bowel.

Meanwhile, bilirubin is formed by the breakdown of heme into unconjugated (indirect) bilirubin which is then bound to albumin and circulated to the hepatocyte where it undergoes conjugation (direct bilirubin) and gets excreted into the biliary system. Jaundice develops when there is a build-up of bilirubin in the serum due to a disruption in one of the steps on this pathway. Fractionating the bilirubin into direct and indirect can help to elicit the differential. A rise in the indirect bilirubin can occur when there is (1) an increase in heme breakdown from hemolysis or from resorption of a hematoma, (2) an inability of the hepatocyte to uptake the bilirubin, or (3) decreased bilirubin conjugation due to a genetic defect (Gilbert or Crigler-Najjar syndrome) or medications. Direct bilirubin elevation happens when there is (1) an inability to properly export conjugated bilirubin into the bile ducts, termed as intrahepatic cholestasis, which can occur with genetic defects (Rotor or Dubin-Johnson syndrome), medications, or sepsis, or (2) there is an obstruction in the bile ducts from a stone, stricture, or mass. Damage to the hepatocyte can also impair metabolism of bilirubin and cause either or both direct and indirect bilirubin elevations.

Prevention

Although there are a broad range of causes that may account for liver chemistry elevations, some causes of liver diseases (and thus liver test elevations) can be prevented with proper discussion and screening. Patients should be counseled on moderate alcohol consumption, optimization of weight and metabolic risk factors, use of clean needles and barrier protection, and avoidance of hepatotoxic medications, herbal and dietary supplements, or ingestion of poisonous mushrooms or foods infected by aflatoxin. Screening should be

considered in patients who have first degree relatives with hereditary liver diseases particularly those with hereditary hemochromatosis, Wilson disease, and alpha-1 anti-trypsin deficiency. Immunization to hepatitis A and B should be routinely assessed and provided if not immune. Those who will receive immunosuppression must be checked for evidence of current or past hepatitis B infection to prevent hepatitis B flare or reactivation.

Clinical Findings

A. Symptoms & Signs

The presentation for abnormal liver tests can range from the asymptomatic patient to the jaundiced and pruritic patient. The importance of a careful history and physical examination cannot be overemphasized.

Patients should be asked about the presence of nonliver associated symptoms that can sometimes help to clue the differential diagnosis. These symptoms include viral prodrome (consider viral hepatitis), autoimmune symptoms (consider autoimmune hepatitis), right sided volume overload (consider hepatic congestion), orthostasis (consider hepatic ischemia), and new abdominal distention (consider ascites or an enlarging lesion).

Regardless of symptoms, all patients should be asked about any history of prior liver test elevations; any temporal association with medication changes (eg, prescriptions, antibiotics, supplements, herbal and dietary supplements), alcohol use, viral exposures, travel, hypotension, pregnancy; any diagnosis of metabolic syndrome, autoimmune disorders, hematologic disease, heart failure, hypotension, inflammatory bowel disease; and any family history of liver diseases.

Table 39–1 summarizes the specific information to be obtained from patients presenting with elevated liver tests.

A physical exam should not only look for stigmata of chronic liver disease but also for signs of acute liver failure and for evidence to support a liver injury etiology. The presence of encephalopathy or asterixis in a patient without underlying chronic liver disease should raise the suspicion for acute liver failure. Signs of chronic liver disease include spider angiomata, palmar erythema, gynecomastia, ascites, hepatomegaly, splenomegaly, and asterixis. Potential causes of liver injury that can be found on exam include hypotension, vasopressor use, blood borne exposures (needle tracks, tattoos, piercing, scars), and right sided heart failure (jugular venous distention, lower extremity edema, pulmonary edema).

B. Laboratory Findings

It is imperative to recognize that ALT, AST, alkaline phosphatase, and bilirubin are liver-associated laboratory parameters that do not reflect liver function despite often being lumped together under the misleading term of "liver function tests" (LFTs). Rather, liver function is primarily measured using

Table 39–1. Specific information to obtain from patients with abnormal liver tests.

Risk Factors and Associations to Inquire About	Liver Disease to Consider
Medications, antibiotics, supplements, herbs, teas, vitamins, home remedies, acetaminophen, mushrooms	Drug-induced liver injury Drug-induced autoimmune hepatitis Acetaminophen overdose Mushroom poisoning
Immunosuppressive medications	Hepatitis B Cytomegalovirus Epstein-Barr virus Herpes simplex virus Varicella zoster virus Drug-induced liver injury
Autoimmune disorders: Hashimoto thyroiditis, rheumatoid arthritis, type 1 diabetes mellitus, celiac disease, lupus erythematosus	Autoimmune hepatitis Primary biliary cholangitis Celiac disease
Inflammatory bowel disease	Primary sclerosing cholangitis Nonalcoholic fatty liver disease Drug-induced liver injury
Alcohol use disorder	Alcohol-related hepatitis
Metabolic syndrome: Obesity, hypertension, hyperlipidemia, type 2 diabetes mellitus	Nonalcoholic fatty liver disease
Viral exposures: Tattoos, piercing, intravenous drug use, intranasal cocaine use, blood transfusions, unprotected intercourse with high risk individual, needlestick exposure, shared razors or toothbrush, surgery, homelessness, travel, unsanitary food handling	Hepatitis A Hepatitis B Hepatitis C Hepatitis D Hepatitis E
Travel and exposure to animals	Hepatitis A Hepatitis E Tick borne illnesses Leptospirosis
Pregnancy including immediate post-partum	Hyperemesis gravidarum Intrahepatic cholestasis of pregnancy HELLP syndrome Acute fatty liver of pregnancy Choledocholithiasis Parvovirus Hepatitis E Undiagnosed chronic liver disease
Heart failure	Hepatic congestion Iron overload Amyloidosis
Hypotension	Ischemic hepatitis
Hematologic diseases	Secondary iron overload Sickle cell hepatopathy Hepatitis B Hepatitis C Graft versus host disease (if post bone marrow transplant) Veno-occlusive disease (if with ascites or weight gain) Amyloidosis Drug-induced liver injury

(Continued)

Table 39–1. Specific information to obtain from patients with abnormal liver tests. (Continued)

Risk Factors and Associations to Inquire About	Liver Disease to Consider
Solid organ transplants	Graft versus host disease Hepatitis B Hepatitis E Cytomegalovirus Epstein Barr virus Drug-induced liver injury
Diabetes mellitus type 1	Glycogenic hepatopathy
Diabetes mellitus type 2	Non-alcoholic fatty liver disease Diabetic hepatosclerosis
Autoimmune pancreatitis Retroperitoneal fibrosis	IgG4 related disease
Sarcoidosis	Hepatic sarcoidosis
Intestinal failure and/or long-term total parenteral nutrition	Intestinal failure associated liver disease
Family history of liver disease	Hepatitis B Hepatitis C Hereditary iron overload Wilson disease Alpha-1 anti-trypsin deficiency Non-alcoholic fatty liver disease Lysosomal acid lipase deficiency Celiac disease Cystic fibrosis Congenital hepatic fibrosis Progressive familial intrahepatic cholestasis Benign recurrent intrahepatic fibrosis
Symptoms to Inquire About	**Liver Disease to Consider**
Viral prodrome (fevers, rash, respiratory symptoms)	Acute viral hepatitis (not only hepatotropic viruses)
Autoimmune symptoms (fatigue, joint pain)	Autoimmune hepatitis
Right-sided volume overload (dyspnea, weight gain, peripheral edema)	Hepatic congestion
Orthostasis (lightheadedness, syncope)	Ischemic hepatitis
Abdominal pain	Choledocholithiasis Cholangitis Hepatic abscess Peritonitis
New abdominal distention	Ascites Enlarging abdominal lesion

INR and albumin. The presence of encephalopathy and an INR ≥1.5 in a patient without chronic liver disease should prompt urgent evaluation for acute liver failure. Those with chronic liver disease may have concomitant findings of thrombocytopenia, hypoalbuminemia, and macrocytosis.

Interpreting liver tests requires recognition of the pattern, severity, and acuity as each type can provide a different diagnostic path. Predominant elevations in ALT and AST suggest hepatocellular injury while those in alkaline phosphatase or bilirubin indicate cholestasis. For those with hepatocellular injury, an ALT or AST of 19–25 IU/L for females and 29–33 IU/L for males are considered the ULN. Using these cut-offs, the severity of a hepatocellular injury can be defined as borderline (<2X ULN), mild (2–5X ULN), moderate (5–15X ULN), or severe (>15X ULN). The R factor, (defined as ALT ÷ ULN ALT) / (alkaline phosphatase ÷ ULN alkaline phosphatase), can be used to guide the type of liver injury with >5 hepatocellular, 2 to 5 mixed, and <2 cholestatic. An isolated or out of proportion AST should prompt checking creatine kinase (CK) levels to rule out rhabdomyolysis as the source. In rare situations, cardiac causes and macro-AST should be considered. For those with an isolated elevated alkaline phosphatase, a 5′ nucleotidase should be checked to confirm that the alkaline phosphatase is hepatic in etiology and not secondary to the bone, placenta, or bowel. Other less specific tests are gamma glutamyl peptidase (GGT) and alkaline phosphatase fractionation. For those with an isolated bilirubin elevation, fractionation should be performed to determine whether it is predominantly direct or indirect with the latter prompting a hemolysis workup.

Laboratory tests that can be obtained during the workup for abnormal liver tests are guided by the history, exam, and liver test pattern. Table 39–2 summarizes a selection of diagnostic tests by etiology.

Of note, a few diagnoses can be entertained with high probability based on the pattern of liver test abnormalities. Herpes simplex virus hepatitis should be presumed in a critically ill patient with aminotransferases to the thousands with a disproportionately low bilirubin. Shock liver should be strongly considered in a patient with a hypotensive episode with aminotransferases in the thousands that rapidly improve with restoration of perfusion. Wilson disease must be considered in a young patient with an alkaline phosphatase to bilirubin ratio less than 4 and an AST to ALT ratio of at least 2. Alcohol-related hepatitis should be considered in a patient with recently increased alcohol ingestion, macrocytosis, leukocytosis, and an AST to ALT ratio of at least 2 with aminotransferase levels generally no higher than a few hundred.

C. Imaging Studies

An abdominal ultrasound can help rule out the presence of a hepatobiliary mass, biliary stricture, and choledocholithiasis. When clinical suspicion remains high for one of these diagnoses despite a negative ultrasound, magnetic resonance cholangiopancreatography or endoscopic ultrasound may need to be performed. The abdominal ultrasound can also characterize the presence of chronic liver disease by describing liver nodularity, periumbilical collaterals, and splenomegaly. In cases where patients have ascites, a Doppler study should be requested to rule out Budd-Chiari syndrome and an echocardiogram obtained to evaluate cardiac causes of portal hypertension.

Vibration-controlled transient elastography and magnetic resonance elastography are relatively new noninvasive methods for quantifying hepatic fibrosis in patients without hepatic congestion, ascites, or pregnancy. As liver test elevations and imaging studies do not always correlate with underlying hepatic fibrosis, elastography can help to characterize whether patients have underlying chronic liver disease.

If the clinical suspicion for chronic liver disease, portal hypertension, or biliary obstruction remains high and the imaging study is negative or discordant with the clinical history and exam, further diagnostic or therapeutic interventions should be considered.

▶ Differential Diagnosis

The diagnosis and selection of diagnostic tests for abnormal liver tests can be narrowed by first recognizing the liver enzyme elevations as hepatocellular or cholestatic and using information obtained from a thorough history and physical (Figure 39–1).

A. Hepatocellular Pattern

Patients with aminotransferase elevations should be evaluated by the acuity and severity of the liver enzymes. Those with moderate or severe acute liver injury should be assessed for acute viral hepatitis, autoimmune hepatitis, drug induced liver injury, ischemic hepatitis, Wilson disease, liver diseases of pregnancy, choledocholithiasis, and rarely infiltrative disease. Budd-Chiari syndrome should be entertained if ascites is present.

Borderline and mild acute or chronic liver enzymes elevations should prompt consideration for drug-induced liver injury, chronic viral hepatitis, alcohol-associated hepatitis, nonalcoholic steatohepatitis, autoimmune hepatitis, iron overload, Wilson disease, alpha-1-antitrypsin deficiency, congestive hepatopathy, and hepatobiliary lesions. Some rare causes include abnormal thyroid function, adrenal insufficiency, celiac disease, sickle-cell disease, tick-borne diseases, infiltrative diseases, cystic fibrosis, lysosomal acid lipase deficiency, and congenital hepatic fibrosis.

Those with isolated AST elevations should be evaluated for rhabdomyolysis, cardiac disease, and macro-AST.

B. Cholestatic Pattern

Cholestasis can be characterized by elevations in the bilirubin and/or alkaline phosphatase. Those with an isolated

Table 39–2. Select diagnostic tests that can be considered during workup for abnormal liver tests.

Liver Disease Entity	Diagnostic Tests
Alcohol related liver disease	Blood alcohol level Ethyl glucuronide Ethyl sulfate Phosphatidylethanol
Alpha-1 anti-trypsin disease	Alpha-1 anti-trypsin phenotype
Acetaminophen overdose	Acetaminophen level (may be undetectable by time of liver injury)
Autoimmune hepatitis	Immunoglobulin G Anti-nuclear antibody Smooth muscle or actin antibody Liver-kidney microsomal antigen Soluble liver antigen
Budd Chiari syndrome	Abdominal ultrasound with Doppler study Magnetic resonance imaging
Celiac disease	Tissue transglutaminase IgA (assuming no IgA deficiency)
Choledocholithiasis	Abdominal ultrasound Magnetic resonance cholangiopancreatography Endoscopic ultrasound
Hepatic congestion	Transthoracic echocardiogram
Hepatic lesion	Abdominal ultrasound Magnetic resonance cholangiopancreatography Endoscopic ultrasound
Iron overload	Transferrin saturation Ferritin
Ischemic hepatitis	Transthoracic echocardiogram
Primary biliary cholangitis	Anti-mitochondrial antibody
Primary sclerosing cholangitis	Magnetic resonance cholangiopancreatography IgG4
Secondary sclerosing cholangitis	Magnetic resonance cholangiopancreatography IgG4
Viral hepatitis	Hepatitis A IgM Hepatitis B surface antigen Hepatitis B core IgM Hepatitis B PCR Hepatitis C PCR Hepatitis D PCR Hepatitis E IgM Hepatitis E PCR Epstein Barr virus PCR Cytomegalovirus PCR Herpes simplex PCR Varicella zoster PCR Parvovirus PCR Adenovirus PCR
Wilson disease	Ceruloplasmin 24-hour urine copper excretion Slit lamp examination

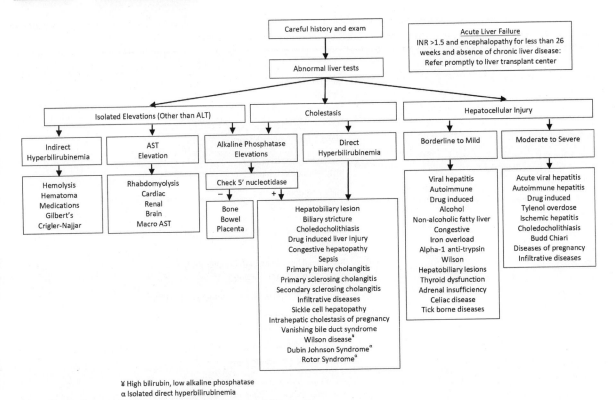

¥ High bilirubin, low alkaline phosphatase
α Isolated direct hyperbilirubinemia

▲ **Figure 39–1.** Diagnostic algorithm for abnormal liver tests.

indirect hyperbilirubinemia should undergo a hemolysis workup which if negative could suggest Gilbert syndrome in the absence of any hematoma or associated medication. Patients with cholestasis involving an isolated direct bilirubin or alkaline phosphatase elevation, with the latter confirmed by an elevated 5′ nucleotidase, should undergo abdominal imaging to exclude biliary obstruction from choledocholithiasis, strictures, and compression from a mass or adjacent structure. The absence of biliary dilatation should lead to consideration of medications/supplements, infection, and hepatic congestion. Sometimes alcohol related liver disease and nonalcoholic fatty liver disease can be associated with alkaline phosphatase elevations. A mitochondrial antibody assay should also be checked in those with chronic alkaline phosphatase elevations. In select situations, less common diagnoses should be considered such as infiltrative diseases (lymphoma, metastatic cancer, amyloidosis, sarcoidosis), intrahepatic cholestasis of pregnancy, sickle-cell disease, and vanishing bile duct syndrome. In cases where there is concern for biliary ischemia from hepatic artery thrombosis, the hepatic artery should be assessed with Doppler. Additionally, alkaline phosphatase elevations in liver transplant recipients may be suggestive of chronic ductopenic rejection. Recurrent episodes of cholestasis without association to medications or to the aforementioned diagnoses may lead

to consideration of benign recurrent intrahepatic cholestasis and progressive familial intrahepatic cholestasis.

▶ Complications

Undiagnosed and untreated liver test elevations over time may lead to the development of cirrhosis or in some cases acute liver failure.

▶ Treatment

The treatment of liver test elevations and hyperbilirubinemia depends on the underlying cause.

▶ Prognosis

The prognosis is dependent upon the etiology of the liver test elevations and whether there is underlying advanced hepatic fibrosis and/or portal hypertension on laboratory testing and imaging.

▶ When to Refer & Admit

The degree and pattern of abnormal liver tests do not necessarily correlate with the urgency for referral or admission. Any patient with signs of acute liver failure (INR ≥1.5, hepatic encephalopathy, duration less than 26 weeks, and typically no chronic liver disease) should be promptly admitted to a liver transplant center for expedited evaluation and treatment. Patients with liver test elevations of unclear etiology, prolonged chronicity, or features of chronic liver disease should be referred to a hepatologist. As most causes of liver disease and fibrosis can be assessed with noninvasive testing, it may be prudent to consult with a hepatologist before pursuing a liver biopsy. In general, a liver biopsy should be used to confirm or rule out a diagnosis if there is discordance

with noninvasive testing and if that information would affect treatment for the patient.

Kwo PY, Cohen SM, Kim JK. ACG Clinical Guideline: evaluation of abnormal liver chemistries. *Am J Gastroenterol.* 2017;112(1):18–35. [PMID: 27995906]

Newsome PN, Cramb R, Davison SM, et al. Guidelines on the management of abnormal liver blood tests. *Gut* 2018;67(1):6–19. [PMID: 29122851]

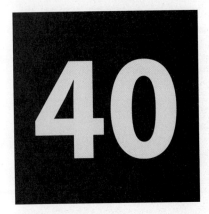

Acute Liver Failure

Anna Rutherford, MD, MPH

ESSENTIALS OF DIAGNOSIS

▶ Drugs, toxins, viral hepatitis, and hypoperfusion are the most common causes of acute liver failure (ALF).

▶ Laboratory findings may confirm the cause and severity of presentation.

▶ Consider acetaminophen toxicity in all patients, even without a history of toxic ingestion, particularly when serum aminotransferase levels are very high (>1000 IU).

▶ Depending on interval between time of ingestion and level drawn, acetaminophen levels may not be elevated even in cases of overdose.

▶ Rapid diagnostic and psychiatric evaluation is required at presentation.

General Considerations

ALF is the rapid deterioration of liver function in a patient without pre-existing liver disease. The most widely accepted definition of ALF includes evidence of coagulation abnormality (international normalized ratio [INR] ≥1.5), and encephalopathy in a patient without pre-existing liver disease and with a hepatic illness of less than 26 weeks' duration. ALF is a rare condition with an incidence of one to six cases per million per year in the developed world and affecting approximately 2000 people in the United States each year.

The US Acute Liver Failure Study Group (ALFSG) was formed in 1998 as a consortium of centers aimed at capturing nationwide data on ALF. Results of 2614 patients enrolled from January 1998 to March 2019 found that the most common causes of ALF were acetaminophen (46%), indeterminate (12%), idiosyncratic drug reactions (11%), and viral hepatitis A or B (9%).

Currently in the United States, spontaneous survival for all etiologies of ALF is approximately 45% without liver transplantation. The outcome of ALF, however, varies by etiology

with favorable prognoses being found with acetaminophen overdose, hepatitis A, and ischemia, and poor prognoses with other drug-induced ALF, hepatitis B, and indeterminate cases.

Lee WM, Larson AM, Stravitz RT. AASLD position paper: the management of acute liver failure: update 2011. *Hepatology*. 2012;55:965–967.

Stravitz RT, Lee WM. Acute liver failure. *Lancet*. 2019;394: 869–881. [PMID: 31498101]

Clinical Findings

ALF is a multisystem disorder, comprised of the acute onset of jaundice in a previously healthy person and the rapid onset of altered mental status accompanied by laboratory evidence of coagulopathy and acute hepatic injury.

A. Signs & Symptoms

Jaundice is a common physical examination finding on initial presentation, often prompting medical attention by the patient, but when minimal and the patient presents with altered mental status, the diagnosis of ALF may be delayed. The evaluation of mental status is the most critical component of the physical examination both initially and throughout the clinical course. Right upper quadrant tenderness may or may not be present. An enlarged liver on physical exam or imaging may been found in early viral hepatitis, malignant infiltration, congestive heart failure, or acute Budd-Chiari syndrome.

Careful history taking is a critical component of the initial assessment as it may elicit the etiology of ALF. Evaluation should include a review of all possible exposures to viral infection, drugs, and toxic ingestions, as well as risk factors for underlying chronic liver disease. If the patient has an advanced grade of encephalopathy, history should be obtained from family members.

Table 40–1. Initial laboratory evaluation in acute liver failure.[a]

Complete blood count
Complete metabolic panel (include magnesium, phosphate)
Prothrombin time/INR
Arterial blood gas
Lactate
Ammonia
Amylase, lipase
Viral hepatitis studies (anti-HAV IgM, HBsAg, HBcAB IgM, HBV viral load, anti-HEV IgM, anti-HCV Ab, HCV RNA, HSV IgM, VZV, EBV, CMV)
Acetaminophen level
Ceruloplasmin
Autoimmune markers (ANA, ASMA, IgG levels)
HIV
Pregnancy test in females

[a]ANA, antinuclear antibody; ASMA, antismooth muscle antibody; CMV, cytomegalovirus; EBV, Epstein-Barr virus; HAV, hepatitis A virus; HBcAb, hepatitis B core antibody; HBsAg, hepatitis B surface antigen; HBV, hepatitis B virus; HCV, hepatitis C virus; HEV, hepatitis E virus; HSV, herpes simplex virus; IgG, immunoglobulin G; IgM, immunoglobulin M; INR, international normalized ratio; VZV, varicella zoster virus.
Adapted with permission from Lee WM, Stravitz RT, Larson AM. Introduction to the revised American Association for the Study of Liver Diseases Position Paper on acute liver failure 2011, *Hepatology* 2012;55(3):965–967.

B. Laboratory Evaluation

Initial laboratory analysis should aim to determine the cause of ALF, the severity of presentation, and associated complications (Table 40–1).

Liver biopsy, usually done via the transjugular route due to coagulopathy, may be indicated when certain conditions such as autoimmune hepatitis, malignant infiltration of the liver, lymphoma, or herpes simplex virus are suspected or the etiology of injury is unclear. Ongoing daily laboratory monitoring should include INR, complete metabolic panel, and complete blood count.

▶ Complications

The initial injury in ALF results in the death of hepatocytes, leading to a systemic inflammatory response syndrome (SIRS) and multiorgan dysfunction. Significant neurologic, cardiopulmonary, and renal sequelae are associated with ALF, with cerebral edema and intracranial hypertension being the most serious of these complications. Acute renal failure complicates ALF in 30–50% of patients and can be a sign of poor prognosis, though mortality is most commonly related to neurologic dysfunction and infection.

▶ Treatment

A. General Management Concerns

ALF often involves the rapid deterioration of mental status and the potential for multiorgan failure and therefore,

patients should be managed in the intensive care unit. Table 40–2 outlines general treatment recommendations for intensive care management of patients with ALF according to specific potential complications. For patients not at a transplant center, the possibility of rapid progression of ALF makes early consultation with a transplant facility critical. Accordingly, plans for transfer to a transplant center should begin in patients with abnormal mentation or any indication of neurologic compromise.

Early institution of antidotes or specific therapy may prevent the need for liver transplantation and reduce the likelihood of poor outcome. *N*-acetylcysteine (NAC) is the antidote for acetaminophen-induced ALF, but some data suggest intravenous NAC improves transplant-free survival in non–acetaminophen induced liver failure due to its antioxidant and immunologic effects. Other measures appropriate for specific causes of ALF are described in detail later in this chapter.

Bernal W, Wendon J. Acute liver failure. *N Engl J Med.* 2013;369:2525–2534. [PMID: 24369077]

Flamm SL, Yang YX, Singh S, et al. American Gastroenterological Association Institute Guidelines for the Diagnosis and Management of Acute Liver Failure. *Gastroenterology.* 2017;152:644–647. [PMID: 28056348]

Lee WM, Hynan LS, Rossaro L, et al. Intravenous *N*-acetylcysteine improves transplant-free survival in early stage non-acetaminophen acute liver failure. *Gastroenterology.* 2009;137:856–864. [PMID: 19524577]

Wendon J, Cordoba J, Dhawan A, et al. EASL Clinical Practical Guidelines on the management of acute (fulminant) liver failure. *J Hepatol.* 2017;66:1047–1081. [PMID: 28417882]

B. Management of Specific Complications

1. Neurologic complications—Hepatic encephalopathy in ALF can range from minor confusion to coma and cerebral edema, and its presence, even mild in severity, indicates poor prognosis. Patients should be carefully and regularly assessed to follow progression of encephalopathy as severity correlates with the occurrence of cerebral edema and intracranial hypertension (Table 40–3). The pathophysiology behind the development of encephalopathy and cerebral edema is not completely understood, but it is thought that systemic and local inflammation and circulating neurotoxins such as ammonia play a role in astrocyte swelling, with the risk of intracranial hypertension significantly increasing with a sustained ammonia level of over 200 μmol/L.

Goals of management in early encephalopathy (grade I/II) should involve minimizing severity and preventing progression. Sepsis, gastrointestinal bleeding, hypoglycemia, hypoxemia, and electrolyte abnormalities can worsen encephalopathy and should be appropriately managed. Stimulation and overhydration can cause elevations in intracranial pressure (ICP) and should be avoided. Unmanageable agitation may be treated with short-acting benzodiazepines

Table 40–2. Intensive care in acute liver failure.

Complication	Assessment/Monitoring	Management
Central nervous system		
Encephalopathy	Careful/regular neurologic examination Check ammonia CT scan to rule out other causes of altered mental status Screen for sepsis	Grade III/IV: Endotracheal intubation Avoid sedatives Hypertonic saline (serum sodium 145–155 mmol/L) Consider lactulose
Intracranial hypertension/ cerebral edema	Intracranial pressure monitoring	Elevate head of bead Immediate treatment of seizures Hypertonic saline (serum sodium 145–155 mmol/L) Mannitol Hyperventilation (transient effect)
Cardiovascular system		
Hypotension	Pulmonary artery catheterization Echocardiogram	Treatment according to etiology Volume replacement if depleted Vasopressors—norepinephrine first line Inotropic support for low cardiac output and right ventricular failure
Respiratory system		
Risk of aspiration	Monitor level of consciousness	Intubation if mental status altered
Gastrointestinal/Hepatic system		
Hepatic dysfunction	Serial biochemical testing Serial coagulation testing	Intravenous N-acetylcysteine Treat etiology of ALF if possible
Stress ulceration		Prophylaxis with proton pump inhibitor or H-2 blocker
Renal system		
Renal dysfunction	Serial biochemical testing	Avoid nephrotoxic agents Volume replacement Renal replacement therapy Renal dosing of medications
Hematologic system		
Coagulopathy	Serial coagulation testing	Vitamin K × at least 1 dose FFP for invasive procedures or active bleeding Recombinant activated factor VII for invasive procedures Platelet transfusion for invasive procedures or platelets <10,000/mm^3
Metabolic system		
Hypoglycemia, electrolyte imbalance	Serial biochemical testing	Replacement of electrolytes, glucose Fluid adjustment Nutritional support (enteral feeding if possible)
Immunologic system		
Sepsis	Frequent monitoring	Surveillance cultures Consider prophylaxis if worsening clinical condition Prompt treatment of infection

ALF, acute liver failure; CT, computed tomography; FFP, fresh frozen plasm.
Data from Lee WM, Stravitz RT, Larson AM. Introduction to the revised American Association for the Study of Liver Diseases Position Paper on acute liver failure 2011, *Hepatology* 2012;55(3):965–967.

Table 40–3. Grades of encephalopathy.

Grade	Description
I	Changes in behavior with minimal change in level of consciousness
II	Gross disorientation, drowsiness, possibly asterixis, inappropriate behavior
III	Marked confusion, incoherent speech, sleeping most of the time but arousable to vocal stimuli
IV	Comatose, unresponsive to pain, decorticate or decerebrate posturing

Adapted from Conn HO, Leevy CM, Vlahcevic ZR, et al: Comparison of lactulose and neomycin in the treatment of chronic portal-systemic encephalopathy. A double blind controlled trial, *Gastroenterology* 1977;72(4 Pt 1):573–583.

in small doses, but may mask the severity of encephalopathy, limiting the value of neurologic evaluation. Standard medications used to treat hyperammonemia in patients with cirrhosis, such as Lactulose and nonabsorbable antibiotics (eg, Rifaximin) have never been tested in ALF, however they seem intuitively reasonable, and are commonly used.

In a large cohort of patients with ALF, continuous renal replacement therapy for those with oliguria, volume overload or hyperammonemia (>150 mmol/L) provided a reduction in serum ammonia level and improvement in transplant free survival. L-Ornithine-L-aspartate detoxifies ammonia to glutamine in muscle, but in a large randomized controlled trial, did not lower circulating ammonia levels, reduce the severity of encephalopathy, or improve survival.

For patients who progress to grade III–IV encephalopathy, care should be focused on prevention of cerebral edema and intracranial hypertension. The cause of intracranial hypertension in ALF is likely multifactorial, combining cytotoxic brain edema due to an increase in cerebral blood volume and cerebral blood flow due to inflammation and toxic products of the diseased liver. Cerebral edema inside the cranial vault raises ICP and decreases cerebral perfusion assessed by cerebral perfusion pressure (CPP; defined as mean arterial pressure minus ICP). Patients with cerebral edema may have systemic hypertension and bradycardia (Cushing reflex), increased muscle tone followed by decerebrate rigidity and posturing, abnormal papillary reflexes (usually dilation), and finally brainstem respiratory patterns and apnea. Brain herniation from elevated ICP is the immediate cause of death in 35% of patients with ALF, and 15–20% of patients listed for transplantation die from increased ICP. Cerebral edema is rarely seen in patients with grade I–II encephalopathy, but incidence increases to 65–75% in patients with grade IV coma and is the leading cause of death in these patients.

Intubation for airway protection is generally required for patients with grade III–IV encephalopathy. In order to maintain adequate CPP, optimization of blood pressure is essential. Both arterial hypertension and hypotension can compromise CPP, and therefore the use of sedation or vasopressors, respectively, may be necessary. Propofol has been suggested for sedation because it may reduce cerebral blood flow. Factors that increase ICP need to be avoided, including high positive end-expiratory pressure, frequent movements, neck vein compression, fever, arterial hypertension, hypoxia, coughing, sneezing, seizures, head-lowered position, and respiratory suctioning. The head of the bed should be elevated to 30 degrees, and electrolytes, blood gases, glucose, and neurologic status are monitored frequently.

The use of ICP monitoring in ALF patients is the most accurate method of monitoring for intracranial hypertension as clinical signs of elevated ICP are not always present, and neurologic changes such as pupillary dilation or decerebrate posturing often occur only late in the course. The risks of ICP monitoring in ALF patients include bleeding and infection, with subdural and intraparenchymal monitors demonstrating greater reliability, but increased rates of complications when compared with epidural catheters. A survival benefit with the use of ICP monitoring has not been shown, but the goal is to maintain ICP below 20–25 mm Hg and CPP above 50 mm Hg. Evidence of elevated ICP such as pupillary abnormalities, decerebrate posturing, or monitoring suggesting ICP above 20–25 mm Hg and CPP below 50–60 mm Hg, should prompt intervention.

Seizure is common in patients with ALF, although presentation is often subclinical and likely due to use of sedatives and paralytics in intubated patients. Seizures aggravate intracranial hypertension and should therefore be promptly controlled with phenytoin or levetiracetam. Small clinical trials using prophylactic phenytoin have shown no mortality benefit and unclear impact on cerebral edema or prevention of seizures.

Mannitol, in doses of 0.5–1 g/kg IV, has been demonstrated to decrease cerebral edema in the short term and improve survival. The efficacy of mannitol in patients with ICP may be affected by acute renal failure and oliguria. The dose may be repeated as needed as long as serum osmolality has not exceeded 320 mOsm/L. In order to be able to use mannitol repeatedly, fluid can be taken off with hemofiltration, which by itself reduces ICP. Prophylactic administration of mannitol is not indicated.

Hypertonic saline has been studied with one randomized study suggesting that it could delay onset of intracranial hypertension in patients with high-grade encephalopathy. Although no survival benefit has been demonstrated with hypernatremia, it is currently recommended as a prophylactic measure in patients at high risk for developing cerebral edema.

Hypothermia slows whole body metabolism, therefore lowering production and cerebral uptake of ammonia. Small studies have shown a benefit with reduction of body temperature to 34°C, specifically as a bridge to liver transplantation. More recently a small randomized trial showed that reduction of body temperature to 33–34°C was no more beneficial in improving survival or preventing cerebral edema than a normothermic body temperature of 36°C.

Hyperventilation has also been shown to cause quick reductions in ICP, but the effect is short-lived and therefore may be of therapeutic benefit only in situations of life-threatening intracranial hypertension to prevent herniation.

Barbiturate agents such as thiopental or pentobarbital may be considered when severe intracranial hypertension does not respond to other measures. However, in practice, the use of pentobarbital coma has largely been replaced with therapeutic hypothermia to decrease brain metabolism. Additionally, propofol is used more commonly given its pharmacokinetics are not altered in liver failure.

Acharya SK, Bhatia V, Sreenivas V, et al. Efficacy of L-ornithine L-aspartate in acute liver failure: a double-blind, randomized, placebo controlled study. *Gastroenterology*. 2009;136:2159–2168. [PMID: 19505424]

Bernal W, Hall C, Karvellas CJ, et al. Arterial ammonia and clinical risk factors for encephalopathy and intracranial hypertension in acute liver failure. *Hepatology*. 2007;46:1844–1852. [PMID: 17685471]

Bernal W, Murphy N, Brown S, et al. A multicentre randomized controlled trial of moderate hypothermia to prevent intracranial hypertension in acute liver failure. *J Hepatology*. 2016:65:273–279. [PMID: 26980000]

Cardosi FS, Gottfried M, Tjiois S, et al. Continuous renal replacement therapy is associated with reduced serum ammonia levels and mortality in acute liver failure. *Hepatology*. 2018;67:711–720. [PMID: 28859230]

Karvellas CJ, Fix OK, Battenhouse H, et al. Outcomes and complications of intracranial pressure monitoring in acute liver failure: a retrospective cohort study. *Crit Care Med*. 2014;42:1157–1167. [PMID: 24351370]

Mohsenin V. Assessment and management of cerebral edema and intracranial hypertension in acute liver failure. *J Crit Care*. 2013;28:783–791. [PMID: 23683564]

Murphy N, Auzinger G, Bernal W, et al. The effect of hypertonic sodium chloride on intracranial pressure in patients with acute liver failure. *Hepatology*. 2002;39:464–470. [PMID: 14767999]

Vaquero J, Fontana R, Larson AM, et al. Complications and use of intracranial pressure monitoring in patients with acute liver failure and severe encephalopathy. *Liver Transpl*. 2005;11:1581–1589. [PMID: 16315300]

Wijdicks EF, Nyberg SL. Propofol to control intracranial pressure in fulminant hepatic failure. *Transplant Proc*. 2002;34:1220–1222. [PMID: 12072321]

2. Cardiovascular complications—Increased cardiac output and low systemic vascular resistance are seen in ALF similarly to other critical illnesses. Intravascular volume depletion may also be present due to poor oral intake from altered mental status. Hypotension should be treated preferentially with fluid challenge, but systemic vasopressor support should be used if fluid replacement fails to maintain mean arterial pressure of 60–75 mm Hg. There is little evidence supporting the use of any specific fluid for volume support in ALF, and the choice should be determined by biochemical parameters. The role of albumin has not been investigated in ALF. Norepinephrine may be the optimal vasopressor to augment organ perfusion and preserve hepatic blood flow. The addition of vasopressin and its analogues may enhance the effects of norepinephrine, but should be used with caution as one study reported cerebral vasodilation and increased ICH in encephalopathic patients. Relative adrenal insufficiency occurs in more than 50% of patients with ALF, and may contribute to cardiovascular collapse. There are no mortality studies looking at the benefit of giving physiologic doses of hydrocortisone to ALF patients with vasopressor resistant shock, however one study has suggested use of steroids decreases vasopressor requirements and prolongs time to death.

Seetharam A. Intensive care management of acute liver failure: considerations while awaiting liver transplantation. *J Clin Transl Hepatol*. 2019;7:384–391. [PMID: 31915608]

Stravitz RT, Kramer AH, Davern T, et al. Intensive care of patients with acute liver failure: recommendations of the U.S. Acute Liver Failure Study Group. *Crit Care Med*. 2007;35:2498–2508. [PMID: 17901832]

Wendon J, Cordoba J, Dhawan A, et al. EASL Clinical Practical Guidelines on the management of acute (fulminant) liver failure. *J Hepatol*. 2017;66:1047–1081. [PMID: 28417882]

3. Pulmonary complications—Pulmonary edema and pulmonary infections are commonly seen in patients with ALF. Mechanical ventilation may be required but positive end-expiratory pressure can worsen cerebral edema and decrease hepatic blood flow.

4. Coagulopathy and gastrointestinal bleeding—Impaired hepatic synthesis of clotting factors, increased consumption of factors, low-grade fibrinolysis, and intravascular coagulation are typical of ALF. Thrombocytopenia is common and platelets may also be dysfunctional. Despite these features of abnormal hemostasis, bleeding complications in patients with ALF are uncommon (<10%). The prophylactic correction of INR with fresh frozen plasma is not recommended as transfusion may not appropriately correct INR, there are risks of volume overload, and INR is a useful prognostic marker to follow the patient's clinical course. Vitamin K (5–10 mg subcutaneously) should be given to treat an abnormal prothrombin time regardless of a patient's nutritional status. Replacement therapy with fresh frozen plasma or platelets are recommended only in the setting of hemorrhage or prior to an invasive procedure. Administration of recombinant factor VIIa should be considered prior to high-risk bleeding procedures such as liver biopsy or ICP monitor placement. A hemoglobin target for transfusion is 7 g/dl. Proton pump inhibitors and H-2 receptor blockers are shown to reduce risk of gastrointestinal bleeding in ALF patients.

Stravitz RT, Ellerbe C, Drukalski V, et al. Bleeding complications in acute liver failure. *Hepatology.* 2018;67:1931–1942. [PMID: 29194678]

Wendon J, Cordoba J, Dhawan A, et al. EASL Clinical Practical Guidelines on the management of acute (fulminant) liver failure. *J Hepatol.* 2017;66:1047–1081. [PMID: 28417882]

5. Renal failure—Acute kidney injury is common in patients with ALF and imparts important prognostic information, but rarely results in chronic kidney disease. Prevention of renal failure by ensuring adequate systemic blood pressure, treating infections, and avoiding nephrotoxic agents is important. Intravascular volume deficits are often present on admission and volume replacement is required. Acute renal failure may occur due to dehydration, hemodynamic changes similar to hepatorenal syndrome, or acute tubular necrosis. Renal failure may be even more common with acetaminophen overdose or other toxic ingestions due to direct nephrotoxicity causing acid-base disturbances and lactic acidosis. Prompt fluid resuscitation with crystalloids for low arterial pressure, or colloids in hepatorenal syndrome along with midodrine and octreotide, have been suggested. If renal dysfunction, fluid balance, and metabolic derangements necessitate renal replacement, continuous renal replacement therapy should be used for hemodynamic and metabolic stability.

Tujios SR, Hynan LS, Vazquez MA, et al. Risk factors and outcomes of acute kidney injury in patients with acute liver failure. *Clin Gastroenterol Hepatol.* 2015;13:352–359. [PMID 25019700]

6. Nutrition, electrolytes, and metabolic derangements—ALF is a high catabolic state, and adequate nutrition is essential. Caloric goal for patients should be approximately 25–30 kcal/kg/day. In patients with grade I or II encephalopathy, enteral feeding should be initiated early. Parenteral nutrition should be used only if enteral feeding is contraindicated as it increases the risk of infection. Severe restriction of protein should be avoided: 60 g/day of protein is a reasonable recommendation for patients with ALF.

Multiple electrolyte abnormalities are common in ALF. Correction of hypokalemia is essential as hypokalemia increases renal ammonia production, potentially exacerbating encephalopathy. Hyponatremia is a poor prognostic indicator, and levels above 125 mEq/L are desirable as hyponatremia can precipitate cerebral swelling. Hypophosphatemia is especially common in patients with acetaminophen-induced ALF and in those with intact renal function. Hypoglycemia occurs in many patients with ALF and is often due to depletion of hepatic glycogen stores and impaired gluconeogenesis. Plasma glucose concentration should be monitored and euglycemia should be maintained with continuous glucose infusion or insulin.

Plaut M, Bernal W, Dasarthy S, et al. ESPEN Guideline on clinical nutrition in liver disease. *Clin Nutr.* 2019;38:485–521. [PMID: 30712783]

7. Infection—Infection remains one of the leading causes of mortality in patients with ALF. Defective cellular and humoral immunity as well as presence of indwelling catheters, coma, broad-spectrum antibiotics, and medications that suppress immunity all predispose to infection. Localizing symptoms of infection such as fever and sputum production are frequently absent, and the only clue to an underlying infectious process may be worsening clinical status. Bacterial infections have been documented in 60–80% of ALF patients, most commonly pneumonia (50%), urinary tract infections (22%), IV catheter induced bacteremia (12%) or spontaneous bacteremia (16%). Prophylactic antibiotics or antifungals have not been shown to improve survival in ALF, but regular surveillance cultures (blood, urine, sputum, and ascites) should be performed in all patients, and consideration of treatment upon progression of encephalopathy, clinical signs of infection or elements of SIRS. Fungal infections occur in about one-third of ALF patients, particularly those with a prolonged intensive care unit course.

C. Liver Transplantation

Before availability of liver transplantation for patients with ALF, overall mortality from ALF approached 80%. Less than 10% of liver transplants performed each year are in patients with ALF. In studies in both the United States and Europe, about 25% of patients with ALF receive a liver transplant, contributing to a decrease in overall mortality from ALF to about 33%. One year survival post liver transplant for ALF is greater than 80%. In both the United States and Europe patients with ALF are listed Status 1a, ahead of patients who are listed for chronic liver disease, because of the high risk of 7 day mortality.

Current United Network for Organ Sharing (UNOS) criteria for priority (Status 1A) listing are (1) onset of any degree of hepatic encephalopathy within 8 weeks of onset of acute liver injury; (2) absence of pre-existing liver disease; (3) in the intensive care unit (ICU); and (4) requiring either mechanical ventilation, renal dialysis, or with severe coagulopathy (INR 2.0).

Reuben A, Tillman H, Fontana R, et al. Outcomes in adults with acute liver failure between 1998 and 2013: an observational cohort study. *Ann Intern Med.* 2016;164:724–732. [PMID: 27043883]

D. Liver Support Systems

Liver support systems attempt to support the patient until recovery or serve as a bridge to liver transplantation. These support systems fall into two main categories: noncell based systems which include plasmapheresis, plasma exchange, albumin dialysis and charcoal based hemabsorption, and bioartificial liver support systems which incorporate living hepatocytes or hepatic tissue. Although many liver support systems appear to be safe and have some biologic effect, none are approved for use in patients with ALF and are currently used only in the context of randomized clinical trials.

E. Prognosis

Due to the scarcity of organs and the importance of the timing and decision regarding transplantation in a rapidly progressive disease, the ability to assess prognosis in ALF is critical. The most important determinant of short-term (3 weeks) outcome appears to be the etiology of ALF. In patients with acetaminophen overdose, hepatitis A virus infection, shock liver, or pregnancy-related ALF, short-term survival without transplantation is 50% or greater. Patients with other etiologies of ALF including drug induced liver injury, hepatitis B, Wilson disease and indeterminate etiology have a survival rate of less than 25% without transplantation.

Various prognostic models exist, mostly taking patient's age, degree of encephalopathy, and coagulopathy into account, but no model is adequately sensitive or specific. The traditional King's College Hospital criteria (Table 40–4) have been the most commonly used and most frequently tested of the numerous proposed criteria for determining prognosis in all etiologies of ALF. King's College Hospital Criteria has a sensitivity of 61% and specificity of 86% for identifying who will benefit from a liver transplantation. A MELD score of >32 has a sensitivity of 79% and specificity of 71% in predicting who is unlikely to survive without liver transplantation. Other scores that may also predict mortality in patients with ALF include the Sequential Organ Failure Assessment (SOFA score) and the Clichy criteria.

Bernal W, Hyyrlainen A, Gera A, et al. Lessons from a look-back in acute liver failure? A single centre experience of 3300 patients. *J Hepatology.* 2013;59:74–80. [PMID: 23439263]

Shakil AO. Predicting the outcome of fulminant hepatic failure. *Liver Transpl.* 2005;11:1028–1030. [PMID: 16123964]

SPECIFIC CAUSES OF ACUTE LIVER FAILURE

1. Acetaminophen

The most common cause of ALF in developed countries is acetaminophen toxicity, which causes about 46% of cases of ALF in North America and 65% of cases in the United Kingdom. These numbers may underestimate the contribution of acetaminophen to ALF, as one study using a acetaminophen detection assay found 20% of ALF patients with indeterminate etiology to have acetaminophen-containing protein adducts released from dying hepatocytes. Actaminophen has a dose-related toxicity, and most ingestions leading to ALF exceed 10 g/day. Approximately half of cases of ALF from acetaminophen are due to intentional overdoses, taking a large quantity of acetaminophen at a single timepoint with suicidal intent. Unintentional overdoses occur when patients take excessive doses of acetaminophen over several days,

Table 40–4. Potentially helpful indicators[a] of poor (transplant-free) prognosis in patients with acute liver failure.

Etiology	Idiosyncratic drug injury Acute hepatitis B (and other nonhepatitis A viral infections) Autoimmune hepatitis Mushroom poisoning Budd-Chiari syndrome Indeterminate cause Wilson disease
Coma grade on admission	III or IV

King's College criteria	**Acetaminophen-induced ALF:**
	• Arterial lactate >3.0 mmol/L after adequate fluid resuscitation
	  Arterial pH <7.3 (following adequate volume resuscitation) irrespective of coma grade
	  OR
	• PT >100 seconds (INR 6.5) +serum creatinine >300 mol/L (3.4 mg/dL) in patients with grade III/IV encephalopathy
	Non–acetaminophen-induced ALF:
	• PT >100 seconds (INR >6.5) and encephalopathy present (irrespective of grade)
	  OR
	• Any 3 of the following, irrespective of coma grade:
	  –Drug toxicity, Wilson disease, indeterminate cause of ALF
	  –Age <10 or >40
	  –Jaundice to coma interval >7 days
	  –PT >50 seconds (INR 3.5)
	  –Serum bilirubin >300 mol/L (17 mg/dL)

ALF, acute liver failure; INR, international normalized ratio; PT, prothrombin time.

[a]None of these factors, with the exception of Wilson disease and possibly mushroom poisoning, are either necessary or sufficient to indicate the need for immediate liver transplantation.

Adapted with permission from Lee WM, Stravitz RT, Larson AM. Introduction to the revised American Association for the Study of Liver Diseases Position Paper on acute liver failure 2011, *Hepatology* 2012;55(3):965–967.

often paired with narcotics such as hydrocodone, specifically for pain relief.

▶ Clinical Findings

Acetaminophen induced ALF is characterized by extreme elevations of serum aminotransferases (often >10,000 IU/ml), normal bilirubin levels, metabolic acidosis, elevated serum lactate, hypoglycemia and acute kidney injury. Patients have a rapidly progressive multiorgan failure and hepatic encephalopathy, which can progress from mild encephalopathy to coma in just a few hours.

Treatment

If ingestion is suspected within a few hours of presentation, activated charcoal (1 g/kg orally) may be useful up to 3–4 hours after ingestion and does not reduce the effectiveness of oral *N*-acetylcysteine (NAC). The administration of NAC, which replenishes glutathione stores, is recommended in any patient with ALF in whom acetaminophen overdose is suspected. Although early administration enhances efficacy, some benefits have been shown even when NAC is given as late as 36 hours, and possibly even 48 hours, after ingestion. NAC can be given orally 140 mg/kg followed by 70 mg/kg every 4 hours for 17 doses. Intravenous administration is given as 150 mg/kg loading dose over 15 minutes, followed by maintenance at 50 mg/kg for over 4 hours and then 100 mg/kg over 16 hours. No studies have shown any difference between oral and intravenous routes of administration. Allergic reactions to NAC may be treated with antihistamines and epinephrine for bronchospasm or discontinuation if necessary.

Prognosis

In data from the ALFSG, among 1195 patients with acetaminophen-induced ALF, 72% survived, 65% survived without transplantation, and 9% underwent transplantation. Patients with unintentional overdose will often have more severe illness on presentation due to delay in seeking medical attention, but outcomes appear to be similar between patients with intentional and unintentional overdose once the patient develops ALF.

Lee WM, Larson A, Stravitz RT. AASLD Position Paper: The Management of Acute Liver Failure: Update 2011. *Hepatology.* 2012;55:965–967.

Reddy KR, Ellerbe C, Schilsky M, et al. Determinants of outcome among patients with acute liver failure listing for liver transplantation in the United States. *Liver Transpl.* 2016;22:505–515. [PMID: 26421889]

Stravitz RT, Lee WM. Acute liver failure. *Lancet.* 2019;394:869–881. [PMID: 31498101]

2. Viral Hepatitis

A. Hepatitis A

Hepatitis A is transmitted fecal-orally, with high incidence of infection associated with poor hygiene and sanitation. ALF is rare in hepatitis A (<1% cases), but some studies suggest that women, the elderly, and patients with underlying liver disease may be at greater risk of morbidity and mortality with acute infection. Since the introduction of hepatitis A vaccine in 1995 and the recommendations for routine early childhood immunization, reported cases in the United States have declined by more than 85%, and therefore the incidence of hepatitis A–associated acute liver failure has also declined. Patients with ALF from hepatitis A have a transplant free survival of 51%.

Rezende G, Roque-Afonso AM, Samuel D, et al. Viral and clinical factors associated with the fulminant course of hepatitis A infection. *Hepatology.* 2003;38:613–618. [PMID: 12939587]

Taylor RM, Davern T, Munoz S, et al. Fulminant hepatitis A virus infection in the United States: incidence, prognosis, outcomes. *Hepatology.* 2006;44:1589–1597. [PMID: 17133489]

B. Hepatitis B

Acute hepatitis B infection is the most common viral cause of ALF, accounting for 8% of cases overall. Outside of United States and United Kingdom, it is one of the most important causes of ALF, representing nearly 30% of ALF in parts of Europe, Asia, sub-Saharan Africa, and the Amazon basin. About two-thirds of the cases of ALF due to hepatitis B are caused by new infections, or delta superinfection, and the remainder are caused by reactivation of chronic hepatitis B infection or prior hepatitis B infection in the setting of chemotherapy or immune modulation.

Reactivation is associated with higher risk of progression to liver failure, and therefore patients who are hepatitis B surface antigen positive and are to begin immunosuppression are recommended to receive antiviral therapy throughout treatment and for 6–12 months after completion of immunosuppressive therapy.

Mortality from ALF from hepatitis B is higher than hepatitis A or E infection. Lamivudine, entecavir, tenofovir, telbivudine, and adefovir, commonly used to treat chronic hepatitis B, have also been used in ALF, but the data are equivocal.

Anastasiou OE, Widera M. Westhaus, et al. Clinical outcome and viral genome variability of hepatitis B virus-induced acute liver failure. *Hepatology.* 2019;69:993–1003. [PMID: 30229977]

Dao DY, Seremba E, Ajmera V, et al. Use of nucleoside (tide) analogues in patients with hepatitis B related acute liver failure. *Dig Dis Sci.* 2012;57:1348–1357. [PMID: 22198704]

Terrault NA, Lok ASF, McMahon BJ, et al. Update on prevention, diagnosis, and treatment of chronic hepatitis B: AASLD 2018 hepatitis B guidance. *Hepatology.* 2018;67:1560–1500. [PMID: 29405329]

C. Hepatitis C

The role of hepatitis C infection in ALF is controversial. Studies from Japan and India report the presence of anti-hepatitis C virus antibody or hepatitis C virus RNA among patients with ALF, but studies in France, the United States, and the United Kingdom have not shown hepatitis C to be a significant cause of ALF.

D. Hepatitis D

Hepatitis B/hepatitis D coinfection is associated with a more severe acute hepatitis than hepatitis B infection alone. Hepatitis D virus is cleared if hepatitis B virus is cleared. Hepatitis D superinfection in a chronic hepatitis B patient can also manifest as acute hepatitis, and usually results in chronic hepatitis D. In the United States, infection with hepatitis D virus is reported to account for fewer than 10% of all cases of ALF related to hepatitis B virus.

Price J. An update on hepatitis B, D, and E viruses. *Top Antivir Med.* 2014;21:157–163. [PMID: 24531556]

E. Hepatitis E

Hepatitis E occurs in epidemics in which a high incidence of ALF is seen, particularly in pregnant women, the elderly and patients with chronic liver disease from another etiology. In pregnancy, infection is most common in the third trimester and the fatality rate approaches 40%. Vertical transmission can result in ALF in neonates as well. Hepatitis E has only rarely been identified in the United States, but should be considered in anyone with recent travel to endemic areas such as Russia, Pakistan, Mexico, or India or who is immuno-compromised. Treatment is generally supportive and overall outcomes are good.

EASL Clinical Practice Guidelines on hepatitis E virus infection. *J Hepatol.* 2018;68:1256–1271. [PMID: 29609832]

Kamar N, Bendall R, Legrand-Abravanel F, et al. Hepatitis E. *Lancet.* 2012;379:2477–2488. [PMID: 22549046]

F. Other Viral Hepatitides

Cytomegalovirus, Epstein-Barr virus, parvovirus B19, herpes simplex virus 1 and 2, and human herpes virus 6 are occasionally implicated as causes of ALF. ALF related to herpes-virus infection is usually associated with immunosuppressive therapy or pregnancy, although reports in healthy individuals do exist. Patients present with anicteric hepatitis and are often critically ill. Skin lesions are present in only about 50% of cases, making diagnosis more difficult and often reliant on liver biopsy. Treatment should be initiated with acyclovir for suspected or documented cases. Varicella virus has been rarely implicated in ALF and can also be treated with acyclovir.

Adenovirus-induced ALF is rare, but multiple cases have been reported after allogeneic stem cell transplantation, liver transplantation, chemotherapy, and renal transplantation. It has an aggressive clinical course and poor prognosis.

Lee WM, Stravitz RT, Larson AM. Introduction to the revised American Association for the Study of Liver Diseases Position Paper on Acute liver failure 2011. *Hepatology.* 2012;55:965–967. [PMID: 22213561]

Nakazawa H, Ito T, Makishima H, et al. Adenovirus fulminant hepatic failure: disseminated adenovirus disease after unrelated allogeneic stem cell transplantation for acute lymphoblastic leukemia. *Intern Med.* 2006;45:975–980. [PMID: 16974062]

3. Non–Acetaminophen Drug Toxicity

Many drugs produce idiosyncratic ALF (Table 40–5), often leading to safety-related withdrawal from the market. In the United States about 11% of ALF cases are attributed to idiosyncratic drug-induced hepatotoxicity other than acetaminophen. Only 10% of all patients with drug induced liver injury develop ALF.

Antimicrobials account for over 50% of ALF from drug induced liver injury, including antituberculous drugs (particularly isoniazid), antibiotics (nitrofurantoin and ketoconazole), anti-epileptics (phenytoin and valproate), nonsteroidal anti-inflammatory drugs, and a wide variety of other medications as well as herbal medicine products and nutritional supplements.

Table 40–5. Drugs that may cause idiosyncratic liver injury leading to acute liver failure.

Single Agents Associated with Hepatotoxicity	
Allopurinol	Labetalol
Amiodarone	Lisinopril
Amphetamines/ecstasy	Metformin
Dapsone	Methyldopa
Diclofenac	Nefazodone
Didanosine	Nicotinic acid
Disulfiram	Ofloxacin
Efavirenz	Phenytoin
Etoposide	Propylthiouracil
Flutamide	PZA
Gemtuzumab	Quetiapine
Halothane	Statins
Imipramine	Sulfonamides
Isoflurane	Tolcapone
Isoniazid	Troglitazone
Ketoconazole	Valproic acid
Combination Agents with Enhanced Toxicity	
Amoxicillin–clavulanate	
Rifampin–isoniazid	
Trimethoprim–sulfamethoxazole	
Herbal Products/Dietary Supplements Associated with Hepatotoxicity	
Kava Kava	
Herbalife	
Hydroxycut	
Comfrey	
Senecio	
Greater celandine	
He Shon Wu	
LipoKinetix	
Ma Huang	

Adapted with permission from Lee WM, Stravitz RT, Larson AM. Introduction to the revised American Association for the Study of Liver Diseases Position Paper on acute liver failure 2011, *Hepatology* 2012;55(3):965–967.

Clinical Findings

Identification of drug-induced ALF requires careful history taking, including all medications, over-the-counter preparations, vitamin supplements, herbal supplements, and health foods. Peripheral eosinophilia, skin rash, and fever may be seen when associated with hypersensitivity; however, many cases of drug-induced hepatotoxicity are nonallergic and idiosyncratic. Aminotransferase levels are often only moderately elevated (in contrast with acetaminophen-induced liver failure).

Treatment

Patients with non–acetaminophen drug-induced ALF have a poor outcome overall, with only about 25% recovering spontaneously, and a 60–80% mortality rate without liver transplantation. The outcome of drug-induced ALF is predicted by the degree of liver dysfunction, but not by the class of drugs, drug injury pattern, age, gender, obesity, or timing of cessation of drug use.

Initial treatment of drug-induced liver disease includes supportive care, exclusion of other causes of liver injury, and withdrawal of the offending agent. Corticosteroids are not indicated unless there is evidence of a hypersensitivity reaction.

Hillman L, Gottfried M, Whitsett M, et al. Clinical features and outcomes of complementary and alternative medicine induced acute liver failure and injury. *Am J Gastroenterol.* 2016;111: 958–965. [PMID:27045922]

Reuben A, Koch DG, Lee WM. Drug-induced acute liver failure: results of a U.S. multicenter, prospective study. *Hepatology.* 2010;52:2065–2076. [PMID: 20949552]

4. Mushroom Poisoning

Mushroom poisoning is common in Western Europe, with 50–100 fatal cases reported yearly. *Amanita phalloides* is the most common species implicated. ALF is preceded by muscarinic symptoms such as profuse sweating, vomiting, and diarrhea. Diagnosis should be suspected in patients with a history of severe vomiting, diarrhea, and abdominal cramping within hours to a day of ingesting wild mushrooms. Gastric lavage and activated charcoal via nasogastric tube to remove stomach contents and to decrease the toxin in the enterohepatic circulation has been used, although there are no definitive studies of usefulness. The cholera-type diarrhea seen most commonly as an effect of phalloidin during the first 24 hours of illness can produce a profound metabolic alkalosis requiring vigorous fluid resuscitation and electrolyte replacement. Penicillin G, in doses of 250,000–1,000,000 units/kg/day, is used as treatment and is believed to work by displacing amanitin from plasma protein-binding sites and allowing for increased renal excretion. Sibilin (milk thistle) also has cytoprotective abilities against amatoxin. Both antidotes are used commonly despite no controlled trial demonstrating benefit.

Patients should be considered for liver transplantation as very low rates of spontaneous survival have been reported. Importantly, encephalopathy is not always present in severe cases and should not be an absolute prerequisite for deciding on transplantation.

Kieslichova E, Frankova S, Protus M, et al. Acute liver failure due to Amanita Phalloides poisoning: therapeutic approach and outcome. *Transplant Proc.* 2018;50:192–197. [PMID: 29407307]

Yongzhuang Y, Liu Z. Management of Amanita Phalloides poisoning: a literature review and update. *J Crit Care.* 2018;45:17–22. [PMID: 29627659]

5. Autoimmune Hepatitis

Most patients with autoimmune hepatitis exhibit clinical features of chronic hepatitis, but some present with ALF or an acute-on-chronic presentation. Diagnosis of ALF due to autoimmune hepatitis can be difficult, and other causes need to be ruled out. Autoantibodies may be absent, but autoantibodies can also be positive with other causes of liver disease such as drug-induced ALF. Liver biopsy is often needed to confirm a diagnosis. Treatment with steroids may be effective if given early, however once a patient has developed ALF, steroids are often ineffective and may predispose a patient to septic complications. ALF caused by autoimmune hepatitis has poor outcomes without liver transplantation (spontaneous survival <15%).

Stravitz RT, Lefkowitch JH, Fontana RJ, et al. Autoimmune acute liver failure: proposed clinical and histological criteria. *Hepatology.* 2011;53:517–526. [PMID: 21274872]

6. Wilson Disease

ALF is rare in Wilson disease and appears to be more common in women. It is frequently associated with a Coombs negative hemolytic anemia as hepatocyte necrosis results in the massive release of copper ions into the circulation. Clinical signs include jaundice, hemolytic anemia, and renal failure. Diagnosis can be difficult because ceruloplasmin, serum copper, urinary copper, and even liver biopsy with copper staining can be unreliable. As with autoimmune hepatitis, patients may have evidence of cirrhosis and still present with signs of ALF when rapid deterioration occurs. Kayser-Fleischer rings are present in 50% of patients presenting with ALF due to Wilson disease. Findings suggestive of the disease include very high bilirubin level (>20 mg/dL), markedly decreased serum albumin and cholesterol levels, decreased serum alkaline phosphatase, decreased uric acid, and a serum AST greater than ALT (at least 2.2:1) due to hemolysis. A high bilirubin (mg/dL) to alkaline phosphatase (IU/L) ratio (>4) is also a reliable indicator of Wilson disease in this setting.

ALF due to Wilson disease is nearly always fatal without transplantation, making early identification and immediate listing for transplant critical. Treatment to acutely lower serum copper and limit further hemolysis should include continuous hemofiltration, plasmapheresis, or plasma exchange. Penicillamine is not recommended in ALF as there is a risk of hypersensitivity.

Ferenci P, Czlonkowska A, Stremmel W, et al. EASL Clinical Practice Guidelines: Wilson's Disease. *J Hepatol.* 2012;56:671–685. [PMID: 22340672]

Palumbo SC, Schilsky ML. Clinical Practical Guidelines in Wilson Disease. *Ann Transl Med.* 2019;7(suppl 2):S65. [PMID: 31179302]

Roberts EA, Schilsky ML. American Association for the Study of Liver Diseases. Diagnosis and treatment of Wilson disease: an update. *Hepatology.* 2008;47:2089–2111. [PMID: 18506894]

7. Malignancy & Vascular Causes

Vascular causes of ALF include portal vein thrombosis, hepatic vein thrombosis, veno-occlusive disease, and ischemic hepatitis. Ischemic liver injury produces marked aminotransferase elevations, centrilobular necrosis, and ALF often with concurrent renal failure, myocardial infarction, cardiac arrest, cardiomyopathy, congestive heart failure, hypovolemia, and pulmonary embolism. Drug-induced hypotension or hypoperfusion causing ALF can be observed with long-acting niacin, cocaine, or methamphetamine.

Budd-Chiari syndrome or acute hepatic vein thrombosis can also present as ALF and often is due to an underlying hypercoagulable condition. Abdominal pain, ascites, hepatomegaly and lactic acidosis are often present. The diagnosis should be confirmed by imaging. Transjugular intrahepatic portosystemic shunt, surgical decompression, portocaval shunt, or thrombolysis may be beneficial in patients with acute Budd-Chiari syndrome. Transplantation may be required in patients who do not respond to venous decompression or in whom significant liver failure develops. It is important to rule out underlying malignancy prior to transplantation.

Malignant infiltration may cause ALF. Massive hepatic enlargement may be seen. Diagnosis should be made by imaging and biopsy, and treatment for the underlying disease is indicated. Common causes include breast cancer, small cell lung cancer, lymphoma, and melanoma. Transplantation is not an option in these patients.

Northup PG, Garcia-Pagan JC, Garcia-Tsao G, et al. Vascular liver disorders, portal vein thrombosis, and procedural bleeding in patients with liver disease: 2020 Practice Guidance by the American Association for the Study of Liver Diseases. *Hepatology.* 2021;71:366–413. [PMID: 33219529]

Parekh J, Matei VM, Canas-Coto A, et al. Budd Chiari syndrome causing acute liver failure: a multicenter case series. *Liver Transpl.* 2017;23:135–142. [PMID: 27656864]

8. Pregnancy

Viral hepatitis is the most common cause of ALF in pregnancy and accounts for 40% of jaundice. The outcome of ALF related to hepatitis E virus infection in pregnancy is poor. Supportive care is advocated, and termination, caesarean, or discouragement of breast feeding are not indicated. Pregnancy can also increase the risk of ALF due to herpesvirus infection, which should be treated with acyclovir. Acute fatty liver of pregnancy (AFLP) occurs during the third trimester and occasionally presents as ALF. It is characterized by sudden onset of jaundice and coagulopathy, altered mental status, hypoglycemia, and elevated transaminases but not to the extent seen in acute viral or drug-related hepatitis. Steatosis documented by imaging or biopsy supports the diagnosis of AFLP. Rapid delivery is the treatment, but in 40% of cases the fetus dies before delivery. Fatty liver of pregnancy can be treated with transplantation if prompt recovery does not follow delivery. Alternatively, HELLP syndrome, which involves very high aminotransferase levels, hemolysis, thrombocytopenia, hypertension, proteinuria, and preeclampsia, occurs in 0.1–0.6% of all pregnancies and in 4–12% of women with severe preeclampsia. The only definitive treatment is emergent delivery along with antepartum stabilization of hypertension and disseminated intravascular coagulation (DIC), seizure prophylaxis, and fetal monitoring.

Casey LC, Fontana RJ, Aday A, et al. Acute liver failure (ALF) in pregnancy: how much is pregnancy related? *Hepatology.* 2020;72:1366–1377. [PMID: 21991493]

9. Indeterminate Cause

Other rare causes of ALF include giant cell hepatitis or arteritis, amebic abscesses, disseminated tuberculosis, sepsis, heat stroke, and hemophagocytic lymphohistiocytosis (HLH). The cause of ALF is indeterminate in nearly 12% of adult patients in the United States. Indeterminate ALF typically carries a poor prognosis, with a spontaneous survival rate less than 25%. Several reports have implicated a variety of viruses in indeterminate ALF including togaviruses, paramyxoviruses, herpes simplex virus, SEN virus, and hepatitis C virus. The presence of many of these viruses has been discovered later by PCR, after results of routine serologic testing were negative.

Viral Hepatitis

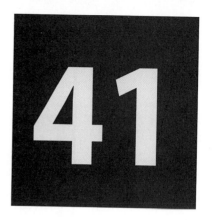

Anne F. Liu, MD
Stephen D. Zucker, MD

ESSENTIALS OF DIAGNOSIS

► Hepatitis A and E, which are transmitted by the fecal-oral route, are self-limited and rarely cause chronic infection.

► Hepatitis B, C, and D are acquired percutaneously or sexually; all can result in chronic infection.

► Infection with hepatitis D occurs only in a host with concurrent hepatitis B.

► All five hepatitis viruses can cause acute liver failure.

► Diagnostic tests appropriate to different clinical situations detect specific viral antigens and antibodies in serum by sensitive immunoassay, and viral DNA/RNA by sensitive amplification assays (eg, polymerase chain reaction [PCR]).

General Considerations

Although hepatitis viruses have been characterized extensively, knowledge of the pathogenesis, diagnosis, and treatment of chronic viral hepatitis continues to evolve. Sensitive and specific assays are available for all five forms (A–E) of viral hepatitis (Table 41–1). Nevertheless, approximately 5–10% of cases of apparent acute infectious hepatitis are unable to be attributed to any of the readily identifiable viral hepatidities, and nearly 50% of cases of acute liver failure cannot be attributed to a specific cause. Whether additional unidentified viruses cause acute or chronic liver disease remains an unanswered question. This chapter focuses on clinical features of the five known hepatitis viruses, hepatitis A through E, that are responsible for the majority of recognized cases of acute and chronic viral hepatitis (Table 41–2).

Clinical Findings

A. Acute Viral Hepatitis

1. Symptoms and signs—Symptoms of acute viral hepatitis are nonspecific, but have been categorized into four main phases: (1) incubation/preclinical, (2) prodromal, (3) icteric, and (4) resolution/convalescent. The initial period of time when the patient becomes infected, but remains asymptomatic, is referred to as the incubation/preclinical phase. During the prodrome phase, vague symptoms such as malaise, fatigue, nausea, anorexia, and arthralgias appear. Fever, if present, is usually low-grade. As the disease progresses, pruritus, dark urine, yellowing of the conjunctiva, and jaundice are hallmarks of the icteric phase. Jaundice is more common in adults and predicts immunologic clearance of the virus, whereas infants and young children are more prone to experience anicteric asymptomatic infection which may progress to chronic hepatitis. Patients who progress to the resolution/convalescent phase develop protective antibodies that not only facilitate clearance of the infection, but also prevent reinfection from occurring.

2. Laboratory findings—In any acute viral hepatitis, serum aminotransferase levels typically exceed 500 units/L and often 1000 units/L, with the alanine aminotransferase (ALT) characteristically higher than the aspartate aminotransferase (AST). Elevation of aminotransferase levels begins in the prodromal phase and precedes the rise in bilirubin level in patients with icteric hepatitis. Serum alkaline phosphatase typically is normal, or only mildly elevated. Serum bilirubin may be normal (anicteric cases) or elevated (icteric cases), but albumin and prothrombin time are generally normal unless the acute hepatitis is sufficiently severe to impair hepatic synthetic function. In most instances, bilirubin is divided fairly equally between conjugated and unconjugated fractions; values above 20 mg/dL that persist late into the course of acute viral hepatitis are more likely to be associated with

Table 41–1. Serologic diagnosis of viral hepatitis.

	IgM Anti-HAV	HBsAg	HBeAg	IgM Anti-HBc	IgG Anti-HBc	Anti-HBs	Anti-HBe	HBV DNA	Anti-HCV	Anti-HDV	IgM Anti-HEV
Acute hepatitis A	+	−	−	−	−	−	−	−	−	−	−
Acute hepatitis B	−	+	+	+	−	−	−	>20,000	−	−	−
HBeAg-reactive chronic hepatitis B											
Replicative phase	−	+	+	−	+	−	−	>20,000	−	−	−
Chronic HBV flare	−	+	+	+	−	−	−	>2000	−	−	−
HBeAg-negative chronic hepatitis B											
Chronic HBV flare	−	+	−	+	−	−	−	>2000	−	−	−
Inactive hepatitis B carrier	−	+	−	−	+	−	+	±	−	−	−
Precore mutant	−	+	−	+	±	−	±	>2000	−	−	−
Precore	−	+	−	−	+	−	+	>2000	−	−	−
Resolved hepatitis B	−	−	−	−	+	+	+	−	−	−	−
Posthepatitis B vaccine	−	−	−	−	−	+	−	−	−	−	−
Acute or chronic hepatitis C	−	−	−	−	−	−	−	−	+	−	−
Acute or chronic hepatitis D	−	+	±	−	±	−	±	−	−	+	−
Acute hepatitis E	−	−	−	−	−	−	−	−	−	−	+

Anti-HAV, antibody to hepatitis A virus; anti-HBc, antibody to hepatitis B core antigen; anti-HBe, antibody to hepatitis B e antigen; anti-HBs, antibody to hepatitis B surface antigen; anti-HCV, antibody to hepatitis C virus; anti-HDV, antibody to hepatitis D virus; anti-HEV, antibody to hepatitis E virus; HBeAg, hepatitis B e antigen; HBsAg, hepatitis B surface antigen; IgG, immunoglobulin G; IgM, immunoglobulin M.

Table 41–2. Properties & clinical characteristics of viruses.

	Hepatitis A	Hepatitis B	Hepatitis C	Hepatitis D	Hepatitis E
Size	27 nm	42 nm	32 nm	36 nm	27–34 nm
Length	7.5 kb	3.2 kb	10 kb	1.7 kb	7.6 kb
Genome	ssRNA	ds/ssDNA	ssRNA	ssRNA	ssRNA
Family	Picornaviridae	Hepadnaviridae	Flaviviridae	Deltaviridae	Caliciviridae
Incubation	14–49 days	30–180 days	14–160 days	21–42 days	21–63 days
Transmission	Fecal-oral, sexual	Percutaneous, sexual, perinatal	Percutaneous, (especially injection drug use), sexual and perinatal (rare but increased in HIV co-infection)	Percutaneous, sexual	Fecal-oral
Vaccine	Available	Available	None	None (but hepatitis B vaccine protects against acute hepatitis D)	Available in China since 2011, unavailable outside of China
Severity of acute illness	Usually mild, particularly in children, 0.1% fulminant	Adults: 70% subclinical, 30% clinical, 1% fulminant Newborn: subclinical	Usually subclinical, 1% severe	May be fulminant in 20–25% coinfection, rare in superinfection	0.1–1% fulminant; 15–25% during pregnancy with 20% mortality
Chronic infection	None, regardless of age	90% neonatal, 50% infants, 20% children, 5% adults	60–85% regardless of age	2% with HBV coinfection, >90% with HBV superinfection	May occur in immunocompromised hosts post solid organ transplant or with hematologic malignancies

HBV, hepatitis B virus.

severe disease. Prolongation of the international normalized ratio (INR) above 1.7 should raise concern and prompt close monitoring of the patient for worsening hepatic function and impending hepatic failure. Neutropenia and lymphopenia are transient and followed by a relative lymphocytosis. A mild and diffuse elevation of the γ-globulin fraction is common, especially in patients with acute hepatitis A.

3. Imaging findings—Abdominal imaging is generally unnecessary as findings are nonspecific (eg, hepatomegaly, periportal edema), except in the setting of cholestasis (as can occur with hepatitis A and E) where ultrasonography may be helpful in excluding extrahepatic biliary tract obstruction.

4. Histologic evaluation—Liver biopsy is rarely necessary in acute viral hepatitis.

B. Chronic Viral Hepatitis

1. Symptoms and signs—Chronic viral hepatitis is often asymptomatic, and patients can be unaware of their condition for decades. The diagnosis typically is established incidentally, on routine screening, or when progression to advanced liver disease results in manifestations of hepatic dysfunction.

2. Laboratory findings—Serum aminotransferase levels are characteristically elevated to a variable degree, either continuously or in a fluctuating pattern, although occasional patients may manifest liver enzymes that are persistently within the normal range. The level of ALT is usually higher than the AST, unless the patient has underlying cirrhosis, when AST levels tend to be more elevated. Laboratory values that reflect hepatic function (bilirubin, albumin, INR) are usually normal, unless hepatic decompensation ensues.

3. Imaging findings—Abdominal ultrasound, computed tomography (CT), or magnetic resonance imaging (MRI) are useful to evaluate liver morphology, and to assess for the existence of varices, ascites, splenomegaly, or other signs of portal hypertension. Patients with cirrhosis are at increased risk for hepatocellular carcinoma (HCC) and should undergo regular imaging every 6 months as part of routine screening.

4. Histologic evaluation—Given the ready availability of robust serologic testing, improved accuracy of noninvasive methods for assessing hepatic fibrosis (eg, elastography), and a plethora of highly effective medical therapies, obtaining liver histology is rarely necessary. Liver biopsy generally is reserved for diagnostically challenging situations.

Differential Diagnosis

A. Acute Viral Hepatitis

The principal causes of an acute rise in aminotransferase levels are infections, drug- or toxin-induced liver injury, hepatic ischemia, and autoimmune hepatitis. A presentation that involves a prodromal illness would support an infectious etiology. In addition to the standard viral hepatidities, other nonhepatitis viruses, such as cytomegalovirus, Epstein-Barr virus, herpes simplex, varicella zoster, and coxsackie viruses, can cause in an acute viral syndrome with elevated serum aminotransferase levels. Toxoplasmosis and leptospirosis also share clinical features with acute hepatitis. While most drug-induced liver injury is asymptomatic, several medications and herbal remedies can produce a picture similar to that of acute viral hepatitis; therefore, taking a careful drug history is important. In alcoholic hepatitis, serum aminotransferase levels rarely rise above 300 units/L and generally with a serum AST that exceeds the serum ALT by a 2:1 ratio. Ischemic hepatitis almost invariably occurs in the setting of a readily apparent cause of systemic hypotension. Autoimmune hepatitis should always be considered in the differential diagnosis of patients, particularly women, who present with acute hepatitis in the absence of an alternative explanation.

B. Chronic Viral Hepatitis

The differential diagnosis of chronic elevations in aminotransferases is broad. In addition to chronic viral hepatitis, metabolic (eg, nonalcoholic fatty liver disease, hereditary hemochromatosis, α_1-antitrypsin deficiency, Wilson disease), drugs/toxin-induced (alcohol, medications, herbals), and immune-mediated (autoimmune hepatitis, primary sclerosing cholangitis, celiac disease) disorders should be considered. Biochemical and serologic testing, abdominal imaging and, occasionally, liver histopathology can aid in establishing the diagnosis in most instances.

HEPATITIS A

ESSENTIALS OF DIAGNOSIS

▶ Infection with hepatitis A is acquired via the fecal-oral route and causes a self-limited hepatitis that resolves spontaneously.

▶ Unique clinical aspects include relapsing infection and a protracted cholestatic phase.

▶ The diagnosis of acute hepatitis A infection depends on the detection of immunoglobulin M (IgM) antibodies to the hepatitis A virus (IgM anti-HAV).

▶ The development of an immunoglobulin G (IgG) anti-HAV, which occurs subsequent to the IgM response, is protective and provides lifelong immunity.

General Considerations

Hepatitis A virus (HAV) is a 27-nm nonenveloped RNA virus (genus *Hepatovirus*) that is transmitted through ingestion of contaminated water or food (eg, shellfish, strawberries, onions). The incubation period ranges between 2 and 6 weeks. The duration of viremia is short, approximately 5–7 days, and chronic infection does not occur. Infection is most prevalent in the setting of insufficient sanitation. Hepatitis A is endemic in developing countries, where most individuals are infected as children, generally by the age of 10. In the United States, incidence rates have declined to 2.6/100,000 population following the initiation of routine vaccination of children in high-risk regions, although there remain periodic outbreaks in adults.

Pathogenesis and Histologic Features

As is true for all hepatitis viruses, viral replication of HAV occurs primarily within hepatocytes. Hepatitis A is not believed to be cytopathic, with liver cell damage primarily resulting from host immune cell–mediated cytotoxicity. Histologically, necroinflammatory changes and mononuclear cell infiltrates are prominent in periportal areas, although focal lobular necrosis with ballooning and apoptosis of hepatocytes also are regular features. HAV antigen can be demonstrated on immunohistochemical staining, manifesting as fine granules in the cytoplasm of hepatocytes and Kupffer cells. In the cholestatic phase of disease, centrilobular cholestasis may be severe. Serum neutralizing antibodies protect against HAV infection.

Clinical Findings

Over 70% of adults infected with HAV develop symptoms while, conversely, 70% of infections in young children are asymptomatic. The most frequent complaints are of abrupt onset fatigue, malaise, right upper quadrant or epigastric discomfort, nausea, vomiting, and anorexia. Within several days to a week, patients may also experience jaundice and dark urine, the development of which generally heralds a diminution in the early symptomatology. Patients are contagious during the incubation period and for a week after jaundice appears, with marked viral shedding in the stool. Jaundice typically peaks within 2 weeks, and full clinical and biochemical recovery generally occurs within 2–3 months.

Up to 5% of patients may experience a protracted *cholestatic phase* of acute hepatitis A infection, with jaundice, pruritus, acholic stools, and diarrhea that can persist for over 3 months. Biochemically, patients manifest marked elevations in total bilirubin (>10 mg/dL) and alkaline phosphatase, with normal to modestly elevated aminotransferases. There is no specific treatment aside from controlling pruritus, as cholestasis resolves spontaneously without long-term sequelae. In addition, 10% of patient may recover both symptomatically and biochemically from the initial infection, only to experience a relapse of hepatitis. Relapse of hepatitis C generally occurs within 6 months of the original infection, and typically is milder than the initial episode. Rare instances of multiple relapses have been described.

Hepatitis A rarely can cause acute liver failure (<1% of acute hepatitis A infections), from which transplant free survival is approximately 70%. As patients with pre-existing liver disease are at increased risk of acute liver failure from hepatitis A, it is recommended that patients with liver disease be vaccinated to prevent infection. Although extraordinarily rare, reports suggest that acute hepatitis A may trigger autoimmune hepatitis in susceptible individuals.

Prevention

General measures to prevent the spread of HAV include establishment of a safe water supply and proper environmental measures. Available vaccines against hepatitis A are extraordinarily safe and have a protective efficacy of 94–100% after two doses administered at least 6 months apart. Immunoglobulin is safe and effective against HAV infection as both pre- and post-exposure prophylaxis. Given within 10–14 days of exposure, immunoglobulin has an efficacy of 85%. In the absence of concomitant active immunization, the passive protection offered by immunoglobulin lasts only a few months.

Treatment

Treatment of hepatitis A is largely supportive and involves discontinuation of potentially hepatotoxic medications and curtailment of alcohol intake. Neither bed rest nor dietary restrictions are effective. Most patients do not require hospitalization unless clinical and/or laboratory findings suggest impending acute liver failure.

Course & Prognosis

The overall case fatality rate for HAV infection is very low (~0.3–0.8%), although higher in adults older than age 60 (2.6%). Hepatitis A does not cause chronic infection, and individuals cannot become reinfected following recovery.

Abutaleb A, Kottilil S. Hepatitis A: epidemiology, natural history, unusual clinical manifestations, and prevention. *Gastroenterol Clin North Am.* 2020;49:191–199. [PMID: 32389358]

Foster MA, Hofmeister MG, Kupronis BA, et al. Increase in hepatitis A virus infections – United States, 2013-2018. *MMWR Morb Mortal Wkly Rep.* 2019;68:413–415. [PMID: 6542191]

Lemon SM, Ott JJ, Van Damme P, et al. Type A viral hepatitis: a summary and update on the molecular virology, epidemiology, pathogenesis and prevention. *J Hepatol.* 2018;68:167–184. [PMID: 28887164]

Shouval D. The history of hepatitis A. *Clin Liver Dis.* 2020;15: 12–23. [PMID: 33042523]

HEPATITIS B

ESSENTIALS OF DIAGNOSIS

▶ Hepatitis B is acquired by percutaneous or parenteral exposure, or by vertical transmission. Spontaneous clearance is common in immunocompetent adults, while persistent, chronic infection is the norm in neonates (immune tolerance).

▶ The diagnosis of hepatitis B relies on the presence of hepatitis B surface antigen (HBsAg) in the serum.

▶ Presence of IgM antibodies to hepatitis B core antigen (anti-HBc) indicates recent infection (previous 6 months) or, occasionally, reactivation of a chronic infection.

▶ Hepatitis Be antigen (HBeAg) appears early in the course of infection and is associated with high viral replication and ongoing liver injury.

▶ Replacement of HBeAg by antibody to HBeAg (anti-HBe) is associated with suppression of viral replication and reduced liver injury. It can herald spontaneous viral clearance.

▶ In patients with precore mutations (HBeAg-negative chronic hepatitis B), HBV DNA levels fluctuate, and anti-HBe is detectable in serum.

▶ Antibodies to HBsAg (anti-HBs) are protective against infection. The presence of isolated anti-HBs is consistent with vaccine-induced immunity, while antibodies to both surface and core proteins (anti-HBs, anti-HBc, and anti-HBe) indicate prior HBV infection.

General Considerations

It is estimated that approximately 2 billion people have been infected with the hepatitis B virus (HBV), constituting over 20% of the world population, with more than 240 million people harboring active disease. The highest rates of chronic HBV (8–25%) are in East Asia, the Pacific Islands, and sub-Saharan Africa where the predominant mode of transmission is perinatally and by horizontal spread between young children. In the United States, the prevalence of chronic HBV is

0.1–0.2% (~2 million individuals) and most HBV infections occur in adolescence and early adulthood through sexual and percutaneous (via injection drug use) routes.

Pathogenesis

HBV is a partially double-stranded DNA virus (*hepadnavirus type 1*) that replicates via reverse transcription through an RNA intermediate. Although HBV is strongly hepatotropic, viral sequences, including HBV replicative intermediates, are present in extrahepatic tissues (lymph nodes, peripheral blood mononuclear cells), which is why hepatitis B invariably recurs following liver transplantation. The HBV genome contains four open reading frames that encode four major proteins: (1) the S gene codes for the envelope protein, HBsAg; (2) the C gene encodes the nucleocapsid proteins hepatitis B core antigen (HBcAg) and hepatitis B e antigen (HBeAg); (3) the P (or pol) gene codes for the DNA polymerase that catalyzes transcription and reverse transcription steps involved in viral replication; and (4) the X gene codes for the X protein, a protein that upregulates the transcription of host cellular and viral genes (including other viruses such as HIV).

The envelope protein, HBsAg, is the primary marker of HBV infection. In the hepatocyte, high levels of HBsAg expression can be recognized histologically by a "ground-glass" appearance of the cytoplasm. The error prone HBV polymerase creates the genetic variability of the virus, including genotype, sub-genotypes, and viral quasi-species (a closely related set of viral variants). Ten HBV genotypes (A–J) and nearly 40 sub-genotypes have been identified, the prevalence of which varies geographically. Genotype A is found in North America, Europe, South-East Africa, and India; genotypes B and C in Asia and Oceania; genotype D (the most widely distributed) in North America, North Africa, Europe, the Middle-East, and Oceania; genotype E in West Africa; genotype F in South America; and genotypes G and H in Central and South America. Genotypes I and J are thought to be genotype C recombinants. Variations in the viral genome can lead to drug resistance, immune and vaccine escape mutants, and an inability to express nonessential viral proteins (eg, HBeAg), and specific genotypes have been associated with more rapid disease progression, enhanced risk of HCC, and likelihood of response to interferon therapy.

The C region has two initiation codons leading to two gene transcripts (precore and core), the translation of which result in two protein products, the HBeAg and the HBcAg. The HBeAg is a nonparticulate protein that circulates in serum and is indicative of active viral replication. HBeAg directly correlates with infectivity and liver injury. HBcAg is expressed on 27-nm nucleocapsid core particles localized to the hepatocyte nucleus and, to a lesser degree, the hepatocyte surface membrane, but is not found in serum. HBcAg is a target of the host immune response to infection, which is critical to the pathogenesis liver injury. HBcAg and HBeAg have considerable amino acid homology and immune cross-reactivity at the T-cell level.

Antibodies to HBcAg (anti-HBc) appears at the onset of clinical hepatitis, shortly after the appearance of HBsAg. During acute hepatitis B, anti-HBe appears as clinical symptoms and aminotransferase levels are waning, marking a transition to lower viral replication, reduced infectivity, and less liver injury. HBeAg-negative variants result from mutations in the precore region of the C gene, leading to a failure of HBeAg synthesis. Patients who harbor this "precore mutation" will be HBeAg negative, yet continue to manifest active viral replication and ongoing liver inflammation.

Liver injury associated with HBV infection is the product of innate and adaptive immune responses, the latter of which are affected by CD8+ cytotoxic T cells directed at liver membrane complexes of host histocompatibility antigens and HBcAg. The clinical outcome of HBV infection depends on the balance between viral activity and the host immune response; however, other than certain clinical features (eg, age, infection at birth, immunocompetence), what distinguishes those who recover from those who progress to chronic infection remains poorly defined. In perinatally acquired infection, the presence of HBV on hepatocytes in the context of an immature neonatal immune system combine to produce a high level of immunologic tolerance to the virus, which can persist for extended periods of time or even indefinitely. In this circumstance, there is no cytotoxic T-cell response against HBV, so no clinical illness ensues; however, development of a chronic infection is almost invariable (>90%). In contrast, in adults who develop acute hepatitis B, the cytotoxic T-cell response generally is robust and efficient, which leads to acute liver injury and, typically, viral clearance and recovery. Chronicity after clinically apparent acute hepatitis B in healthy, immunocompetent adults occurs in fewer than 5% of cases.

A. Hepatocellular Carcinoma

Chronic infection with HBV is strongly linked to the development of HCC, with a prevalence of up to 50% in patients with cirrhosis as a result of lifelong infection acquired perinatally (see Chapter 49 on Liver Neoplasms). It appears that viral integration into the host genome is required for oncogenesis, although no consistent sites of integration have been identified. Liver cell turnover associated with chronic inflammation likely contributes to the pathogenesis of HCC, as do genetic and environmental factors.

B. Hepatitis B Virus Variants

1. Precore mutants or HBeAg-negative chronic HBV infection—A precore nucleotide or core-promoter mutation can lead to premature termination of the precore protein, preventing production of HBeAg. HBeAg-negative HBV infection is found more frequently in HBV genotypes other than genotype A, and its prevalence was concentrated initially in Mediterranean countries. Currently, HBeAg-negative chronic hepatitis B is the predominant form of chronic hepatitis B in Europe and represents a growing proportion (~40%) of chronic hepatitis B infections in the United States. Wild-type (HBeAg-positive) chronic hepatitis B is associated with higher levels of HBV replication ($\geq 10^6$ virions/mL) than HBeAg-negative chronic hepatitis B ($\leq 10^5$ virions/mL), whereas HBeAg-negative chronic hepatitis B is more likely to be associated with fluctuating levels of HBV DNA and aminotransferase activity. As HBeAg-negative patients with chronic infection cannot manifest HBeAg seroconversion as a treatment end point, therapy duration remains undefined.

2. S mutants—A mutation in the S gene has been reported in infants who are born to HBV-infected mothers, but acquire HBV infection after vaccination, and also in liver transplant recipients who develop breakthrough reinfection while receiving hepatitis B immunoglobulin (HBIG). These mutations alter the antigenicity of the HBV envelope, thereby evading neutralizing anti-HBs. Fortunately, the frequency of such mutations—and their public health impact—is limited.

3. P mutants—Mutations in the polymerase gene are associated with resistance to the antiviral agents lamivudine, adefovir, and telbivudine. As these agents are no longer utilized as first-line anti-viral therapy, there is minimal clinical impact.

► Clinical Findings

A. Acute Hepatitis B

The incubation period of acute hepatitis B ranges from 4 weeks to 6 months, with a median of approximately 3 months. Clinical symptoms are similar to other forms of acute viral hepatitis (eg, fatigue, anorexia, jaundice). Aminotransferase elevations are the biochemical hallmark of illness. In 5–10% of patients with acute hepatitis B, a serum sickness-like syndrome with arthralgias, rash, angioedema, and, rarely, proteinuria and hematuria may develop in the prodromal phase. In children, hepatitis B may rarely present as anicteric hepatitis associated with a nonpruritic papular rash on the face, buttocks, and limbs (papular acrodermatitis of childhood).

B. Chronic Hepatitis B

Progression from acute to chronic hepatitis can be heralded by the persistence of anorexia, weight loss, and fatigue, although most patients with chronic hepatitis B are asymptomatic. Hepatomegaly and splenomegaly may be detectable on physical exam, while typical laboratory findings include persistence of HBsAg, detectable HBeAg (in the absence of a precore mutation), and elevations of aminotransferase, bilirubin, and globulin levels. Patients with high levels of viremia may develop immune complex deposition that can rarely manifest as arthritis, Henoch-Schönlein purpura, generalized vasculitis (polyarteritis nodosa), glomerulonephritis, pericarditis/myocarditis, pancreatitis, transverse myelitis, and peripheral neuropathy. Typical histologic features of chronic hepatitis B include the presence of lymphocyte-predominant portal inflammation, and the variable presence of fibrosis depending on duration and severity of disease. Ground glass hepatocytes, indicative of robust production HBsAg, may be observed. Patients who develop anti-HBe typically have normal aminotransferase levels and no to minimal activity on liver biopsy.

C. Serologic Assays

The diagnosis of HBV infection relies on the presence of HBsAg. The presence of high titer IgM antibodies to HBcAg (anti-HBc) is helpful in distinguishing acute versus chronic infections, with the presence of IgM anti-HBc generally indicative of an infection onset within the previous 6 months. However, anti-HBc IgM can occasionally reappear in the setting of a hepatitis flare during a chronic infection. HBeAg appears early during acute hepatitis B when viral replication is at peak levels. In self-limited infections, HBeAg is replaced within 2–3 months by antibody to HBeAg (anti-HBe). In patients chronically infected with wild-type HBV, the presence of HBeAg is indicative of a highly replicative phase of illness, where levels of HBV DNA generally exceed 10^6 virions/mL, the risk of transmission is high, and liver injury is ongoing. Patients may subsequently develop anti-HBe, leading to a low level of viral replication (HBV DNA $\leq 10^3$ virions/mL) and minimal liver inflammation. Patients in this phase are sometimes referred to as "inactive carriers." In patients with precore mutations (HBeAg-negative chronic hepatitis B), HBV DNA levels range between undetectable and 10^5 virions/mL and anti-HBe is present in the serum. These patients may or may not have ongoing liver injury.

In chronic hepatitis B, anti-HBc is of the IgG class except in the rare situation of viral reactivation when anti-HBc IgM may reappear transiently. As anti-HBs is protective against infection, antibodies to both surface and core proteins (anti-HBs, anti-HBc, and anti-HBe) are indicative prior HBV infection with subsequent clearance, while the presence of an isolated anti-HBs is consistent with vaccine-induced immunity. An isolated positive IgG anti-HBc may represent a remote prior HBV infection (with subsequent waning of anti-HBs titers) or a false-positive result. The term "occult hepatitis B" is used to describe patients with negative HBsAg and ongoing, generally low-level, viremia. While most commonly observed in individuals with a history of injection drug use and/or with HIV infection, the clinical significance remains unclear.

► Prevention

Vaccination against hepatitis B is an extremely safe and effective way to prevent disease. The standard 3 dose recombinant vaccine, which was 71–90% effective in adults and nearly 100% in newborns, was supplanted in February 2018 by the HepB-CpG vaccine for individuals over 18 years of age. This new vaccine is comprised of recombinant HBsAg mixed with a synthetic oligonucleotide containing CpG motifs that stimulate innate immunity through the Toll-like receptor-9 (TLR9). The HepB-CpG vaccine, given in two doses 4 weeks apart, is more efficacious (seroprotection rate 90–100%) and has a favorable safety profile compared to existing vaccines. The shorter, two-dose regimen (4 weeks apart) produces earlier seroprotection, improved adherence, and higher immunogenicity (especially in populations with poor response rates), making this an important therapeutic option in hepatitis B vaccination.

Currently, the US Public Health Service recommends universal vaccination against hepatitis B of all neonates and prepubertal teenagers. HBV vaccination also is recommended for immunocompromised patients, hemodialysis patients, and patients with coexisting chronic liver disease. High-risk populations, including health care workers, injection drug users, residents of chronic care facilities, incarcerated individuals, and those with high-risk sexual exposures should be vaccinated as well (Table 41–3). Currently, routine booster immunization is not recommended, although it may be prudent in immunosuppressed persons who have lost detectable anti-HBs, or in immunocompetent persons who sustain HBsAg inoculation after losing detectable antibody (although this subgroup appears to be protected even after loss of detectable anti-HBs through an anamnestic response).

▶ Treatment

A. Acute Liver Failure Secondary to Hepatitis B

In patients with acute liver failure secondary to hepatitis B, intensive care in a specialized unit with early consideration of liver transplantation reduces mortality. Transplant-free survival for acute liver failure from hepatitis B is estimated at 25%. Treatment with oral nucleoside or nucleotide agents (described below) may be of benefit. As reinfection of the liver allograft with HBV is universal, measures should be taken to prevent recurrent hepatitis in patients undergoing liver transplantation (see later discussion).

B. Chronic Hepatitis B

The objectives of treatment for chronic hepatitis B are to suppress HBV replication, reduce liver injury, and decrease the risk of HCC. Among the end-points of therapy are (1) reduction in circulating HBV DNA, preferably to levels undetectable by highly sensitive amplification assays; (2) HBeAg seroconversion (loss of HBeAg and acquisition of anti-HBe) in individuals with HBeAg-positive chronic hepatitis B; (3) normalization of ALT levels; and (4) improvement in liver histology (reduction in the grade of necroinflammatory activity and limiting progression of, or even improving, the stage of hepatic fibrosis). Data suggest that successful antiviral therapy has the potential to prevent or delay progression to cirrhosis, hepatic decompensation, and/or HCC. Recommendations for patients with chronic hepatitis B who are candidates for treatment are summarized

Table 41–3. Indications for vaccination against hepatitis A & B.

Hepatitis A
- At least 2 weeks prior to travel to countries with high or intermediate endemicity of infection, including Africa, Southeast Asia, the Mediterranean basin, Eastern Europe, the Middle East, Mexico, Central and South America, and parts of the Caribbean
- Household members and other close contacts of adopted children arriving from regions of moderate and high hepatitis A endemicity
- All children at age 1 (12–23 months) as part of routine vaccinations
- Men who have sex with men and others with high-risk sexual behaviors
- Users of injection and noninjecting drugs of abuse
- Persons with occupational risk for infection (eg, food handlers, child-care workers, laboratory workers exposed to hepatitis A or stool specimens, or people working with nonhuman primates)
- Persons with chronic liver disease including chronic viral hepatitis, particularly hepatitis C, in whom hepatitis A may be severe
- Susceptible persons who receive clotting factor concentrates, especially solvent detergent treated preparations
- Military personnel
- Populations with cyclic outbreaks of hepatitis A

Hepatitis B
- All children at birth (before discharge from hospital) and continued thereafter as part of routine childhood vaccinations
- Unvaccinated children <19 years of age
- At birth (along with simultaneous hepatitis B immune globulin) for babies born to HBsAg-positive mothers
- Health care workers and emergency personnel
- Public safety workers with exposure to blood in the workplace
- Clients and staff of institutions for the developmentally disabled, day care centers, and schools
- Hemodialysis patients and staff
- Patients with end-stage renal disease
- Persons who have clotting factor disorders and who receive clotting factor concentrates
- Household contacts and sexual partners of persons with chronic hepatitis B
- Adoptees from countries where hepatitis B infection is endemic
- Children who are Alaskan natives or Pacific islanders or residents in households of first-generation immigrants from countries in which hepatitis B is endemic
- International travelers spending >6 months in endemic areas and who may have close contact with local population or who are likely to have blood exposure from or sexual exposure with the local population
- Men who have sex with men
- HIV-infected persons
- Sexually active heterosexual men or women who have recently acquired other sexually transmitted diseases, who are sex workers, or who have multiple sexual partners
- Residents and staff of correctional facilities and residential group homes
- Persons with chronic liver disease, including chronic hepatitis C
- Persons born in countries with a prevalence of hepatitis B infection ≥2%
- Persons age <60 with diabetes mellitus

HBsAg, hepatitis B surface antigen.

Table 41–4. Recommendations for treatment of chronic hepatitis B.

HBeAg	HBV DNA	ALT	Treatment Strategy
Positive	>20,000 IU/mL	≤2 × ULN	Low efficacy of treatment If ALT <ULN, observe every 3–6 months for ALT and HBV DNA If ALT 1–2 × ULN: • Consider biopsy for age >40, family history of HCC • Treat if biopsy shows substantial inflammation ≥A3 or any fibrosis ≥F2
	>20,000 IU/mL	>2 × ULN	Treat with any of recommended agents (Of the oral antiviral agents, entecavir and tenofovir are favored over earlier-generation drugs with lower barriers to resistance; PEG-IFN has supplanted standard IFN) Liver biopsy optional
Negative	>20,000 IU/mL	>2 × ULN	Treat with any of recommended agents (Of the oral antiviral agents, entecavir and tenofovir are favored over earlier-generation drugs with lower barriers to resistance; PEG-IFN has supplanted standard IFN) Liver biopsy optional
	>2000 IU/mL	1–2 × ULN	Consider biopsy Treat if substantial inflammation ≥A3 or any fibrosis ≥F2
	<2000 IU/mL	<ULN	No treatment Observe (inactive carrier) every 3 months for 1 year for ALT and HBV DNA then every 6–12 months if remains inactive phase

ALT, alanine aminotransferase; HBeAg, hepatitis B e antigen; HBV, hepatitis B virus; HCC, hepatocellular carcinoma; IFN, interferon; PEG-IFN, pegylated interferon; ULN, upper limit of normal.

in Table 41–4; eight therapies are approved (interferon-α2b, PEG–IFN–α2a, lamivudine, adefovir, telbivudine, entecavir, tenofovir disoproxil fumarate [TDF], and tenofovir alafenamide [TAF]) but only four of them are recommended for treatment of chronic hepatitis B (summarized in Table 41–5).

1. PEG–IFN–α2a—PEG–IFN–α2a 180 μg weekly for 48 weeks is the only pegylated interferon approved for the treatment of chronic hepatitis B in the United States. For HBeAg-positive patients, the most definitive trial involved a comparison of 48 weeks of PEG–IFN–α2a monotherapy versus lamivudine monotherapy versus combination therapy. Twenty-four weeks after completion of therapy, seroconversion was highest (32%) in the PEG–IFN–α2a monotherapy arm. In this study, and a similar study of HBeAg-negative patients, a small proportion of PEG–IFN–α2a–treated subjects experienced HBsAg seroconversion during (in the HBeAg-negative trial) or after (in the HBeAg-positive trial) therapy. However, the 48 weekly injections are associated with substantial side-effects and require frequent clinical and laboratory monitoring. As oral agents are very well tolerated, and similar HBeAg seroconversion rates are achieved when oral therapy is extended out to 18–24 months, it is the rare patient who chooses to receive PEG–IFN–α2a for treatment of hepatitis B.

2. Entecavir—Entecavir, a carbocyclic analog of 2′-deoxyguanosine, inhibits HBV replication at three steps: priming of the HBV polymerase, reverse transcription of the negative-strand HBV DNA from the pregenomic RNA, and synthesis of the positive-strand HBV DNA. It is substantially more potent than lamivudine and adefovir. At an oral dose of 0.5 mg daily, entecavir has been shown to suppress HBV DNA by almost 7 $\log_{10}$ copies/mL in HBeAg-positive patients and 5.2 $\log_{10}$ copies/mL in HBeAg-negative patients. Among the 21% of HBeAg-positive patients who underwent HBeAg seroconversion during the first year of therapy and who stopped treatment at 48 weeks, 70% remained HBeAg negative. In HBeAg-negative patients, the majority relapse if treatment is stopped after 1 year.

In nucleoside-naïve patients, entecavir has a very high barrier to viral resistance, which has not been encountered during the first year of therapy and emerged in only 1.2% of patients through year 6. On the other hand, cross-resistance does occur between entecavir and other L-nucleosides (eg, lamivudine, telbivudine). In lamivudine-resistant patients, subsequent entecavir resistance is seen in 7% of patients at 1 year, 16% of patients at 2 years, and 51% of patients after 5 years. Therefore, while entecavir is favored above other L-nucleosides as a first-line therapy for treatment-naïve patients, entecavir is not recommended for treatment of lamivudine-resistant hepatitis B.

3. Tenofovir disoproxil fumarate—TDF, a nucleotide analogue structurally similar to adefovir that inhibits reverse transcription of HBV RNA to DNA, was first approved for the treatment of HIV infection, either alone or in combination with emtricitabine. At an oral dose of 300 mg daily, TDF is highly effective against hepatitis B, and resistance has not been encountered in treatment-naïve patients through year 6

Table 41–5. Approved preferred antiviral therapy among treatment-naïve patients with HBeAg-positive chronic hepatitis B.

	PEG–IFN-α2a 180 mcg QW	Entecavir 0.5 mg daily	Tenofovir Disoproxil Fumarate 300 mg daily	Tenofovir Alafenamide 25 mg daily
HBeAg positive				
% HBV DNA suppression	30–42%	61%	76%	73%
% HBeAg loss	32–36%	22–25%	NA	22%
% HBeAg seroconversion	29–36%	21–22%	21%	18%
% ALT normalization	34–52%	68–81%	68%	NA
% HBsAg loss (1 year)	2–7%	4–5%	8%	1%
HBeAg negative				
% HBV DNA suppression	43%	90–91%	93%	90%
% ALT normalization	59%	78–88%	76%	81%
% HBsAg loss (1 year)	4%	0–1%	0%	<1%
Histology improvement	38%	72%	74%	NA
Resistance	None	0% year 1, 1.2% through year 6	0% year 6	NA

ALT, alanine aminotransferase; HBeAg, hepatitis Be antigen; IFN-α, interferon-α; NA, not available; PEG–IFN-α, pegylated interferon α.

of monitoring. Currently, either entecavir or tenofovir is considered first-line oral therapy for treatment-naïve patients with chronic hepatitis B, with no added clinical benefit conferred by the use of the medications in combination. While adefovir and tenofovir are cross-resistant, tenofovir is first-line treatment for chronic hepatitis B in patients with lamivudine resistance.

4. Tenofovir alafenamide—TAF, at an oral dose of 25 mg daily, is noninferior to TDF in the treatment of chronic hepatitis B. However TAF, presumably due to the lower effective dose, has been associated with a decreased risk of nephrotoxicity and reduced rates of bone mineral loss as compared with TDF.

5. Other therapies—Combination pills containing emtricitabine and TDF or TAF, which are licensed for treatment of HIV infection, have the potential advantage of combination, non–cross-resistant L-nucleoside and nucleotide analog therapy, but the superiority of this combination has yet to be shown versus tenofovir monotherapy. Innovative antiviral approaches including RNA interference, antisense molecules that interrupt transcription or translation of HBV DNA or HBV RNA, or non-HBV–specific immunomodulatory therapies are currently under study.

C. Special Situations

1. HBV-HIV coinfection—It is generally recommended that an antiretroviral regimen containing tenofovir (typically tenofovir in combination with emtricitabine) be utilized in patients coinfected with HBV and HIV. Entecavir monotherapy is not recommended in patients who are not coincidently receiving antiretroviral therapy due to concerns about emergence of HIV resistance.

2. HBV-HDV coinfection—Refer to the later discussion of hepatitis D.

3. HBV-HCV coinfection—Limited information is available to guide treatment in this setting, although it appears that antiviral therapy directed against the hepatitis C virus (HCV) in coinfected patients yields similar response rates to those infected with hepatitis C alone. While patients co-infected with HBV and HCV tend to manifest low levels of HBV replication, rebound activation of HBV has been described during hepatitis C treatment. Therefore, patients not already on therapy for hepatitis B should be monitored closely (eg, liver enzymes, HBV DNA) while on and after completion of HCV antiviral therapy, and hepatitis B treatment initiated promptly if HBV activation is noted to occur.

4. Immunosuppressive therapy—Patients with chronic hepatitis B have a nontrivial (10–50%) risk of reactivation following human stem cell transplantation (HSCT) or after initiation of long-term immunosuppressive therapy. Agents that have been associated with reactivation include corticosteroids (≥10 mg/d for ≥4 weeks), B-cell depleting agents (eg, rituximab), anthracycline derivatives (eg, doxorubicin),

TNF-inhibitors (eg, infliximab), cytokine/integrin inhibitors (eg, abatacept), tyrosine kinase inhibitors (eg, imatinib), and proteasome inhibitors (eg, bortezomib). Clinically severe, and even fatal, HBV reactivation can occur, reflected initially by increases in serum HBV DNA and ALT. Prophylactic first-line antiviral therapy (entecavir, TAF, TDF) should be administered to any patient with a positive HBsAg prior to the onset of immunosuppressive therapy. It also is generally recommended that HSCT patients, or individuals receiving B-cell depleting regimens, who have a negative HBsAg but positive anti-HBc receive antiviral prophylaxis. Treatment should continue for a minimum of 6–12 months after completion of therapy, and patients should be monitored regularly for HBV DNA and liver enzymes during treatment and after withdrawal of antiviral therapy.

D. Liver Transplantation

Liver transplantation is an effective treatment for decompensated cirrhosis or acute liver failure secondary to hepatitis B. HBV-associated liver disease remains the seventh leading indication for liver transplantation in the United States, comprising 4–5% of cases. Due to the presence of extrahepatic viral reservoirs, nearly all patients relapse post-transplantation in the absence of prophylaxis. In patients who are HBsAg positive prior to liver transplant, viral recurrence can be effectively prevented by the administration of short-term high-dose HBIG perioperatively and postoperatively, combined with long-term oral antiviral therapy. Recent data suggest that use of HBIG is unnecessary when newer, more potent antiviral agents (ie, entecavir, tenofovir) are utilized, except in liver recipients who are co-infected with HIV or HDV. Transplant recipients who receive an organ from a donor who is anti-HBc positive also should receive long-term antiviral prophylaxis.

An unusual clinical form of aggressive hepatitis B (or hepatitis C), termed fibrosing cholestatic hepatitis (FCH), has been described in untreated immunocompromised patients, particularly following solid organ transplantation. FCH is characterized by a rapidly rising bilirubin, with only mild-to-moderate elevations in aminotransferase levels, and can rapidly progress to liver failure, with jaundice, hepatic encephalopathy, and coagulopathy occurring within weeks to months of onset. Histologically, FCH is characterized by marked hepatocyte ballooning, ductular reaction, cholestasis, and extensive periportal and/or perisinusoidal fibrosis with minimal inflammation. It is postulated that these histologic features are the result of a direct cytopathic effect of high levels of viral replication within liver cells, as evidenced by intense HBcAg staining.

E. Postexposure Prophylaxis

For neonates born to infected mothers and any person with a percutaneous or sexual exposure, early HBIG administration achieves immediate high-level circulating anti-HBs (passive immunization). Simultaneously, active immunization with hepatitis B vaccine also is recommended.

Course & Prognosis

Healthy, immunocompetent young adults who develop an acute HBV infection have a favorable course, with the vast majority (95–99%) exhibiting complete recovery. In contrast, rates of chronic infection are much higher in neonates (> 90%), young children (~50%), and immunocompromised adults (>50%), such as organ-transplant recipients, HIV-positive individuals, or persons receiving immunosuppressive chemotherapy. The case fatality rate for acute hepatitis B is low (~0.1%), but increases with age and associated comorbid systemic illnesses. Hepatitis B accounts for approximately half of all cases of acute liver failure caused by viral hepatitis.

Patients chronically infected with hepatitis B who have high levels of viral replication are at increased risk of developing cirrhosis, hepatic decompensation, and HCC. In HBV-endemic regions, HCC is the leading cause of cancer-related death. While HCC can occur in the absence of advanced hepatic fibrosis, cirrhosis is present in 70–80% of HBV-related HCC. The estimated incidence of HCC is 0.06–0.3% per year in asymptomatic carriers, 0.5–0.8% per year in patients with active viral replication and ongoing hepatitis, and 1.5–6.6% per year in those with cirrhosis. In addition to cirrhosis, other risk factors for HCC in patients with chronic hepatitis B include male sex, a family history of HCC, a positive HBeAg, a high viral load, HBV genotype C, and coinfection with hepatitis C. Presently, it is recommended that all patients chronically infected with hepatitis B who have cirrhosis or a family history of HCC undergo routine screening for HCC every 6 months with abdominal ultrasound with or without alfa-fetoprotein measurement. Guidelines also suggest that chronically infected Asian men over the age of 40 and Asian women over the age of 50, as well as well as African and North American blacks beginning at younger ages, should undergo HCC screening. Due to questions of cost-effectiveness, it remains a topic of debate whether younger patients infected with HBV at an early age (who also are at increased risk for HCC) should undergo routine screening.

EASL clinical practice guidelines: management of chronic hepatitis B. J Hepatol. 2012;57:167–185. [PMID: 22436845]

EASL 2017 clinical practice guidelines on the management of hepatitis B virus infection. J Hepatol. 2017;67:370–398. [PMID: 28427875]

Myint A, Tong MJ, Beaven SW. Reactivation of hepatitis B virus: a review of clinical guidelines. Clin Liver Dis. 2020;15:162–167. [PMID: 32395244]

Rajoriya N, Combet C, Zoulim F, et al. How viral genetic variants and genotypes influence disease and treatment outcome of chronic hepatitis B. Time for an individualised approach? J Hepatol. 2017;67:1281–1297. [PMID: 28736138]

Te H, Doucette K. Viral hepatitis: guidelines by the American Society of Transplantation Infectious Diseases Community of Practice. *Clin Transplant.* 2019;33:e13514. [PMID: 30817047]

Terrault NA, Lok AS, et al. Update on prevention, diagnosis, and treatment of chronic hepatitis B: AASLD 2018 hepatitis B guidance. *Hepatology.* 2018;67:1560–1599. [PMID 29405329]

Xiao SY, Lu L, Wang HL. Fibrosing cholestatic hepatitis: clinicopathologic spectrum, diagnosis and pathogenesis. *Int J Clin Exp Pathol.* 2008;1:396–402. [PMID: 18787628]

HEPATITIS C

 ESSENTIALS OF DIAGNOSIS

► Hepatitis C virus (HCV) is usually acquired by percutaneous exposure and frequently leads to chronic infection.

► Enzyme immunoassay (EIA) for antibody to hepatitis C virus (anti-HCV) usually indicates ether an ongoing infection or a prior exposure, but can be falsely positive, particularly in individuals without risk factors.

► The presence HCV RNA in the serum is indicative of active infection with HCV, and is usually detectable 7–14 days after exposure.

► With the advent of accurate noninvasive measures of hepatic fibrosis, liver biopsy is rarely necessary.

General Considerations

Hepatitis C (HCV) is the most common blood-borne infection in the United States, with an estimated 2.4 million people harboring an active infection. Although the demographics are changing rapidly in light of the widespread availability of direct acting antiviral (DAA) agents, hepatitis C remains the leading cause of chronic liver disease, and among the top three indications for liver transplantation in the United States. The majority of new cases are in patients aged 20–39 years, driven in large part by injection drug use as a result of the opioid epidemic. Current guidelines recommend universal one-time, opt-out HCV screening for all adults 18 years and older, and HCV testing is also recommended for persons younger than age 18 if they exhibit behaviors or have exposures associated with increased HCV transmission risk. Periodic HCV testing is recommended for individuals with ongoing behaviors, exposures and/or conditions, including men with HIV who have unprotected sex with men and for all people who use intravenous drugs. Additional groups at risk for HCV infection include individuals who received blood transfusions prior to 1992 (when serologic screening of donor blood began), hemodialysis patients, Vietnam-era veterans, and health care workers.

The prevalence of HCV infection is extremely high in persons with repeated exposures, such as those with hemophilia who received factor VIII infusions before HCV screening was initiated (74–90%) and intravenous drug users (72–90%). Acquisition by health care workers as a result of a single needlestick is uncommon (≤3%). Perinatal transmission occurs in approximately 5% of infants born to HCV-infected mothers, independent of the route of delivery. Sexual transmission of HCV is generally low (~1% in stable, monogamous sexual partners) and, not infrequently, other concurrent risk factors are identified. However, in the sexually promiscuous, those with sexually transmitted diseases, and sex workers, the risk of transmission has been estimated to be as high as 10%. Sporadic HCV infection, in which the mode of transmission is unknown, accounts for approximately 10% of cases, although it is speculated that many of these are attributable to remote intravenous drug use.

Pathogenesis

HCV is a single-stranded, 9600 base-pair RNA virus (genus *Hepacivirus*). The genome encodes core and envelope structural proteins at the 5′ end, and five nonstructural proteins critical for viral replication (including a helicase, protease, and RNA polymerase) at the 3′ end. Six major HCV genotypes have been identified, which are further subdivided into subtypes (1a, 1b, 2a, etc.) of which over 50 have been described. Considerable variation exists in the geographic distribution of HCV genotypes. In the United States, approximately 70% of patients are infected with genotype 1 and the other 30% with genotypes 2 and 3. Genotype analysis is not predictive of the outcome, and has become less important in the era of highly effective, pan-genotypic antiviral agents.

In addition to its genotypic diversity, the heterogeneity of HCV is augmented by a multitude of circulating viral quasispecies (or swarm), reflecting the hypervariability of regions of the HCV envelope proteins that arise as a product of evolutionary changes in response to the host immunologic response. This viral diversity accounts for the limited ability of the host to mount durable neutralizing antibodies leading to a high likelihood (~85%) of HCV persistence (chronic infection) after an acute exposure. This also explains the difficulty in developing an effective hepatitis C vaccine.

Compared with HBV, levels of HCV in serum are lower (up to 10^5–10^6, rarely 10^7 virions/mL), and HCV antigens are not detectable in blood. The clinical features of acute and chronic hepatitis C are similar to those of hepatitis B, except that acute hepatitis C tends to be milder and progression to chronicity the norm, rather than the exception. Histologic features characteristic of chronic hepatitis C include a dense, lymphocytic portal inflammatory infiltrate with an appearance similar to a lymphoid follicle and hepatocellular steatosis. Liver injury associated with HCV infection is believed to be immunologically mediated. Differences in the diversity and robustness of cytolytic T-cell responses appear to be critical for the uncommon patient with spontaneous recovery from acute hepatitis C. Notably, variants in the cytokine *IL28B* gene have not only been shown to influence responsiveness to interferon-based antiviral therapy, but also the likelihood of recovery from acute HCV infection. Over 50% of patients with the favorable C/C haplotype experience self-limited acute HCV infection, while ~80% of those with the unfavorable T/T haplotype progress to chronic infection.

Clinical Findings

A. Acute HCV Infection

In the vast majority of cases, acute hepatitis C is asymptomatic and goes unrecognized by the patient. Jaundice, fatigue, fever, nausea, vomiting, and right upper quadrant discomfort can occur, usually within 2–12 weeks of exposure and lasting 2–12 weeks in duration. The diagnosis is established by demonstration of circulating HCV RNA, as antibodies to HCV can take up to 12 weeks to manifest.

B. Chronic HCV Infection

Chronic hepatitis C is frequently asymptomatic. ALT values typically fluctuate in a "saw-tooth" type pattern. Symptoms of chronic infection, when they do manifest, are generally nonspecific, and include fatigue, malaise, arthralgias, and anorexia. Extrahepatic manifestations of chronic hepatitis C, which develop in as many as 15% of patients, include such immune-complex disorders as essential mixed cryoglobulinemia, membranoproliferative glomerulonephritis, and leukocytoclastic vasculitis. Other associated extrahepatic disorders include thyroiditis, lichen planus, and porphyria cutanea tarda.

C. Serologic Assays

Initial screening for chronic infection with HCV is with the EIA for anti-HCV, which is indicative of prior exposure or ongoing infection. The contemporary third-generation enzyme immunoassay (EIA) detects antibodies to recombinant antigens from the core, NS3, NS4, and NS5 proteins. False-positive EIA tests can occur, and are most often encountered in populations with a low prior probability of infection, such as healthy blood donors or patients with immunologic disorders that result in nonspecific cross-reactive antibodies. Distinctions between IgM and IgG anti-HCV are not clinically helpful; therefore, assays for IgM anti-HCV are not available. False-negative tests are seen most often in immunocompromised patients, including hemodialysis patients and organ allograft recipients.

HCV RNA assays confirm the presence or absence of an active HCV infection, and can quantify levels of viral RNA in the serum. HCV RNA is generally detectable within 7–14 days following exposure. Quantitation of HCV RNA is based on World Health Organization–standardized international units (IU) per milliliter. Current highly sensitive PCR assays have a broad dynamic range with a lower limit of detection of under 10 IU/mL.

D. Liver Biopsy

Due to the ease of serologic diagnosis and the ready availability of a number of noninvasive modalities capable of accurately quantifying hepatic fibrosis, liver biopsy is rarely necessary for patients with chronic hepatitis C.

Prevention

Because injection drug users represent the largest reservoir of HCV infection in the United States, prevention of high-risk, drug-related behaviors is the most effective way to prevent new infections. Currently, an effective preventive vaccine against hepatitis C is not available, and prospects for successful development of a vaccine remain distant (see the discussion of pathogenesis, earlier).

Treatment

The goal of treatment is to eradicate the infection and thereby prevent disease progression and complications. Eradication has been defined as a sustained virologic response (SVR), which is the absence of HCV RNA in the serum (as demonstrated by the most sensitive amplification assay) 12 weeks following completion of antiviral therapy. An SVR is associated with improved histologic findings in up to 94% of patients, including a reduced histologic activity index and improvement in fibrosis stage. Clinically, achievement of an SVR correlates with a reduced risk of progression to cirrhosis, hepatic failure, or death. Patients with cirrhosis who achieve SVR manifest a marked reduction in the risk of hepatic decompensation, liver-related mortality, liver transplantation, and HCC.

A. Direct Acting Antiviral Therapies

Antiviral therapy for chronic hepatitis C has evolved dramatically over the past 20 years. Current antiviral agents for treatment of HCV infection consist of small-molecule inhibitors, which can be categorized on the basis of the target of action. They are well-tolerated (thus routine monitoring is not required) and highly effective, with rates of SVR ranging from 90% to 100%. While a few genotype-specific DAA regiments remain, most current treatment regimens are pan-genotypic. The selection of treatment and duration is primarily determined by prior treatment experience and/or the presence of decompensated cirrhosis. Presently, for adults with chronic hepatitis C without cirrhosis who are treatment-naïve, the recommended regimens are: sofosbuvir (NS5B inhibitor) and velpatasvir (NS5A inhibitor) for a 12-week course or glecaprevir (NS3/4A protease inhibitor) and pibrentasvir (NS5A inhibitor) for an 8-week course. For adults who have been treated but did not achieve SVR, there is concern for the potential selection of resistance-associated substitutions (RASs), particularly in the viral NS5A protein. Those who have experienced treatment failure with a sofosbuvir-based regimen, the recommendation is retreatment with 12 weeks of sofosbuvir, velpatasvir, and voxilaprevir (NS3/4A protease inhibitor). Ribavirin may be added if the patient has genotype 3 and cirrhosis. However, with the ongoing development and approval of newer generations of antiviral therapy, HCV treatment is evolving too rapidly to rely on convened conferences of experts. Since 2014, guidelines for management of HCV infection have been released jointly by the American Association for the Study of Liver Diseases (AASLD) and the Infectious Diseases Society of America (IDSA). These recommendations, which are updated continually, can be accessed at www.hcvguidelines.org.

B. Special Treatment Considerations

1. Acute Hepatitis C—Patients who test positive for HCV Ab and RNA should receive immediate antiviral therapy, as opposed to monitoring for 6 months to assess for spontaneous clearance.

2. Renal impairment—Currently for patients with chronic kidney disease (CKD), no dose adjustments are required in recommended DAA regimens with the exception of ribavirin, which may require a dose reduction in patients with CKD stage 3–5.

3. Decompensated cirrhosis—Patients with chronic hepatitis C and cirrhosis, with Model for End-Stage Liver Disease (MELD) score >20 or a history of decompensating events, may benefit from liver transplantation. Before initiating antiviral therapy in these individuals, referral to a hepatologist is advised. Although reinfection of the donor liver allograft with HCV is universal, antiviral therapy in patients with decompensated cirrhosis can be associated with substantial morbidity. As treatment of hepatitis C in liver transplant recipients is straightforward, it may be preferable to wait until after the patient undergoes transplantation to initiate therapy in certain circumstances.

C. Other Aspects of Disease Management

Because of a reported risk of increased morbidity and mortality associated with acute hepatitis A superinfection in patients with chronic hepatitis C, it is recommended that susceptible patients (IgG anti–HAV negative) be vaccinated against hepatitis A. Similarly, because of the risk of hepatitis B when superimposed on chronic hepatitis C, patients who are susceptible to HBV infection (eg, HBsAg-, anti–HBs-, anti–HBc-negative) are advised to be vaccinated against hepatitis B. Excessive and frequent alcohol consumption promotes progression of chronic hepatitis C; therefore, patients should be advised to have very modest alcohol consumption or to abstain from alcohol use entirely. HCV risk reduction by advising patients to abstain from and seeking counseling for IV drug use also is recommended. Hepatic steatosis, obesity, and insulin resistance promote progression of fibrosis in hepatitis C; therefore, interventions that reverse the metabolic

syndrome and lead to weight reduction are worthwhile. Finally, screening for HCC is recommended for patients with cirrhosis. Abdominal ultrasound with or without alpha fetoprotein measurement every 6 months is advised.

▶ Course & Prognosis

Cirrhosis develops in approximately 20% of patients with long-standing (20–25 years) of chronic hepatitis C if left untreated. Progression to cirrhosis is more common in persons infected at older ages (particularly men), who drink more than 50 g of alcohol daily, and who are coinfected with HIV. Among patients with cirrhosis and chronic infection with HCV, HCC develops at a rate estimated at 1% per year, with a cumulative incidence of 7% of over the course of 10 years. Conversely, HCC rarely occurs in patients with chronic hepatitis C in the absence of advanced fibrosis. Successful antiviral therapy in patients with chronic hepatitis C reduces substantially, but does not eliminate, the risk of HCC; therefore, it is recommended that HCC screening should continue in patients with cirrhosis even after achievement of a SVR.

A. Children

Children who are infected with HCV are more likely to clear the virus spontaneously, to have milder hepatitis, and to progress less frequently to cirrhosis. In one study of German children who acquired hepatitis C genotype 1 as a result of cardiac surgery during infancy, 45% cleared the virus spontaneously, and, at a mean of 21 years after infection, only 3 of 17 had histologic evidence of advanced liver disease.

B. HCV-HIV

Coinfection with HCV and HIV is common, with estimates that 25% of HIV-infected persons in the Western world have concomitant HCV infection. Approximately 6% of HIV-infected persons with chronic hepatitis C fail to demonstrate detectable anti-HCV; therefore, HCV RNA should be tested in HIV-positive patients with unexplained liver disease. Since the advent of highly active antiretroviral therapy in 1996, liver disease has become an increasingly important cause of morbidity and mortality in patients with HIV/AIDS. In addition, HIV infection accelerates the course of HCV infection. In one series, cirrhosis developed within 15 years in 25% of coinfected patients, compared with only 6.5% of those who had HCV infection alone. Patients with HCV-HIV coinfection respond as well as patients with HCV monoinfection to current HCV antiviral regimens. However, expert consultation is recommended to help determine the appropriate HIV and HCV antiviral combinations to avoid adverse interactions.

C. HCV-HBV

Coinfection with HCV and HBV increases the risk and rate of development of cirrhosis and HCC, relative to those observed in patients infected with either virus alone. In coinfected patient's undergoing treatment for hepatitis C, hepatitis B viral levels can rise dramatically, so close monitoring is advised (see section on hepatitis B above).

American Association of the Study of Liver Diseases and the Infectious Diseases Society of America. Recommendations for testing, managing, and treating hepatitis C. http://www.hcvguidelines.org/.

Hofmeister MG, Rosenthal EM, Barker, LK, et al. Estimating prevalence of hepatitis C virus infection in the United States, 2013-2016. *Hepatology*. 2019;69:1020–1031. [PMID 30398671]

Lim JK. Management of hepatitis C in special populations: HIV coinfection, renal disease, and decompensated cirrhosis. *Clin Liver Dis*. 2020;16:29–31. [PMID: 32714521]

Pearlman B. Management of hepatitis C-infected patients after sustained virological response. *Clin Liver Dis*. 2020;16:20–24 [PMID: 32714519]

Rabaan AA, Al-Ahmed SH, Bazzi AM, et al. Overview of hepatitis C infection, molecular biology, and new treatment. *J Infect Public Health*. 2020;13:773–783. [PMID: 31870632]

HEPATITIS D

 ESSENTIALS OF DIAGNOSIS

▶ Infection with the hepatitis D virus (HDV) occurs only in the presence of HBV and is detected by demonstrating anti-HDV in the serum. Distinguishing IgM versus IgG anti-HDV is not clinically useful.

▶ HDV RNA detected in serum by molecular hybridization or PCR assays is helpful in confirming the diagnosis.

▶ Testing for IgM and IgG anti-HBc helps distinguish between acute, simultaneous HBV-HDV coinfection (IgM anti–HBc-positive), and acute HDV superinfection in patients with chronic HBV infection (IgG anti–HBc-positive).

General Considerations

As the HDV uses the hepatitis B surface antigen (HBsAg) as its envelope protein, hepatitis D can only infect individuals who are co-infected with hepatitis B. On a worldwide basis, an estimated 62–72 million people with chronic hepatitis B harbor a concomitant infection with HDV, with the highest prevalence in Mongolia, the Amazon basin, West Africa, the Mediterranean basin, and Eastern Europe. Transmission can occur through sexual contact and through blood and blood-derived products; vertical transmission is rare. In endemic regions transmission of HDV is perpetuated by close personal contact (ie, within families), while in nonendemic areas, such as the United States, the virus is transmitted primarily by percutaneous route (ie, injection drug users and their sexual contacts).

Pathogenesis

Originally termed "delta agent," hepatitis D is a unique hepatitis virus with the smallest known genome (1.7 kb) of any animal RNA virus. The 36-nm HDV virion comprises an RNA genome, a single HDV-encoded antigen, and a lipoprotein envelope that is provided by HBV. Hence, HDV requires the simultaneous presence of HBV for complete virion assembly and secretion and can be acquired either through simultaneous acute HBV-HDV coinfection (which is limited by the duration of the HBV infection) or HDV superinfection of a person with chronic hepatitis B, (whereby the HDV infection almost invariably becomes chronic). HDV characteristically causes suppression of HBV replication, so patients exhibit low-level, or even undetectable, HBV DNA. In acute HDV infection, characteristic histologic findings in the liver include microvesicular steatosis and granular eosinophilic necrosis, while chronic hepatitis D generally manifests as nonspecific necroinflammatory activity. HDV antigen (HDVAg) can be identified in hepatocyte nuclei by immunohistochemical staining.

There are eight distinct HDV genotypes with up to 40% sequence divergence (I–VIII) and specific clinical features of hepatitis D seem to cluster in distinct geographic areas. Genotype I is most common in the Western world, including the United States, and Africa, where acute HDV is more likely to be fulminant, and chronic infection is more likely to progress rapidly to cirrhosis. Genotype II is predominantly an Eastern genotype and is thought to be less pathogenic than genotype I. Genotype III is seen almost exclusively in Central and South America, where HDV superinfection in persons with underlying chronic hepatitis B tends to be associated with severe hepatitis ("Labrea fever").

Clinical Findings

A. Acute HBV-HDV Coinfection

Acute coinfection with hepatitis B and D is characterized by prominent liver inflammation, which can be severe with hepatocellular necrosis. Acute liver failure is reported in approximately 5% of coinfection outbreaks in injection drug users, a rate that is approximately 10 times higher than observed in patients who develop acute hepatitis B alone. However, the majority of HBV-HDV coinfections are self-limited, with spontaneous clearance of both viruses.

B. Chronic HBV-HDV Infection

Chronic coinfection is generally the result of acute HDV superinfection of a patient with underlying chronic hepatitis B. In chronic HBV-HDV infection, HDV viremia persists, although generally at levels lower than is encountered during the period of acute infection. On liver biopsy, necroinflammatory findings are similar to that seen with chronic HBV infection alone, although, on average, the activity is more severe. Episodes that resemble acute hepatitis can also mark the course in chronic coinfection. Labrea fever is an unusual form of delta hepatitis described in the Amazon basin where superinfection can result in acute liver failure, with jaundice, fever, and black vomitus.

C. Serologic Assays

HDV infection is detected by demonstrating the presence of anti-HDV. While distinction between IgM and IgG anti-HDV is of limited clinical utility, testing for IgM and IgG anti-HBc can aid in distinguishing between acute, simultaneous HBV-HDV coinfection (IgM anti–HBc-positive), and HDV superinfection in someone already harboring chronic HBV infection (IgG anti–HBc-positive). The nucleocapsid HDV protein is always encapsulated within an envelope of HBsAg; therefore, HBsAg is always positive while circulating levels of HDVAg are undetectable (hence, HDVAg assays are not commercially available). HDV RNA can be detected in serum by either molecular hybridization or PCR assays, which is helpful in confirming the diagnosis and in monitoring viremia during a course of antiviral therapy.

▶ Prevention

Because hepatitis D requires the presence of HBV infection, HDV can be prevented by vaccinating susceptible persons against hepatitis B and using standard precautions against hepatitis B infection. There is no effective vaccine against HDV.

▶ Treatment

Oral agents used to suppress HBV replication are not effective for treatment of hepatitis D. While there are ongoing efforts to develop targeted antiviral agents that are effective against hepatitis D, none exist as of present, and IFN-α remains the only licensed drug for treatment of HDV. PEG–IFN-α monotherapy for 12 months has been shown to result in a 43% SVR, with no additional benefit from simultaneous administration ribavirin. Patients with decompensated cirrhosis resulting from chronic hepatitis D are acceptable candidates for liver transplantation. Currently, with efficient antiviral therapy to prevent recurrent HBV infection of the liver allograft, recurrent hepatitis D after transplantation is uncommon.

▶ Course & Prognosis

A. Acute HBV-HDV Coinfection

Acute coinfection resolves spontaneously in 80–95% of cases, paralleling clearance of HBV without which HDV infection cannot persist. However, in 2–20% of cases, acute liver failure can develop, with case fatality rates approaching 5%. In addition, 2–5% of cases of acute HBV-HDV coinfection result in chronic infection.

B. Acute HDV Superinfection

Unlike acute coinfection, HDV superinfection results in chronic HDV-HBV in the vast majority of cases. Similar to acute coinfection, acute HDV superinfection can cause acute liver failure, with mortality exceeding 20% in some studies. Hepatitis D superinfection rarely resolves unless HBV infection resolves.

C. Chronic HBV-HDV Infection

While some patients with chronic HBV-HDV infection can manifest very mild liver disease, chronic hepatitis D is considered one of the more severe form of chronic viral hepatitis, with faster progression to cirrhosis and an increased risk of hepatic decompensation. It has been estimated that 10–15% of patients infected chronically with HDV develop cirrhosis within 5 years of from infection onset. Overall, the pattern of disease progression appears to vary with geography, genotype, and mode of transmission. Slowly progressive, mild disease is more common in endemic areas. On the other hand, HDV-associated disease appears to be more severe in nonendemic areas, where injection drug use is the main form of transmission.

Caviglia GP, Rizzetto M. Treatment of hepatitis D: an unmet medical need. *Clin Microbiol Infect.* 2020;26(7):824–827. [PMID: 32120043]

Cheung A, Kwo P. Viral hepatitis other than A, B, and C: evaluation and management. *Clin Liver Dis.* 2020;24:405–419. [PMID: 32620280]

Mentha N, Clément S, Negro F, et al. A review on hepatitis D: from virology to new therapies. *J Adv Res.* 2019;17:3–15. [PMID: 31193285]

Stockdale AJ, Kreuels B, Henrion MYR, et al. The Global Prevalence of Hepatitis D virus infection: systemic review and meta-analysis. *J Hepatol.* 2020;73:523–532. [PMID: 32335166]

HEPATITIS E

 ESSENTIALS OF DIAGNOSIS

▶ Hepatitis E virus (HEV) is primarily transmitted by the fecal oral route and causes a self-limited infection, except in rare instances when chronic infection can occur in immunocompromised patients.

▶ The diagnosis of acute HEV is established by demonstrating the presence of serum IgM antibody to hepatitis E virus (anti-HEV) by immunoassay or HEV RNA by PCR.

▶ IgM anti-HEV is detectable for only a few months after acquisition of HEV, and IgG anti-HEV remains detectable for ~1 year.

▶ HEV hepatitis can be particularly severe among pregnant women.

▶ A vaccine has been developed that is effective in preventing hepatitis E, but this vaccine is not available in the United States.

General Considerations

Like hepatitis A, the HEV is transmitted predominantly through the fecal-oral route. HEV is endemic to the Indian subcontinent, Central America, Africa, northwest China, and the Central Asian Republics (the former Soviet Union), where most reported outbreaks of infection have been related to the consumption of fecally contaminated drinking water. In countries where HEV infection is not endemic, the virus accounts for less than 1% of cases of acute viral hepatitis, and is primarily observed in travelers returning from endemic regions. Unusual for an enteric virus, HEV is not readily spread via person-to-person transmission.

There are four major genotypes of HEV (plus a fifth in nonhuman hosts). Genotypes 1 and 2, common in endemic areas, are relatively virulent and account for the clinically apparent, often severe disease in these regions. The highest attack rate occurs in young adults, a subpopulation that ordinarily would be immune to enterically transmitted endemic agents, and hepatitis can be particularly severe among pregnant women. Genotypes 3 and 4 predominate in nonendemic areas, such as the United States. They are relatively nonvirulent and commonly associated with inapparent infection. As these genotypes can infect pigs, it is hypothesized that the 20% prevalence of antibodies to HEV in the US population is attributable to exposure to a low pathogenicity swine reservoir.

Pathogenesis

HEV is a small, 27–34 nm, nonenveloped spherical, 7600-base-pair single-stranded, positive sense RNA virus (genus *Hepacivirus*). Transmission is through the fecal-oral route, and, like other hepatitis viruses, the main target cells are hepatocytes. Despite substantial genomic variability, all genotypes share at least one major serologically cross-reactive epitope, thereby permitting the development of an effective vaccine.

Clinical Findings

The incubation period for hepatitis E ranges from 2 to 10 weeks. The clinical course of acute hepatitis E is similar to that of acute hepatitis A, but generally more severe. Acute hepatitis E has an insidious onset, most commonly beginning with a several-day prodromal phase consisting of a flu-like illness with fever, abdominal pain, nausea and vomiting, dark urine, clay-colored stools, diarrhea, and, in a small proportion of cases, a transient macular skin rash. The prodromal phase is followed by the development of frank jaundice (in icteric cases), pronounced elevation of aminotransaminase

and bilirubin levels. In a proportion of patients with cholestatic features, the alkaline phosphatase may also be elevated. Histologically, cholestasis with rosette formation and a polymorphonuclear leukocyte lobular infiltrate is observed. Acute hepatitis E can be very severe in pregnant women, in whom the mortality rate can reach 15–25%. Like hepatitis A, HEV was initially thought to only cause acute, self-limited infections. However, chronic infections have been identified in immunocompromised individuals, most commonly organ-transplant recipients, patients receiving chemotherapy, and those with HIV-infection. The diagnosis of HEV is established by demonstrating the presence of serum IgM anti-HEV by immunoassay or HEV RNA by PCR. IgM anti-HEV becomes undetectable within a few months of infection, and even IgG anti-HEV does not persist much beyond 1 year.

Prevention

Prophylactic measures to minimize the occurrence of HEV infection include improved sanitation and sanitary handling of food and water. Boiling water appears to reduce the risk of infection. Because person-to-person transmission is rare, isolation of affected patients is not indicated. Postexposure immunoglobulin has not been shown to confer protection against HEV. Recently, a recombinant polypeptide vaccine was shown to be effective in a randomized, double-blind, placebo-controlled trial. This vaccine is utilized in endemic regions, but is not yet available in the United States.

Treatment

Treatment of acute HEV is largely supportive (see the discussion of hepatitis A treatment earlier in this chapter). In patients who have developed chronic HEV infection, reducing or withdrawing immunosuppressive therapy can help stimulate spontaneous viral clearance. Chronic hepatitis E also has been found to be susceptible to antiviral therapy, including PEG-IFN, ribavirin, or a combination, although no randomized, controlled trials have been conducted. In a study of 59 solid organ recipients with chronic HEV infection, a median ribavirin dose of 600 mg daily for a median duration of 3 months yielded a SVR rate of 78%.

Course & Prognosis

Acute HEV infection is self-limited, with an illness usually lasting 1–4 weeks, although a subsequent cholestatic phase can persist for 2–6 months. Acute liver failure can occur, with an overall case fatality rate of 0.1–4%. Pregnant women appear particularly susceptible to developing acute liver failure, with mortality rates approaching 15–25%, primarily in the third trimester. This has led to the recommendation that pregnant women avoid traveling to regions where HEV is endemic. Other conditions that increase susceptibility to severe disease include an underlying liver disorder and malnutrition.

Hoofnagle JH, Nelson KE, Purcell RH. Current concepts: hepatitis E. *N Engl J Med*. 2012;367:1237–1244. [PMID: 23013075]

Kamar N, Izopet J, Tripon S, et al. Ribavirin for chronic hepatitis E virus infection in transplant recipients. *N Engl J Med*. 2014;370:1111–1120. [PMID: 24941183]

Oechslin N, Moradpour D, Gouttenoire J. On the host side of the hepatitis E virus life cycle. *Cells*. 2020;9(5):1294. [PMID: 32456000]

Unzueta A, Rakela J. Hepatitis E infection in liver transplant recipients. *Liver Transpl*. 2014;20:15–24. [PMID: 24123928]

Velavan TP, Pallerla SR, Johne R, et al. Hepatitis E: an update on One Health and clinical medicine. *Liver Int*. 2021;41:1462–1473. [PMID: 33960603]

Autoimmune Liver Disorders

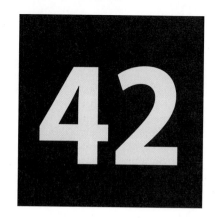

42

Michael Li, MD, MPH

Stephen D. Zucker, MD

AUTOIMMUNE HEPATITIS

ESSENTIALS OF DIAGNOSIS

▶ Autoimmune hepatitis (AIH) is characterized by hepatocellular liver injury in the presence of autoantibodies and elevated serum immunoglobulin G (IgG) levels.

▶ Women are disproportionately affected.

▶ Classic histologic findings are a prominent plasma cell infiltrate with interface hepatitis.

▶ The diagnosis is based on a constellation of clinical features, biochemical abnormalities, serologic tests, and liver histology.

▶ Overlap syndromes include features of other chronic liver disorders (eg, primary biliary cholangitis, primary sclerosing cholangitis).

General Considerations

AIH is an immune-mediated chronic inflammatory disorder of the liver that is typically characterized by the presence of elevated serum IgGs and circulating autoantibodies. When severe, the immune cell-induced inflammatory reaction within the liver can lead to hepatocellular necrosis and collapse or, when protracted, progressive fibrosis leading to cirrhosis. AIH occurs in all races and at all ages, but disproportionately affects women with a 4:1 female to male preponderance. A personal history of autoimmunity and family history of AIH confer an increased likelihood of disease. The prevalence of AIH in the United States and Europe is approximately 30 per 100,000 population, constituting 2–3% of pediatric and 4–6% of adult liver transplant candidates.

Liberal R, Zen Y, Mieli-Vergani G, Vergani D. Liver transplantation and autoimmune liver diseases. *Liver Transpl.* 2013;19: 1065–1077. [PMID: 23873751]

Mieli-Vergani G, Vergani D, Czaja AJ, et al. Autoimmune hepatitis. *Nat Rev Dis Primers.* 2018;4:18017. [PMID: 29644994]

Tunio HA, Mansoor E, Sheriff MZ, et al. Epidemiology of autoimmune hepatitis (AIH) in the United States between 2014 and 2019: a population based national study. *J Clin Gastroenterol.* 2021;55(10):903–910. [PMID: 33074948]

Pathogenesis

The pathogenesis of AIH remains poorly understood, although there appear to be both genetic and environmental influences. It is believed that susceptible individuals have a genetic predisposition, and that a triggering event ultimately leads to an immunologic process directed against hepatocytes. Among the proposed inciting factors are toxins, medications, and infectious agents, although none have been convincingly proven. Possible mechanisms include molecular mimicry (immune responses to antigens from viruses such as HCV and the herpesvirus family becoming directed against structurally similar self-proteins) and loss of self-tolerance. AIH occurs in 10–20% of patients with the Autoimmune-Endocrinopathy-Candidiasis-Ectodermal Dystrophy (APECED) syndrome, an autosomal recessive disorder caused by mutations in the autoimmune response modulator gene AIRE (which provides instructions for making a protein called the autoimmune regulator).

Classification

AIH is classified into two distinct subtypes based on the clinical presentation and presence of specific autoantibodies. Type 1 or "classic" AIH is characterized by a positive antinuclear (ANA) and/or anti-smooth muscle (ASMA) antibodies, the latter with specificity to F-actin. These antibodies are detected in 80% and 63% of patients, respectively. This is the most common form of AIH, and has been linked to HLA DRB 10301 (DR3) and DRB 10401 (DR4). Type 2 AIH, which accounts for only 5–10% of cases, is typically diagnosed in childhood. Anti-liver/kidney microsomal type 1 (ALKM-1) antibodies and/or antibodies directed against liver cytosol antigen type 1 (ALC-1) have low sensitivity, but high specificity for type 2 AIH, which has been linked to HLA DRB 10701. Notably, the presence of any of these autoantibodies is not diagnostic, as they can be present in a variety of other conditions.

Certain forms of drug-induced liver injury (DILI) can manifest AIH-like features, including circulating autoantibodies, elevated immunoglobulin levels, and liver histology demonstrating a lymphoplasmacytic portal infiltrate with interface activity. Medications associated with an autoimmune-type hepatic injury include minocycline, nitrofurantoin, HMG-CoA reductase inhibitors (statins), α-methyl DOPA, hydralazine, and anti–TNF-α agents (eg, infliximab, adalimumab). Resolution after discontinuation of the medication is common; however, some patients require corticosteroid therapy to induce remission.

Assis DN. Immunopathogenesis of autoimmune hepatitis. *Clin Liver Dis.* 2020;15:129–132. [PMID: 32257125]

Chascsa DM, Ferré EMN, Hadjiyannis Y, et al. APECED-associated hepatitis: clinical, biochemical, histological and treatment data from a large, predominantly American cohort. *Hepatology.* 2021;73:1088–1104. [PMID: 32557834]

de Boer YS, Kosinski AS, Urban TJ, et al. Features of autoimmune hepatitis in patients with drug-induced liver injury. *Clin Gastroenterol Hepatol.* 2017;15:103–112. [PMID: 27311619]

Sebode M, Weiler-Normann C, Liwinski T, Schramm C. Autoantibodies in autoimmune liver disease: clinical and diagnostic relevance. *Front Immunol.* 2018;9:609. [PMID: 29636752].

Zhang WC, Zhao FR, Chen J, Chen WX. Meta-analysis: diagnostic accuracy of antinuclear antibodies, smooth muscle antibodies and antibodies to a soluble liver antigen/liver pancreas in autoimmune hepatitis. *PLoS One.* 2014;9(3):e92267. [PMID: 24651126]

▶ Clinical Findings

A. Symptoms & Signs

There is a wide spectrum of presentation for AIH, ranging from asymptomatic elevations in liver enzymes, to acute liver failure, to complications of cirrhosis. Symptomatic patients typically endorse nonspecific complaints such as fatigue, right upper quadrant abdominal discomfort, and anorexia. Physical examination can range from unremarkable to stigmata of chronic liver disease, including hepatosplenomegaly, jaundice, ascites, and hepatic encephalopathy.

B. Laboratory Findings

Patients with AIH manifest a predominantly hepatocellular pattern of liver injury, with mild to marked elevation in aminotransferases and generally modest elevations in alkaline phosphatase. The diagnosis of AIH should be considered in all patients with acute or chronic elevations in alanine aminotransferase (ALT) and aspartate aminotransferase (AST) of undetermined cause, including patients with acute severe hepatitis. All adult patients suspected of having AIH should have ANA, ASMA, and IgG levels obtained. ALKM-1 and ALC-1 are of higher utility in patients presenting in childhood or adolescence, given their association with type 2 AIH.

C. Histologic Findings

Liver histology should be obtained in all patients suspected of having AIH. While there are no pathognomonic histologic features, the presence of a plasma cell-rich lymphoplasmacytic infiltrate with interface activity is considered highly typical of AIH. While nonspecific, lobular hepatitis with bridging necrosis is not infrequently encountered in cases with more severe liver inflammation. Bile duct injury or granulomas should not be present in the common form of AIH.

D. Diagnostic Criteria

A personal history or family history of autoimmune disorders increase the likelihood of AIH. Common associations include autoimmune thyroid disease, Sjögren's (sicca) syndrome, rheumatoid arthritis or nondestructive polyarthropathy, inflammatory bowel disease, systemic lupus erythematosus, and celiac disease. A careful medication and herbal/dietary supplement history should be obtained in order to exclude a drug-induced autoimmune-type liver injury. Serologic testing to evaluate for viral hepatitis, inherited disorders of the liver (eg, Wilson disease, hemochromatosis, α1-antitrypsin deficiency), and primary biliary cholangitis (PBC) should be obtained. As there is no single test that is pathognomonic, the diagnosis of AIH is based on a constellation of clinical findings, biochemistries, serologic tests, and histologic features. Several scoring systems for AIH have been developed to aid in diagnostic decision-making, one of which is shown in Table 42–1. According to this nomogram, a score of ≥7 implies a high-likelihood of AIH, with an 81% sensitivity and a 99% specificity. Among patients in whom the diagnosis is uncertain, a strong biochemical response to corticosteroids can inform the diagnosis.

Geller SA. Autoimmune hepatitis: histopathology. *Clin Liver Dis.* 2014;3:19–23. [PMID: 31236264]

Lucey MR, Vierling JM. Clinical presentation and natural history of autoimmune hepatitis. *Clin Liver Dis.* 2014;3:9–11. [PMID: 30992880]

Vergani D, Mieli-Vergani. Autoimmune hepatitis: diagnostic criteria and serologic testing. *Clin Liver Dis.* 2014;3:38–41. [PMID: 31236268]

Table 42-1. Simplified diagnostic criteria for autoimmune hepatitis (AIH).

Variable	Result	Score[a]
ANA or SMA	1:40	1
ANA or SMA or LKM or SLA	1:80 1:40 Positive	2[b]
IgG	>Upper normal limit >1.10 times upper normal limit	1 2
Liver histology (evidence of hepatitis is a necessary condition)	Compatible with AIH Typical AIH	1 2
Absence of viral hepatitis	Yes	2 TOTAL: 6: probable AIH 7: definite AIH

[a]Scores from criteria above are summed. Prior to steroid therapy a definite diagnosis requires a score 7, while a probable diagnosis requires a score of 6 or higher.
[b]Addition of points achieved for all autoantibodies (maximum, 2 points). For details, see reference cited in the following text.
AIH, autoimmune hepatitis; ANA, antinuclear antibody; IgG, immunoglobulin G; LKM, liver kidney microsomal (antibody); SLA, soluble liver antigen; SMA, smooth muscle antibody.
Reproduced with permission from Hennes EM, Zeniya M, Czaja AJ, et al. Simplified criteria for the diagnosis of autoimmune hepatitis. *Hepatology.* 2008;48(1):169–176.

Treatment

The goal of treatment for AIH is to achieve complete biochemical and histologic remission in order to prevent disease progression. While society guidelines differ with regard to the indications for initiating therapy, in general, all patients with active AIH, symptomatic disease, or advanced fibrosis should receive therapy. Indeed, substantial regression of fibrosis has been reported in patients with cirrhosis following successful treatment. While the benefits of immunosuppressive therapy in asymptomatic older patients with mild activity on liver biopsy is debated, the fluctuating nature of the disease and the nontrivial risk of progression of subclinical disease make it imperative that untreated patients, at a minimum, undergo regular monitoring.

Predniso(lo)ne (0.5–1 mg/kg/day) is the first line treatment for AIH. Higher initial doses of corticosteroids can induce more rapid remission, but at the expense of increased steroid-related side-effects. For maintenance of remission, azathioprine (which is metabolized to 6-mercaptopurine [6-MP]) should be commenced, generally 2 weeks after initiation of corticosteroids. The initial azathioprine dose is 50 mg/day, which can be progressively increased to a target dose of 1–2 mg/kg/day depending on biochemical response.

Societies have advocated for routinely assessing the activity of thiopurine methyltransferase (TPMT), the enzyme that catalyzes the degradation of 6-MP, prior to initiating azathioprine. However, despite theoretical concerns about slow metabolizers, neither the presence of the low-activity TPMT allele nor testing for 6-MP metabolite levels have been found to reliably predict azathioprine efficacy or toxicity in clinical studies. Hence, close monitoring of all patients following initiation of azathioprine is mandatory, particularly cell counts to detect drug-induced cytopenias. In patients who are intolerant of azathioprine, mycophenolate mofetil (MMF) at 2 g/day in divided dose, appears to be an effective alternative. Budesonide (a glucocorticoid with a high first-pass hepatic clearance) can be considered for remission induction in patients without cirrhosis who have co-morbidities that could be exacerbated by prednisone, although long-term data on safety and efficacy in AIH are lacking. The goal of treatment is to achieve corticosteroid-free complete biochemical remission (normal liver tests) along with histologic resolution.

While most patients with AIH will achieve remission with conventional therapy, the remaining 10–15% likely represent a group of individuals with either poor compliance, refractory AIH, or variant/overlap syndromes. For refractory AIH, up titration of prednisone and azathioprine (to a target of 2–2.5 mg/kg/day) can be effective. Addition of a calcineurin inhibitor (eg, cyclosporin, tacrolimus) to the medical regimen can be considered should liver enzymes remain elevated. Other immunosuppressive agents with anecdotal evidence for efficacy in refractory AIH include sirolimus, cyclophosphamide, methotrexate, infliximab, and rituximab. The goal of treatment remains biochemical remission with complete steroid withdrawal whenever possible. Variant syndromes involving overlap with primary biliary cholangitis (AIH/PBC) or primary sclerosing cholangitis (AIH/PSC), while uncommon, should be considered whenever response to standard therapy is suboptimal (see below).

Liver Transplantation for AIH

Indications for performing a liver transplant in patients with AIH include acute liver failure and decompensated cirrhosis. While liver transplantation is highly effective, AIH recurs in 20–25% of patients at a mean of 4.6 years post-transplant. Most patients with recurrent AIH respond to the reintroduction of corticosteroids and azathioprine. Additionally, "*de novo*" AIH develops in 2–7% of patients undergoing liver transplantation for a range of nonimmunologic liver diseases, and generally is responsive to standard AIH management.

Heneghan MA, Allan, ML, Bornstein JD, et al. Utility of thiopurine methyltransferase genotyping and phenotyping, and measurement of azathioprine metabolites in the management of patients with autoimmune hepatitis. *J Hepatol.* 2006;45:584–591. [PMID: 16876902]

Liberal R, Zen Y, Mieli-Vergani G, et al. Liver transplantation and autoimmune liver diseases. *Liver Transplant.* 2013;19:1065–1077. [PMID: 23873751]

Lohse AW, Chazouillères O, Dalekos G, et al. EASL Clinical Practice Guidelines: autoimmune hepatitis. *J Hepatol.* 2015;63(4):971–1004. [PMID: 26341719]

Mack CL, Adams D, Assis DN, et al. Diagnosis and management of autoimmune hepatitis in adults and children: 2019 practice guidance and guidelines from the American Association for the Study of Liver Diseases. *Hepatology.* 2019;10.1002/hep.31065. [PMID: 31863477]

Sebode M, Hartl J, Vergani D, et al. Autoimmune hepatitis: from current knowledge and clinical practice to future research agenda. *Liver Int.* 2018;38:15–22. [PMID: 28432836]

▶ Prognosis

Outcomes are excellent in those patients with AIH who achieve biochemical and histologic remission. Even among those with cirrhosis, reversal of hepatic fibrosis and improvement in decompensating events (ascites, jaundice, coagulopathy) have been observed with effective long-term treatment. There remains debate as to whether patients who achieve complete normalization of aminotransferases and serum IgG levels should undergo confirmation of histological remission. Noninvasive monitoring by elastography may supplant liver biopsy. Patients with AIH generally require permanent maintenance therapy, as treatment withdrawal is achievable only in a small fraction of patients (~10%). Tapering of immunosuppression should be undertaken only after a minimum of 3 years of continuous therapy, with at least 2 years of complete biochemical remission. Predictors of successful treatment withdrawal include an ALT less than half of the upper limit of normal, an IgG level below 12 g/L, and a histological disease activity (HAI) score ≤3. When attempting to withdraw immunosuppression, dosing should be reduced in a stepwise fashion with close monitoring of liver tests. Flares should be treated aggressively and preclude further drug withdrawal. Relapses typically occur within the first 12 months of discontinuing immunosuppression, although late relapses have been described, highlighting the importance of continuous long-term monitoring of patients. Standard screening for hepatocellular carcinoma in patients with AIH and cirrhosis is advised.

Dhaliwal HK, Hoeroldt BS, Dube AK, et al. Long-term prognostic significance of persisting histological activity despite biochemical remission in autoimmune hepatitis. *Am J Gastroenterol.* 2015;110:993–999. [PMID: 26010310]

Gleeson D. Long-term outcomes of autoimmune hepatitis. *Clin Liver Dis.* 2019;14:24–28. [PMID: 31391933]

Hartl J, Ehlken H, Sebode M, et al. Usefulness of biochemical remission and transient elastography in monitoring disease course in autoimmune hepatitis. *J Hepatol.* 2018;68:754–763. [PMID 29180000]

Tansel A, Katz LH, El-Serag HB, et al. Incidence and determinants of hepatocellular carcinoma in autoimmune hepatitis: a systematic review and meta-analysis. *Clin Gastroenterol Hepatol.* 2017;15:1207–1217. [PMID: 28215616]

Van den Brand FF, Snijders RJALM, de Boer YS, et al. Drug withdrawal in patients with autoimmune hepatitis in long-term histological remission: a prospective observational study. *Eur J Int Med.* 2021;90:30–36. [PMID: 33865679]

▶ AIH Overlap Syndromes

There are variants of the autoimmune liver disease in which serologic and clinical characteristics overlap with other forms of immune-mediated liver disorders, with a prevalence of under 10%.

A. Autoimmune Hepatitis/Primary Biliary Cholangitis (AIH/PBC) Overlap

In the majority of patients with AIH/PBC overlap, serologic testing is positive for antimitochondrial antibodies (AMA), but histologic features of AIH are present on liver biopsy. These patients generally respond to standard AIH therapy. A separate subset of patients have cholestatic biochemistries, but are negative for AMA and positive for ANA and/or ASMA with histologic findings consistent with PBC. Approximately half of these patients will respond to ursodeoxycholic acid (UDCA) and are thought to represent an AMA-negative form of PBC. Those that fail to achieve biochemical improvement with UDCA will frequently respond to the addition of corticosteroids/azathioprine. The Paris criteria can facilitate the diagnosis of AIH/PBC overlap syndrome, with two out of the three criteria for both AIH and PBC features yielding a sensitivity and specificity of 92% and 97%, respectively (Table 42–2).

B. Autoimmune Hepatitis/Primary Sclerosing Cholangitis (AIH/PSC) Overlap

Patients with AIH/PSC overlap syndrome have serologic findings suggestive of AIH but radiographic and histologic findings suggestive of PSC. (see chapter on primary sclerosing cholangitis).

Table 42–2. Paris criteria for the diagnosis of AIH/PBC overlap syndrome.

Primary Biliary Cholangitis	Autoimmune Hepatitis
Two of the following criteria: - ALP > 2-fold ULN or GGT > 5-fold ULN - Positive AMA (> 1:40) - Florid duct lesion on liver biopsy	**Mandatory:** Moderate to severe interface hepatitis **At least one additional criteria:** - ALT > 5-fold ULN - IgG > 2-fold ULN or positive ASMA (> 1:40)

ALP, alkaline phosphatase; GGT, gamma-glutamyl transferase; ULN, upper limit of normal.

Freedman BL, Danford CJ, Patwardhan V, Bonder A. Treatment of overlap syndromes in autoimmune liver disease: a systematic review and meta-analysis. *J Clin Med.* 2020;9:1449. [PMID: 32414025]

Kerkar N, Chan A. Autoimmune hepatitis, sclerosing cholangitis, and autoimmune sclerosing cholangitis or overlap syndrome. *Clin Liver Dis.* 2018;22:689–702. [PMID: 30266157]

To U, Silveira M. Overlap syndrome of autoimmune hepatitis and primary biliary cholangitis. *Clin Liver Dis.* 2018;22:603–611. [PMID: 30259856]

PRIMARY BILIARY CHOLANGITIS

 ESSENTIALS OF DIAGNOSIS

▶ Most patients with PBC are asymptomatic at the time of diagnosis, but may eventually develop symptoms, most commonly fatigue and pruritus.

▶ Consider PBC in any patient (particularly women) with an unexplained isolated elevation in alkaline phosphatase of liver origin.

▶ AMAs have 95% sensitivity for PBC and are central to the diagnosis.

General Considerations

PBC, previously termed primary biliary cirrhosis, is a chronic, cholestatic immune-mediated liver disease characterized by destruction of the small intrahepatic bile ducts. PBC is predominantly a disorder of women, with a female:male ratio of 9:1. The typical age of onset is in the 5th decade of life. The disease is most prevalent in northern Europe and the United States. Patients most commonly present as asymptomatic, with an isolated elevation in the serum alkaline phosphatase. Antimitochondrial autoantibodies (AMA) are a hallmark of PBC, and are found in approximately 95% of cases. The targets of these autoantibodies are a family of 2-oxo-acid dehydrogenases, specifically the E2 subunits of the pyruvate dehydrogenase complex (PDC-E2). Liver histology is characterized by T-cell–mediated destruction of the septal and intralobular bile ducts.

Carey EJ, Ali AH, Lindor KD. Primary biliary cirrhosis. *Lancet.* 2015;386:1565–1575. [PMID: 26530622]

Louie JS, Grandhe S, Matsukuma K, et al. Primary bilirubin cholangitis: a brief overview. *Clin Liver Dis.* 2020;15:100–104. [PMID: 32257120]

Pathogenesis

A. Genetic Factors

Evidence for the role of genetic factors in the pathogenesis of PBC include the 100-fold higher prevalence of the disease in first-degree relatives as compared with the general population. In monozygotic twins, PBC has the highest reported concordance rate (62.5%) of any autoimmune disease. Several candidate genes have been correlated with PBC, including certain HLA haplotypes and variants at loci along the interleukin-12 pathway, which is implicated in CD4+ T-cell activation (Figure 42–1).

B. Environmental Factors

It is theorized that molecular mimicry initiates an autoimmune response in an individual genetically predisposed to developing PBC. Several candidate environmental triggers with homology to human mitochondrial proteins (particularly PDC-E2) have been proposed, including infectious agents (eg, *Escherichia coli*) and chemical exposures (eg, cosmetics). Geographical clustering of PBC cases support the existence of pathogenetic environmental factors.

Tanaka A, Leung PS, Gershwin ME. Environmental basis of primary biliary cholangitis. *Exp Biol Med.* 2018;243:184–189. [PMID: 29307284]

Webb GJ, Siminovitch KA, Hirschfield GM. The immunogenetics of primary biliary cirrhosis: a comprehensive review. *J Autoimmun.* 2015;64:42–52. [PMID: 26250073]

Clinical Findings

A. Symptoms & Signs

Over half of patients diagnosed with PBC are asymptomatic at the time of presentation. The most common symptom is fatigue (50–80%), with pruritus and/or right upper quadrant abdominal pain reported in 20% of cases. Additional associated symptoms include sicca syndrome (dry eyes, dry mouth) and arthralgias. The physical examination is usually normal in early-stage disease, with signs of hepatomegaly, splenomegaly, ascites, xanthelasmas and jaundice heralding advanced liver disease.

B. Laboratory Findings

PBC is commonly diagnosed during workup for an isolated, elevation in alkaline phosphatase (ALP) incidentally discovered on laboratory testing. In this situation, it is prudent to confirm that the ALP is of hepatobiliary origin by obtaining a γ-glutamyl transferase (GGT), 5′-nucleotidase, or by fractionation of the ALP. Notably, histologically-confirmed PBC rarely has been identified in individuals with normal ALP levels. Nearly all patients with PBC have an elevated AMA titer, which has a sensitivity and specificity of approximately 95%. However, AMA titers do not correlate with disease severity, nor is an elevated AMA perfectly specific for PBC, as it can be found in up to 20% of patients with AIH and other immune disorders. In patients with a positive AMA and a cholestatic biochemical profile (ALP above 1.5 times the upper limit of normal; ULN) in the absence of a markedly elevated AST (less

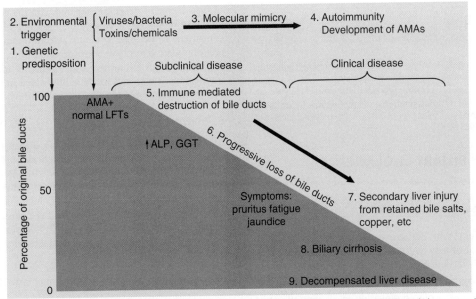

▲ **Figure 42–1.** Pathogenesis and natural history of primary biliary cholangitis (PBC). It is believed that genetically susceptible patients may develop autoimmunity through molecular mimicry if exposed to specific environmental triggers, with the primary target of the resultant antimitochondrial antibodies being pyruvate dehydrogenase E2 complex (PDC-E2). Through an as yet undetermined process, this leads to a persistent T-cell–mediated destruction of the intrahepatic bile ducts. Untreated, this destructive process eventually destroys a critical percentage of bile ducts and secondary injury from retained bile salts ensues. Injury progresses to biliary cirrhosis and eventually to decompensated liver disease. ALP, alkaline phosphatase; AMA, antimitochondrial antibody; GGT, γ-glutamyl transferase; LFTs, liver function tests.

than 5 times the ULN), liver biopsy generally is not required to establish the diagnosis of PBC. Conversely, patients suspected of having PBC but who are AMA-negative, do require liver histology. Obtaining titers for anti-gp210 and anti-sp100 autoantibodies also can be helpful, as they have high specificity for PBC.

C. Histologic Findings

Typical liver histology in PBC demonstrates nonsuppurative cholangitis involving the small- and/or medium-sized bile ducts. The presence of florid bile duct lesions (a bile duct at the center of a dense lymphocytic infiltrate) is pathognomonic for PBC, but is uncommonly encountered. A lymphocyte-predominant portal infiltrate with poorly formed epithelioid granulomas is frequently observed. The liver is not involved uniformly in PBC, a fact that increases the likelihood of sampling variability.

Beretta-Piccoli BT, Stirnimann G, Mertens J, et al. Primary biliary cholangitis with normal alkaline phosphatase: a neglected clinical entity challenging current guidelines. *J Autoimmun.* 2021;116:102578 [PMID: 33229138]

Namisaki T, Fujinaga Y, Moriya K, et al. The association of histological progression with biochemical response to ursodeoxycholic acid in primary biliary cholangitis. *Hepatol Res.* 2021;51:31–38. [PMID: 33210415]

Takamura M, Matsuda Y, Kimura N, et al. Changes in disease characteristics of primary biliary cholangitis: an observational retrospective study from 1982 to 2016. *Hepatol Res.* 2021;51:166–175. [PMID: 33126288]

▶ Treatment

A. Ursodeoxycholic Acid

UDCA, at a dose of 13–15 mg/kg/day, is the first-line therapy for PBC. It is well tolerated, with mild diarrhea or modest weight gain being the most common side-effects. The mechanism of action of UDCA remains unknown, but it has been shown to improve liver biochemistries and transplant-free survival. A number of predictive models based on biochemical (eg, alkaline phosphatase, total bilirubin, albumin, platelets) response to UDCA at one-year of treatment have been developed. Of these, the GLOBE and UK-PBC scoring systems appear to have the best prognostic performance. Those patients who achieve a complete response to UDCA (as determined by these scoring systems) generally have a normal life expectancy as long as they remain on treatment. Patients with a suboptimal response are at risk for disease progression and are anticipated to benefit from the addition of another agent to their treatment regimen.

B. Obeticholic Acid

Obeticholic acid (OCA), starting at a dose of 5 mg daily and increasing to a maximum of 10 mg daily based on biochemical response, is approved as monotherapy for patients who are unable to tolerate UDCA, or in combination with UDCA in patients who experience an inadequate response. Like UDCA, OCA is a choleretic agent; however, in contrast to UDCA, OCA acts as an agonist for the farnesoid X receptor (FXR). While OCA is effective in reducing serum ALP levels in patients with PBC, long-term outcomes data are lacking. Dose-dependent pruritus is the most common side-effect of OCA, leading to treatment discontinuation in up to 10% of patients. As OCA has been associated with hepatic decompensation in individuals with advanced liver disease (Child-Pugh class B or C), its use should be avoided in these patients. OCA treatment is contraindicated in patients with decompensated cirrhosis and in patients with evidence of portal hypertension.

C. Fibrates

There is emerging evidence that fibrates, which are currently approved as lipid-lowering agents, may be effective in treating PBC. Fibrates downregulate bile acid synthesis, and studies of bezafibrate in combination with UDCA in PBC patients with an inadequate response to UDCA monotherapy, have shown improvement in serum ALP. An added benefit of bezafibrate is that, in contrast with OCA, it has been observed to improve pruritus. While long-term studies are ongoing, the American Association for the Study of Liver Diseases suggests that fibrates can be considered in patients with PBC who fail UDCA treatment. Notably, fibrates have not been studied in patients with decompensated liver disease.

D. Liver Transplantation

Liver transplantation is reserved for patients with PBC who develop decompensated cirrhosis. While recurrence of PBC post-transplant has been reported to occur in up to 30% of patients, due to the slow rate of disease progression, this rarely impacts long-term outcomes, which are quite good.

E. Symptomatic Therapies

1. Pruritus—Cholestyramine and colestipol are resins that bind to bile acids and increase fecal excretion. They are reasonably effective and are considered first-line agents. As these bile sequestrants bind to and block intestinal absorption of UDCA and OCA, it is critical to educate patients regarding the need to separate the dosing of these medications by at least 2–4 hours. Second-line agents for pruritus are rifampin (150 mg twice daily) and oral opioid receptor antagonists. Selective serotonin reuptake inhibitors (eg, sertraline) and gabapentin also may be of some benefit for treatment of pruritus. Antihistamines have little role aside from use as a sleep aid. Plasmapheresis has been effective in truly refractory cases. (A detailed discussion of the management of pruritus can be found in the chapter on primary sclerosing cholangitis.)

2. Fatigue—This symptom can be incapacitating, even in patients with early-stage PBC. Unfortunately, no medication has been reliably proven to improve fatigue, and there is no recommended therapy at this time. Superimposed treatable causes of fatigue, such as depression and sleep apnea, should be considered and addressed.

3. Osteopenia/osteoporosis—Approximately one-third of patients with PBC develop osteoporosis, and it is recommended that bone density be checked every 2–3 years. Calcium and vitamin D supplementation, particularly in peri- or post-menopausal women should be offered. Bisphosphonate therapy is appropriate in patients who are found to be osteoporotic.

4. Hyperlipidemia—Although serum cholesterol is typically elevated in PBC, patients are not at increased risk of atherosclerosis. This finding is explained, in part, by the presence of high levels of high-density lipoprotein and also by the presence of a unique subfraction of low-density lipoproteins, called lipoprotein X, that exert antiatherogenic properties. Hence, only those PBC patients with a personal or strong family history of atherosclerotic disease require lipid-lowering agents. When indicated, statin drugs can be used safely in patients with PBC as long as standard monitoring for hepatotoxicity is performed.

5. Fat-soluble vitamin deficiency—Deficiency of fat-soluble vitamins occurs in patients with PBC, particularly those with advanced stage disease. Vitamin A deficiency can occur in up to one-third of patients and cases of night blindness have been reported. Fat-soluble vitamin levels should be checked every 3 years and supplemented as needed.

Beuers U, Boberg KM, Chapman RW, et al. EASL Clinical Practice Guidelines: the diagnosis and management of patients with primary biliary cholangitis. *J Hepatol.* 2017;67(1):145–172. [PMID: 28427765]

Efe C, Taşçilar K, Henriksson I et al. Validation of risk scoring systems in ursodeoxycholic acid-treated patients with primary biliary cholangitis. *Am J Gastroenterol.* 2019;114:1101–1108. [PMID: 31241547]

Hirschfield GM, Dyson, JK, Aleander GJM et al. The British Society of Gastroenterology/UK-PBC primary biliary cholangitis treatment and management guidelines. *Gut.* 2018;67:1568–1594. [PMID: 29593060]

Lindor KD, Bowlus CL, Boyer J, Levy C, Mayo M. Primary biliary cholangitis: 2018 practice guidance from the American Association for the Study of Liver Diseases. *Hepatology.* 2019;69:394–419. [PMID: 30070375]

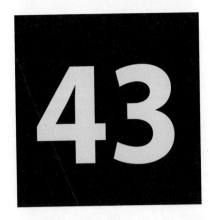

Metabolic Liver Diseases

Alexander S. Vogel, MD

Benjamin Smith, MD

HEMOCHROMATOSIS

ESSENTIALS OF DIAGNOSIS AND TREATMENT

▶ Hemochromatosis classically refers to *HFE*-mediated genetic iron overload, but several alternatively mediated genetic iron overload syndromes have been described.

▶ C282Y is the major mutation and H63D the minor mutation of the *HFE* gene; individuals with two copies of C282Y or one copy of both mutations (compound heterozygote) are at risk for iron overload.

▶ Excess iron deposition in tissues leads to end-organ damage; advanced hemochromatosis typically involves the liver first and may also involve the pancreas, heart, pituitary gland, as well as other organs.

▶ Most patients are identified by laboratory screening or family history and are asymptomatic at diagnosis.

▶ Symptomatic patients usually present with nonspecific complaints of fatigue, arthralgias, and abdominal pain.

▶ Screening studies include serum iron/total iron-binding capacity (abnormal if >45%) and serum ferritin (abnormal if >200 μg/L in women, >250 μg/L in men); if either test is positive, genetic testing should be pursued.

▶ Liver biopsy to assess iron concentration and hepatic iron index is indicated if serum ferritin is >1000 μg/dL or liver tests are abnormal.

▶ Early diagnosis (precirrhotic stage) and treatment, which is usually phlebotomy, is associated with a normal life expectancy.

▶ General Considerations

Eighty percent of clinically established cases of hemochromatosis worldwide and over 90% of cases in the United States result from the autosomal-recessive inheritance of two copies of the major mutation (C282Y) of the *HFE* gene. Individuals with this genotype are described as C282Y homozygotes. Prevalence estimates of homozygosity for the C282Y mutation in populations of Northern European descent are 1 in 260 persons. In Caucasian populations, 10–15% are heterozygotes, possessing one copy of the major mutation. One copy of the H63D mutation, the minor mutation of the *HFE* gene, may be found in 15–40% of Caucasian populations. About 4% of cases of hemochromatosis result from the inheritance of one copy of the major mutation, C282Y, and one copy of the minor mutation, H63D, with these individuals being described as compound heterozygotes. The majority of compound heterozygotes will not develop clinically significant iron overload with the risk estimated to be 200 times less than in C282Y homozygotes. H63D homozygotes typically do not develop clinically significant iron overload. Individuals with this genotype may have an elevated transferrin saturation, but an elevated ferritin should prompt a search for secondary causes of iron overload. Mutations in the *HFE* gene are believed to have originated more than 6000 years ago amid Celtic or Viking ancestry. It has been postulated that the mutation may have had a potential selective advantage, preventing iron deficiency in the setting of scarce resources such as red meat.

Phenotypic expression of these altered gene states is variable and, as a result, the proportion of patients who go on to develop clinically significant hemochromatosis remains uncertain. It has been estimated that 38–50% of C282Y homozygotes will develop iron overload, but only 10–33% will manifest hemochromatosis-related morbidity. Men are much more likely than women to develop iron overload-related disease (28% vs 1%), which is attributed to increased dietary iron consumption in men as well as iron losses in women during menstruation. Ethnicity also plays an important role in prevalence; in the United States, the majority of patients are of Caucasian ancestry while the disease is rarely seen in African Americans, Mexican Americans, and Asian Americans. Globally, the majority of patients in Europe are of Caucasian ancestry, and low rates are seen in Asia, the Middle East and Africa. There are relatively high rates of iron overload syndromes found in sub-Saharan Africa but these are not due to C282Y mutations (instead secondary to SLC40A1 variants). The majority of individuals who develop end-organ damage likely have cofactors such as significant alcohol intake or nonalcoholic steatohepatitis (NASH). Overall, secondary causes of iron overload are still more common than primary iron overload syndromes.

Allen KJ, Gurrin LC, Constantine CC, et al. Iron-overload-related disease in HFE hereditary hemochromatosis. N Engl J Med. 2008;358:221–230. [PMID: 18199861]

Brissot P, Pietrangelo A, Adams PC, et al. (2018). Haemochromatosis. Nat Rev Dis Primers. 2018;4(1):18016. [PMID: 29620054]

▶ Pathogenesis

A. Normal Iron Metabolism

The quantity of total body iron is closely regulated and is estimated to be approximately 3 g in women and 5 g in men. Most of this iron is incorporated into red blood cells. The remainder is stored in the liver and a small amount in skeletal muscle. Almost all iron absorption occurs in the duodenum. After iron is absorbed, it circulates bound to the carrier protein transferrin for distribution to tissues. In addition to taking up inorganic iron in this way, the duodenal enterocytes may also take up iron in the form of heme.

Most of the circulating iron is taken up within sites of erythropoiesis, where it is incorporated into hemoglobin by developing erythrons. The liver serves as a storage reservoir for iron and then releases iron back into circulation as needed. As red blood cells senesce, they are phagocytosed by macrophages which then process and release iron for recycling into newly developing cells at a controlled rate.

The amount of iron absorbed from food can be upregulated quickly when excess iron is lost or utilized, such as through menstruation, pregnancy, or gastrointestinal bleeding. Small amounts of iron, on the order of 1–2 mg daily, are lost as cells of the gastrointestinal and urogenital tracts are shed. Via menstruation, an additional 1–2 mg of iron is lost daily by women during their reproductive years. However, the human body has no effective physiologic mechanism for excreting excess iron. The duodenal enterocytes must correctly sense or be signaled to absorb enough iron to replace losses but no more.

The duodenal enterocytes, hepatocytes, and macrophages all play important roles in iron homeostasis. Multiple systemic and intestinal factors influence iron absorption. Systemic factors include the level of body iron stores, erythropoietic activity, hemoglobin concentration, and oxygen saturation as well as the presence or absence of inflammatory cytokines. Intestinal factors include pancreatic insufficiency and disturbances in pH. Disorders of iron metabolism develop when disease states overwhelm the homeostatic mechanisms. For example, infections or chronic inflammation induce iron sequestration by macrophages and signal a decrease of iron absorption, leading to the anemia of chronic disease. Conversely, disorders of erythropoiesis, such as the thalassemias, release signals promoting iron absorption by developing erythrons that overwhelm the inhibitory signals generated by excessive accumulation of iron stores.

Sharma N, Butterworth J, Cooper BT, et al. The emerging role of the liver in iron metabolism. Am J Gastroenterol. 2005;100:201–206. [PMID: 15654801]

B. Hereditary Hemochromatosis

In hereditary hemochromatosis (HHC), one or more genetic mutations lead to excess iron absorption relative to body iron stores. The excess iron is stored in the liver initially but, if unrecognized and untreated, the iron may deposit in multiple end organs when hepatic storage is saturated, leading to the phenotypic expressions of the disease. Iron spillover has been observed once total body stores reach 4.5 g with hepatic levels in excess of 400 µg/g of tissue.

In 1996, Feder and colleagues published the discovery of a candidate gene for hemochromatosis located on the short arm of chromosome 6, now called HFE. As noted earlier, two mutations are now recognized. The major mutation results from a tyrosine substitution for cysteine at the 282 amino acid position on the gene and is abbreviated as C282Y. The minor mutation results from an aspartate substitution for histidine at the 63rd amino acid position and is abbreviated as H63D.

Feder JN, Gnirke A, Thomas W, et al. A novel MHC class I-like gene is mutated in patients with hereditary hemochromatosis. Nat Genet. 1996;13:399–408. [PMID: 8696333]

C. Pathophysiology of Iron Overload in HHC

While the full mechanism of iron overload in HHC is not completely understood, the overall pathway that leads from HFE gene mutations to eventual phenotypic iron overload is better characterized at this time.

The key regulator of iron absorption has been shown, in a variety of studies, to be hepcidin, which is produced by the liver. In normal iron homeostasis, hepcidin serves as a counterregulatory protein – as iron absorption and stores increase, hepcidin levels increase, leading to decreased iron absorption and thus levels. Hepcidin appears to work via several targets. The primary target is ferroportin, the main iron exporter from mammalian cells such as duodenal enterocytes.

When hepcidin binds to ferroportin at the basolateral cell surface of enterocytes, this leads to ferroportin internalization and degradation. This, in turn, limits iron export from enterocytes, leading to accumulation of iron within these cells and decreased iron absorption. Reticuloendothelial macrophages also have ferroportin receptors, and the effects of hepcidin here are thought to be similar.

In HH, an inappropriately low hepcidin level appears to result from a cascade of events that starts with *HFE* mutations. The low hepcidin levels lead to increased intestinal iron absorption, but unlike in normal iron homeostasis, hepcidin levels remain low despite increasing iron stores, resulting in ongoing iron accumulation. The iron, which accumulates in many tissues over years, including the liver, heart, pancreas and pituitary causes damage to these tissues, leading to the phenotypic presentation of HH; the mechanism of this tissue damage over time is not yet completely understood but thought to be potentially related to free radicals (Figure 43–1).

Adams PC. Hepcidin in hemochromatosis: the message or the messenger? *Hepatology.* 2014;59:749–750. [PMID: 23996780]

Bardou-Jacquet E, Philip J, Lorho R, et al. Liver transplantation normalizes serum hepcidin level and cures iron metabolism alterations in HFE hemochromatosis. *Hepatology.* 2014;59: 839–847. [PMID: 23775519]

Bridle KR, Frazer DM, Wilkins SJ, et al. Disrupted hepcidin regulation in HFE-associated hemochromatosis and the liver as a regulator of body iron homoeostasis. *Lancet.* 2003;361:669–673. [PMID: 12606179]

Fleming RE, Bacon BR. Orchestration of iron homeostasis. *N Engl J Med.* 2005;352:1741–1744. [PMID: 15858181]

Nemeth E, Tuttle MS, Powelson J, et al. Hepcidin regulates cellular iron efflux by binding to ferroportin and inducing its internalization. *Science.* 2004;306:2090–2093. [PMID: 15514116]

Park CH, Valore EV, Waring AJ, et al. Hepcidin, a urinary antimicrobial peptide synthesized in the liver. *J Biol Chem.* 2001;276:7806–7810. [PMID: 11113131]

Pietrangelo A. Hereditary hemochromatosis: pathogenesis, diagnosis and treatment. *Gastroenterology.* 2010;139:393–408. [PMID: 20542038]

Roy CN, Enns CA. Iron homeostasis: new tales from the crypt. *Blood.* 2000;96:4020–4027. [PMID: 11110669]

Weinstein DA, Roy CN, Fleming MD, et al. Inappropriate expression of hepcidin is associated with iron refractory anemia: implications for the anemia of chronic disease. *Blood.* 2002;100:3776–3781. [PMID: 12393428]

Wu XG, Wang Y, Wu Q, et al. HFE interacts with the BMP type I receptor ALK3 to regulate hepcidin expression. *Blood.* 2014;124:1335–1343. [PMID: 24904118]

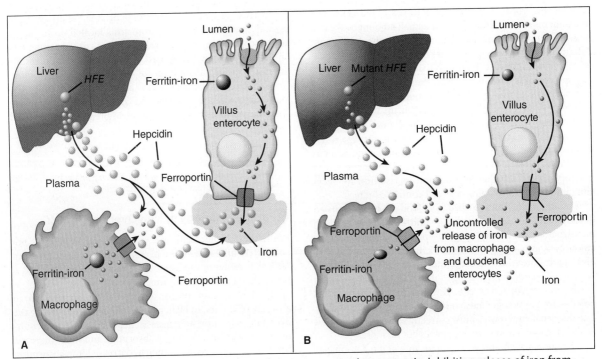

▲ **Figure 43–1.** Hepcidin model. Hepcidin normally functions as a regulatory protein, inhibiting release of iron from villus enterocytes and macrophages, which in turn inhibits iron absorption. **A.** Normal. **B.** *HFE*-related hemochromatosis. (Adapted with permission from Pietrangelo A. Hereditary hemochromatosis—a new look at an old disease, *N Engl J Med* 2004;350(23):2383–2397.)

D. Factors Predisposing to Phenotypic Expression

The fact that only a small percentage of C282Y homozygotes develop signs and symptoms of iron overload suggests that other genetic and environmental modifiers are present. Perhaps other proteins influencing hepcidin expression may compensate for the effects of the *HFE* mutation.

Much higher rates of cirrhosis have been observed in patients with HHC who consume more than 60 g of alcohol per day. It is believed that alcohol and iron deposition may act synergistically to promote fibrosis through increased oxidative stress and hepatic stellate cell activation. Investigations into the mechanism of action of alcohol on exacerbating disease activity have demonstrated downregulation of hepcidin activity as well as increased C/EBPα, DMT-1, and ferroportin expression in animal models.

The long-recognized gender disparity in the phenotypic expression of at-risk *HFE* genotypes may be in part explained by the role of testosterone in iron regulation, in addition to increased iron losses in women via menstruation. Testosterone appears to suppress hepcidin expression by enhancing epidermal growth factor signaling in the liver.

Latour C, Kautz L, Besson-Fournier C, et al. Testosterone perturbs systemic iron balance through activation of epidermal growth factor receptor signaling in the liver and repression of hepcidin. *Hepatology.* 2014;59:683–694. [PMID: 23907767]

Stickel F, Buch S, Zoller H, et al. Evaluation of genome-wide loci of iron metabolism in hereditary hemochromatosis identifies PCSK7 as a host risk factor of liver cirrhosis. *Hum Mol Genet.* 2014;23:3883–3890. [PMID: 24556216]

E. Non-*HFE* Hemochromatosis

Although *HFE* mutations are responsible for the great majority of cases of hemochromatosis worldwide, the commercial availability of testing for *HFE* mutations soon identified individuals and subpopulations with significant iron overload in the absence of these mutations. Three other gene mutations have been identified that cause autosomal-recessive iron overload with a phenotype very similar to that of *HFE*-related hemochromatosis. They are the *HJV* gene on chromosome 1, the *HAMP* gene on chromosome 19, and the *TfR2* gene on chromosome 7. All three mutations decrease hepcidin levels and lead to a primarily hepatocellular deposition of excess iron (Table 43–1).

The term *juvenile hemochromatosis* was first used in 1979 to describe an overload syndrome that resembled *HFE*-related hemochromatosis but with iron loading and end-organ damage at an early age. This form of severe hemochromatosis appears to be caused by mutations in either the *HJV* or *HAMP* genes. Hemojuvelin (the product of HJV), is believed to modulate hepcidin expression. Mutations in *HJV* appear to be more common than mutations of the *HAMP* gene, which encodes hepcidin itself. *HAMP* mutations may lead to severe and potentially fatal iron overload before age 30, corroborating the critical role of hepcidin in iron homeostasis.

TfR2 mutations lead to a milder form of iron overload similar to *HFE*. *TfR2* is a receptor on the surface of hepatocytes which senses levels of diferric transferrin in the portal blood with the potential mechanism by which *TfR2* mutations lead to low hepcidin levels and iron overload being through incorrect sensing of blood iron levels.

Mutations in ferroportin, the target of hepcidin in duodenal enterocytes and macrophages can also lead to autosomal-dominant iron overload. One mutation inactivates ferroportin and leads to retention of iron in duodenal enterocytes and macrophages, called ferroportin disease, leading to a reticuloendothelial distribution of iron within the macrophage populations of the liver, spleen, and bone marrow. Circulating levels of iron tend to be lower than in *HFE*-related hemochromatosis with a high serum ferritin but normal or low transferrin saturation. Since the parenchymal cells of the affected end organs do not accumulate iron in ferroportin disease, there is minimal end-organ damage, and aggressive

Table 43–1. OMIM classification of primary iron overload syndromes.

OMIM	Implicated Gene	Gene Product	Hepcidin Level	Pattern of Inheritance	Potential for Organ Damage	Hepatic Iron Deposition
Type 1	*HFE*, 6p21.3	HFE	Low	AR	Variable	Parenchymal
Type 2A	*HJV*, 1q21	Hemojuvelin	Low	AR	High	Parenchymal
Type 2B	*HAMP*, 19q13.1	Hepcidin	Absent	AR	High	Parenchymal
Type 3	*TfR2*, 7q22	Transferrin receptor 2	Low	AR	Variable	Parenchymal
Type 4	*SLC40A1*, 2q32	Ferroportin	High	AD	Low	Reticuloendothelial

AD, autosomal dominant; AR, autosomal recessive; OMIM, Online Mendelian Inheritance in Man database.
Data from the OMIM database and Pietrangelo A. Hereditary hemochromatosis—a new look at an old disease, *N Engl J Med* 2004; 350(23):2383–2397.

phlebotomy can actually lead to iron-restricted anemia. Ferroportin disease is the second most common cause of inherited hyperferritinemia after hemochromatosis caused by *HFE* mutations. The second ferroportin mutation partially disables the interaction between ferroportin and hepcidin, leading to hepcidin resistance. This leads to effects similar to low levels of hepcidin with a primarily hepatocellular distribution of iron similar to *HFE*-related disease.

Recognition of these different genes, and the influence of their proteins on iron metabolism, has led to a new classification of iron overload syndromes in the Online Mendelian Inheritance in Man (OMIM) database (see Table 43–1).

The relative importance of the different proteins on hepcidin expression and therefore iron metabolism is reflected by the severity of iron overload that develops in their absence: mutations in the *HJV* (or *HAMP*) gene lead to an early development of severe iron overload, whereas either *HFE* or *TfR2* mutations alone lead to a milder phenotype that develops later in life, if at all. It is now apparent not only that mutations in multiple genes may lead to the hemochromatosis phenotype but also that various combinations of mutations may be responsible for the variable presentation of the disease.

The rate at which iron accumulates in the different types of hemochromatosis affects the phenotype. Mutations in the hemojuvelin and HAMP genes typically lead to overtly symptomatic disease before age 20 affecting the heart and endocrine organs. The liver is relatively spared. On the other hand, the gradual accumulation of iron that typically occurs with *HFE* and *TfR2* mutations, leads to minimally symptomatic disease that affects the liver first and uncommonly affects the other end organs. Intermediate phenotypes may occur with other combinations of mutations.

Merryweather-Clarke AT, Cadet E, Bomfor A, et al. Digenic inheritance of mutations in HAMP and HFE results in different types of hemochromatosis. *Hum Mol Genet*. 2003;12:2241–2247. [PMID: 12915468]

Pietrangelo A. Hereditary hemochromatosis—a new look at an old disease. *N Engl J Med*. 2004;350:2383–2397. [PMID: 15175440]

▶ Clinical Findings

A. Symptoms & Signs

Iron overload is typically an insidious process. Patients are commonly asymptomatic until 10–20 g of iron stores have accumulated in parenchymal tissues. Diagnosis is typically made earlier in men, as iron overload is often delayed by menstrual losses and decreased dietary intake in women. As a result, while men are typically diagnosed in the fourth to fifth decade of life, women are diagnosed on average a decade later. As the use of screening laboratory measures has increased, more patients are now being diagnosed in an asymptomatic stage.

1. Presentation—Clinical manifestations of iron overload include unexplained fatigue, arthralgias, weight loss, abdominal pain, and reduced libido. Identification of the most common genetic abnormalities associated with HHC has led increasingly to diagnosis in asymptomatic individuals.

HHC can lead to iron deposition within multiple organ sites. Complications by organ system are reviewed in the following text.

2. Liver—Elevated liver enzymes, hepatomegaly, or cirrhosis is present in greater than 95% of patients with clinically advanced HHC. Liver manifestations usually do not begin until liver stores become saturated (6–7 g). The majority of deaths related to HHC (89%) are attributable to complications of cirrhosis. Overall, the risk of hepatocellular carcinoma (HHC) in patients with HCC who develop cirrhosis is 20–200 times that of the general population (5% annual risk after the development of cirrhosis). Pathologically, the presence of "iron-free" nodules on histologic examination has correlated with onset of HHC.

With treatment, elevations in liver function tests and hepatomegaly are reversible. No strong evidence currently exists with respect to the reversibility of cirrhosis and the resultant complications related to portal hypertension with treatment.

3. Cardiac—Iron deposition within cardiac tissue can lead to either dilated cardiomyopathy or a mixed dilated-restrictive picture. Conduction disturbances such as atrial fibrillation or sick sinus syndrome have also been linked with HHC. The extent of cardiac involvement is highly variable and does not necessarily correlate with the extent of other organ involvement. Dysrhythmias and cardiomyopathy are the leading cause of sudden death in patients with iron overload.

With phlebotomy, both the cardiomyopathy and dysrhythmias associated with iron deposition can be reversed, albeit to a variable extent.

4. Endocrine—Diabetes mellitus and hypogonadism are the most commonly described endocrinopathies associated with HHC secondary to iron deposition in the pancreas and pituitary respectively. The prevalence of *HFE* gene mutations is significantly increased in type 1 diabetes whereas the prevalence of *HFE* gene mutations in type 2 diabetes is similar to the general population. The onset of diabetes has been described in up to 65% of patients with symptomatic iron overload. The mechanism is believed to be twofold: both direct damage to pancreatic islet cells by iron deposition as well as increased insulin resistance due to higher circulating iron levels. The incidence of diabetes is increased in patients with a family history of diabetes, suggesting that a genetic predisposition is at least partially responsible. Unlike the cardiac disturbances, once diabetes has developed in the setting of HHC it is often nonreversible despite therapy for iron overload.

Reduced secretion of gonadotropin as a result of iron interference in the hypothalamic-pituitary axis can lead to hypogonadism. This is the second most common form of endocrinopathy associated with HHC and can present as impotence, amenorrhea, and reduced libido, as well as osteoporosis. Secondary hypothyroidism is a less common form of endocrinopathy seen in men with HHC. Patients who develop hypo-gonadism or hypothyroidism often require lifelong hormone supplementation.

5. Arthropathy—Twenty to seventy percent of symptomatic patients present with complaints of arthropathy. Classically, the second and third metacarpophalangeal and proximal interphalangeal joints of the hands are involved. In addition, the wrists, shoulders, knees, and ankles can be affected. Radiographically, joint space narrowing is accompanied by squared-off bone ends and hook-like osteophytes. These changes resemble those of calcium pyrophosphate crystal deposition disease (pseudogout). It has been difficult to tease apart the contribution of HHC to arthropathy given the relatively high prevalence of joint disease in the general population. Significant improvement in symptoms is not often observed with treatment of the underlying iron overload.

6. Skin—The classic metallic or slate-gray hue described as "bronzing" is a result of increased melanin in the dermis. In addition, direct iron deposition in the dermis contributes to the gray appearance. Although best appreciated by examining the volar (unexposed) portion of the forearms, additional sites of involvement include the face, neck, dorsum of the hands, lower legs, and genital regions. Cutaneous atrophy, flattening of the nails, and loss of body hair have also been described. Estimates of the prevalence of bronzing in symptomatic individuals range from 18–47%. Data are sparse with respect to changes in pigmentation with phlebotomy therapy.

7. Infection—There are certain bacteria, known as siderophilic bacteria, which have increased virulence in the setting of iron overload (including secondary to HHC). The main organisms within this group are two gram negative bacteria – *Yersinia enterocolitica* and *Vibrio vulnificus*. Both are traditionally foodborne with *Yersinia* often transmitted via livestock and *Vibrio* via uncooked fish, mollusks and crustaceans. Raw seafood should be avoided by patients with HHC and iron overload.

B. Laboratory Findings

1. General approach—Patients suspected of iron overload, based on either symptoms or routine laboratory testing, should undergo a thorough history and review of systems. Emphasis should be placed on eliciting symptoms suggesting involvement of the gastrointestinal, cardiac, endocrine, and rheumatologic systems. Because the C282Y homozygous state does not necessarily translate into clinical disease, the diagnosis of HHC is determined by a combination of genetic, serologic, and clinical features. Current diagnostic markers include gene analysis, iron studies, liver biopsy, and response to therapy.

2. Serum iron studies—Initial evaluation usually begins with serologic testing of iron studies. The transferrin saturation is regarded as the single best screening test for HHC. Although widely accepted as an accurate marker of the genetic defect in *HFE*-associated hemochromatosis, there is controversy over the optimal cutoff level. Previously suggested levels include transferrin saturation of 45% or higher, 55% and higher, and 60% and higher, as thresholds. With increasing thresholds, sensitivity decreases as specificity increases. However, the transferrin saturation does not reflect the extent of hepatic iron stores. The unsaturated iron-binding capacity (UIBC) has also been examined as a single test for screening patients for HHC with similar results to the transferrin saturation.

Serum ferritin is an index of the body's iron stores with a high sensitivity but a relatively low specificity. Although the ferritin level is typically greatly elevated in HHC, ferritin may also be elevated as an acute phase reactant in additional inflammatory states in the absence of the genetic disease, notably alcohol-associated liver disease, NASH, and chronic hepatitis C. Combined measurement of the percent transferrin saturation and serum ferritin provides a simple means to exclude patients from further analysis. We generally apply a combination threshold of transferrin saturation >45% with a ferritin >200 μg/L for women and >250 μg/L for men. If either is elevated in the absence of a known inflammatory condition, further genetic testing for HHC is indicated.

3. Other labs—Initial studies suggest that serum hyaluronic acid levels appear to correlate well with the degree of hepatic fibrosis in HHC patients with advanced disease. If these data are corroborated, it would provide another noninvasive tool for assessing fibrosis and cirrhosis.

C. Imaging Studies & Special Tests

1. Liver biopsy—Liver biopsy provides information relevant to the diagnosis and staging of hemochromatosis. First, sampling of liver tissue provides documentation of fibrosis or cirrhosis. Second, it allows for evaluation of additional causes of liver disease. Finally, biopsy allows for determination of the hepatic iron index (a ratio of hepatic iron concentration to age of the patient). An index >1.9 is highly supportive of HHC and helps to distinguish this from alcohol-associated liver disease.

With the widespread availability of genetic testing, liver biopsy for diagnostic purposes is now reserved for cases in which either genetic testing is unavailable or non–*HFE*-related iron overload is suspected in patients with suggestive iron studies but a normal *HFE* gene analysis. Current guidelines from the United States also recommend biopsy in C282Y homozygotes or C282Y/H63D compound heterozygotes with a serum ferritin level greater than 1000 and abnormal liver enzymes. In Europe, hepatomegaly or age greater than 40 have also been suggested as additional criteria. If none of these indicators of chronic liver disease are present, studies have suggested that the presence of significant fibrosis or cirrhosis is unlikely and liver biopsy may be deferred, provided treatment to deplete iron stores is initiated. The presence of abnormal liver enzymes and hepatomegaly at any age are indications to pursue a biopsy. Younger C282Y homozygotes with normal iron studies can defer biopsy with repeat testing of iron studies every 5 years. European guidelines suggest a ferritin measurement annually.

2. Quantitative phlebotomy—Although not providing information with respect to the extent of disease, quantitative phlebotomy can be used to diagnose iron overload. The calculated iron storage can be assessed by determining the number of phlebotomies required to produce iron deficiency. Four phlebotomy sessions of 500 mL each will remove approximately 1 g of iron. Calculated iron storage greater than 5 g is considered abnormal.

3. Imaging studies—Noninvasive imaging techniques can be useful as part of an algorithm for the diagnosis and staging of HHC. In general, noninvasive imaging is useful for advanced disease but is not feasible for screening of early disease.

Magnetic resonance imaging (MRI) studies have found a relatively high concordance between MRI and liver biopsy with respect to detection of hepatic iron levels. MRI also has the ability to distinguish parenchymal from mesenchymal iron overload and to detect iron-free neoplastic nodules. MRI, of the liver or heart, can be helpful in classifying hepatic iron levels in a noninvasive manner.

Transient elastography, with either ultrasound or MRI, has shown promise for the detection of advanced fibrosis and cirrhosis. Similarly, the superconducting quantum interference device susceptometer (SQUID) enables an in vivo measurement of hepatic iron that appears to be quantitatively equivalent to liver biopsy measurement of hepatic iron. The technique has not yet been validated for HHC patients.

4. Genetic testing—Discovery of the *HFE* gene, and the C282Y and H63D mutations, has revolutionized the diagnosis of HHC. Genetic testing for these mutations should be undertaken in any patient with documentation of iron overload based on the results of laboratory testing. The results of genetic testing, however, must be combined with a patient's clinical presentation as penetrance of the genetic defect is variable, in some recent estimates below 1%. Genetic testing is not recommended for the general population. However, it should be considered in patients with porphyria cutanea tarda (due to sensitivity to body iron levels in this condition), chondrocalcinosis, HCC, or type 1 diabetes mellitus.

5. Screening for HHC—

A. FAMILY SCREENING—Screening of first-degree relatives of C282Y homozygotes is universally recommended. Siblings have a 1 in 4 to 1 in 2 chance of inheriting the mutation, depending on whether the parents are homozygous or heterozygous for the mutation. Children of C282Y homozygotes have an approximately 1 in 20 chance of inheriting two copies of the C282Y mutation.

Once an individual is identified with hemochromatosis, his or her spouse should be genotyped if the couple has more than one child. If the spouse has at least one copy of the major or minor mutation, then the children should undergo *HFE* gene testing. It is more cost-effective to directly genotype an only child. Genetic screening of family members is preferred over phenotypic screening methods due to improved efficiency, as biochemical iron overload is not always present initially. Screening of first- to third-degree relatives of carriers may detect up to 40% of at-risk individuals.

B. POPULATION-BASED SCREENING—HHC satisfies many of the criteria set forth by the US Preventative Services Task Force and World Health Organization to determine diseases appropriate for population screening. HHC has adequate prevalence with a prolonged latent phase. In addition, treatment for the disease has been shown to be widely successful in forestalling associated complications that, if untreated, can be associated with significant morbidity and mortality. Moreover, testing for hemochromatosis is relatively inexpensive, widely available, and reliable.

Issues that have hindered acceptance of widespread screening guidelines for HHC have included varying case definitions, relatively low phenotypic expression, concerns about discrimination (ie, insurance coverage) for *HFE* patients who do not phenotypically express, as well as disagreement over the cost-effectiveness of general population screening.

Bacon BR, Adams PC, Kowdley KV, et al. Diagnosis and management of hemochromatosis: 2011 practice guideline by the American Association for the Study of Liver Diseases. *Hepatology*. 2011;54:328–343. [PMID: 21452290]

European Association for the Study of the Liver. EASL clinical guidelines for HFE hemochromatosis. *J Hepatol*. 2010;53:3–22. [PMID: 20471131]

Qaseem A, Aronson M, Fitterman N, et al. Screening for hereditary hemochromatosis: a clinical practice guideline from the American College of Physicians. *Ann Intern Med*. 2005;143:517–521. [PMID: 16204164]

▶ Treatment

Phlebotomy is the mainstay of treatment for iron overload. Initiation of therapeutic phlebotomy has been demonstrated to have significant survival benefit in patients with and without cirrhosis; phlebotomy should be started in those with an appropriate HH genotype, and either serum ferritin of at least 500 ng/mL (some recommend at least 1000 ng/mL), evidence of increased tissue iron on MRI (or biopsy) or evidence of tissue injury. The main contraindication to phlebotomy is severe anemia. Every four phlebotomy treatments remove approximately 1 g of iron. Although an optimal regimen has not been specified, early and rapid depletion of iron stores is the goal of therapy. Weekly phlebotomy is generally instituted in the early phase of treatment, with frequent monitoring of the hemoglobin as well as ferritin levels. In most cases, the therapeutic goal is a serum ferritin level less than 50 µg/L with some societies recommending even lower ferritin goals.

After initial depletion of iron stores, maintenance phlebotomy can be performed. A CBC and ferritin level should be checked in the months after induction phlebotomy is completed. If there is evidence of rising ferritin levels (without an alternative explanation) then maintenance phlebotomy should be pursued with a target ferritin range of 50–100 ng/mL; often this requires phlebotomy every 2–4 months. Some patients may reaccumulate iron very slowly, perhaps due to decreased iron absorption in the setting of proton pump inhibitor therapy or iron loss from chronic nonsteroidal anti-inflammatory drug (NSAID) use. If iron loss is suspected, appropriate investigation should be pursued, guided by the clinical circumstances. Maintaining appropriate follow-up is the key to avoiding the damaging long-term effects of iron deposition, avoiding cirrhosis, and improving overall survival.

With the general success and relatively low cost of phlebotomy, chelation therapy for HHC is rarely necessary. Subcutaneous desferrioxamine (1–2 g daily infused over 8 hours) is typically used when phlebotomy is contraindicated or in the case of specific cardiac disease that can be improved with aggressive iron depletion.

Certain lifestyle modifications are also important to counsel all patients with HHC about. Limiting alcohol consumption is important in protecting against worsening of liver related morbidity. From a dietary perspective, the major recommendation to patients is to avoid vitamins and supplements that include supplemental iron. Finally, in those with advanced hepatic fibrosis, it is important to screen patients for HCC, with ultrasound every 6 months.

▶ **Summary**

HFE-related hemochromatosis is the most common autosomal-recessive disorder in Caucasians with an incidence of approximately 1:260 persons. It remains underdiagnosed, although early diagnosis and treatment to deplete iron stores before the development of cirrhosis is associated with a normal life expectancy. In patients with cirrhosis at the time of diagnosis, depletion of hepatic iron stores reduces insulin requirement in patients with diabetes and improves survival when compared to untreated patients. The discovery of HFE has led to a rapid evolution of our understanding and management of this disease.

It now appears that hepcidin is the key regulator of iron homeostasis, influenced by multiple proteins, including HFE, TfR2, and HJV. Mutations in multiple genes may lead to the hemochromatosis phenotype. The unifying feature is iron overload that begins with early expansion of the plasma iron compartment, resulting from inappropriate release of iron from villus enterocytes and macrophages. Progressive parenchymal iron deposition ensues with the potential for severe organ damage.

The phenotypic expression of hemochromatosis may be influenced by multiple other host and environmental factors. For example, C282Y homozygotes experience increased rates of cirrhosis and a poorer prognosis when faced with added insults to the liver such as alcohol or NASH. In addition, patients with both HHC and hepatitis C have been found to be less responsive to treatment with combination interferon and ribavirin.

Areas for future investigation include further elucidation of the molecular mechanisms of action of hepcidin and the proteins that influence its production, including HFE, TfR2, HJV, and possibly others. Testing for the multiple genes implicated in the hemochromatosis phenotype may become commercially available in the foreseeable future. Potential therapeutic applications of our rapidly expanding knowledge of iron metabolism include administration of exogenous hepcidin, also known as hepcidin mimetics or minihepcidins, for the treatment of iron overload and hepcidin antagonists to treat anemia associated with chronic inflammatory states.

Camaschella C. Treating iron overload. *N Engl J Med.* 2013;368: 2325–2327.

Niederau C, Fischer R, Sonnenberg A, et al. Survival and causes of death in cirrhotic and in noncirrhotic patients with primary hemochromatosis. *N Engl J Med.* 1985;313:1256–1262. [PMID: 4058506]

Yen AW, Fancher TL, Bowlus CL. Revisiting hereditary hemochromatosis: current concepts and progress. *Am J Med.* 2006;119: 391–399. [PMID: 16651049]

WILSON DISEASE

 ESSENTIALS OF DIAGNOSIS

▶ Autosomally inherited disorder of copper metabolism first described by Samuel Alexander Kinnier Wilson in 1912.

▶ Estimated prevalence of the disease is 1 in 30,000 individuals.

▶ Genetic defect is a mutation in a P-type copper-dependent ATPase, ATP7B.

▶ Copper deposition in many tissues, with liver and neuropsychiatric disease the most prominent manifestations.

▶ Wilson disease should be considered in any young person with unexplained chronic hepatitis or cirrhosis, patients with family history of cirrhosis and in patients with a Coombs-negative hemolytic anemia. A diagnostic clue is the presence of a low alkaline phosphatase level, characteristic of Wilson disease.

▶ Diagnosis is challenging and requires measurement of serum ceruloplasmin levels, measurement of urinary copper, and an ophthalmic examination; all three tests are necessary as only 40% of patients have abnormalities in all three.

▶ Liver biopsy is often necessary to confirm the diagnosis and stage severity of disease.

General Considerations

Wilson disease is a rare disease of impaired biliary excretion of copper. It is an autosomal-recessive disorder with prevalence of approximately 1 in 30,000 persons. The defective gene is on chromosome 13 and has been identified as a copper-dependent P-type ATPase. Copper is a cofactor for many proteins and is obtained through dietary consumption. On average, humans consume between 1 and 5 mg/day of copper, far in excess of the daily physiologic requirement of around 0.9 mg/day. Copper absorption occurs in the small intestine (duodenum and proximal jejunum). Copper enters the portal circulation, mainly bound to albumin, and then is used for synthetic processes in the liver. Most excess copper is secreted into bile for subsequent fecal elimination with a minority excreted in the urine.

Ala A, Walker AP, Ashkan K, et al. Wilson's disease. *Lancet.* 2007;369:397–408. [PMID: 17276780]

Pathogenesis

The defective gene, *ATP7B*, encodes a transmembrane protein with two important physiologic roles: (1) transport of copper across the canalicular membrane into the biliary tract, and (2) transport of copper into the trans-Golgi network, where it complexes with apoceruloplasmin to form ceruloplasmin which is an acute phase reactant and copper-binding protein. When *ATP7B* is absent, copper accumulates within the lysosomes in the cell and is absent in the biliary secretions. This leads to accumulation of hepatocellular copper. Additionally, because copper is required for stability of ceruloplasmin, its serum half-life is markedly decreased in persons with Wilson disease. The low level of ceruloplasmin in patients with Wilson disease accounts for its use as a screening test.

Clinical Findings

Wilson disease is a disease of young people, manifesting with liver disease most commonly in the second and the third decades of life, with mean age at diagnosis of 13. It is unusual for Wilson disease to manifest after the age of 40 and when it does, neurologic complications are often the principal presenting symptoms. Copper deposition in hepatic tissue can lead to a spectrum of liver disease including chronic hepatitis, fulminant Wilson disease, and cirrhosis.

A. Chronic Hepatitis

Young patients presenting with Wilson disease may experience flares of hepatitis with spontaneous remission. These flares may be asymptomatic and a high level of awareness is necessary to prevent a delay in diagnosis and the development of cirrhosis and the other clinical manifestations of the disease are noted below.

B. Fulminant Disease

In fulminant Wilson disease there are marked elevations in serum transaminase levels, with the AST level often greater than the ALT (additional AST is present as a result of accompanying Coombs-negative hemolytic anemia). The serum alkaline phosphatase is characteristically below normal. The serum uric acid can also be low as a result of copper deposition in the kidneys leading to renal tubular acidosis and uricosuria. A coombs negative hemolytic anemia often accompanies acute liver failure; this is due to release of copper ions from hepatocyte necrosis and subsequent disruptive effects on the red blood cell membrane from excess free copper. Jaundice and liver failure invariably result, and the survival is almost always dependent on the patient undergoing liver transplantation.

C. Cirrhotic Disease

A more indolent form of liver disease results in cirrhosis. Patients may present with compensated disease or have significant evidence of hepatic dysfunction by the time of diagnosis. Peripheral stigmata or chronic liver disease such as palmar erythema and spider angiomata are often present. Clinical features of portal hypertension such as splenomegaly and ascites may be present.

D. Other Disease Manifestations

In addition to liver disease, patients with Wilson disease may have neurologic and psychiatric manifestations amongst the presenting features in 40–50% of patients. The resulting clinical manifestations occur as a result of copper deposition in many parts of the brain, including but not limited to the putamen, globus pallidus, caudate, and thalamus. Associated neurologic disorders include (1) a Parkinson-like movement disorder, (2) ataxia, (3) dystonia, and (4) tremors. A wing-beating tremor of the upper extremities and micrographia are other noteworthy manifestations of this disease. Patients often experience incoordination (eg, in writing, painting, playing the piano; rapid deterioration can ensue over a few months). Psychiatric manifestations may also occur and occasionally can dominate the presentation, with decline in performance status (eg, worsening school grades), mood and behavioral changes.

In addition to the liver and central nervous system, copper is deposited at other sites, leading to a range of disease manifestations. Deposition in the eye can result in Kayser-Fleischer rings and sunflower cataracts; both are visible on slit-lamp examinations. The former is a golden-brown pigment in the outside rim of the cornea, whereas the later is visualized as multicolored cataracts. Sunflower cataracts do not result in impaired vision. Deposition of copper also occurs in the kidneys, predominantly in the proximal tubules, where a Fanconi-like syndrome may manifest. Proximal renal tubular acidosis and nephrolithiasis are possible consequences. Chondrocalcinosis, osteomalacia, and osteoarthritis are also

Table 43–2. Clinical spectrum of Wilson disease.

Affected Organ	Clinical Manifestations
Liver	Chronic hepatitis Cirrhosis Fulminant liver failure
CNS	Spasticity and rigidity Ataxia Dystonia Tremors Behavioral changes Decreased performance status
Ophthalmic	Kayser-Fleischer rings Sunflower cataracts
Hematologic	Coombs-negative hemolytic anemia
Renal	Proximal renal tubular acidosis Nephrolithiasis Aminoaciduria Hypouricemia
Musculoskeletal	Chondrocalcinosis Osteoarthritis Osteomalacia Osteoporosis

CNS, central nervous system.

common in patients with Wilson disease. Table 43–2 summarizes the clinical spectrum of Wilson disease.

E. Diagnostic Tests

The diagnosis of Wilson disease is often challenging but is based on a combination of astute clinical suspicion and laboratory data. The disease should be suspected in any young person who presents with unexplained, chronic active hepatitis, or cirrhosis. Serum ceruloplasmin may be normal in approximately 20% of patients with Wilson disease because ceruloplasmin is an acute phase reactant and levels go up in pro-inflammatory states including chronic active hepatitis. Regardless, the initial screening test is the measurement of serum ceruloplasmin.

In patients with low ceruloplasmin or in whom there is a high-degree of clinical suspicion for Wilson disease, additional tests are needed for confirmation. These include slit-lamp examinations to look for Kayser-Fleischer rings and 24-hour urinary copper collection; a 24-hour urine copper of greater than 40 μg would be considered a positive test if Kayser-Fleischer rings are present and a level greater than 100 μg would be considered a positive test if Kayser-Fleischer rings are absent. Abnormalities in all three tests—low ceruloplasmin, Kayser-Fleischer rings on slit-lamp examination, and elevated urinary copper levels—are present in only about 40% of patients but would be diagnostic for Wilsons disease. However, in patients with

neuro-psychiatric manifestations of Wilson disease, 98% have Kayser-Fleischer rings.

When there is diagnostic uncertainty, a liver biopsy is sometimes necessary and may show histologic evidence of copper deposition within the liver. In addition, measurement of the hepatic tissue content of copper can show elevated copper levels (normally ~40 μg copper/g dry liver vs >250 μg copper/g dry liver in Wilson disease).

Increasingly, genetic testing has been adopted in patients with diagnostic uncertainty and in screening family members of those diagnosed with Wilson disease and where the specific mutations are known. While the genetic locus is known, a multitude of mutations that have been identified with the most common mutation, H1069Q, only present in approximately 30% of patients with Wilson disease. The majority of patients are compound heterozygotes and thus one mutation is suggestive of Wilson and two mutations more strongly indicates a diagnosis of Wilson.

The Leipzig scoring system with weighted points has also been created to help with diagnosis. Variables in the model include clinical manifestations (neuro-psychiatric manifestations, Kayser-Fleischer rings), biochemical testing (ceruloplasmin levels, presence of hemolytic anemia, urine copper levels and hepatic copper levels on biopsy), and mutational analysis (testing for ATP7B mutations).

Cho YH, Dong-Wook J, Sang-Yeoup L, et al. A case of Wilson's disease in patient with mildly elevated liver enzymcs. *Korean J Fam Med.* 2011;32(3):205–208. [PMID: 22745856]

Ferenci P, Caca K, Loudianos G, et al. Diagnosis and phenotypic classification of Wilson disease. *Liver Int.* 2003;23(3):139–142. [PMID: 12955875]

Ferenci P, Czlokowska A, Merle U, et al. Late-onset Wilson's disease. *Gastroenterology.* 2007;132:1294–1298. [PMID: 17433323]

Lin LJ, Wang DX, Ding NN, et al. Comprehensive analysis on clinical features of Wilson's disease: an experience over 28 years with 133 cases. *Neurol Res.* 2014;36(2):157–163. [PMID: 24107488]

Page RA, Davie CA, MacManus D, et al. Clinical correlation of brain MRI and MRS abnormalities in patients with Wilson disease. *Neurology.* 2004;63:638–643. [PMID: 15326235]

Roberts EA, Schilsky ML. Diagnosis and treatment of Wilson's disease: an update. *Hepatology.* 2008;47:2089–2111. [PMID: 18506894]

▶ Differential Diagnosis

The differential diagnosis of Wilson disease includes acute and chronic hepatitides and depends on the form of presentation. In patients with fulminant Wilson disease, acute toxic injury, acute viral hepatitis, acute vascular hepatic injury, and autoimmune hepatitis (AIH) should be considered. For those presenting with chronic hepatitis, considerations should include toxic injury, chronic viral hepatitis, nonalcoholic fatty liver disease, other inherited liver disorders, and AIH.

Table 43–3. Treatment of Wilson disease.

Agent	Initial Dose	Maintenance Dose	Comment
Penicillamine	Adult: 250–500 mg/day to maximum of 1200–1500 mg/day in 2–4 divided doses Children: 20 mg/kg/day	Adult: 750–1000 mg/day in 2 divided doses	Give 1 hour before or 2 hours after eating Many possible acute-onset and delayed side effects Monitor: complete blood count, proteinuria Give vitamin B$_6$, 50 mg weekly
Trientine	Adult: 1200–800 mg/day in 2–3 divided doses Children: 20 mg/kg/day	Adult: 900–1200 mg/day in 2–3 divided doses	Give 1 hour before or 2 hours after eating Fewer side effects than penicillamine Safety in pregnancy unclear
Zinc	150 mg (elemental) in 3 divided doses	Same	Safe in pregnancy Some preparations may cause gastrointestinal upset

▶ Treatment

Treatment of nonfulminant Wilson disease is geared toward mobilizing and eliminating accumulated tissue copper (Table 43–3). At the same time, attempts should be made to prevent further excess copper absorption through the gastrointestinal tract. The first goal is accomplished by the use of chelating agents such as D-penicillamine and trientine. These agents bind tissue copper and then lead to elimination through the urinary tract. The second goal is enabled by Zinc therapy and dietary modification

D-Penicillamine is the drug of choice, although its use is sometimes limited by side effects. These include allergic hypersensitivity reactions, proteinuria, immunosuppression, and a plethora of dermatologic changes. D-Penicillamine also interferes with the metabolism of pyridoxine, so it is customary to co-prescribe vitamin B$_6$.

The majority of patients respond favorably to D-penicillamine therapy and dramatic but slow improvement of neurologic symptoms can ensue. Effectiveness of chelation therapy is often tracked by closely monitoring urine copper levels. In patients who are unable to tolerate D-penicillamine, trientine should be used. Zinc, which competes with copper for intestinal absorption and therefore reduces the amount of copper that can be absorbed, is also a widely used therapeutic choice. Recent studies suggest that zinc monotherapy is not as effective as the chelating agents in preventing hepatic deterioration in patients with Wilson disease; however, zinc can have a role in maintenance therapy once chelation has been used to decrease copper stores. For those patients in whom zinc is used, many preparations are available, and gastrointestinal upset has been associated especially with the acetate form. A new medication, Ammonium tetrathiomolybdate, is currently under investigation and may disrupt the current treatment paradigm based on the results of a clinical trial currently underway.

In addition to pharmacologic maintenance therapy, dietary instructions should stress the avoidance of foods that are rich in copper. These foods include liver, chocolate, shellfish, and nuts. Since the disease is inherited as an autosomal-recessive trait and characterized by a high consanguinity rate, all siblings, children, and blood relatives of a patient with Wilson disease should be appropriately screened.

In patients with fulminant hepatic failure, medical therapy is usually ineffective and liver transplantation is the definitive treatment. Outcomes for patients with fulminant hepatic failure or cirrhosis secondary to Wilson disease who undergo liver transplantation are excellent. Furthermore, liver transplantation is thought to be curative for Wilson disease and no further targeted therapy is required for Wilson after transplantation.

Arnon R, Annunziato R, Schilsky M, et al. Liver transplantation for children with Wilson disease: comparison of outcomes between children and adults. *Clin Transplant.* 2011;25(1):E52–E60. [PMID: 20946468]

Roberts EA, Schilsky ML. Diagnosis and treatment of Wilson's disease: an update. *Hepatology.* 2008;47:2089–2111. [PMID: 18506894]

Weiss KH, Gotthardt DN, Klemm D, et al. Zinc monotherapy is not as effective as chelating agents in the treatment of Wilson's Disease. *Gastroenterology.* 2011;140:1189–1198.

α$_1$-ANTITRYPSIN DEFICIENCY

ESSENTIALS OF DIAGNOSIS

▶ Autosomal codominant disease resulting from defects in the *SERPINA1* gene.

▶ Produces a spectrum of disease; liver, lung, hematologic, and dermatologic manifestations are possible.

▶ Liver complications most often result from deposition of a poorly degradable mutant of α$_1$-antitrypsin (α$_1$-AT) in hepatocytes.

▶ Diagnosis is through measurement of serum α_1-AT levels followed by pi-typing for mutant alleles.

▶ Liver biopsy shows characteristic PAS-positive granules that are resistant to diastase.

General Considerations

α_1-AT deficiency is an autosomal codominant disease that affects about 1 in 2000–5000 persons. It is most common in people of northern European descent.

Stoller JK, Aboussouan LS. Alpha1-antitrypsin deficiency. *Lancet.* 2005;365:2225–2236. [PMID: 15978931]

Pathogenesis

α_1-AT is a elastase inhibitor. To date more than 100 mutant alleles of the culprit *SERPINA1* gene have been identified and implicated in lung, liver, or hematologic disease. The alleles are characterized phenotypically on the basis of their migration on pH gradient gels, with faster migrating variants, A (anodal), to slower migrating variants, Z. Individuals with ZZ alleles have severe deficiency of α_1-AT.

Functionally, α_1-AT alleles can be categorized into four major groups:

1. Normal, with α_1-AT levels of greater than 80 mg/dL.
2. Deficiency alleles characterized by serum α_1-AT levels of less than 80 mg/dL or decreased activity (eg, Z alleles). The Z allele is the most common deficiency variant, accounting for 95% of all α_1-AT deficiency. A single mutation of lysine to glutamate at position 342 is responsible.
3. Null variants in which there is a complete lack of circulating α_1-AT.
4. Dysfunctional variants in which the mutant protein results in a novel function, such as the *Pittsburgh* allele, which acts as a thrombin inhibitor (Table 41–7).

The pathogenesis of pulmonary disease in patients with α_1-AT deficiency, often early onset emphysema, is driven by the lack of the α_1-AT elastase inhibitor which leads to increased elastase activity and lung destruction; therefore, it is a loss of function that leads to pulmonary disease. In contrast to this, liver disease is caused by accumulation of Z-type α_1-AT molecule polymers in hepatocytes, and is not related to the actual function of α_1-AT. For instance, in patients with null-null mutations (no α_1-AT produced), they are at highest risk of lung manifestations but do not develop liver disease as there is no protein to accumulate in hepatocytes (Table 43–4).

Lomas DA, Mahadeva R. Alpha 1-antitrypsin polymerization and the serpinopathies: pathobiology and prospects for therapy. *J Clin Invest.* 2002;110:1585–1590. [PMID: 12464660]

Teckman JH, Jain A. Advances in Alph-1-antitrypsindeficiency liver disease. *Curr Gastroenterol Rep.* 2014;16:367.

Clinical Findings

A. Symptoms & Signs

α_1-AT deficiency causes several significant chronic clinical problems, including emphysema, which occurs mostly in the fourth and fifth decades of life as a result of unopposed activity of leukocyte elastase. This lung disease is accelerated in patients who smoke. A second clinical entity is panniculitis, which is characterized by the appearance of painful cutaneous nodules at sites of trauma. Additionally, a coagulopathy can occur in persons who have the *Pittsburgh* allele, as noted earlier, due to its antithrombin effects.

Chronic liver disease, unlike the associated lung disease, occurs due to accumulation of an insoluble and nondegraded mutant protein within hepatocytes. The spectrum of liver abnormalities includes chronic hepatitis, cirrhosis, and HCC. Among the patients with chronic hepatitis, the risk of cirrhosis has been estimated at between 12% and 50%. More than 25% of those with neonatal hepatitis die in the first decade of life and presenting symptoms vary but can include hepatomegaly, jaundice, ascites, and bleeding.

B. Laboratory Findings

Evaluation of α_1-AT levels is usually the first step in the diagnostic workup of patients with suspected α_1-AT deficiency. For individuals with low circulating levels of α_1-AT, pi-typing

Table 43–4. α_1-AT phenotypes & corresponding α_1-AT serum levels.

Phenotype	Level (mg/dL)	Risk of Lung Disease	Risk of Liver Disease
PiMM	104–250	Normal	Normal
PiMZ	60–180	Generally normal	Slightly increased
PiSS	78–170	Generally normal	Normal
PiSZ	40–119	Slightly increased	Slightly increased
PiZZ	13–36	High	High
Null-null	0.0	High	No risk

is then performed to look for abnormal alleles that might lead either to lack of or for abnormal forms of α_1-AT. Caution should be used in interpreting α_1-AT levels in settings of acute inflammation as it is an acute phase reactant and thus maybe falsely elevated in such conditions. The gold standard for diagnosis of α_1-AT deficiency is the analysis of the phenotype of the α_1-AT protein in the patient's serum. For patients with liver disease, histologic evaluation of the liver biopsy samples shows the presence of globules that are periodic acid-Schiff–positive and diastase-resistant.

American Thoracic Society/European Respiratory Society statement: standards for the diagnosis and management of individuals with alpha-1 antitrypsin deficiency. *Am J Respir Crit Care Med.* 2003;168:818–900. [PMID: 14522813]

Differential Diagnosis

The differential diagnosis is the same as for the other forms of chronic hepatitis discussed earlier. α_1-AT deficiency should be considered in certain patients with emphysema (young patients, those without a history of smoking, basilar pattern), those with unexplained liver disease, or in those with a family history of liver or lung disease.

Treatment

Management of α_1-AT deficiency is based on screening, treating, and preventing complications of end-stage liver disease such as variceal bleeding, malnutrition, ascites, and HCC. Patients should be counselled to avoid smoking and alcohol. Screening for HCC is unclear. HCC can occur in patients with α_1-AT deficiency with or without cirrhosis. It is recommended to perform HCC screening every 6 months with ultrasound for all patients with α_1-AT deficiency with cirrhosis. Some guidelines suggest annual ultrasound for HCC screening in patients with α_1-AT deficiency without cirrhosis. For patients with emphysema, recombinant α_1-AT can be used. However, the only effective therapy for advanced cirrhosis secondary to α_1-AT deficiency is transplantation.

A potential future therapy, carbamazepine, is currently in human trials. In a mouse model of liver disease caused by aggregates of misfolded α_1-AT in liver, the burden of misfolded protein and the degree of liver fibrosis can be reduced by the use the autophagy-enhancing drug carbamazepine.

Hidvegi T, Ewing M, Hale P, et al. An autophagy-enhancing drug promotes degradation of mutant alpha1-antitrypsin Z and reduces hepatic fibrosis. *Science.* 2010;329:229–232. [PMID: 20522742]

Perlmutter D. Alpha-1-antitrypsin deficiency: importance of proteasomal and autophagic degradative pathways in disposal of liver disease-associated protein aggregates. *Annu Rev Med.* 2011;62:333–345. [PMID: 20707674]

Sandhaus RA, Turino G, Brantly ML, et al. The diagnosis and management of alpha-1 antitrypsin deficiency in the adult. *Chronic Obstr Pulm Dis.* 2016;3(3):668–682. [PMID 28490420]

Alcohol-Associated Liver Disease

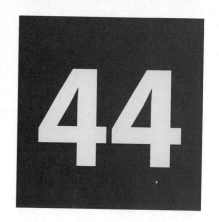

Alexander S Vogel, MD

Gyorgy Baffy, MD, PhD

ESSENTIALS OF DIAGNOSIS

▶ Harmful alcohol consumption is defined as more than 4 drinks on any single day or more than 14 drinks per week for men, while for women the threshold is more than 3 drinks on any single day or more than 7 drinks per week.

▶ In the United States, a standard drink is defined as any drink that contains about 14 g of pure ethyl alcohol.

▶ More than 60% of adult Americans consume alcohol in a more or less regular fashion, and it is estimated that 18 million Americans have an alcohol use disorder.

▶ The spectrum of alcohol-associated liver disease ranges from steatosis to cirrhosis, while alcohol-associated hepatitis may occur episodically as acute or acute-on-chronic liver injury.

▶ Virtually everyone with excessive alcohol intake has steatosis, while 10–15% of the affected population develop cirrhosis and 10–35% develop one or more episodes of symptomatic alcohol-associated hepatitis.

▶ Patients with alcohol-associated liver disease are at increased risk of hepatocellular carcinoma with an incidence rate of 1–2% per year among patients with cirrhosis.

▶ Alcohol-induced liver injury is suggested by moderately increased serum aspartate aminotransferase (AST) and alanine aminotransferase (ALT) levels with an AST/ALT ratio exceeding 2.0.

General Considerations

Alcohol (ethyl alcohol, ethanol, CH_3CH_2OH) is one of the most common hepatotoxic agents and humans have consumed it since prehistoric times. Alcohol-associated liver disease develops in virtually everyone who is engaged in excessive use of alcohol, although the severity of hepatic injury may vary considerably. While steatosis is almost always present, alcohol-associated liver disease evolves into cirrhosis in 10–15% of those that have sustained heavy alcohol use. Patients with advanced alcohol-associated liver disease are also at risk of hepatocellular carcinoma, which may develop with an annual risk of 1–2%. The natural course of alcohol-associated liver disease may be complicated by episodes of symptomatic alcohol-associated hepatitis, which occurs in 10–35% of patients with excessive alcohol consumption. This wide spectrum of alcohol-associated liver disease outcomes is a result of the complex interplay between variables including the amount of alcohol consumed, the pattern of drinking, individual genetic predisposition, and the presence of comorbidities.

A. Epidemiology

In the United States, the population aged 15 years and older had an annual per capita alcohol consumption of 9.2 L of pure alcohol between 2008 and 2010. More than 60% of adult Americans consume alcohol in a more or less regular manner and it is estimated that 18 million Americans have an alcohol use disorder, classified as either abuse or dependence. Epidemiologic studies have established a dose-effect relationship between alcohol intake and alcohol-induced liver damage. While any amount of alcohol could have adverse health effects, epidemiologic evidence supports recommendations for a threshold amount of regularly consumed alcohol above which the risk of physical and mental health impairment is increased. In the United States, harmful alcohol consumption has been defined as more than 4 drinks on any single day or more than 14 drinks per week for men, while for women the threshold is more than 3 drinks on any single day or more than 7 drinks per week. In this schema, a standard drink denotes any drink that contains about 14 g of pure alcohol.

B. Societal Costs

Alcohol consumption has a profound economic and health impact, with more than 200 health conditions and an estimated 5.1% of the global burden of disease attributable to the consumption of alcohol. In 2016, the World Health Organization estimated that 3 million fatalities, or 5.3% of all deaths world-wide, were linked to harmful use of alcohol. Alcohol represents the third largest cause of disability in the United States with an estimated overall cost exceeding $234 billion or 2.7% of the GDP in 2012. Furthermore, as of 2019, with prevalence of alcohol-associated liver disease rising and improved therapies for hepatitis C, alcohol-associated liver disease is now the leading etiology of liver disease for those on the liver transplant waitlist.

Moon AM, Yang JY, Barritt AS, et al. Rising mortality from alcohol-associated liver disease in the United States in the 21st century. *Am J Gastroenterol*. 2020;115:79–87. [PMID: 31688021]

O'Shea RS, Dasarathy S, McCullough AJ. Alcoholic liver disease. *Hepatology*. 2010;51:307–328. [PMID: 20034030]

Shirazi F, Singal AK, Wong RJ. Alcohol-associated cirrhosis and alcoholic hepatitis hospitalization trends in the United States. *J Clin Gastroenterol*. 2021;55(2):174–179. [PMID: 32520887]

Singal AK, Arora S, Wong RJ, Satapathy SK, Shah VH, Kuo YF, Kamath PS. Increasing burden of acute-on-chronic liver failure among alcohol-associated liver disease in the young population in the United States. *Am J Gastroenterol*. 2020;115:88–95. [PMID: 31651447]

Wong RJ, Singal AK. Trends in liver disease etiology among adults awaiting liver transplantation in the United States, 2014-2019. *JAMA Network Open*. 2020;3(2):e1920294. [PMID: 32022875]

World Health Organization. Global status report on alcohol and health, 2018. Geneva, Switzerland, 2018.

▶ Pathogenesis

A. Risk Factors & Comorbidities

In most cases, excessive alcohol consumption is associated with steatosis only, suggesting the importance of individual risk factors in the development of advanced liver disease such as alcohol-associated hepatitis and cirrhosis. Sex, race, ethnicity, and socioeconomic factors appear to have a major impact on the degree of alcohol-induced hepatotoxicity. Ample evidence indicates that women are more susceptible to the hepatotoxic effects of alcohol than are men, and this has been linked to gender differences in the metabolism of alcohol. In women, higher body fat content results in lower volume of distribution and delayed elimination of alcohol, while lower gastric acetaldehyde dehydrogenase activity may allow increased delivery of alcohol to the portal circulation. Several observations suggest the role of race and ethnicity in the severity and progression of alcohol-associated liver disease. For instance, mortality rates of alcohol-associated cirrhosis in the United States are highest among white Hispanic

males and black non-Hispanic females. Importantly, socioeconomic factors may contribute to these ethnic differences by affecting at-risk drinking behavior and limiting access to health care.

Twin studies in which alcohol-associated cirrhosis was more prevalent among monozygotic than dizygotic twin pairs support the role of genetic factors in alcohol-associated liver disease. Individual susceptibility to alcohol-induced hepatotoxicity may be modified by single nucleotide polymorphisms (SNPs) of genes involved in the regulation of alcohol metabolism, lipid storage and utilization, oxidative stress and inflammation, and the development of addiction.

Harmful effects of excessive alcohol consumption may be significantly enhanced by the presence of coexisting chronic liver disease, resulting in faster disease progression and worse disease outcomes. Alcohol-associated liver disease increasingly co-occurs with nonalcoholic fatty liver disease (NAFLD) due to the dramatically rising prevalence of obesity and diabetes. Among 1604 French patients with biopsy-proven alcohol-associated liver disease, those that were overweight or obese for at least 10 years had an independently increased risk of developing cirrhosis with an odds ratio of 2.5. In an American single-center study, diabetes was associated with a 10-fold higher risk of developing hepatocellular carcinoma among individuals with heavy alcohol consumption. Similarly, the pathogenic synergy between alcohol and chronic hepatitis C can result in increased hepatitis C virus (HCV) replication, impaired dendritic cell function, and diminished interferon response, supporting the emergence of HCV quasispecies and promoting increased rates of fibrosis and hepatocarcinogenesis.

Alcohol consumption appears to also increase the risk of acetaminophen-induced liver injury. This is because alcohol augments the accumulation of N-acetyl-p-benzoquinoneimine (NAPQI), the hepatotoxic metabolite of acetaminophen, by stimulating its production via the cytochrome P450 isoenzyme 2E1 (CYP2E1) and blocking its elimination by depleting intracellular glutathione stores. It is therefore recommended that the daily dose of acetaminophen should not exceed 2 g for those who drink alcohol. Similar dose reduction is advisable in the setting of cirrhosis even in the absence of ongoing alcohol consumption.

B. Alcohol Metabolism

Alcohol is mostly metabolized in the liver into the highly toxic acetaldehyde by cytosolic alcohol dehydrogenase (ADH) and to a lesser extent by the microsomal ethanol oxidizing system (MEOS). Acetaldehyde is a highly toxic molecule that may covalently bind to various macromolecules and activate the innate immune response by novel epitopes of protein adducts and other damage-associated molecular patterns (DAMPs). Moreover, mitochondrial catabolism of acetaldehyde shifts the redox balance and interferes with lipid utilization pathways, leading to hepatic steatosis. Microsomal oxidation of alcohol occurs primarily through CYP2E1, which is markedly

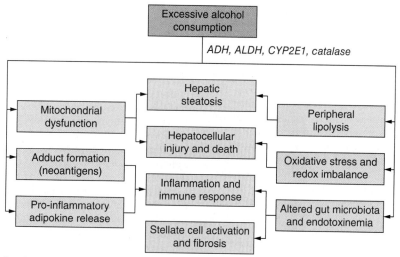

▲ **Figure 44–1.** Pathophysiology of alcohol-associated liver disease. This schematic diagram illustrates molecular mechanisms promoted by the intake and metabolism of alcohol in the liver, adipose tissue, and gastrointestinal tract (*Purple boxes*), contributing to characteristic pathologic changes in alcohol-associated liver disease (*gray boxes*).

induced by chronic alcohol consumption and contributes to the generation of intracellular free oxygen radicals.

Chronic alcohol consumption interferes with insulin-mediated regulation of peripheral lipolysis, contributing to hepatic lipid accumulation. Moreover, metabolism of alcohol by enteral bacteria may increase local acetaldehyde levels and weaken the integrity of mucosal tight junctions, promoting intestinal permeability and increasing the absorption of endotoxin or lipopolysaccharide (LPS). The increased portal levels of LPS and other pathogen-associated molecular patterns (PAMPs) then activate Kupffer cells and contribute to the liver inflammatory response. Major mechanisms in the pathophysiology of alcohol-associated liver disease are summarized in Figure 44–1.

Albano E. Role of adaptive immunity in alcoholic liver disease. *Int J Hepatol.* 2012;2012:893026. [PMID: 22229098]

Beier JI, McClain CJ. Mechanisms and cell signaling in alcoholic liver disease. *Biol Chem.* 2010;391:1249–1264. [PMID: 20868231]

Cederbaum AI. Alcohol metabolism. *Clin Liver Dis.* 2012;16:667–685. [PMID: 23101976]

Chen P, Schnabl B. Host-microbiome interactions in alcoholic liver disease. *Gut Liver.* 2014;8:237–241. [PMID: 24827618]

Grittner U, Kuntsche S, Graham K, Bloomfield K. Social inequalities and gender differences in the experience of alcohol-related problems. *Alcohol Alcohol.* 2012;47:597–605. [PMID: 22542707]

Hassan MM, Hwang LY, Hatten CJ, et al. Risk factors for hepatocellular carcinoma: synergism of alcohol with viral hepatitis and diabetes mellitus. *Hepatology.* 2002;36:1206–1213. [PMID: 12395331]

Stickel F, Hampe J. Genetic determinants of alcoholic liver disease. *Gut.* 2012;61:150–159. [PMID: 22110053]

► Clinical Findings

A. Symptoms & Signs

Steatosis is by far the most common manifestation of alcohol-associated liver disease, with few clinically discernible findings. Severe fatty infiltration of the liver may cause fatigue, anorexia, nausea, and right upper quadrant abdominal discomfort. Persistent exposure of the liver to the hepatotoxic effects of alcohol can lead to the development of cirrhosis. This process usually takes many years or decades and the insidious progression may occur without significant clinical features. However, once established, cirrhosis is associated with a multitude of clinical symptoms and signs. Patients may complain of fatigue, anorexia, weakness, insomnia, decreased sexual drive, peripheral neuropathy, and fluid retention with lower extremity edema and increased abdominal girth. Physical examination often reveals palmar erythema, spider nevi, Dupuytren contracture, atrophic glossitis, parotid gland enlargement, gynecomastia, testicular atrophy, and peripheral muscle wasting.

Development of portal hypertension in alcohol-associated cirrhosis is indicated by splenomegaly, ascites, and the formation of portosystemic collaterals in the form of gastroesophageal or rectal varices and the presence of engorged veins in the abdominal wall arranged either in a palisade pattern or centered at the umbilicus ("*caput Medusae*"). Occasionally alcohol-associated cirrhosis only comes to clinical attention at a more advanced stage in the form of a major health event, such as acute hepatic encephalopathy, gastrointestinal bleeding from varices, spontaneous bacterial peritonitis, and hepatorenal syndrome. Importantly, these clinical and diagnostic features are not specific to alcohol-associated liver disease and may occur in cirrhosis of any etiology.

B. Laboratory Findings & Imaging Studies

Liver function tests typically remain normal in alcohol-induced steatosis with the exception of mild elevations in serum levels of AST, ALT, and γ-glutamyl transpeptidase. Macrocytic anemia may also be seen in patients with alcohol abuse due to multiple mechanisms including nutritional deficiencies and the effect of alcohol on bone marrow function. Similarly, alcohol-associated cirrhosis may reveal limited laboratory findings and preserved synthetic function in the early and compensated stages. Progression of alcohol-associated cirrhosis results in worsening synthetic dysfunction and increasingly severe manifestations of portal hypertension that can be monitored by the Child-Turcotte-Pugh score, a composite index of the functional stage calculated from the serum albumin, serum bilirubin, prothrombin time, quantity of ascites, and degree of hepatic encephalopathy or the Model for End-stage Liver Disease (MELD) score which is a composite of serum bilirubin, prothrombin time, and creatinine with or without sodium.

Right upper quadrant ultrasound may confirm the presence of fatty liver and exclude other causes of abnormal liver tests in a patient with excessive use of alcohol. At more advanced stages, abdominal imaging studies may reveal cirrhosis by describing a small, nodular liver and the presence of portosystemic collaterals. Elastography can also be used to assess for increased liver stiffness which is often suggestive of underlying fibrosis. Hepatocellular carcinoma typically presents as an arterially enhancing mass with delayed hypointensity ("washout") on magnetic resonance imaging or hepatic protocol "triple-phase" computed tomography scans. This highly sensitive and specific diagnostic feature obviates the need for histologic confirmation of hepatocellular carcinoma in the majority of cases.

C. Histologic Assessment

The histologic presence of fibrosis or early cirrhosis is an important determinant of the long-term prognosis in alcohol-associated liver disease. While liver biopsy remains the "gold standard," this diagnostic approach is rarely needed today as many reliable noninvasive markers have become available to estimate the degree of fibrosis. Imaging methods for additional assessment of liver fibrosis include ultrasound-based and magnetic resonance elastography. These methods have been repeatedly validated in chronic liver disease of various origins.

Chrostek L, Panasiuk A. Liver fibrosis markers in alcoholic liver disease. *World J Gastroenterol.* 2014;20:8018–8023. [PMID: 25009372]

Lucey MR. Alcohol-associated cirrhosis. *Clin Liver Dis.* 2019;23(1): 115–126. [PMID: 30454826]

Moreno C, Mueller S, Szabo G. Non-invasive diagnosis and biomarkers in alcohol-related liver disease. *J Hepatol.* 2019;70:273–283. [PMID: 30658728]

Tsochatzis EA, Bosch J, Burroughs AK. Liver cirrhosis. *Lancet.* 2014;383:1749–1761. [PMID: 24480518]

▶ Differential Diagnosis

It may be challenging to identify alcohol as the primary cause of liver disease in a given patient. Major factors that complicate the diagnosis include recall bias, surreptitious drinking, variable definitions of excess alcohol consumption, and the presence of overlapping liver conditions. While fatty liver has numerous causative factors, NAFLD is by far the most important condition to consider in the differential diagnosis of alcohol-induced steatosis. Careful clinical history taking to address the extent and regularity of alcohol consumption, identification of components of the metabolic syndrome, and measurement of cytokines and cell death markers may help distinguish between alcohol-related and other etiologies. However, as the prevalence of NAFLD parallels the obesity epidemic, co-occurrence of the two conditions is becoming increasingly common. Disease entities that should be considered in the differential diagnosis of various manifestations of alcohol-associated liver disease are listed in Table 44–1.

Sowa JP, Atmaca O, Kahraman A, et al. Non-invasive separation of alcoholic and non-alcoholic liver disease with predictive modeling. *PLoS One.* 2014;9:e101444. [PMID: 24988316]

Subramaniyan V, Chakravarthi S, Jegasothy R, et al. Alcohol-associated liver disease: a review on its pathophysiology, diagnosis and drug therapy. *Toxicol Rep.* 2021;8:376–385. [PMID: 33680863]

Table 44–1. Differential diagnosis of alcohol-associated liver disease.

Form of Alcohol-associated Liver Disease	Condition with Similar Appearance
Alcohol-associated steatosis	Isolated ("simple") nonalcoholic fatty liver Drug-induced steatosis Chronic hepatitis C
Alcohol-associated hepatitis	Nonalcoholic steatohepatitis Acute hepatitis B or C Choledocholithiasis Chronic pancreatitis with obstructive jaundice Pancreatobiliary neoplasms Drug-induced liver injury Wilson disease

Alcohol-associated cirrhosis	Cirrhosis associated with any of the following:
	  Nonalcoholic fatty liver disease
	  Chronic hepatitis B or C
	  Hereditary hemochromatosis
	  Primary biliary cirrhosis
	  Autoimmune hepatitis

▶ Treatment

A. Management of Alcohol Use Disorder

Abstinence has remarkable benefits in altering the course of alcohol-associated liver disease as there is good evidence that discontinuation of alcohol consumption may halt the progression of cirrhosis and result in longer survival. It is therefore absolutely critical to aim for sustained abstinence. Patients with at-risk drinking can be identified by asking how often they have exceeded the daily threshold of moderate- or "low"-risk drinking in the previous year. A useful approach to screen for alcohol misuse is the AUDIT-C questionnaire, which develops a score based on the following three questions: (1) how often did you have a drink containing alcohol in the past year?, (2) how many drinks containing alcohol did you have on a typical day when you were drinking in the past year?, and (3) how often did you have six or more drinks on one occasion in the past year? A positive score is highly suggestive of harmful alcohol use. The AUDIT-C has been found to perform better than the CAGE questionnaire in screening for alcohol misuse. Successful rehabilitation from alcohol addiction is difficult and usually requires mental health expertise and complex cognitive-behavioral modification strategies delivered in structured and stepwise programs. However, the essential first step is identifying at-risk patients via routine screening when patients interface with the medical field.

There are a number of potential pharmacotherapeutic options available for managing alcohol dependence and relapse prevention. The three FDA-approved agents for alcohol use disorders are disulfiram (an acetaldehyde dehydrogenase inhibitor), naltrexone (an opioid receptor antagonist), and acamprosate (an N-methyl-D-aspartate receptor antagonist). Of these, only acamprosate is not metabolized by the liver and is generally thought to be safe in those with underlying liver disease. Another agent, baclofen (a gamma-aminobutyric acid type b receptor agonist) is the only agent that has been tested via a randomized controlled trial specifically in those with alcohol use disorder and alcohol-associated cirrhosis; in this trial baclofen was shown to have a modest benefit with increased rates of achieving and maintaining abstinence. Current guidance suggests that one can consider either acamprosate or baclofen in patients with alcohol-associated liver disease for relapse prevention.

B. Lifestyle Modification & Other Measures

There are no specific dietary recommendations in alcohol-associated liver disease with the exception of keeping a healthy, balanced diet and observing salt restriction once cirrhosis is diagnosed. This lifestyle modification is important in the setting of cirrhosis due to increased sodium avidity and fluid retention, with the ultimate risk of ascites formation and development of the hepatorenal syndrome. While one should avoid the intake of large amounts of protein for fear of hepatic encephalopathy, significant protein restriction is counterproductive in the setting of impaired nutrition and sarcopenia typically seen in cirrhosis. Regular physical exercise may help prevent or delay peripheral muscle wasting.

In more advanced stages of cirrhosis, medical therapy is mostly supportive and follows established protocols. These include the use of nonselective β-blockers for the primary prophylaxis of esophageal variceal bleeding; combination of loop diuretics (eg, furosemide) and aldosterone antagonists (eg, spironolactone) in patients with ascites for managing fluid retention; and administration of lactulose with or without rifaximin for the prevention and management of hepatic encephalopathy.

C. Liver Transplantation

In advanced stages of cirrhosis, liver transplantation is the ultimate hope for survival with regained quality of life. Currently, alcohol-associated liver disease and NAFLD are the most common indications for liver transplantation. Liver transplants performed in alcohol-associated cirrhosis yield survival rates that routinely exceed 95% in the first year. However, long-term survival rates can be much less favorable, which is likely related to recurrent alcohol use, smoking, cardiovascular complications, and de novo malignancies. Unfortunately, 20–50% of transplanted patients resume some degree of drinking (so-called "slips") and 10–15% will eventually return to heavy drinking, causing disease recurrence and jeopardizing allograft survival. Careful assessment of a patient's addiction history is critical in the selection process and close monitoring post-transplant is essential.

D. Screening for Hepatocellular Carcinoma

Cirrhosis secondary to alcohol-associated liver disease has long been associated with increased risk of hepatocellular carcinoma, although the incidence rates are significantly less than those seen in chronic hepatitis C. A Danish study analyzed a nationwide cohort of 8482 patients with alcohol-associated cirrhosis and found that the yearly incidence of hepatocellular carcinoma was no more than 1%, which is less than the risk threshold of 1.5% per year recommended by major professional societies to justify liver cancer screening. Of note, several recent reports have given evidence that the development of hepatocellular carcinoma is influenced by synergistic effects of alcohol consumption with the HCV as well as with obesity and diabetes, findings which may have implications for future screening guidelines.

Addolorato G, Mirijello A, Barrio P, Gual A. Treatment of alcohol use disorders in patients with alcoholic liver disease. *J Hepatol.* 2016;65:618–630. [PMID: 27155530]

Bradley KA, DeBenedetti AF, Wolk RJ, Williams EC, Frank D, Kivlahan DR. AUDIT-C as a brief screen for alcohol misuse in primary care. *Alcohol Clin Exp Res.* 2007;31:1208–1217. [PMID: 17451397]

Crabb DW, Im GY, Szabo G, Mellinger JL, Lucey MR. Diagnosis and treatment of alcohol-associated liver diseases: 2019 practice guidance from the American Association for the Study of Liver Diseases. *Hepatology*. 2020;71(1):306–333. [PMID: 31314133]

Cotter TG, Rinella M. Nonalcoholic fatty liver disease 2020: the state of the disease. *Gastroenterology*. 2020;158:1851–1864. [PMID: 32061595]

Goldberg D, Ditah IC, Saeian K, et al. Changes in the prevalence of hepatitis C virus infection, nonalcoholic steatohepatitis and alcoholic liver disease among patients with cirrhosis or liver failure on the waitlist for liver transplantation. *Gastroenterology*. 2017;152:1090–1099. [PMID: 28088461]

Jepsen P, Ott P, Andersen PK, Sorensen HT, Vilstrup H. Risk for hepatocellular carcinoma in patients with alcoholic cirrhosis: a Danish nationwide cohort study. *Ann Intern Med*. 2012;156: 841–847, W295. [PMID: 22711076]

Lucey MR, Singal AK. Integrated treatment of alcohol use disorder in patients with alcohol-associated liver disease: an evolving story. *Hepatology*. 2020;71:1891–1893. [PMID: 32171034]

Morgan TR, Mandayam S, Jamal MM. Alcohol and hepatocellular carcinoma. *Gastroenterology*. 2004;127:S87–S96. [PMID: 15508108]

Alcohol-associated Hepatitis

Symptomatic alcohol-associated hepatitis occurs in up to one-third of patients with excess alcohol consumption. Alcohol-associated hepatitis is an acute illness that typically develops in response to the consumption of persistently large amounts of alcohol (>120 g/day) for a considerable amount of time. Alcohol-associated hepatitis can occur as a single or recurrent episode at any stage of alcohol-associated liver disease.

A. Symptoms & Signs

Clinically significant alcohol-associated hepatitis commonly presents with jaundice, fever, nausea, anorexia, generalized edema, and right upper quadrant abdominal pain with tender hepatosplenomegaly. In severe cases, in particular if complicated by cirrhosis, synthetic and vascular liver health may precipitously deteriorate, resulting in coagulopathy, ascites formation, variceal bleeding, and hepatic encephalopathy. Alcohol-associated hepatitis may be complicated by acute renal injury and multiorgan failure, resulting in 30-day mortality rates that reach 60%.

B. Laboratory Findings & Imaging Studies

Serum transaminase levels are elevated in symptomatic alcohol-associated hepatitis, but they rarely exceed 300 units/L. The ratio of AST and ALT is usually greater than 2.0, a pattern known as the de Ritis quotient. It is caused by the preferential release of mitochondrial AST and a diminished presence of ALT due to pyridoxal 5'-phosphate deficiency, and is highly suggestive of alcohol-induced hepatotoxicity. Serum bilirubin levels may become markedly elevated in alcohol-associated hepatitis as a result of direct hepatocellular damage, although

intrahepatic cholestasis may also develop indicated by simultaneously increasing alkaline phosphatase levels. Elevated leukocytosis is also often present on presentation, likely secondary to inflammation but can also be secondary to concomitant infection. Rapidly declining serum albumin and prolonged prothrombin time indicate a guarded prognosis. Similarly, deterioration of renal function may herald the development of hepatorenal syndrome, multiorgan failure, and poor outcomes.

Right upper quadrant ultrasound may help in excluding biliary obstruction, assess the degree of portal hypertension, and inform about focal liver lesions, portal vein thrombosis, or ascites. Upper endoscopy is indicated if gastrointestinal hemorrhage is suspected and can evaluate for the presence of variceal or nonvariceal sources of bleeding. The diagnosis of alcohol-associated hepatitis typically relies on the clinical history, physical findings, and laboratory studies, making histologic confirmation unnecessary. If necessary, liver biopsy is typically obtained by transjugular approach to decrease the risk of bleeding. Histologic features of alcohol-associated hepatitis include steatosis, pericellular fibrosis, neutrophilic lobular inflammation, and degenerative changes in hepatocytes (including Mallory-Denk bodies and ballooning).

C. Prognostic Indicators

One of the earliest prognostic tools to predict short-term mortality in severe alcohol-associated hepatitis is the Maddrey discriminant function (MDF), based on the serum bilirubin level and prothrombin time. Patients with an MDF of 32 and greater are at high risk of dying and may benefit from the use of corticosteroids. Reevaluation after 1 week of treatment by the Lille score identifies patients who remain unresponsive to corticosteroids, suggested by a Lille score of >0.45, and may need therapeutic alternatives such as liver transplantation. Additional prognostic indicators developed to assist the risk assessment in alcohol-associated hepatitis are listed in Table 44–2.

D. Supportive & Medical Therapy

Management of severe alcohol-associated hepatitis is complex and requires a multidisciplinary approach. Complete abstinence from alcohol is essential in the treatment of alcohol-associated hepatitis and in mild cases it may be sufficient. By contrast, mortality from severe alcohol-associated hepatitis may reach 60% within 1 month after initial presentation. Disease severity in alcohol-associated hepatitis must be therefore stratified to guide appropriate management decisions. Corticosteroids remain the cornerstone of medical treatment for a patient with severe alcohol-associated hepatitis, defined by the MDF reaching 32 or by the onset of hepatic encephalopathy. Earlier randomized controlled trials found that oral administration of 40 mg prednisolone or the equivalent intravenous dose of 32 mg methylprednisolone daily for 28 days significantly improves short-term (28-day) survival, while corticosteroids have no or little impact on longer-term

Table 44–2. Prognostic models in the evaluation of alcohol-associated hepatitis.

Scoring System	Variables	Advantages and Limitations
MDF	PT, serum bilirubin	Widely accepted, simple
Glasgow	Age, BUN, WBC, serum bilirubin, INR	May predict long-term outcome if recalculated on day 6–9
MELD	Serum bilirubin, INR, serum creatinine	Reference score for liver transplantation referral
ABIC	Age, serum bilirubin, INR, serum creatinine	Lacks broad validation
Lille	Age, serum bilirubin, serum albumin, PT, change in serum bilirubin on day 7	Day 7 score allows assessment of response to corticosteroids

BUN, blood urea nitrogen; INR, international normalized ratio; MDF, Maddrey discriminant function; MELD, model for end-stage liver disease; PT, prothrombin time; WBC, white blood cell.

mortality rates. More recently, even short-term survival benefits of corticosteroid in severe alcohol-associated hepatitis have been questioned. Contraindications to corticosteroid administration include uncontrolled infections, acute kidney injury (with a creatinine of >2.5 mg/dL), multiorgan failure or shock and uncontrolled upper gastrointestinal bleeding; it is important to rule out these potential barriers to corticosteroids early in the clinical course to avoid unnecessary delay in therapy. Another potentially efficacious treatment is the glutathione-repleting agent N-acetylcysteine (40 mg/day intravenously for 5 days). Studies have suggested that N-acetylcysteine, in conjunction with corticosteroid therapy, has a survival benefit over corticosteroids alone.

Additional therapeutic attempts with propylthiouracil, pentoxifylline, antioxidants, infliximab, and etanercept have failed to improve the outcomes of patients with alcohol-associated hepatitis. In fact, administration of the anticytokine agents infliximab and etanercept resulted in increased rates of severe systemic infections and higher mortality, making these drugs contraindicated in alcohol-associated hepatitis. Recent investigational agents for the treatment of severe cases include interleukin-22, the pan-caspase inhibitor emricasan, and antibodies developed against LPS and the interleukin-1 receptor. An algorithm for the management of alcohol-associated hepatitis is shown in Figure 44–2.

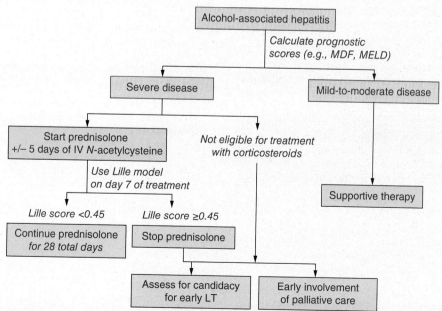

▲ **Figure 44–2.** Management of alcohol-associated hepatitis. This algorithm illustrates major decision steps in the prognostication and treatment of alcohol-associated hepatitis with variable severity. Prednisone is usually given at a dose of 40 mg PO daily for 4 weeks followed by rapid tapering within 4 weeks. Pentoxifylline is usually given at a dose of 400 mg PO three times a day for 4 weeks. MDF, Maddrey discriminant function; MELD, Model for end-stage liver disease.

E. Liver Transplantation

The place of liver transplantation in the management of life-threatening alcohol-associated hepatitis resistant to corticosteroids remains controversial but is becoming more widely accepted. While prior guidelines for liver transplantation in the United States required a 6-month abstinence from alcohol, a practice still widely used for patients with alcohol-associated cirrhosis, patients with symptomatic alcohol-associated hepatitis are often automatically ineligible given their poor survival rates at even 30 days. This stance has been challenged by several studies that found significantly higher survival rates after liver transplantation in severe alcohol-associated hepatitis refractory to medical therapy compared to the control group and similar relapse rates to patients transplanted for alcohol-associated cirrhosis that had achieved at least 6-months of sobriety prior to transplantation. Based on this increasing body of evidence, liver transplantation is being increasingly considered for select patients with a first episode of severe alcohol-associated hepatitis.

A comprehensive psychosocial evaluation of all patients being considered for early liver transplantation in alcohol-associated hepatitis is essential, with only very select patients being listed; in one major study close to 90% of medication nonresponders were not listed for transplantation secondary to poor psychosocial profiles. New risk scores are now being developed to aid in patient screening and selection. One risk assessment tool, studied specifically in patients that underwent early liver transplantation for alcohol-associated hepatitis, is the sustained alcohol use post-liver transplant (SALT) score which looks at the following variables: greater than 10 drinks/day at initial presentation (4 points), multiple prior rehabilitation attempts (4 points), prior alcohol-associated legal issues (2 points), and prior illicit substance use (1 point). Patients with a score of less that 5 were found to have a 95% negative predictive value for sustained alcohol use following liver transplantation. An alternative score, created for all patients with alcohol-associated liver disease (not just hepatitis) is the harmful alcohol use post-liver transplant (HALT) score. The four variables include age at liver transplantation, non-alcohol-related criminal history, pretransplant abstinence period (greater than vs less than 6 months) and drinks per day (greater than vs less than 10 drinks per day).

The result is a probability of harmful alcohol relapse after liver transplantation. Ongoing research is needed in determining which patients should be listed for liver transplantation and how best to minimize the risk of harmful alcohol use post-transplant.

Asrani SK, Trotter J, Lake J, et al. Meeting Report: The Dallas Consensus Conference on liver transplantation for alcohol associated hepatitis. *Liver Transpl.* 2020;26(1):127–140. [PMID: 31743578]

Botros M, Sikaris KA. The de ritis ratio: the test of time. *Clin Biochem Rev.* 2013;34:117–130. [PMID: 24353357]

Chayanupatkul M, Liangpunsakul S. Alcoholic hepatitis: a comprehensive review of pathogenesis and treatment. *World J Gastroenterol.* 2014;20:6279–6286. [PMID: 24876748]

Crabb DW, Im GY, Szabo G, Mellinger JL, Lucey MR. Diagnosis and treatment of alcohol-associated liver diseases: 2019 Practice guidance from the American Association for the Study of Liver Diseases. *Hepatology.* 2020;71:306–333. [PMID: 31314133]

Degré D, Stauber RE, Englebert G, et al. Long-term outcomes in patients with decompensated alcohol-related liver disease, steatohepatitis and Maddrey's discriminant function <32. *J Hepatol.* 2020;72:636–642. [PMID: 31954208]

Lee BP, Vittinghoff E, Hsu C, et al. Predicting low risk for sustained alcohol use after early liver transplant for acute alcoholic hepatitis: the sustained alchol use post-liver transplant score. *Hepatology.* 2019;69:1477–1487. [PMID: 30561766]

Louvet A, Naveau S, Abdelnour M, et al. The Lille model: a new tool for therapeutic strategy in patients with severe alcoholic hepatitis treated with steroids. *Hepatology.* 2007;45:1348–1354. [PMID: 17518367]

Lucey MR, Mathurin P, Morgan TR. Alcoholic hepatitis. *N Engl J Med.* 2009;360:2758–2769. [PMID: 19553649]

Mathurin P, Moreno C, Samuel D, et al. Early liver transplantation for severe alcoholic hepatitis. *N Engl J Med.* 2011;365:1790–1800. [PMID: 22070476]

Mellinger JL, Stine JG. Early liver transplantation for severe alcoholic hepatitis. *Dig Dis Sci.* 2020;65:1608–1614. [PMID: 32107678]

Satapathy SK, Thornburgh C, Heda R, et al. Predicting harmful alcohol relapse after liver transplant: the HALT score. *Clin Transplant.* 2020;34:e14003. [PMID: 32506677]

Thursz MR, Richardson P, Allison M, et al. Prednisolone or pentoxifylline for alcoholic hepatitis. *N Engl J Med.* 2015;372:1619–1628. [PMID: 25901427]

Nonalcoholic Fatty Liver Disease

Anne F. Liu, MD

Kathleen Viveiros, MD

ESSENTIALS OF DIAGNOSIS

▶ Nonalcoholic fatty liver disease (NAFLD) is the term that represents a broad spectrum of diseases ranging from simple steatosis to nonalcoholic steatohepatitis (NASH) and steatofibrosis.

▶ NAFLD is commonly associated with the metabolic syndrome, obesity, type 2 diabetes, and dyslipidemia; 80% of patients with the metabolic syndrome have NAFLD.

▶ Patients generally present without clinical symptoms but with mild aminotransferase elevations; NAFLD is the most common cause of increased serum aminotransferase levels in the United States.

▶ NAFLD is a clinical diagnosis after exclusion of other causes of liver disease.

▶ Vibration-controlled transient elastography (VCTE) and magnetic resonance elastography (MRE) are useful for detection.

▶ Liver biopsy is currently required to distinguish NASH from NAFL.

▶ General Considerations: Definitions

NAFLD is the overarching term and ranges from fatty liver to steatohepatitis to cirrhosis. In fact, NAFLD encompasses the entire spectrum in individuals without significant alcohol consumption, steatogenic medication use, or hereditary disorders. Nonalcoholic Fatty Liver (NAFL) is defined as the presence of ≥5% hepatic steatohepatitis without evidence of hepatocellular injury (in the form of hepatocyte ballooning) or fibrosis. In NAFL, there is often minimal risk of progression to cirrhosis and liver failure. NASH is defined as the presence of ≥5% hepatic steatosis with inflammation and hepatocyte injury that can have fibrosis and progress to cirrhosis, liver failure, and liver cancer. NASH cirrhosis is the presence of cirrhosis with current or previous histological evidence of steatosis or steatohepatitis. Cryptogenic cirrhosis is the presence of cirrhosis without any obvious etiologies.

Whereas the histopathology of NAFLD is similar to that of alcohol-related liver disease, the etiology is quite distinct. Significant data from basic and clinical research have demonstrated that the metabolic underpinnings of NAFLD are rooted in insulin resistance. Indeed, NAFLD is commonly associated with other manifestations of insulin resistance including obesity, essential hypertension, type 2 diabetes mellitus, low levels of high-density lipoprotein (HDL), hypertriglyceridemia, and less commonly polycystic ovarian disease, or hypothyroidism. Although early studies suggested it to be a benign condition, it is now apparent that NAFLD has become a major cause of liver-related morbidity and mortality.

A. Epidemiology

The absence of signs and symptoms, combined with a lack of sensitive and specific diagnostic tests, makes it difficult to estimate the prevalence of NAFLD. Elevated liver enzymes are not sensitive for detecting NAFLD and the invasive nature of liver biopsy is a limitation to the use of histopathology as the gold standard for diagnosis. Although likely an underestimate for these reasons, the prevalence of NAFLD in the United States is considered to be between 32% and 40% of the general population. Global estimates are approximately 25%. In a meta-analysis of NAFLD articles estimating global prevalence published from 1989 to 2015, the highest prevalence of NAFLD is in the Middle East (32%), followed by South America (30%). Determining the prevalence of NASH is limited by the need for liver biopsy for diagnosis, however, is estimated to be 7–30% in those with NAFLD. In studies looking at the overall NASH prevalence in biopsy-proven NAFLD patients, the prevalence is higher, ranging from 33% to 59%, which is expected given the selection group.

Population-based studies reveal that NAFLD is more common in men than women. It is more common in Hispanics compared with whites; and, more common in whites than blacks. A common polymorphism in the gene encoding patatin-like phospholipase domain-containing protein 3 (*PNPLA3*) is strongly associated with presence of NAFLD (in some racial and ethnic groups) as well as the histopathologic severity of NAFLD. *PNPLA3* encodes for a protein called adiponutrin which has homologies to enzymes linked to lipid metabolism. It is assumed that the prevalence of NAFLD will increase over time in parallel with the growing epidemic of obesity and diabetes. Obesity is present in 51% of patients with NAFLD and 82% with NASH. Of particular concern is that NAFLD is increasing in the pediatric population, with prevalence estimated at around 3% of children and 29–38% of obese children based on ALT elevation and autopsy studies. There is also higher risk in children in these subpopulations: male gender, diabetes, obstructive sleep apnea, and panhypopituitarism.

Buzzetti E, Pinzani M, Tsochatzis E. The multiple-hit pathogenesis of non-alcoholic fatty liver disease (NAFLD). *Metabolism.* 2016;65(8):1038–1048. [PMID: 26823198]

Chalasani N, Younossi Z, Lavine JE, et al. The diagnosis and management of nonalcoholic fatty liver disease: practice guidance from the American Association for the Study of Liver Diseases. *Hepatology.* 2018;67:328–357.

Ciardullo S, Perseghin G. Prevalence of NAFLD, MAFLD and associated advanced fibrosis in the contemporary United States population. *Liver Int.* 2021;41(6):1290–1293. [PMID: 33590934]

Cohen JC, Horton JD, Hobbs HH. Human fatty liver disease: old questions and new insights. *Science.* 2011;332:1519–1523. [PMID: 21700865]

Cotter, TG. Rinella, M. Nonalcoholic fatty liver disease 2020: the state of the disease. *Gastroenterology.* 2020;158(7):1851–1864. [PMID: 32061595]

Krawczyk M, Portincasa P, Lammert F. PNPLA3-associated steatohepatitis: toward a gene-based classification of fatty liver disease. *Semin Liver Dis.* 2013;33:369–379. [PMID: 24222094]

Vos MB, Abrams SH, Barlow SE, et al. NASPGHAN Clinical Practice Guideline for the Diagnosis and Treatment of Nonalcoholic Fatty Liver Disease in Children: Recommendations from the Expert Committee on NAFLD (ECON) and the North American Society of Pediatric Gastroenterology, Hepatology and Nutrition (NASPGHAN). *J Pediatr Gastroenterol Nutr.* 2017;64(2):319–334. [PMID: 28107283]

Younossi ZM, Koenig AB, Abdelatif D, Fazel Y, Henry L, Wymer M. Global epidemiology of nonalcoholic fatty liver disease-Meta-analytic assessment of prevalence, incidence, and outcomes. *Hepatology.* 2016;64(1):73–84. [PMID: 26707365]

Zou B, Yeo YH, Nguyen VH, Cheung R, Ingelsson E, Nguyen MH. Prevalence, characteristics and mortality outcomes of obese, nonobese and lean NAFLD in the United States, 1999-2016. *J Intern Med.* 2020;288(1):139–151. [PMID: 32319718]

B. Association of NAFLD with the Metabolic Syndrome, Obesity, Diabetes, & Hyperlipidemia

Insulin resistance represents the most important risk factor for the development of NAFLD. Because insulin resistance is also the hallmark of the metabolic syndrome, it is

not surprising that there is a close mechanistic link between NAFLD and the metabolic syndrome. Metabolic syndrome is generally defined as the coexistence of three or more of the following findings: (1) increased waist circumference (>102 cm in men and >88 cm in women), (2) hypertriglyceridemia ≥150 mg/dL, (3) hypertension with systolic blood pressure ≥130 mmHg or diastolic blood pressure ≥85 mmHg, (4) elevated fasting plasma glucose ≥110 mg/dL, and (5) low HDL cholesterol level <40 mg/dL in men and <50 mg/dL in women. Approximately 80% of patients with metabolic syndrome have NAFLD. Patients who have NAFLD and metabolic syndrome have a threefold risk for NASH compared with NAFLD alone. It is possible that steatosis may simply characterize the hepatic manifestation of the metabolic syndrome. However, ethnic differences in NAFLD prevalence are still observed in patients with the metabolic syndrome or obesity, indicating that additional genetic factors play key roles.

There is also a close association of NAFLD with obesity. The prevalence of obesity in patients with NAFLD is reported to vary from 30% to 100%. In obese patients (body mass index [BMI] ≥30 kg/m² in non-Asian ethnicity, ≥27 kg/m² in Asian ethnicity according to WHO) the risk of NAFLD is elevated fivefold. Importantly, the frequency of NASH also varies in proportion to weight. The prevalence of NASH is 3% in the lean population but rises to 19% in obesity and to nearly 50% in morbidly obese individuals. Consistent with the close relationship of NAFLD with the metabolic syndrome, NAFLD is more common in individuals with an abdominal concentration of fat, even at lower BMIs.

The prevalence of NAFLD is high in the type 2 diabetic population (50%), and the prevalence of type 2 diabetes in NAFLD patients ranges from 10% to 75%. The prevalence of NAFLD appears to increase as a continuous function of fasting plasma glucose. Importantly, NASH is disproportionately represented in type 2 diabetics, with significant fibrosis and cirrhosis present in approximately 20% of patients. In hyperlipidemic patients, the overall prevalence of fatty liver is 50%, with hypertriglyceridemia and mixed dyslipidemia conferring a fivefold increased risk of NAFLD. The prevalence of hyperlipidemia associated with NAFLD varies from 20% to 90%. In keeping with a strong link to the metabolic syndrome, low HDL cholesterol levels are also commonly observed in patients with NAFLD. Emerging evidence suggests that hypertension is linked to NAFLD through its relationship to insulin resistance with activation of the sympathetic nervous system and renal sodium retention.

Artunc F, Schleicher E, Weigert C, Fritsche A, Stefan N, Häring HU. The impact of insulin resistance on the kidney and vasculature. *Nat Rev Nephrol.* 2016;12(12):721–737. [PMID: 27748389]

Jichitu A, Bungau S, Stanescu AMA, et al. Non-alcoholic fatty liver disease and cardiovascular comorbidities: pathophysiological links, diagnosis, and therapeutic management. *Diagnostics (Basel).* 2021;11(4):689. [PMID: 33921359]

Tarantino G, Finelli C. What about non-alcoholic fatty liver disease as a new criterion to define metabolic syndrome? *World J Gastroenterol*. 2013;19:3375–3384. [PMID: 3683675]

Tota-Maharaj R, Blaha MJ, Zeb I, et al. Ethnic and sex differences in fatty liver on cardiac computed tomography: the multi-ethnic study of atherosclerosis. *Mayo Clin Proc*. 2014;89:493–503. [PMID: 24613289]

▶ Pathogenesis

Current concepts indicate that insulin resistance is the primary metabolic defect leading to NAFLD (Figure 45–1). This leads to an influx into the liver of free (ie, nonesterified) fatty acids that are liberated from adipose tissues due to a failure of insulin to suppress hormone-sensitive lipase. In addition, elevated insulin and glucose levels associated with insulin resistance promote continued synthesis of triglycerides in the liver. These two sources of triglycerides result in lipid-engorged hepatocytes (ie, macrovesicular hepatic steatosis alone). The presence of NAFLD appears to be a relatively innocuous occurrence, and it does not appear that progressive liver injury necessarily ensues. Although many patients with NAFLD have coexisting type 2 diabetes, this is not uniformly true. Indeed, steatosis and insulin resistance may be present in the absence of other components of the metabolic syndrome.

A common, but not uniformly accepted hypothesis suggests that NASH evolves as a progression from NAFLD.

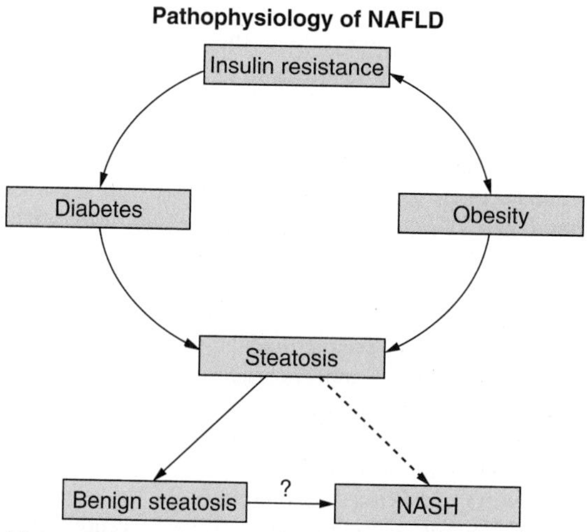

Pathophysiology of NAFLD

▲ **Figure 45–1.** Insulin resistance is the foundation of hepatic steatosis. Type 2 diabetes is a consequence of insulin resistance, but obesity can also result in insulin resistance. As indicated by the question mark, it is not known whether there is progression of benign steatosis to nonalcoholic steatohepatitis (NASH). NAFLD, nonalcoholic fatty liver disease. (Reproduced with permission from Parekh S, Anania FA. Abnormal lipid and glucose metabolism in obesity: implications for nonalcoholic fatty liver disease, *Gastroenterology*. 2007;132(6):2191–2207.)

In this regard, the presence of NAFLD represents a first "hit." According to this theory, NASH develops due to additional "hits" whereby hepatocytes laden with triglycerides are vulnerable to further insult. Free fatty acids and hyperinsulinemia potentiate lipid peroxidation and the release of hydroxy free radicals, which directly injure hepatocytes by recruitment of necroinflammatory mediators. Chronic liver injury sustained over time will then lead to activation of hepatic stellate cells, creating the potential for hepatic fibrosis.

In certain animal models of NASH, altered gut flora leads to further production of fatty acids, increased small bowel permeability and increased absorption of fatty acids into the portal vein which are potent agonists for inflammatory pathways and release of proinflammatory cytokines such as tumor necrosis factor-α (TNF-α) production, with the subsequent release of interleukins. Interestingly, the same mechanisms appear to be pathogenic in alcoholic hepatitis and produce quite similar histopathologic lesions. The combination of oxidative stress and necroinflammatory cytokines is associated with compromised mitochondrial function, which impairs electron transport and depletes adenosine triphosphate. This renders hepatocytes incapable of handling the enhanced oxidative stress. In this setting, the increased oxidative stress may overwhelm the intrinsic antioxidant capacity of the liver. Intracellular free fatty acids within the liver also promote endoplasmic reticulum stress and mitochondrial damage, which lead to increase lipid synthesis and hepatocyte apoptosis via activation of c-Jun N-terminal kinase (JNK).

The majority of patients with NAFLD, but a lesser fraction of those with NASH, never progress to fibrosis, which results from a complex series of molecular events in response to all types of liver injury. However, in the setting of excess oxidative stress, stellate cells in the liver may become activated, and this results in increased deposition of extracellular matrix. Excess extracellular matrix eventually disrupts normal signal transduction between cells and the matrix on which they rest, as well as the normal flow of nutrients and blood in the liver sinusoids. The result is a wound-healing response that can compromise liver function and promote the development of portal hypertension.

Adiponectin, also known as adipocyte complement–related protein (ACRP30), is a hormone produced by omental fat. Adiponectin is produced primarily in adipose tissues, in addition to the brain and muscles. It stimulates glucose utilization and fatty acid oxidation in the liver by activating adenosine monophosphate–activated protein kinase (AMPK). Adiponectin is correlated positively with insulin sensitivity and negatively with intra-abdominal fat. Adiponectin gene expression and secretion are decreased in obesity and are lower in patients with insulin resistance, type 2 diabetes, and other conditions associated with the metabolic syndrome than in age- and sex-matched controls. Adiponectin levels measured in patients with NAFLD or NASH were found to be lower than those in age- and sex-matched controls and correlate negatively with hepatic fat. Low levels of adiponectin expression may predispose patients to the progression to NASH.

Birkenfeld AL, Shulman GI. Nonalcoholic fatty liver disease, hepatic insulin resistance, and type 2 diabetes. *Hepatology*. 2014;59:713–723. [PMID: 23929732]

Buzzetti E, Pinzani M, Tsochatzis E. The multiple-hit pathogenesis of non-alcoholic fatty liver disease (NAFLD). *Metabolism*. 2016;65(8):1038–1048. [PMID: 26823198]

Cheung O, Sanyal AJ. Recent advances in nonalcoholic fatty liver disease. *Curr Opin Gastroenterol*. 2010;26:202–208. [PMID: 20168226]

Schuppan D, Schattenberg JM. Non-alcoholic steatohepatitis: pathogenesis and novel therapeutic approaches. *J Gastroenterol Hepatol*. 2013;28(suppl 1):68–76. [PMID: 23855299]

▶ Clinical Findings

A. Symptoms & Signs

Most patients with NAFLD present because abnormal serum aminotransferase levels are discovered incidentally in panels of laboratory tests sent for screening purposes or for thoracic and abdominal imaging for reasons other than suspected liver disease. In general, patients with NAFLD are asymptomatic. If present, symptoms tend to be nonspecific and constitutional but may include right upper quadrant discomfort. On physical examination, associated findings are limited to hepatomegaly.

Because NAFLD is a diagnosis of exclusion, historical information is important. Several risk factors that increase the likelihood of NAFLD may be elicited in the history. Importantly, alcohol use must be limited to qualify as NAFLD, so that the maximum rate of alcohol intake is two standard drinks per day (140 g ethanol/week) for men, and one standard drink per day (70 g ethanol/week) for women. Other important risk factors for NAFLD include age, obesity, dyslipidemia, and type 2 diabetes. A family history of diabetes, obesity, and liver disease without a clear etiology provides important cues.

B. Laboratory Findings

Modest elevations of alanine aminotransferase (ALT) and aspartate aminotransferase (AST) are typically present at levels in the range of two- to threefold the upper limit of normal. However, ALT and AST can range up to 10 times the upper limit of normal in NAFLD. The AST/ALT ratio is typically less than 1.0, and this helps to distinguish NAFLD from alcoholic liver disease (ALD). Because NAFLD is very common in the general population, it is also important to exclude other common and uncommon causes of elevated aminotransferase levels. These include causes of macrovesicular steatosis such as: hepatitis C genotype 3, excessive alcohol consumption, Wilson's Disease, lipodystrophy, starvation, parenteral nutrition, abetalipoproteinemia and causes of microvesicular steatosis such as: Reye's syndrome, acute fatty liver of pregnancy, HELLP syndrome, and inborn errors of metabolism. Medications that can cause steatosis also need to be considered, such as amiodarone, methotrexate, tamoxifen, corticosteroids, mipomersen, lomitapide, valproate, and antiretrovirals. It will also be important to exclude autoimmune hepatitis, hemochromatosis, thyroid disease, and α_1-antitrypsin deficiency. It is often useful to obtain a fasting lipid profile and plasma glucose concentration. Patients with biopsy-proven NASH are more likely to have higher levels of AST and ALT, alkaline phosphatase, γ-glutamyl transpeptidase and insulin resistance. Estimates of insulin resistance can be made using the homeostatic model assessment of insulin resistance (HOMA-IR), which is a method for assessing β-cell function and insulin resistance from glucose and insulin concentrations.

Chalasani N, Younossi Z, Lavine JE, et al. The diagnosis and management of nonalcoholic fatty liver disease: practice guidance from the American Association for the Study of Liver Diseases. *Hepatology*. 2018;67:328–357. [PMID: 28714183]

Neuschwander-Tetri BA, Clark JM, Bass NM, et al. Clinical, laboratory and histological associations in adults with non-alcoholic fatty liver disease. *Hepatology*. 2010;52:913–924. [PMID: 20648476]

C. Imaging Studies

Imaging studies play a key role in the diagnosis of NAFLD. The mainstay is ultrasonography, which reveals a diffuse echogenic pattern in the setting of hepatic fat accumulation. Ultrasound is also the least invasive imaging modality and is relatively inexpensive. The sensitivity for ultrasound detection of NAFLD is in the range of 60–90%, with specificity around 90%. These numbers depend on the degree of fat infiltration and will decline in mild cases of NAFLD. In the setting of morbid obesity, sensitivity and specificity of ultrasound are also reduced due to body habitus. CT is a reasonable but more costly imaging modality for detecting hepatic fatty infiltration, which appears as a low radiographic attenuation of the liver when compared with the attenuation of the spleen or paraspinal region. The sensitivity of CT for detecting NAFLD approaches 90%.

The ultrasound-based technique of VCTE, commonly delivered by the FibroScan device, has recently gained approval for estimating the degree liver fibrosis in both adults and children, and this may prove useful as an adjunct to the clinical assessment of NAFLD. AUROC for advanced fibrosis detection was 0.93. The sensitivity is 95% and specificity 77%. However there have been some cohorts with various failure rates, including 10.5% in a Japanese cohort and 2.6% in the US multi-national cohort.

MRE is an emerging technique to assess liver fibrosis. This is achieved by MRI of the liver after shear waves are induced by an external vibrating compression device.

The VCTE performed equally to MRE for identifying fibrosis stage 3 and 4 only. MRI-proton-density-fat fraction (PDFF) is an imaging modality that produces quantitative assessment of liver fat used in clinical trials on drug trials to assess for anti-steatotic effects.

Bonder A, Afdhal N. Utilization of FibroScan in clinical practice. *Curr Gastroenterol Rep.* 2014;16:372. [PMID: 24452634]

Caussy C, Reeder SB, Sirlin CB, Loomba R. Noninvasive, quantitative assessment of liver Fat by MRI-PDFF as an endpoint in NASH Trials. *Hepatology.* 2018;68(2):763–772. [PMID: 29356032]

Nozaki Y, Fujita K, Wafa K, et al. Deficiency of eNOS exacerbates early-stage NAFLD pathogenesis by changing fat distribution. *BMC Gastroenterol.* 2015;15:177. [PMID: 26678309]

Vuppalanchi R, Siddiqui MS, Hallinan EK. Transient elastography is feasible with high success rate for evaluation of non-alcoholic fatty liver disease (NAFLD) in a multicenter setting. *Hepatology.* 2015;62:1290A. [PMID: 20158692]

D. Calculations

There are several different calculations that have served as clinical decision aids. The NAFLD fibrosis score (NFS) is based on age, BMI, hyperglycemia, albumin, platelet count, and AST/ALT ratio. In a meta-analysis of 13 studies with 3064 patients, NFS had a high AUROC of 0.85 for advanced fibrosis prediction accuracy. Score of <-1.455 has a sensitivity of 90% and specificity of 50% in excluding advanced fibrosis. Score of >0.676 has a sensitivity of 67% and specificity of 97% to identify advanced fibrosis.

Other scoring systems include the FIB4 index which includes: platelets, age, ALT, and AST. Score of <1.45 is unlikely to have advanced fibrosis and a score of >3.25 is likely to have advanced fibrosis. The Enhanced Liver Fibrosis (ELF) panel includes matrix turnover proteins hyaluronic acid, tissue inhibitor of metalloproteinase 1, and N-terminal procollagen III-peptide. It has an AUROC of 0.90 with 80% sensitivity and 90% specificity for advanced fibrosis detection. Currently the panel is only used in Europe. The NFS and FIB-4 were comparable to the MRI elastography (MRE) for predicting advanced fibrosis in patients with biopsy-proven NAFLD.

Musso G, Gambino R, Cassader M, et al. Meta-analysis: natural history of non-alcoholic fatty liver disease (NAFLD) and diagnostic accuracy of non-invasive tests for liver disease severity. *Ann Med.* 2011;43:617–659. [PMID: 21039302]

E. Liver Biopsy

The value of liver biopsy in the management of NAFLD is controversial. Histologic features that can be appreciated in NAFLD include hepatocellular steatosis and balloon degeneration, mixed inflammatory-cell infiltrates, necrosis, glycogen nuclei, and Mallory hyaline. Liver biopsy can also assess degree of fibrosis. An important limitation of liver biopsy is that sampling error can be substantial, leading to both over-estimation and underestimation of degree of disease severity and fibrosis. Although liver biopsy is the only procedure that can distinguish between simple steatosis and NASH, its value in clinical practice remains uncertain. NASH accounts for a relatively small fraction of patients when compared with the high prevalence of NAFL in the population. Therefore, most patients will have steatosis alone by biopsy, and this carries a favorable prognosis. Moreover, there are no approved therapies for NAFL or NASH, so distinguishing between these two entities would not likely influence management. On the other hand, histopathology does provide prognostic information by determining fibrosis with better accuracy than noninvasive methods. In addition, biopsy can exclude other causes of underlying liver disease with approved medical therapy, such as autoimmune hepatitis. Eliminating treatable causes of liver inflammation by liver biopsy may become even more important as the prevalence of obesity and diabetes increase in the population.

Papastergiou V, Tsochatzis E, Burroughs AK. Non-invasive assessment of liver fibrosis. *Ann Gastroenterol.* 2012;25:218–231. [PMID: 3959378]

Rowe IA. Decision making for liver biopsy in NASH, not so FAST? *Lancet Gastroenterol Hepatol.* 2020;5(4):332–334. [PMID: 32027859]

▶ Treatment

Although both the prevalence and pathophysiology of NAFLD have increased, therapies for this common condition remain very limited. At present, there are no reliable evidence-based treatments. Efforts to develop effective management strategies, including improving insulin resistance, reducing oxidative stress in the liver and treating associated metabolic comorbidities of obesity, hyperlipidemia, and diabetes are based on current understanding of NAFLD pathogenesis. Current approaches include both weight loss and pharmacotherapies.

A. Weight Loss

Considering the strong association among obesity, NAFLD, and type 2 diabetes, it is logical that improving insulin resistance would represent the cornerstone of therapy for NAFLD. Because rapid weight loss can induce or exacerbate NASH, gradual weight loss constitutes the main objective. Gradual weight loss can be achieved through therapeutic lifestyle modifications, pharmacologic treatment, and bariatric surgery.

1. Therapeutic lifestyle modifications—Lifestyle modifications are generally accepted as beneficial for the treatment of NAFLD. Because weight loss through reduced caloric intake and increased physical activity improves insulin resistance, it is logical to think it would also lead to improvements in NAFLD. A 2020 American Gastroenterology Association position paper on NAFLD advocated weight loss as the first-line intervention in patients with NAFLD and provides evidence-based lifestyle interventions for the treatment of NASH. In obese patients with biopsy-proven NASH, a ≥10% reduction in weight over 12 months led to significant improvements in liver histopathology compared with controls. In patients with type 2 diabetes, an 8% reduction in weight was associated with 25% greater reduction in hepatic steatosis compared with controls as measured by MRI spectroscopy.

Patients who exercise more than 150 minutes/week or increase their activity level by >60 minutes/week were shown to have a reduction in aminotransferase levels in a Korean NAFLD cohort. As for NASH, patients with ≥6 Metabolic Equivalent of task (METs) activity had a benefit in fibrosis. There have also been studies combining diet (restricted to 750 kcal/day) with exercise (200 minutes/week) that have shown improvement in fibrosis.

Hallsworth K, Adams LA. Lifestyle modification in NAFLD/NASH: facts and figures. *JHEP Rep*. 2019;1(6):468–479. [PMID: 32039399]

Kistler KD, Brunt EM, Clark JM, et al. Physical activity recommendations, exercise intensity and histological severity of nonalcoholic fatty liver disease. *Am J Gastroenterol*. 2011;106;460–468. [PMID: 21206486]

Lazo, M, Solga SF, Horska A, et al. Effect of a 12-month intensive lifestyle intervention on hepatic steatosis in adults with type 2 diabetes. *Diabetes Care*. 2010;33:2156–2163. [PMID: 20664019]

Promrat K, Kleiner DE, Niemeier HM, et al. Randomized controlled trial testing the effects of weight loss on nonalcoholic steatohepatitis. *Hepatology*. 2010;51:121–129. [PMID: 19827166]

Sung KC, Ryu S, Lee JY. Effect of exercise on the development of new fatty liver and the resolution of existing fatty liver. *J Hepatol*. 2016;65:791–797. [PMID: 27255583]

Vilar-Gomez E, Martinez-Perez Y, Calzadilla-Bertot L. Weight loss through lifestyle modification significantly reduces features of nonalcoholic steatohepatitis. *Gastroenterology*. 2015;149: 367–378. [PMID: 25865049]

Viveiros K. The role of lifestyle modifications in comprehensive non-alcoholic fatty liver disease treatment. *Clin Liver Dis (Hoboken)*. 2021;17(1):11–14. [PMID: 33552479]

Younossi ZM, Corey KE, Lim JK. AGA clinical practice update on lifestyle modification using diet and exercise to achieve weight loss in the management of nonalcoholic fatty liver Disease: expert review. *AGA Clinical Practice Updates*. 2020;160(3): 912–918. [PMID: 33307021]

2. Pharmacologic weight reduction—Appreciating that weight loss through therapeutic lifestyle modifications is not always successful, pharmacologic options are frequently sought. Orlistat reduces the absorption of dietary triglycerides by inhibiting gastric and pancreatic lipase. In randomized trials compared with dietary changes alone, orlistat reduced weight modestly over a 1-year period by 4–8 lb.

This was accompanied by significant reductions in blood pressure and plasma cholesterol, with improved glucose control. Orlistat has been studied for the treatment of NAFLD in small case series and pilot studies. Significant weight reductions achieved using orlistat have been associated with improvements in liver enzymes and hepatic fat on ultrasound. Improvements in liver histology appear to require approximately 9% reductions in body weight. Limitations to the use of orlistat include dyspepsia, bloating, diarrhea, and steatorrhea; decreased absorption of fat-soluble vitamins; as well as a requirement for three times daily dosing.

Patel AA, Torres DM, Harrison SA. Effect of weight loss on nonalcoholic fatty liver disease. *J Clin Gastroenterol*. 2009;43:970–974. [PMID: 19727004]

Younossi ZM, Reyes MJ, Mishra A, Mehta R, Henry L. Systematic review with meta-analysis: non-alcoholic steatohepatitis—a case for personalised treatment based on pathogenic targets. *Aliment Pharmacol Ther*. 2014;39:3–14. [PMID: 24206433]

3. Bariatric surgery—Surgery to promote weight loss is considered for obese patients who are unable to lose weight by therapeutic lifestyle modifications. Current evidence suggests that bariatric surgery is beneficial for many morbidly obese patients with NAFLD. Bariatric surgery includes procedures that restrict caloric intake and those that promote malabsorption of nutrients. For obese patients to qualify for bariatric surgery, their BMI must generally exceed 40. Patients may also be candidates if their BMI exceeds 35 and if they suffer from a significant obesity-related disease.

Depending on the type of procedure, bariatric surgery achieves sustained weight loss (defined as the percentage of the pounds above ideal body weight), in many cases with resolution of type 2 diabetes, hypertension, dyslipidemia, and the metabolic syndrome. NAFLD largely improves in patients who undergo bariatric surgery, with reduced steatosis, inflammation, and fibrosis all reported in several studies that utilized different surgical approaches. In a direct comparison Roux-en-Y gastric bypass proved superior to adjustable gastric banding for the improvement of NASH, an effect that was primarily attributable to greater weight loss. Whereas bariatric surgery appears to be generally safe, it is not currently considered as primary therapy for NASH, but rather an option in the context of other comorbidities that would justify the overall surgical risk. Bariatric surgery in patients with NASH cirrhosis does not have a well-established safety and efficacy profile but in general mortality will be higher in those with decompensated cirrhosis over compensated cirrhosis and over those without cirrhosis.

Caiazzo R, Lassailly G, Leteurtre E, et al. Roux-en-Y gastric bypass versus adjustable gastric banding to reduce nonalcoholic fatty liver disease: a 5-year controlled longitudinal study. *Ann Surg*. 2014;260:893–898. [PMID: 25379859]

Corrado RL, Torres DM, Harrison SA. Review of treatment options for nonalcoholic fatty liver disease. *Med Clin North Am.* 2014;98:55–72. [PMID: 25379859]

B. Medical Management

1. Current therapies—Because insulin resistance is central to pathogenesis, attention has been focused on antidiabetic agents that reduce insulin resistance as therapies for NAFL and NASH. Although metformin showed initial promise in laboratory animals, results in human trials have not born this out. The thiazolidinediones (TZDs), rosiglitazone, and pioglitazone, have met with more success. These drugs activate the nuclear hormone receptor peroxisome proliferator-activated receptor γ (PPARγ). A fundamental mechanism whereby PPARγ agonists work is to increase insulin sensitivity by enhancing adiponectin production in subcutaneous and visceral fat. TZDs have proven effective in the treatment of type 2 diabetes, although weight gain is a well-recognized side effect. The PIVENS trial compared pioglitazone versus vitamin E versus placebo for the treatment of nondiabetic patients with NASH. This was a phase 3, multicenter, randomized, placebo-controlled, double-blind clinical trial of pioglitazone or vitamin E (α-tocopherol) for the treatment of adults without diabetes who had biopsy-confirmed NASH. It was found that pioglitazone treatment reduced hepatic steatosis and lobular inflammation but did not achieve the primary endpoint of the trial (ie, improvement in histologic features of NASH, as assessed with the use of a composite of standardized scores for steatosis, lobular inflammation, hepatocellular ballooning, and fibrosis). Vitamin E 800 IU/day is an antioxidant that proved superior to placebo for the treatment of NASH in adults without diabetes in the PIVENS trial.

Based on a strong association between NAFLD and dyslipidemia, particularly elevated triglyceride and low HDL cholesterol concentrations in plasma, the use of lipid-lowering agents has been tested in pilot studies. In general, the use of statins and fibrates has led to improvements in serum transaminases. However, mixed results and limited histopathologic data preclude recommending these therapies for the treatment of NAFLD. Because patients with NAFLD are at increased risk of adverse cardiovascular events, it is important to point out that the use of statins does not appear to carry any additional risk of hepatotoxicity in these patients.

Bays H, Cohen DE, Chalasani N, Harrison SA. An assessment by the Statin Liver Safety Task Force: 2014 update. *J Clin Lipidol.* 2014;8:S47–S57. [PMID: 24793441]

Chalasani N, Younossi Z, Lavine JE, et al. The diagnosis and management of non-alcoholic fatty liver disease: practice guideline by the American Association for the Study of Liver Diseases, American College of Gastroenterology, and the American Gastroenterological Association. *Hepatology.* 2012;55:2005–2023. [PMID: 22488764]

Sanyal AJ, Chalasani N, Kowdley KV, et al. Pioglitazone, vitamin E, or placebo for nonalcoholic steatohepatitis. *N Engl J Med.* 2010;362:1675–1685. [PMID: 20427778]

2. Emerging therapies—Novel therapies have begun to show promise in the management of NAFLD. The recently available antidiabetic incretin mimetics liraglutide and exenatide, which act as glucagon-like peptide-1 (GLP-1) receptor agonists, have demonstrated promise in NASH, but further studies are needed to establish efficacy and which mechanism(s) of action are important to resolving steatosis. Obeticholic acid is a derivative of the bile acid chenodeoxycholic acid and a potent agonist of the farnesoid X receptor (FXR). This nuclear hormone receptor is a liver-enriched transcription factor that modulated bile acid metabolism, insulin sensitivity, and inflammation. A recent randomized clinical trial has demonstrated considerable promise for this agent in the management of NASH. The same study has also raised some concern due to increased plasma concentrations of LDL cholesterol, which could increase cardiovascular risk. Obeticholic acid was associated with hyperlipidemia and pruritus. Ongoing studies should clarify this issue. Another promising agent is Elafibranor, a dual PPARα/δ agonist, which improved NASH over 1 year. Of note, there was an increase in creatinine levels that was transient. Other emerging agents include chemokine receptor antagonists, antifibrotic agents, G-protein–coupled receptor 5 (GPCR5) agonists, ursodeoxycholic acid, omega-3 fatty acids, and fatty acid–bile acid conjugates.

Mells JE, Anania FA. The role of gastrointestinal hormones in hepatic lipid metabolism. *Semin Liver Dis.* 2013;33:343–357. [PMID: 24222092]

Neuschwander-Tetri BA, Loomba R, Sanyal AJ, et al. Farnesoid X nuclear receptor ligand obeticholic acid for non-cirrhotic, non-alcoholic steatohepatitis (FLINT): a multicentre, randomised, placebo-controlled trial. *Lancet.* 2015;385:956–965. [PMID: 25468160]

Ratziu V. Starting the battle to control non-alcoholic steatohepatitis. *Lancet.* 2015;385:922–924. [PMID: 25468161]

Course & Prognosis

A challenging aspect in the care of patients with NAFLD is predicting natural history (Figure 45–2). At present, there are no agreed upon biomarkers that permit the clinician to determine prognosis accurately. Rather, histopathology is required to predict which patients with NAFLD are likely to progress to cirrhosis. Progression of liver disease is dependent on the degree of damage that is present on a liver biopsy specimen. Hepatocellular steatosis in the absence of inflammation and fibrosis suggests the NAFL will not progress and that the clinical course will be benign. By contrast, the presence of steatohepatitis and more advanced fibrosis portend a worse prognosis, with increased likelihood of progression to cirrhosis.

Natural History of NAFLD

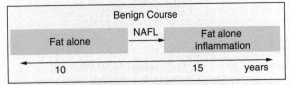

Benign Course

| Fat alone | NAFL → | Fat alone inflammation |

10   15   years

Aggressive Course

| Fat alone inflammation ballooning degeneration | NASH → | Fat alone fibrosis Mallory bodies |

10   15   years

Up to 23% may progress to cirrhosis; 5% risk
of hepatocellular carcinoma

▲ **Figure 45–2.** The natural history of nonalcoholic fatty liver disease depends on histopathology. Nonalcoholic fatty liver (NAFL) progresses very slowly, if at all, when fat alone is present on liver biopsy. By contrast, the presence of nonalcoholic steatohepatitis (NASH) is associated with a more accelerated progression to fibrosis. (Reproduced with permission from Parekh S, Anania FA. Abnormal lipid and glucose metabolism in obesity: implications for nonalcoholic fatty liver disease, *Gastroenterology*. 2007;132(6):2191–2207.)

Whereas the overall prevalence of NAFLD approximates 20% of the population, only about 10% of these individuals (ie, 5–8% of adults in the United States) have NASH. Approximately 20% of patients with NASH will progress to cirrhosis.

Although the overall risk of cirrhosis due to NAFLD is modest, certain groups are at particular risk. Important risk factors for NASH include obesity, diabetes, and advanced age. In the setting of morbid obesity, steatosis is present in up to 90% of patients, with NASH in up to 40% and advanced fibrosis or cirrhosis in the range of 13–14%. The prevalence of NAFLD in diabetic patients is approximately 50%, with disproportionately high representation of NASH. Fibrosis or cirrhosis is present in up to 20% of diabetic patients. Patients with morbid obesity and diabetes have hepatic steatosis at rates of nearly 100%, of which 50% have NASH and 19%

have cirrhosis. Age is also a negative prognostic indicator, with markedly increased rates of fibrosis (10-fold) in NASH patients older than 45 years (40%) compared with only 4% of NASH patients younger than 45 years.

Assessments of prognosis in NAFLD patients may also be guided by the demographics of cryptogenic cirrhosis. Prior to the appreciation of NAFLD as a disease entity, the pathophysiologic basis of cirrhosis in many patients was characterized as cryptogenic. It is now considered likely that 67–75% of these individuals suffered from NASH, which led to cirrhosis and liver biopsies that had progressed beyond the point at which the etiology could be discerned. Indeed, patients with cryptogenic cirrhosis are more likely to exhibit features of the metabolic syndrome. In patients awaiting liver transplantation due to cryptogenic cirrhosis, there was increased prevalence of obesity and diabetes compared with matched controls. NASH may occur even following liver transplantation for cryptogenic cirrhosis, as has been described in patients with the diagnosis of NASH that come to transplantation.

Hepatocellular carcinoma is now recognized as a potential complication of NAFLD that progresses to NASH with cirrhosis but may also occur in the absence of advanced liver disease in a very small subset. This risk is compounded when diabetes is present, suggesting the possibility that chronic hyperinsulinemia may provide a carcinogenic stimulus.

Overall, up to 40% of patients with cirrhosis attributable to NASH will die of liver disease–related complications or will receive a liver transplant. NAFLD cirrhosis is now the leading indication for liver transplantation in the United States.

Starley BQ, Calcagno CJ, Harrison SA. Nonalcoholic fatty liver disease and hepatocellular carcinoma: a weighty connection. *Hepatology*. 2010;51:1820–1832. [PMID: 20432259]

Younossi ZM, Corey KE, Lim JK. AGA clinical practice update on lifestyle modification using diet and exercise to achieve weight loss in the management of nonalcoholic fatty liver disease: expert eeview. *AGA Clinical Practice Updates*. 2020;160(3): 912–918. [PMID: 33307021]

Zezos P, Renner EL. Liver transplantation and non-alcoholic fatty liver disease. *World J Gastroenterol*. 2014;20:15532–15538. [PMID: 20432259]

Complications of Cirrhosis: Ascites & Hepatic Encephalopathy

46

Jordan Sack, MD, MPH

Kathleen Viveiros, MD

ESSENTIALS OF DIAGNOSIS

▶ The complications of cirrhosis include hepatic encephalopathy, ascites, and variceal hemorrhage which indicate worsening liver function and survival.

▶ Optimal control of the underlying cause of cirrhosis and prevention of secondary causes of hepatic inflammation may prevent cirrhosis complications.

▶ Hepatic encephalopathy is a clinical diagnosis and is managed with lactulose, rifaximin, and avoidance of precipitants.

▶ Common precipitants of hepatic encephalopathy are infection, gastrointestinal bleeding, hypovolemia, acute kidney injury, electrolyte derangements, and medications.

▶ Patients with cirrhosis and ascites should undergo a diagnostic paracentesis to confirm the etiology at least initially and should be regularly evaluated for spontaneous bacterial peritonitis even if asymptomatic.

▶ Ascites is treated with a low salt added diet and diuresis; refractory cases may be managed with large volume paracentesis or transjugular intrahepatic portosystemic shunt (TIPS).

▶ Hepatorenal syndrome must be considered in those with both ascites and renal failure and should be treated with volume expansion and vasoconstriction.

▶ Patients with cirrhosis-related complications should be followed by a hepatologist with a low threshold for liver transplant evaluation.

INTRODUCTION

The complications of cirrhosis include the development of hepatic encephalopathy, ascites, and variceal hemorrhage. The presence of any one of these decompensating events indicates worsening liver function and reduced patient survival. These episodes are often precipitated by continued liver disease progression leading to worsening hepatic fibrosis, inflammation, and portal hypertension; though other triggers of decompensation such as hepatocellular carcinoma, infection, and thrombosis within the liver vasculature may contribute. Clinicians should focus on preventing these complications by treating the underlying cause(s) of cirrhosis and promoting preventative measures. When one of these liver-related complications occurs, timely diagnosis and treatment are essential for patient recovery, and strong consideration should be given for transplant referral.

In this chapter, we will focus on hepatic encephalopathy and ascites including spontaneous bacterial peritonitis and hepatorenal syndrome. Variceal hemorrhage is addressed in the chapter on portal hypertension.

GENERAL CONSIDERATIONS

Prevention of Decompensation

An important way to prevent the development of liver related decompensation in a patient with cirrhosis is to have good control of the underlying cause of cirrhosis and to prevent secondary insults. Patients should be advised to abstain from alcohol, to optimize any risk factors for nonalcoholic fatty liver disease, to refrain from high risk activities involving exchange of bodily fluids, and to avoid hepatoxic medications. Screening for hepatocellular carcinoma every 6 months and immunization to both hepatitis A and B are important as cancer or acute hepatitis can trigger decompensation in patients with cirrhosis.

Prognosis after Decompensation

Patients with cirrhosis and no liver-related complications have a median life expectancy of over 12 years which is reduced to 1.5 years after developing a liver-related decompensation.

The prognosis further depends on what precipitated the liver complication and whether this can be controlled sufficiently to prevent recurrent or additional complications. Given the morbidity and mortality associated with cirrhosis complications, patients who develop new liver related decompensation should seek prompt medical attention and be referred for potential liver transplant evaluation. In some cases, palliative care involvement may be warranted.

ASCITES

▶ Pathogenesis

The liver is perfused both by the venous and arterial systems from the portal vein and hepatic artery with blood passing through the hepatic sinusoids before leaving through the central vein and subsequently the hepatic vein. These hepatic sinusoids are normally fenestrated which enables fluid to move out into the hepatic capsule and peritoneal cavity where it is resorbed by the lymphatics.

Portal hypertensive ascites develops when there is increased pressure at or beyond the hepatic sinusoids, leading to preferential output through the fenestrated hepatic sinusoids that exceeds the rate of drainage by the lymphatic system. The increased resistance formed by hepatic fibrosis in patients with cirrhosis is a common cause of portal hypertensive ascites, though it is important to recognize that hepatic vein thrombosis, hepatic congestion, and hepatic tumor burden can also cause portal hypertensive ascites by increasing hepatic sinusoidal pressure–and as such these causes should be ruled out. This process of portal hypertensive ascites formation from increased hepatic resistance is also intertwined with increased portal in-flow caused by inflammatory cytokines that promote splanchnic vasodilation, hyperdynamic circulation, and retention of sodium through activation of the renin-angiotensin-aldosterone system and upregulation of vasopressin. Hepatic hydrothorax can occur in those who have a defect in the diaphragm, allowing for preferential movement of ascites into the pleural space. Though less common, nonportal hypertensive etiologies of ascites may occur in patients with cirrhosis from lymphatic disruption, malignancy, or tuberculosis–and in these cases the formation of ascites is not related to the hepatic sinusoids. Patients with cirrhosis and ascites can develop additional complications including spontaneous bacterial peritonitis and hepatorenal syndrome. Spontaneous bacterial peritonitis typically occurs in a patient with portal hypertensive ascites caused by cirrhosis as the ascitic fluid is usually low in protein, and therefore there are fewer antimicrobial proteins such as complement to counter bacterial gut translocation. Hepatorenal syndrome occurs in patients with refractory ascites who have low effective arterial volume as a consequence of significant splanchnic and systemic vasodilatation caused by portal hypertension and is often accelerated by a secondary insult such as infection. These vascular changes lead to increased stimulation of the renin-angiotensin-aldosterone system and vasopressin that are unable to counteract the low effective arterial volume, causing severe vasoconstriction of the afferent arterioles in the kidneys and subsequent renal failure.

Hepatorenal syndrome is a diagnosis of exclusion and requires the presence of portal hypertensive ascites, acute kidney injury (defined as an increase in serum creatinine by 0.3 mg/dL from baseline within 48 hours or a 50% increase from baseline within 7 days), and lack of improvement in creatinine despite a 48-hour trial of 1g/kg of 25% albumin and cessation of diuresis. It further requires the exclusion of hypovolemia, shock, nephrotoxic substances, and intrinsic renal disease (defined as proteinuria [>500 mg/24 hours], microhematuria [>50 red blood cells/high power field], or abnormal renal ultrasound). Patients who fulfill these criteria are now defined as having hepatorenal syndrome-acute kidney injury (HRS-AKI), which replaces the former term of hepatorenal syndrome type 1. This change in definition allows for sooner treatment of hepatorenal syndrome by using acute kidney injury criteria (defined as an increase in serum creatinine by 0.3 mg/dL from baseline within 48 hours or a 50% increase from baseline within 7 days) instead of requiring a doubling of creatinine to greater than 2.5 mg/dL within 2 weeks. Given its high mortality, HRS-AKI should be promptly diagnosed and treated. The former definition of hepatorenal syndrome type 2 is now reclassified as hepatorenal syndrome-non acute kidney injury (HRS-NAKI) which is defined as having a GFR <60 mL/min in the absence of other causes of kidney disease and it is further stratified by whether this has occurred for more or less than 3 months.

Table 46–1 outlines the new definitions for hepatorenal syndrome.

Table 46–1 Hepatorenal syndrome criteria.

HRS-AKI	HRS-NAKI

1. Cirrhosis with ascites
2. Acute kidney injury
  a. Serum creatinine increase by ≥0.3 mg/dL from baseline within 48 hours
  OR
  b. Serum creatinine increase by 50% from baseline within 7 days (or closest known prior baseline)
3. No response to 2 day challenge of 1 g/kg of 25% albumin and diuretic cessation
4. Absence of shock
5. Absence of nephrotoxic medications and contrast
6. No intrinsic kidney disease
  a. Absence of proteinuria (>500 mg/day)
  b. Absence of microhematuria (>50 RBC/HPF)
  c. Normal renal ultrasound
	1. Does not meet criteria for HRS-AKI
	2. Estimated GFR <60 mL/min
	3. Absence of other potential causes of kidney disease

GFR, glomerular filtration rate; HPF, high power field; HRS-AKI, hepatorenal syndrome-acute kidney injury; HRS-NAKI, hepatorenal syndrome-non acute kidney injury; RBC, red blood cell.

Prevention

New onset ascites from cirrhosis may be prevented by adhering to general liver preventative measures outlined earlier and by encouraging adherence to a low sodium diet. Recurrent ascites may be avoided with low salt diet, diuretics, or a TIPS. Primary prophylaxis to prevent the first episode of spontaneous bacterial peritonitis is recommended for patients who have an ascitic protein less than 1.5 g/dL and advanced liver disease (defined as Child-Pugh score ≥9 and bilirubin ≥3 mg/dL) or renal dysfunction (defined as serum creatinine ≥1.2 mg/dL, blood urea nitrogen ≥25 mg/dL, or sodium ≤130 mEq/L). Shorter courses of prophylactic antibiotics are recommended for gastrointestinal hemorrhage (7-day course) or ascitic protein less than 1.0 g/dL (for duration of hospitalization). Patients with a history of spontaneous bacterial peritonitis should be maintained on antibiotics for secondary prophylaxis.

Clinical Findings

A. Symptoms & Signs

Patients with ascites often report weight gain, abdominal distention, abdominal pressure, bloating, or early satiety. Those with spontaneous bacterial peritonitis may have abdominal pain or fevers but are often asymptomatic. Those with hepatic hydrothorax typically have shortness of breath.

A physical exam usually reveals ascites once there is at least 500 mL of ascites. Patients often have abdominal distention which can sometimes be mistaken for other causes of abdominal distention such as obesity, pregnancy, ileus, or stool burden. The abdomen should be examined for shifting dullness on percussion, a fluid wave, and any umbilical or ventral hernias. Those with hepatic hydrothorax will have dullness on percussion and decreased breath sounds and may be hypoxic. The presence of jugular venous distention may suggest a cardiac cause of the ascites. Peripheral edema should be noted as it can help guide the choice of diuretics.

B. Laboratory Findings

Patients with cirrhosis and new onset ascites should undergo an initial diagnostic paracentesis in order to calculate a serum ascites albumin gradient (SAAG) [serum albumin minus ascitic albumin] and to check the ascitic protein, ascitic white blood cell count with differential, ascitic red blood cell count, and ascitic culture. In select cases additional studies such as cytology may be obtained. In rare cases when there is concern for ascites caused by a bile duct leak, pancreatic duct leak, or urinary tract leak, ascitic testing can be performed for bilirubin, amylase, and creatinine, respectively.

A SAAG greater than or equal to 1.1 g/dL is generally consistent with portal hypertension. The presence of a borderline SAAG slightly above or below 1.1 g/dL does not necessarily rule in or rule out portal hypertension. Careful attention should also be made to the timing of when the serum and ascitic albumin values were collected and whether the serum albumin could have been falsely elevated by administering albumin around the time of the blood draw. Ascitic neutrophils of 250 or higher with a positive culture is consistent with spontaneous bacterial peritonitis while a negative culture is termed culture negative neutrocytic ascites. If the ascites is bloody, a correction may be required to properly calculate the number of ascitic neutrophils and is done by subtracting one ascitic neutrophil for every 250 ascitic red cells that are present. The presence of a positive culture with fewer than 250 ascitic neutrophils is reported as non-neutrocytic bacterascites. Ascitic cultures growing more than one bacterial species should raise concern for secondary peritonitis from a bowel perforation. A low ascitic glucose and elevated ascitic lactate dehydrogenase can also suggest secondary peritonitis.

As patients with spontaneous bacterial peritonitis may be asymptomatic and a delay in diagnosis and treatment is associated with high mortality, all patients with ascites who present for therapeutic paracentesis or seek medical attention should have diagnostic paracentesis with cell count performed to rule out an ascitic infection. Patients with hepatic hydrothorax should be managed similarly with a diagnostic thoracentesis and the presence of an infection would be termed spontaneous bacterial empyema.

Those with refractory ascites may develop hepatorenal syndrome with the clinical criteria and required laboratory testing discussed earlier and shown in Table 46–1.

C. Imaging Studies

Patients with new onset ascites should undergo imaging of both the liver and hepatic vein to assess for any hepatic mass or hepatic vein thrombosis. Sometimes imaging can help to confirm the diagnosis of ascites when it is too small to detect clinically or difficult to distinguish from another cause of a distended abdomen. Imaging typically starts with a liver ultrasound with dopplers and cross-sectional imaging is subsequently obtained if needed. For those with hepatic hydrothorax, a chest x-ray should be performed. In cases where a cardiac cause of the ascites is suspected, a transthoracic echocardiogram should be performed.

Differential Diagnosis

The differential diagnosis for abdominal distention includes causes other than ascites such as obesity, stool burden, pregnancy, tumor, large hernia, ileus, or bowel obstruction. These causes can usually be elicited by a physical exam but sometimes imaging is warranted. Once ascites is confirmed in a patient with cirrhosis, the most likely etiology is portal hypertensive ascites from the increased pressure caused by hepatic fibrosis and splanchnic vasodilation, though it is important to entertain other causes of ascites. As mentioned earlier, diagnostic paracentesis with SAAG and ascitic protein can help delineate most etiologies. A SAAG equal to or greater than 1.1 g/dL suggests portal hypertensive ascites.

A low ascitic protein (<2.5 mg/dL) is indicative of cirrhosis whereas a high ascitic protein (≥2.5 mg/dL) may suggest a noncirrhotic etiology such as hepatic congestion, hepatic vein thrombosis, or hepatic vein stenosis and should be corroborated with imaging. In select situations, sinusoidal obstruction syndrome and mixed causes should be considered. It is important to obtain a cell count to rule out spontaneous bacterial peritonitis even in the asymptomatic patient with ascites. A SAAG less than 1.1 g/dL should lead to consideration of nonportal hypertensive causes of ascites such as peritoneal carcinomatosis, pancreatic duct leak, nephrotic syndrome, lymphatic disruption, and inflammatory diseases. In those cases, additional diagnostic tests may be indicated such as ascitic amylase, triglyceride, and cytology. A similar diagnostic approach of obtaining SAAG, protein, and cell count should be done for those with a hepatic hydrothorax.

Table 46–2 provides the differential diagnosis when performing a diagnostic paracentesis.

▶ Complications

The complications of ascites include spontaneous bacterial peritonitis and hepatorenal syndrome which are associated with significant morbidity and mortality. Spontaneous bacterial peritonitis and its variates such as culture negative neutrocytic ascites and spontaneous bacterial empyema can occur in asymptomatic patients which makes prompt diagnosis and treatment essential when patients with ascites seek medical attention. Hepatorenal syndrome must be considered in patients with portal hypertensive ascites who develop acute kidney injury that is not responsive to a fluid or albumin challenge, diuretic cessation, and occurs in the absence of shock, nephrotoxic substances, and intrinsic renal disease– as outlined in Table 46–1.

▶ Treatment

Portal hypertensive ascites can often be managed with a low salt added diet and diuresis. Dietary counseling about salt intake is important as dietary indiscretion is common. Overly restrictive salt intake should be avoided as this can limit overall caloric and protein intake which are important for building muscle mass. Fluid restriction is not necessary unless the patient has severe hyponatremia. The main diuretic for treating ascites is spironolactone since it is an aldosterone antagonist which counteracts one of the main physiologic mechanisms that contribute to ascites formation. If painful gynecomastia develops, eplerenone can be substituted. Furosemide alone may not be effective for removing ascites and should be reserved to treat concurrent peripheral edema. Patients should undergo close monitoring of electrolyte, renal function, and weight changes with initiation and titration of diuresis. Over-diuresis should be avoided as it can precipitate renal failure and hepatic encephalopathy. Patients may sometimes develop muscle cramping with diuresis

Table 46–2 Differential to consider based on diagnostic paracenteses findings.

SAAG ≥1.1 with Protein ≥2.5
Hepatic congestion
Thrombosis of hepatic vein or inferior vena cava
Stenosis of hepatic vein or inferior vena cava
Sinusoidal obstruction syndrome
Nodular regenerative hyperplasia or hepatoportal sclerosis
Mixed causes
SAAG ≥1.1 with Protein <2.5
Cirrhosis
Nodular regenerative hyperplasia or hepatoportal sclerosis
Mixed causes
SAAG <1.1
Malignancy
Tuberculosis
Inflammatory/Rheumatologic diseases
Nephrotic syndrome
Ascitic neutrophils ≥250
Spontaneous bacterial peritonitis (positive ascitic culture)
Culture negative neutrocytic ascites (negative ascitic culture)
Ascitic neutrophils <250
Non-neutrocytic bacterascites
Ascitic bilirubin >Serum bilirubin
Bile duct leak
Ascitic amylase > Serum amylase
Pancreatic duct leak
Ascitic creatinine > Serum creatinine
Urinary tract leak

SAAG, serum ascites albumin gradient.

which can be treated with diuretic reduction, electrolyte correction, and/or quinine.

In cases of tense ascites, large volume paracentesis can be performed followed by initiation of diuresis along with a low salt added diet to prevent recurrence of the ascites. With refractory ascites caused by diuretic intolerance or diuretic resistance, diuresis will not be feasible and large volume paracenteses will need to be scheduled on a regular basis ranging from weekly to monthly depending on how quickly the patient reaccumulates fluid. As removal of more than 5 L of ascites increases the risk of post paracentesis circulatory dysfunction, 8 grams of 25% albumin should be administered for every liter of ascites removed beyond 5 L with typically no more than 10 liters removed at one time. Cell counts should be routinely obtained to rule out the presence of spontaneous bacterial peritonitis as some patients may be asymptomatic. In patients with refractory ascites who have low MELD scores (generally less than 18 on the MELD score calculator that does not correct for sodium), low bilirubin (usually <3 mg/dL), good cardiac function, minimal hepatic encephalopathy, and no liver lesions, a TIPS can be considered. Patients should be counseled on the potential complications of TIPS including procedural-related bleeding, infection, hepatic encephalopathy, and decreased liver function. Drainage devices for removing ascites should be reserved for patients focused on palliative measures as these drains often lead to peritonitis.

Those with hepatic hydrothorax can be managed similarly with low salt added diet, diuresis, and as needed thoracentesis with cell counts. These are often more difficult to manage as respiratory symptoms can recur with small re-accumulation of fluid in the pleural space. TIPS may sometimes be helpful in treating hepatic hydrothorax. Chest tubes and drainage catheters should be avoided given their predisposition to infection.

Spontaneous bacterial peritonitis and its variants including culture negative neutrocytic ascites and spontaneous bacterial empyema should be treated with a third-generation cephalosporin for 5 days with an infusion of 25% albumin at day 1 (1.5 g/kg) and day 3 (1 g/kg) and with temporary cessation or dose reduction of nonselective beta blockers as needed to optimize hemodynamics and reduce the risk of hepatorenal syndrome. In patients who have frequent hospitalizations and antibiotic use, there should be a low threshold to initiate broad spectrum antimicrobial therapies while waiting for the initial ascitic cell count and culture. A lack of clinical improvement by day 3 or the presence of atypical or drug resistant organisms necessitates a repeat paracentesis to assess for improvement in the cell count and absence of any growth on ascitic cultures. Those who have persistent peritonitis or have multiple organisms on ascitic cultures should undergo cross-sectional imaging and surgical consultation promptly to rule out bowel perforation. Secondary prophylaxis with ciprofloxacin daily or sulfamethoxazole/trimethoprim daily should be instituted after completing treatment. Secondary prophylaxis is continued indefinitely until there is resolution of ascites.

Hepatorenal syndrome should be treated with the goal of improving renal function by reversing renal vasoconstriction and splanchnic vasodilation. Treatment entails volume expansion with albumin and vasoconstrictive therapy using midodrine and octreotide to improve systemic hemodynamics. Terlipressin (not available in the United States) and norepinephrine are alternative vasoconstrictive therapies that can be considered. Diuretics, nonselective beta blockers, nephrotoxic substances, and large volume paracentesis should be avoided. If patients have discomfort from tense

ascites, a limited paracentesis removing 1–2 L can be performed with albumin repletion. It is also important to identify and treat triggers for hepatorenal syndrome which are often from infection or bleeding. The duration of treatment is dependent upon the improvement (or lack of improvement) in renal function with vasoconstrictive therapies and whether maximal dosage has been achieved. Lack of response may warrant initiation of hemodialysis as a bridge to liver transplantation and palliative care discussions. In select situations TIPS placement may be considered. Given the poor prognosis associated with hepatorenal syndrome, it is important to consider referral to a liver transplant center in patients who would otherwise be potentially suitable candidates and in some cases to involve palliative care.

Table 46–3 outlines the current treatments for ascites, spontaneous bacterial peritonitis, and hepatorenal syndrome.

▶ When to Admit

Those with recurrent ascites that are mild may be able to be managed as an outpatient with close coordination with the patient and the patient's support system. Patients with tense ascites, symptomatic ascites, spontaneous bacterial peritonitis,

Table 46–3 Current management of ascites, spontaneous bacterial peritonitis, hepatorenal syndrome.

Ascites
Low salt added diet
Diuresis primarily with spironolactone (furosemide can be added for peripheral edema)
Large volume paracentesis
Transjugular intrahepatic portosystemic shunt
Liver transplantation
Drainage catheter (only in palliative setting)
Spontaneous bacterial peritonitis
Prompt antibiotic treatment
25% albumin infusion (Day 1: 1.5 g/kg and Day 3: 1 g/kg)
Secondary antibiotic prophylaxis after completing treatment
Hepatorenal syndrome
Cessation of diuretics
Avoidance of nephrotoxic agents
25% albumin infusion
Vasoconstrictive therapy with midodrine and octreotide or norepinephrine
Hemodialysis
Liver transplantation

or renal failure concerning for hepatorenal syndrome should be promptly hospitalized for urgent evaluation. Referral to a hepatologist for management and for liver transplant evaluation should be considered.

HEPATIC ENCEPHALOPATHY

▶ Pathogenesis

Hepatic encephalopathy develops when toxins produced by gut bacteria are not sufficiently cleared by the liver, accumulate in the systemic circulation, and cross the blood brain barrier. These toxins often entail nitrogenous products including ammonia. The failure to sufficiently clear toxins usually results from poor liver function and is often compounded by a second insult such as infection, bleeding, hypovolemia, acute kidney injury, electrolyte derangements, constipation, and/or sedative medications. Portosystemic shunts are another cause of encephalopathy and these may occur de-novo with portal hypertension. Less common causes of encephalopathy and hyperammonemia that should be considered in atypical cases are acquired urea cycle defects, carnitine deficiency, medications especially valproic acid, and infection from urease producing bacteria.

▶ Prevention

While there are no specific treatments that prevent the first episode of hepatic encephalopathy, adhering to general liver preventative measures outlined earlier can help avoid hepatic encephalopathy. It is also important to minimize triggers of hepatic encephalopathy by avoiding bleeding, hypovolemia, acute kidney injury, electrolyte derangements, infection, constipation, and sedating medications. Subsequent episodes of hepatic encephalopathy may be prevented with lactulose and/or rifaximin as well as avoidance of precipitants.

▶ Clinical Findings

A. Symptoms & Signs

Hepatic encephalopathy can manifest as a wide spectrum of neuropsychiatric abnormalities. Patients may have minimal hepatic encephalopathy which requires psychometric testing for diagnosis or they may present with personality change, disorientation, lethargy, somnolence, or be comatose–which can be graded clinically from zero to four using West Haven criteria. The presence of asterixis in a patient with cirrhosis is highly suggestive of hepatic encephalopathy, but its absence does not rule out the diagnosis. Any focal neurological deficit warrants consideration of another acute cause such as stroke or intracranial hemorrhage.

Table 46–4 outlines the West Haven criteria for grading hepatic encephalopathy.

Table 46–4 West Haven criteria for hepatic encephalopathy.

Grade	Manifestations
0 (Minimal)	Abnormal psychometric tests but no obvious abnormalities in consciousness, personality, or behavior
1	Trivial lack of awareness, short attention span, reversed day-night sleep cycle
2	Lethargy, disorientation, personality change, inappropriate behavior
3	Somnolence to semistupor, confusion, response to noxious stimuli preserved
4	Coma; no response to noxious stimuli

B. Laboratory Findings

Ammonia levels in patients with cirrhosis do not necessarily correlate with the presence, severity, or resolution of hepatic encephalopathy. Instead, clinical assessment of hepatic encephalopathy should be utilized. A one-time ammonia level may be useful to help guide the clinical suspicion for hepatic encephalopathy when evaluating a patient with altered mental status of unclear etiology. In that situation, an arterial ammonia level is preferred over a venous ammonia level. It should be noted that hyperammonemia can be caused by etiologies other than cirrhosis such as portosystemic shunts, urea cycle defects, organic acidemia, carnitine deficiency, urease producing bacteria, medications, and acute liver failure.

Patients with cirrhosis who present with hepatic encephalopathy should undergo testing to evaluate for potential triggers such as electrolyte derangements, acute kidney injury, gastrointestinal bleeding, sepsis, and substance use. Laboratory testing should consist of a basic metabolic profile, complete blood count, blood cultures, urinalysis, urine culture, diagnostic paracentesis or thoracentesis (if there is a sufficient amount of fluid that can be sampled from the ascites or hepatic hydrothorax percutaneously without obstruction by other organs), and toxicology panels.

C. Imaging Studies

Imaging can be useful for identifying potential causes of hepatic encephalopathy and for ruling out other causes of altered mental status. An abdominal ultrasound and chest x-ray evaluate for the presence of ascites and hepatic hydrothorax as an infection of either fluid collection can cause encephalopathy. These radiographic studies also assess for other causes of infection such as pneumonia. In cases where patients have recurrent episodes of hepatic encephalopathy, cross-sectional imaging with contrast (as tolerated by renal function) can help evaluate for the presence of de-novo or congenital portosystemic shunts. Imaging of the head may

Table 46–5 Precipitants of hepatic encephalopathy.

Infection
Gastrointestinal bleeding
Hypovolemia (eg, over-diuresis, diarrhea)
Acute kidney injury
Electrolyte derangements (eg, hyponatremia, hypokalemia)
Medications (eg, narcotics, sedatives)
Constipation
Noncompliance with lactulose and/or rifaximin
Portosystemic shunts (de novo, congenital, or TIPS)
TIPS: transjugular intrahepatic portosystemic shunt

Table 46–6 Select differential for hepatic encephalopathy and hyperammonemia.

Hepatic Encephalopathy	Hyperammonemia
Electrolyte derangements (eg, hypoglycemia)	Hepatic encephalopathy (in setting of cirrhosis)
Substance intoxication	Portosystemic shunt
Substance withdrawal	Acute liver failure
Stroke	Urea cycle defect
Intracranial bleeding	Organic acidemia
Seizures	Carnitine deficiency
Psychiatric disorders	Medications (eg, valproic acid)
Dementia	Infection (urease producing bacteria)
Nutritional deficiencies	Renal failure

be useful to rule out an acute intracranial process especially when focal neurological deficits are present.

Table 46–5 lists common precipitants of hepatic encephalopathy.

Differential Diagnosis

The differential diagnosis of hepatic encephalopathy is broad and includes electrolyte derangements, substance intoxication, substance withdrawal, stroke, intracranial bleeding, seizures, psychiatric disorders, and dementia. As mentioned earlier, once the diagnosis of hepatic encephalopathy is established, it is important to develop a wide differential for what triggered the encephalopathy including infection, gastrointestinal bleeding, hypovolemia, acute kidney injury, electrolyte derangements, constipation, sedative medications, and portosystemic shunts. Medication noncompliance with lactulose or rifaximin should always be considered a diagnosis of exclusion. Similarly, hyperammonemia in a noncirrhotic patient does not necessarily imply liver-related hepatic encephalopathy as this finding can occur from portosystemic shunts, acquired urea cycle defects, carnitine deficiency, medications, and from sepsis related to urease producing bacteria.

Table 46–6 provides the differential to consider for both hepatic encephalopathy and hyperammonemia.

Treatment

The primary treatment of hepatic encephalopathy is to treat the underlying precipitant if feasible and to use a medication that lowers urease producing colonic bacteria in order to reduce the amount of ammonia that enters the blood circulation. First line treatment after the first episode of hepatic encephalopathy is lactulose which should be titrated to achieve three to four soft bowel movements per 24-hour period. In cases where the patient is unable to safely take oral medications due to encephalopathy, lactulose can be administered through an enteral tube or a tap water enema can be given rectally. Although lactulose is the preferred laxative because of its ability to reduce ammonia generation by increasing colonic acidity, it can cause abdominal bloating and discomfort for some patients and can be substituted for an alternative laxative such as polyethylene glycol 3350. After resolution of hepatic encephalopathy, lactulose should be continued for secondary prophylaxis and all potential triggers of hepatic encephalopathy should be avoided.

If the patient has a second episode of hepatic encephalopathy, the evaluation for a potential trigger should be repeated and rifaximin 550 mg twice daily added to both the treatment and prophylaxis regimen. If hepatic encephalopathy continues to be persistent in the absence of any known triggers, uncommon causes such as portosystemic shunts should be ruled out. Medication compliance should be reinforced with the patient and the patient's support system with plans made to address any treatment barriers. Nutrition counseling with a goal of a daily caloric intake of 35–40 kcal/kg and daily protein intake of 1.2–1.5 g/kg is important as increased skeletal muscle mass may allow for myocyte metabolism of ammonia into glutamine, thus potentially improving hepatic encephalopathy. The addition of oral zinc sulfate 220 mg daily to the treatment and prophylaxis regimen can be considered when patients have zinc deficiency or refractory hepatic encephalopathy. Several studies are exploring the feasibility of using fecal microbiota transplantation to treat hepatic encephalopathy and this may become a future treatment option. Until then, liver transplantation may need to be considered in refractory cases.

Table 46–7 outlines the current treatment options for hepatic encephalopathy.

When to Admit

Those with mild hepatic encephalopathy may be able to be managed as an outpatient with close coordination with the patient and his or her support system. Patients with severe or

Table 46–7 Current management of hepatic encephalopathy.

Control of underlying precipitant
Nutrition with adequate caloric and protein intake
Lactulose titrated for 3–4 soft bowel movements per 24 hour period
Rifaximin
Zinc
Clinical trials (eg, fecal microbiota transplant)
Liver transplantation

refractory hepatic encephalopathy should be promptly hospitalized for urgent evaluation. Potential triggers of hepatic encephalopathy from infection and bleeding must be assessed and treated quickly. Referral to a hepatologist for management and for liver transplant evaluation should be considered.

Acharya C, Bajaj JS. Current management of hepatic encephalopathy. *Am J Gastroenterol.* 2018;113(11):1600–1612. [PMID: 30002466]

Adebayo D, Neong SF, Wong F. Ascites and hepatorenal syndrome. *Clin Liver Dis.* 2019;23(4):659–682. [PMID: 31563217]

Aithal GP, Palaniyappan N, China L, et al. Guidelines on the management of ascites in cirrhosis. *Gut.* 2021 Jan;70(1):9–29. [PMID: 33067334]

Biggins SW, Angeli P, Garcia-Tsao G, et al. Diagnosis, evaluation, and management of ascites, spontaneous bacterial peritonitis and hepatorenal syndrome: 2021 Practice Guidance by the American Association for the Study of Liver Diseases. *Hepatology.* 2021 Aug;74(2):1014–1048. [PMID: 33942342]

Simonetto DA, Gines P, Kamath PS. Hepatorenal syndrome: pathophysiology, diagnosis, and management. *BMJ.* 2020;370:m2687. [PMID: 32928750]

Vilstrup H, Amodio P, Bajaj J, et al. Hepatic encephalopathy in chronic liver disease: 2014 Practice Guideline by the American Association for the Study of Liver Diseases and the European Association for the Study of the Liver. *Hepatology.* 2014;60(2):715–735. [PMID: 25042402]

Portal Hypertension & Esophageal Variceal Hemorrhage

47

Kathleen Viveiros, MD

Marvin Ryou, MD

ESSENTIAL CONCEPTS

▶ Either nonselective β-blockers or esophageal variceal ligation are first-line treatment for primary prophylaxis of variceal hemorrhage in patients with medium to large esophageal and high-risk small varices.

▶ Endoscopic variceal ligation (EVL) is an alternative to pharmacologic therapy for patients intolerant to β-blockers.

▶ Management of acute variceal hemorrhage includes resuscitation to conservative PRBC transfusion thresholds, antibiotic prophylaxis, use of vasoactive agents, and endoscopic treatment with band ligation. Early transjugular intrahepatic portosystemic shunt (TIPS) should be considered for high-risk patients.

▶ Balloon tamponade or an esophageal stent can be used as a bridge to TIPS or surgical shunt therapy.

▶ The combination of a nonselective β-blocker and esophageal variceal ligation is first-line treatment for prevention of recurrent variceal hemorrhage.

▶ Hepatic venous pressure gradient (HVPG) measurements aid in prognosis and therapy.

▶ TIPS, surgical shunt procedures, or liver transplantation are treatment options for patients who do not respond to medical therapy.

▶ Gastric varices that are cardiofundal in location (isolated gastric varices Type I and gastroesophageal varices Type II) are best treated with endoscopic ultrasound (EUS) guided injection therapy with hemostatic coils and/or cyanoacrylate glue or direct endoscopic injection with glue. Gastroesophageal varices Type I (esophageal varices extending into the lesser curvature) can be treated as esophageal varices (banding ligation) or injection therapy.

▶ TIPS is the preferred rescue procedure for uncontrolled variceal bleeding and can be first-line therapy for high-risk patients.

▶ Portal hypertensive gastropathy (PHG) is usually mild to moderate and bleeding can be chronic or acute.

▶ Chronic bleeding from PHG is treated with β-blockers or TIPS based on the severity of hemorrhage.

▶ General Considerations

Chronic liver disease and cirrhosis are among the leading causes of mortality in the United States. Cirrhosis is further defined into two clinically important categories: compensated and decompensated cirrhosis. The distinction between these two stages reflects the presence or absence of cirrhosis complications resulting from clinically significant portal hypertension (defined by a HVPG of ≥10 mm Hg). The main decompensating events of cirrhosis are development of ascites, hepatic encephalopathy or variceal hemorrhage. Portal hypertension and its consequences are progressively debilitating complications of cirrhosis (Table 47–1). Variceal hemorrhage, spontaneous bacterial peritonitis, and the hepatorenal syndrome are chiefly responsible for the high morbidity and mortality rates in patients with cirrhosis.

Esophageal varices develop at a rate of 7–8% per year in patients with compensated cirrhosis. Progression from small to large sized varices happens at a rate of 10–12% per year. In patients with compensated cirrhosis, the presence of varices can be found in 30–40% and can be present in up to 80% of patients with decompensated cirrhosis. Variceal hemorrhage occurs in 25–35% of patients with cirrhosis and large esophagogastric varices. The majority of bleeding episodes occur within the first year of diagnosis of varices. Bleeding from esophageal varices is associated with 15–20% early mortality and accounts for one-third of all deaths. If no long-term therapy is instituted after control of acute hemorrhage,

Table 47–1. Causes of portal hypertension.

	Presinusoidal	Sinusoidal or Mixed
Infectious (other than hepatitis)	Schistosomiasis	—
Toxin-mediated	Azathioprine Chronic arsenic ingestion Vinyl chloride	Methotrexate Alcoholic hepatitis Hypervitaminosis A
Cirrhotic	Early biliary cirrhosis	Chronic hepatitis Alcoholic cirrhosis Cryptogenic cirrhosis Primary biliary cirrhosis Nonalcoholic steatohepatitis
Autoimmune, oncologic, primary fibrotic	Sarcoidosis Myeloproliferative diseases Congenital hepatic fibrosis Early primary sclerosing cholangitis	Incomplete septal fibrosis Nodular regenerative hyperplasia Primary sclerosing cholangitis
Vascular	Splenic vein thrombosis Portal vein thrombosis Cavernous transformation of the portal vein Extrinsic compression of the portal vein	—
Other	Idiopathic portal hypertension	—

Reproduced with permission from Bayles TM, Diehl AM: *Advanced Therapy in Gastroenterology and Liver Disease*. Shelton, CT: BC Decker; 2005.

60–70% of patients will experience recurrent variceal hemorrhage. Most of these episodes occur within 6–24 months of the index bleed.

Pathogenesis

Portal hypertension develops as a result of two main factors: (1) an increase in intrahepatic resistance, and (2) an increase in portal blood flow. In cirrhosis, the initiating event is an increase in hepatic and portocollateral resistance. The increased resistance occurs, in part, from sinusoidal encroachment, collagen deposition, vascular tree pruning, and nodular regeneration. These elements, together with the overexpression of endogenous vasoconstrictors (eg, endothelins and leukotrienes) and the underproduction of endogenous vasodilators (primarily nitric oxide), are responsible for the increase in intrahepatic and portocollateral resistance. Systemic vasodilation follows with the increased release of neurohormonal vasodilators (eg, nitric oxide, glucagon, tumor necrosis factor, prostaglandins, and other cytokines) and results in a hyperdynamic circulatory system. This is further complicated by angiogenesis, which increases splanchnic blood flow, exacerbates portal pressure elevation, induces neovascularization, and enhances the development of portosystemic collateral circulation including the development of esophageal varices. These factors also lead to the development of nonvariceal complications of portal hypertension including the development of ascites, hydrothorax, and the hepatorenal syndrome. The goal of therapy is to interrupt the process by decreasing portal venous blood flow and/or intrahepatic and portocollateral resistance.

Bosch J, Abraldes JG, Fernandez M, et al. Hepatic endothelial dysfunction and abnormal angiogenesis: new targets in the treatment of portal hypertension. *J Hepatol.* 2010;53:558–567. [PMID: 20561700]

Garcia-Tsao G, Abraldes JG, Berzigotti A, Bosch J. Portal hypertensive bleeding in cirrhosis: risk stratification, diagnosis, and management: 2016 practice guidance by the American Association for the study of liver diseases. *Hepatology.* 2017;65(1):310–335. [PMID: 27786365]

Natural History of Cirrhosis

Cirrhosis is no longer considered a static entity but may progress from a compensated state to a decompensated state, with the prognosis varying with the stage. This progression is dynamic, not necessarily relentless and potentially reversible. In a classic review by D'Amico et al. involving 843 patients, the estimated 1-year mortality was 1% for stage 1, 3.4% for stage 2, 20% for stage 3, and 57% for stage 4 (**Figure 47–1**). Median survival for compensated cirrhosis was >12 years compared to 2 years for decompensated cirrhosis.

D'Amico G, Garcia-Tsao G, Pagliaro L. Natural history and prognostic indicators of survival in cirrhosis: a systematic review of 118 studies. *J Hepatol.* 2006;44:217–231. [PMID: 16298014]

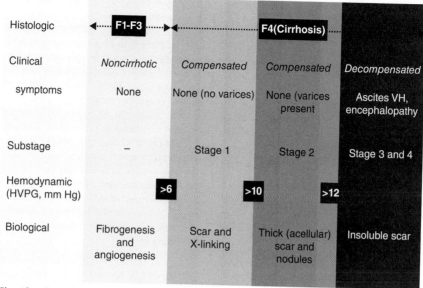

Histologic	◄······ F1-F3 ·····► ◄····················· F4(Cirrhosis) ·····················►			
Clinical	Noncirrhotic	Compensated	Compensated	Decompensated
symptoms	None	None (no varices)	None (varices present	Ascites VH, encephalopathy
Substage	–	Stage 1	Stage 2	Stage 3 and 4
Hemodynamic (HVPG, mm Hg)	>6		>10	>12
Biological	Fibrogenesis and angiogenesis	Scar and X-linking	Thick (acellular) scar and nodules	Insoluble scar

▲ **Figure 47–1.** Classification of cirrhosis, from a compensated stage to decompensated stages. (Adapted with permission from Garcia-Tsao G, Friedman S, Iredale J, et al. Now there are many (stages) where before there was one: in search of a pathophysiological classification of cirrhosis, *Hepatology* 2010;51(4):1445–1449.)

Garcia-Tsao G, Friedman S, Iredale J, et al. Now there are many stages where before there was one: in search of a pathophysiological classification of cirrhosis. *Hepatology.* 2010;51:1445–1449.

► Clinical Findings

A. Symptoms & Signs

Patients with cirrhosis have symptoms that are nonspecific for the presence of portal hypertension. Physical findings in cirrhosis that may suggest the presence of portal hypertension include muscle wasting, spider angiomata, jaundice, splenomegaly, ascites, abdominal collateral vessels, and an altered mental status.

B. Laboratory Findings

Laboratory findings include hyperbilirubinemia, hypoalbuminemia, thrombocytopenia, and a prolonged prothrombin time. Other abnormalities that may coexist include anemia, elevated creatinine level, and hyponatremia. Although the presence of these abnormalities may indicate the presence of portal hypertension, these values often remain normal in patients with compensated or early cirrhosis.

C. Noninvasive Studies for Predicting Cirrhosis

Radiographic studies that strongly suggest cirrhosis include a small, nodular liver, ascites, splenomegaly, intra-abdominal varices, or portal and hepatic vein thrombosis; however, no test is considered a diagnostic gold standard. The current best test for diagnosing cirrhosis is liver biopsy. However,

transient elastography as a noninvasive alternative has excellent predictive value for diagnosing cirrhosis and hepatic decompensation.

1. Abdominal ultrasound—Abdominal ultrasound findings that support a diagnosis of cirrhosis include a nodular liver, with increased echogenicity. In patients with more advanced cirrhosis and portal hypertension, findings of ascites, splenomegaly, and intra-abdominal varices may be detected. Unfortunately, ultrasonography is limited by interoperator variability, with a diagnostic accuracy of 85–91%. The addition of portal and hepatic vein flow Doppler images enables the assessment of hemodynamic changes that occur with cirrhosis. The reversal of portal vein flow occurs with increased hepatic resistance. This resistance results in the diversion of flow from the portal vein through portosystemic collaterals. This mechanism has been shown to be present in patients with advanced portal hypertension. Interoperator variability, patient position, phase of respiration, cardiac output, and timing of meals limit the accuracy of Doppler ultrasound.

2. Computed tomography scan and magnetic resonance imaging—These imaging studies are limited in their ability to detect changes associated with early cirrhosis but can accurately demonstrate later changes in liver architecture, ascites, and varices. Computed tomography angiography and magnetic resonance angiography can assess portal vein patency. Magnetic resonance elastography is very good for evaluating liver and spleen stiffness and identifies patients with cirrhosis and esophageal varices. However, performance of this test is not yet recommended for routine clinical evaluation.

3. Transient elastography

Transient elastography (Fibroscan®) is a technique that uses pulse-echo ultrasound to measure liver stiffness as a way of detecting fibrosis. This method of measuring fibrosis is reported to have a low interobserver variability and correlates well with the severity of fibrosis and the presence of portal hypertension. It is probably the best noninvasive test for determining the presence of cirrhosis. Spleen stiffness can be measured by either transient elastography or acoustic radiation force impulse imaging. However, the heterogeneity of the results precludes its value for routine clinical practice.

Asrani SK, Talwalkar JJA, Kamath PS, et.al. Role of magnetic resonance elastography in compensated and decompensated liver disease. *J Hepatol.* 2014;60:934–939. [PMID: 24362072]

Bonder A, Afdhal N. Utilization of FibroScan in clinical practice. *Curr Gastroenterol Rep.* 2014;16(2):372. [PMID: 24452634]

Castera L, Le Bail B, Roudot-Thoraval F, et al. Early detection in routine clinical practice of cirrhosis and oesophageal varices in chronic hepatitis C: comparison of transient elastography (Fibroscan) with standard laboratory tests and non-invasive scores. *J Hepatol.* 2009;50:59–68. [PMID: 19013661]

Singh S, Fujii LL, Murad MH, et al. Liver stiffness is associated with risk of decompensation, liver cancer, and death in patients with chronic liver disease: a systematic review and meta-analysis. *Clin Gastroenterol Hepatol.* 2013;11:1573–1584. [PMID: 23954643]

D. Noninvasive Predictors of Esophageal Varices

Current practice guidelines recommend endoscopic screening for the presence of esophageal varices in most patients with cirrhosis. If varices are not present, screening endoscopy should be repeated in 2–3 years or sooner if there is evidence of hepatic decompensation. Wireless capsule endoscopy has been compared with conventional upper endoscopy (EGD) in identifying and characterizing esophageal varices. High sensitivity and specificity have been reported for the ability of wireless capsule endoscopy to determine the presence of esophageal varices (84–96% accuracy), the size of esophageal varices, and the presence of red wale signs. The potential benefits of capsule endoscopy include decreased study time, better patient tolerance, avoidance of intravenous conscious sedation, and possibly decreased costs. Wireless capsule endoscopy is not currently recommended for clinical care as it is limited by inability to insufflate the esophagus, difficulty in measuring the length of varices, and image quality artifacts.

Several studies have attempted to identify noninvasive predictors of esophageal varices. A low platelet count is associated with the presence of varices, although the discriminating threshold for the presence of varices ranges between 68,000 and 160,000/mm². Studies have found that patients with esophageal varices have a lower mean platelet count and a greater rate of reduction of platelets over time compared with those who did not have varices. Noninvasive serum markers (indices combining a number of biochemical tests)

have been useful in identifying cirrhotic patients in whom the risk of developing clinically significant esophageal varices is low. However, their positive or negative predictive values are insufficient to avoid screening endoscopy. Other noninvasive findings, such as splenomegaly, enlarged portal vein diameter greater than 13 mm on ultrasound imaging, and advanced Child-Pugh class, have not been reproducible predictors of esophageal varices.

The exception to noninvasive measures approved for variceal screening in cirrhosis is Fibroscan. Patients with a liver stiffness <20 kilopascals (kPa) measured by transient elastography and a platelet count >150,000/mm³ were very unlikely to have high-risk varices (<5%) and thus, endoscopy can be safely avoided. Fibroscan is readily available and used in office settings as well as academic medical centers. The use of Fibroscan with platelet count parameters in compensated cirrhosis patients may circumvent approximately 20–25% of screening EGDs.

Garcia-Tsao G, Abraldes JG, Berzigotti A, Bosch J. Portal hypertensive bleeding in cirrhosis: Risk stratification, diagnosis, and management: 2016 practice guidance by the American Association for the study of liver diseases. *Hepatology.* 2017;65(1):310–335. [PMID: 27786365]

Lapalus MG, Ben Soussan E, Gaudric M, et al. Esophageal capsule endoscopy vs EGD for the evaluation of portal hypertension: a French prospective multicentre comparative study. *Am J Gastroenterol.* 2009;104:1112–1118. [PMID: 19337246]

Qamar AA, Grace ND, Groszmann RJ, et al; Portal Hypertension Collaborative Group. Platelet count is not a predictor of the presence of development of gastroesophageal varices in cirrhosis. *Hepatology.* 2008;47:153–159. [PMID: 18161700]

Sebastiani G, Tempesta D, Fattovich G, et al. Prediction of oesophageal varices in hepatic cirrhosis by simple serum non-invasive markers: results of a multicenter, large-scale study. *J Hepatol.* 2010;53:630–638. [PMID: 20615567]

E. Invasive Studies to Measure Portal Hypertension: Hepatic Venous Pressure Gradient

HVPG measurements obtained by angiography provide information for diagnosis, prognosis, and management of portal hypertension. The HVPG is the difference between the wedged or occluded hepatic vein pressure and the free hepatic vein pressure. Normal portal pressure (HVPG) ranges from 1 to 5 mm Hg with greater than 5 mm Hg indicating the presence of portal hypertension. In patients with sinusoidal cirrhosis, the HVPG accurately predicts the portal venous pressure gradient. An HVPG equal to or greater than 10 mm Hg identifies patients with clinically significant portal hypertension and is predictive of the development of varices. Pharmacologically reducing the HPVG more than 10% at 1 year compared with the baseline measurement significantly lowers the risk of developing varices. Similarly, a 10% increase in HPVG significantly increases the risk of developing varices.

Determining a patient's HPVG also predicts variceal bleeding, development of hepatic decompensation, development of hepatocellular carcinoma, determination of response to clinical treatment, and estimations of patient survival. Variceal bleeding can occur in patients with HVPG greater than 12 mm Hg. In patients with acute or ongoing bleeding, an HVPG greater than 20 mm Hg is associated with early rebleeding or uncontrolled bleeding, longer intensive care unit stays, prolonged hospital stays, higher transfusion requirements, and a lower probability of survival.

Patients achieving a reduction in HVPG to less than 12 mm Hg or a reduction in HVPG of 20% after pharmacologic therapy are less likely to develop recurrent esophagogastric variceal bleeding, ascites, spontaneous bacterial peritonitis, hepatorenal syndrome, and hepatic encephalopathy. Unfortunately, only 35–45% of treated patients respond with a 20% decrease in HVPG. Patients, who do not achieve an HVPG of less than 12 mm Hg, or a 20% reduction from their baseline HVPG after pharmacologic treatment, have a high risk for recurrent variceal bleeding and a greater risk of developing complications of portal hypertension and a higher probability of death. Repeat HPVG measurements obtained 1–3 months after initiating treatment help guide therapeutic decisions such as their candidacy for TIPS to mitigate their risk of recurrent variceal bleeding.

A promising new method for measuring the portal pressure gradient (PPG) is through EUS guided direct measurement of the portal vein and hepatic vein. This method using an FDA-approved device appears feasible and safe, and a multicenter registry study is underway. With direct portal pressure measurement, EUS-guided PPG can potentially assess post-sinusoidal, sinusoidal, and pre-sinusoidal causes of portal hypertension.

Abraldes JG, Tarantino I, Turnes J, et al. Hemodynamic response to pharmacological treatment of portal hypertension and long-term prognosis of cirrhosis. *Hepatology.* 2003;37:902–908. [PMID: 12668985]

Huang JY, Samarasena JB, Tsujino T, et al. EUS-guided portal pressure gradient measurement with a simple novel device: a human pilot study. *Gastrointest Endosc.* 2017;85:996–1001. [PMID: 27693644]

Ripoll C, Groszmann R, Garcia-Tsao G, et al. Hepatic venous pressure gradient predicts clinical decompensation in patients with compensated cirrhosis. *Gastroenterology.* 2007;133:481–488. [PMID: 17681169]

▶ Treatment

A. Goal & Options

Treatment of portal hypertension includes pharmacologic management aimed at decreasing portal pressure and endoscopic therapy aimed at obliterating esophageal varices. When medical treatment fails, shunt procedures can be used to decompress high portal pressure. The goal of treatment is to interrupt the process that leads to the development of varices, and other complications of portal hypertension including the development of ascites, hepatic encephalopathy, and the hepatorenal syndrome.

De Franchis R. Revising consensus in portal hypertension: report of the Baveno V consensus workshop on methodology of diagnosis and therapy in portal hypertension. *J Hepatol.* 2010;53:762–768. [PMID: 20638742]

Garcia-Tsao G, Bosch J. Management of varices and variceal hemorrhage in cirrhosis. *N Engl J Med.* 2010;362:823–832. [PMID: 20200386]

1. Pharmacologic therapy—Nonselective β-blockers (propranolol, nadolol, and carvedilol) are the cornerstones of long-term management in patients with portal hypertension (Table 47–2). β-Blockers work by decreasing cardiac output by blocking β$_1$-receptors and by vasoconstricting splanchnic vessels via blockade of β$_2$-receptors, thereby leaving unopposed

Table 47–2. Drugs used in the management of portal hypertension.

Drug	Class of Drug	Starting Dose	Maximum Dose
Propranolol	Nonselective β-blocker	20–40 mg twice daily	640 mg/day
Nadolol	Nonselective β-blocker	40 mg daily	320 mg/day
Timolol	Nonselective β-blocker	10 mg daily	40 mg/day
Carvedilol	Nonselective β-blocker with intrinsic anti-α-adrenergic activity	6.25 mg daily	12.5 mg/day
Isosorbide mononitrate	Long-acting nitrate	20 mg daily	240 mg/day
Spironolactone	Aldosterone antagonist	25 mg daily	400 mg/day
Furosemide	Loop diuretic	40 mg daily	80 mg/day
Octreotide	Splanchnic vasoconstrictor	50 μg bolus, followed by 50 μg/h	50 μg/h
Norfloxacin	Quinolone antibiotic	400 mg twice daily	—

α-adrenergic activity. Unfortunately, not all patients respond to maximally tolerated doses of β-blockers. In patients who fail to show a reduction in HPVG, there is often an increase in portocollateral resistance. The long-acting nitrate isosorbide mononitrate, when used in conjunction with β-blockers, has been shown to counteract this increase in portocollateral resistance. Oral nitrates may cause systemic hypotension, which limits their clinical usefulness. Carvedilol, a nonselective β-blocker with intrinsic anti–α$_1$-adrenergic activity, produces a greater reduction in the HVPG than nonselective β-blockers given as monotherapy and has been shown to be well tolerated in clinical trials.

The use of β-blockers in patients with cirrhosis is limited by their side-effect profile, which includes hypotension, fatigue, lethargy, depression, and dyspnea in patients with associated pulmonary disease. Due to concomitant diseases such as reactive airway disease, congestive heart failure, bradycardia, and heart block, 15–20% of patients are unable to take β-blockers. An additional 15% of patients discontinue the drug because of intolerable side effects. In patients who are candidates for β-blocker therapy, dose titration should be adjusted to patient tolerance.

Terlipressin, an analog of vasopressin, and somatostatin and its analogs, octreotide, vapreotide, and lanreotide, have been the agents used for the management of acute variceal bleeding. These vasoconstrictive drugs act by decreasing splanchnic blood flow, resulting in a lowering of portal pressure, and by decreasing splanchnic hyperemia. Vasopressin is no longer used because of its significant side-effect profile.

Terlipressin has a milder side-effect profile than vasopressin, and it does not appear to alter renal excretion of sodium. Its intravenous half-life is 4 hours, and its use results in a 21% decrease in HVPG. Randomized controlled trials comparing terlipressin with a placebo or no pharmacologic treatment in patients with acute variceal hemorrhage have demonstrated a significant survival benefit for terlipressin. It is safer and more effective than either vasopressin or vasopressin plus nitroglycerin.

Somatostatin has been shown to decrease portal pressure in patients with portal hypertension. It works by inhibiting vasodilatory peptides from the gastrointestinal tract that have been shown to contribute to the maintenance of portal hypertension. Due to its short half-life (2 minutes), somatostatin is used as a continuous infusion after an initial bolus to treat acute variceal hemorrhage.

The somatostatin analogs, namely octreotide, lanreotide, and vapreotide, have similar pharmacologic properties to somatostatin.

Octreotide, which is used widely in the United States, is thought to act through the inhibition of the vasodilator glucagon. The intravenous half-life of octreotide, like that of somatostatin, is short; therefore, it is given as a bolus followed by a continuous infusion. Although intravenous octreotide may decrease portal pressure and bleeding from esophageal varices, its use has not been shown to improve overall

survival. Similarly, vapreotide in combination with endoscopic therapy has been shown to decrease bleeding from esophageal varices more effectively than endoscopic therapy alone, but without a benefit in survival.

Together with a low-sodium diet, continuous spironolactone (100 mg/day) treatment results in a modest decrease in portal pressure. The efficacy and safety of losartan and irbesartan, angiotensin II receptor blockers, in lowering portal pressure have been established in Child-Pugh class A patients but the risk of systemic hypotension and renal failure precludes their use in patients with decompensated cirrhosis. Randomized controlled trials with established clinical endpoints are needed to establish clinical efficacy.

Unfortunately, none of these drugs have been approved by the Food and Drug Administration (FDA) specifically for the treatment of variceal hemorrhage. Some have FDA approval for other indications (octreotide) and are widely used for control of variceal bleeding. Others are generic (nonselective β-blockers) and approval has not been sought because of the huge expense involved.

Calés P, Masliah C, Bernard B, et al. Early administration of vapreotide for variceal bleeding in patients with cirrhosis. *N Engl J Med*. 2001;244:23–28. [PMID: 11136956]

Groszmann RJ, Garcia-Tsao G, Bosch J, et al; Portal Hypertension Collaborative Group. Beta-blockers to prevent gastroesophageal varices in patients with cirrhosis. *N Engl J Med*. 2005;353: 2254–2261. [PMID: 16306522]

Seo YS, Park SY, Kim MY, et al. Lack of difference among terlipressin, somatostatin and octreotide in control of acute gastroesophageal variceal hemorrhage. *Hepatology*. 2014;60:954–963. [PMID: 24415445]

2. Endoscopic variceal ligation—EVL is a local treatment for varices and does not alter the pathophysiologic processes that lead to their development. As such, even with successful EVL, varices eventually recur. EVL consists of the placement of rubber bands on variceal columns that lead to localized mucosal and submucosal necrosis and replacement of the varix by scar tissue. Band ligation carries the risk of causing esophageal ulcerations that have the potential to bleed.

EVL has replaced sclerotherapy as the endoscopic treatment of choice.

Garcia-Pagán JC, Bosch J. Endoscopic band ligation in the treatment of portal hypertension. *Nat Clin Pract Gastroenterol Hepatol*. 2005;2:526–535. [PMID: 16355158]

3. Radiologic therapy—TIPS was first introduced in the 1980s as an alternative to surgically performed shunts. TIPS should be reserved for patients who fail pharmacologic and endoscopic management for either acute or recurrent variceal bleeding.

Placement of a TIPS bypasses the fibrosed liver and allows for unhindered blood flow between the portal and hepatic veins.

A catheter is inserted into the right internal jugular vein and advanced to the hepatic venous system (usually the right hepatic vein). A needle is then used to cannulate the liver, creating a tract to the portal vein. The transhepatic tract is dilated, and a flexible metal stent is placed, resulting in a shunt between the hepatic and portal veins. Placement of TIPS successfully treats variceal bleeding in greater than 90% of cases and is effective in acutely decreasing portal pressure.

Early complications of TIPS include fever, infection, renal dysfunction, intrahepatic or intraperitoneal hemorrhage, and liver failure. Furthermore, hyperbilirubinemia, secondary to hemolytic anemia, may persist until the TIPS stent is re-epithelialized. Long-term complications from TIPS placement include hepatic encephalopathy and stent occlusion. Over 20% of patients with TIPS will either develop or have worsening hepatic encephalopathy and should be treated with lactulose, neomycin, or rifaximin. Risk factors for developing hepatic encephalopathy include older age, larger stent diameter (10 mm diameter vs 8 mm diameter), and prior episodes of hepatic encephalopathy. Seventy percent of patients who undergo TIPS with noncoated stents will develop stent occlusion within 1 year and 90% by 2 years. Angioplasty or additional stent placement is successful in treating stent occlusion and decreases the reocclusion rate to 10% at 2 years. However, these complication rates are significantly reduced with the use of coated stents which have replaced noncoated stents as standard therapy. Patients treated with TIPS should have Doppler ultrasound surveillance at regular intervals to confirm stent patency, as TIPS dysfunction can result in variceal bleeding. However, angiographic assessment and measurements of portal pressure are more accurate in establishing TIPS dysfunction.

Absolute contraindications to TIPS placement include right heart failure and polycystic liver disease. Relative contraindications include systemic infection, portal vein thrombosis, biliary obstruction, and severe hepatic encephalopathy. Although TIPS can be successfully placed in most patients, placement is associated with a 30-day mortality rate of 3–15% and a procedure-related mortality rate of 2–5%.

Boyer TD, Haskal ZJ; American Association for the Study of Liver Diseases. The role of transjugular intrahepatic portosystemic shunt in the management of portal hypertension. *Hepatology.* 2005;41:386–400. [PMID: 15660434]

Bureau C, Garcia-Pagan JC, Otal P, et al. Improved clinical outcome using polytetrafluoroethylene-coated stents for TIPS: results of a randomized study. *Gastroenterology.* 2004;126:469–475. [PMID: 14762784]

4. Liver transplantation—Variceal hemorrhage alone is not an indication for liver transplantation. However in appropriate candidates as determined by the Model for End-Stage Liver Disease (MELD) scoring system, liver transplantation can result in eliminating the complications of portal hypertension including variceal hemorrhage. Liver transplantation continues to be limited by organ availability.

5. Prevention of portal hypertension—Early treatment with β-blockers prior to the development of complications of portal hypertension has not been shown to halt or delay the progression of portal hypertension. Unfortunately, the results from a large multicenter randomized controlled trial have not supported the use of nonselective β-blockers in the setting prior to the development of clinically significant portal hypertension. However, data from this trial show that measurements of the HVPG predict the development of esophageal varices, hepatic decompensation, and the development of hepatocellular carcinoma.

B. Primary Prophylaxis for Variceal Hemorrhage

1. Nonselective β-blockers—Because of the high morbidity and mortality in patients with cirrhosis associated with acute variceal bleeding, pharmacologic therapy aimed at preventing initial variceal bleeding is paramount (Figure 47–2). Nonselective β-blockers are the only established pharmacologic therapy for primary prophylaxis of variceal bleeding. A meta-analysis of randomized controlled trials has demonstrated their efficacy in decreasing the rates of a first variceal bleed from 24% to 15%. These studies involved primarily patients with Child-Pugh class A and B cirrhosis.

Current practice guidelines on the management of portal hypertension recommend that patients with small varices who are at increased risk of bleeding (red wale sign on endoscopy, hepatic decompensation) should be treated prophylactically with β-blockers. Patients with small varices who are not at high risk may be started on β-blockers, but their long-term efficacy has not been established. All patients with medium- to large-sized varices who are judged to be compliant and are without contraindications to or intolerant of nonselective β-blockers should be treated with these drugs. Therapy must be continued for a lifetime, as the risk of bleeding recurs if treatment is discontinued.

Although combining a long-acting nitrate with a nonselective β-blocker increases the number of hemodynamic responders, it has not resulted in incremental clinical benefit (ie, by preventing initial variceal hemorrhage or leading to improved survival). Similarly, combining spironolactone with β-blockers showed no benefit in decreasing rates of bleeding episodes or survival compared with treatment using β-blockers alone. Current data do not support the use of combination therapy or monotherapy with nitrates for the prevention of a first variceal bleed.

Garcia-Tsao G, Abraldes JG, Berzigotti A, Bosch J. Portal hypertensive bleeding in cirrhosis: risk stratification, diagnosis, and management: 2016 practice guidance by the American Association for the study of liver diseases. *Hepatology.* 2017;65(1): 310–335. [PMID: 27786365]

2. Esophageal variceal ligation—Nonselective β-blockers or esophageal variceal ligation are considered to be first-line therapies for the prevention of initial variceal hemorrhage.

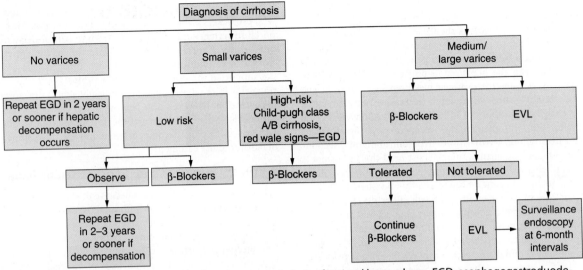

▲ **Figure 47–2.** Management algorithm for primary prophylaxis of variceal hemorrhage. EGD, esophagogastroduodenoscopy; EVL, endoscopic variceal ligation.

However, 15% of patients have absolute or relative contraindications to nonselective β-blockers, and an additional 15–20% are intolerant of β-blocker therapy. EVL is an excellent alternative for these patients.

For patients who undergo esophageal variceal ligation, it is recommended that the procedure be performed every 2–8 weeks until the varices are obliterated. As new varices may develop after eradication treatment, it is important to repeat an upper endoscopy in 3–6 months after the first documentation of eradicated varices and continue surveillance for varices every 6–12 months thereafter.

Meta-analyses have shown a benefit for EVL over β-blocker therapy in preventing first variceal hemorrhage, but EVL is associated with more serious side effects such as ulcer formation, post-procedural dysphagia, sedation risks and bleeding and offers no survival advantage. Randomized controlled trials of EVL have been limited by a short duration of follow-up. The studies with the largest number of patients and the longest follow-up have failed to show a difference between EVL and nonselective β-blockers, either for the prevention of initial variceal bleeding or for survival. Combination therapy using β-blockers plus EVL compared with EVL alone has not been shown to decrease the risk of first variceal hemorrhage and is associated with increased side effects. Unlike EVL, which is a local treatment, nonselective β-blockers have been shown to reduce the incidence of nonvariceal complications of portal hypertension.

There is no role for endoscopic sclerotherapy, TIPS, surgical shunts, or liver transplantation in the primary prophylaxis of variceal hemorrhage.

dela Peña J, Brullet E, Sanchez-Hernández R, et al. Variceal ligation plus nadolol compared with ligation for prophylaxis of variceal rebleeding: a multicenter trial. *Hepatology.* 2005;41:572–578. [PMID: 15726659]

Garcia-Tsao G, Sanyal AJ, Grace ND, et al; Practice Guidelines Committee of the American Association for the Study of Liver Diseases; Practice Parameters Committee of the American College of Gastroenterology. Prevention and management of gastroesophageal varices and variceal hemorrhage in cirrhosis. *Hepatology.* 2007;46:922–938. [PMID: 17879356]

Gonzalez R, Zamora J, Gomez-Camarero J, et al. Meta-analysis: combination endoscopic and drug therapy to prevent variceal rebleeding in cirrhosis. *Ann Intern Med.* 2008;149:109–122. [PMID: 18626050]

Lo GH, Lai KH, Cheng JS, et al. Endoscopic variceal ligation plus nadolol and sucralfate compared with ligation alone for the prevention of variceal bleeding: a prospective, randomized trial. *Hepatology.* 2000;32:461–465. [PMID: 10960435]

C. Acute Variceal Hemorrhage

Patients with acute variceal bleeding may present with hematemesis, melena, or hematochezia. The initial management includes immediate resuscitation, administration of prophylactic antibiotics and vasoactive agents, and endoscopy (Figure 47–3). It is important to consider elective intubation in patients with active bleeding to protect the airway from aspiration, especially if there is concomitant hepatic encephalopathy.

1. Resuscitation—Resuscitative measures should be aimed at replacing blood volume to a goal hemoglobin of 7–9 g/dL with a transfusion threshold of 7 g/dL, thereby avoiding

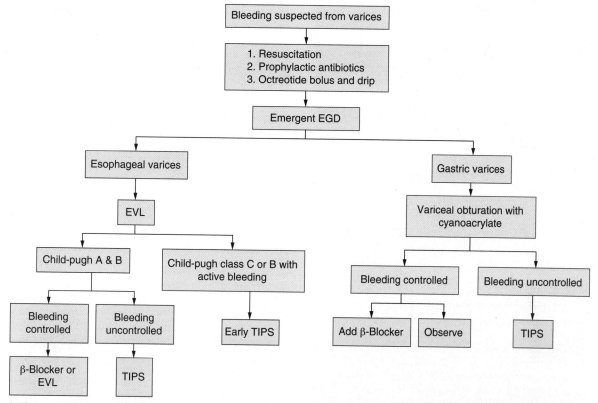

▲ **Figure 47–3.** Management algorithm for acute variceal hemorrhage. EGD, esophagogastroduodenoscopy; EVL, endoscopic variceal ligation; TIPS, transjugular intrahepatic portosystemic shunt.

increases in portal pressure and potential exacerbation of variceal bleeding associated with aggressive transfusion. Correcting thrombocytopenia and coagulopathy have not been shown to improve survival from an acute variceal bleed. Nonetheless, transfusing platelets in order to increase levels to greater than 50,000 and transfusing fresh frozen plasma or recombinant factor VII to reverse coagulopathy might be beneficial in the acute setting. The excessive use of saline should be avoided in resuscitation, as it can worsen portal hypertension, precipitate the formation of ascites and lead to volume overload.

2. Antibiotic prophylaxis—Infection in the setting of acute variceal bleeding is associated with early rebleeding and a high mortality rate. Patients with bleeding from varices are at high risk of developing infection, including spontaneous bacterial peritonitis. Short-term duration of antibiotics for 7 days should be administered to all patients with cirrhosis and acute variceal bleeding. Ceftriaxone (1 g/day) IV is superior to norfloxacin in patients with severely decompensated cirrhosis and is the antibiotic of choice in this setting.

3. Vasoactive agents—As soon as variceal hemorrhage is suspected, administration of vasoactive agents should be initiated. These agents include terlipressin, vasopressin and somatostatin or its analogs and provide adjunct therapy to EVL by lowering the portal pressures in the acute setting. All agents can safely be continued for 2–5 days except for vasopressin which should only be used for 24 hours. Terlipressin has fewer side effects than vasopressin and is the only pharmacologic agent that may have a survival benefit in patients with acute variceal hemorrhage.

Octreotide has been shown to have equal efficacy to sclerotherapy in controlling bleeding. It is safe with very few side effects and can be used continuously for up to 5 days. However, its use has been associated with tachyphylaxis, and its vasoactive effects may be transient. When combined with endoscopic therapy, octreotide improves management of acute bleeding compared with EVL alone, but without a survival benefit.

A recent multicenter prospective trial comparing terlipressin, somatostatin, and octreotide found them to be equally effective in controlling acute variceal bleeding and preventing early rebleeding episodes.

β-Blockers should not be administered during an active bleed, due to the physiologic blunting of heart rate in the setting of hypotension.

4. Endoscopic therapy—Endoscopic evaluation should occur as soon as possible and within the first 12 hours of a patient presenting with an acute variceal bleed. In addition to confirming the source of bleeding, endoscopic treatments are successful in controlling hemorrhage in 90% of cases. EVL is the procedure of choice. The combination of EVL and a somatostatin analog has been shown to be more effective than either EVL or a pharmacologic agent, given as monotherapy, and is the treatment of choice.

5. Balloon tamponade—Balloon tamponade is 80% effective in immediate control of hemorrhage from esophagogastric varices. However, serious complications occur when the balloon is left inflated for more than 24 hours. The complications, which occur in 20% of cases, include aspiration, esophageal ulceration and necrosis, and esophageal perforation. Balloon tamponade is best utilized as a short-term bridge to TIPS or liver transplantation.

6. Esophageal stent—A randomized controlled trial demonstrated that self-expandable esophageal covered metal stents (SX-ELLA Danis; Ella-CS, Hradec Kralove, Czech Republic) have greater efficacy (66%) with less serious adverse events (15%) compared to balloon tamponade (efficacy 20%; SAE 47%) in the control of esophageal variceal bleeding in treatment failures. This particular stent is currently unavailable in the US, although other through-the-scope covered esophageal stents have been introduced. Some expert centers now favor use of esophageal stents over balloon tamponade for refractory variceal bleeding. Trials for esophageal stents as initial therapy in high risk patients are planned.

7. Transjugular intrahepatic portosystemic shunt—TIPS is used to manage variceal bleeding when endoscopic and pharmacologic treatments fail. In 90% of cases of uncontrolled bleeding, TIPS is successful in stopping bleeding. Predictors of early mortality for the use of TIPS include creatinine greater than 1.7 mg/dL, bilirubin greater than 5 mg/dL, a Child-Pugh score greater than 12 and an APACHE II score greater than 18.

The use of polytetrafluoroethylene-coated stents results in significantly less stent dysfunction and lower clinical relapse rates. Patients receiving coated stents, compared with those receiving uncoated stents, had lower rates of recurrent bleeding and hepatic encephalopathy after 2 years of follow-up. Recent studies have shown that the early use of TIPS with coated stents in patients at high risk for treatment failure (ie, Child-Pugh class C patients or Child-Pugh class B patients with active bleeding at endoscopy) is associated with a decrease in treatment failure and in mortality.

Bureau C, Garcia-Pagan JC, Otal P, et al. Improved clinical outcome using polytetrafluoroethylene coated stents for TIPS: results of a randomized study. *Gastroenterology*. 2004;126:469–475. [PMID: 14762784]

Escorsell À, Pavel O, Cárdenas A, et al.; Variceal Bleeding Study Group. Esophageal balloon tamponade versus esophageal stent in controlling acute refractory variceal bleeding: a multicenter randomized, controlled trial. *Hepatology*. 2016;63(6):1957–1967. [PMID: 26600191]

Garcia-Pagan JC, Caca K, Bureau C, et al. Early use of TIPS in patients with cirrhosis and variceal bleeding. *N Engl J Med*. 2010;362:2370–2379. [PMID: 20573925]

Garcia-Tsao G, Abraldes JG, Berzigotti A, Bosch J. Portal hypertensive bleeding in cirrhosis: risk stratification, diagnosis, and management: 2016 practice guidance by the American Association for the study of liver diseases. *Hepatology*. 2017;65(1):310–335. [PMID: 27786365]

Reverter E, Tandon P, Augustin S, et al. A MELD-based model to determine risk of mortality among patients with acute variceal bleeding. *Gastroenterology*. 2014;146:412–419. [PMID: 24148622]

D. Prevention of Recurrent Variceal Hemorrhage

Once the acute bleed has been controlled, secondary prevention of rebleeding is paramount. First-line therapy for prevention of recurrent variceal hemorrhage is the combination of pharmacologic therapy and EVL. For patients who fail to respond to medical therapy, TIPS, surgical shunts, or urgent liver transplantation for appropriate candidates who meet listing criteria are options.

Pharmacologic treatment for prevention of recurring variceal hemorrhage is initiated by administration of a nonselective β-blocker, titrated to tolerance. β-Blockers have been shown to decrease rates of rebleeding from 63% to 42% and to decrease mortality from 27% to 20%. The hemodynamic goal of β-blocker therapy is to decrease the HVPG by greater than 20% or to a level less than 12 mm Hg (Figure 47–4). Achieving this goal has been shown to reduce rebleeding rates to less than 15%.

If patients are unable to tolerate β-blockers, EVL is the preferred endoscopic treatment to prevent recurrent variceal hemorrhage. Although EVL is more effective than sclerotherapy at preventing rebleeding, the risk of rebleeding after EVL remains high, reaching 30–50% at 2 years. The combination of a nonselective β-blocker and EVL has been shown to result in a decreased rate of variceal rebleeding, a lower transfusion requirement, a lower recurrence of esophageal varices, and a trend toward improved survival. However, there are slightly increased side effects with combination therapy. Current guidelines recommend combination therapy as the treatment of choice for prevention of variceal rebleeding.

EVL sessions should be performed every 1–4 weeks until complete variceal obliteration is achieved. Once varices are eradicated, continued surveillance every 3–6 months then 6–12 months thereafter is required to screen for recurrent varices.

In patients who do not respond to pharmacologic or endoscopic therapy, alone or in combination, decompression of the portal system by use of TIPS with coated stents is the next option. Liver transplantation provides the only

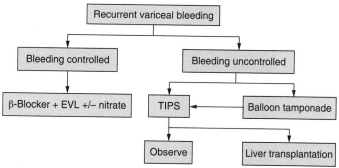

▲ **Figure 47–4.** Prevention of recurrent variceal hemorrhage. EVL, endoscopic variceal ligation; TIPS, transjugular intrahepatic portosystemic shunt.

definitive treatment for rebleeding as it directly addresses the underlying liver pathology that leads to portal hypertension and the formation of varices. Variceal bleeding is one of the clinical hallmarks of decompensated cirrhosis and warrants consideration for evaluation for liver transplantation in the appropriate candidate.

Numerous meta-analyses have demonstrated that TIPS is more effective than endoscopic therapy in preventing rebleeding from varices. The drawback of TIPS is an increase in hepatic encephalopathy and the lack of a survival benefit. Endoscopic and pharmacologic therapy remains the first-line therapy for prevention of rebleeding, with TIPS reserved as a rescue therapy.

GASTRIC VARICES

▶ General Considerations

Gastric varices are present in 20% of patients with portal hypertension and account for 10–15% of variceal bleeds. Gastric varices can occur alone or in combination with esophageal varices. Although the risk of bleeding from gastric varices is lower than that from esophageal varices, gastric variceal hemorrhage can be more severe than esophageal variceal bleeding and are associated with higher rates of rebleeding (between 34% and 89%). Gastric varices are more common in patients with extrahepatic portal vein obstruction than in patients with cirrhosis.

A. Etiology

Management depends on the underlying etiology of the gastric varix; therefore, it is important to identify the cause of the varix before treatment. Varices that develop from portal hypertension have been treated with EVL, administration of vasoactive agents or cyanoacrylate glue, or TIPS (see Figure 47–3). Varices that develop after splenic vein thrombosis or stenosis, leading to isolated left-sided portal hypertension, are best treated with splenectomy or splenic artery embolization.

B. Classification

Gastric varices are classified according to their anatomic location in the stomach and their relationship to esophageal varices. Isolated type 1 gastric varices (GOV1) extend from esophageal varices to the lesser curvature of the stomach. As such, they should be treated similarly to esophageal varices (ie, using EVL). Isolated type 2 gastric varices (GOV2) extend from esophageal varices to the gastric fundus. IGV1 are located in the fundus, whereas IGV2 are located elsewhere in the stomach. Risk factors for gastric variceal bleeding include location in the fundus (GOV2, IGV1), size larger than 5 mm, presence of endoscopic red wale signs, and Child-Pugh class C cirrhosis.

Unlike esophageal varices, gastric varices can bleed with HVPG less than 12 mm Hg. This is thought to be the result of a higher prevalence of spontaneous shunting (gastrorenal shunts), which decreases portal pressure but does not decrease the reversal of flow in splenic veins that result in gastric varices.

▶ Treatment

A. Pharmacologic Therapy

Given the high morbidity and mortality from gastric variceal bleeds, it is reasonable to treat patients empirically with vasoactive agents shown to improve bleeding outcomes in esophageal variceal hemorrhage. Similarly, nonselective β-blockers have been used for prevention of recurrent variceal bleeding.

B. Endoscopic Therapy

Endoscopy is essential for identifying gastric varices. However, because these varices can lie deep in the submucosa, standard endoscopy can underestimate their true prevalence. Most gastric varices that bleed are close to the mucosal surface and are readily identifiable.

EVL is associated with a high rate of rebleeding for GOV2 and IGV1 varices. Its use should be limited to GOV1 varices. Endoscopic variceal obturation refers to the injection of adhesive and glue agents into a varix. Tissue adhesives, including *N*-butylcyanoacrylate, isobutyl-2-cyanoacrylate, and thrombin, have resulted in better control of initial gastric variceal bleeding for GOV2 and IGV1 varices than EVL. Furthermore, gastric variceal obturation with *N*-butylcyanoacrylate has a lower rate of rebleeding and an overall survival benefit compared with EVL. Documented side effects from use of glue include fever, sepsis, retroperitoneal abscess formation, and distal embolization. Embolic complications to cerebral arteries, pulmonary arteries, coronary arteries, renal veins, and inferior vena cava have been documented. The only agent (off label) available in the United States is 2-octyl-cyanoacrylate (Dermabond). The use of thrombin injections has been reported to be effective in controlling gastric variceal bleeding but the data are limited, and more studies are needed.

Recently, EUS guided interventions including coil injection have emerged as a promising treatment modality for gastric varices with high technical and clinical success rates (>90%) and lower rates of adverse events (5% for coils, up to 20% with glue) and recurrent bleeding (15% at 1 year). EUS-guided injection of synthetic glues like cyanoacrylate appears superior to direct endoscopic injection. EUS-guided injection of combination therapy with coils plus glue appears superior to coil or glue monotherapy, possibly because of a synergistic hemostatic effect and lower volume of glue injected. Absorbable gelatin sponge (Gelfoam) and thrombin have also been used in lieu of glue. Prospective comparative studies are required.

If endoscopic therapy fails, placement of a Linton-Nachlas tube or Sengstaken-Blakemore tube can be lifesaving as a temporizing procedure. Balloon tamponade should only be used as a bridge to more definitive therapy (TIPS or liver transplantation), because of its associated complications.

Lo GH, Lai KH, Cheung JS, et al. A prospective, randomized trial of butyl cyanoacrylate injection versus band ligation in the management of bleeding gastric varices. *Hepatology.* 2001;33:1060–1064. [PMID: 11343232]

Ramesh J, Limdi JK, Sharma V, et al. The use of thrombin injections in the management of bleeding gastric varices: a single-center experience. *Gastrointest Endosc.* 2008;68:877–882. [PMID: 18534583]

Tan PC, Hou MC, Lin HC, et al. A randomized trial of endoscopic treatment of acute gastric variceal hemorrhage: N-butyl-2-cyanoacrylate injection versus band ligation. *Hepatology.* 2006;43:690–697. [PMID: 16557539]

C. Endovascular Treatments

Hemorrhage control using minimally invasive endovascular treatments such as TIPS or balloon-occluded retrograde transvenous obliteration (BRTO) can be achieved in more than 90% of cases. These endovascular treatments, however, is recommended after one failed attempt of endoscopic management of gastric variceal bleeding or after early rebleeding. BRTO requires the presence of a gastrorenal or splenorenal shunt in order to obliterate the gastric varices. BRTO tends to have lower rates of rebleeding and hepatic encephalopathy compared to TIPS. Ultimately, the choice between TIPS and BRTO depends on anatomic considerations and local expertise.

Garcia-Pagan JC, Barrufet M, Cardenas A, Escorsell A. Management of gastric varices. *Clin Gastronterol Hepatol.* 2014;12:919–928. [PMID: 23899955]

PORTAL HYPERTENSIVE GASTROPATHY

PHG describes the endoscopic appearance of gastric erythema with a whitish mosaic-like pattern that is found in 51–98% of patients with cirrhotic and noncirrhotic portal hypertension. In part, PHG develops as a result of increased resistance to portal flow, but there is no linear correlation between the development of PHG and the level of portal pressures. The development of PHG has been correlated with the duration and severity of liver disease, presence and size of gastroesophageal varices, and previous eradication of varices by banding or sclerotherapy. The pathogenesis of PHG is not clearly understood, but it may be related to the overproduction of nitric oxide, which results in capillary dilation, or increased levels of vascular endothelial growth factor, which results in increased angiogenesis.

PHG is characterized by mucosal congestion, with dilated capillaries and venules in the mucosa and submucosa of the stomach. Endoscopically, the gastric mucosa appears erythematous and edematous, with a characteristic mosaic pattern, often described as a snakeskin appearance. In PHG, the gastric mucosa is friable and may have associated hemorrhagic spots. The gastric mucosa in patients with PHG bleeds easily on contact and is more susceptible to damage by noxious stimuli such as bile acids, aspirin, and nonsteroidal anti-inflammatory drugs. PHG is most prominent in the gastric body and fundus but may be noted diffusely. Several endoscopic classification systems for PHG have been proposed but there is no consensus on the best system.

Patients with PHG typically present with chronic anemia and more rarely with acute blood loss. An estimated 8% of upper gastrointestinal hemorrhage in patients with cirrhosis is due to PHG bleeding and tends to occur in patients with severe PHG. Mortality from PHG bleeding is reported to be very low.

First-line treatment for PHG includes medical therapies aimed at decreasing gastric blood flow (eg, β-blockers, octreotide, vasopressin). Small studies have shown efficacy of propranolol in decreasing rates of chronic and recurrent bleeding from PHG. If medical therapy is not tolerated or fails to reduce bleeding rates, TIPS may be beneficial. Endoscopic therapy has not been shown to be effective.

Surgical shunts or liver transplantation are not recommended for the treatment of PHG, and endoscopic therapy has no proven benefit or safety profile. It remains to be seen how advances in argon plasma coagulation, cryotherapy, and photodynamic therapy may evolve in the future as therapeutic options for PHG.

Gjeorgjievski M, Cappell M. Portal hypertensive gastropathy: a systematic review of the pathophysiology, clinical presentation, natural history and therapy. *World J Hepatol.* 2016;8(4): 231–262. [PMID: 26855694]

Primignani M, Carpinelli L, Preatoni P, et al. Natural history of portal hypertensive gastropathy in patients with liver cirrhosis. The New Italian Endoscopic Club for the Study and Treatment of Esophageal Varices (NIEC). *Gastroenterology.* 2000;119: 181–187. [PMID: 10889167]

Sarin SK, Shahi HM, Jain M, et al. The natural history of portal hypertensive gastropathy: influence of variceal eradication. *Am J Gastroenterol.* 2000;95:2888–2893. [PMID: 11051364]

IDIOPATHIC PORTAL HYPERTENSION

Idiopathic portal hypertension is characterized by portal hypertension in the absence of cirrhosis. Pathologic findings include portal fibrosis, nodular regenerative hyperplasia, phlebosclerosis, and sinusoidal dilatation. Clinically, patients develop esophageal varices as the most common complication of portal hypertension. Ascites and hepatic encephalopathy are less frequent complications. Management of variceal hemorrhage is the same as for patients with cirrhosis. The prognosis is generally good with a low mortality.

FUTURE TREATMENT TRENDS

Over the past 30 years, major advances in pharmacologic and endoscopic therapy for primary and secondary prophylaxis of variceal hemorrhage, together with a better understanding of resuscitative measures, have led to a marked improvement in the morbidity and mortality associated with variceal hemorrhage. Early mortality from variceal bleeding has been reduced by 50% to its present 15%. The advent of TIPS as a rescue procedure has reduced surgical shunts to a footnote. Future research will be directed toward finding alternative drugs for patients who cannot tolerate or do not benefit from the use of β-blockers. Carvedilol and simvastatin are included in the most recent guidelines and have promising futures. Recent interest has centered on drugs that inhibit angiogenesis or are antifibrogenic, but evaluation of their clinical efficacy has not reached large-scale clinical trials. Transient elastography is excellent for the diagnosis of cirrhosis and portal hypertension but is not sensitive enough to detect changes in portal pressure induced by pharmacologic therapy to help guide management. A noninvasive test is needed that will give information similar to that now obtained by measurements of the HVPG for the diagnosis, prognosis, and management of patients with cirrhosis and portal hypertension.

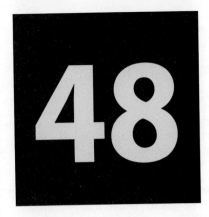

Drug-Induced Liver Injury

48

Michael Li, MD, MPH

Gyorgy Baffy, MD, PhD

ESSENTIALS OF DIAGNOSIS

▶ Clinical, laboratory, and histological manifestations of drug-induced liver injury (DILI) are often indistinguishable from those of liver disease caused by other etiologies.

▶ A remarkable array of therapeutic drugs has been shown to cause liver damage across a broad range of manifestations. There are no specific diagnostic tests that establish the presence of DILI; therefore, the diagnosis is often one of exclusion.

▶ A drug-induced etiology should be considered in any patient who develops acute hepatitis with elevated aminotransferases (hepatocellular injury) or jaundice associated with pruritus and elevated alkaline phosphatase and bilirubin levels (cholestatic injury).

▶ Diagnosis of DILI involves a careful and thorough drug history, excluding underlying liver disease (eg, viral hepatitis, biliary obstruction, alcohol-associated liver disease, or nonalcoholic fatty liver disease [NAFLD]), and characterizing the pattern (hepatocellular, cholestatic, or mixed) and timing of the liver injury and comparing those features to what has been reported in the literature for the suspected drug exposure.

▶ Improvement following discontinuation of a drug suspected to have caused liver injury (deceleration) is often helpful in the diagnosis, as is recurrence of the liver injury if the patient is rechallenged with the same offending agent.

▶ General Considerations

A frequent task facing clinicians is determining whether elevations in liver biochemical studies (eg, aminotransferases, bilirubin, or alkaline phosphatase) may have been caused by

a drug. The problem of separating DILI from abnormalities related to the underlying disease process may be challenging (and often impossible). Identification is especially difficult if the patient has underlying viral hepatitis, alcohol-associated liver disease, NAFLD, or a malignancy which involves the liver.

Adverse drug reactions are widespread and manifold (Figure 48–1). Almost all therapeutic drugs in current use have been suggested as a cause of some liver-related abnormalities, most often asymptomatic elevations of aminotransferases. DILI can be classified as either intrinsic (predictable and dose-dependent) or idiosyncratic (unpredictable and not dose-dependent).

While idiosyncratic DILI is quite rare (less than 1 in 10,000 patients who take medications), it accounts for the majority of all DILI cases and therefore the diagnosis of DILI can be difficult. Overall, DILI is the most common cause of acute liver failure in the developed world. In addition, several drugs with proven efficacy have been withdrawn from the market following postrelease approval by the FDA with rates of idiosyncratic DILI ranging from 1% to 10%. The economic consequences resulting from the removal of an approved drug from the market or even markedly restricting its use are tremendous as are the costs uselessly expended in the development of a new agent which fails late in the preapproval process. The key challenge is to improve the methods by which the risk of DILI from a specific drug is assessed (and hopefully predicted) so that effective plans to minimize the risk are in place.

The National Institute of Diabetes and Digestive and Kidney Diseases (NIDDK) publishes a database of medications known to cause liver injury called LiverTox (http://livertox.nih.gov); this site is updated regularly and is a helpful resource for clinicians seeking more information regarding the frequency, pattern, and management of liver injury attributable to specific drugs. In addition, the Drug-Induced Liver Injury Network (DILIN) was established by the NIDDK to analyze cases of liver injury caused by drugs, supplements, and herbal products. In a large prospective study, the DILIN

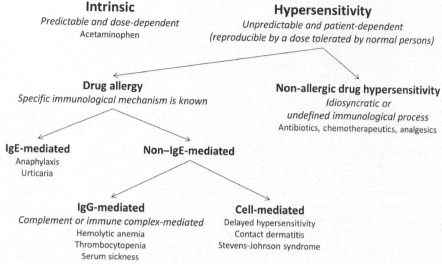

Intrinsic
Predictable and dose-dependent
Acetaminophen

Hypersensitivity
Unpredictable and patient-dependent
(reproducible by a dose tolerated by normal persons)

Drug allergy
Specific immunological mechanism is known

Non-allergic drug hypersensitivity
Idiosyncratic or
undefined immunological process
Antibiotics, chemotherapeutics, analgesics

IgE-mediated
Anaphylaxis
Urticaria

Non–IgE-mediated

IgG-mediated
Complement or immune complex-mediated
Hemolytic anemia
Thrombocytopenia
Serum sickness

Cell-mediated
Delayed hypersensitivity
Contact dermatitis
Stevens-Johnson syndrome

▲ **Figure 48–1.** Classification of adverse drug reactions.

found that the most common class of medication to cause DILI is antimicrobials (45%) followed by herbal and dietary supplements (16%).

Transient biochemical changes induced by most drugs typically occur in patients in whom there are no symptoms or signs suggesting liver injury. In most of these occurrences, the usually minor elevations in serum transaminase levels subside as the liver adapts to the newly introduced agent. The mechanisms leading to these adaptations remain obscure. It is often difficult to determine the threshold of tolerance (risk-benefit factor) for mild to moderate changes in biochemical tests caused by drugs that are acceptable in order to provide effective treatment of serious illnesses. The frequency of

hepatotoxicity may be affected by age, alcohol use, concomitant chronic liver disease, patterns of use (short courses vs long-term administration), sex, ethnicity, and genetic factors that regulate metabolism and the immune responses to the drug or its metabolic products. Furthermore, transport of specific drugs into hepatocytes from the blood and from hepatocytes into bile depends on genetically influenced transporters (Figure 48–2).

Evidence of clinically apparent severe liver injury from an approved drug is uncommon. However, it must be noted that clinically significant events may not occur during the preapproval development during which a relatively limited (several thousand) number of patients are exposed. Evidence of

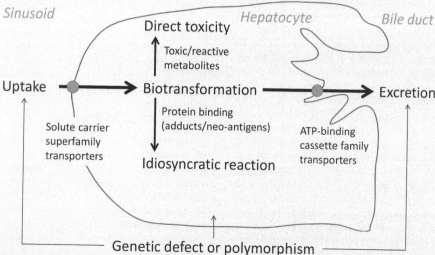

▲ **Figure 48–2.** Hepatocellular drug transport and metabolism.

liver injury may be recognized only after the drug is already on the market and large numbers of patients with variable backgrounds (eg, age, other drugs, alcohol use, weight) have been treated. A challenge for further research is to identify more precisely those factors that determine why an agent well tolerated by thousands of patients may cause a devastating injury in a select few.

DILI is usually indistinguishable (clinically and histologically) from liver injury of other causes and the clinician's suspicion and persistence is paramount in making the correct diagnosis. Careful attention must be given to the time of onset, duration of therapy, and nature of the hepatic injury, as well as consideration of the roles of other drugs being concurrently taken that may enhance production or accumulation of reactive intermediates or interfere with drug transport. The increasing focus of drug metabolites eliciting the innate immune responses should eventually lead to more effective ways to assess risk and aid in diagnosis. In general, clinical scenarios of liver injury that do not seem to follow the textbook or "make sense" are always suspicious for drug-induced mechanisms.

Most clinicians prescribe a relatively limited panel of drugs. It is essential that the clinician become familiar with the hepatic risk profile and patterns of manifestation of these preferred medications. Resolution of DILI upon withdrawal of a drug may identify it as the causative factor. Polypharmacy, including the use of over-the-counter medications, supplements, and herbal products, is a major challenge in the diagnosis as it may be difficult to decide which agent or agents is the likely culprit and should be removed first when evidence of liver injury is found.

Traditionally, DILI has been classified as predominantly hepatocellular (elevated aminotransferase levels) or predominantly cholestatic (elevated alkaline phosphatase and bilirubin levels). With some drugs, there are elements of both patterns of injury, leading to a category of a mixed reaction. While certain drugs may have a somewhat specific "signature" with regard to the onset, type, and outcomes of DILI, this distinction is often blurred and unreliable. Cholestatic disorders range from mild elevations of bilirubin and alkaline phosphatase levels inadvertently found on routine laboratory testing to symptomatic cholestatic syndromes with jaundice and pruritus that may resemble primary biliary cholangitis or primary sclerosing cholangitis. NAFLD is a widely prevalent liver condition associated with mild-to-moderate elevation of serum transaminases, predominantly ALT, in about 20% of the cases. If performed, liver biopsy in NAFLD reveals macrovesicular or microvascular steatosis with variable degree of cell injury, inflammation, and fibrosis. Drugs that cause mitochondrial injury (eg, valproate, tetracycline, nucleotide reverse transcriptase inhibitors, aspirin) may lead to microvesicular steatosis. Several drugs (eg, phenylbutazone and allopurinol) have been implicated in hepatic granulomatous inflammation indistinguishable from those found in a variety of infections and sarcoidosis.

Liver injury induced by herbal preparations and dietary supplements is an increasing problem that may cause significant or even fatal liver injury. Besides the fact that the main ingredients of these products may have intrinsic hepatotoxicity, they may not have proper dose labeling and may be contaminated by unknown compounds. Sometimes it is difficult to ascertain where and how these herbal or dietary supplements (HDS) have been produced. Moreover, obtaining an accurate history from the patient of the use of herbal products and dietary supplements is often extremely difficult.

Andrade RJ, Chalasani N, Björnsson ES, et al. Drug-induced liver injury. *Nat Rev Dis Primers.* 2019;5(1):58. [PMID: 31439850]

Chalasani N, Bonkovsky HL, Fontana R, et al. Features and outcomes of 899 patients with drug-induced liver injury: the DILIN prospective study. *Gastroenterology.* 2015;148(7):1340–1352.e7. [PMID: 25754159]

Goldberg DS, Forde KA, Carbonari DM, et al. Population-representative incidence of drug-induced acute liver failure based on an analysis of an integrated health care system. *Gastroenterology.* 2015;148(7):1353–1361.e3. [PMID: 25733099]

Kullak-Ublick GA, Andrade RJ, Merz M, et al. Drug-induced liver injury: recent advances in diagnosis and risk assessment. *Gut.* 2017;66(6):1154–1164. [PMID: 28341748]

LiverTox: Clinical and Research Information on Drug-Induced Liver Injury [Internet]. Bethesda (MD): National Institute of Diabetes and Digestive and Kidney Diseases; 2012-. Available from: https://www.ncbi.nlm.nih.gov/books/NBK547852/

► Clinical Findings

A. Symptoms & Signs

Early symptoms associated with drug-induced liver injuries are nonspecific and include loss of appetite, fatigue, and occasionally discomfort in the right upper quadrant of the abdomen. There may be few clinical signs or symptoms suggesting liver injury, even in a patient who has biochemical and histologic evidence indicating significant involvement of the liver. These are the same symptoms and patterns of abnormalities that may be found in patients who have chronic viral hepatitis B or C or alcohol-associated liver disease. With a few drugs (eg, phenytoin), there is the concomitant presence of fever or rash consistent with hypersensitivity mechanisms.

B. Laboratory Findings

While the most common presentation of DILI is an acute hepatocellular injury, it can also present with nearly any pattern or degree of biochemical derangements. For agents that are known to cause DILI, the NIDDK LiverTox database describes their typical patterns of injury based on the available evidence and can be a useful tool for clinicians who are evaluating a suspected case of DILI. Elevations in serum autoimmune markers such as antinuclear antibody may be seen in patients with an autoimmune hepatitis-like reaction, while peripheral eosinophilia may be present in patients who develop a hypersensitivity reaction. Typical laboratory tests to obtain include aminotransferases, alkaline phosphatase, bilirubin and, in cases of more severe liver injury, prothrombin time to screen for development of liver failure.

C. Liver Biopsy

There are no histologic findings that are diagnostic of DILI as a whole or even for hepatotoxicity caused by specific agents. Often, the utility of a liver biopsy is in ruling out underlying etiologies of liver disease. As liver biochemistries can be split broadly into hepatocellular and cholestatic patterns, histology often is correlated with these distinctions. Patients with elevated alkaline phosphatase and bilirubin can be expected to have histologic evidence of cholestatic injury, which can range from cholestasis and bile plugging to portal inflammation and bile duct injury and/or proliferation. On the other hand, patients with markedly elevated aminotransferases are likely to have predominantly hepatocellular injury on histology, with lobular inflammation and hepatocyte necrosis.

▶ Differential Diagnosis

The development of reliable tests to detect hepatitis A to E has made the task of excluding viral hepatitis relatively straightforward. Other etiologies of viral hepatitis can also be ruled out with serological testing in the appropriate clinical setting (HSV and VZV in acutely ill patients with markedly elevated aminotransferases, EBV and CMV in patients with a more cholestatic pattern of injury). The finding of anti-mitochondrial antibodies in a patient who has biochemical evidence of cholestasis and jaundice supports the diagnosis of primary biliary cholangitis over a drug-induced syndrome that resembles the disorder. Autoimmune hepatitis may be suspected based on serological markers of autoimmunity and typical histologic findings though some drugs can cause an autoimmune hepatitis-like reaction that may be difficult to distinguish. Other etiologies of chronic liver disease including primary sclerosing cholangitis, alcohol-associated liver disease, NAFLD, hemochromatosis, and Wilson's disease may need to be considered when searching for DILI as an exclusionary diagnosis; as stated previously, liver biopsy may be more helpful in ruling out these chronic conditions rather than being diagnostic for DILI. It is important to remember that patients with liver disorders of all types may develop superimposed DILI, which may have a more robust manifestation and worse clinical outcomes in patients with advanced liver disease and decreased hepatic reserve.

While DILI most often occurs as an acute or subacute disease, chronic liver injury may also develop based on hypersensitivity mechanisms. Generally, drugs that cause chronic changes in the liver have been taken for extended intervals and the manifestations develop late in the course of therapy. Several drugs cause chronic hepatitis syndromes that may be difficult to differentiate from autoimmune hepatitis.

The histologic changes may also be indistinguishable from autoimmune hepatitis. Well-established agents that cause a pattern of chronic hepatitis include minocycline, nitrofurantoin, and methyldopa. There is a risk that chronic steroid therapy is initiated in patients while administration of the offending drug continues. Occasionally, chronic hepatitis may present as insidious progressive hepatic failure in a patient who develops hepatosplenomegaly and evidence of portal hypertension or ascites.

Chalasani NP, Hayashi PH, Bonkovsky HL, et al. ACG Clinical Guideline: the diagnosis and management of idiosyncratic drug-induced liver injury. *Am J Gastroenterol.* 2014;109(7):950–967. [PMID: 24935270]

Kleiner DE, Chalasani NP, Lee WM, et al. Hepatic histological findings in suspected drug-induced liver injury: systematic evaluation and clinical associations. *Hepatology.* 2014;59(2):661–670. [PMID: 24037963]

Leise MD, Poterucha JJ, Talwalkar JA. Drug-induced liver injury. *Mayo Clin Proc.* 2014;89(1):95–106. [PMID: 24388027]

▶ Treatment

The vast majority of drug-induced elevations of serum aminotransferases occur in individuals who are minimally symptomatic or asymptomatic and require no treatment beyond identification and withdrawal of the causative agent. Removal of the inciting agent is generally followed by resolution of the biochemical abnormalities over several days to weeks.

With some drugs that cause symptomatic hepatitis, careful evaluation and often hospitalization to allow careful monitoring is required. Clinical trials have established that significant hepatocellular injury and impaired bilirubin excretion capacity (in the absence of alkaline phosphatase elevation that would indicate a cholestatic component) follow Hy's law predicting that serum ALT elevation three times over the upper limit of normal along with a 2-fold bilirubin elevation can identify patients at high risk for adverse outcomes. If drug-induced acute liver failure occurs, the patient should be viewed as a candidate for liver transplantation and quickly referred to a transplant center. While the role of glucocorticoids has not definitely been established in the treatment of DILI, they have often been used in cases where DILI is accompanied by hypersensitivity reactions, as seen with the formerly widely used anesthetic halothane or diphenylhydantoin.

In cases of self-resolving DILI, serum levels of aminotransferases, bilirubin and alkaline phosphatase may normalize within 1–2 weeks following the removal of the offending drug (deceleration phase). However, this resolution may be protracted with drugs whose parent compound or metabolic products have accumulated in the hepatocytes. The longer these abnormalities persist, the greater the possibility that permanent hepatic injury will develop or that the diagnosis of DILI was not correct. Rechallenge with a suspected drug to establish a diagnosis of DILI should not be considered as it is neither ethical nor safe and may result in severe or fatal escalation of liver injury, though in cases where there are multiple possible offending agents it may be reasonable to perform a carefully-monitored trial of restarting the lowest-risk medications first if they are deemed clinically necessary and there are no reasonable alternative drugs.

DRUGS OF SPECIAL INTEREST

1. Acetaminophen

Acetaminophen hepatotoxicity is the most frequent cause of acute liver failure in the United States and is likely the cause of (or a major contributor to) elevations of aminotransferases found on routine evaluations. Ingestion of excessive amounts of acetaminophen (>10–15 g over a 24-hour period), often used in suicidal attempts, predictably leads to liver injury ranging from elevated aminotransferases to acute liver failure followed by death or the need for liver transplantation. In therapeutic doses (up to 4 g/day), acetaminophen is usually safe and well tolerated unless administered to patients with advanced liver disease or combined with alcohol consumption. Patients often underestimate or understate the amount of acetaminophen ingested, especially since acetaminophen is present in many widely used combination products. In an effort to reduce the risk of unintentional acetaminophen overdose, the FDA has therefore limited the strength of acetaminophen when combined with prescription drug products (mostly given with opioids) to 325 mg per dose and has added boxed warnings regarding the possibility of liver failure.

The safety margin for acetaminophen in patients who are regular users of alcohol appears to be diminished, and these individuals are at increased risk of developing acetaminophen-induced liver injury, particularly after ingestion of repeated supratherapeutic doses. Therapeutic use of up to 4 g/day in these patients appears safe. Chronic use of alcohol may induce changes in levels of CYP2E1 (the major cytochrome P450 enzyme involved in the metabolism of both ethanol and acetaminophen) yielding an excess amount of the reactive acetaminophen metabolite N-acetyl-p-benzoquinoneimine (NAPQI). In addition, alcohol may deplete hepatocellular levels of the antioxidant glutathione, impeding the neutralization of NAPQI by glutathione transferase and further promoting liver injury (Figure 48–3).

N-acetylcysteine, which repletes hepatic glutathione stores, has been shown to be very effective in reducing the extent of hepatic injury from acetaminophen though it must be administered promptly as it has a narrow therapeutic window; prompt treatment with N-acetylcysteine within 8 hours following aminotransferase elevation is therefore preferred. A nomogram can assist clinicians in making a decision regarding initiation of N-acetylcysteine based on serum acetaminophen concentration and time since last ingestion, and both intravenous and oral regimens are effective and available.

Chiew AL, Gluud C, Brok J, Buckley NA. Interventions for paracetamol (acetaminophen) overdose. *Cochrane Database Syst Rev.* 2018;2(2):CD003328. [PMID: 29473717]

LiverTox: Clinical and Research Information on Drug-Induced Liver Injury [Internet]. Bethesda (MD): National Institute of Diabetes and Digestive and Kidney Diseases; 2012-. Acetaminophen. [Updated 2016 Jan 28]. Available from: https://www.ncbi.nlm.nih.gov/books/NBK548162/

Yan M, Huo Y, Yin S, Hu H. Mechanisms of acetaminophen-induced liver injury and its implications for therapeutic interventions. *Redox Biol.* 2018;17:274–283. [PMID: 29753208]

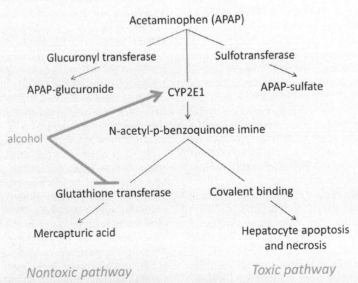

▲ **Figure 48–3.** Hepatic acetaminophen metabolism and the impact of alcohol.

2. Amoxicillin–Clavulanate

Hepatotoxicity from the extensive use of combination amoxicillin and clavulanic acid is widely recognized and attributed to clavulanic acid. Amoxicillin given alone is one of the safest antibiotics in common usage and patients who develop liver injury from amoxicillin-clavulanate can typically be given amoxicillin alone if necessary. The frequency of clinically apparent hepatic injury from amoxicillin–clavulanate is low (~1 in every 2000 prescriptions), although as millions of prescriptions are filled yearly, it is among the most frequently identified drugs causing liver injury, implicated in 10% of DILI cases in the DILIN Prospective Study.

The range of clinical and laboratory manifestations of DILI associated with amoxicillin-clavulanate is broad. The drug is generally used as short-duration therapy (7–10 days). However, manifest liver injury is often delayed for days to weeks after initiation of therapy and may occur well after its completion. In these cases, the causative role of amoxicillin–clavulanate can remain overlooked. Liver injury from amoxicillin–clavulanate is typically cholestatic, though some patients will present with a mixed hepatocellular-cholestatic pattern. Signs of hypersensitivity (rash and fever) can occur, but the most common presentation is nonspecific symptoms followed by a pruritic jaundice with a gradual and complete resolution of the process over several days to weeks. Advancing age and prolonged therapy are factors associated with the development of cholestatic injury from amoxicillin–clavulanate. A few instances of severe hepatocellular injury leading to death or the need for transplantation have been reported.

Chalasani N, Bonkovsky HL, Fontana R, et al. Features and outcomes of 899 patients with drug-induced liver injury: the DILIN prospective study. *Gastroenterology*. 2015;148(7):1340–1352.e7. [PMID: 25754159]

deLemos AS, Ghabril M, Rockey DC, et al. Amoxicillin-clavulanate-induced liver injury. *Dig Dis Sci*. 2016;61(8):2406–2416. [PMID: 20394749]

LiverTox: Clinical and Research Information on Drug-Induced Liver Injury [Internet]. Bethesda (MD): National Institute of Diabetes and Digestive and Kidney Diseases; 2012-. Amoxicillin-Clavulanate. [Updated 2016 Mar 30]. Available from: https://www.ncbi.nlm.nih.gov/books/NBK548517/

3. Isoniazid

Isoniazid (INH) has been recognized as an established cause of liver injury for the past six decades since the drug was introduced as the mainstay therapy for tuberculosis. In the DILIN Prospective Study, 5% of DILI cases were attributed to INH; liver injury from INH is even more frequent in Asia and approaches 25% of DILI cases. Elevations of aminotransferase levels are found in 10–20% of patients who receive INH, usually within several weeks of beginning treatment. In most patients, INH-induced aminotransferase elevations are not associated with clinical symptoms and often return to normal with ongoing therapy. ALT elevations greater than five times the upper limit of normal are a reasonable threshold for discontinuing INH. Patients above the age of 50 appear to be at higher risk of hepatotoxicity as are those with preexisting liver disease. A cholestatic pattern of liver injury may predict worse outcomes with death or need for liver transplantation in up to 10% of jaundiced patients.

The principal mechanism underlying INH-induced DILI is not entirely understood. A metabolic intermediate of INH with toxic effects has not been definitively established but is likely a hydrazine derivative. Genetic polymorphisms of the genes for N-acetyltransferase and CYP2E1, both of which have important roles in the metabolism of INH, have been shown to influence susceptibility. Awareness of the risk of INH-induced liver injury and regular biochemical monitoring in patients receiving the drug have proven effective in identifying evidence of hepatic injury early, at a time when withdrawal of the drug usually leads to resolution.

Chalasani N, Bonkovsky HL, Fontana R, et al. Features and outcomes of 899 patients with drug-induced liver injury: the DILIN prospective study. *Gastroenterology*. 2015;148(7):1340–1352.e7. [PMID: 25754159]

LiverTox: Clinical and Research Information on Drug-Induced Liver Injury [Internet]. Bethesda (MD): National Institute of Diabetes and Digestive and Kidney Diseases; 2012-. Isoniazid. [Updated 2018 Apr 5]. Available from: https://www.ncbi.nlm.nih.gov/books/NBK548754/

Low EXS, Zheng Q, Chan E, Lim SG. Drug induced liver injury: East versus West - a systematic review and meta-analysis. *Clin Mol Hepatol*. 2020;26(2):142–154. [PMID: 31816676]

4. Statins

The era of the widespread and long-term use of statin drugs to lower low-density lipoprotein and cholesterol levels through inhibition of HMG-CoA began in the 1980s and statins now are among the most frequently prescribed drugs. In fact, statins are increasingly administered to patients with chronic liver disease including NAFLD and compensated cirrhosis, based on their overall impact on lipid metabolism and potential benefits on sinusoidal homeostasis and portal hypertension. Increases of aminotransferase levels to more than three times the upper limit of normal occur in 1–3% of patients receiving statins. The extent of the elevations appears dose-related and there is some evidence suggesting that certain statins (atorvastatin, simvastatin) are more frequently implicated in causing hepatotoxicity. In the DILIN Prospective Study, statins were the cause of 2% of DILI cases.

Statin-induced aminotransferase elevations are usually noted within weeks to months of initiating the therapy, and the increases may be linked in some as-yet undetermined way to the extent of changes in lipids. There have been remarkably few instances of clinically significant DILI reliably attributed to statins. Outcomes of statin-associated liver injury are generally favorable. The risk of statin-induced acute liver failure is less than one in 1 million patients, and cases of statin-induced significant liver injury are rare in large series of patients with acute liver failure. Death or need for liver transplantation appear to be similarly rare.

The mechanism of statin-related hepatotoxicity remains unclear. There may be two separate causes of elevated liver chemistries. Initially, mild and self-limited aminotransferase elevations are not uncommon following the start of statin treatment and may be related to a toxic metabolite. Usual practice is to continue therapy unless transaminase levels exceed three times the upper normal limit. There is no evidence to suggest that routine liver test monitoring following the initiation of statin treatment is necessary, and statins are safe to use even in patients with chronic underlying liver disease. Adaptation may explain why these liver enzyme elevations usually reverse spontaneously. More severe liver injury may be due to failure of adaptation or are potentially immune-mediated, as there have been cases of an autoimmune-like hepatitis induced by statin therapy. Nevertheless, even patients who experience severe hepatotoxicity (aminotransferase levels rising to above 10 times the upper limit of normal or persisting at above 5 times the upper limit of normal) typically experience spontaneous resolution of their liver injury following statin discontinuation, and subsequent administration of statins at a lower dose or a different statin compound with lower hepatotoxicity risk can be considered depending on the clinical context.

Björnsson ES. Hepatotoxicity of statins and other lipid-lowering agents. *Liver Int.* 2017;37(2):173–178. [PMID: 27860156]

Chalasani N, Bonkovsky HL, Fontana R, et al. Features and outcomes of 899 patients with drug-induced liver injury: the DILIN prospective study. *Gastroenterology.* 2015;148(7):1340–1352.e7. [PMID: 25754159]

Chang CH, Chang YC, Lee YC, Liu YC, Chuang LM, Lin JW. Severe hepatic injury associated with different statins in patients with chronic liver disease: a nationwide population-based cohort study. *J Gastroenterol Hepatol.* 2015;30(1):155–162. [PMID: 25041076]

LiverTox: Clinical and Research Information on Drug-Induced Liver Injury [Internet]. Bethesda (MD): National Institute of Diabetes and Digestive and Kidney Diseases; 2012-. Statins. [Updated 2017 Aug 5]. Available from: https://www.ncbi.nlm.nih.gov/books/NBK548067/

5. Herbal Agents & Dietary Supplements

Hepatic injury from a variety of HDS have been associated with hepatotoxicity. In most instances, these products have not been well characterized chemically and have not been subjected to clinical trials. As a combined group, HDS are one of the most common causes of DILI, further highlighting the importance of obtaining a thorough medication and supplement history. Sixteen percent of liver injury cases in the DILIN Prospective Study were attributed to HDS, with approximately one-third of these related to body building products. However, data regarding specific agents is limited;

in the same study, no single specific HDS agent was in the top 25 most common causes of DILI and most agents were only implicated in single isolated cases. HDS products frequently contain multiple ingredients and due to limited regulatory requirements only rarely list ingredient concentrations and sources, which further complicates efforts to characterize liver injury related to these agents.

A significant proportion of HDS-related DILI cases in the United States can be attributed to anabolic steroids which are thought to be illicitly added to performance enhancing products. Anabolic steroids are associated with an acute cholestatic pattern of liver injury, generally months following their first use. This bland cholestasis can present with minimally elevated aminotransferases and markedly elevated levels of bilirubin (often reaching levels above 40 mg/dL) and alkaline phosphatase with associated jaundice and pruritus. The mechanism of injury is unclear, though may be related to a deficiency of bile salt transporter proteins. However, despite the severity of cholestatic injury, outcomes are usually good and death or need for liver transplant are rare. There is no treatment for cholestatic injury associated with anabolic steroids although for pruritus, symptomatic treatment with ursodiol or cholestyramine is reasonable.

Herbal products like green tea extract, black cohosh, and kava are widely used for a variety of purposes around the world. In the DILIN Prospective Study, 49 of the 97 implicated HDS products were available for testing and over half of them contained catechins, a group of chemical compounds in green tea that have antioxidant properties. However, catechins have also been shown to be hepatotoxic in animal models and may be implicated in many cases of liver injury caused by herbal products. In addition, tea extracts and other herbal agents may be contaminated with unknown herbs or illicit addition of conventional drugs such as statins, nonsteroidal anti-inflammatory medications, and 5-phosphodiesterase inhibitors. Liver injury due to these agents can have variable presentations, though most are hepatocellular and self-limited. As in other cases of DILI, a cholestatic pattern of injury may be associated with worse clinical outcomes.

Regulatory issues continue to pose a significant challenge to characterization of liver injury from HDS products. The most important lesson for clinicians is that a thorough history of HDS products must be obtained in every case of abnormal liver tests.

Chalasani N, Bonkovsky HL, Fontana R, et al. Features and outcomes of 899 patients with drug-induced liver injury: the DILIN prospective study. *Gastroenterology.* 2015;148(7):1340–1352.e7. [PMID: 25754159]

LiverTox: Clinical and Research Information on Drug-Induced Liver Injury [Internet]. Bethesda (MD): National Institute of Diabetes and Digestive and Kidney Diseases; 2012-. Androgenic Steroids. [Updated 2020 May 30]. Available from: https://www.ncbi.nlm.nih.gov/books/NBK548931/

Navarro VJ, Khan I, Björnsson E, Seeff LB, Serrano J, Hoofnagle JH. Liver injury from herbal and dietary supplements. *Hepatology.* 2017;65(1):363–373. [PMID: 27677775]

Zheng EX, Navarro VJ. Liver injury from herbal, dietary, and weight loss supplements: a review. *J Clin Transl Hepatol.* 2015;3(2):93–98. [PMID: 26357638]

6. Immune Checkpoint Inhibitors

In the last decade, cancer pharmacotherapy has been transformed by the introduction of immune checkpoint inhibitors (ICIs), which work to prevent tumor cells from evading T-cell mediated immune defenses. Unfortunately, ICI therapy is often complicated by immune-related adverse events, off-target inflammatory responses that can affect almost any organ system including commonly the gastrointestinal tract and liver. Approximately 10% of patients treated with single-agent ICI therapy will develop elevated liver enzymes of any degree, and 1–2% will experience aminotransferase elevations at least five times the upper limit of normal. Liver tests should be monitored routinely during ICI treatment.

While patients who develop ICI hepatitis can have elevated levels of alkaline phosphatase and/or bilirubin, there is a predominantly hepatocellular pattern. Typically, liver injury will occur weeks to months following the initiation of ICI therapy. Unlike many other causes of DILI, ICI-induced hepatitis is eminently treatable by discontinuation of ICI therapy and initiation of high-dose (up to 1–2 mg/kg/day) of systemic glucocorticoids; additional immunosuppressive therapy with mycophenolate mofetil, azathioprine, or tacrolimus can be considered if there is an inadequate biochemical response to steroid treatment. Following normalization of liver enzymes, steroids are typically tapered over the course of 4–6 weeks.

Brahmer JR, Lacchetti C, Schneider BJ, et al. Management of immune-related adverse events in patients treated with immune checkpoint inhibitor therapy: American Society of Clinical Oncology Clinical Practice Guideline. *J Clin Oncol.* 2018;36(17):1714–1768.

Haanen JBAG, Carbonnel F, Robert C, et al. Management of toxicities from immunotherapy: ESMO Clinical Practice Guidelines for diagnosis, treatment and follow-up. *Ann Oncol.* 2018;29(suppl 4):iv264–iv266.

Michot JM, Bigenwald C, Champiat S, et al. Immune-related adverse events with immune checkpoint blockade: a comprehensive review. *Eur J Cancer.* 2016;54:139–148.

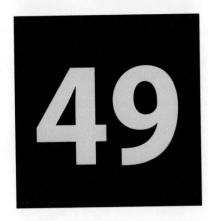

Liver Neoplasms

49

Nikroo Hashemi, MD, MPH

General Considerations

The increased use of imaging modalities—ultrasound, computed tomography (CT), and magnetic resonance imaging (MRI)—over the past few decades has led to an increase in the detection of hepatic masses. In patients without cirrhosis or a history of extrahepatic malignancies, most of these lesions are benign. Diagnosis is generally made on the basis of radiographic appearance, and only in rare equivocal cases histologic analysis is required. In patients with chronic advanced liver disease or cirrhosis, the detection of a hepatic mass often raises suspicion of a primary liver cancer, requiring additional diagnostic (including histologic) and therapeutic interventions and/or surveillance.

Liver lesions can be classified on the basis of appearance (cystic or solid) and histologic composition (hepatocellular or biliary). They can also be classified based on malignant potential (benign or malignant), and when, malignant, they can be classified based on origin of the cancerous cells (primary or secondary/metastatic). In adults, malignant tumors are more common than benign tumors and metastatic lesions account for the majority of liver neoplasms. The differential diagnosis of liver lesions includes benign lesions (eg, hemangioma, focal nodular hyperplasia [FNH], adenoma, focal regenerative hyperplasia, simple hepatic cysts, polycystic liver disease, bile ductular cystadenoma, and bile ductular hamartomas) and malignant lesions (eg, primary hepatocellular cancer, cholangiocarcinoma, metastatic tumors, and lymphoma).

Venkatesh SK, Chandan V, Roberts LR. Liver masses: a clinical, radiologic, and pathologic perspective. *Clin Gastroenterol Hepatol.* 2014;12:1414–1429. [PMID: 24055987]

BENIGN LIVER TUMORS

ESSENTIALS OF DIAGNOSIS

▶ Cavernous hemangiomas, FNH, hepatic adenomas (HAs), and nodular regenerative hyperplasia are the most common benign tumors of the liver.

▶ Cavernous hemangiomas are usually asymptomatic and can be identified by their classic appearance on CT and MRI.

▶ FNH is common in young women and can be identified by the presence of a central stellate scar on CT or MRI.

▶ HAs are common in women of childbearing age, especially after prolonged oral contraceptive use. Because hemorrhage, rupture or malignant transformation can occur, they may require surgically excision if large or enlarging.

▶ Nodular regenerative hyperplasia is associated with many systemic illnesses. Patients present with signs of portal hypertension. Radiographic characteristics are nonspecific, and histologic evaluation shows no fibrosis.

In clinical practice, the most commonly encountered lesions are cavernous hemangiomas, FNH, HA, and nodular regenerative hyperplasia.

EASL Clinical Practice Guidelines on the management of benign liver tumours. *J Hepatol.* 2016;65(2):386–398. [PMID: 27085809]

Grazioli L, Ambrosini R, Frittoli B, et al. Primary benign liver lesions. *Eur J Radiol.* 2017;95:378–398. [PMID: 28987695]

Marrero JA, Ahn J, Reddy KR. American College of Gastroenterology. ACG clinical guideline: the diagnosis and management of focal liver lesions. *Am J Gastroenterol.* 2014;109:1328–1347. [PMID: 25135008]

1. Cavernous Hemangiomas

General Considerations

Hemangiomas are the most common primary liver tumors, with a prevalence of 5% in imaging series and 20% of autopsies. They are typically discovered incidentally during evaluation of nonspecific abdominal complaints. Female to male ratio is 1.2–6:1. They can be diagnosed at any age but are mostly diagnosed in females between ages 30 and 50. They vary in size from a few millimeters to greater than 20 cm. Even when they are large, most patients are asymptomatic. There is no risk of malignant transformation (Figure 49–1).

Clinical Findings

Hepatic hemangiomas are often found incidentally on abdominal imaging and very frequently seen on surgical specimens resected for other reasons. Hemangiomas measuring 10 cm or more, referred to as "giant hemangiomas," may be symptomatic, including pain and features of an inflammatory reaction syndrome and consumptive coagulopathy named Kasabach-Merritt syndrome (KMS) with thrombocytopenia and purpura. The diagnostic modalities available include ultrasound, CT, and MRI. Ultrasound has sensitivity of 60–70% and specificity of 60–80% for detection of hemangiomas. Because of nonspecific findings on ultrasound, contrast-enhanced CT or MRI is often necessary for diagnosis of cavernous hemangiomas.

On CT scan, the lesions are characterized by progressive enhancement during the arterial phase that begins at the periphery of the lesion and progresses inward. The intensity of enhancement during this arterial phase resembles that of the aorta. Small hemangiomas are difficult to diagnose on contrast-enhanced CT because of inability to detect the stepwise enhancement seen in larger lesions. Because of this apparent homogenous enhancement, they may resemble hypervascular liver masses. Overall, the sensitivity of contrast-enhanced CT for diagnosis of cavernous hemangiomas is estimated at around 90%, with specificity of around 90%.

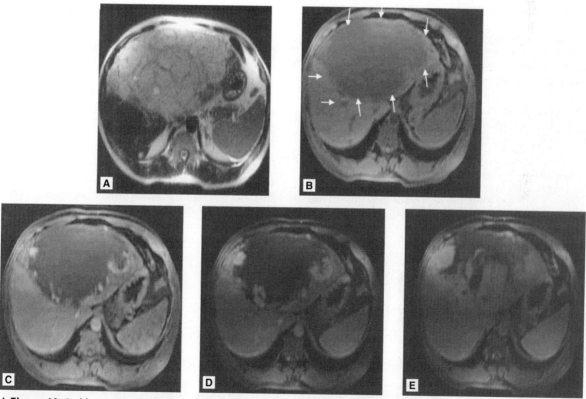

▲ **Figure 49–1.** Magnetic resonance images of a 25-cm giant hemangioma of the left hepatic lobe. The lesion is very bright on the T2-weighted image (**A**) but dark on the T1 precontrast image (**B**). Dynamic postgadolinium images show gradual nodular enhancement from the periphery to the center of the lesion on early arterial (**C**), late arterial (**D**), and delayed phase views (**E**). Arrows in B indicate the area of the hemangioma. (Reproduced with permission of Dr Cheryl Sadow, Department of Radiology, Brigham and Women's Hospital.)

On MRI, cavernous hemangiomas appear hypodense on T1-weighted images, hyperdense on T2, and with gadolinium they show the classic peripheral enhancement with progressive inward enhancement (see Figure 49–1).

Treatment

Most hepatic hemangiomas are asymptomatic. They are usually discovered during abdominal imaging for unrelated symptoms. Treatment is usually not necessary. Imaging follow-up is not required for typical hemangioma. There is no relationship between the size of hemangioma and complications and little relationship with symptoms. Pregnancy and oral contraceptives are not contraindicated. It is debatable if patients with large lesions or those with mild symptoms benefit from surgery. Surgical resection is rarely indicated except with KMS.

2. Focal Nodular Hyperplasia

General Considerations

FNH is the second most common benign liver tumor seen in 0.9% of the population. FNH is more common in women, occurring with a frequency of 9:1 and usually present between ages 30 and 50. Lesions are most often solitary and smaller than 5 cm, but they may be larger. FNH are multiple in 20–30% of patients and are associated with liver hemangioma in 20% of cases.

Pathogenesis

FNH is thought to represent a polyclonal hepatocyte proliferation in response to increased blood flow in an intrahepatic anomalous artery and may be associated with other conditions characterized by arterial damage, such as hereditary hemorrhagic telangiectasia. Given the higher incidence in women, a correlative link has been made to the use of oral contraceptive pills (OCPs). However, pregnancy and OCPs have not been demonstrated to play a role in development or progression of FNH.

Clinical Findings

In more than 70% of patients with FNH, lesions are detected incidentally. In the remaining patients, symptoms (especially right upper quadrant discomfort) prompt evaluation. FNH can be classified into two broad categories: the more prevalent classic FNH, and the nonclassic FNH. Classic lesions are nodular, vascular lesions with bile duct proliferation. Radiographically, the lesions are often identified by the presence of a central scar; however, 95% of nonclassic lesions lack this feature. Histologically, the lesions are well circumscribed with proliferating hepatocytes and Kupffer cells. A central vascular scar is invariably present in the classic form of FNH.

- Ultrasound can be used for the diagnosis of FNH. The central scar is seen in only 20% of ultrasounds. Doppler imaging shows increased blood flow with a pattern of abnormal blood vessels that emanate radially from a central feeding artery ("spoke-wheeling"). Because ultrasound is not considered the preferred diagnostic modality to rule out FNH, additional imaging with CT or MRI is recommended. MRI has highest diagnostic performance overall, with a higher sensitivity than US and CT and specificity ~100%.

- On contrast-enhanced CT, the lesion is isodense with the liver on precontrast and postcontrast images but shows homogenous enhancement during the arterial phase, along with the central scar (Figure 49–2). Figure 49–3 shows the typical MRI features of FNH. Hepatobiliary MR contrast agents are taken up by hepatoctyes and excreted into bile ductules of the tumor, highlighting the hepatocellular origin of the lesions. The lesion is isointense in T2-weighted images with a bright central scar (see Figure 49–3A). It is isointense or hypointense with a central dark scar on T1-weighted images (see Figure 49–3B), homogenously vascular except for the central scar in the arterial phase (see Figure 49–3C), isointense in the portal phase (see Figure 49–3D), and shows subsequent delayed

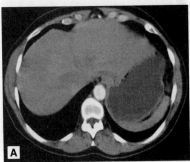 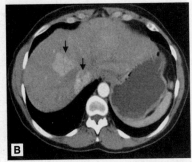 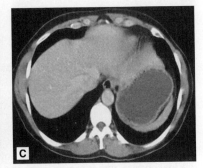

▲ **Figure 49–2.** Computed tomographic scans of focal nodular hyperplasia. The lesions are barely visible in the early arterial phase image (**A**) and not visible in the postvenous phase (**C**) but can be detected as two homogenous hypervascular images in the late arterial phase with contrast (**B**, *arrows*). A central scar is present. (Reproduced with permission of Dr Cheryl Sadow, Department of Radiology, Brigham and Women's Hospital.)

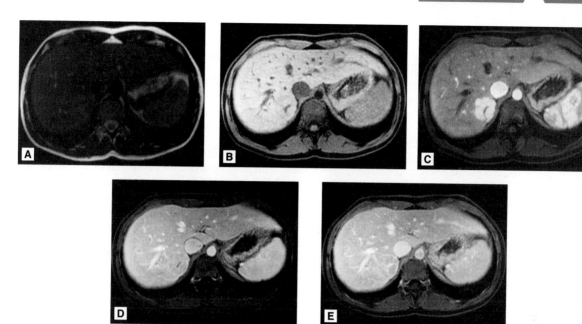

▲ **Figure 49–3.** Magnetic resonance images of focal nodular hyperplasia. The lesion is isointense with the liver on the T2-weighted image, but a bright scar is visible (**A**). On the T1-weighted precontrast image, the lesion remains isointense to slightly hypointense with liver, but a dark central scar is visible (**B**). Dynamic postgadolinium T1 image shows a homogenous hypervascular lesion except for a dark central scar (**C**). The lesion becomes isointense in the portovenous phase (**D**), with delayed enhancement of the central scar (**E**). Arrows indicate the location of the lesion. (Reproduced with permission of Dr Cheryl Sadow, Department of Radiology, Brigham and Women's Hospital.)

enhancement of the central scar (see Figure 49–3E). Gadobenate (GD-BOPTA) or gadoxetate (Eovist) contrast enhanced MRI increases the sensitivity (92–96%) and specificity (91–100%) to differentiate FNH from HA.

Treatment

The size of FNH is stable over time in the vast majority of cases. Majority are asymptomatic and complications are extremely rare. A slow incidental increase in size is not cause for concern in cases with a solid diagnosis. A conservative approach is recommended in the absence of symptoms given the rarity of complications. There is a correlation between FNH and symptoms therefore treatment is rarely indicated even if symptomatic. Treatment is only pursued in exceptional cases (pedunculated, expanding, exophytic). Resection is the treatment of choice in these cases; nonsurgical treatments reserved for those unfit for resection. There is no indication for discontinuing oral contraceptives and follow-up during pregnancy is not required.

Perrakis A, Demir R, Muller V, et al. Management of the focal nodular hyperplasia of the liver: evaluation of the surgical treatment comparing with observation only. *Am J Surg.* 2012;204:689–696. [PMID: 22578408]

Rifai K, Mix H, Krusche S, et al. No evidence of substantial growth progression or complications of large focal nodular hyperplasia during pregnancy. *Scand J Gastroenterol.* 2013;48:88–92. [PMID: 23110461]

Suh CH, Kim KW, Kim GY, et al. The diagnostic value of Gd-EOB-DTPA-MRI for the diagnosis of focal nodular hyperplasia: a systematic review and meta-analysis. *Eur Radiol.* 2015;25:950–960. [PMID: 25537979]

3. Hepatic Adenomas

General Considerations & Pathogenesis

HA is approximately 10 times less common than FNH and is frequently diagnosed in women ages 35–40 years, with a female:male ratio of 10:1. The major risk factors are OCP use, glycogen storage diseases, diabetes, and androgen use. Among patients who use OCPs there is a 30-fold increase in prevalence of HAs. The recent increase in the HA prevalence is noticeably associated with the rising prevalence of obesity and the metabolic syndrome. The tumors are usually solitary and increase in size during states of enhanced estrogen levels, such as pregnancy and OCP use (see Figure 9–33). Of note, hepatic adenomatosis is a distinct entity from HAs. Although the former syndrome is characterized by the presence of multiple HAs, there is no association with OCP use, and it occurs equally in men and women. In addition, laboratory data usually show an elevated alkaline phosphatase level.

▶ Clinical Findings

HAs encompass various types of clonal benign hepatocellular proliferations including several molecular subtypes associated with specific morphological features. The course of HA diagnosed in women is more often benign, while HA diagnosed in men have a significantly higher incidence of malignant transformation, partly reflecting the differences in molecular subtypes. The beta-catenin mutated subtype (10–15%) has the highest risk for malignant transformation, is over represented in males and is also associated with androgenic steroids and familial polyposis. The hepatocyte nuclear factor 1 alpha mutated (HNF1a) subtype (30–40%) is almost always seen in females, 90% are due to biallelic inactivating somatic mutations associated with OCP use and 10% are due to germline mutations associated with MODY (maturity onset DM of the young) and adenomatosis. The inflammatory subtype (50%)

has the highest risk of intratumoral bleeding and is associated with obesity and alcohol use.

Pathologic evaluation of HAs shows a smooth, well-circumscribed, hypervascular and rarely encapsulated tumor. On histology, adenomas are characterized by sheets of hepatocytes supplied by "naked" arteries (no bile ductules, portal tracts, and central veins). The lesion often has a high fat and glycogen content, and necrosis and frank hemorrhage may be present.

Ultrasonographic evaluation can show a hyperechoic mass due to the intracellular fat, with areas that are hypoechoic as a result of hemorrhage. In the absence of contrast, CT usually shows a lesion hypodense to the liver parenchyma if there is no intramural blood. With contrast there is brisk, early enhancement as a result of the vascular nature of the tumor followed by an equally brisk washout due to arteriovenous shunting. On MRI, HAs appear as hyperintense lesions on T2-weighted images (Figure 49–4A). On post-gadolinium images, they show early arterial enhancement that rapidly washes out (Figure 49–4B and C). Adenomas have no uptake

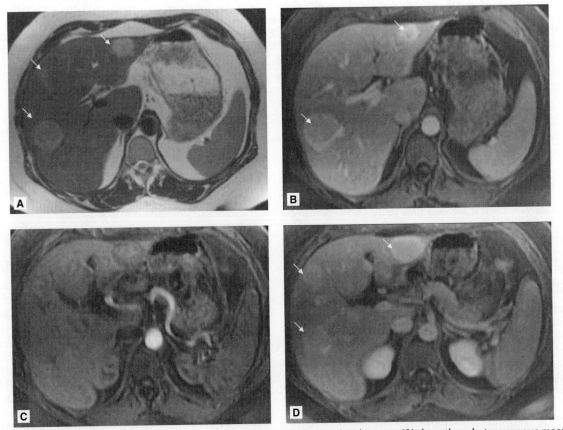

▲ **Figure 49–4.** Magnetic resonance images of hepatic adenoma: T2-weighted images (**A**) show three heterogenous masses (*arrows*). Dynamic postgadolinium T1 images show early arterial enhancement (**B** and **C**) with washout in the delayed image (**D**). (Reproduced with permission of Dr Koenraad Mortele, Department of Radiology, Beth Israel Deaconess Medical Center.)

of contrast agents with hepatobiliary excretion (gadoxetate) in the delayed hepatobiliary phase and can therefore be differentiated from FNH which retain the contrast in the delayed phase.

In approximately 20% of cases, HAs are detected during radiographic imaging for unrelated issues in asymptomatic patients. The clinical implications of HAs are bleeding (1/3 within mass, 2/3 into abdomen) which occurs in larger lesions (≥5 cm) with a mortality up to 25–30% and malignant transformation with an overall risk of 4.2% and the vast majority (>95%) occurring in lesions ≥5 cm.

Complications & Treatment

Unlike the other benign hepatic lesions, HAs produce significant associated morbidity. The lesion can lead to life-threatening hemorrhage resulting from tumor necrosis and rupture. In addition, HAs have the potential for malignant transformation. Men are more likely to have a malignancy associated with HA likely related to the higher prevalence of beta-catenin mutated type among males. Although adenomas may be discovered incidentally, right upper abdominal pain resulting from encroachment on neighboring tissues or from necrosis can also occur. Shock from hemorrhage resulting from rupture is a life-threatening emergency that requires emergent resuscitation and surgical therapy. Surgical resection is recommended in symptomatic patients, men (regardless of size), lesions >5 cm or growing ≥20% diameter, and any instance of proven β-catenin mutation. Radiofrequency ablation has also been shown to a treatment option for HAs in patients who are not surgical resection candidates.

Chang CY, Hernandez-Prera JC, Roayaie S, et al. Changing epidemiology of hepatocellular adenoma in the United States: review of the literature. Int J Hepatol. 2013;2013:604860. [PMID: 23509632]

Dokmak S, Belghiti J. Will weight loss become a future treatment of hepatocellular adenoma in obese patients? Liver Int. 2015;35:2228–2232.[PMID: 26216699]

Nault JC, Bioulac-Sage P, Zucman-Rossi J. Hepatocellular benign tumors from molecular classification to personalized clinical care. Gastroenterology. 2013;144:888–902. [PMID: 23485860]

4. Nodular Regenerative Hyperplasia
General Considerations

This is a disorder characterized by benign proliferation of hepatocytes, resulting in nodules that range in size from 0.1 to 1 cm. It is associated with many systemic diseases, including rheumatoid arthritis, Felty syndrome, Raynaud phenomena, myeloproliferative diseases, lupus erythematosus, polyarthritis nodosa, hereditary hemorrhagic telangiectasia, and amyloidosis, as well as with anabolic steroid use.

Clinical Findings

Patients often present with marked signs of portal hypertension, esophageal varices, upper gastrointestinal bleeding, thrombocytopenia, and ascites. Radiologic appearance is nonspecific, showing multiple nodules throughout the liver that can be confused with cirrhosis. On histology, nodular regenerative hyperplasia is defined by micronodular transformation of the liver parenchyma, with central hyperplasia, an atrophic rim, and no fibrosis.

Treatment

Treatment focuses on management of the complications of associated portal hypertension and hepatic dysfunction, as discussed in Chapters 46–49.

Gottardi AD, Rautou PE, Schouten J, et al. VALVIG group. Porto-sinusoidal vascular disease: proposal and description of a novel entity. Lancet Gastroenterol Hepatol. 2019;4(5):399–411. [PMID: 30957754]

HEPATOCELLULAR CARCINOMA

 ESSENTIALS OF DIAGNOSIS

► Accounts for ~90% of primary liver cancer.

► Predisposing conditions include cirrhosis from any cause, chronic hepatitis B, and possibly hepatitis C and nonalcoholic steatohepatitis (NASH) with advanced fibrosis.

► Screening and surveillance programs for early detection use ultrasound with or without AFP every 6 months.

► Multiphase contrast CT or MRI of suspicious lesions can identify typical radiographic characteristics.

► Biopsy may be required to establish the diagnosis.

General Considerations

Hepatocellular carcinoma (HCC) is now the fifth most common cancer in the world and the third cause of cancer related mortality as estimated by the World Health Organization. In North America, HCC has an incidence of approximately 2.1 in 100,000 persons. In the United States, HCC is the fastest growing cause of cancer-related death and mortality rates have been increasing over the past three decades. In addition, a recent study using the SEER registry projects that the incidence of HCC will continue to rise until 2030, with the highest increase in Hispanics, followed by African Americans and then Caucasians, with a decrease noted among Asian Americans. The increase in incidence of HCC in the United States is attributed primarily to the hepatitis C virus (HCV) epidemic. Recent data have also shown that nonalcoholic fatty liver disease (NAFLD) and the metabolic syndrome contribute numerically more to the burden of HCC than any other risk factor including HCV infection, which is due primarily to the high prevalence of NAFLD in the population overall.

Of all cases of HCC worldwide, 83% are diagnosed in less developed regions of the world with the highest annual incidence rates in eastern Asia and sub-Saharan Africa. During the past few decades the average age at occurrence of cancer has decreased. Older age, male sex, advanced cirrhosis, and active liver disease predict HCC irrespective of the underlying cause of liver disease.

A. Predisposing Conditions

The presence of cirrhosis represents a key risk factor for the development of HCC. The prevalence of cirrhosis among patients with HCC has been estimated to be 85–95%, and the HCC incidence rate among patients with cirrhosis has been shown to be 2–4% per year. Therefore, patients with cirrhosis constitute a high-risk group for efforts at prevention and early detection. The fact that patients with HCC have underlying liver disease impacts the management and therapeutic options substantially.

1. Hepatitis B—The annual incidence rate of HCC in patients with hepatitis B ranges between 0.2% and 8% depending on the presence of cirrhosis and disease activity. Older age groups appear to be at the highest risk of developing HCC. Asians, Africans, and patients with hepatitis B virus (HBV) infections acquired through vertical transmission are also at increased risk of developing HCC. In contrast, North Americans and Europeans with hepatitis B have a lower incidence of HCC, with various cohorts reporting rates of 0–0.46% per year. The difference in HCC rates may be related to the acquisition of the HBV infection later in life among non-Asian and non-African patients. Interestingly, among Asian patients who lose the HBV surface antigen, the risk of HCC remains unchanged. Based on the increased risk of HCC among HBV-infected patients, surveillance is recommended (Table 49–1).

2. Hepatitis C—The 5-year cumulative incidence of HCC among patients with HCV-related cirrhosis has been reported to be 17–30%. All patients with hepatitis C and cirrhosis should undergo surveillance. Patients with bridging fibrosis (F3) have a higher risk of HCC but it remains unclear if this risk is high enough to warrant screening.

3. Alcoholic liver disease—The 5-year cumulative incidence of HCC in patients with alcoholic liver disease without associated hepatitis B and C is 8%. However, infection with HBV or HCV further increases the risk of developing HCC.

4. Nonalcoholic steatohepatitis—The annual incidence of HCC in patients with NASH with advanced fibrosis or cirrhosis (F3–F4) is 2.6%. Diabetes mellitus and obesity both commonly associated with NASH have been found to be associated with HCC.

Table 49–1. Recommended surveillance for patients at risk for hepatocellular carcinoma (level III[a]).

Hepatitis B Carriers
Asian males >40 years
Asian females >50 years
All cirrhotic hepatitis B carriers
Family history of HCC
Africans >20 years
For noncirrhotic hepatitis B carriers not listed above, risk of HCC varies depending on severity of underlying liver disease and current and past hepatic inflammatory activity; patients with high HBV DNA concentrations and those with ongoing hepatic inflammatory activity remain at risk for HCC
Non-Hepatitis B Cirrhosis
Hepatitis C
Alcoholic cirrhosis
Genetic hemochromatosis
Primary biliary cirrhosis
Although the following groups have an increased risk of HCC no recommendations for or against surveillance can be made because lack of data precludes assessment of whether surveillance would be beneficial:
• α₁-Antitypsin deficiency
• Nonalcoholic steatohepatitis
• Autoimmune hepatitis

HBV, hepatitis B virus; HCC, hepatocellular carcinoma.

[a]American Association for the Study of Liver Diseases level III: opinion of respected authorities, descriptive epidemiology.

Reproduced with permission from Bruix J, Sherman M; Practice Guidelines Committee, American Association for the Study of Liver Diseases. Management of hepatocellular carcinoma, *Hepatology*. 2005;42(5):1208–1236.

5. Genetic or inherited liver diseases—Patients with hemochromatosis who develop cirrhosis have an increased 5-year cumulative incidence of HCC that is reported to be 21%. In contrast, in Wilson disease and α₁-antitrypsin deficiency and cirrhosis, the incidence rates of HCC are currently unknown but thought to be >1.5% per year. Lastly, patients with hereditary tyrosinemia can develop HCC and in one study, primary liver cancers occurred in up to 37% of patients.

6. Autoimmune hepatitis and primary biliary cholangitis—HCC surveillance of patients with primary biliary cholangitis who are cirrhotic is recommended based on a study that shows an incidence similar to that of patients with HCV cirrhosis. The association between autoimmune hepatitis and HCC is not clear, but case reports have illustrated the occurrence of HCC in such patients with cirrhosis. Surveillance of patients with autoimmune liver disease and cirrhosis is recommended.

7. Other conditions—Aflatoxin, produced by *Aspergillus flavus*, is clearly associated with HCC, particularly among patients infected with HBV.

8. Fibrolamellar hepatocellular carcinoma—This tumor, which is a distinct primary HCC, tends to occur in patients without cirrhosis who are in their 20s–40s. The long-term prognosis is generally good with either resection or transplantation.

Chayanupatkul M, Omino R, Mittal S, et al. Hepatocellular carcinoma in the absence of cirrhosis in patients with chronic hepatitis B virus infection. *J Hepatol.* 2017;66(2):355–362. [PMID: 27693539]

El-Serag HB. Epidemiology of viral hepatitis and hepatocellular carcinoma. *Gastroenterology.* 2012;142(6):1264–1273. e1. [PMID: 22537432]

Kulik L, El-Serag HB. Epidemiology and management of hepatocellular carcinoma. *Gastroenterology.* 2019;156(2):477–491. [PMID: 30367835]

Makarova-Rusher OV, Altekruse SF, McNeel TS, et al. Population attributable fractions of risk factors for hepatocellular carcinoma in the United States. *Cancer.* 2016;122:1757–1765. [PMID: 26998818]

Mittal S, El-Serag HB, Sada YH, et al. Hepatocellular carcinoma in the absence of cirrhosis in United States veterans is associated with nonalcoholic fatty liver disease. *Clin Gastroenterol Hepatol.* 2016;14(1):124–131. e1. [PMID: 26196445]

Perumpail RB, Wong RJ, Ahmed A, Harrison SA. Hepatocellular carcinoma in the setting of non-cirrhotic nonalcoholic fatty liver disease and the metabolic syndrome: US experience. *Dig Dis Sci.* 2015;60(10):3142–3148. [PMID: 26250831]

Petrick JL, Braunlin M, Laversanne M, et al. International trends in liver cancer incidence, overall and by histologic subtype, 1978-2007. *Int J Cancer.* 2016;139:1534–1545. [PMID: 27244487]

Petrick JL, Kelly SP, Altekruse SF, et al. Future of Hepatocellular Carcinoma Incidence in the United States Forecast Through 2030. *J Clin Oncol.* 2016;34(15):1787–1794. [PMID: 27044939]

Thrift AP, El-Serag HB, Kanwal F. Global epidemiology and burden of HCV infection and HCV-related disease. *Nat Rev Gastroenterol Hepatol.* 2017;14(2):122. [PMID: 27924080]

Younossi ZM, Koenig AB, Abdelatif D, Fazel Y, Linda H, Wymer M. Global epidemiology of nonalcoholic fatty liver disease-Meta-analytic assessment of prevalence, incidence, and outcomes. *Hepatology.* 2016;64(1):73–84. [PMID: 26707365]

B. Screening & Surveillance

The goal of surveillance and screening is to reduce mortality. Liver societies including American Association of the Study of Liver Diseases (AASLD) and European Association for the Study of the Liver (EASL) recommend surveillance of adults with cirrhosis because it improves overall survival. It is not possible to determine which type of surveillance test, ultrasound (US) alone or the combination of US plus alpha-fetoprotein (AFP) leads to a greater improvement in survival. Despite these recommendations, studies have reported that fewer than 20% of cirrhosis patients with a new diagnosis of HCC underwent regular surveillance. Surveillance is recommended in the patients' groups identified in Table 49–1.

In the one large-scale study performed to date, from China, 18,816 HBV carriers were randomized to either surveillance with ultrasound and α-fetoprotein every 6 months or no monitoring. A 37% decrease in HCC-related mortality was noted in those who were screened compared with the unscreened cohort. The 1-, 3-, and 5-year survival rates in the screened group were 66%, 53%, and 46% compared with rates of 31%, 7%, and 0%, respectively, in the control group. There are no randomized controlled trials of surveillance in patients with cirrhosis. However, several observational cohort studies evaluating surveillance in patients with cirrhosis have shown improved 3-year survival, compared to no surveillance. In countries with nationwide surveillance programs, most HCCs are diagnosed in early stages and amenable to curative treatments.

Although it is well established that US should be part of surveillance, it is unknown whether the addition of biomarkers such as AFP allows for improved survival. The AASLD suggests surveillance using US, with or without AFP, every 6 months. It remains unclear whether other serum biomarkers in addition to AFP complement US, such as des-gamma carboxy prothrombin, AFP L3, and other novel serum tests.

A lesion of >1 cm on US should trigger recall procedures for the diagnosis of HCC. If using AFP with US then an AFP >20 ng/mL should trigger recall procedures for diagnosis of HCC. Unlike most other malignancies, diagnosis of HCC can be established noninvasively, and treatment may be initiated based on imaging alone, without confirmatory biopsy. The rationale is that in patients with cirrhosis, the pretest probability of HCC is sufficiently high, and the pretest probability of lesions that may mimic HCC at imaging is sufficiently low such that a lesion meeting HCC imaging criteria can be assumed reliably and confidently to be HCC. Although there is strong consensus that the imaging diagnosis of HCC requires multiphasic imaging, there is not agreement about which diagnostic imaging test to use. Commonly used methods in clinical practice include multiphasic CT with extracellular agents, multiphasic MRI with extracellular agents (gadolinium-based compounds that stay in the extracellular space and permit characterization of blood flow), and multiphasic MRI with gadoxetate disodium (Eovist), a specific gadolinium-based compound that accumulates in hepatocytes and permits characterization of hepatocellular "function" in addition to blood flow. HCC radiological hallmark is arterial hypervascularity and venous/late phase washout. The AASLD recommends diagnostic evaluation for HCC with either multiphasic CT or multiphasic MRI because of similar diagnostic performance characteristics.

Forner A, Reig M, Bruix J. Hepatocellular carcinoma. *Lancet.* 2018;391:1301–1314. [PMID: 29307467]

Marrero JA, Kulik LM, Sirlin C, et al. Diagnosis, staging and management of hepatocellular carcinoma: 2018 practice guidance by the American Association for the Study of Liver Diseases. *Hepatology.* 2018;68(2):723–750. [PMID: 29624699]

Clinical Findings

A. Symptoms & Signs

Patients with compensated liver disease who are diagnosed with HCC during routine surveillance are often asymptomatic at presentation. However, any patient with compensated cirrhosis who suddenly develops signs and symptoms of worsening hepatic function or portal hypertension should undergo appropriate studies to exclude the development of HCC.

Symptoms may be related to the cancer patients including right upper quadrant pain, weight loss, fatigue, anorexia, jaundice, and pruritus. Patients may also present with signs of liver decompensation including variceal hemorrhage, ascites, or hepatic encephalopathy. Physical examination findings often show stigmata of portal hypertension and cirrhosis. Occasionally, tender and firm hepatomegaly may be present. In patients suspected of having HCC who present with peritoneal signs, hemoperitoneum should be suspected as a consequence of hemorrhage related to the tumor. Additional clinical findings may be secondary to associated paraneoplastic syndromes, including hypercholesterolemia, cryoglobulinemia, carcinoid syndrome, hypercalcemia, dysfibrinogenemia, erythrocytosis, and hypoglycemia.

B. Diagnostic Approach

With the exception of AFP, laboratory testing is generally not very useful and radiographic studies are required to make a diagnosis. The diagnosis of HCC can be made using a combination of radiographic, laboratory, or pathologic studies. The size of the tumor influences the diagnostic evaluation.

1. Lesions larger than 1 cm—A nodule greater than 1 cm in size that fulfills the radiographic hallmark for HCC (early arterial enhancement and washout in delayed phase) on multiphasic CT or MRI is HCC and a biopsy to confirm the diagnosis is not required for clinical purposes. However, if characteristics of HCC are not seen on the initial multiphasic radiographic study, then a second CT or MRI study (whichever was not performed initially) is recommended. If typical HCC characteristics are seen on the follow-up study, then the diagnosis of HCC is confirmed. If the second study still does not confirm the diagnosis of HCC, a biopsy is recommended. If a negative biopsy result is obtained in an individual with risk factors for HCC (eg, chronic HBV infection or cirrhosis), then short-term follow-up with MRI or CT is recommended to ensure stability of the lesion and a repeat biopsy should be considered.

2. Lesions smaller than 1 cm—These lesions have a very low probability of being HCC. The AASLD recommends an ultrasound every 3 months for up to 2 years and if no growth is documented, reverting to typical HCC surveillance guidelines thereafter. Alternatively, if the lesion enlarges, additional diagnostic testing with CT, MRI, or biopsy is recommended.

3. Metastases—Many patients with HCC have invasion of the portal and hepatic veins and inferior vena cava, and/or metastases to the portal, pancreatic, and para-aortic lymph nodes. Other sites of metastasis include the lung, bone, myocardium, and adrenal gland. Imaging by Doppler ultrasound, contrast-enhanced CT, or MRI can be used to identify a thrombus in the major vessels and for nodal involvement. Chest CT is requited for initial HCC staging at the time of diagnosis.

Differential Diagnosis

The differential diagnosis of HCC is very broad and includes benign and malignant lesions. Among these are cholangiocarcinoma, HA, hemangioma, FNH, cystic neoplasms, metastatic tumors, peliosis hepatis, and lymphoma.

Treatment

Therapeutic management of HCC is influenced by the tumor size and extent, underlying liver function, and the patient's performance status. The Barcelona Clinic Liver Cancer (BCLC) criteria may offer the most prognostic information because it includes an assessment of tumor burden, liver function, and patient performance status, and thereby, has been endorsed by the societies that specialized in liver disease. The prognostic ability of the BCLC has been validated in European, American, and Asian populations. The value of the BCLC is in its ability to stratify the survival of patients with HCC among the sub-strata of 0, A, B, C and D, and therefore, it can be easily applied directly to patient care (Figure 49–5). Treatment options include resection, liver transplantation, percutaneous ablation, transarterial embolization, chemotherapy, and radiation.

Heimbach JK, Kulik LM, Finn RS, et al. AASLD Guidelines for the treatment of hepatocellular carcinoma. *Hepatology*. 2018;67(1):358–380. [PMID: 28130846]

Kim SY, An J, Lim Y-S, et al. MRI with liver-specific contrast for surveillance of patients with cirrhosis at high risk of hepatocellular carcinoma. *JAMA Oncol*. 2017;3(4):456–463. [PMID: 27657493]

Singal AG, Pillai A, Tiro J. Early detection, curative treatment, and survival rates for hepatocellular carcinoma surveillance in patients with cirrhosis: a meta-analysis. *PLoS Med*. 2014;11(4):e1001624. [PMID: 24691105]

A. Resection

Surgical resection is the treatment of choice for non-cirrhotic HCC (5% in West, 40% in Asia), or in Child A cirrhosis without clinically significant portal hypertension. Five year survival after resection is 30–50%. There is no size cut-off for tumor diameter if there is a sufficient functional liver remnant. When large volume of resection is anticipated such as with >3 segments, portal vein embolization is performed to increase the size of the contralateral lobe.

After resection, the 5-year recurrence rate is approximately 70%. Microvascular invasion is the most important predictor of recurrence and is present in up to 90% of tumors

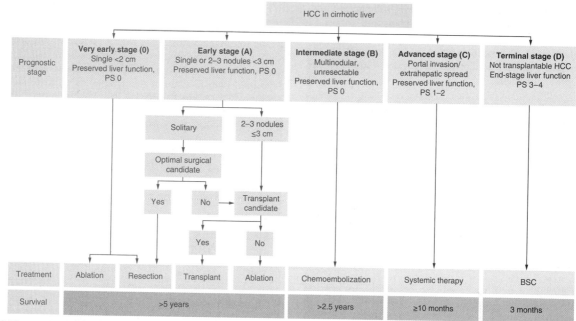

▲ **Figure 49–5.** Modified BCLC staging system and treatment strategy. BCLC, Barcelona Clinic Liver Cancer; BSC, Best Supportive Care; HCC, hepatocellular carcinoma. (Reproduced with permission from Bruix J, Sherman M; Practice Guidelines Committee; American Association for the Study of Liver Diseases: Management of hepatocellular carcinoma, *Hepatology* 2005;42(5):1208–1236.)

greater than 5 cm. Other predictors are tumor differentiation, macro vascular invasion, and the presence of satellite nodules. A large randomized controlled trial of adjuvant sorafenib showed no effect on HCC recurrence thus, adjuvant therapy is not usually recommended.

Bruix J, Takayama T, Mazzaferro V, et al. Adjuvant sorafenib for hepatocellular carcinoma after resection or ablation (STORM): a phase 3, randomised, double-blind, placebo-controlled trial. *Lancet Oncol.* 2015;16(13):1344–1354. [PMID: 26361969]

Tabrizian P, Jibara G, Schrager B, Schwartz M, Roayaie S. Recurrence of hepatocellular cancer after resection: patterns, treatments, and prognosis. *Ann Surg.* 2015;261(5):947–955. [PMID: 25010665]

B. Liver Transplantation

Both cadaveric and live donor liver transplantation have been used in patients with HCC. Based on the Milan criteria (single HCC <5cm or ≤3 tumors ≤3 cm without vascular invasion or distant metastases), carefully chosen patients with HCC who undergo liver transplantation have a 5-year survival rate of 70% and recurrence <15%. The United Network for Organ Sharing (UNOS) has created a priority system for such patients. Priority (exemption) Model for End-Stage Liver Disease (MELD) scores are given to single T2 tumor 2–5 cm or up to 3 tumors each up to 3 cm. For patients who meet these criteria, a MELD score equivalent to Median MELD at Transplant minus 3 (MMaT – 3) is awarded 6 months after listing for liver transplantation. Listed patients require multiphase imaging and AFP every 3 months until they receive a transplant. Patients whose HCC progress beyond MC while on the waitlist should be put on hold, and considered for downstaging. Patients developing macrovascular invasion or extrahepatic spread should be delisted.

Patients with HCC tumor burden just outside UNOS criteria have been shown to successfully undergo liver transplantation with careful patient selection. To meet University of California San Francisco (UCSF) or extended criteria, there can be one lesion not greater than 6.5 cm or up to three tumors ≤4.5 cm, the total tumor volume ≤8 cm. For patients who successfully undergo downstaging the HCC from UCSF criteria to Milan criteria and then undergo liver transplantation, the 5-year survival is approximately 80%.

In many regions, the wait time for transplant can be long even with the priority MELD system, extending up to 12 months or more. Most centers with wait times greater than 6 months practice some form of bridging therapy. For patients with small tumors, percutaneous ablative techniques using either microwave, cryoablation, or radiofrequency ablation, can be considered. For patients with multiple or larger tumors, transarterial chemoembolization or radioembolization can also be considered. The AASLD suggests bridging to transplant in patients listed for liver transplantation within T2 (Milan) criteria to decrease progression of disease and subsequent dropout from the waiting list but does not recommend one form of liver-directed therapy over another for the purposes of bridging.

Mazzaferro V, Regalia E, Doci R, et al. Liver transplantation for the treatment of small hepatocellular carcinomas in patients with cirrhosis. *N Engl J Med.* 1996;334:693–700. [PMID: 8594428]

Yao FY, Mehta N, Flemming J, et al. Downstaging of hepatocellular cancer before liver transplant: long-term outcome compared to tumors within Milan criteria. *Hepatology.* 2015;61(6): 1968–1977. [PMID: 25689978]

Yao FY, Xiao L, Bass NM, et al. Liver transplantation for hepatocellular carcinoma: validation of the UCSF-expanded criteria based on preoperative imaging. *Am J Transplant.* 2007;7: 2587–2596. [PMID: 17868066]

C. Percutaneous Ablation

Image-guided ablative techniques use tumor destruction using microwave, radiofrequency or cryoablation. These are most often performed percutaneously by interventional radiologists. Ablation is used as curative therapy for very early HCC (solitary tumors smaller than 2 cm), bridging therapy in patients listed for liver transplantation, for downstaging in order to become eligible for liver transplantation and for palliation. Ablation is the standard of care for early small HCCs not suitable for surgery, where the 5-year survival rate is 80–90% and equivalent to resection.

Lencioni R, Crocetti L. Local-regional treatment of hepatocellular carcinoma. *Radiology.* 2012;262(1):43–58. [PMID: 2219065]

D. Transarterial Chemoembolization

Transarterial chemoembolization (TACE) is the intra-arterial infusion of a cytotoxic agent such as doxorubicin and cisplatin followed by embolization of the tumor-feeding blood vessels results in a strong cytotoxic and ischemic effect. TACE achieves partial responses in 15–55% of patients, and significantly delays tumor progression and macrovascular invasion. TACE is the standard of care for intermediate stage (BCLC B). Patients with advanced liver disease are at greater risk of morbidity and mortality related to liver failure with the procedure. Therefore patients should be carefully selected to ensure adequate liver reserve. Patients should have relatively well-preserved liver function (mostly Child A or B7 without ascites).

Survival rates appear to be around 20–60% at 2 years with this intervention. Side effects related to the procedure include liver failure, chemotherapeutic side effects, and postembolization syndrome related to hepatic artery occlusion.

Parikh ND, Waljee AK, Singal AG. Downstaging hepatocellular carcinoma: a systematic review and pooled analysis. *Liver Transplant.* 2015;21:1142–1152. [PMID: 25981135]

E. Transarterial Radioembolization

Transarterial Radioembolization (TARE or Y90) has had a greater role in the management of HCC. It involves the delivery of ß-emitting microspheres that provide local, high-dose tumor radiation. Major risk is radiation hepatitis and lung deposition (99mTc-albumin scintigraphy to confirm <20% shunting). TARE may provide similar or better results than TACE including treating multiple tumors, large tumor burden, segmental or lobar portal vein thrombosis, down-staging to allow radical therapy in cases exceeding Milan criteria. Compared to TACE, TARE is associated with longer time to progression, less abdominal pain, fewer treatment sessions, and improved quality of life. TACE and TARE have shown similar overall survival in retrospective studies.

Salem R, Gordon AC, Mouli S, et al. Y90 Radioembolization significantly prolongs time to progression compared with chemoembolization in patients with hepatocellular carcinoma. *Gastroenterology.* 2016;151(6):1155–1163. [PMID: 27575820]

F. Chemotherapy

Sorafenib, an oral multi-tyrosine kinase inhibitor, is the standard systemic therapy for HCC based on the landmark SHARP trial. It is the first drug to show survival benefit in advanced HCC (10.7 months in sorafenib group, 7.9 months in placebo group). Serious side effects were rare, and common side effects included diarrhea, fatigue, and hand-foot skin reaction. Since then, multiple other systemic therapies have shown survival in HCC. These are summarized in Figure 49–6.

Llovet JM, Ricci S, Mazzaferro V, et al; SHARP Investigators Study Group. Sorafenib in advanced hepatocellular carcinoma. *N Engl J Med.* 2008;359:378–390. [PMID: 18650514]

Abou-Alfa GK, Meyer T, Cheng AL, et al; Cabozantinib in Patients with Advanced and Progressing Hepatocellular Carcinoma. *N Engl J Med.* 2018;379(1):54–63. [PMID: 29972759]

Bruix J, Qin S, Merle P, et al; Regorafenib for patients with hepatocellular carcinoma who progressed on sorafenib treatment: a randomised, double-blind, placebo-controlled, phase 3 trial. *Lancet.* 2017;389(10064):56–66. [PMID: 27932229]

Faivre S, Raymond E, Boucher E, et al; Safety and efficacy of sunitinib in patients with advanced hepatocellular carcinoma: an open-label, multicentre, phase II study. *Lancet Oncol.* 2009;10(8):794–800. [PMID: 19586800]

Zhu AX, Finn RS, Edeline J, et al; Pembrolizumab in patients with advanced hepatocellular carcinoma previously treated with sorafenib: a non-randomised, open-label phase 2 trial. *Lancet Oncol.* 2018;19(7):940–952. [PMID: 29875066]

G. Immunotherapy

Anti PD-1 monoclonal antibodies have been studied as a systemic treatment for HCC. Nivolumab has been approved by FDA as a second line agent for advanced HCC. Median overall survival in sorafenib-experienced patients was 16.7 months

Study	Treatment	Control	Primary Endpoint	Hazard Ratio	Reference
SHARP	Sorafenib	Placebo	OS	0.69 (0.55–0.87; *p* <0.001)	Llovet et al., 2008
Asia-Pacific	Sorafenib	Placebo	OS	0.68 (0.50–0.93; *p* =0.014)	Cheng Lancet 2009
REFLECT	Lenvatinib	Sorafenib	OS (non-inferior)	0.92 (0.79–1.06)	Kudo Lancet 2018
RESORCE	Regorafenib	Placebo	OS	0.63 (0.50–0.79; *p* <0.0001)	Bruix Lancet 2017
CELESTIAL	Cabozantinib	Placebo	OS	0.76 (0.63–0.92; *p*=0.0049)	Abou-Alfa ASCO GI 2018

▲ **Figure 49-6.** Systemic therapies with a survival benefit in HCC. HCC, hepatocellular carcinoma.

CHOLANGIOCARCINOMA

 ESSENTIALS OF DIAGNOSIS

▶ Risk factors include biliary and liver diseases (eg, primary sclerosing cholangitis [PSC] in the West, liver flukes in the East, choledocholithiasis, hepatolithiasis, choledochal cysts, and HCV cirrhosis).

▶ Diagnosis usually requires abdominal imaging and tissue sampling either by percutaneous biopsy or endoscopic retrograde cholangiopancreatography (ERCP).

▶ Associated with a poor prognosis.

General Considerations

Although the incidence of cholangiocarcinoma is increasing globally, it remains a rare cancer with an incidence of approximately 8 per million persons.

The risk factors for cholangiocarcinoma include PSC, choledocholithiasis, hepatolithiasis, choledochal cyst, Caroli disease, bile duct adenoma, thorotrast, HCV cirrhosis, chronic parasitic infection, and typhoid carrier state. Age and smoking are also risk factors. However, most patients have no risk factors.

Shaib Y, El-Serag HB. The epidemiology of cholangiocarcinoma. *Semin Liver Dis.* 2004;24:115–125. [PMID: 15192785]

Clinical Findings

Patients with intrahepatic cholangiocarcinoma present with large intrahepatic masses with or without metastases. Patients with extrahepatic (perihilar or distal) cholangiocarcinoma may present with symptoms of biliary obstruction.

Cross-sectional abdominal imaging with either CT or MRI is required. ERCP with cytologic brushing of the biliary tree may be required for extrahepatic tumors. The role of serologic testing is not entirely clear, but of the many markers, CA 19-9 is most frequently used. A CA 19-9 level >100 U/mL has a 65–75% sensitivity and a 85–95% specificity for cholangiocarcinoma; a CA 19-9 level >1000 predicts metastases.

Malhi H, Gores GJ. Cholangiocarcinoma: modern advances in understanding a deadly old disease. *J Hepatol.* 2006;45:856–867. [PMID: 17030071]

Patel AH, Harnois DM, Klee GG, et al. The utility of CA 19-9 in the diagnoses of cholangiocarcinoma in patients without primary sclerosing cholangitis. *Am J Gastroenterol.* 2000;95:204–207. [PMID: 10638584]

Differential Diagnosis

The differential diagnosis is similar to that of HCC (see earlier discussion).

Treatment

The best treatment option in cholangiocarcinoma is surgical resection, but even when patients are carefully selected, the 5-year survival rate is only 20–45%. The absence of positive lymph nodes, a clear resection margin (>1 cm), lack of vascular invasion, and single lesions are the predictors of good response to surgery. Patients with compromised liver function, PSC, and bilobar involvement are not candidates for surgical resection. Patients with intrahepatic and distal cholangiocarcinoma are not candidates for liver transplantation. Early experience with liver transplantation for unresectable hilar cholangiocarcinoma was poor, with 5 year overall survival of 23% and recurrence rate of 51%. Neoadjuvant chemotherapy and radiation followed by exploratory laparotomy to confirm downstaging of hilar cholangiocarcinoma and subsequent liver transplantation has been associated with a good prognosis with 1, 3, and 5 year survival of 91%, 81%, and 74%, respectively. Otherwise, there appears to be minimal response to chemotherapy and radiation in this disease.

Most patients who present with cholangiocarcinoma are not candidates for curative therapy but require palliation. Biliary obstruction is a common complication of this disease, and decompression using endoscopic, percutaneous, or surgical approaches is often necessary. There is interest in photodynamic and radiofrequency ablation therapies, but further confirmatory studies are needed.

Prognosis

Overall, the prognosis is poor. Most patients develop liver failure or biliary complications, resulting in a dismal 5-year survival rate of approximately 5%.

Murad SD, Kim WR, Harnois DM, et al. Efficacy of neoadjuvant chemoradiation, followed by liver transplantation, for peri-hilar cholangiocarcinoma at 12 US centers. *Gastroenterology.* 2012;143:88–98. [PMID: 22504095]

Rea DJ, Heimbach JK, Rosen CB, et al. Liver transplantation with neoadjuvant chemoradiation is more effective than resection for hilar cholangiocarcinoma. *Ann Surg.* 2005;242:451–458. [PMID: 16135931]

Silva MA, Tekin K, Aytekin F, et al. Surgery for hilar cholangiocarcinoma: a 10-year experience of a tertiary referral centre in the UK. *Eur J Surg Oncol.* 2005;31:533–539. [PMID: 15922889]

Sudan D, DeRoover A, Chinnakotla S, et al. Radiochemotherapy and transplantation allow long-term survival for nonresectable hilar cholangiocarcinoma. *Am J Transplant.* 2002;2:774–779. [PMID: 12243499]

Yeh CN, Yan YY, Yeh TS, et al. Hepatic resection of the intraductal papillary type of peripheral cholangiocarcinoma. *Ann Surg Oncol.* 2004;11:606–611. [PMID: 15172934]

Zamora-Valdes D, Heimbach JK. Liver Transplant for cholangiocarcinoma. *Gastroenterol Clin North Am.* 2018;47(2):267–280. [PMID: 29735023]

METASTATIC LIVER DISEASE

General Considerations

Liver metastases are the most frequent malignant liver masses. Metastasis to the liver is most commonly seen with colorectal, gastric, pancreatic, renal, and neuroendocrine malignancies. It is uncommon for patients with cirrhosis to develop liver metastases. However, in a patient without cirrhosis with a liver lesion, there must be a strong degree of suspicion for metastatic liver disease.

Clinical Findings

Patients may be asymptomatic who are found to have liver lesions either incidentally or during surveillance imaging for the primary tumor. Most patients present with symptoms related to the underlying malignancy. In patients with a high burden of metastatic disease, liver failure may occur. Patients may present with jaundice, portal hypertensive bleeding, ascites, and hepatic encephalopathy.

Imaging may identify a single or more often multiple liver lesions. Most lesions are found to be hypoechoic on ultrasound or hypovascular on MRI or CT scan. Hypovascular metastases are generally from gastrointestinal cancer. Conversely, hypervascular metastases are generally from renal cell, breast, melanoma, thyroid, and neuroendocrine malignancies.

Differential Diagnosis

The differential diagnosis is similar to that of HCC (see earlier discussion).

Treatment

The primary objective to treat metastatic liver disease is to treat the primary malignancy. For patients with solitary or limited lesions, surgical resection may be considered. Ablation, transarterial chemoembolic and radioembolic treatment, and stereotactic radiation may also be considered for patients with low burden of metastatic liver disease. In one study that assessed patients with colorectal metastases to the liver, the 3-year survival rate for surgical resection was 73% and for ablation was 37%. Systemic chemotherapy combined with TARE can be used for diffuse liver metastases.

Abdalla EK, Vauthey JN, Ellis LM, et al. Recurrence and outcomes following hepatic resection, radiofrequency ablation, and combined resection/ablation for colorectal liver metastases. *Ann Surg.* 2004;239:818–824. [PMID: 15166961]

Albrecht T, Hohmann J, Oldenburg A, et al. Detection and characterization of liver metastases. *Eur Radiol.* 2004;14(suppl 8): P25–P33.

Liver Transplantation

Jordan Sack, MD, MPH

Nikroo Hashemi, MD, MPH

ESSENTIALS OF DIAGNOSIS

▶ Alcohol related liver disease, non-alcoholic fatty liver disease, and hepatocellular carcinoma are leading etiologies for liver transplantation in the United States.

▶ Liver transplant referral should be considered for acute liver failure or advanced chronic liver disease when the limits of medical therapy have been reached.

▶ Multidisciplinary evaluations focusing on medical, surgical, psychiatric, and social components are required prior to listing patients for transplantation.

▶ Liver transplantation is predominantly performed using deceased donor livers in the United States. Model for End-Stage Liver Disease score is used for prioritizing patients on the liver transplant waiting list. Some liver diseases and complications may qualify for exception scores. Waitlist time is also affected by blood type.

▶ Average 1-year survival after liver transplant is about 91% in the United States.

▶ Early liver transplant complications include primary graft dysfunction, acute cellular rejection, infections, vascular thrombosis, biliary leaks, and biliary strictures.

▶ Late (> 1st year) modifiable risk factors associated with higher mortality include hypertension, diabetes, renal insufficiency, and smoking.

▶ Patients should be monitored for long term immunosuppression side effects including metabolic syndrome, cardiovascular disease, chronic kidney disease, and malignancies.

General Considerations

A. Background

Liver transplantation has radically changed the management of patients with chronic liver disease and acute liver failure.

Following the first liver transplant in 1963, numerous medical, surgical, and technical breakthroughs were required before transplantation became a viable therapy in liver disease. The 1-year survival rate remained low at 25% until the introduction of cyclosporine as a long-term immunosuppressant in the 1980s. Improvements in patient selection, refinements in surgical techniques, addition of novel immunosuppressive agents including mycophenolate mofetil, sirolimus, tacrolimus, azathioprine, and effective anti-infective treatment and prophylaxis, have resulted in an average 5-year survival rate of 75%.

In 2020, over 13,000 liver transplant candidates were added to the waiting list. Nearly 9,000 patients were transplanted that year and about 2,400 died waiting for a transplant or became too sick for transplant. The leading etiologies for liver transplantation are alcohol related liver disease, non-alcoholic fatty liver disease, and hepatocellular carcinoma (HCC).

B. Role of UNOS

The United Network for Organ Sharing (UNOS) is a nonprofit scientific organization based in Virginia that is responsible for matching donors to recipients and coordinating the organ transplantation process.

Since 2002, UNOS has used the Model for End-Stage Liver Disease (MELD) score (range 6–40), calculated by the patient's serum bilirubin, international normalized ratio, and creatinine, to prioritize the need for liver transplantation. The MELD score was updated in 2016 to include serum sodium. As shown in Figure 50–1, the 90-day survival of patients decreases with higher MELD scores. The risks of deceased donor liver transplantation in patients with MELD <15 outweigh its benefits in most circumstances. Consequently, a MELD score ≥15 is recommended to list most patients with liver disease.

The time to liver transplant relies primarily upon the patient's UNOS MELD score which typically corresponds with their natural MELD score. Patients may be able to receive a UNOS MELD score that is higher than their natural MELD score if they can qualify for exception points.

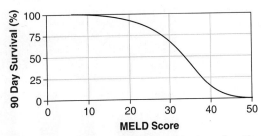

▲ **Figure 50–1.** Estimated 90-day survival as a function of the Model for End-Stage Liver Disease (MELD) score. INR, international normalized ratio. (Reproduced with permission from Wiesner R, Edwards E, Freeman R, et al; Model for end-stage liver disease (MELD) and allocation of donor livers, *Gastroenterology* 2003;124(1):91–96.)

These exception criteria help patients who have certain diagnoses and complications that carry significant morbidity and mortality without liver transplantation but are not reflected by the natural MELD score. Patients can obtain standard exception scores by fulfilling the requirements set by the Organ Procurement and Transplant Network (OPTN). Less commonly, an appeal can be made on a case-by-case basis to the National Liver Review Board (NLRB) for exception scores in situations that do not meet the OPTN requirements.

Until recently, UNOS had allocated deceased donor livers using 58 donation service areas and 11 transplant regions. To reduce geographic inequities, the system was recalibrated in February 2020 so that deceased donor livers are allocated incrementally within a 500-mile nautical range from the donor hospital starting with the highest priority designations on the waitlist followed by decreasing MELD scores until a match has been made.

It is important to recognize that there are other factors that UNOS incorporates when allocating livers which can affect time to transplant—such as blood type compatibility, liver size suitability, type of donor livers, and region of listing. These factors may potentially help patients who have MELD scores that are not high enough for transplantation. Since donor and recipient blood type compatibility is preferred, having blood types B and AB may be favorable in some situations as there are fewer listed candidates with those blood types. Furthermore, depending on the patient's circumstances, patients may accept a higher risk deceased donor liver or may consider multi-listing in another region where the patient's MELD score would be higher than that region's median MELD score for transplantation. Additionally, some patients who have a living liver donor may be candidates for living donor transplantation and can bypass the UNOS waitlist.

INDICATIONS FOR TRANSPLANTATION

There are numerous indications for liver transplantation which can be categorized as acute liver failure, chronic liver disease, and other less common causes, as listed in Table 50–1. It is important to be aware of the wide indications for liver transplantation and how exception points, blood type, type of deceased donor liver, and living donation can help patients who have relatively lower MELD scores.

Table 50–1. Indications for liver transplantation.

Acute Liver Failure[a]	Chronic Liver Disease	Other
Acute fatty liver of pregnancy	Alcohol related liver disease	Alagille syndrome
Acute viral hepatitis	Alpha 1 antitrypsin disease	Allograft cirrhosis
Acetaminophen overdose	Autoimmune hepatitis	Biliary atresia
Amanita phalloides	Budd Chiari syndrome	Congenital hepatic fibrosis
Autoimmune hepatitis	Chronic hepatitis B	Cystic fibrosis[b]
Budd Chiari syndrome	Chronic hepatitis C	Erythropoietic protoporphyria
Drug-induced	Hereditary hemochromatosis	Familial amyloid polyneuropathy[b]
Hepatectomy	Non-alcoholic fatty liver disease	Progressive familial intrahepatic cholestasis
Wilson's disease	Non-cirrhotic portal hypertension	Hepatic adenomas
	Primary biliary cholangitis	Hepatic artery thrombosis[a]
	Primary sclerosing cholangitis	Hepatic epithelioid hemangioendothelioma
	Secondary sclerosing cholangitis	Hereditary hemorrhagic telangiectasia
	Wilson disease	Metastatic neuroendocrine tumors
		Polycystic liver disease
	Liver Complications:	Primary graft failure[a]
	- hepatocellular carcinoma[b]	Primary hyperoxaluria[b]
	- hepatopulmonary syndrome[b]	Urea cycle defect or organic acidemia[b]
	- porto-pulmonary hypertension[b]	

[a]May qualify for high priority listing.
[b]May qualify for standard exception scores.

1. Chronic Liver Disease

Chronic liver disease decompensation from jaundice, ascites, variceal hemorrhage, or hepatic encephalopathy is the most common indication for liver transplantation.

Until the recent development of direct acting antivirals, hepatitis C virus (HCV) was the leading liver disease etiology for liver transplantation in the United States. Presently, alcohol related liver disease, non-alcoholic fatty liver disease, and HCC are the top three causes for liver transplantation in the United States.

Generally, patients transplanted for chronic liver disease have good transplant outcomes regardless of etiology except for hereditary hemochromatosis which may be attributable to iron related cardiomyopathy. Until approximately 20 years ago, transplantation of patients infected with hepatitis B virus (HBV) was controversial. The near universal recurrence of HBV generally resulted in early graft loss. A major advance in the field of transplantation was the introduction of hepatitis B immunoglobulin (HBIG) and antiviral therapy with nucleoside and nucleotide analogs. As these interventions have resulted in a dramatic improvement in transplant outcomes, liver failure and/or HCC related to HBV infection is now a well-accepted indication for liver transplantation with a good prognosis. While there is concern that patients with alcohol related liver disease are high-risk candidates for poor outcomes after liver transplantation, graft loss from recurrent alcohol abuse is uncommon. Most transplant centers recommend a six-month period of abstinence from alcohol before considering a patient for liver transplantation; however, the "6-month" rule is not required by UNOS and is a poor predictor of alcohol use in the first 12 months after liver transplantation. American and European liver societies recommend considering liver transplantation as a salvage therapy for carefully selected patients with severe alcoholic hepatitis not responding to medical therapy and have favorable psychosocial profiles.

Some complications of chronic liver disease—specifically HCC, hepatopulmonary syndrome, and portopulmonary hypertension—may qualify for standard exception points if they meet OPTN criteria. This approach is particularly useful when the patient's natural MELD is not high.

For patients with HCC, the requirement for receiving standard exception points is a T2 lesion—defined as a solitary tumor at least 2 cm and no greater than 5 cm or two to three tumors each less than 3 cm in size with one at least 1 cm (Milan criteria). The 5-year survival rate in this group of patients has been reported to be 70%. Patients with HCC tumor burden beyond Milan criteria have been shown to successfully undergo liver transplantation with careful patient selection if they are downstaged to within Milan. Therefore, patients meeting University of California San Francisco (UCSF) criteria (single tumor >5 and ≤8 cm or multifocal tumors with total size not exceeding 8 cm) are eligible for exception points if they undergo successful tumor downstaging to fall within the Milan criteria.

2. Acute Liver Failure

Acute liver failure is life threatening without transplantation if the etiology of the acute liver failure cannot be reversed. Patients presenting with acute liver failure qualify for high priority listing if they fulfill specific OPTN criteria. A detailed review of acute liver failure is provided in a separate chapter.

3. Other Etiologies

There are other less common indications for liver transplantation some of which qualify for standard MELD exception points including cystic fibrosis, primary hyperoxaluria, and familial amyloid polyneuropathy. Another consideration for liver transplantation are urea cycle disorders and some of these patients who are transplanted may be able to donate their native liver to another liver transplant candidate, which is called domino liver transplantation. Other indications for liver transplantation include metastatic neuroendocrine tumors, polycystic liver disease, and hereditary hemorrhagic telangiectasia—if conservative therapies fail. Living donor transplantation should be considered in these patients if they are unable to acquire exception points as they are unlikely to have a high MELD score in the absence of significant liver decompensation.

PRETRANSPLANT EVALUATION

The evaluation of patients for liver transplantation candidacy occurs in a multidisciplinary setting and involves hepatologists, transplant surgeons, anesthesiologists, infectious disease physicians, psychiatrists, social workers, nutritionists, financial coordinators, and other subspecialists as needed.

Several diagnostic tests and procedures are used to evaluate patients; these are listed in Table 50–2. Upon completion of an evaluation, patients are presented at a recipient selection committee to discuss the patient and to determine whether the patient is eligible to be placed on the waitlist for liver transplantation.

1. Hepatology Evaluation

The hepatologist assesses disease severity/prognosis, confirms the diagnosis, and optimizes management of the liver disease.

2. Transplant Surgery Evaluation

The transplant surgeon confirms the need for transplantation, identifies technical challenges, and discusses donor options including deceased donation, living donation, and extended criteria donation.

3. Cardiopulmonary Evaluation

Cardiopulmonary complications are leading causes of liver transplant mortality. Meticulous cardiopulmonary evaluation is required in every patient being considered for liver

Table 50–2. Liver transplant candidate evaluation.

Laboratory Testing
Liver tests and serologies
Type and screen
HIV testing
QuantiFERON gold test
Viral hepatitis A, B, C, D, and E serologies
Cytomegalovirus, Epstein-Barr virus, Herpes simplex virus serologies
Vaccination serologies

Imaging
Hepatic cross-sectional imaging with contrast
Chest radiograph
Electrocardiogram
Echocardiogram +/− stress test

Malignancy Evaluation
Colonoscopy (based on age and family risk)
Cervical cancer screening (for women)
Mammogram (for women)
Prostate-specific antigen assay (for men)
Skin assessment

Clearances Needed
Hepatology
Financial
Psychosocial
Transplant surgery
Infectious disease
Cardiology
Nutrition
Other subspecialties as needed (Anesthesia, Nephrology, Hematology, Oncology, etc)

transplantation. All patients require a transthoracic echocardiogram to assess cardiac function and pulmonary hypertension. Patients who are older or have comorbidities are also required to obtain a cardiac stress test. If there is concern for coronary disease, pulmonary hypertension, or other cardiopulmonary diseases, additional testing is warranted.

4. Psychosocial Evaluation

A comprehensive social evaluation of the candidate by a transplant social worker is needed before listing. Strong social support is necessary after liver transplantation to ensure that the patient has the resources to monitor for complications and to ensure compliance with medications and medical appointments.

Patients who have psychiatric illness or alcohol or substance use disorders require further evaluation by a transplant psychiatrist. These patients are at risk of relapse and should demonstrate insight into how their addiction has contributed to their liver disease, should take initiative to participate in a formal program, and should show commitment to maintaining sobriety and a substance-free lifestyle. While most transplant centers require alcohol abstinence for 6 months prior to listing, some waive this requirement for

select patients with severe alcoholic hepatitis given the high 1-month mortality. Consideration may be given to those who present with a first episode of alcohol related liver decompensation, were not previously counseled on the deleterious effects of alcohol on the liver, were influenced by a life-changing event that can be addressed with psychiatric support, show motivation to stop drinking and to participate in programs, and have a strong social support system.

5. Infectious Disease Evaluation

Given the risk of infectious complications in patients taking immunosuppression, a thorough evaluation for infection risk is warranted. This evaluation should include testing for human immunodeficiency virus, cytomegalovirus immunoglobulin G (IgG), Epstein-Barr virus (EBV) IgG, herpes simplex virus IgG, and syphilis. Patients should undergo evaluation for *Mycobacterium tuberculosis* infection. Patients from regions in which strongyloidiasis, schistosomiasis, and histoplasmosis are endemic should undergo serologic evaluation and prophylactic treatment as deemed appropriate by the transplant infectious disease team. This team also provides input on pretransplant vaccinations and peri-operative anti-infective medications.

6. Nephrology Evaluation

Patients with abnormal renal function should be evaluated by a transplant nephrologist to determine whether a combined liver kidney transplant is warranted. Patients may be eligible for a simultaneous liver-kidney transplant if they have (1) chronic kidney disease with glomerular filtration rate (GFR) less than 60 mL/min for the previous 90 days and a current GFR ≤30 mL/min, or (2) have sustained acute kidney injury with GFR less than 25 mL/min and/or dialysis at least weekly for the past 6 weeks. Less common indications for simultaneous liver kidney transplant is the presence of hyperoxaluria, familial non-neuropathic systemic amyloid, or methylmalonic aciduria. Additionally, patients with severe hyponatremia warrant nephrology and anesthesia guidance peri-operatively to minimize the risk of central pontine myelinolysis.

7. Other Subspecialties

Depending on the patient's medical comorbidities, other subspecialists may be asked to evaluate the patient's suitability for liver transplantation. A common scenario is the need for a hematologist or oncologist to comment on whether a prior malignancy is in remission and the risk of recurrence with immunosuppression.

CONTRAINDICATIONS

There is no actual policy to define absolute contraindications to liver transplantation. However, there are many relative contraindications that vary on a case-by-case basis at different centers (Table 50–3).

Table 50–3. Contraindications to liver transplantation.

Absolute Contraindications	Relative Contraindications
Advanced cardiopulmonary disease that is not correctable	Age >70 years
Acquired immunodeficiency syndrome	Body mass index >40
Active nonhepatobiliary malignancy (except neuroendocrine tumors)	Cholangiocarcinoma
Anatomic abnormalities that preclude liver transplantation	Hepatocellular carcinoma beyond Milan criteria
Hemangiosarcoma	Human immunodeficiency virus (can consider HIV donor liver)
Hepatocellular carcinoma with metastatic spread	Superior mesenteric vein thrombosis (may require multi-visceral transplant)
Lack of adequate social support	
Nonadherence with medical care	
Uncontrolled bacteremia or fungemia not primarily from the hepatobiliary system	

Table 50–4. Components of the liver donor evaluation.

Selection of donor
ABO compatibility
Brain dead donor with satisfactory blood pressure and oxygenation
Liver size compatible with hepatic cavity of recipient
Factors affecting donor selection
Pre-existing liver disease
Diabetes mellitus
Uncontrolled hypertension
Active malignancy, excluding brain tumors
Active bacterial, viral, or fungal infection
Active alcohol or substance abuse
Morbid obesity

LISTING & DONOR LIVER OPTIONS

After patients have been listed for liver transplant, they are put on the waitlist for a deceased brain donor (DBD) liver. As mentioned earlier, the time to transplant is dependent upon the UNOS MELD which often corresponds with the natural MELD score unless the recipient qualifies for standard exception points or high priority listing. Factors that can further influence the waitlist time are blood type compatibility, liver size suitability, types of donor liver, and region of listing.

To reduce the waiting time, patients may have the option of choosing other types of deceased donor livers which might carry a higher risk of graft injury. These types of livers are termed as expanded criteria donors (ECD) which includes donation after cardiac death (DCD), donors older than 70 years, graft steatosis, and prolonged cold and warm ischemia times.

An alternative option for reducing the waiting time is living donor liver transplantation (LDLT) which may be useful for those who have a relatively low MELD score and are unlikely to achieve a higher MELD score naturally or through exception points. This option is best served for candidates who have relatively preserved hepatic function and have a potential living donor.

TRANSPLANTATION PROCEDURES

Surgical options for liver transplantation have undergone significant changes since the first human operation by Dr. Starzl in 1963. Currently, liver transplantation is performed orthotopically using cadaveric or living donors.

1. Donor Suitability & Procurement

Deceased Donors

After a patient has been matched for a deceased donor, the surgical team carefully evaluates the quality of the donor liver before considering procurement. This is particularly relevant for ECD livers. The surgeons will assess the cause of patient demise, hemodynamic instability, age, metabolic syndrome risk factors, substance abuse risk factors, and will also test for HIV, HBV, and HCV. If abnormal liver enzymes are found, a biopsy of the donor liver may be considered to ensure that advanced histopathologic changes are not present. Table 50–4 summarizes the important components of the evaluation of the donor liver.

Living Donors

LDLT was initiated in children in 1989 and the first adult case in the United States was in 1998. Typically, adult patients receive the right lobe (2/3 mass of liver) while pediatric patients receive the left lobe, though this is dependent upon the amount of liver volume required for a recipient. The major goal of LDLT is to reduce waitlist mortality. However, LDLT still comprises <5% of adult liver transplants in the United States. Living donor grafts usually come from people who have a connection with the recipient, though some come from altruistic donors or as part of a domino transplant. Living donors are evaluated by a separate liver transplant team from the recipient. Extreme care is taken to ensure that the donor understands the risk of donation, is not coerced into donation, and is healthy enough to undergo the surgery. Donors are assessed for blood type compatibility, suitable liver anatomy, liver diseases, and comorbidities. Donor safety is paramount. Donor morbidity is 15–25% and is related to vascular and biliary complications. The risk of donor death is 0.5%. LDLT is best for patients who are less sick (generally MELD 15–20), are well enough to tolerate a partial liver graft, and have an anticipated prolonged waitlist time.

2. Transplantation

Orthotopic liver transplantation is the most commonly used technique. The method of procurement depends on whether the liver is acquired after brain death, cardiac death, or living donation. The procuring and recipient surgical teams coordinate their procedure times to minimize both cold ischemia time (time from cooling of liver graft after donor procurement until re-warming prior to transplantation in recipient) and warm ischemia time (time from re-warming graft until anastomosis to the recipient). Recently, there has been increased interest in oxygenated machine perfusion to reduce ischemia related injury to the graft. After donor procurement, the recipient surgical team removes the native liver with careful dissection. The graft is then placed with anastomoses made to the recipient portal vein, hepatic artery, common bile duct, and hepatic vein or inferior vena cava. It is important to be cognizant of how and where each of those anastomoses are made as they can vary based on the anatomy of the donor and recipient.

COMPLICATIONS

Complications from liver transplantation can occur early or late and can be related to the graft, surgical procedure, or medical sequelae. Most complications occurring immediately after transplantation are technical and related to the surgery.

1. Primary Graft Nonfunction

Primary graft nonfunction occurs in about 5% of liver transplants and is caused by ischemia reperfusion injury. There is an increased risk for this diagnosis with advanced donor liver age, donor liver steatosis, prolonged cold ischemia time, donation after cardiac death, blood type incompatibility, and liver size incompatibility. The typical presentation is graft failure in the absence of vascular complications and there is often minimal bile output. This is a true emergency and the patient needs to be urgently listed for re-transplantation. Supportive care and aggressive medical therapy for infectious and hemodynamic complications are needed while awaiting re-transplantation.

2. Vascular Complications

Vascular complications develop in about 8% of liver transplants. Hepatic artery thrombosis or stenosis are the most common vascular complications and must be considered when there is graft failure, biliary strictures, or sepsis. Presentations can range from asymptomatic liver test elevations to graft failure. Risk factors include technical complications during the transplant, low donor size to recipient size ratio, immunologic factors, clotting abnormalities, smoking, and infection. Hepatic artery thrombosis or stenosis can be detected with imaging using ultrasound doppler, cross-sectional studies, or angiograms. It can be treated using interventional radiology techniques or surgical revisions. Patients may require listing for re-transplantation.

Less common vascular complications include portal vein or hepatic outflow stenoses which should be suspected when there is persistent or new onset ascites. These are typically managed with angioplasty or stenting by interventional radiology and sometimes require surgical revision.

3. Biliary Complications

Biliary complications after liver transplantation include bile leaks and biliary strictures and occur in up to 20% of recipients, typically in the first few months after transplantation.

Bile leaks occur most commonly in the early perioperative period at the site of the cystic duct or biliary anastomosis. Depending on the patient's anatomy and clinical factors, interventions for biliary strictures or leaks may involve endoscopic retrograde cholangiopancreatography (ERCP), percutaneous transhepatic cholangiography, surgical re-anastomosis, or conversion to Roux-en-Y loop.

A biliary stricture is suspected when the patient has cholestatic liver tests and is typically confirmed by imaging with ultrasound or magnetic resonance cholangiopancreatography. Anastomotic strictures may be related to surgical technique or ischemia. Most can be managed with ERCP and biliary stenting. Rare cases need surgical Roux-en-Y hepaticojejunostomy revision. Non-anastomotic strictures may also be related to ischemia due to hepatic artery thrombosis. Other risk factors include DCD donors, ABO incompatibility, Roux-en-Y reconstruction, prolonged cold ischemia time, primary sclerosing cholangitis, and post-transplant CMV infection. Re-transplantation may be warranted in select cases.

4. Rejection

A. Prevention of Allograft Rejection

For the graft to survive and function in the recipient, the recipient's immune system needs to be adequately suppressed, particularly in the early post-transplant period. A typical immunosuppression protocol is shown in Table 50–5. The protocol varies by transplant center but the principles remain the same and are individually tailored to the patient based on their clinical issues and immunosuppressive side effects. Table 50–6 lists the common side effects of the various immunosuppressant medications.

Corticosteroids are used for their potent anti-inflammatory effects in suppressing IL-1, IL-2, IL-6, tumor necrosis factor, and interferon-γ. Cyclosporine and tacrolimus are calcineurin inhibitors that suppress IL-2–dependent T-cell proliferation. Mycophenolate mofetil and azathioprine inhibit B-cell and T-cell proliferation by interfering with purine synthesis. Sirolimus interrupts IL-2 receptor signaling pathways and is generally not used as a first-line immunosuppressant because of initial concerns for hepatic artery thrombosis and impaired wound healing but later use may be beneficial in patients with malignancy.

B. Allograft Rejection

One of the most common complications after transplantation is allograft rejection. There are three forms of rejection: acute T-cell mediated rejection (TCMR), chronic ductopenic rejection (CDR), and antibody mediated rejection (AMR).

Table 50–5. Sample transplant immunosuppression protocol.

Month	Tacrolimus or Cyclosporine: Therapeutic Range[a]	Mycophenolate Mofetil	Prednisone
0–1	T: 10–15 mg/dL C: 250–300 ng/dL	M: 1 g twice daily	Taper by 10 mg orally daily until at 10 mg daily
1–3	T: 8–12 mg/dL C: 200–250 ng/dL	M: 1 g twice daily	Reduce to 5 mg daily
3–6	T: 7–10 mg/dL C: 150–200 ng/dL	M: 0.5 g twice daily	Off unless transplanted for autoimmune hepatitis or ongoing TCMR
6–12+	T: 4–6 mg/dL C: 50–100 ng/dL	Off	Off unless transplanted for autoimmune hepatitis or ongoing TCMR

C, cyclosporine; M, mycophenolate mofetil; T, tacrolimus; TCMR, T-cell mediated rejection.
[a]Dose titrated to trough levels

1. Acute T-cell mediated rejection—Acute rejection or TCMR is encountered in about 10–30% of recipients and usually within the first year. It is triggered by recipient T cell recognition of donor allo-antigens presented on recipient antigen presenting cells (APCs) or recognition of endogenous antigens presented on donor APCs. Acute rejection typically occurs in the setting of immunosuppression reduction, nonadherence, or interaction with other medications. Patients are often asymptomatic with abnormal liver tests and sub-therapeutic immunosuppression trough levels. While performing a workup for TCMR, it is important to also rule out biliary strictures, vascular complications, or infection. Depending on the severity of liver test elevations, patients may warrant a liver biopsy to confirm the diagnosis. Histopathologic changes of TCMR include mixed portal and lobular infiltrate, arteriolar and ductular injury, endotheliitis, and ductopenia. It is treated with pulse glucocorticoid therapy along with optimization of immunosuppressants, typically using a calcineurin inhibitor. Steroid refractory cases may require additional immunosuppressive therapies such as anti-thymocyte globulin. It is important to restart anti-infective prophylaxis when administering high dose glucocorticoids.

2. Chronic ductopenic rejection—CDR may occur in the setting of severe or recurrent rejection episodes, but often has an indolent course. The rate has decreased to <5% of recipients with improved immunosuppression from using calcineurin inhibitors, particularly tacrolimus. The pathogenesis of chronic rejection is not entirely understood. It usually manifests with cholestatic liver tests and is diagnosed by liver biopsy which is characterized by obliterative arteriopathy and bile duct injury and loss effecting >50% of the portal tracts. CDR is managed by optimizing immunosuppression with tacrolimus. Left untreated, it can lead to allograft cirrhosis over many months to years.

3. Antibody mediated rejection—AMR is rare and is caused by donor specific antibodies (DSAs). Preformed

Table 50–6. Common side effects of immunosuppressants.

Drug Class	Drug Name	Side Effect
Calcineurin inhibitors	Cyclosporine	Nephrotoxicity, hypertension, hypercholesterolemia, gingival hyperplasia, hirsutism
	Tacrolimus	Nephrotoxicity, diabetes mellitus type two, hypertension, neurotoxicity (including tremor, seizure, headaches), nausea, vomiting
Corticosteroids	Prednisone	Hyperglycemia, hypertension, peptic ulcer disease, osteoporosis, bruising, cataracts, myopathy, depression, psychosis
Antimetabolites	Mycophenolate mofetil Mycophenolic acid Azathioprine	Nausea, vomiting, diarrhea, bone marrow suppression
mTOR inhibitors	Sirolimus Everolimus	Hyperlipidemia, wound dehiscence, hepatic artery thrombosis, bone marrow suppression
Antibody	Antithymocyte globulin	Cytokine release syndrome

DSAs can cause hyperacute rejection leading to acute liver failure when there is graft blood type incompatibility which is an exceedingly rare occurrence. De-novo DSAs can occur in isolation or in conjunction with TCMR or CDR. It can be diagnosed by performing DSA testing or by performing C4d staining on liver biopsy. Treatment typically entails treating the underlying TCMR or CDR but sometimes DSA depleting therapies such as plasmapheresis, intravenous immunoglobulin, bortezomib, or rituximab are warranted.

5. Post-transplantation Lymphoproliferative Disorder

Post-transplantation lymphoproliferative disorder (PTLD) is a heterogeneous group of hematologic disorders of polyclonal or monoclonal lymphoid and nonlymphoid organs affecting nodal and particularly extranodal sites. It is a serious complication after transplantation and occurs in 2–4% of liver transplant recipients. Risk factors include age >50 years, severity of immunosuppression, and use of antilymphocyte antibodies. The majority of cases are associated with EBV, leading to B cell proliferation in the setting of depressed T cell function associated with immunosuppression. The clinical presentation of PTLD is broad, ranging from symptoms suggestive of mononucleosis to those consistent with lymphoma or related to an affected organ. Extranodal involvement of the liver, brain, gastrointestinal tract, and bone marrow is common. Seventy-seven percent of patients with PTLD presented with extranodal disease.

The treatment requires reducing immunosuppression, which may be effective in inducing a long complete response rate in 20–50%. Antiviral therapy in EBV-positive PTLD may also be considered. Anti CD-20 antibodies, radiation therapy, or surgery is used in patients who do not improve with reduction of immunosuppression or have more aggressive disease at initial presentation.

INFECTION AFTER LIVER TRANSPLANTATION

Infection risk among transplant recipients is related to the exposure to pathogens and the net state of immunosuppression. Additionally, disrupted integrity of the mucocutaneous and epithelial barriers, instrumentation, diabetes, and immunomodulating viruses contribute to overall infection risk. The typical pattern of infection is shown in Figure 50–2.

1. Bacterial & Fungal Infections

Patients are at risk of bacterial and fungal infection during and after liver transplantation. Careful attention must be made to minimize the risk of iatrogenic infections. Antibiotics are often administered perioperatively. Antifungal prophylaxis is often warranted during the first month of transplant especially for those at higher risk for fungal infection. Risk factors for fungal infection are typically prolonged

or complicated liver transplant, intra-operative blood transfusions, any repeat abdominal operation including washout or re-transplantation, use of antibiotics prior to transplantation, and transplantation for acute liver failure.

2. Pneumocystis carinii

Infection with *Pneumocystis carinii* pneumonia (PCP) is rare in the transplant setting because prophylaxis against PCP is practiced by all transplant centers. In the absence of prophylaxis, the incidence of PCP is 10–12%. The standard regimen is to use single-strength trimethoprim–sulfamethoxazole (TMP-SMZ) daily typically between 3 and 12 months (depending on the transplant center) and longer in patients with HIV. Atovaquone can be considered in patients with insensitivity to TMP-SMZ. An additional benefit of TMP-SMZ is the decreased risk of toxoplasmosis, *Listeria monocytogenes*, and *Nocardia asteroides*.

3. Cytomegalovirus

Cytomegalovirus (CMV) is the most important pathogen affecting patients after liver transplantation. The virus can be either acquired after transplantation from the donor or reactivated in the recipient by immunosuppression (Table 50–7). Most centers require antiviral prophylaxis with the duration dependent on the status of CMV infection in the donor and recipient as well as the amount of immunosuppression.

Clinical CMV infection can manifest itself in many ways. The presentation can be in the form of leukopenia, thrombocytopenia, pneumonitis, gastroenteritis, pancreatitis, colitis, dermatitis, neuritis, or ophthalmitis. It is commonly diagnosed by serum polymerase chain reaction amplification or by tissue biopsy. In addition to its direct effect, CMV is also associated with an increased risk of acute and chronic rejection, PTLD, and recurrent HCV. Treatment consists of antiviral therapy with the assistance of the infectious disease team until viral clearance is achieved.

LONG-TERM MEDICAL CARE AFTER LIVER TRANSPLANTATION

Patients who undergo liver transplantation remain at greater risk of developing common medical problems seen in the general population.

1. Diabetes Mellitus

The incidence of post-transplant diabetes mellitus is between 4% and 20%. This risk is often related to underlying metabolic syndrome and the use of tacrolimus, cyclosporine, or prednisone. Prospective studies have shown a significant increased incidence of hyperglycemia after administration of these agents. The treatment includes diet, weight loss, oral hypoglycemic agents, and insulin.

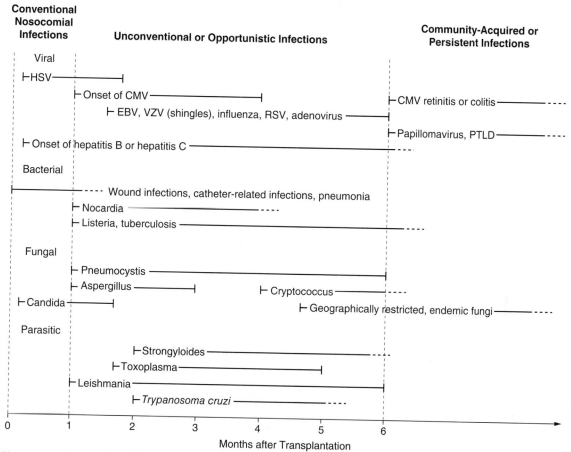

▲ Figure 50–2. Usual sequence of infections after organ transplantation. Exceptions to the usual sequence of infections after transplantation suggest the presence of unusual epidemiologic exposure or excessive immunosuppression. CMV, cytomegalovirus; EBV, Epstein-Barr virus; HSV, herpes simplex virus; PTLD, post-transplantation lymphoproliferative disease; RSV, respiratory syncytial virus; VZV, varicella-zoster virus. Zero indicates the time of transplantation. Solid lines indicate the most common period for the onset of infection; dotted lines and arrows indicate periods of continued risk at reduced levels. (Adapted with permission from Rubin RH, Wolfson JS, Cosimi AB, et al: Infection in the renal transplant recipient, *Am J Med.* 1981;70(2):405–411.)

Table 50–7. Antiviral prophylaxis for cytomegalovirus (CMV).

CMV Status	Risk	Prophylaxis
Donor negative/recipient negative	Low	Valacyclovir (typically 1 month)
Donor negative/recipient positive	Moderate	Valgancyclovir (typically 3 months)
Donor positive/recipient positive	Moderate	Valgancyclovir (typically 3 months)
Donor positive/recipient negative	High	Valgancyclovir (typically 6 months)

2. Hypertension

Hypertension is a common occurrence after transplantation and is likely a result of age and the use of calcineurin inhibitors. Standard antihypertensive regimens are efficacious in patients post-transplantation. Nifedipine is the agent of choice, and β-blockers are second-line agents.

3. Hyperlipidemia

Hyperlipidemia is a common occurrence after liver transplantation and is usually related to calcineurin inhibitors or mammalian target of rapamycin (mTOR) inhibitors. Weight loss and dietary changes are recommended; if these strategies are unsuccessful, treatment with an HMG CoA inhibitor is recommended. For patients with hypertriglyceridemia, fish oil and fibric acid derivatives should be considered.

4. Renal Insufficiency

The incidence of chronic renal failure after solid organ transplantation is about 7–21% among nonrenal transplant recipients. It is often associated with older age, diabetes mellitus, hypertension, and use of calcineurin inhibitors. Strategies to prevent renal failure are limited by the need to use a calcineurin inhibitor to prevent rejection. In patients with mild renal insufficiency, treatment options may entail lowering the calcineurin inhibitor trough goal or transitioning to an alternative immunosuppressant. Some patients develop renal failure within the first year of liver transplantation. Recently a safety net was made to prioritize kidney transplantation in liver transplant recipients who are registered on the kidney transplant waitlist 60–365 days after liver transplantation and either require chronic hemodialysis or have a GFR <20 mL/min.

5. Osteoporosis

Pretransplant bone disease resulting from impaired vitamin D absorption in cholestatic liver disease, low calcium intake and activity, use of diuretics for ascites, and prednisone for autoimmune hepatitis is common. Inactivity after the transplant procedure and the use of high doses of steroids further accelerate bone loss. Consequently, post-transplant osteoporosis is a major cause of morbidity in patients undergoing transplantation. All patients should receive calcium and vitamin D supplementation after transplantation. Bone densitometry testing is recommended and bisphosphonates prescribed if osteoporosis is noted.

6. Pregnancy

As liver transplant outcomes have improved and patients have achieved normalization of sex hormones, pregnancy among liver transplant recipients has been increasing over the past few decades with 40% of these pregnancies unplanned. Since intensive immunosuppressive and prophylactic medications can adversely affect male and female reproductive organs as well as fetus health, it is recommended that family planning be discussed to avoid conception until liver transplant recipients are at least 1-year post-transplant and are without rejection or other transplant-related complications. When liver transplant recipients are ready to conceive, immunosuppression is continued to minimize the risk of rejection and graft failure; however teratogenic medications such as mycophenolate mofetil are discontinued or substituted beforehand. Because transplantation is associated with an increased incidence of premature and low-birth-weight infants, pregnant liver transplant recipients should be managed by an obstetrician who specializes in high-risk pregnancy.

7. Neurologic Conditions

Chronic headaches, tremors, or seizures can be observed with calcineurin inhibitors and may require dose modification or an alternative immunosuppressant.

8. Psychiatric Conditions

Depression and anxiety are common after transplantation and should be treated. Among patients who had substance or alcohol abuse prior to transplant, continued participation in relapse prevention programs is critical in the post-transplant setting to prevent recurrent liver disease.

9. Malignancy

Liver transplant recipients are at an increased risk of cancer which is driven by age, immunosuppression, prior cancer history, prior liver disease, and family history. The incidence of malignancy is between 11% and 20% up to 10 years after liver transplantation.

It is important that all patients adhere to cancer screening based on age and family history risk while also having proper follow up for any previous history of cancer or precancerous lesions. Some liver diseases warrant continued surveillance after transplantation. Patients transplanted for primary sclerosing cholangitis and have inflammatory bowel disease remain at increased risk of colon cancer. Additionally, those who had HCC may require continued surveillance with cross-sectional imaging and alpha fetoprotein (AFP), with the frequency of testing dependent on the extent of disease on explant. It is helpful to take note of whether the tumor was AFP producing. Furthermore, immunosuppression can predispose to skin and oropharyngeal cancer. Careful attention should be made to monitor for the development of post-transplant lymphocytic disease (PTLD).

Table 50–8 outlines cancer screening in patients after liver transplantation.

PROGNOSIS & DISEASE RECURRENCE

Over the past decade, the prognosis for patients who undergo liver transplantation has improved considerably. Most patients do not have liver-related morbidity but rather have complications from long-standing immunosuppression. It is important to note that while some liver diseases such as metabolic disorders and amyloidosis are cured by transplantation, others can recur (Table 50–9). Furthermore, some liver diseases may progress to allograft cirrhosis and about 15% of patients may require re-transplantation during their lifetime.

1. Recurrent Hepatitis C

Recurrent HCV is almost universal after transplantation. Older donor age, female gender, HIV co-infection, and use of steroids and high-intensity regimens to treat acute rejection are predictors of severe recurrence. However, with the

Table 50–8. Cancer screening after liver transplantation.

Cancer	Recommended Screening
Skin and oropharyngeal cancer	Self-examinations, and routine physician and dental examinations
Colon cancer	Age, personal risk, and family risk determined colonoscopy (annual if primary sclerosing cholangitis)
Lung cancer	CT Chest based on smoking risk
Breast cancer	Age and family risk determined mammography
Cervical cancer	Age-appropriate pap smear
Prostate cancer	Age and family risk determined testing
Hepatocellular carcinoma	CT and AFP frequency determined based on recurrence risk
Post-transplant lympho-cytic disease	Physician monitoring

recent advent of direct acting antiviral therapies that have high efficacy in viral eradication, HCV has not only become a less common indication for transplantation but also is no longer a contraindication for graft use. With the recent rise in drug overdoses, the number of donor grafts that are hepatitis C infected have increased. These can now be given to both HCV infected and uninfected recipients with direct acting antiviral therapy typically started within several months after transplantation.

2. Recurrent Hepatitis B

The incidence of HBV recurrence has been very low since the development of antiviral nucleoside and nucleotide therapies

that can suppress HBV replication pretransplant and with the use of HBIG peri-transplant. Patients are maintained on life-long antiviral therapy with tenofovir or entecavir after transplant. The duration of HBIG therapy varies by transplant center and typically entails maintaining a hepatitis B surface antibody level greater than 500 IU/mL. Patients with HBV recurrence must resume HCC screening.

3. Recurrent Nonalcoholic Fatty Liver Disease

The incidence of recurrent non-alcoholic steatohepatitis is up to 40% after transplantation. Patients frequently gain weight gain and develop diabetes mellitus type two, hyperlipidemia, and hypertension—usually as a consequence of immunosuppression and increased enteral intake. Patients should be counseled on appropriate weight goals and lifestyle modifications with diet and exercise. Close collaboration with an internist is warranted to optimize risk factors for metabolic syndrome.

4. Recurrent Alcohol-related Liver Disease

Risk factors for alcohol relapse after liver transplant include poor social support, family history of alcohol abuse, and alcohol abstinence for <6 months before transplant. In a meta-analysis, relapse rates were 2.5 cases/100 patient/year with heavy alcohol use and 5.6 cases/100 patient/year with any alcohol use. However, recidivism has not been shown to decrease patient or graft survival. It is important for these patients to maintain lifelong alcohol sobriety and to participate in alcohol cessation programs and therapy. Five-year patient and graft survivals are similar for alcohol and nonalcohol etiologies. Survival >5 years is worse in alcohol related liver disease due to increased risk for cardiopulmonary disease, cerebrovascular events, and de novo malignancy especially oropharyngeal and lung cancer.

Table 50–9. Recurrence & 5-year survival rates after liver transplantation.

Etiology of Disease	Recurrence Rate	5-Year Survival	5-Year Graft Survival
Hepatitis C	>90%	70%	57%
Hepatitis B	<5% with prophylaxis	79%	68%
Hepatocellular carcinoma	8–15%	52%	46%
Primary biliary cholangitis	11–23%	86%	73%
Primary sclerosing cholangitis	9–47%	86%	73%
Autoimmune hepatitis	16–46%	77%	68%
Alcohol-induced cirrhosis	<5%	72%	65%
Nonalcoholic steatohepatitis	11–38%	73%	66%

Reproduced with permission from Kotlyar DS, Campbell MS, Reddy KR. Recurrences of diseases following orthotopic liver transplantation, *Am J Gastroenterol* 2006;101(6):1370–1378.

5. Recurrent Autoimmune Hepatitis

Autoimmune hepatitis recurs in 8–12% of patients within the first year after liver transplantation and 36–68% after 5 years. Risk factors include HLA DR3 or DR4, high-grade inflammation in the native liver, and suboptimal immunosuppression. Liver biopsy in conjunction with biochemical markers are needed for diagnosis of recurrence which should be distinguished from acute rejection or de novo autoimmune hepatitis which refers to new autoimmune hepatitis in a patient transplanted for reasons other than autoimmune hepatitis. To minimize the risk of recurrent autoimmune hepatitis, patients are usually maintained on low dose oral glucocorticoid therapy indefinitely. Although the rate of acute and chronic rejection is often higher in these patients compared to other liver diseases, there is no significant impact on overall survival.

6. Recurrent Primary Biliary Cholangitis

Primary biliary cholangitis (PBC) has been reported to recur in 11–42% of patients but has not been associated with decreased graft or patient survival. As serologies are not helpful in establishing the diagnosis, a liver biopsy is required and the findings must be distinguished from CDR. Prophylactic ursodiol to prevent PBC recurrence is a reasonable and safe strategy.

7. Recurrent Primary Sclerosing Cholangitis

The incidence of recurrent primary sclerosing cholangitis is 10–37% within 5 years after liver transplantation and may require re-transplantation. It is important to distinguish recurrent primary sclerosing cholangitis from anastomotic strictures, ischemia related nonanastomotic strictures, and CDR. Risk factors include HLA-DRB1*08, male gender, inflammatory bowel disease with intact colon, recurrent or steroid-resistant rejection, need for chronic steroids, and cholangiocarcinoma. The diagnosis should be suspected in patients who had definitive primary sclerosing cholangitis pretransplant and have biliary structuring and beading occurring more than 90 days after transplant or have consistent findings on biopsy of the transplanted liver.

Abu-Gazala S, Olthoff KM. Current status of living donor liver transplantation in the United States. *Annu Rev Med.* 2019;70:225–238. [PMID: 30355261]

Bodzin AS, Baker TB. Liver transplantation today: where we are now and where we are going. *Liver Transpl.* 2018;24(10):1470–1475. [PMID: 30080954]

Chascsa DM, Vargas HE. The gastroenterologist's guide to management of the post-liver transplant patient. *Am J Gastroenterol.* 2018;113(6):819–828. [PMID: 29748558]

Heimbach JK. United States liver allocation. *Curr Opin Organ Transplant.* 2020;25(2):104–109. [PMID: 32142481]

Lucey MR, Terrault N, Ojo L, et al. Long-term management of the successful adult liver transplant: 2012 practice guideline by the American Association for the Study of Liver Diseases and the American Society of Transplantation. *Liver Transpl.* 2013; 19:3–26. [PMID 23281277]

Ma M, Falloon K, Chen PH, et al. The role of liver transplantation in alcoholic hepatitis. *J Intensive Care Med.* 2019;34(4):277–291. [PMID: 29879862]

Martin P, DiMartini A, Feng S, Brown R, Fallon M. Evaluation for liver transplantation in adults: 2013 practice guideline by the American Association for the Study of Liver Diseases and the American Society of Transplantation. *Hepatology.* 2014;59:1144–1165. [PMID: 24716201]

OPTN: Organ Procurement and Transplantation Network Policy; Policy 9: Allocation of Livers and Liver-Intestines. April 1, 2021. [PDF file] Retrieved from https://optn.transplant.hrsa.gov/media/1200/optn_policies.pdf

Sarkar M, Brady CW, Fleckenstein J, et al. Reproductive health and liver disease: Practice Guidance by the American Association for the Study of Liver Diseases. *Hepatology.* 2021;73(1):318–365. [PMID: 32946672]

Singal AK, Ong S, Satapathy SK, Kamath PS, Wiesner RH. Simultaneous liver kidney transplantation. *Transpl Int.* 2019;32(4):343–352. [PMID: 30548094]

Primary Sclerosing Cholangitis & Congenital Disorders of the Biliary System

Marvin Ryou, MD
Stephen D. Zucker, MD

ESSENTIALS OF DIAGNOSIS

▶ Primary sclerosing cholangitis (PSC) is an inflammatory, fibrosing, and obliterative disease of the intra- and/or extrahepatic bile ducts.

▶ A typical biochemical feature is an elevated serum alkaline phosphatase level.

▶ The diagnostic hallmark is multifocal stricturing of the intra- and/or extrahepatic bile ducts on magnetic resonance cholangiography (MRC) or endoscopic retrograde cholangiography (ERC)

▶ Characteristic histologic findings include fibrous obliteration of small bile ducts with concentric replacement by connective tissue in an "onion skin" pattern.

▶ Patients with PSC and congenital cystic disease of the biliary system have an increased risk of developing cholangiocarcinoma.

General Considerations: Primary Sclerosing Cholangitis

PSC is a progressive inflammatory, sclerosing, and obliterative process involving the medium-sized and large intra- and/or extrahepatic bile ducts. The mean age at presentation is 40 years, with a 2:1 male predominance. Approximately 70–80% of patients with PSC have underlying inflammatory bowel disease, primarily ulcerative colitis (75–80%). Conversely, 5–10% of patients with inflammatory bowel disease will develop PSC. The course of PSC is highly variable and independent of the underlying inflammatory bowel disease. Median transplant-free survival for patients with PSC is 13–21 years. There presently is no approved medical therapy that has been shown to alter the natural history of the disease. Approximately 15% of patients with PSC will go on to liver transplantation, the principal indications being decompensated cirrhosis, recurrent cholangitis, and/or cholangiocarcinoma. Patients with PSC also are at increased risk of adenocarcinoma of the gallbladder and colon.

Boonstra KB, Weersma RK, van Erecum KJ et al. Population-based epidemiology, malignancy risk, and outcome of primary sclerosing cholangitis. *Hepatology.* 2013;144:1357–1374. [PMID: 23775876]

Chapman RW. Update on primary sclerosing cholangitis. *Clin Liver Dis.* 2017;9:107–110. [PMID 30992971]

Lazaridis KN, LaRusso NF. Primary sclerosing cholangitis. *N Engl J Med.* 2016;375:1161–1170. [PMID 27653566]

Pathogenesis

Data suggest that PSC is a complex polygenic immune-mediated disorder. Genome-wide association studies have identified at least 19 separate disease loci (primarily immune-related) and demonstrate that PSC manifests a distinct genetic profile from either ulcerative colitis or Crohn's disease. Patients with PSC also exhibit unique alterations in the enteric microbiome, which is postulated to trigger immune-mediated injury to the biliary epithelium. A proposed mechanism is that altered intestinal permeability leads to an increase in migration of bacteria and/or toxins into the portal circulation. Additional potential contributing factors to bile duct injury in PSC are an enrichment of bile in hydrophobic (toxic) bile acids, aberrant T-cell homing to the biliary epithelium, and recurrent infections in the biliary tract. That PSC recurs in up to 20% of patients following liver transplantation supports that factors external to the liver drive disease development.

Dean G, Hanauer S, Levitsky J. The role of intestine in the patho-genesis of primary sclerosing cholangitis: evidence and thera-peutic implications. *Hepatology*. 2020;72:1127–1138. [PMID: 32394535]

Ji SG, Juran BD, Mucha S, et al. Genome-wide association study of primary sclerosing cholangitis identifies new risk loci and quan-tifies the genetic relationship with inflammatory bowel disease. *Nat Genet*. 2017;49:269–273. [PMID: 27992413]

► Clinical Findings

A. Symptoms & Signs

Patients with PSC are often asymptomatic at the time of diag-nosis and are typically identified by a persistent cholestatic pattern of liver enzymes in the setting of underlying inflam-matory bowel disease. Symptomatic patients generally pres-ent with signs and symptoms of biliary obstruction, including right upper quadrant abdominal pain, pruritus, jaundice, or cholangitis (when concurrent fever is present).

B. Laboratory Findings

Patients with PSC typically manifest a cholestatic pattern of liver enzymes, with a disproportionate elevation in serum alkaline phosphatase. Aminotransferases (ALT and AST) also can be elevated. A small proportion of patients with PSC may exhibit normal alkaline phosphatase levels, highlight-ing the need for a high index of suspicion. A persistently low alkaline phosphatase (less than 1.5 times the upper limit of normal) has been associated with better clinical outcome. There currently are no known serological assays that are diagnostic for PSC.

C. Imaging Studies

MRC is considered the modality of choice for establishing the diagnosis of PSC, with a sensitivity of 0.86 and speci-ficity of 0.94. Characteristic findings include multifocal biliary duct stricturing (ie, beading) and peripheral prun-ing of the intrahepatic ducts (Figure 51–1). Most patients (~85%) have both intrahepatic and extrahepatic bile duct strictures, while 10–15% have isolated intrahepatic duct involvement, and 2–4% manifest only extrahepatic bili-ary disease. Due to the risk of pancreatitis or cholangitis, ERC is reserved for indeterminate cases or for situations where therapeutic intervention is required (eg, dilatation of a dominant stricture, stone extraction, assessment for pos-sible cholangiocarcinoma).

Approximately 10% of patients have isolated involvement of peripheral biliary ductules and will demonstrate no chol-angiographic abnormalities, a condition termed "small-duct PSC." In these patients, the diagnosis is established by liver biopsy in conjunction with other clinical features (eg, persis-tent elevation in serum alkaline phosphatase in a patient with underlying inflammatory bowel disease).

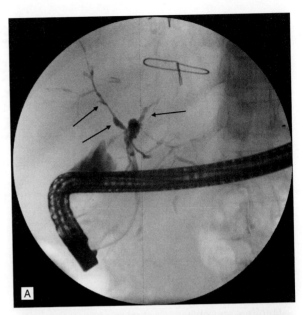

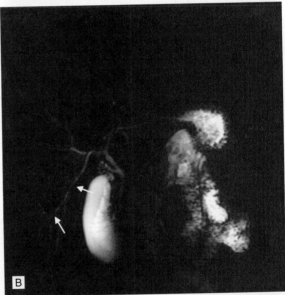

▲ **Figure 51–1.** Imaging findings. **A.** ERCP demonstrating stricturing and beading of the intrahepatic ducts (*arrows* denote stricturing). **B.** MRCP showing stricturing (*arrows*) of the biliary tree. (Reproduced with permission of Dr. John R. Saltzman, Brigham and Women's Hospital.)

D. Histologic Findings

The most characteristic histologic abnormality in PSC is fibrous obliteration of small bile ducts, with concentric periductal "onion skin" fibrosis (Plate 99). However, this distinctive finding is uncommon, with nonspecific portal mononuclear cell infiltration and associated bile duct injury being the most often encountered histologic pattern. For this reason, liver biopsy generally is unnecessary in diagnosing PSC unless small-duct PSC or an overlap with autoimmune hepatitis is suspected (see below). Histologic staging (1–4) is according to the Metavir classification system.

Gochanour E, Jayasekera C, Kowdley K. Primary sclerosing cholangitis: epidemiology, genetics, diagnosis, and current management. *Clin Liver Dis.* 2020;15:125–128. [PMID: 32257124]

▶ Differential Diagnosis

There are several disorders that can present with similar biochemical and imaging findings to PSC, including secondary sclerosing cholangitis, immunoglobulin G4 (IgG4)–associated cholangitis, overlap syndrome with autoimmune hepatitis, primary biliary cholangitis, ischemic cholangiopathy, papillary tumors of the biliary system, cholangiocarcinoma, cholangiolithiasis, and HIV cholangiopathy.

A. Small Duct Primary Sclerosing Cholangitis

Small duct PSC has all the clinical, biochemical, and histopathological features of PSC, but with normal findings on cholangiography. Small duct PSC is found in 5–15% of patients with PSC (more commonly in children), and is associated with a significantly better long-term prognosis, with longer transplant-free survival and a lower incidence of cholangiocarcinoma. However, this may (at least in part) reflect lead-time bias, as up to 20% of patients with small duct PSC progress to large duct involvement within 8 years of diagnosis. Hence, regular monitoring of these patients is required.

Angulo P, Maor-Kendler Y, Lindor KD. Small duct primary sclerosing cholangitis: a long-term follow-up. *Hepatology.* 2002;35:1494–1500. [PMID: 12029635]

Björnsson E, Olsson R, Bergquist A, et al. The natural history of small-duct primary sclerosing cholangitis. *Gastroenterology.* 2008;134:975–980. [PMID: 18395078]

B. IgG$_4$-Associated Cholangitis

IgG4-associated cholangitis (IAC) is the biliary manifestation of IgG4-related disease, a systemic fibroinflammatory condition. It is the most common extrapancreatic manifestation of autoimmune pancreatitis type 1, although IAC can be isolated to the biliary system in 8% of cases. IAC has a male predominance and patients typically present in the fifth and sixth decades with obstructive jaundice (70–80% of cases), weight loss, and abdominal pain. Classic imaging features include long multifocal biliary strictures with mild upstream dilatation, and proximal biliary disease with diffuse pancreatic swelling and a thin, narrowed pancreatic duct. Serum IgG4 concentrations are increased (>1.4 g/L) in 65–80% of patients at the time of diagnosis, although this degree of

elevation can be seen up to 25% of those with other inflammatory, autoimmune, and malignant conditions. Serum IgG4 levels greater than 5.6 g/L are considered highly specific but are less sensitive for IAC. Histologic features include a lymphoplasmacytic infiltrate, obliterative phlebitis, and storiform fibrosis, with more than 10 IgG4-positive cells per high powered field. However, an abundance of IgG4-positive cells can be seen in PSC or cholangiocarcinoma so, in the absence of other histologic features, this finding in and of itself is insufficient to establish the diagnosis of IAC. In its early inflammatory phase, IAC is highly responsive to corticosteroids; therefore, it is important to establish the diagnosis expeditiously as delays in treatment can lead to irreversible fibrosis with organ failure (see Chapter 30 for a detailed discussion of autoimmune pancreatitis).

Culver EL, Barnes E. IgG4-related sclerosing cholangitis. *Clin Liver Dis.* 2017;10:9–16. [PMID: 30992751]

Madhusudhan KS, Das P, Gunjan D, et al. IgG4-related sclerosing cholangitis: a clinical and imaging review. *Am J Radiol.* 2019;213:1221–1231. [PMID: 31509439]

C. Primary Sclerosing Cholangitis-Autoimmune Hepatitis (PSC-AIH) Overlap Syndrome

Patients with PSC-AIH overlap syndrome have overt cholangiographic abnormalities characteristic of PSC, but with serologic (elevated ANA, ASMA, and/or IgG, with negative AMA) and histologic (interface hepatitis) findings consistent with autoimmune hepatitis. It is a rare syndrome that has mainly been described in children, adolescents, and young adults. Manifestations are uncommonly sequential, with patients first presenting with features of AIH before subsequently developing biliary abnormalities later in the disease course. PSC-AIH overlap should be considered in patients with autoimmune hepatitis who respond poorly to immunosuppressive therapy, particularly in the setting of an elevated alkaline phosphatase and/or underlying inflammatory bowel disease, although IgG4-associated sclerosing cholangitis also is a diagnostic consideration (see above).

Bunchorntavakul C, Reddy KR. Diagnosis and management of overlap syndromes. *Clin Liver Dis.* 2015;19:81–97. [PMID: 25454298]

Floreani A, Rizzoto ER, Ferrera F, et al. Clinical course and outcome of autoimmune hepatitis/primary sclerosing cholangitis overlap syndrome. *Am J Gastroenterol.* 2005;100:1515–1522. [PMID: 15984974]

Trivedi PJ, Hirschfield GM. Review article: overlap syndromes and autoimmune liver disease. *Aliment Pharmacol Ther.* 2012;36:517–533. [PMID: 22817525]

D. Acquired Immunodeficiency Syndrome

Biliary tract lesions in patients with AIDS can involve cholangiographic changes similar to PSC, such as: (1) diffuse involvement of the intrahepatic bile ducts alone,

555575555

555555555

(2) involvement of both intrahepatic and extrahepatic bile ducts, (3) ampullary stenosis, and/or (4) stricture of the intrapancreatic portion of the common bile duct. Infectious organisms that have been associated with these biliary abnormalities include *Cryptosporidium parvum*, cytomegalovirus, microsporidia (primarily *Enterocytozoon bieneusi*), *Isospora*, and *Histoplasma capsulatum*.

year, with a cumulative incidence of 6–11% at 10 years and 20% at 30 years. The presence of concomitant ulcerative colitis, underlying cirrhosis, and male sex are associated with an increased likelihood of cholangiocarcinoma. Patients with PSC have a lifetime risk of gallbladder cancer of approximately 2%. Despite little supportive data, professional societies and expert opinion recommend screening for cholangiocarcinoma and gallbladder cancer with MRC or ultrasonography (with or without serum CA 19-9) every 6–12 months.

Due to a high risk of inducing cholangitis and/or pancreatitis, ERC is reserved for therapeutic biliary intervention. Indications for endoscopic evaluation (eg, EUS, ERC) include increasing cholestatic biochemistries, new onset jaundice, fever, right upper-quadrant pain, pruritus, or concerning imaging findings. Routine administration of prophylactic antibiotics prior to performing ERC is recommended in patients with PSC in order to prevent bacteremia and/or cholangitis. Brush cytology should be performed when biliary strictures are encountered, with fluorescence *in situ* hybridization (FISH) or targeted biopsy (via cholangioscopy or transhepatic image-guided) employed in situations with a high suspicion for cholangiocarcinoma. Similar to patients without PSC, the presence of cirrhosis warrants HCC screening every 6 months.

B. Colorectal Cancer

The risk of colorectal cancer is significantly increased in patients with PSC and ulcerative colitis or Crohn's colitis. In such patients, surveillance colonoscopy with biopsies should be carried out at 1–2 year intervals. In all patients with a new diagnosis of PSC and no previous history or symptoms of inflammatory bowel disease, a full colonoscopy with biopsies generally is recommended.

C. Pruritus

As with other cholestatic conditions, a common symptom encountered in patients with PSC is pruritus. Unfortunately, the treatment of pruritus is hampered by an incomplete understanding of its causes. Bile acids, endogenous opioids, and lysphosphatidic acid (LPA) have all been implicated in the pathogenesis of the pruritus of cholestasis, and pharmacologic therapy has been targeted to modulate these potential mediators. Bile acid sequestrants (eg, colestipol, cholestyramine) at a dose of 4 g to a maximum of 16 g daily in two divided doses can be helpful in reducing pruritus in a substantial proportion of patients, with pills tending to be better tolerated than powder form. In patients that fail bile acid sequestrants, oral rifampin (150–300 mg twice daily) can be helpful, presumably by decreasing LPA through suppression of the LPA-generating enzyme, autotaxin. The opioid antagonist naltrexone (12.5–50 mg daily) can improve pruritus of cholestasis, but should be avoided in patients receiving opioid therapy. Sertraline (75–100 mg daily) improves

pruritus in some patients as well. Despite a lack of efficacy data, antihistamines (eg, hydroxyzine, diphenhydramine) are frequently administered to patients with pruritus; however, their benefit is primarily through sedation rather than exerting a direct impact on itching.

D. Gallstone Disease/Cholangitis

Patients with PSC are at increased risk of developing cholelithiasis, with gallstones reported in approximately 25% of patients. However, bile stasis as a consequence of biliary stricturing can lead to spontaneous bacterial cholangitis in the absence of cholelithiasis or choledocholithiasis. In patients who experience recurrent bouts of cholangitis, early initiation of or chronic administration of prophylactic antibiotics can prevent severe infections and bacteremia.

E. Fat-soluble Vitamin Malabsorption

Advanced PSC can result in decreased secretion of conjugated bile salts into the small intestine, leading to impaired absorption of fat-soluble vitamins (A, D, E, K) and, rarely, steatorrhea. Hence, patients with PSC have an increased risk of *hepatic osteodystrophy*, with osteopenia and/or osteoporosis most commonly involving the lumbar spine, iliac crest, and femur. The incidence of osteoporosis in PSC ranges from 4% to 10%. It is recommended that patients should receive repletion of vitamin D and undergo bone densitometry at diagnosis, and at 2–3 year intervals thereafter.

Aabakken L, Karlsen TH, Albert J, et al. Role of endoscopy in primary sclerosing cholangitis: European Society of Gastrointestinal Endoscopy (ESGE) and European Association for the Study of the Liver (EAL) clinical guideline. *Endoscopy*. 2017;49:588–608. [PMID: 28420030]

Bowlus CL, Lim JK, Lindor KD. AGA clinical practice update on surveillance for hepatobiliary cancers in patients with primary sclerosing cholangitis: expert review. *Clin Gastroenterol Hepatol*. 2019;17:2416–2422. [PMID: 31306801]

Goode EC, Clark AB, Mells GF, et al. Factors associated with outcomes of patients with primary sclerosing cholangitis and development and validation of a risk scoring system. *Hepatology*. 2019;69:2120–2135. [PMID: 30566748]

Sanjel B, Shim WS. Recent advances in understanding the molecular mechanisms of cholestatic pruritus: a review. *Biochim Biophys Acta Mol Basis Dis*. 2020;1866:165958. [PMID: 32896605]

Weismüller TJ, Trivedi PJ, Bergquist A, et al. Patient age, sex, and inflammatory bowel disease phenotype associate with course of primary sclerosing cholangitis. *Gastroenterology*. 2017;152:1975–1984. [PMID: 28274849]

General Considerations: Congenital Cystic Diseases of the Biliary System

Bile duct cysts are rare congenital abnormalities of the biliary tree characterized by cystic dilatation of the extrahepatic and/or intrahepatic bile ducts. Congenital cystic diseases of the biliary system comprise approximately 1% of all benign

Table 51-1. Todani classification of choledochal cysts.

Type	Subtype	Description	Incidence	Anatomy
I		Cystic dilatation of the common bile duct	50–85%	
	IA	Diffuse dilatation		
	IB	Focal dilatation		
	IC	Fusiform dilatation		
II		Diverticulum of the extrahepatic biliary tree	<2%	
III		Cystic dilatation of the intraduodenal common bile duct (choledochocele)	4–5%	
IV		Multiple cysts of the intrahepatic and extrahepatic biliary tree	10–15%	
	IVA	Both intra- and extrahepatic		
	IVB	Extrahepatic only		
V		Isolated intrahepatic biliary cystic disease (Caroli's disease)	Rare	

bile duct disorders. While typically diagnosed in infancy or childhood, approximately 20% of patients will present in adulthood. It is more commonly encountered in women, with a female to male ratio of approximately 3:1. The most serious complication of congenital biliary cysts is cholangiocarcinoma, with an estimated incidence of approximately 10% in adult patients. Additional complications include hepatolithiasis, cholangitis, pancreatitis, and hepatic fibrosis.

Pathogenesis

While the etiology of biliary cysts is speculative, the leading hypothesis is that extrahepatic cysts result from an anomalous bilio-pancreatic junction (common channel longer than 10–15 mm, pancreatico-biliary junction proximal to the sphincter of Oddi) which allows for reflux of pancreatic secretions into the biliary tree. This persistent reflux of pancreatic juice is thought to lead to chronic inflammation and secondary biliary ductal dilatation. In contrast, intrahepatic biliary cysts are believed to be caused by embryological malformations of the ductal plate which, when involving small interlobular bile ducts, results in congenital hepatic fibrosis, while involvement of large ducts leads to Caroli's disease (which has been associated with mutations in the PKHD1 gene).

Classification

Cystic disorders of the biliary system are classified by the site (extrahepatic and/or intrahepatic), extent (segmental or complete), and shape (cystic or saccular, fusiform) of the cysts (Table 51–1).

Clinical Findings

A. Symptoms & Signs

In adults, the most common symptoms of biliary cysts are right upper quadrant pain and recurrent cholangitis, except for choledochoceles (type III) which are usually asymptomatic. The diagnosis is typically established by abdominal imaging, most commonly MRCP.

B. Symptoms & Signs

Due to the high risk of cholangiocarcinoma within the cyst wall, total excision with Roux-en-Y hepaticojejunostomy typically is recommended for the treatment of types I and IV biliary cysts. Due to a low risk of malignancy, symptomatic choledochoceles (type III) are managed by endoscopic sphincterotomy or transduodenal sphincteroplasty with cyst excision. Treatment of Caroli's disease is confounded by the intrahepatic (and frequently diffuse) nature of the cysts, and the relatively low lifetime risk of cholangiocarcinoma (~7% incidence). For focal disease that is symptomatic, hepatic lobectomy can provide long-term benefit. On the other hand, liver transplantation is required if hepatic involvement is diffuse.

Jabłońska, B. Biliary cysts: etiology, diagnosis and management. *World J Gastroenterol.* 2012;18:4801–4810. [PMID: 23002354]

Mabrut JY, Bozio G, Hubert C, et al. Management of congenital bile duct cysts. *Dig Surg.* 2010;27:12–18. [PMID: 20357466]

Ten Hove, A, de Meijer, VE, Huluscher JBF, de Kleine RHJ. Meta-analysis of risk of developing malignancy in congenital choledochal malformation. *Br J Surg.* 2018;105:482–490. [PMID: 29480528]

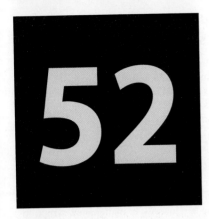

Gallstone Disease

Stephen D. Zucker, MD

ESSENTIALS OF DIAGNOSIS

▶ Major risk factors for cholesterol gallstones include age >50, female sex, Native American or Mexican ethnicity, genetic predisposition, family history, pregnancy and parity, estrogens, obesity, and the metabolic syndrome.

▶ Gallstones are often found incidentally during abdominal ultrasonography, which has >95% sensitivity for cholesterol stones ≥1.5 mm.

▶ In ~80% of cases gallstones remain asymptomatic; in symptomatic patients, biliary colic is almost always present, often radiating to the right scapula or shoulder.

▶ Laparoscopic cholecystectomy is indicated in patients with symptomatic gallstones.

▶ Major complications of gallstone disease requiring treatment are acute cholecystitis, choledocholithiasis, obstructive jaundice, cholangitis, and pancreatitis.

▶ Acute cholangitis caused by an obstructing gallstone should be treated by endoscopic removal of the stone under antibiotic coverage as soon as possible.

General Considerations

Gallstone disease represents a considerable health burden in Western industrialized countries, with a prevalence of 10–15% and a 5-year incidence of 2–4%. In the United States, approximately 600,000 cholecystectomies are performed annually at a cost of approximately $6.5 billion. Both genetic and environmental factors have been shown to play a role in the development of gallstone disease. The clinical manifestations of gallstones include episodic abdominal pain, acute cholecystitis, obstructive jaundice, cholangitis, and pancreatitis.

In Western industrialized countries, the vast majority of gallstones are comprised principally of cholesterol; hence, cholelithiasis can be regarded primarily as a disturbance of cholesterol elimination. A complex solubilizing system is required to keep cholesterol in solution in the bile. If this system fails, or if its capacity is exceeded by hypersecretion of cholesterol, cholesterol precipitates within the gallbladder, and gallstones may develop.

Pathogenesis

There are two major classes of gallstones. Cholesterol stones, which account for more than 85% of all gallstones in Western countries, are comprised primarily of cholesterol with variable admixtures of calcium salts, bile pigments, proteins, and fatty acids. Pigment stones comprise the remaining 15% of gallstones and are principally composed of calcium bilirubinate, with a cholesterol content of less than 20%. Pigment stones are further subdivided into black pigment stones, which develop in the gallbladder, and brown pigment stones, which form within the biliary system.

A. Cholesterol Stones

Because cholesterol has poor aqueous solubility, bile acids and phospholipids are required for adequate solubilization of cholesterol in the bile, through the formation of mixed micelles (Figure 52–1). When the cholesterol concentration in bile exceeds the solubilizing capacity of bile acids and phospholipids (termed cholesterol supersaturation), unstable cholesterol-rich vesicles aggregate into large multilamellar vesicles, from which cholesterol crystals precipitate. If not expeditiously expelled from the gallbladder, these crystals become entrapped in gallbladder mucin gel, where they grow and agglomerate to form stones.

While an excess of biliary cholesterol in relation to its carriers (phospholipids and bile acids) is a *sine qua non* for the formation of cholesterol gallstones, cholesterol supersaturation alone is not sufficient for stone formation. Indeed, nearly 50% of adults manifest supersaturated bile over the course of a day, yet only a minority develop gallstones. Bile stability,

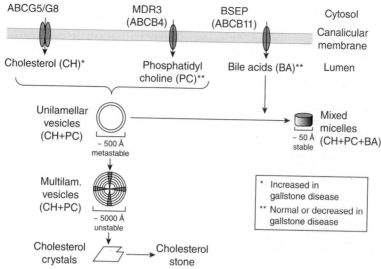

▲ Figure 52–1. Biliary secretion and solubilization of cholesterol. Cholesterol is secreted by the ABC-binding cassette (ABC) transporter ABCG5/G8, phosphatidylcholine by the multidrug-resistance p-glycoprotein 3 (MDR3; ABCB4), and bile acids by the bile salt export pump (BSEP; ABCB11). Cholesterol and phosphatidylcholine reach the bile as metastable unilamellar vesicles, which are converted into water-soluble stable mixed micelles by the bile acids. If the secretion of cholesterol into bile exceeds the solubilizing capacity of bile acids and phospholipids, cholesterol-rich vesicles remain, which aggregate into large unstable multilamellar vesicles from which cholesterol crystals precipitate. These crystals may aggregate and form cholesterol stones. Recent evidence indicates that a variant in the hepatocanalicular cholesterol transporter gene *ABCG8* contributes to the risk of cholesterol gallstone formation (for details see text).

mediated by inhibitors and promoters of cholesterol crystal nucleation, as well as gallbladder stasis, are essential factors in the pathogenesis of cholesterol gallstones:

1. Cholesterol supersaturation—The supersaturation of bile with cholesterol may result from hypersecretion of cholesterol, hyposecretion of bile acids and/or phospholipids, or a combination of both. The transport of biliary lipids from the hepatocyte into the bile canaliculus is mediated by several key canalicular membrane transport proteins (Figure 52–1), including the cholesterol transporter (ABCG5/ABCG8), the bile salt export pump (BSEP; ABCB11), and the multidrug resistance p-glycoprotein 3 (MDR3; ABCB4) which translocates phosphatidylcholine across the canalicular membrane. *Cholesterol hypersecretion* is the most common cause of bile supersaturation. It may result from enhanced synthesis of cholesterol, increased hepatic uptake of endogenous (via low-density lipoproteins) or exogenous (via chylomicrons) cholesterol, and/or augmented canalicular transport of cholesterol into bile. An inappropriately low rate of cholesterol 7α-hydroxylation, the rate-limiting step in the conversion of cholesterol to bile acids, also can increase cholesterol secretion into bile. Additionally, reduced enterohepatic cycling of bile acids as a result of impaired ileal uptake with resultant fecal loss can play a role by decreasing the bile acid pool.

2. Destabilization of bile—Most individuals with supersaturated bile do not develop gallstones because the time

necessary for cholesterol crystals to nucleate and grow exceeds the duration of time the bile is held in the gallbladder. The stability of phospholipid-cholesterol vesicles depends not only on the cholesterol concentration, but also on the balance between inhibitors and promoters of cholesterol crystal formation. A principal protein that promotes cholesterol nucleation is gallbladder mucin, a mixture of glycoproteins that layers at the mucosal surface of the gallbladder wall (Figure 52–2). Release of mucin is stimulated by deoxycholic acid. The influence of promoting and inhibiting factors on the appearance of crystals in bile is termed the "nucleation time," which is much shorter in gallbladder bile from patients with cholesterol gallstones than in equally supersaturated gallbladder bile from normal subjects.

3. Stasis of bile in the gallbladder—If the gallbladder emptied all supersaturated bile completely before crystals had formed, stones would not be able to grow. Hence, prolonged retention of bile within the gallbladder is another important prerequisite for lithogenesis. A high percentage of patients with gallstones manifest impaired gallbladder emptying. Studies of gallbladder motility using ultrasonography have shown that patients with gallstones have increased fasting and residual gallbladder volume, and that fractional emptying of the gallbladder is diminished (Figure 52–3). The incidence of gallstones is increased in conditions associated with reduced or infrequent gallbladder emptying, such as fasting, parenteral nutrition, or pregnancy, and in patients

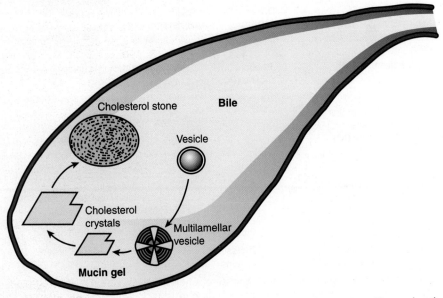

▲ **Figure 52–2.** Formation, growth, and aggregation of cholesterol crystals in the mucin gel layered at the mucosal surface of the gallbladder wall (for details see text).

using drugs that inhibit gallbladder motility (eg, octreotide, loperamide). Gallbladder hypomotility during fasting results from lack of gallbladder stimulation; consequently, the risk of stone formation during parenteral nutrition can be decreased by administration of cholecystokinin. During pregnancy, both the fasting volume and the residual volume of the gallbladder rise with serum progesterone, which inhibits smooth muscle contractility and impairs emptying.

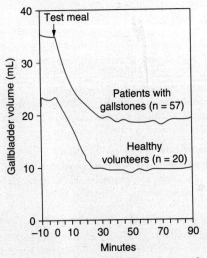

▲ **Figure 52–3.** Impaired gallbladder emptying after a test meal in patients with gallstones measured by ultrasonography. (Data from Paumgartner G, Pauletzki J, Sackmann M. Ursodeoxycholic acid treatment of cholesterol gallstone disease. *Scand J Gastroenterol Suppl.* 1994;204:27–31.)

B. Pigment Stones

Pigment stones are comprised primarily of bilirubin and form when appreciable levels of unconjugated bilirubin, which is poorly water soluble, are present within the bile. Bilirubin is conjugated in the liver by the 1A1 isoform of the enzyme UDP-glucuronosyltransferase (UGT1A1) to form the water-soluble bilirubin diglucuronide, which is secreted across the bile canaliculus by the multidrug resistance-associated protein 2 (MRP2; ABCC2). Pigment stones are sub-categorized as *black pigment stones*, which principally consist of calcium bilirubinate and form in the gallbladder. They occur in patients who have chronic hemolytic states (eg, sickle cell anemia), cirrhosis, Gilbert syndrome, or cystic fibrosis, all of which lead to augmented levels of unconjugated bilirubin in the bile (Table 52–1). There also is an increased incidence of black pigment stones in patients with bile salt malabsorption (eg, ileal disease, ileal resection), which increases solubilization of bilirubin in the colon, thereby enhancing its enterohepatic cycling.

Brown pigment stones are comprised of calcium salts and unconjugated bilirubin, with varying amounts of cholesterol

Table 52–1. Major risk factors for pigment stones.

Associated conditions
Chronic hemolysis
Pernicious anemia
Liver cirrhosis
Cystic fibrosis
Chronic biliary tract infections
Biliary parasites
Ileal disease/Crohn's disease Ileal resection or bypass

and protein. They result from the generation of unconjugated bilirubin within the biliary system through the action of the bacterial enzymes β-glucuronidase, phospholipase A1, and conjugated bile acid hydrolase, which act to deconjugate bilirubin glucuronides. Brown pigment stones typically form in the setting of bile stasis and chronic infection of the biliary system, as seen in patients with strictures (eg, primary sclerosing cholangitis, ischemic cholangiopathy), parasitic disorders (eg, Clonorchis sinensis, Ascaris lumbricoides), or congenital abnormalities (eg, Caroli's disease).

Gurusamy KS, Davidson BR. Gallstones. *BMJ.* 2014;348:g2669. [PMID: 24755732]

Lammert F, Gurusamy K, Ko CW, et al. Gallstones. *Nat Rev Dis Primers.* 2016;2:16024. [PMID: 27121416]

Portincasa P, Moschetta A, Palasciano G. Cholesterol gallstone disease. *Lancet.* 2006;368:230–239. [PMID: 16844493]

C. Epidemiology & Genetics Gallstones

In the third National Health and Nutrition Examination Survey (NHANES III), a large cross-sectional epidemiologic study of the U.S. population, the overall prevalence of gallstones in the United States was 7.9% in men and 16.6% in women, with a progressive increase after age 20. The prevalence was high in Mexican Americans (men: 8.9%, women: 26.7%), intermediate for non-Hispanic whites (men: 8.6%, women: 16.6%), and low for African Americans (5.3% in men, 13.9% in women). Overall gallstone prevalence rates in Europe, as ascertained from large abdominal ultrasound surveys of adults aged 30–69, are similar to those in the NHANES III study. The prevalence of gallstone disease is lower in Asian populations (ranging from 3% to 15%) and very low (<5%) in Africans. Certain ethnic groups appear particularly susceptible to gallstones, with a prevalence exceeding 75% among Native Americans in the western United States.

Epidemiologic surveys and family clustering point to a critical role of genetics in determining susceptibility to gallstones. For example, in the Swedish population, the genetic contribution to the pathogenesis of symptomatic gallstone disease has been estimated to be approximately 25%. Associations between multiple lithogenic gene variants and gallstone formation have been identified, indicating that cholelithiasis is a polygenic complex disease. Genome-wide association studies (GWAS) have found that a single nucleotide polymorphism (amino acid substitution p.D19H) in the hepatic cholesterol transporter ABCG8 (which is present in 5–9% of most populations studied) constitutes the most frequent genetic risk factor for cholesterol gallstones. Notably, women older than 60 years who are homozygous for the p.D19H variant have a 13% 10-year risk of symptomatic gallstone disease versus a 2–4% risk in noncarriers. With regard to pigment stones, several candidate susceptibility genes that predispose to enhanced enterohepatic cycling of bilirubin have been identified, and gallstone prevalence has been strongly associated with the *UGT1A1* promoter variant in patients with cystic fibrosis or sickle cell disease.

Although the predisposition to gallstone formation appears to be polygenic in the vast majority of individuals, rare forms of monogenic gallstone disease exist. For example, the low phospholipid-associated cholelithiasis (LPAC) syndrome characterized by early-onset (age <40 years) cholesterol gallstones is caused by mutations in the gene encoding the canalicular phospholipid transporter (ABCB4), leading to extremely low phosphatidylcholine levels in bile. Additional rarer polymorphisms in canalicular transporters (ABCG5, ABCB11) and other metabolic genes (CYP7A1, SLUT21, GCKR, TM4SF4, ABCC7, NPC1L1) also have been shown to confer an increased likelihood of gallstone formation, with higher risks in individuals possessing polymorphisms in multiple susceptibility genes. Counterintuitively, the *UGT1A1* Gilbert polymorphism has been associated with both pigment and cholesterol gallstones, suggesting a potential role for bilirubin as a cholesterol nucleation factor.

D. Risk Factors for Gallstones

Risk factors for the development of cholesterol gallstones are detailed in Table 52–2. The prevalence of gallstones is nearly

Table 52–2. Major risk factors for cholesterol gallstones.

General
Increasing age
Female sex
Family history
Diet
High calorie intake
Low fiber intake
High refined carbohydrates
High glycemic load
Prolonged total parenteral nutrition
Lifestyle
Prolonged fasting
Rapid weight loss
Weight cycling
Pregnancy and parity
Physical inactivity
Associated conditions
Obesity
Metabolic syndrome
Non-alcoholic fatty liver disease
Cirrhosis
Spinal cord injury
Gastrectomy
Medications
Hormone-replacement therapy/oral contraceptives
Octreotide
Fibrates
Calcineurin inhibitors

twice as high in women as in men and increases with age such that 38% of women and 22% of men manifest gallstones by age 90. The sex difference in gallstone prevalence is principally explained by endogenous estrogens, which increase biliary cholesterol secretion and, hence, cholesterol saturation of bile. Pregnancy further augments the risk of gallstones through the added effect of progesterone, which reduces bile salt secretion and impairs gallbladder emptying. While there is a stepwise increase in gallstone prevalence with parity, up to 60% of gallstones can resolve postpartum. Obese individuals ingest and synthesize more cholesterol leading to hypersecretion into bile. Conversely, rapid weight loss induces gallstone formation as a result of decreased bile salt secretion, enhanced cholesterol mobilization, and diminished gallbladder contractility.

An increased risk of black pigment stones is observed when there are elevated circulating levels of unconjugated bilirubin. This occurs in the setting of enhanced bilirubin production (eg, hemolytic anemia, ineffective erythropoiesis), impaired bilirubin conjugation (eg, Crigler-Najjar syndrome), or augmented enterohepatic cycling of bilirubin (eg, ileal resection). Brown pigment stones form in the setting of abnormal biliary drainage, as seen with biliary strictures (eg, primary sclerosing cholangitis) and congenital bile duct abnormalities (eg, Caroli's disease).

Attili AF, De Santis A, Capri R, et al. The natural history of gallstones: the GREPCO experience. The GREPCO Group. *Hepatology*. 1995;21:655–660. [PMID: 7875663]

Everhart JE, Khare M, Hill M, et al. Prevalence and ethnic differences in gallbladder disease in the United States. *Gastroenterology*. 1999;117:632–639. [PMID: 10464139]

Katsika D, Grjibovski A, Einarsson C, et al. Genetic and environmental influences on symptomatic gallstone disease: a Swedish study of 43,141 twin pairs. *Hepatology*. 2005;41:1138–1143. [PMID: 15747383]

Poupon R, Rosmorduc O, Boelle PY, et al. Genotype-phenotype relationships in the low-phospholipid-associated cholelithiasis syndrome: a study of 156 consecutive patients. *Hepatology*. 2013;58:1105–1110. [PMID: 23533021]

Rebholz C, Krawczyk M, Lammert F. Genetics of gallstone disease. *Eur J Clin Invest*. 2018;48:e12935. [PMID: 29635711]

Schafmayer C, Hartleb J, Tepel J, et al. Predictors of gallstone composition in 1025 symptomatic gallstones from Northern Germany. *BMC Gastroenterol*. 2006;6:36. [PMID: 17121681]

▶ Clinical Features

A. Symptoms & Signs of Gallstone Disease

Gallstones are frequently asymptomatic and are often discovered incidentally during cross-sectional abdominal imaging. As incidentally discovered gallstones remain asymptomatic in nearly 80% of cases, the mere presence of cholelithiasis is not an indication for intervention. The most common symptom of cholelithiasis is biliary colic, with only 10% of symptomatic patients presenting with cholecystitis, obstructive jaundice, or pancreatitis as the initial manifestation of gallstone disease. Biliary colic results from obstruction of the cystic duct, leading to distention of the viscus which induces pain that typically is described as a severe, steady ache or fullness in the epigastrium or right upper quadrant, frequently radiating to the interscapular area, right scapula, or shoulder. The onset of pain is sudden and persists for 15 minutes to 5 hours, subsiding gradually. There may be concomitant nausea (with or without vomiting) and diaphoresis. A nocturnal onset that awakens the patient from sleep is common. While 30% of patients do not experience a second episode after the first bout of biliary colic, the majority suffer from recurrent attacks of pain, with a complication rate of 1–3% per year. If there are no further episodes of biliary colic within 5 years after the first attack, the natural history of the patient may be regarded as that of asymptomatic gallstone disease.

It is important to remember that not all abdominal symptoms in patients with cholelithiasis are caused by gallstones, as evidenced by the fact that 40% of patients who undergo cholecystectomy do not experience resolution of abdominal discomfort. Nonspecific gastrointestinal symptoms, such as belching, heartburn, and bloating in the absence of biliary pain should not be attributed to gallstones without considering other diagnostic possibilities (eg, gastroesophageal reflux disease and peptic ulcer disease). In patients with gallstones and upper abdominal pain, the odds of pain relief following cholecystectomy increases progressively from 25% to 75% with each additional feature: (1) pain frequency is once a month or less; (2) initial onset of pain is within 1 year; (3) pain lasts for 30 minutes to 24 hours; and (4) pain most frequently occurs in the evening or at night. *Symptomatic gallstone disease* is called *uncomplicated* if it is characterized by episodes of biliary pain of less than 5 hours with no other manifestations. *Complicated gallstone disease* should be suspected if an episode of biliary pain persists beyond 5 hours and/or clinical or laboratory findings of acute cholecystitis, acute biliary pancreatitis, biliary obstruction, or symptoms and signs of other complications develop.

B. Laboratory & Imaging Studies

1. Ultrasonography—Abdominal ultrasonography is the method of choice for the diagnosis of cholelithiasis (see Figure 9–35), with a sensitivity greater than 95% for the detection of gallstones 1.5 mm or more in diameter. The characteristic finding is a mobile echogenic focus within the gallbladder lumen that displays an acoustic shadow and moves in a gravity-dependent fashion with changes in the patient's position. The gravity-dependent mobility of the echogenic foci allows differentiation from gallbladder polyps. Ultrasonography also provides information about the presence of a thickened gallbladder wall and pericholecystic fluid, which can be signs of acute cholecystitis. In combination with a sonographic Murphy sign, defined as maximal abdominal tenderness from pressure of the ultrasound probe over the visualized gallbladder, ultrasonography has high sensitivity (94%) and specificity (78%) for the diagnosis of acute cholecystitis. While bile duct dilatation can indicate bile duct obstruction from choledocholithiasis, ultrasonography offers a low to moderate sensitivity for identifying bile duct stones. Functional ultrasonography can provide additional information about gallbladder emptying and cystic duct patency.

2. Computed tomography (CT)—CT is occasionally useful for the detection or exclusion of gallstones, especially if calcified, but it is less sensitive and more expensive than ultrasound and requires exposure to radiation. It is useful for evaluation of suspected biliary pancreatitis or complicated acute cholecystitis when abscess or perforation is suspected.

3. Magnetic resonance imaging (MRI) and magnetic resonance cholangiopancreatography (MRCP)—MRI is not recommended for screening for gallstones, but MRCP is useful for visualizing the biliary and pancreatic ducts, with a sensitivity of 85% for detection of bile duct stones. MRCP is used as an alternative to endoscopic retrograde cholangiopancreatography (ERCP) to exclude bile duct stones in the preoperative screening of patients undergoing laparoscopic cholecystectomy, if there is a low to intermediate level of suspicion for choledocholithiasis.

4. Endoscopic ultrasound—This is the most sensitive method for the detection of ampullary stones.

5. Endoscopic retrograde cholangiopancreatography—ERCP is the method of choice for the extraction of bile duct stones.

6. Hepatobiliary scintigraphy—Cholecystoscintigraphy has an approximate 95% sensitivity for detecting acute cholecystitis. While HIDA (hepatoiminodiacetic acid) has long been used as a generic term for cholescintigraphy, 99mTc-disofenin (diisopropyl-IDA; DISIDA) or 99mTc-mebrofenin (bromotriethyl-IDA; BIDA) has supplanted HIDA as imaging agents due to higher liver extraction (useful up to serum bilirubin levels as high as 25–30 mg/dL) and more rapid biliary clearance. Notably, this test has no role in the detection of gallstones or choledocholithasis.

Lammert F, Neubrand MW, Bittner R, et al. S3-guidelines for diagnosis and treatment of gallstones. German Society for Digestive and Metabolic Diseases and German Society for Surgery of the Alimentary Tract. *Z Gastroenterol.* 2007;45:971–1001. [PMID: 17874360]

Rickes S, Treiber G, Mönkemüller K, et al. Impact of the operator's experience on value of high-resolution transabdominal ultrasound in the diagnosis of choledocholithiasis: a prospective comparison using endoscopic retrograde cholangiography as the gold standard. *Scand J Gastroenterol.* 2006;41:838–843. [PMID: 16785198]

Thistle JL, Longstreth GF, Romero Y, et al. Factors that predict relief from upper abdominal pain after cholecystectomy. *Clin Gastroenterol Hepatol.* 2011;9:891–896. [PMID: 21699805]

Verma D, Kapadia A, Eisen GM, et al. EUS vs MRCP for detection of choledocholithiasis. *Gastrointest Endosc.* 2006;64:248–254. [PMID: 16860077]

Ziessman HA. Hepatobiliary scintigraphy in 2014. *J Nucl Med.* 2014;55:1–9. [PMID: 24744445]

▶ Differential Diagnosis

The differential diagnosis of acute right upper quadrant and/or epigastric abdominal discomfort is broad. In addition to gallstone disease and its complications (see below), gastroesophageal reflux disease, peptic ulcer disease, hepatitis, gastroparesis, gastric outlet obstruction, nonulcer dyspepsia, pancreatitis, and mesenteric venous outflow obstruction are diagnostic considerations.

▶ Complications

A. Acute Cholecystitis

Acute cholecystitis is the most frequent complication of gallstone disease. In 90% of cases, acute cholecystitis is caused by a transient or permanent obstruction of the cystic duct by a gallstone, resulting in an inflammatory response to the mechanical, chemical, and/or bacterial insults. Increased intraluminal pressure and distention of the gallbladder can further lead to ischemia of the mucosa and the wall of the gallbladder. Bacterial infection occurs in 50–85% of patients with acute cholecystitis, generally later in the course. The most common organisms are *Escherichia coli*, *Klebsiella*, *Streptococcus*, and *Clostridium* species.

Acute cholecystitis typically begins as an attack of biliary pain that progressively worsens. Most patients have experienced previous episodes of biliary pain. When cholecystitis develops, the pain becomes more localized to the right upper quadrant. Signs of peritoneal inflammation, such as increased pain with jarring, or pain on deep inspiration, may develop. Nausea and vomiting are frequent. Low-grade fever is usually present, but high-grade fevers, shaking chills, and/or rigors can occur.

Physical examination of patients with acute cholecystitis reveals right upper quadrant tenderness. Usually, there is marked tenderness and inhibition of inspiration on deep palpation under the right subcostal margin (Murphy sign). An enlarged, tense gallbladder is palpable in about one-third of patients, often associated with a stone in the neck of the gallbladder (see Figure 9–37).

Mild to moderate leukocytosis is common. Serum bilirubin and serum liver enzymes are frequently normal, but may be mildly elevated in some patients. Substantial elevations in liver tests suggest bile duct obstruction (choledocholithiasis), or Mirizzi syndrome, an uncommon complication in which a gallstone becomes impacted in the neck of the gallbladder or cystic duct causing compression of the common bile duct and obstructive jaundice. In 10–30% of the patients with acute cholecystitis, particularly if presentation or intervention is delayed, severe complications such as gallbladder gangrene, empyema, perforation, or biliary enteric fistula can occur (see below).

Chronic cholecystitis is a lingering inflammation of the gallbladder wall that results from repeated attacks of acute and subacute cholecystitis or mechanical irritation of the gallbladder mucosa by gallstones. It may progress from asymptomatic to symptomatic.

B. Choledocholithiasis

Passage of gallbladder stones into the common bile duct occurs in approximately 10–15% of patients with cholelithiasis. In up to 25% of elderly patients who undergo cholecystectomy, gallstones are discovered in the common duct. The large majority of these are cholesterol stones that originate in the gallbladder. Stones that primarily form in the bile ducts are typically pigment stones (see "Pathogenesis," earlier). An exception is the formation of cholesterol gallstones in the bile ducts of patients with an ABCB4 gene defect causing impaired biliary phospholipid secretion. Most patients with common bile duct stones present with biliary pain accompanied by abnormal liver tests, with or without jaundice. Major complications of choledocholithiasis are obstructive jaundice, cholangitis, pancreatitis, and (when protracted) secondary biliary cirrhosis.

The presentation of acute obstruction of the common bile duct by a gallstone usually includes biliary pain, similar to the pain of cystic duct obstruction, and—if of sufficient duration—is followed by jaundice. Most patients with obstruction have elevated liver enzymes (alanine aminotransferase [ALT], aspartate aminotransferase [AST]) in the acute phase of obstruction. In the later course, ALT and AST decrease toward normal even if the obstruction persists, whereas alkaline phosphatase rises followed by bilirubin elevation and, eventually, jaundice.

Transcutaneous abdominal ultrasonography has only moderate diagnostic accuracy for the detection or exclusion of bile duct stones. Sensitivities ranging from 38% to 82% have been reported. If the diameter of the common bile duct is larger than 6 mm, the presence of a bile duct stone should be considered. Determination of γ-glutamyl transferase (GGT), alkaline phosphatase, ALT, and serum bilirubin levels can be helpful in this situation (Table 52–3).

Table 52–3. Criteria for simultaneous choledocholithiasis in patients with gallbladder stones.

High probability for simultaneous bile duct stones
- Common bile duct dilated (>6–8 mm) + hyperbilirubinemia + elevated GGT, alkaline phosphatase and/or ALT
- Common bile duct >10 mm in presence of gallbladder stones
- Direct evidence of stone in bile ducts by ultrasound
Low probability for simultaneous bile duct stones
- Common bile duct not dilated
- GGT, alkaline phosphatase, and ALT within normal limits

ALT, alanine aminotransferase; GGT, γ-glutamyl transferase.

If ultrasonography is nondiagnostic, clinical symptoms and signs should guide further diagnostic measures. If there is high suspicion for choledocholithiasis, endoscopic retrograde cholangiography (ERC) is indicated because it permits simultaneous therapeutic intervention (endoscopic papillotomy and stone extraction). The sensitivity and specificity of ERC for the detection of bile duct stones is greater than 90%. However, routine ERC prior to laparoscopic cholecystectomy is not recommended, as the prevalence of choledocholithiasis in patients with gallbladder stones is low, ranging from 5% to 15%, and the risk of ERC is nontrivial. In situations where the index of suspicion for choledocholithiasis is intermediate, endoscopic ultrasound or MRCP (see Figure 9–36) should be considered prior to performing an ERC. A meta-analysis of five randomized controlled studies reported similar sensitivity (93% vs 85%) and specificity (96% vs 93%) of endoscopic ultrasound and MRCP for identification of bile duct stones. Endoscopic ultrasound has the advantage of permitting the rapid transition to therapeutic ERC if choledocholithiasis is encountered.

C. Ascending Cholangitis

The characteristic presentation of ascending cholangitis includes biliary pain (typically in the right upper quadrant and/or epigastrium), jaundice, and spiking fevers with chills. These clinical features, termed Charcot's triad, have a 36% specificity and 93% specificity for cholangitis. Leukocytosis is typical, and blood cultures are positive in about 75% of cases, the most common organisms being E. coli (25–50%), Klebsiella (15–20%), enterococcus (10–20%), and Enterobacter (5–10%).

D. Biliary Pancreatitis

Biliary pancreatitis occurs when gallstones pass through the ampulla of Vater leading to ampullary spasm, fibrosis, and obstruction with consequent biliopancreatic reflux. In patients with gallstones, 4–8% will ultimately develop biliary pancreatitis, which can be the first manifestation of gallstone disease. A serum lipase greater than three times the upper limit of normal is a main diagnostic criteria. The most common liver enzyme abnormality is the ALT level, with a three-fold elevation having a positive predictive value of approximately 95% in diagnosing biliary pancreatitis.

E. Biliary Fistula

Bilioenteric fistulas are spontaneous communications between the biliary system and the gastrointestinal tract that develop in 1–2% of patients with gallstones. The most common clinical manifestations are ascending cholangitis or a bile acid malabsorption syndrome similar to postcholecystectomy, although patients can be asymptomatic. In approximately 60% of cases, the fistulas are located between the gallbladder and the duodenum. Passage of large stones through a fistula can cause gastric outlet obstruction as a result of impaction in the proximal duodenum (Bouveret syndrome), or gallstone ileus should the gallstone become lodged in the terminal ileum. In the absence of prior biliary intervention, aerobilia (air in the biliary system) on cross-sectional imaging is a suggestive finding.

▶ Treatment

A. Surgical Therapy

1. Asymptomatic gallstones—Prophylactic cholecystectomy in individuals with asymptomatic gallstones is not recommended because the risks of biliary colic, biliary complications, and/or gallbladder cancer are low. Sixty to eighty percent of individuals with asymptomatic gallstones remain asymptomatic over follow-up periods as long as 25 years. The probability of developing symptoms within the first 5 years after diagnosis is 2–4% per year, decreasing to 1–2% per year thereafter. Treatment of patients with asymptomatic gallstones does not prolong life expectancy because the likelihood of biliary complications (0.1–0.3% per year) is counterbalanced by the operative risk. Moreover, the overall costs of expectant management (cholecystectomy performed only when symptoms occur) are lower than those of a prophylactic operative approach. This dictum remains true in patients with diabetes mellitus, in whom asymptomatic gallstones also are low risk.

Prophylactic cholecystectomy has been recommended for individuals with a porcelain gallbladder, a rare condition where the inner wall of the gallbladder becomes hardened and calcified as a result of chronic inflammation (see Figure 9–38), because of an increased risk of gallbladder carcinoma. However, recent studies have found the associated risk of malignancy in patients with porcelain gallbladder to be substantially lower than originally thought, raising debate about surgical versus conservative management and leading some to advocate for noninvasive monitoring of asymptomatic patients with serial abdominal ultrasound. Routine prophylactic cholecystectomy for patients undergoing bariatric surgery is no longer recommended due to a low likelihood of subsequent biliary complications and an increased risk of postoperative complications.

2. Symptomatic gallstones—In addition to analgesic therapy, patients with symptomatic gallstones should be offered elective laparoscopic cholecystectomy as it provides a permanent cure and is cost-effective when compared with open cholecystectomy. Currently, over 93% of all cholecystectomies are initiated by laparoscopy, with approximately 4–7% necessitating conversion to an open procedure. A meta-analysis of randomized studies comparing laparoscopic and open cholecystectomy found identical complication rates but, on the average, a 3-day shorter hospital stay and a 3-week shorter convalescence for the former. In patients with liver cirrhosis (Child class A or B) and portal hypertension, laparoscopic cholecystectomy also appears to be superior to open cholecystectomy.

3. Preoperative diagnostic studies—Preoperative ultrasonography should be performed, not only to diagnose gallbladder stones, but also for detection of potential complications. Preoperative determination of liver enzymes (alkaline phosphatase, aminotransferases) and serum bilirubin also is helpful to assess the likelihood of concurrent choledocholithiasis or pre-existing liver disease. Predictors of bile duct stones include a common bile duct diameter greater than 6–8 mm and elevated alkaline phosphatase and serum bilirubin levels. In patients with acute cholecystitis, an ALT >3 times the upper limit of normal, an elevated alkaline phosphatase, and a common bile duct diameter >6 mm had a 78% sensitivity for choledocholithiasis. In case of uncertainty, an endoscopic ultrasound or an MRCP can be considered.

Buxbaum JL, Abbas Fehmi SM, Sultan S, et al. ASGE guideline on the role of endoscopy in the evaluation and management of choledocholithiasis. *Gastrointest Endosc.* 2019;89:1075–1105. [PMID: 30979521]

Chisholm PR, Patel AH, Law RJ, et al. Preoperative predictors of choledocholithiasis in patients presenting with acute calculous cholecystitis. *Gastrointest Endosc.* 2019;89:977–983. [PMID: 30465770]

Lam R, Zakko A, Petrov JC, et al. Gallbladder disorders: a comprehensive review. *Dis Mon.* 2021;67(7):101130. [PMID: 33622550]

Rumsey S, Winders J, MacCormick AD. Diagnostic accuracy of Charcot's triad: a systematic review. *ANZ J Surg.* 2017;87: 232–238. [PMID: 28213923]

Van Geenen EJM, van der Peet DL, Bhagirath P, et al. Etiology and diagnosis of acute biliary pancreatitis. *Nat Rev Gastroenterol Hepatol.* 2010;7:495–502. [PMID: 20703238]

Williams E, Beckingham I, El Sayed G, et al. Updated guidelines on the management of common bile duct stones (CBDS). *Gut.* 2017;66:765–782. [PMID: 28122906]

B. Nonsurgical Therapy

1. Oral bile acid dissolution—In selected patients who have gallbladder stones with mild and infrequent episodes of biliary pain and in the absence of other complications, gallstone dissolution with ursodeoxycholic acid (UDCA) can be considered. UDCA reduces cholesterol saturation and produces a lamellar liquid crystalline phase in bile that allows for the dispersion of cholesterol from stones. In carefully selected patients with radiolucent (noncalcified) stones that are smaller than 5–10 mm in diameter and with a functioning gallbladder, UDCA (10–15 mg/kg/day orally) can induce complete resolution of gallstones in up to 50%. However, stone dissolution is slow, requiring as long as 18 months to achieve. Gallstones larger than 15 mm rarely dissolve, and pigment stones are not responsive to UDCA. Following completion of therapy, stones recur in 30–50% of patients within 3–5 years, which is why UDCA treatment generally is limited to those who refuse or are poor candidates for cholecystectomy.

2. Extracorporeal shock wave lithotripsy—Following the introduction of laparoscopic cholecystectomy, this nonsurgical therapeutic modality has been abandoned mainly because of high rates of stone recurrence (11–29% at 2 years, 60–80% at 10 years). Extracorporeal shock wave lithotripsy has maintained a limited role in the treatment of bile duct stones resistant to endoscopic extraction.

3. Medical prophylaxis of cholesterol gallstones—UDCA can prevent gallstone formation in obese patients during rapid weight loss (>1.5 kg/week). A minimal dose of 500 mg/day is recommended until constant body weight is attained.

May GR, Sutherland LR, Shaffer EA. Efficacy of bile acid therapy for gallstone dissolution: a meta-analysis of randomized trials. *Aliment Pharmacol Ther.* 1993;7:139–148. [PMID: 8485266]

Paumgartner G, Pauletzki J, Sackmann M. Ursodeoxycholic acid treatment of cholesterol gallstone disease. *Scand J Gastroenterol Suppl.* 1994;204:27–31. [PMID: 7824875]

Shiffman ML, Kaplan GD, Brinkman-Kaplan V, et al. Prophylaxis against gallstone formation with ursodeoxycholic acid in patients participating in a very-low-calorie diet program. *Ann Intern Med.* 1995;122:899–905. [PMID: 7755224]

Stokes CS, Gluud LL, Casper M, et al. Ursodeoxycholic acid and diets higher in fat prevent gallbladder stones during weight loss: a meta-analysis of randomized controlled trials. *Clin Gastroenterol Hepatol.* 2014;12:1090–1100.

C. Interventional Management of Gallstone Complications

1. Cholecystitis—Patients with acute cholecystitis should undergo early elective laparoscopic cholecystectomy, ideally within 24–72 hours of hospital admission. A large European randomized multicenter trial of immediate (within 24 hours of admission) versus delayed laparoscopic cholecystectomy, demonstrated a lower morbidity (11.6% vs 34.4%) and shorter length of stay (5.4 vs 10.0 days) in the early intervention group, with no difference in conversion rates to open cholecystectomy. Two large observational studies came to similar conclusions, while a more recent meta-analysis of 77 case-control studies showed that laparoscopic cholecystectomy within 72 hours was associated with decreased mortality, fewer complications (bile duct injuries, wound infections), lower conversion rates, reduced length of stay, and less blood loss.

From admission until operation the patient should be kept NPO with intravenous hydration and careful control of serum electrolytes. Administration of antibiotics targeting gram negative and anaerobic organisms (eg, piperacillin/tazobactam, cefoxitin, cefotaxime, ceftriaxone with metronidazole, ciprofloxacin or levofloxacin with metronidazole) generally is recommended; although, subsequent definitive surgery is necessary as antibiotic treatment alone fails acutely in over 20% of cases. Continuing antibiotics beyond the day of surgery has not been shown to alter postoperative infection rates.

While percutaneous drainage of the gallbladder (cholecystostomy) is an option for patients considered to be at high operative risk, this intervention should be entertained very selectively as it is associated with substantial morbidity. A recent randomized controlled trial comparing laparoscopic cholecystectomy versus percutaneous cholecystostomy in 142 high-risk patients (Apache II score ≥7) found similar mortality, but significantly higher rates of major complications (65% vs 12%), need for reintervention (66% vs 12%), recurrence of biliary disease (53% vs 5%), and prolonged length of hospital stay (9 vs 5 days) in the cholecystostomy group. Percutaneous catheter removal should only be performed if cystic duct patency has been established by cholangiography and sufficient time has elapsed to ensure that the fistulous tract has matured (generally 3 months) or, alternatively, if the patient becomes a candidate for definitive surgical management. Endoscopic ultrasound guided directed drainage of the gallbladder is a new option generally reserved for patients who are poor candidates for other interventions.

If cholecystectomy cannot be performed within 1–5 days of presentation (eg, delayed diagnosis, medical comorbidities), it is generally performed within 6 weeks after the acute cholecystitis has subsided. Complications of cholecystitis, such as diffuse peritonitis with suspected perforation, gangrene, or empyema require nuanced surgical management.

Bagla, P, Sarria, JC, Riall TS. Management of acute cholecystitis. *Curr Opin Infect Dis.* 2016;29:508–513. [PMID: 27429137]

Gutt CN, Encke J, Koninger J, et al. Acute cholecystitis: early versus delayed cholecystectomy, a multicenter randomized trial (ACDC study, NCT00447304). *Ann Surg.* 2013;258:385–393.

Loozen CS, van Santvoort HC, van Duijvendijk P, et al. Laparoscopic cholecystectomy versus percutaneous catheter drainage for acute cholecystitis in high-risk patients (CHOCOLATE): multicentre randomized clinical trial. *BMJ.* 2018;363:k3965. [PMID: 30297544]

Papi C, Catarci M, D'Ambrosio L, et al. Timing of cholecystectomy for acute calculous cholecystitis: a meta-analysis. *Am J Gastroenterol.* 2004;99:147–155. [PMID: 14687156]

Van Dijk AH, de Reuver PR, Tasma TN, et al. Systematic review of antibiotic treatment for acute calculous cholecystitis. *BJS.* 2016;103:797–811. [PMID: 27027851]

2. Choledocholithiasis—Data on the natural history of symptomatic choledocholithiasis indicate that recurrent colic occurs in more than 50% of the patients and complications in nearly 25%; hence, symptomatic bile duct stones should be removed. Asymptomatic bile duct stones appear to be more benign than symptomatic stones, with long-term retrospective studies suggesting a 17% incidence of complications at 5 years and a 20% rate of spontaneous passage. Conversely, patients with asymptomatic choledocholithiasis have a substantially increased risk of post-ERCP complications (14–32%), presumably due to the high likelihood of a non-dilated common bile duct leading to more difficult and prolonged cannulation times. These data suggest that decision-making regarding biliary stone extraction in patients with asymptomatic choledocholithiasis should be individualized.

Patients with symptomatic bile duct stones who have undergone prior cholecystectomy should be offered endoscopic stone extraction. If endoscopic transpapillary therapy is not possible or fails, percutaneous transhepatic intervention or surgical therapy may be employed. Patients with simultaneous gallbladder and bile duct stones benefit from therapeutic splitting, with ERC performed either before or after cholecystectomy. If the probability of simultaneous choledocholithiasis is high, preoperative endoscopic papillotomy (EPT) and stone extraction are preferred in most hospitals. EPT and cholecystectomy should not be performed on the same day to exclude complications of EPT before surgery. If the probability of choledocholithiasis is low, preoperative ERC should not be the standard; rather—depending on availability—less-invasive diagnostic procedures can be considered. Both endosonography and MRC have high sensitivity and specificity for the detection of bile duct stones. In centers with high expertise, laparoscopic cholecystectomy may be combined with intraoperative cholangiogram and laparoscopic removal of common duct stones if present.

After successful endoscopic or percutaneous removal of bile duct stones in patients with cholelithiasis, cholecystectomy should be performed. This recommendation is based on a study that randomized patients to expectant management versus early laparoscopic cholecystectomy following endoscopic sphincterotomy and clearance of choledocholithiasis. Within a median follow-up of approximately 5 years, 24% of patients with the gallbladder left *in situ* returned with further biliary events (cholangitis, acute cholecystitis, biliary pain, jaundice) as compared with only 7% (cholangitis, biliary pain) in the cholecystectomy group. Cholecystectomy should be performed early, preferably during the same hospital admission. A randomized study showed that recurrent biliary events occurred in 17 out of 47 patients (36%) whose laparoscopic cholecystectomy was delayed for 6–8 weeks, but in only 1 out of 49 patients who underwent early laparoscopic cholecystectomy within 72 hours after endoscopic sphincterotomy.

Buxbaum JL, Abbas Fehmi SM, Sultan S, et al. ASGE guideline on the role of endoscopy in the evaluation and management of choledocholithiasis. *Gastrointest Endosc.* 2019;89:1075–1105. [PMID: 30979521]

Nawara H, Ibrahim R, Abounozha S, et al. Best evidence topic: should patients with asymptomatic choledocholithiasis be treated differently from those with symptomatic or complicated disease? *Ann Med Surg (Lond).* 2021;62:150–153. [PMID: 33520213]

Reinders JS, Goud A, Timmer R, et al. Early laparoscopic cholecystectomy improves outcomes after endoscopic sphincterotomy for choledochocystolithiasis. *Gastroenterology.* 2010;138: 2315–2320. [PMID: 20206179]

Schiphorst AH, Besselink MG, Boerma D, et al. Timing of cholecystectomy after endoscopic sphincterotomy for common bile duct stones. *Surg Endosc.* 2008;22:2046–2050. [PMID: 18270768]

3. Cholangitis—Patients with acute cholangitis caused by an obstructive gallstone should undergo urgent endoscopic removal of the stone (emergently in patients with sepsis). A randomized study has shown a significant advantage of an endoscopic versus a surgical approach with regard to complications and mortality. Immediate systemic antibiotic therapy is indicated to prevent septic complications (see section on Cholecystitis for antibiotic selection). If stone extraction fails, a biliary stent should be placed.

Lai EC, Mok FP, Tan ES, et al. Endoscopic biliary drainage for severe acute cholangitis. *N Engl J Med.* 1992;326:1582–1586. [PMID: 1584258]

4. Biliary pancreatitis—While most cases of acute gallstone pancreatitis are mild and resolve spontaneously, in the absence of cholangitis, patients should be managed expectantly (NPO, intravenous fluids, analgesics) regardless of severity. A recent randomized trial involving patients with severe gallstone pancreatitis found no benefit of urgent ERCP with sphincterotomy over conservative treatment with regard to major complications or mortality. In the presence of cholangitis, biliary stone extraction within 24 hours is indicated. After resolution of acute pancreatitis, cholecystectomy and removal of residual bile duct stones should be performed prior to discharge from the hospital.

Schlepers NJ, Hallensleben ND, Besselink MG, et al. Urgent endoscopic retrograde cholangiopancreatography with sphincterotomy versus conservative treatment in predicted severe acute gallstone pancreatitis (APEC): a multicentre randomized controlled trial. *Lancet.* 2020;396:167–176. [PMID: 32682482]

Van Baal MC, Besselink MG, Bakker OJ, et al. Timing of cholecystectomy after mild biliary pancreatitis: a systematic review. *Ann Surg.* 2012;255:860–866. [PMID: 22470079]

Zhong FP, Wang K, Tan XQ, et al. The optimal timing of laparoscopic cholecystectomy in patients with mild gallstone pancreatitis: a meta-analysis. *Medicine (Baltimore).* 2019;98:e17429. [PMID: 31577759]

Index

Note: Page numbers followed by *f* and *t* indicate figures and tables, respectively.

for pancreatic cystic neoplasms,
416–417
for rectal cancer, 473
technique for, 470
Fissures, in Crohn's disease, 51, 51*f*
Fistula
aortoenteric, 283
aortoesophageal, 463
biliary, 644–645
biliary-vascular, 434
bilioenteric, 644
colovaginal, 332
colovesical, 332
in Crohn's disease. *See* Crohn's
disease, fistulas associated with
in diverticulitis, 332
enterobiliary, 482
enteropancreatic, 482
gastrocolic, 297*t*
jejunocolic, 297*t*
obstetric, 98
perianal, 143, 144*f*
Fistula-in-ano, 48
Fistulotomy, 49
FIT. *See* Fecal immunochemical testing
Flatulence, 370*t*
Flexible sigmoidoscopy
for colorectal cancer screening, 347
for inflammatory bowel disease in
pregnancy, 101
for lower gastrointestinal bleeding,
379
in pregnancy, 117
FLIP. *See* Functional luminal imaging
probe
Flumazenil, 115
Fluoroquinolones
in pregnancy, 103*t*
traveler's diarrhea treated with, 74
Yersinia illnesses treated with, 62
Fluticasone, for eosinophilic esophagitis,
224
FMT. *See* Fecal microbiota transplant
FNH. *See* Focal nodular hyperplasia
FOBT. *See* Fecal occult blood testing
Focal nodular hyperplasia, 149, 150*f*,
608*f*–609*f*, 608–609
FODMAPS, 249, 253, 310, 370
Foley catheter, 467
Follicle-associated epithelium, 14
Follicular helper cells, 14
Food bolus impaction, 465–466, 468
Food intolerances
in functional dyspepsia, 249
irritable bowel syndrome versus,
370
Forceps, for foreign body removal, 466,
467*f*

Foreign bodies
blunt, 465
button batteries, 465
classification of, 464–466
clinical findings of, 462–464
colorectal, 463, 466
drug packages as, 465
endoscopic removal of, 465–466
esophageal, 463, 463*f*
Foley catheter for, 467
food bolus impaction, 465–466, 468
forceps for, 466, 467*f*
gastric, 463
general considerations for, 462
imaging of, 464, 464*f*
magnets, 465
metallic, 465
overtubes for, 466–467, 467*f*
rectal, 463, 466
removal of, 466–468
sharp and pointed, 464*f*, 464–465
small bowel, 463
snares for, 466, 467*f*
toxic, 465
treatment of, 464–468, 467*f*
Foreign body hood, 467*f*, 467–468
FPC. *See* Familial pancreatic cancer
Fructose intolerance, 369
Fulminant Wilson disease, 556
Functional abdominal pain syndrome, 2
Functional biliary sphincter disorder,
438
Functional constipation, 367
Functional dyspepsia
algorithm for, 251*f*
antidepressants for, 254
antinociceptive agents for, 255
antisecretory agents for, 254
buspirone for, 255
causes of, 247, 248*t*
classification of, 247
clinical findings of, 250–252
complementary and alternative
medical therapy for, 256
course of, 256
definition of, 247
diagnostic evaluation for, 250–252
dietary factors in, 249, 253
differential diagnosis of, 252–253
duodenal eosinophilia as cause of,
250
epidemiology of, 247–248
esophagogastroduodenoscopy
evaluations for, 251
food intolerances in, 249
gastric scintigraphy for, 252–253
gastroesophageal reflux disease and,
248, 252

gastrointestinal motility disorders as
cause of, 248–249, 252–253
general considerations for, 247
Helicobacter pylori as cause of, 249,
251–252, 254–255
infections that cause, 253
irritable bowel syndrome and, 253
management of, 251*f*
medications that cause, 248*t*
microbiome alterations as cause of,
249
pancreatobiliary disease and, 252
pathogenesis of, 248–250
peptic ulcer disease and, 252
pharmacotherapy for, 253–256
physical examination findings in, 250
prognosis for, 256
promotility agents for, 254–255, 255*t*
proton pump inhibitors for, 254
psychiatric disorders as cause of, 250,
256
Rome IV criteria for, 247, 248*t*
signs and symptoms of, 250
small intestinal bacterial overgrowth
and, 253
treatment of, 253–256
upper gastrointestinal malignancy as
cause of, 250*t*, 252
visceral hypersensitivity as cause of,
249
Functional gallbladder disorder, 438
Functional luminal imaging probe, 209,
215
Fundic gland polyps, 357
Fungal infections
diarrheal diseases caused by, 72–73
after liver transplantation, 626, 627*f*
Furosemide, for portal hypertension,
589*t*

G
Gabapentin, 255, 265
Gallbladder
bile stasis in, 639, 640*f*
carcinoma of, 155, 156*f*
disorders of, 437–438
endoscopic ultrasound-guided
drainage of, 484
hypomobility in, 640
porcelain, 155, 156*f*, 645
Gallstone(s)
cholesterol, 638–639, 640*f*, 641*t*, 646
composition of, 638
imaging of, 153–154, 154*f*
in pregnancy, 110, 116
prevalence of, 641
risk factors for, 641*t*, 641–642
ursodeoxycholic acid for, 645